The American Psychiatric Association Publishing

TEXTBOOK OF
SUBSTANCE
USE DISORDER
TREATMENT

SIXTH EDITION

The American Psychiatric Association Publishing

TEXTBOOK OF
SUBSTANCE USE DISORDER TREATMENT

SIXTH EDITION

EDITED BY

Kathleen T. Brady, M.D., Ph.D.
Frances R. Levin, M.D.
Marc Galanter, M.D.
Herbert D. Kleber, M.D.

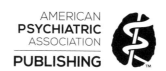

AMERICAN
PSYCHIATRIC
ASSOCIATION
PUBLISHING

Copyright © 2021 American Psychiatric Association Publishing

ALL RIGHTS RESERVED

Sixth Edition

Manufactured in the United States of America on acid-free paper
25 24 23 22 21   5 4 3 2 1

American Psychiatric Association Publishing
800 Maine Avenue SW
Suite 900
Washington, DC 20024-2812
www.appi.org

Library of Congress Cataloging-in-Publication Data
Names: Brady, Kathleen, 1952– editor. | Levin, Frances R., editor. | Galanter, Marc, editor. | Kleber, Herbert D., editor. | American Psychiatric Association Publishing, issuing body.
Title: The American Psychiatric Association Publishing textbook of substance use disorder treatment / edited by Kathleen T. Brady, Frances R. Levin, Marc Galanter, Herbert D. Kleber.
Other titles: American Psychiatric Publishing textbook of substance abuse treatment | Textbook of substance use disorder treatment
Description: Sixth edition. | Washington, DC : American Psychiatric Association Publishing, [2021] | Preceded by American Psychiatric Publishing textbook of substance abuse treatment. Fifth edition. Washington, DC : American Psychiatric Publishing, 2015. | Includes bibliographical references and index.
Identifiers: LCCN 2020046613 (print) | LCCN 2020046614 (ebook) | ISBN 9781615372218 (hardcover ; alk. paper) | ISBN 9781615373536 (ebook)
Subjects: MESH: Substance-Related Disorders—therapy | Behavior, Addictive—therapy
Classification: LCC RC564 (print) | LCC RC564 (ebook) | NLM WM 270 | DDC 362.29—dc23
LC record available at https://lccn.loc.gov/2020046613
LC ebook record available at https://lccn.loc.gov/2020046614

British Library Cataloguing in Publication Data
A CIP record is available from the British Library.

In Memoriam: Herbert D. Kleber, M.D.

We are dedicating this Sixth Edition *Textbook* to the memory of Dr. Herbert D. Kleber, who passed away on October 5, 2018. From 1994 on, Dr. Kleber coedited the first five editions of this *Textbook*, embodying in it his command of the research base and the clinical practice of addiction medicine, which he had achieved over five decades of leadership in the field. His particular contribution was his support of empirical research to drive substance use disorder treatment. He thereby firmly established the credibility of this research in the discipline of medical practice overall, as well as its central role in the country's approach to combating this leading public health problem.

Dr. Kleber began his career in addiction medicine while serving in the U.S. Public Health Service's first narcotic treatment center, in Lexington, Kentucky. He drew on his experience there to establish the drug dependence program at Yale University, where he framed the concept of an academic center focused on substance use disorders that combined research, education, and progressive clinical care. He thereby created a setting for training a generation of academic leaders who now serve across the country and worldwide.

Among his many accomplishments, Dr. Kleber was a pioneering influence in developing new solutions to the practical problems of substance use disorder treatment in the New Haven community. Given these achievements and his academic leadership, he was asked to serve as Deputy Director for Demand Reduction at the White House Office of National Drug Control Policy, where he had an important impact on improving treatment for one of the country's most highly compromised populations.

Dr. Kleber later went on to take the lead in establishing the Substance Abuse Division (now the Division on Substance Use Disorders) at Columbia University, where he wedded a major academic setting to a policy institute. There, he framed innovative approaches to understanding and treating the diversity of substance use disorders, from alcohol to opiates, psychostimulants, and marijuana. For all of these contributions, among his many honors, he was elected to the Institute of Medicine (now called the National Academy of Medicine). He will be sorely missed by many as a major leader and mentor in the addiction field.

Kathleen Brady, M.D., Ph.D.
Frances R. Levin, M.D.
Marc Galanter, M.D.

Contents

PART IV
Nonpharmacotherapeutic
Treatment Modalities

PART V
Public Health Issues

PART VI
Special Populations

PART VII
Psychiatric Comorbidity in Substance-Related Disorders

PART VIII
Special Topics

Contributors

Elie G. Aoun, M.D.
Assistant Professor of Psychiatry, Columbia University, New York, New York

Sudie Back, Ph.D.
Professor, Department of Psychiatry and Behavioral Sciences, Medical University of South Carolina, Charleston; Staff Psychologist, Ralph H. Johnson VA Medical Center, Charleston, South Carolina

Kelly S. Barth, D.O.
Associate Professor, Departments of Psychiatry and of Internal Medicine, Medical University of South Carolina, Charleston, South Carolina

Neal L. Benowitz, M.D.
Professor of Medicine Emeritus, Program in Clinical Pharmacology, Division of Cardiology, Department of Medicine; Center for Tobacco Control Research and Education, University of California San Francisco

Carlos Blanco, M.D., Ph.D., M.S.
Director, Division of Epidemiology, Services, and Prevention Research, National Institute on Drug Abuse, Bethesda, Maryland

Ron Borland, Ph.D., FASSA
Deputy Director, Melbourne Centre for Behaviour Change, and Professor of Psychology in Health Behaviour, Melbourne School of Psychological Sciences, The University of Melbourne, Victoria, Australia

Sarah Bowen, Ph.D.
Associate Professor, School of Graduate Psychology, College of Health Professions, Pacific University, Hillsboro, Oregon

David Braak, M.D. Candidate
Medical student, College of Medicine, Medical University of South Carolina, Charleston, South Carolina

Kathleen T. Brady, M.D., Ph.D.
Director, South Carolina Clinical and Translational Research Center; Distinguished University Professor; Associate Dean, Clinical and Translational Research, Medical University of South Carolina, Department of Psychiatry and Behavioral Sciences, Clinical Neuroscience Division, Charleston, South Carolina

Alyssa Braxton, M.D.
Addiction Psychiatry Fellow, Medical University of South Carolina, Charleston

Timothy D. Brewerton, M.D.
Affiliate Professor, Department of Psychiatry and Behavioral Sciences, Medical University of South Carolina, Charleston

Christina Brezing, M.D.
Assistant Professor of Clinical Psychiatry, Division on Substance Use Disorders, Columbia University Irving Medical Center, New York City

Mary F. Brunette, M.D.
Associate Professor of Psychiatry, Department of Psychiatry, Geisel School of Medicine at Dartmouth, Hanover, New Hampshire

Alan J. Budney, Ph.D.
Director, Treatment Development and Evaluation Core, The Center for Technology and Behavioral Health, Geisel School of Medicine, Dartmouth College, Hanover, New Hampshire

Michael Capata, M.D.
Addiction Psychiatry Fellow, Medical University of South Carolina, Charleston, South Carolina

Kenneth M. Carpenter, Ph.D.
Research Scientist, Division on Substance Use Disorders, New York State Psychiatric Institute; Director of Training, CMC:Foundation for Change, New York, New York

Kathleen M. Carroll, Ph.D.
Albert E Kent Professor of Psychiatry, Yale University School of Medicine, New Haven, Connecticut

Vamsee Chaguturu, M.D.
Assistant Professor, Rutgers Robert Wood Johnson Medical School, New Brunswick, New Jersey

Katrina E. Champion, Ph.D.
Senior Research Fellow, The Matilda Centre for Research in Mental Health and Substance Use, The University of Sydney, Sydney, Australia

Sandra D. Comer, Ph.D.
Professor of Neurobiology (in Psychiatry), Department of Psychiatry, Division on Substance Use Disorders, Columbia University Irving Medical Center and the New York State Psychiatric Institute, New York City

Wilson M. Compton, M.D., M.P.E.
Deputy Director, National Institute on Drug Abuse, National Institutes of Health, Bethesda, Maryland

Nina Cooperman, Psy.D.
Associate Professor, Division of Addiction Psychiatry, Rutgers Robert Wood Johnson Medical School, Piscataway, New Jersey

Linda B. Cottler, Ph.D., M.P.H., FACE
Associate Dean for Research, College of Public Health and Health Professions; Dean's Professor, Department of Epidemiology, Colleges of Public Health and Health Professions and Medicine, University of Florida, Gainesville

K. Michael Cummings, Ph.D., M.P.H.
Professor, Department of Psychiatry and Behavioral Sciences, Medical University of South Carolina, Charleston, South Carolina

Elias Dakwar, M.D.
Associate Professor, Department of Psychiatry, Columbia University Irving Medical Center and the New York State Psychiatric Institute, New York City

Jeffrey J. DeVido, M.D., M.T.S., FASAM
Chief, Addiction Services, Department of Health and Human Services, Behavioral Health and Recovery Services, Marin County, California, San Rafael, California; Behavioral Health Clinical Director, Partnership HealthPlan of California; Assistant Professor, Department of Psychiatry, University of California, San Francisco

Elise E. DeVito, Ph.D.
Associate Research Scientist in Psychiatry, Yale University School of Medicine, New Haven, Connecticut

Ellen L. Edens, M.D., M.P.E., M.A.
Associate Fellowship Director, Addiction Psychiatry; Associate Professor, Department of Psychiatry, Yale School of Medicine, New Haven, Connecticut

Nady el-Guebaly, M.D., D.Psych., D.P.H.
Professor Emeritus, Psychiatry, University of Calgary, Calgary, Alberta, Canada

Skye Fitzpatrick, Ph.D.
Assistant Professor, Department of Psychology, York University, Toronto, Ontario, Canada

Timothy Fong, M.D.
Professor of Psychiatry, Addiction Psychiatry, Jane and Terry Semel Institute for Neuroscience and Human Behavior, David Geffen School of Medicine at UCLA, Los Angeles, California

Marc Galanter, M.D.
Research Professor of Psychiatry Department of Psychiatry, New York University School of Medicine, New York, New York

Joel Gelernter, M.D.
Foundations Fund Professor of Psychiatry and Professor of Genetics, and Neuroscience, Yale University School of Medicine, New Haven; and Psychiatric Genetics Laboratory Chief, VA CT Healthcare Center, West Haven, Connecticut

David A. Gorelick, M.D., Ph.D., DLFAPA, FASAM
Professor of Psychiatry, University of Maryland School of Medicine, Baltimore

Kevin M. Gray, M.D.
Professor, Department of Psychiatry and Behavioral Sciences, Medical University of South Carolina, Charleston

Alan I. Green, M.D.
Raymond Sobel Professor and Chair Emeritus, Department of Psychiatry, and Professor, Department of Molecular and Systems Biology, Geisel School of Medicine at Dartmouth, Hanover, New Hampshire

Shelly F. Greenfield, M.D., M.P.H.
Professor of Psychiatry, Harvard Medical School, Boston, Massachusetts; Kristine M. Trustey Endowed Chair in Psychiatry and Chief Academic Officer, McLean Hospital;

Chief, Division of Women's Mental Health; Director, Clinical and Health Services Research and Education, Division of Alcohol, Drugs & Addiction, McLean Hospital, Belmont, Massachusetts

Noah R. Gubner, Ph.D.
Research Scientist, Department of Psychiatry and Behavioral Sciences, University of Washington School of Medicine, Seattle

Constance Guille, M.D.
Associate Professor, Department of Psychiatry and Behavioral Sciences and Ob/Gyn; Director, Women's Reproductive Behavioral Health Program, Medical University of South Carolina, Charleston

Karen J. Hartwell, M.D.
Associate Professor, Medical University of South Carolina, Charleston, South Carolina

Deborah S. Hasin, Ph.D.
Professor of Epidemiology, Department of Psychiatry, Columbia University Irving Medical Center; Research Scientist, New York State Psychiatric Institute, New York City

Markus Heilig, M.D., Ph.D.
Professor, Center for Social and Affective Neuroscience, BKV, Linköping University, Linköping, Sweden

Grace Hennessy, M.D.
Clinical Assistant Professor of Psychiatry; Program Director, Addiction Psychiatry Fellowship, New York University School of Medicine; Director, Substance Abuse Recovery Program, VA New York Harbor Healthcare System, New York Campus, New York

Denise A. Hien, Ph.D.
Director and Professor, Center of Alcohol and Substance Use Studies, Graduate School of Applied and Professional Psychology, Rutgers University–New Brunswick, Piscataway, New Jersey; Adjunct Senior Research Scientist, Division on Substance Use Disorders, Columbia University Irving Medical Center, New York City

Elizabeth F. Howell, M.D., M.S., DLFAPA, DFASAM
Associate Professor of Psychiatry (Clinical); Training Director, Addiction Psychiatry Fellowship; Training Director, Addiction Medicine Fellowship; Education Director, Program for Addiction Research, Clinical Care, Knowledge, and Advocacy (PARCKA); Department of Psychiatry, University of Utah Health, Salt Lake City, Utah

Amber Jarnecke, Ph.D.
Research Assistant Professor, Addiction Sciences Division, Department of Psychiatry and Behavioral Sciences, Medical University of South Carolina, Charleston

Christopher M. Jones, Pharm.D., Dr.P.H.
CAPT, U.S. Public Health Service; Deputy Director, National Center for Disease Control and Prevention, Centers for Disease Control and Prevention, Atlanta, Georgia

Jennifer L. Jones, M.D.
Assistant Professor, Medical University of South Carolina, Charleston

Jermaine D. Jones, Ph.D.
Associate Professor of Clinical Neurobiology (in Psychiatry) and Research Scientist IV, Department of Psychiatry, Division on Substance Use Disorders, Columbia University Irving Medical Center and the New York State Psychiatric Institute, New York City

Tamar A. Kaminski, B.S.
Clinical Research Coordinator, Pediatric Psychopharmacology Program, Division of Child and Adolescent Psychiatry, Massachusetts General Hospital, Boston

Gen Kanayama, M.D., Ph.D.
Associate Director, Biological Psychiatry Laboratory, McLean Hospital; Research Associate, Department of Psychiatry, Harvard Medical School, Boston, Massachusetts

Edward J. Khantzian, M.D.
Professor of Psychiatry, Harvard Medical School, Boston, Massachusetts

Jeremy D. Kidd, M.D., M.P.H.
Postdoctoral Fellow in Substance Abuse Research, Columbia University Irving Medical Center and the New York State Psychiatric Institute, New York City

Therese K. Killeen, Ph.D., A.P.R.N.
Research Professor, Addiction Science Division, Department of Psychiatry and Behavioral Sciences, Medical University of South Carolina, Charleston

Brian D. Kiluk, Ph.D.
Associate Professor of Psychiatry, Yale University School of Medicine, New Haven, Connecticut

Hyoun S. Kim, M.A.
Ph.D. candidate, University of Calgary, Calgary, Alberta, Canada

Jungjin Kim, M.D.
Staff Psychiatrist, McLean Hospital, Harvard Medical School, Belmont, Massachusetts

Herbert D. Kleber, M.D.[‡]
Professor of Psychiatry and Director, Division on Substance Abuse (now the Division on Substance Use Disorders), Columbia University Irving Medical Center and the New York State Psychiatric Institute, New York City

George F. Koob, Ph.D.
Director, National Institute on Alcohol Abuse and Alcoholism, National Institutes of Health, Bethesda, Maryland

Thomas R. Kosten, M.D.
Jay H. Waggoner Chair and Professor of Psychiatry and Neuroscience, Baylor College of Medicine, Michael E. DeBakey VA Medical Center, Menninger Department of Psychiatry and Behavioral Sciences, Houston, Texas

Farren R.R. Larson, M.A.
At the time of this work, Ms. Larson was a research assistant in the Department of Translational Epidemiology, New York State Psychiatric Institute, New York, New York

---

[‡] Deceased.

Cameron S. Laue, B.A.
Doctoral student, School of Graduate Psychology, College of Health Professions, Pacific University, Hillsboro, Oregon

Charles J. Levin, B.A.
Medical student, Rutgers Robert Wood Johnson Medical School, New Brunswick, New Jersey

Frances R. Levin, M.D.
Kennedy-Leavy Professor of Psychiatry and Director, Substance Abuse Fellowship Program, Department of Psychiatry, Columbia University Irving Medical Center; Chief, Division on Substance Use Disorders, New York State Psychiatric Institute, New York City

Sarah E. Lord, Ph.D.
Director, Dissemination and Implementation Core, Center for Technology and Behavioral Health, Geisel School of Medicine, Dartmouth College, Hanover, New Hampshire

Robert Malcolm, M.D.
Professor of Psychiatry, Family Medicine, and Pediatrics, Medical University of South Carolina, Charleston

Lisa A. Marsch, Ph.D.
Director, The Center for Technology and Behavioral Health, Geisel School of Medicine, Dartmouth College, Hanover, New Hampshire

Jenna L. McCauley, Ph.D.
Assistant Professor of Psychiatry and Behavioral Sciences, Medical University of South Carolina, Charleston, South Carolina

A. Thomas McLellan, Ph.D.
Emeritus Professor of Psychology in Psychiatry, Perelman School of Medicine, University of Pennsylvania, Philadelphia, Pennsylvania

Aimee McRae-Clark, Pharm.D.
Professor, Department of Psychiatry and Behavioral Sciences, Medical University of South Carolina; Research Health Scientist, Ralph H. Johnson VA Medical Center, Charleston, South Carolina

Souparno Mitra, M.D.
Resident in Psychiatry, Bronxcare Health System, Icahn School of Medicine at Mount Sinai, Bronx, New York

Larissa J. Mooney, M.D.
Associate Clinical Professor, UCLA Department of Psychiatry and Biobehavioral Sciences; Chief, Greater Los Angeles VA Substance Use Disorders Section, UCLA Integrated Substance Abuse Programs, Los Angeles, California

Mudassir Mumtaz, B.S.
Medical student, Sophie Davis Biomedical Education Program, City University of New York (CUNY) School of Medicine, New York, New York

Hugh Myrick, M.D.
ACOS, Mental Health Service Line, Ralph H. Johnson VAMC Associate Professor of Psychiatry; Vice Chair, Psychiatry Practice Plan; Director, Military Sciences Division, Medical University of South Carolina, Charleston

Nicola C. Newton, Ph.D.
Associate Professor, The Matilda Centre for Research in Mental Health and Substance Use, The University of Sydney, Sydney, Australia

Andrea Norcini Pala, Ph.D.
Associate Research Scientist, Social Intervention Group (SIG), Columbia School of Social Work, New York, New York

Sonya Norman, Ph.D.
Professor, University of California San Diego School of Medicine, San Diego; Director, PTSD Consultation Program, National Center for PTSD, San Diego, California

Edward Nunes, M.D.
Professor of Clinical Psychiatry, Division on Substance Use Disorders, Columbia University Irving Medical Center and the New York State Psychiatric Institute, New York City

Mayumi Okuda, M.D.
Director, Gambling Disorders Clinic, Department of Psychiatry, Division on Substance Use Disorders, Columbia University Irving Medical Center and the New York State Psychiatric Institute, New York City

Nancy Petry, Ph.D.‡
Professor of Medicine, Calhoun Cardiology Center, University of Connecticut Health Center, Farmington, Connecticut

Renato Polimanti, Ph.D.
Assistant Professor, Department of Psychiatry, Yale University School of Medicine, New Haven; and VA CT Healthcare Center, West Haven, Connecticut

Harrison G. Pope Jr., M.D.
Director, Biological Psychiatry Laboratory, McLean Hospital; Professor of Psychiatry, Department of Psychiatry, Harvard Medical School, Boston, Massachusetts

Katherine Pruzan, Psy.D.
Director of Evaluation Services, The Center for Motivation and Change, New York, New York

Richard A. Rawson, Ph.D.
Research Psychologist, Vermont Center for Behavior and Health, Department of Psychiatry, University of Vermont, Burlington, Vermont; Professor Emeritus, UCLA Department of Psychiatry and Biobehavioral Sciences, Los Angeles, California

Robert H. Remien, Ph.D.
Professor of Psychology (in Psychiatry), Department of Psychiatry; Director, HIV Center for Clinical and Behavioral Studies, and Associate Director, Division of Gender,

‡ Deceased.

Sexuality, and Health, Columbia University Irving Medical Center and the New York State Psychiatric Institute, New York City

Richard K. Ries, M.D.
Professor of Psychiatry and Director of Addictions Division, Department of Psychiatry, University of Washington School of Medicine, Seattle, Washington

Amanda T. Roten, M.D.
Assistant Professor, Department of Psychiatry and Behavioral Sciences, Medical University of South Carolina, Charleston

Maria Alejandra Gallo Ruiz, M.D.
Psychiatry Resident, Bronxcare Health Systems, Bronx, New York

Gregory Sahlem, M.D.
Assistant Professor, Department of Psychiatry and Behavioral Sciences, Stanford University, Palo Alto, California

Richard Saitz, M.D., M.P.H., FACP, DFASAM
Chair and Professor, Department of Community Health Sciences, Boston University School of Public Health; Professor of Medicine, Boston University School of Medicine; Physician, Clinical Addiction Research and Education Unit, Section of General Internal Medicine, Grayken Center for Addiction, Boston Medical Center, Boston, Massachusetts

Kristen Schmidt, M.D.
Board Certified Addiction Psychiatrist, Hazelden Betty Ford Foundation, Residential Treatment, Center City, and Intensive Outpatient Programming, St. Paul, Minnesota

Jeffrey D. Schulden, M.D.
Deputy Branch Chief, Epidemiology Research Branch, Division of Epidemiology, Services, and Prevention Research, National Institute on Drug Abuse, Bethesda, Maryland

Elizabeth K.C. Schwartz, M.D., Ph.D.
Assistant Clinical Professor, Department of Psychiatry, Icahn School of Medicine at Mount Sinai, New York, New York

Katherine M. Seavey, B.A.
Research Assistant, The Center for Technology and Behavioral Health, Geisel School of Medicine, Dartmouth College, Hanover, New Hampshire

Brian Sherman, Ph.D.
Assistant Professor, Department of Psychiatry and Behavioral Sciences, Medical University of South Carolina, Charleston, South Carolina

Matisyahu Shulman, M.D.
Assistant Professor of Clinical Psychiatry, Department of Psychiatry, Division on Substance Use Disorders, Columbia University Irving Medical Center and the New York State Psychiatric Institute, New York City

Allison J. Smith, M.D.
Assistant Professor, Department of Psychiatry, Medical University of South Carolina, Charleston, South Carolina

Nathan D.L. Smith, A.L.M.
Ph.D. student, Department of Epidemiology, Colleges of Public Health and Health Professions and Medicine, University of Florida, Gainesville

Mehmet Sofuoglu, M.D., Ph.D.
Professor of Psychiatry, Yale University School of Medicine; Director of New England Mental Illness, Research, Education and Clinical Center (MIRECC), VA Connecticut Healthcare System, Psychiatry, West Haven, Connecticut

Rainer Spanagel, Ph.D.
Professor, Institute of Psychopharmacology, Central Institute of Mental Health, Mannheim, Germany

Peter Steinglass, M.D.
President Emeritus, Ackerman Institute for the Family; Clinical Professor of Psychiatry, Weill Cornell Medical College, New York, New York

Maxine L. Stitzer, Ph.D.
Professor Emerita, Department of Psychiatry and Behavioral Sciences, Johns Hopkins University School of Medicine; Senior Research Scientist, Friends Research Institute, Baltimore, Maryland

Kenneth B. Stoller, M.D.
Associate Professor, Department of Psychiatry and Behavioral Sciences; Director, Johns Hopkins Broadway Center, Johns Hopkins University School of Medicine, Baltimore, Maryland

Eric C. Strain, M.D.
The George E. Bigelow Professor, Department of Psychiatry and Behavioral Sciences, Johns Hopkins University School of Medicine, Baltimore, Maryland

Elizabeth Straus, Ph.D.
Postdoctoral Fellow, Advanced Fellowship in Women's Health, VA San Diego Healthcare System, San Diego; Postdoctoral Fellow, Department of Psychiatry, University of California, San Diego, California

Maria A. Sullivan, M.D., Ph.D.
Executive Medical Director, Medical Affairs, Alkermes, Inc., Waltham, Massachusetts; Associate Professor of Clinical Psychiatry, Department of Psychiatry, Columbia University, New York, New York

Mary M. Sweeney, Ph.D.
Assistant Professor, Department of Psychiatry and Behavioral Sciences, Johns Hopkins University School of Medicine, Behavioral Pharmacology Research Unit, Baltimore, Maryland

Maree Teesson, Ph.D.
Professor, The Matilda Centre for Research in Mental Health and Substance Use, The University of Sydney, Sydney, Australia

Amy VandenBerg, Pharm.D., BCPP
Adjunct Clinical Associate Professor in Pharmacy, University of Michigan, Ann Arbor

Nora D. Volkow, M.D.
Director, National Institute on Drug Abuse, National Institutes of Health, Bethesda, Maryland

Jonathan M. Wai, M.D.
Addiction Psychiatry Fellow, Division on Substance Use Disorders, Columbia University Irving Medical Center and the New York State Psychiatric Institute, New York City

Robert Werner, M.D.
Assistant Professor, Department of Psychiatry, Yale School of Medicine, New Haven, Connecticut

Laurence M. Westreich, M.D.
Clinical Associate Professor of Psychiatry, Division of Alcoholism and Drug Abuse, Department of Psychiatry, New York University School of Medicine, New York

Timothy E. Wilens, M.D.
Chief, Division of Child and Adolescent Psychiatry, Massachusetts General Hospital; Professor of Psychiatry, Harvard Medical School, Boston, Massachusetts

Arthur Robin Williams, M.D., M.B.E.
Assistant Professor, Department of Psychiatry, Division on Substance Use Disorders, Columbia University Irving Medical Center and the New York State Psychiatric Institute, New York City

Jill M. Williams, M.D.
Professor of Psychiatry and Director of the Division of Addiction Psychiatry, Rutgers Robert Wood Johnson Medical School, New Brunswick, New Jersey

Adam D. Wilson, M.S.
Department of Psychology, Center on Alcoholism, Substance Abuse, and Addictions, University of New Mexico, Albuquerque, New Mexico

Tara M. Wright, M.D.
Assistant Chief, Mental Health Service Line, Ralph H. Johnson VAMC Addiction Psychiatry Fellowship Director, Medical University of South Carolina, Charleston

Disclosure of Interests

The following contributors to this textbook have indicated a financial interest in or other affiliation with a commercial supporter, manufacturer of a commercial product, and/or provider of a commercial service as listed below:

Neal L. Benowitz, M.D. Dr. Benowitz serves on a scientific advisor board for Pfizer, which markets smoking cessation medications, and is a consultant to Achieve Life Sciences, which is developing new smoking cessation medications. He has also been a paid expert witness in litigation against tobacco companies, with testimony relating to nicotine addiction.

Kathleen T. Brady, M.D., Ph.D. *Consultant:* Embera Pharmaceuticals.

Timothy D. Brewerton, M.D. *Royalties:* Oxford University Press; *Shareholder:* Monte Nido & Affiliates.

Mary F. Brunette, M.D. In the past 3 years, Dr. Brunette has received funding from the National Cancer Institute and from Alkermes.

Kathleen M. Carroll, Ph.D.   Dr. Carroll is a member of CBT4CBT, LLC, which makes validated versions of cognitive-behavioral therapy available to qualified clinical providers.

Sandra D. Comer, Ph.D.   *Research Support:* Alkermes, Braeburn, Cerecor, Indivior, Medici-Nova, NeRRe Therapeutics, and Omeros; *Consulting:* AstraZeneca, Charleston Labs, Clinilabs, Collegium, Daiichi Sankyo, Depomed, Egalet, Endo, Heptares Therapeutics, Inspirion Delivery Sciences, Janssen, KemPharm, Opiant, Pfizer, and Salix.

Wilson M. Compton, M.D., M.P.E.   Dr. Compton reports ownership of stock in General Electric Co., 3M Co., and Pfizer Inc., unrelated to the submitted work.

Nady el-Guebaly, M.D., D.Psych., D.P.H.   Dr. el-Guebaly was Senior Editor of the *International Society of Addiction Medicine (ISAM) Textbook of Addiction Treatment: International Perspectives* (Springer, 2015).

Joel Gelernter, M.D.   Dr. Gelernter is named as inventor on Patent Cooperation Treaty (PCT) patent application #15/878,640 (titled "Genotype-Guided Dosing of Opioid Agonists"), filed January 24, 2018.

Alan I. Green, M.D.   In the past 4 years, Dr. Green has received funding for research from Janssen, Novartis, and Alkermes and has served on a Data Monitoring Board for Eli Lilly and as an unpaid consultant to Otsuka Alkermes. He is the holder of a U.S. patent (#9044471) related to treatment of alcoholism.

Deborah S. Hasin, Ph.D.   Dr. Hasin received a one-time consulting payment from Alkermes, Inc. Through the grants and contracts office of the Research Foundation for Mental Hygiene, she has also received contracted research study funds from Campbell Alliance for U.S. Food and Drug Administration–mandated studies of the assessment and quality assurance of opioid addiction measures for patients with chronic pain.

Markus Heilig, M.D., Ph.D.   Dr. Heilig has served on scientific advisory boards for Aelis Pharma, BrainsWay Inc, Camurus, and Indivior.

Therese K. Killeen, Ph.D., A.P.R.N.   *Royalties:* Oxford University Press; *Shareholder:* Monte Nido & Affiliates.

Frances R. Levin, M.D.   Dr. Levin receives grant support from the National Institute on Drug Abuse (NIDA), the Substance Abuse and Mental Health Services Administration (SAMHSA), and US WorldMeds, and also serves as a consultant for Major League Baseball. She has served as an unpaid member of scientific advisory boards for Alkermes, Indivior, Novartis, and US WorldMeds but did not personally receive any compensation in the form of cash payments (honoraria/consulting fees), free food or beverages (she declined these in each circumstance), or travel reimbursement.

A. Thomas McLellan, Ph.D.   Dr. McLellan is on the Board of Directors of Indivior, Inc. (pharmaceutical firm making Suboxone and Sublocade); Shatterproof (nonprofit addiction research and advocacy organization); and Recover Together (a for-profit treatment company specializing in office-based treatment in rural settings).

Richard Saitz, M.D., M.P.H., FACP, DFASAM   Dr. Saitz is and has been principal investigator on grants awarded to the Boston Medical Center and Boston University from the National Institutes of Health (NIH)—including the National Institute on Alcohol Abuse and Alcoholism (NIAAA), the National Institute on Drug Abuse (NIDA), and the Substance Abuse and Mental Health Services Administration (SAMHSA)—to study the management of unhealthy substance use, including testing of the accuracy of screening; the efficacy of screening, brief intervention, and referral to treatment; and the effectiveness of integrated care. He has been paid to speak at—or has had travel reimbursed to speak at or to consult for—numerous professional and scientific organizations, all of which are nonprofit entities. In the past 3 years, these engagements have included the following: the American Society of Addiction Medicine (ASAM), RAND, the Research Society on Alcoholism, the *British Medical Journal* (BMJ), the American Medical Association, the Institute for Research and Training in the Addictions, the National Council on Behavioral Healthcare, the International Conference on Treatment of Addictive Behaviors, the International Network on Brief Intervention for Alcohol and other drugs (INEBRIA), Leed Management Consulting, Inc. (for a Harvard University opioid use disorder education program supported by NIDA), the Kaiser Permanente Washington Health Research Institute, the Kaiser Permanente Division of Research, the Kaiser Permanente Center for Health Research Portland, the University of Oregon, the National Committee on Quality Assurance, and numerous universities and hospitals. He is an author and editor for Springer, UpToDate, ASAM, the *Journal of the American Medical Association* (JAMA), the BMJ, and the Massachusetts Medical Society (royalties and/or honoraria). Wolters Kluwer has supported Dr. Saitz's conference travel to an editors' meeting. Systembolaget (a Swedish government agency that aims to minimize alcohol-related problems) provided transportation support and lodging for a presentation on brief intervention at an INEBRIA thematic meeting in 2016. Alkermes provided medication for an NIH-funded trial of alcohol use disorder treatment effectiveness. Dr. Saitz has been paid to serve as an expert witness in malpractice cases related to the management of alcohol and other drug use disorders. He has also served as research consultant for Yale University, Brandeis University, Group Health Inc, Beth Israel–Deaconess Hospital, Charles University (Czech Republic), and other universities. Dr. Saitz spoke at a National Press Foundation event on the terminology of addiction and received no compensation; however, the meeting itself was funded by ASAM, Open Society Foundations, Pew Charitable Trusts, Shatterproof, Hazelden Betty Ford Foundation, and the Addiction Technology Transfer Center Network. Dr. Saitz has served as consultant for the National Committee on Quality Assurance regarding alcohol screening and for the University of Oregon on a systematic review of screening and brief intervention (SBI). He is President of the International Society of Addiction Journal Editors. He is employed by the Boston University School of Public Health.

Laurence M. Westreich, M.D.　　Dr. Westreich serves as the Consultant on Behavioral Health and Addiction to the Commissioner of Major League Baseball and is the Director of Corporate Wellness at Strive Health.

Timothy E. Wilens, M.D.　　Dr. Timothy Wilens is or has been a consultant for Alcobra Pharmaceuticals, Neurovance/Otsuka, and Ironshore Pharmaceuticals. He receives grant funding from the National Institutes of Health (National Institute on Drug Abuse). Dr. Timothy Wilens has published books (*Straight Talk About Psychiatric Medications for Kids* [Guilford Press]) and co-edited books (*ADHD in Adults and Children* [Cambridge University Press]; *Massachusetts General Hospital Comprehensive Clinical Psychiatry* [Elsevier]; and *Massachusetts General Hospital Psychopharmacology and Neurotherapeutics* [Elsevier]). Dr. Wilens is co-owner of a copyrighted diagnostic questionnaire (Before School Functioning Questionnaire [BSFQ]) and has a licensing agreement with Ironshore (BSFQ Questionnaire). Dr. Wilens is employed as Chief, Division of Child and Adolescent Psychiatry, and is Co-Director of the Center for Addiction Medicine at Massachusetts General Hospital. He serves as a clinical consultant to the U.S. National Football League (ERM Associates), U.S. Minor/Major League Baseball, Phoenix/Gavin House, and Bay Cove Human Services.

Jill M. Williams, M.D.　　Dr. Williams has received grant support and CME grant support from Pfizer, and she served as an advisory board member for Prizer in 2016.

The following contributors stated that they had no competing interests during the year preceding manuscript submission:

Elie G. Aoun, M.D.; Carlos Blanco, M.D., Ph.D., M.S.; Kenneth M. Carpenter, Ph.D.; Vamsee Chaguturu, M.D.; Katrina Champion, Ph.D.; Nina Cooperman, Psy.D.; Marc Galanter, M.D.; Kevin M. Gray, M.D.; Shelly F. Greenfield, M.D., M.P.H.; Noah R. Gubner, Ph.D.; Amber Jarnecke, Ph.D.; Jermaine D. Jones, Ph.D.; Tamar Arit Kaminski, B.S.; Gen Kanayama, M.D., Ph.D.; Edward J. Khantzian, M.D.; Jeremy D. Kidd, M.D., M.P.H.; Brian D. Kiluk, Ph.D.; Hyoun S. Kim, M.A.; George F. Koob, Ph.D.; Thomas R. Kosten, M.D.; Farren R. R. Larson, M.A.; Charles J. Levin, B.A.; Aimee McRae-Clark, Pharm.D.; Mudassir Mumtaz, B.S.; Nicola Newton, Ph.D.; Andrea Norcini Pala, Ph.D.; Mayumi Okuda Benavides, M.D.; Harrison G. Pope Jr., M.D.; Katherine Pruzan, Psy.D.; Richard K. Ries, M.D.; Maria Alejandra Gallo Ruiz, M.D.; Jeffrey D. Schulden, M.D.; Matisyahu Shulman, M.D.; Peter Steinglass, M.D.; Maxine L. Stitzer, Ph.D.; Elizabeth Straus, Ph.D.; Maree Teesson, Ph.D.

PART I

The Basis of Substance-Related and Addictive Disorders

CHAPTER 1

Neurocircuitry of Addiction

George F. Koob, Ph.D.
Nora D. Volkow, M.D.

Substance and alcohol use disorders cause an enormous amount of human suffering, loss of productivity, costs to our medical care system, and costs to the economy. This chapter provides a heuristic conceptual framework for alcohol and other substance use disorders, in which we integrate preclinical and clinical advances in the neuroscience of addiction that are pertinent to the prevention and management of these disorders. Conceptualization of addiction as a three-component cycle consisting of a binge/intoxication stage, a withdrawal/negative affect stage, and a preoccupation/ anticipation (craving) stage has allowed identification of key neurocircuits that underlie addiction to alcohol and many other drugs. Each stage of the addiction cycle is hypothesized to represent a different domain of dysfunction that is mediated by a different neurobiological circuit. The binge/intoxication stage involves recruitment of reward neurotransmission in the basal ganglia to drive incentive salience and pathological habits. The withdrawal/negative affect stage involves loss of reward neurotransmission and gain of stress neurotransmission in the extended amygdala to drive the negative emotional state of withdrawal. The preoccupation/anticipation stage involves dysregulation of the prefrontal cortex to drive abnormal executive function and craving. Molecular genetic mediation and epigenetic loads on these same three major neurocircuits are hypothesized to confer environment-dependent and environment-independent vulnerabilities to addiction and thus represent promising targets for the development of novel approaches to strengthen resilience and prevent relapse. Accumulating data show how existing treatments for addiction work on these neurocircuits,

The authors thank Michael Arends for assistance with chapter preparation.

and the growing knowledge base on the neurocircuitry of addiction provides evidence-supported information for the development of novel, science-based approaches to diagnosis, prevention, and treatment. Such advances will facilitate implementation of evidence-based practices in primary care, mental health care, and other health care settings.

Conceptual Framework, Definitions, and Animal Models

Drug addiction can be defined as a chronically relapsing disorder, characterized by the compulsion to seek and take the drug, the loss of control in limiting intake, and the emergence of a negative emotional state (e.g., manifesting as dysphoria, anxiety, irritability)—termed the *dark side* of addiction (Koob and Le Moal 2005)—when access to the drug is prevented. From a diagnostic perspective, the term *addiction* is now encompassed within the term *substance use disorder.* The new (fifth) edition of the *Diagnostic and Statistical Manual of Mental Disorders* (DSM-5; American Psychiatric Association 2013) combined what were previously conceptualized as two separate and hierarchical disorders (substance abuse and substance dependence) into a single construct, defining substance use disorders on a range from mild to moderate to severe. The severity of an addiction depends on how many of the established criteria apply. In this chapter, we use the term *addiction* to correspond to a moderate to severe substance use disorder.

Although much of the early research with animal models focused on the acute rewarding effects of drugs of abuse, the research focus has now shifted to the study of brain changes produced by long-term drug administration, including pathological habit formation, withdrawal-induced negative emotional states, and compromised executive function, that decrease the threshold for relapse. From the perspective of compromised executive function and impairments in the reward motivation circuit, human imaging studies of individuals with substance use disorders have provided compelling insights into the neurobiology of addiction.

Understanding changes at the molecular, cellular, and neurocircuitry levels that mediate the transition from occasional, controlled substance use to loss of control over drug intake with addiction has raised compelling questions about individual differences in vulnerability. Only some substance users transition to compulsive drug taking. The neurobiological factors that influence the wide range of individual variation in response to drugs have received intense research interest. It has been argued that addictions are similar to other chronic relapsing disorders, such as diabetes, asthma, and hypertension, in regard to the limited efficacy of treatment (McLellan et al. 2000). As is the case in other chronic relapsing disorders, individual differences in response to compulsive drug use may reflect differences in the pharmacological actions of the drug, the history of the individual, and genetic and epigenetic factors.

Neurobiological Mechanisms in the Addiction Cycle

Drug addiction has been conceptualized as a cycle of three stages, each representing basic neurocircuitry involved in motivation and each predominantly linked to a specific functional domain and its associated brain functional networks (but with the recognition that brain networks interact with one another) (Koob and Volkow 2010):

1. The *binge/intoxication* stage (mediated by neurocircuitry of the basal ganglia) reflects the rewarding effects of drugs and the ways in which drugs impart motivational significance to cues and contexts in the environment, termed *incentive salience,* which is experienced as "well-being," "high," "euphoria," or "relief," depending on the degree of tolerance to the rewarding effects of the drug. This stage begins the process of developing pathological habits that contribute to addiction.
2. The *withdrawal/negative affect* stage (mediated by neurocircuitry of the extended amygdala and the habenula) reflects the enhanced sensitivity and recruitment of brain stress systems and the loss of reward and motivation, termed a *negative emotional state,* which is experienced as dysphoria, anhedonia, and irritability.
3. The *preoccupation/anticipation* ("craving") stage (mediated by neurocircuitry of the prefrontal cortex) reflects impulsivity and the loss of control over drug taking, termed *loss of executive control,* and the input from the default mode network that reflects the enhanced interoceptive awareness of the desire for the drug, which is experienced as drug craving.

Binge/Intoxication Stage

Drugs of abuse activate brain reward systems. A principal focus of research on the neurobiology of the rewarding effects of abused drugs has been the terminal areas of the ascending mesocorticostriatal dopamine system, notably the nucleus accumbens (Koob 1992) (Figure 1–1). During the *binge/intoxication* stage, large surges of dopamine and the release of opioid peptides have been consistently associated with the reinforcing effects of most addictive drugs. Stimulant drugs (e.g., cocaine, methamphetamine) interact with the terminals of dopamine neurons to increase extracellular dopamine. Other drugs, such as nicotine, alcohol, opioids, and Δ^9-tetrahydrocannabinol, modulate dopamine cell firing through their effects on nicotinic, γ-aminobutyric acid (GABA), opioid, and cannabinoid (predominantly CB_1) receptors, respectively, thus increasing dopamine release. In humans, positron emission tomography (PET) studies have shown that intoxicating doses of alcohol and other drugs release dopamine and opioid peptides into the ventral striatum (Mitchell et al. 2012; Volkow et al. 2007). Such PET imaging studies have also shown that the rapid release of dopamine is associated with the subjective sensation of being "high" (Volkow et al. 2003). However, the specific circuitry associated with drug reward has been broadened to include many neural inputs and outputs that interact with the basal forebrain, particularly the nucleus accumbens, and include not only dopamine and opioid peptides but also GABA, glutamate, serotonin, acetylcholine, and endocannabinoid systems that act at the level of either the ventral tegmental area or the nucleus accumbens (see Figure 1–1). This initial reward response initiates a cascade of neurochemical and neurocircuitry changes that set up the withdrawal/negative affect stage. Additionally, drugs also directly or indirectly interact with cortical brain structures that convey different messages about stimulus response, approach behavior, learning, and decision making.

Drugs of abuse have a profound effect on the response to previously neutral stimuli with which the drugs become paired, a phenomenon called *conditioned reinforce-*

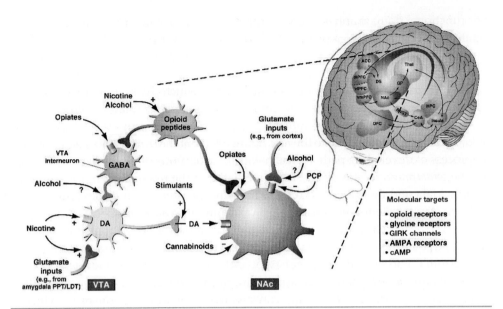

FIGURE 1-1. Neurocircuitry associated with the addiction cycle, part 1: the *binge/intoxication* stage.

To view this figure in color, see Plate 1 in Color Gallery in middle of book.

Reinforcing effects of drugs may engage associative mechanisms and reward neurotransmitters in the nucleus accumbens (NAc) shell and core and then engage stimulus-response habits that depend on the dorsal striatum (DS). Two major neurotransmitters that mediate the rewarding effects of drugs of abuse are dopamine (DA) and opioid peptides. Drugs of abuse, despite diverse initial actions, produce some common effects on the ventral tegmental area (VTA) and the NAc *(inset)*. Stimulant drugs act at DA terminals to either interfere with DA reuptake (cocaine) or increase DA release (methamphetamine). Opioids activate the NAc by inhibiting γ-aminobutyric acid (GABA) interneurons in the VTA, which disinhibit VTA DA neurons. Opioids also act directly on opioid receptors on NAc neurons and converge within some NAc neurons. The actions of other drugs remain more conjectural. Nicotine appears to activate VTA DA neurons directly by stimulating nicotinic acetylcholine receptors on these neurons and indirectly by stimulating nicotinic acetylcholine receptors on glutamatergic nerve terminals that innervate DA cells. Alcohol, by promoting GABA$_A$ receptor function, may inhibit GABAergic terminals in the VTA and hence disinhibit VTA DA neurons. Alcohol may similarly inhibit glutamatergic terminals that innervate NAc neurons. Many additional mechanisms (not shown) are proposed for alcohol. Cannabinoid mechanisms are complex and involve the activation of cannabinoid CB$_1$ receptors (which, like dopamine D$_2$ and opioid receptors, are G$_i$ protein–linked) on glutamatergic and GABAergic nerve terminals in the NAc and on NAc neurons themselves. Phencyclidine (PCP) may act by inhibiting postsynaptic *N*-methyl-D-aspartate (NMDA) glutamate receptors in the NAc. Finally, some evidence indicates that nicotine and alcohol may activate endogenous opioid pathways and that nicotine, alcohol, and other drugs of abuse (such as opioids) may activate endogenous cannabinoid pathways (not shown).

ACC=anterior cingulate cortex; AMPA=α-amino-3-hydroxy-5-methyl-4-isoxazolepropionic acid; BNST= bed nucleus of the stria terminalis; cAMP=cyclic adenosine monophosphate; CeA=central nucleus of the amygdala; dlPFC=dorsolateral prefrontal cortex; GP=globus pallidus; GIRK=G protein–coupled inwardly rectifying K$^+$ (potassium); HPC=hippocampus; OFC=orbitofrontal cortex; PPT/LDT=peduncular pontine tegmentum/lateral dorsal tegmentum; Thal=thalamus; vlPFC=ventrolateral prefrontal cortex; vmPFC= ventromedial prefrontal cortex.

The "Molecular targets" box lists key molecular targets that may convey genetic and epigenetic plasticity to the neurocircuits described in this figure.

Source. Modified with permission from Nestler EJ: "Is There a Common Molecular Pathway for Addiction?" *Nature Neuroscience* 8(11):1445–1449, 2005.

ment (Robbins 1976) that has evolved into what is now known as *incentive salience.* Incentive salience can be defined as the process by which previously neutral stimuli are linked through conditioning to a drug reinforcer and acquire the ability to engender strong motivation to seek the drug, presumably by increasing dopamine activity in the nucleus accumbens in anticipation of the reward. Recordings of the electrical activity of ventral tegmental area dopamine neurons in primates during repeated presentations of rewards and of stimuli associated with rewards showed that dopamine cells at first fired at the initial exposure to the novel reward. With repeated exposure, the neurons decreased firing during reward consumption and instead fired when they were exposed to stimuli that were *predictive* of the reward (Schultz et al. 1997). These results suggested that an increase in phasic dopamine cell firing leads to large and transient short-term increases in dopamine in the presence of stimuli that are predictive of drug reward and become salient by themselves and motivate seeking behaviors. In this way, exposure to drug-related cues in the addicted person results in striatal dopamine release that is associated with craving (Volkow et al. 2006).

Phasic dopamine signaling induced by drug administration then triggers neuroadaptations in basal ganglia circuits. Activation of the ventral striatum leads to the recruitment of striatal–globus pallidal–thalamic–cortical loops that engage the dorsal striatum, resulting in habit formation (Belin et al. 2013) and triggering what is hypothesized to underlie compulsive responding for drugs (Belin and Everitt 2008). Key synaptic changes involve the activation of glutamate in glutamatergic projections from the prefrontal cortex and amygdala to the ventral tegmental area and nucleus accumbens (Scofield et al. 2016; Wolf and Ferrario 2010). Glutamate adaptations that are triggered during the binge/intoxication stage are hypothesized to persist into withdrawal and protracted abstinence and to drive craving during the preoccupation/anticipation stage.

At the molecular and cellular levels in the binge/intoxication stage, different drugs of abuse, even during initial engagement, have been shown to alter the activation of different receptors and their transduction mechanisms, including opioid peptides at opioid receptors (Cahill et al. 2016), alcohol at glycine receptors and G protein–coupled inwardly rectifying potassium (GIRK) channels (Cui and Koob 2017), and psychostimulants at α-amino-3-hydroxy-5-methyl-4-isoxazolepropionic acid (AMPA) receptors (Nestler 2005). Molecular changes within the incentive salience–reward circuitry that may be common to all drugs of abuse include the upregulation of a postsynaptic G_s/cyclic adenosine monophosphate (cAMP)/protein kinase A signaling pathway in the nucleus accumbens that is central to establishing and maintaining the addicted state (Edwards and Koob 2010). Excessive drug use can initiate changes in the expression of certain transcription factors (i.e., nuclear proteins that bind to regulatory regions of genes, thereby regulating their transcription into mRNA), as well as changes in the expression of a wide variety of proteins that are involved in neurotransmission in several key brain regions (Feng and Nestler 2013).

Withdrawal/Negative Affect Stage

The *withdrawal/negative affect* stage consists of key motivational elements, such as chronic irritability, emotional pain, malaise, dysphoria, alexithymia, loss of motivation for natural rewards, and general hypersensitivity to negative emotional states (i.e., hyperkatifeia). Across all major drugs of abuse, drug withdrawal in laboratory animals is characterized by elevations of reward thresholds (i.e., decrease in reward). Decreases in reward neurotransmitters have been hypothesized to reflect a within-system neuroadaptation and are postulated to contribute to negative motivational states associated with acute drug abstinence. Acute and protracted withdrawal from the chronic administration of all major substances of abuse is also associated with increases in stress and anxiety-like responses that contribute significantly to the malaise of abstinence and protracted abstinence (Koob and Le Moal 2005). Human brain-imaging studies have reported decreases in the sensitivity of brain reward circuits to stimulation by natural rewards during the withdrawal/negative affect stage (Garavan et al. 2000).

Chronic drug exposure–induced neurochemical changes in the systems that are implicated in acute drug reward are called *within-system* neuroadaptations in which "the primary cellular response element to the drug…adapt[s] to neutralize the drug's effects; persistence of the opposing effects after the drug disappears…produce[s] the withdrawal response" (Koob and Bloom 1988, p. 720). Such changes include decreases in dopaminergic neurotransmission in the nucleus accumbens during drug withdrawal as measured by in vivo microdialysis in rats (Rossetti et al. 1992). In human brain-imaging studies, amphetamine- or methylphenidate-induced striatal dopamine responses are 50% lower in detoxified abusers and 80% lower in active abusers compared with non-drug-abusing control participants and are accompanied by lower self-reports of the drug's rewarding effects (Martinez et al. 2007; Volkow et al. 1997, 2014). Other within-system changes associated with dependence on drugs and alcohol include decreases in GABAergic activity and increases in N-methyl-D-aspartate (NMDA) glutamatergic neurotransmission in the nucleus accumbens during alcohol withdrawal (Koob and Volkow 2016). In mice that were chronically exposed to nicotine, differential regional changes in nicotinic receptor function in the nucleus accumbens and ventral tegmental area were also reported, implicating $\alpha4\beta2$ nicotinic acetylcholine receptor subtypes (Tolu et al. 2013).

For opioids, many molecular and cellular events contribute to within-system changes in μ-opioid receptor signaling, including alterations of G-protein signaling cascades, receptor desensitization, receptor internalization, transcriptional changes, and structural changes, such as spine remodeling (Cahill et al. 2016). Investigations of one of the major non–G-protein signal transduction pathways for the μ-opioid receptor have identified a key role for the β-arrestin pathway in opioid receptor desensitization and resensitization. These observations suggested that drugs that activate the μ-opioid receptor without activating the β-arrestin signal transduction cascade may have higher analgesic potential and lower tolerance and respiratory depression potential (Raehal et al. 2011); however, more recent data suggest that non-arrestin 3-signaling drugs may retain undesirable constipating and abuse-related effects with repeated exposure, despite their bias for G-protein signaling (Altarifi et al. 2017).

Such changes in neurotransmitter systems that contribute to decreases in reward system function may persist in the form of long-term biochemical changes that contribute to the clinical syndrome of acute withdrawal and protracted abstinence (dysphoria, malaise, depression-like symptoms) and that also may explain the loss of interest in normal, nondrug rewards (i.e., narrowing of the behavioral repertoire toward drugs and drug-related stimuli).

The negative emotional state associated with the withdrawal/negative affect stage also may involve *between-system* neuroadaptations, in which neurochemical systems other than those that are involved in positive rewarding effects of drugs of abuse are recruited or dysregulated by chronic activation of the reward system (Koob and Bloom 1988). The brain stress systems are activated during withdrawal from all drugs of abuse and include neurotransmitter systems such as corticotropin-releasing factor (CRF), dynorphin, norepinephrine, vasopressin, substance P, hypocretin (orexin), and inflammatory cytokines, all of which contribute to the negative emotional states associated with drug withdrawal (Figure 1–2). The concept of *antireward* was developed on the basis of the hypothesis that opponent processes that are a general feature of biological systems also act to limit reward (Koob and Le Moal 1997). A key player in between-system neuroadaptations is the activation of CRF in both the hypothalamic-pituitary-adrenal axis and the extended amygdala, with a common response of elevated adrenocorticotropic hormone, corticosterone, and amygdala CRF during acute withdrawal (Koob et al. 2014; Piazza and Le Moal 1996). During acute withdrawal from all drugs of abuse, CRF increases in the extended amygdala. Critically, CRF receptor antagonists block the anxiety-like and stress-like effects of drug withdrawal as well as excessive drug taking during compulsive drug seeking in animals. Indeed, as tolerance and withdrawal develop, other brain stress systems, such as norepinephrine and dynorphin, are recruited in the extended amygdala and contribute to the development of negative emotional states in withdrawal and protracted abstinence (Koob and Volkow 2016; Koob et al. 2014). κ-Opioid receptor antagonists, when injected into the nucleus accumbens shell, can block the development of compulsive drug seeking in animal models (Koob and Volkow 2016; see Figure 1–2).

Activation of brain stress systems may also drive hypoactivity in brain reward systems. Decreases in the release of dopamine in the nucleus accumbens may also be driven by increases in the activity of both the dynorphin/κ-opioid receptor system in the ventral striatum and CRF in the ventral tegmental area, contributing to the negative emotional state associated with withdrawal and protracted abstinence (Carlezon et al. 2000; Koob et al. 2014). Activation of the habenula is hypothesized to drive a decrease in dopamine neuron firing in the ventral tegmental area that is associated with the failure to receive an expected reward (Hikosaka 2010) and that also may play a role in depression and drug withdrawal (Meye et al. 2017). Thus, the recruitment of brain stress systems in the extended amygdala drives aversive motivational states, and the activation of brain stress systems in the ventral tegmental area and habenula can in turn inhibit dopamine cell firing and dopamine release in the mesolimbic dopamine system, effectively closing the motivational loop on the generation of negative emotional states during withdrawal.

Endogenous antistress systems appear to buffer the brain stress systems and influence vulnerability to the development and perpetuation of addiction. Key neurotransmitters that act in opposition to the brain stress systems include neuropeptide Y, nociceptin, and endocannabinoids (Koob and Volkow 2016) (see Figure 1–2). Thus, the development of enduring aversive emotional states (Leventhal et al. 2008), mediated by overactivation of the stress and antireward systems or underactivation of the antistress systems, may contribute to chronic relapse in drug addiction, in which addicted individuals return to compulsive drug taking long after acute withdrawal (Koob and Le Moal 2008).

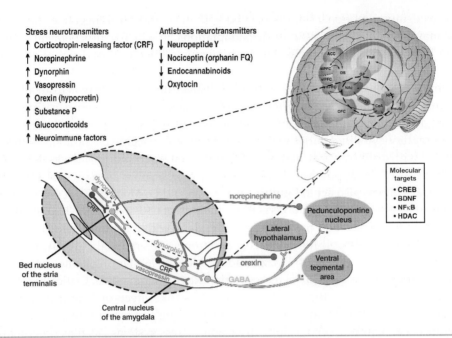

FIGURE 1–2. Neurocircuitry associated with the addiction cycle, part 2: the *withdrawal/ negative affect* stage.

To view this figure in color, see Plate 2 in Color Gallery in middle of book.

The negative emotional state of withdrawal may engage activation of the extended amygdala. The extended amygdala is composed of several basal forebrain structures, including the bed nucleus of the stria terminalis (BNST), the central nucleus of the amygdala (CeA), and possibly a transition area in the medial portion (shell) of the nucleus accumbens (NAc) *(inset)*. Major neurotransmitters in the extended amygdala that are hypothesized to play a role in negative reinforcement are corticotropin-releasing factor (CRF), norepinephrine, and dynorphin. The extended amygdala has major projections to the hypothalamus and the brain stem. The negative emotional state of withdrawal engages activation of the extended amygdala. Neurotransmitter systems engaged in the neurocircuitry of the extended amygdala *(listed at top left)* that convey negative emotional states are indicated by *upward arrows,* and neurotransmitter systems that may buffer negative emotional states *(listed at top center)* are indicated by *downward arrows*. The magnified section *(blue oval enclosed in dashes)* shows the extended amygdala in detail. *Green/blue pathways (see asterisks)* indicate glutamatergic projections.

ACC=anterior cingulate cortex; BDNF=brain-derived neurotrophic factor; CREB=cyclic adenosine monophosphate response element–binding protein; dlPFC=dorsolateral prefrontal cortex; DS=dorsal striatum; GABA=γ-aminobutyric acid; GP=globus pallidus; HDAC=histone deacetylase; HPC=hippocampus; NFκB=nuclear factor κB; OFC=orbitofrontal cortex; Thal=thalamus; vlPFC=ventrolateral prefrontal cortex; vmPFC=ventromedial prefrontal cortex.

The "Molecular targets" box lists key molecular targets that may convey genetic and epigenetic plasticity to the neurocircuits described in this figure.

Source. Adapted from George and Koob 2013 (brain); Koob 2008 (diagram).

In summary, antireward circuits are engaged as neuroadaptations during the development of addiction, producing aversive or stresslike states when the drug is removed (acute withdrawal and protracted abstinence) (Koob and Le Moal 2008). The combination of decreases in reward system function and increases in stress system function in motivational circuits in the ventral striatum, extended amygdala, and habenula is a powerful trigger of negative reinforcement that contributes to compulsive drug-seeking behavior and addiction. Such pro-stress systems are counteracted by "buffer systems" (e.g., neuropeptide Y, nociceptin, endocannabinoids) that act to restore homeostasis in stress circuits in the extended amygdala.

At the molecular level, the activation of transcription factors, such as cAMP response element–binding protein (CREB), has been hypothesized to contribute to symptoms of acute withdrawal and the negative emotional state of withdrawal. An increase in CREB phosphorylation in the nucleus accumbens triggered by use of cocaine or opioids leads to a gain of dynorphin function that causes dysphoria and greater cocaine or morphine intake (Carlezon et al. 2000; Nestler 2012). However, a decrease in CREB phosphorylation in the central nucleus of the amygdala yields a decrease in neuropeptide Y (Pandey et al. 2017). Indeed, the cascade of molecular changes in the central nucleus of the amygdala can be viewed within an epigenetic framework. Following chronic alcohol exposure and subsequent withdrawal, decreases in histone acetylation occur through an increase in histone deacetylase activity and decreases in the expression of brain-derived neurotrophic factor, activity-regulated cytoskeleton-associated protein, and neuropeptide Y in amygdala circuitry, which produce anxiety-like responses (Pandey et al. 2017).

Preoccupation/Anticipation Stage

Relapse after abstinence from drug taking defines addiction as a chronic relapsing disorder and is the domain of the third stage of the addiction cycle: the *preoccupation/ anticipation* stage. Craving is a symptom in the DSM-5 diagnostic criteria for substance use disorder and is a prominent feature of the preoccupation/anticipation stage. However, craving per se as measured in human clinical studies is not always easy to capture (Tiffany et al. 2000). Nevertheless, elements of craving can be defined and are useful for identifying neurobiological mechanisms of relapse and developing medications for treatment.

Executive, top-down control over goal-directed behavior can enhance the flexibility of stimulus–response associations and restrain the power of incentive salience. A key component of the pathophysiology of addiction involves poor inhibitory control and poor executive function, which are mediated by prefrontal cortical regions. For example, selective damage of prefrontal cortical regions induced by chronic intermittent use of alcohol or cocaine can lead to poor decision making, which may perpetuate the addiction cycle (Goldstein and Volkow 2011). Impairments in prefrontal cortex areas can result in dysregulation of reward- and stress-related brain regions and disruptions in higher-order executive functions (e.g., self-control, salience attribution, awareness) (Volkow et al. 2012). Indeed, gray matter volume deficits in specific medial frontal and posterior parietal-occipital brain regions are predictive of relapse risk, suggesting a significant role for gray matter atrophy in poor clinical outcomes in addiction (Rando et al. 2011).

In human brain-imaging studies, craving responses to cues activate an overarching cognitive control network (Volkow and Fowler 2000; Volkow et al. 2011) involving the dorsolateral prefrontal, anterior cingulate, and parietal cortices, all of which support a broad range of executive functions (Niendam et al. 2012). A frontal-cingulate-parietal-subcortical cognitive control network is hypothesized to be consistently recruited across a range of traditional executive function tasks, many of which reveal deficits in humans with alcohol use disorder. Indeed, the most prominent regional target of activation by alcohol-related cues involves the dorsolateral prefrontal cortex, cingulate cortex, and orbitofrontal cortex (Olbrich et al. 2006). Such drug cue–evoked responses are hypothesized to reflect the neural representations of reward and incentive salience constructs (Jasinska et al. 2014). One parsimonious view of the human imaging data that is consistent with animal model data is that a "Go" system in the dorsal prefrontal/cingulate cortex drives impulsivity and craving, and a "Stop" system in the ventromedial prefrontal cortex inhibits impulsivity and craving (Koob and Volkow 2016). From a theoretical perspective, some have hypothesized that competition exists between impulsive and executive function systems that may partially account for self-control failures (Bickel et al. 2012). Studies of mechanisms involved in self-regulation will allow integration of the neuroscience of addiction with developmental processes, socioeconomic status, and comorbidities.

In humans, stress and stressors have long been associated with relapse and the vulnerability to relapse (Marlatt and Gordon 1980). Individuals with an addiction are hypersensitive to pain during substance withdrawal, particularly in the face of negative affect (Jochum et al. 2010). Indeed, the leading precipitant of relapse is negative emotion or affect, including elements of anger, frustration, sadness, anxiety, and guilt (Zywiak et al. 1996).

In animal studies, craving can be divided into three domains: 1) drug seeking that is induced by the drug itself (i.e., drug priming–induced reinstatement), 2) drug seeking that is induced by stimuli that are paired with drug taking (i.e., cue- and context-induced reinstatement), and 3) drug seeking that is induced by an acute stressor or by a state of stress (i.e., stress-induced reinstatement) (Martin-Fardon and Weiss 2013). Neurotransmitter systems that are involved in drug- and cue-induced reinstatement involve a glutamatergic projection from the frontal cortex to the nucleus accumbens that is modulated by dopamine activity in the frontal cortex, basolateral amygdala, and ventral subiculum (Everitt and Wolf 2002) (Figure 1–3). In contrast, the stress-induced reinstatement of drug-related responding in animal models appears to depend on the activation of both CRF and norepinephrine in elements of the extended amygdala (i.e., the central nucleus of the amygdala and the bed nucleus of the stria terminalis) (Shaham et al. 2003). From a theoretical perspective, a cogent argument can be made that addiction involves hyperactivity in the amygdala (impulsive system) and hypoactivity in the prefrontal cortex (reflective system) and that this combination of effects drives emotional (somatic) responses that exaggerate the rewarding effect of available incentives (Verdejo-García and Bechara 2009).

At the molecular level in the preoccupation/anticipation stage, transcription factors, such as CREB and downstream ΔFosB, nuclear factor κB, and cyclin-dependent kinase 5 (CDK5), can alter gene expression and produce long-term changes in protein expression and thus neuronal function (Nestler 2005), including structural changes in the cytoskeleton of neurons via actions on actin (Russo et al. 2010). Indeed, chronic drug exposure can alter the morphology of neurons in dopamine-regulated circuits. For example, in rodents, chronic cocaine, alcohol, or amphetamine administration alters neuronal dendritic branching and spine density in the nucleus accumbens and prefrontal cortex, an adaptation that is thought to play a role in the enhanced incentive motivational value acquired by the drug in addiction (Kroener et al. 2012).

Additionally, growing evidence indicates that epigenetic mechanisms mediate many drug-induced changes in gene expression patterns that lead to structural, synaptic, and behavioral plasticity in the brain (Cadet et al. 2016; Feng and Nestler 2013; Kyzar et al. 2016). The dynamic and often long-lasting changes that occur in the tran-

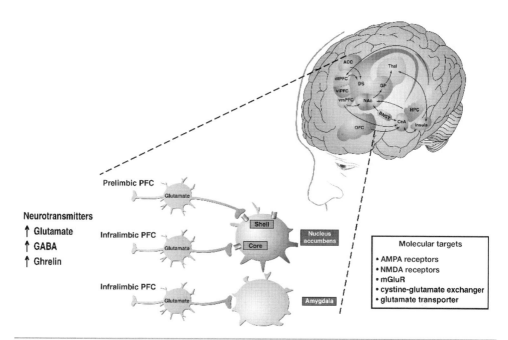

FIGURE 1–3. Neurocircuitry associated with the addiction cycle, part 3: the *preoccupation/anticipation* stage.

To view this figure in color, see Plate 3 in Color Gallery in middle of book.

The preoccupation/anticipation stage involves processing of conditioned reinforcement in the basolateral amygdala and processing of contextual information in the hippocampus (HPC). Executive control depends on the prefrontal cortex (PFC) and includes the representation of contingencies, the representation of outcomes, the presentation of values, and subjective states (i.e., craving and, presumably, feelings) associated with drugs. These subjective states, termed *drug craving* in humans, involve activation of the orbitofrontal cortex (OFC), anterior cingulate cortex (ACC), and temporal lobe, including the amygdala, in functional imaging studies. A major neurotransmitter involved in the preoccupation/anticipation stage is glutamate, which is localized in pathways from the frontal regions and the basolateral amygdala that project to the ventral striatum *(inset).* An increase in the activity of prelimbic and infralimbic cortices in the PFC is hypothesized to initiate and inhibit the reinstatement of drug-seeking behavior. Prelimbic glutamate projections to the nucleus accumbens (NAc) shell are hypothesized to contribute to incentive salience and habit formation. Infralimbic glutamate projections to the NAc core are hypothesized to contribute to the inhibition of drug seeking. Infralimbic glutamate projections to the amygdala are hypothesized to contribute to the inhibition of brain stress systems. A combination of high prelimbic and low infralimbic glutamate activity may drive drug seeking by driving craving and disinhibiting restraints on impulsivity and compulsivity (for a review, see Kalivas 2009).

AMPA=α-amino-3-hydroxy-5-methyl-4-isoxazolepropionic acid; BNST=bed nucleus of the stria terminalis; CeA=central nucleus of the amygdala; dlPFC=dorsolateral prefrontal cortex; DS=dorsal striatum; GABA=γ-aminobutyric acid; GP=globus pallidus; mGLu=metabotropic glutamate; NMDA=N-methyl-D-aspartate; Thal=thalamus; vlPFC=ventrolateral prefrontal cortex; vmPFC=ventromedial prefrontal cortex.

The "Molecular targets" box lists key molecular targets that may convey genetic and epigenetic plasticity to the neurocircuits described in this figure.

Source. Adapted from George and Koob 2013.

scription factors ΔFosB, CREB, and nuclear factor κB after chronic drug administration are particularly interesting because these changes appear to modulate the synthesis of proteins that are involved in key aspects of the addiction phenotype, such as synaptic plasticity (Nestler 2012). Particularly relevant to the preoccupation/anticipation stage are molecular targets involved in glutamate homeostasis, including AMPA receptors; NMDA receptors; metabotropic glutamate receptors 2 and 3 (mGLuR2/3), mGluR1, mGluR5, and mGluR7; the glutamate transporter; and the cystine–glutamate exchanger (Scofield et al. 2016).

Conclusion

Substance use disorders are complex multistage diseases that are characterized by disturbances in three major neurocircuits: the basal ganglia–driven *binge/intoxication* stage, the extended amygdala–driven *withdrawal/negative affect* stage, and the prefrontal cortex–driven *preoccupation/anticipation* stage. In these three domains, neurotransmitter- and neuromodulator-specific neuroplastic changes are seen in multiple neurochemical subsystems, including the ascending mesocorticolimbic dopamine system, CRF in the central nucleus of the amygdala, and corticostriatal glutamate projections. During the binge/intoxication stage, previously neutral stimuli become associated with drug availability, thereby gaining incentive salience and promoting habit formation that fosters excessive drug seeking via increases in dopamine and glutamate neurotransmission. The binge/intoxication stage triggers opponent-process responses in the withdrawal/negative affect stage that are characterized by diminished reward function via dopamine and opioid peptide deficits and an increase in brain stress system activity through the engagement of CRF and dynorphin. Excessive drug intake also drives parallel deficits in executive function via the dysregulation of glutamatergic, GABAergic, and dopaminergic neurochemical systems in the prefrontal cortex, thus perpetuating the dysregulation of reward and stress system function and inducing compulsive drug seeking in the preoccupation/anticipation stage. Additionally, during the preoccupation/anticipation stage, heightened drug cue–induced incentive salience (activated "Go" system) can act against a background of low reward system function and high stress system function (impaired "Stop" system), engaging a powerful combination of positive and negative reinforcement processes that drive pathological drug seeking. Molecular genetic mediation and epigenetic changes in these same three major neurocircuits confer vulnerability to addiction and greater susceptibility to environmental risk factors, thus representing promising targets for the development of novel treatments to strengthen resilience to relapse.

References

Altarifi AA, David B, Muchhala KH, et al: Effects of acute and repeated treatment with the biased mu opioid receptor agonist TRV130 (oliceridine) on measures of antinociception, gastrointestinal function, and abuse liability in rodents. J Psychopharmacol 31(6):730–739, 2017 28142305

American Psychiatric Association: Diagnostic and Statistical Manual of Mental Disorders, 5th Edition. Arlington, VA, American Psychiatric Association, 2013

Belin D, Everitt BJ: Cocaine seeking habits depend upon dopamine-dependent serial connectivity linking the ventral with the dorsal striatum. Neuron 57(3):432–441, 2008 18255035

Belin D, Belin-Rauscent A, Murray JE, et al: Addiction: failure of control over maladaptive incentive habits. Curr Opin Neurobiol 23(4):564–572, 2013 23452942

Bickel WK, Jarmolowicz DP, Mueller ET, et al: Are executive function and impulsivity antipodes? A conceptual reconstruction with special reference to addiction. Psychopharmacology (Berl) 221(3):361–387, 2012 22441659

Cadet JL, McCoy MT, Jayanthi S: Epigenetics and addiction. Clin Pharmacol Ther 99(5):502–511, 2016 26841306

Cahill CM, Walwyn W, Taylor AMW, et al: Allostatic mechanisms of opioid tolerance beyond desensitization and downregulation. Trends Pharmacol Sci 37(11):963–976, 2016 27670390

Carlezon WA Jr, Nestler EJ, Neve RL: Herpes simplex virus-mediated gene transfer as a tool for neuropsychiatric research. Crit Rev Neurobiol 14(1):47–67, 2000 11253955

Cui C, Koob GF: Titrating tipsy targets: the neurobiology of low-dose alcohol. Trends Pharmacol Sci 38(6):556–568, 2017 28372826

Edwards S, Koob GF: Neurobiology of dysregulated motivational systems in drug addiction. Future Neurol 5(3):393–401, 2010 20563312

Everitt BJ, Wolf ME: Psychomotor stimulant addiction: a neural systems perspective. J Neurosci 22(9):3312–3320, 2002 11978805

Feng J, Nestler EJ: Epigenetic mechanisms of drug addiction. Curr Opin Neurobiol 23(4):521–528, 2013 23374537

Garavan H, Pankiewicz J, Bloom A, et al: Cue-induced cocaine craving: neuroanatomical specificity for drug users and drug stimuli. Am J Psychiatry 157(11):1789–1798, 2000 11058476

George O, Koob GF: Control of craving by the prefrontal cortex. Proc Natl Acad Sci U S A 110(11):4165–4166, 2013 23483010

Goldstein RZ, Volkow ND: Dysfunction of the prefrontal cortex in addiction: neuroimaging findings and clinical implications. Nat Rev Neurosci 12(11):652–669, 2011 22011681

Hikosaka O: The habenula: from stress evasion to value-based decision-making. Nat Rev Neurosci 11(7):503–513, 2010 20559337

Jasinska AJ, Stein EA, Kaiser J, et al: Factors modulating neural reactivity to drug cues in addiction: a survey of human neuroimaging studies. Neurosci Biobehav Rev 38:1–16, 2014 24211373

Jochum T, Boettger MK, Burkhardt C, et al: Increased pain sensitivity in alcohol withdrawal syndrome. Eur J Pain 14(7):713–718, 2010 20018536

Kalivas PW: The glutamate homeostasis hypothesis of addiction. Nat Rev Neurosci 10(8):561–572, 2009 19571793

Koob GF: Drugs of abuse: anatomy, pharmacology and function of reward pathways. Trends Pharmacol Sci 13(5):177–184, 1992 1604710

Koob GF: A role for brain stress systems in addiction. Neuron 59(1):11–34, 2008 18614026

Koob GF, Bloom FE: Cellular and molecular mechanisms of drug dependence. Science 242(4879):715–723, 1988 2903550

Koob GF, Le Moal M: Drug abuse: hedonic homeostatic dysregulation. Science 278(5335):52–58, 1997 9311926

Koob GF, Le Moal M: Plasticity of reward neurocircuitry and the "dark side" of drug addiction. Nat Neurosci 8(11):1442–1444, 2005 16251985

Koob GF, Le Moal M: Addiction and the brain antireward system. Annu Rev Psychol 59:29–53, 2008 18154498

Koob GF, Volkow ND: Neurocircuitry of addiction. Neuropsychopharmacology 35(1):217–238, 2010 19710631

Koob GF, Volkow ND: Neurobiology of addiction: a neurocircuitry analysis. Lancet Psychiatry 3(8):760–773, 2016 27475769

Koob GF, Buck CL, Cohen A, et al: Addiction as a stress surfeit disorder. Neuropharmacology 76(pt B):370–382, 2014 23747571

Kroener S, Mulholland PJ, New NN, et al: Chronic alcohol exposure alters behavioral and synaptic plasticity of the rodent prefrontal cortex. PLoS One 7(5):e37541, 2012 22666364

Kyzar EJ, Floreani C, Teppen TL, et al: Adolescent alcohol exposure: burden of epigenetic reprogramming, synaptic remodeling, and adult psychopathology. Front Neurosci 10:222, 2016 27303256

Leventhal AM, Kahler CW, Ray LA, et al: Anhedonia and amotivation in psychiatric outpatients with fully remitted stimulant use disorder. Am J Addict 17(3):218–223, 2008 18463999

Marlatt G, Gordon J: Determinants of relapse: implications for the maintenance of behavioral change, in Behavioral Medicine: Changing Health Lifestyles. Edited by Davidson P, Davidson S. New York, Brunner/Mazel, 1980, pp 410–452

Martin-Fardon R, Weiss F: Modeling relapse in animals. Curr Top Behav Neurosci 13:403–432, 2013 22389178

Martinez D, Narendran R, Foltin RW, et al: Amphetamine-induced dopamine release: markedly blunted in cocaine dependence and predictive of the choice to self-administer cocaine. Am J Psychiatry 164(4):622–629, 2007 17403976

McLellan AT, Lewis DC, O'Brien CP, et al: Drug dependence, a chronic medical illness: implications for treatment, insurance, and outcomes evaluation. JAMA 284(13):1689–1695, 2000 11015800

Meye FJ, Trusel M, Soiza-Reilly M, et al: Neural circuit adaptations during drug withdrawal—spotlight on the lateral habenula. Pharmacol Biochem Behav 162:87–93, 2017 28843423

Mitchell JM, O'Neil JP, Janabi M, et al: Alcohol consumption induces endogenous opioid release in the human orbitofrontal cortex and nucleus accumbens. Sci Transl Med 4(116):116ra6, 2012 22238334

Nestler EJ: Is there a common molecular pathway for addiction? Nat Neurosci 8(11):1445–1449, 2005 16251986

Nestler EJ: Transcriptional mechanisms of drug addiction. Clin Psychopharmacol Neurosci 10(3):136–143, 2012 23430970

Niendam TA, Laird AR, Ray KL, et al: Meta-analytic evidence for a superordinate cognitive control network subserving diverse executive functions. Cogn Affect Behav Neurosci 12(2):241–268, 2012 22282036

Olbrich HM, Valerius G, Paris C, et al: Brain activation during craving for alcohol measured by positron emission tomography. Aust N Z J Psychiatry 40(2):171–178, 2006 16476136

Pandey SC, Kyzar EJ, Zhang H: Epigenetic basis of the dark side of alcohol addiction. Neuropharmacology 122:74–84, 2017 28174112

Piazza PV, Le Moal ML: Pathophysiological basis of vulnerability to drug abuse: role of an interaction between stress, glucocorticoids, and dopaminergic neurons. Annu Rev Pharmacol Toxicol 36:359–378, 1996 8725394

Raehal KM, Schmid CL, Groer CE, et al: Functional selectivity at the μ-opioid receptor: implications for understanding opioid analgesia and tolerance. Pharmacol Rev 63(4):1001–1019, 2011 21873412

Rando K, Hong KI, Bhagwagar Z, et al: Association of frontal and posterior cortical gray matter volume with time to alcohol relapse: a prospective study. Am J Psychiatry 168(2):183–192, 2011 21078704

Robbins TW: Relationship between reward-enhancing and stereotypical effects of psychomotor stimulant drugs. Nature 264(5581):57–59, 1976 12471

Rossetti ZL, Hmaidan Y, Gessa GL: Marked inhibition of mesolimbic dopamine release: a common feature of ethanol, morphine, cocaine and amphetamine abstinence in rats. Eur J Pharmacol 221(2–3):227–234, 1992 1426002

Russo SJ, Dietz DM, Dumitriu D, et al: The addicted synapse: mechanisms of synaptic and structural plasticity in nucleus accumbens. Trends Neurosci 33(6):267–276, 2010 20207024

Schultz W, Dayan P, Montague PR: A neural substrate of prediction and reward. Science 275(5306):1593–1599, 1997 9054347

Scofield MD, Heinsbroek JA, Gipson CD, et al: The nucleus accumbens: mechanisms of addiction across drug classes reflect the importance of glutamate homeostasis. Pharmacol Rev 68(3):816–871, 2016 27363441

Shaham Y, Shalev U, Lu L, et al: The reinstatement model of drug relapse: history, methodology and major findings. Psychopharmacology (Berl) 168(1–2):3–20, 2003 12402102

Tiffany ST, Carter BL, Singleton EG: Challenges in the manipulation, assessment and interpretation of craving relevant variables. Addiction 95 (suppl 2):S177–S187, 2000 11002913

Tolu S, Eddine R, Marti F, et al: Co-activation of VTA DA and GABA neurons mediates nicotine reinforcement. Mol Psychiatry 18(3):382–393, 2013 22751493

Verdejo-García A, Bechara A: A somatic marker theory of addiction. Neuropharmacology 56 (suppl 1):48–62, 2009 18722390

Volkow ND, Fowler JS: Addiction, a disease of compulsion and drive: involvement of the orbitofrontal cortex. Cereb Cortex 10(3):318–325, 2000 10731226

Volkow ND, Wang GJ, Fowler JS, et al: Decreased striatal dopaminergic responsiveness in detoxified cocaine-dependent subjects. Nature 386(6627):830–833, 1997 9126741

Volkow ND, Fowler JS, Wang GJ: The addicted human brain: insights from imaging studies. J Clin Invest 111(10):1444–1451, 2003 12750391

Volkow ND, Wang GJ, Telang F, et al: Cocaine cues and dopamine in dorsal striatum: mechanism of craving in cocaine addiction. J Neurosci 26(24):6583–6588, 2006 16775146

Volkow ND, Wang GJ, Telang F, et al: Profound decreases in dopamine release in striatum in detoxified alcoholics: possible orbitofrontal involvement. J Neurosci 27(46):12700–12706, 2007 18003850

Volkow ND, Wang GJ, Fowler JS, et al: Addiction: beyond dopamine reward circuitry. Proc Natl Acad Sci U S A 108(37):15037–15042, 2011 21402948

Volkow ND, Wang GJ, Fowler JS, et al: Addiction circuitry in the human brain. Annu Rev Pharmacol Toxicol 52:321–336, 2012 21961707

Volkow ND, Tomasi D, Wang GJ, et al: Stimulant-induced dopamine increases are markedly blunted in active cocaine abusers. Mol Psychiatry 19(9):1037–1043, 2014 24912491

Wolf ME, Ferrario CR: AMPA receptor plasticity in the nucleus accumbens after repeated exposure to cocaine. Neurosci Biobehav Rev 35(2):185–211, 2010 20109488

Zywiak WH, Connors GJ, Maisto SA, et al: Relapse research and the Reasons for Drinking Questionnaire: a factor analysis of Marlatt's relapse taxonomy. Addiction 91 (suppl):S121–S130, 1996 8997786

CHAPTER 2

Genetics and Epigenetics of Addiction

Joel Gelernter, M.D.

Renato Polimanti, Ph.D.

The last half-decade or so has seen massive progress in psychiatric genetics. We have exited the age of candidate gene studies. With the benefit of hindsight,
we realize that this is a good thing; most candidate gene findings have not survived
into the current age of unbiased genomewide investigation (Border et al. 2019; Duncan et al. 2019).

Most of this progress is attributable to the use of large samples for genomewide association studies (GWASs) and subsequent analyses based on the results of these
GWASs. Psychiatric traits are genetically complex—that is, they involve many genes,
each of small effect—and for complex traits, large samples are required if we are to
make credible progress. Our ideas of "large" also have shifted. We still occasionally
see published articles describing samples of a few hundred patients as "large." This
may be the case for some areas of investigation, but it is not so for genetics. In the field
of genetics, hundreds or thousands of participants may be adequate to identify the
risk loci of largest effect, but for most traits, this is not the case, and we may need more
than 10,000 subjects; to be called "large," certainly more than 100,000 would be
needed.

Such studies are possible because of the advent of large meta-analysis consortia,
such as the Psychiatric Genomics Consortium (PGC; Sullivan et al. 2018), large biobank
samples such as the UK Biobank (UKB; Collins 2012) and the Million Veteran Program
(MVP; Gaziano et al. 2016), and the direct-to-consumer company 23andMe (Check

This study was supported by National Institutes of Health grants R01 DA12690, R01 AA11330,
R01 AA017535, and R21 DA047527 and by the Department of Veterans Affairs Connecticut
Healthcare Center Mental Illness Research, Education, and Clinical Centers.

Hayden 2017). When traits can be identified that span multiple large-participant collections, sample sizes of more than 1,000,000 subjects are possible (Liu et al. 2019).

These large samples are often crude tools when phenotype is concerned. Investigators have to work with what is available. In the case of meta-analyses, this frequently means use of a lowest-common-denominator phenotype to which every contributing investigator has access. For biobanks, the traits studied must be of medical interest or fall into the broad category of things the originators of the sample thought were useful or interesting. These limitations have been surmountable for psychiatric traits such as schizophrenia and, to a lesser extent, major depressive disorder. These are instructive examples of what can be obtained with adequate data.

For large genetics studies, substance use disorders (SUDs) fall into two categories. The legal substance dependencies—alcohol dependence and nicotine dependence—have benefited from the availability of large biobank samples (Liu et al. 2019). Alcohol and tobacco have such widespread and well-recognized effects on health that information about these two substances is generally collected in any study focused on health outcomes. Alcohol dependence and tobacco dependence (i.e., alcohol use disorder and tobacco us disorder) are also fairly common, and although they are stigmatized, the stigma is not huge. Accordingly, we review a great deal of data on these substances later in this chapter. The situation is very different for the illegal substance dependencies, such as opioid and cocaine use disorder. These are less common than the legal substance dependencies; data are often not collected systematically in biobank samples, and when they are collected, we presume that because of stigma and other factors, the false-negative rate is higher. Thus, genetics studies of the illegal substance dependencies have had to rely mostly on purpose-collected samples (Gelernter et al. 2014b, 2014c) or on samples that used very ad hoc diagnostic criteria. Because funding institutes (public and private) have given only limited support to the recruitment of informative cohorts for these illicit drug dependencies, studies to date tend to be underpowered, replications are difficult to come by, and results are therefore more difficult to interpret than those for alcohol- and nicotine-related traits.

SUDs are inherently different from other psychiatric traits such as schizophrenia, because they include key pharmacogenomic components. This architecture predicts that there may be variants of relatively large effect for these traits. Indeed, a few variants of comparatively large effect have been identified for SUDs and related traits, as is discussed later in this chapter.

With these issues in mind, we now discuss the current state of the art.

Basic Ideas: Genomewide Association Studies and *In Silico* Follow-Up Analyses

GWASs explore genetic variation over the entire genome to identify associations between genetic markers and the trait studied without the requirement of previous biological hypotheses. GWASs have been extremely productive for a range of complex genetic traits. On the basis of the information generated by these large-scale studies, it is possible to gain a better understanding of the molecular basis of complex traits. In particular, it is now clear that the vast majority of common human phenotypes, including disease traits, are highly polygenic (thousands of risk loci) or even omnigenic (i.e., most of the genome is involved in the predisposition to the complex trait of interest) (Boyle et al. 2017). Additionally, psychiatric disorders, such as SUDs, major depressive disorder, and posttraumatic stress disorder, all tend to have effect-size distributions involving a continuum of effects even smaller than that observed in other human diseases (Zhang et al. 2018). This means that—with few exceptions—any single locus can explain very little of the biology of any complex trait. To address this issue, several novel tools specifically designed to leverage polygenic and genomewide information (i.e., data from a limited number of variants and from the entire genome, respectively) have been used to investigate different aspects of the genetics of these traits. Genomewide data can be used to estimate the genetic correlation between complex traits, which is a measure of the genetic components shared by traits (Bulik-Sullivan et al. 2015a). The genetic overlap across complex traits can be used to prepare disease predictions based on polygenic risk scores, wherein an individual's risk is calculated on the basis of the cumulative effect of the risk alleles across the genome—most of which have very small effect individually—weighted for their effects on the phenotype of interest (Zheutlin et al. 2019). Pleiotropy (i.e., the phenomenon by which genetic variants can be associated with multiple phenotypes) is the key phenomenon responsible for the widespread shared liability observed across complex traits. However, it is possible to distinguish two types of pleiotropy: 1) *vertical pleiotropy,* in which genetic variants are associated with a first phenotypic outcome, which then increases the risk of a second phenotypic outcome (or multiple traits); and 2) *horizontal pleiotropy,* in which genetic variants are associated with two or more phenotypic outcomes via independent biological mechanisms. GWAS data can be used to distinguish vertical and horizontal pleiotropy, helping to acquire information about the complex causal networks linking human diseases and phenotypes.

Mendelian randomization is a method that uses the known effects of genetic risk variants to stand in for the biological effects they cause. To date, Mendelian randomization is the most commonly used method of applying genetic instruments (i.e., the known effects of the risk variants) to causal inference (Davey Smith and Hemani 2014). The main advantage of this approach is that genetic variation is randomized in each meiosis and is therefore generally randomized in the human population; so the genetic instruments associated with the risk factors to be tested should not be biased by potential environmental confounders. Other useful GWAS tools can provide information about the biology of the trait of interest. By leveraging external data sets related to tissue- and cell-type-specific transcriptomic profiles and to known molecular pathways, it is possible to understand which are the key biological systems involved by estimating the enrichments of associations observed within genes with a specific transcriptomic profile or within a specific pathway (de Leeuw et al. 2015). Transcriptomic information can be used further to infer the gene expression of the individuals assessed in a GWAS in tissues of interest and to perform a transcriptome-wide association study (Mancuso et al. 2017). Finally, the availability of large independent cohorts, also including biobanks linked to electronic medical records, can permit us to further analyze known risk loci and to conduct association tests with respect to a wide range of phenotypes—that is, we take a risk locus associated with trait *A* and say: this variant has biological activity and some effect on phenotypic outcome; what *other* phenotypic outcomes does this variant affect? This design is also known as a phenomewide association study.

State of the Science for Exemplary Substance-Related Traits

In the following sections, we discuss the current status of research for two SUD traits: alcohol use disorder (and related traits) and opioid use disorder (and related traits). Alcohol use disorder is common, and alcohol is legal; opioid use disorder is less common, and many opioid drugs are consumed illegally. As discussed elsewhere, these differences (common and legal vs. less common and illegal) account for the huge difference in power between the studies conducted so far for these traits.

Alcohol Use Disorder and Related Traits

Alcohol use disorder and related traits provide one of the very few examples of the survival into the current era of candidate gene results based on biology—in this case, because of a strong basis in pharmacogenetics. The main metabolic pathway for alcohol involves metabolism first to acetaldehyde, which is then (through the action of the acetaldehyde dehydrogenases) cleared to acetate. Acetaldehyde is somewhat toxic peripherally and is responsible for the "flushing reaction." The genes that encode several of the acetaldehyde dehydrogenases contain polymorphic variants. Key examples are variants in the alcohol dehydrogenase gene *ADH1B* that increase enzymatic activity and variants in the aldehyde dehydrogenase gene *ALDH2* that decrease enzymatic activity; both kinds of variants increase acetaldehyde accumulation, and both are protective with respect to alcohol intake and alcohol use disorder. The strong relationships between *ALDH2* and *ADH1B* variation and risk for alcohol dependence have been known since very early in the era of molecular markers (Thomasson et al. 1991) and have been persuasively verified in GWASs (Gelernter et al. 2014a; Quillen et al. 2014; Walters et al. 2018; Xu et al. 2015), as has *ALDH2* variation in Asian populations (Gelernter et al. 2018; Quillen et al. 2014). However, with the use of purpose-collected samples, and even PGC meta-analysis (Walters et al. 2018), it was difficult to move beyond these alcohol-metabolizing gene loci.

The use of large biobank samples, with information from electronic health records (EHRs) or survey self-reports, has allowed the field to move beyond these pharmacokinetically acting variants. The MVP is a biobank where participants are U.S. military veterans and users of the Department of Veterans Affairs medical services (Gaziano et al. 2016). To date, two major MVP-based GWASs of alcohol-related traits have been conducted. The first trait studied was *maximum habitual alcohol use* (MaxAlc) (Gelernter et al. 2019), the response to the survey question "In a typical month, what is/was the largest number of drinks of alcohol (beer, wine, and/or liquor) you may have had in one day?" This study included 126,936 European American (EA) and 17,029 African American (AA) participants. As in previous reports, *ADH1B*, on chromosome 4, was the lead locus for both populations; in addition, as in previous reports, different lead single nucleotide polymorphisms (SNPs) were seen in the two populations: for EA participants, rs1229984, and for AA participants, rs2066702. Three additional genome-wide-significant MaxAlc loci were identified in EA participants: one on chromosome 17 at *CRHR1* (corticotropin-releasing hormone receptor 1; the protein product of this gene is involved in stress and immune responses) and two on chromosomes 8 and 10

(Gelernter et al. 2019). When EA and AA data were meta-analyzed, there were two additional genomewide-significant loci. Once sufficiently powered GWAS data are available, *in silico* follow-up analyses become possible; in this case, the follow-up analysis identified a genetic correlation to other alcohol-related traits, smoking-related traits, and many others (Gelernter et al. 2019). The genetic correlation between MaxAlc and alcohol dependence was 0.87, showing that MaxAlc measures something similar to alcohol use disorder, as opposed to being merely a quantity/frequency measure (see below).

Another, larger MVP-based study in a multiancestry sample ($N=274,424$) used EHR diagnostic data to examine alcohol use disorder and the short screening version of the Alcohol Use Disorders Identification Test–Consumption (AUDIT-C), a quantity/frequency measure, to examine alcohol intake (Kranzler et al. 2019). For both traits and for both EA and AA participants, *ADH1B* was the lead locus, and the lead SNPs were the same as those observed in the MaxAlc study (Gelernter et al. 2019). However, this larger study identified 18 genomewide-significant loci overall—five associated with both traits, eight associated with alcohol consumption (AUDIT-C) only, and five associated with alcohol use disorder (EHR diagnosis) only (Kranzler et al. 2019). Again, the *in silico* follow-up analyses were highly informative. The two traits (alcohol use disorder and AUDIT-C alcohol intake) had a genetic correlation of 0.52; genetic correlations for numerous other traits differed significantly for the two traits and showed differing patterns of correlation, with alcohol use disorder tending to be positively correlated with other psychiatric traits and AUDIT-C tending to be positively correlated with some healthy behaviors (Kranzler et al. 2019). Overall, the MVP proved to be a rich resource for gene identification, and these studies each identified several previously unknown alcohol use risk loci.

Large samples for alcohol-related traits such as "drinks per week" have been easier to accumulate than have samples for alcohol use disorder and traits related more closely to pathological dependence—these data have been collected in many studies, including studies primarily concerned with completely different traits. The current largest meta-analysis conducted by the GWAS and Sequencing Consortium of Alcohol and Nicotine Use (GSCAN) for an alcohol-related trait focused on drinks per week and attained a sample size of more than 940,000, with 99 risk loci identified (Liu et al. 2019). As occurred for AUDIT-C, the drinks-per-week trait tended not to show genetic correlation with other pathological psychiatric traits. Although this information greatly advances our understanding of alcohol consumption, its relevance to *pathological* alcohol consumption is less certain.

Overall, these data sources have introduced important issues; the states of the art for genetics of alcohol-related traits differ greatly, both by phenotype (e.g., alcohol use disorder and strongly correlated phenotypes such as MaxAlc [Gelernter et al. 2019] vs. quantity/frequency measures such as the AUDIT-C and drinks per week [Liu et al. 2019]) and by population group (e.g., European ancestry vs. all others). Biobanks typically collect considerable data pertaining to the quantity and frequency of alcohol use (e.g., the AUDIT [Saunders et al. 1993] or the AUDIT-C), and quantity/frequency alcohol measures are recognized as sufficiently medically important to be collected in studies focused on other traits (e.g., cardiac function). Thus, very large samples are available for the study of these kinds of measures, which function as lowest-common-denominator phenotypes (Gelernter 2019; Liu et al. 2019). Before the availability of well-powered studies of these traits, we might have assumed that they would be highly correlated to alcohol use disorder with use of an appropriately defined cutoff. But this is not the case. As discussed earlier, the genetic correlation between quantity/frequency measures and alcohol use disorder is not high (Kranzler et al. 2019; Walters et al. 2018).

Furthermore, these distinct kinds of measures—dependence, on the one hand (medical consequences of alcohol use are a reasonable proxy [see, e.g., Sanchez-Roige et al. 2019]), and frequency of use, on the other—have very different patterns of genetic correlation with other traits, including psychiatric traits, biometric traits, and, for example, educational attainment (Kranzler et al. 2019; Sanchez-Roige et al. 2019). Although alcohol consumption is correlated with medical consequences, these traits are *not* genetically correlated with other psychiatric traits, such as schizophrenia—in contrast to alcohol use disorder. Also, even though many databases collect quantity/ frequency alcohol information, information about alcohol use disorder per se is more sparse. The genetic correlation patterns support the conclusion that alcohol use disorder should nevertheless be a major focus; and this delineation of genetic, and biological, differences between alcohol use quantity/frequency measures, on the one hand (including normal-range drinking), and alcohol use disorder, on the other, is one of the major accomplishments of the research field so far.

Whereas in European populations there are very good sample collections for AUDIT-C and related measures and acceptable (and growing, in the case of MVP) sample collections for alcohol use disorder, the situation for non-European populations, particularly those of African ancestry, is very different—and, accordingly, progress in locus discovery and discovery of biology from GWAS data is also very different. Given that linkage disequilibrium score regression (Bulik-Sullivan et al. 2015b), the main method used at present to detect genetic pleiotropy, can be validly used only with same-population comparators and can be biased when applied to admixed populations, the discovery of correlations with other traits and behaviors for AA participants is also in a very early stage. We need larger samples and methods specifically designed to account for the genetic diversity of admixed populations to study many important traits, each to detect genetic correlation with the others. As discussed earlier, EA and AA populations share the same major risk locus for alcohol-related traits, but a different lead variant is characteristic of each population. Much more research is needed to address the similarities and differences in genetic risk for alcohol-related behaviors across populations.

With large and informative samples, Mendelian randomization becomes a frequently used approach in genetic epidemiology. To understand the biology of alcohol-related traits with respect to major depressive disorder (the two are frequently comorbid), a recent study based on PGC GWAS data investigated the genetic overlap and causal relationships of alcohol dependence, alcohol consumption quantity, and alcohol consumption frequency with major depressive disorder (Polimanti et al. 2019). Findings showed that alcohol consumption frequency and quantity had significant and opposite genetic correlations with major depressive disorder (negative and positive, respectively), whereas Mendelian randomization analysis identified a causal effect of major depressive disorder on alcohol dependence (Polimanti et al. 2019).

Taken overall, however, very substantial advances have been seen in alcohol dependence genetics, many in 2018–2019: identification of numerous replicable risk loci beyond the alcohol-metabolizing enzymes; advances in understanding the phenotypic differences between quantity/frequency measures and dependence; and (following on GWAS results) better understanding of the genetic relation of alcohol-related traits to other traits. Most of this progress has been attributable to work done in large meta-analyses, such as the PGC (Walters et al. 2018) and the GSCAN (Liu et al. 2019), and based in large biobanks, such as the MVP (Gelernter et al. 2019; Kranzler et al. 2019), the UKB (Sanchez-Roige et al. 2019), and 23andMe. The current picture for other addictions reflects the applicability of these data sources closely. In addition, there has been considerable interest in personalized medicine via specific SNPs that may predict medication response; the best-studied example for alcohol use disorder treatment is a possible effect of a variant in *OPRM1*, the gene encoding the μ-opioid receptor, in predicting naltrexone response. This seemed promising at first (Oslin et al. 2003), but findings from subsequent studies (e.g., Gelernter et al. 2007; Oslin et al. 2015) have been inconsistent. It seems likely that single-variant risk-prediction strategies will be insufficient to meet clinical needs for alcohol use disorder pharmacogenomics.

Opioid Use Disorder and Related Traits

Opioid use disorder and related traits show a starkly different pattern of discovery from that for alcohol use disorder. Illegal opioid use disorder is much less common than alcohol use disorder; even in an epidemiologically assessed sample, less information would be available. Biobank samples, however, tend to be biased in favor of higher socioeconomic status and high function—the UKB and 23andMe cohorts have these characteristics. The MVP is somewhat better in this regard but still has relatively little relevant EHR data, reflecting population prevalence and probably also underreporting because of stigma. Therefore, samples of individuals with opioid use disorder must be purpose-collected, and most of our genetic knowledge at this point is based on studies of this kind. To date, no large-scale efforts can approach what has been done with alcohol use disorder.

Three published GWASs of opioid use disorder have yielded genomewide significant loci (Cheng et al. 2018; Gelernter et al. 2014b; Nelson et al. 2016). In the first of these studies, in the Yale–Penn sample (Gelernter et al. 2014b), genomewide significant associations with SNPs from multiple loci were identified, with the most compelling results obtained for genes involved in potassium signaling pathways. Pathway analysis also implicated genes involved in calcium signaling and long-term potentiation (Gelernter et al. 2014b). In this study, the significant findings were seen in AA participants. A GWAS primarily in Australian opioid-dependent patients recruited from methadone and buprenorphine treatment programs provided evidence of associations for multiple variants in *CNIH3* (Nelson et al. 2016). In the most recent investigation (Cheng et al. 2018), also in the Yale–Penn sample, a variant mapped to the *RGMA* locus was identified as significantly associated with opioid use disorder risk in EA participants. Li et al. (2015) also completed a genomewide analysis of copy number variations (CNVs) in a sample that overlapped with the sample of a previous GWAS (Gelernter et al. 2014b). For common CNVs, two deletions and one duplication were significantly associated with opioid dependence genomewide. All of these studies were comparatively small (i.e., involving thousands rather than tens of thousands of affected subjects), and the significant results tended to be in the range of 10^{-8}–10^{-9}

significance; in GWAS terms, when a Bonferroni correction needs to be taken into account to allow for all of the markers in the genome, these results are truly significant but not strongly so. This comparative lack of power means that it is very important that the results be replicated independently, but so far, that has not been possible because of the lack of sample collections worldwide. This low power also means that the opportunity for subsequent analyses, such as studies of genetic correlation and functional annotation, is very limited.

Other studies have looked beyond the opioid use disorder phenotype per se to study other genetically influenced traits related to opioid use. For example, opioid dosing is a very important clinical problem. If we consider opioid substitution therapy and methadone use, for example, under- and overdosing of methadone both carry risks. Another GWAS from the Yale–Penn sample identified a significant association of methadone dose with a variant upstream of *OPRM1* (not the same variant as that studied previously as a candidate variant with respect to naltrexone response) in AA participants (Smith et al. 2017). This finding was subsequently replicated for morphine dose in a pediatric AA population (Smith et al. 2017), albeit in a sample that was very small in the context of complex-trait GWASs. Note that this was a GWAS, not a candidate gene study. Still, because methadone acts directly on the protein product of the implicated gene, *OPRM1*, we can consider that the previous support for this particular locus was very high and that the results are highly provocative but require replication.

If we consider the current state of affairs for opioid use disorder genetics, we find that insufficient effort has been devoted by the research community worldwide to human studies, notwithstanding the current epidemic in the United States. We have some very promising results, but the greater context is one of power limitations that will be impossible to overcome until more human participants can be recruited.

Other Substance Use Disorders

One of the most durable findings in SUD genetics research pertains to nicotine use— that is, the relation between markers mapped to the *CHRNA3/A5/B4* gene cluster and smoking heaviness or dependence (Saccone et al. 2010; Sherva et al. 2010; Tobacco and Genetics Consortium 2010). There have been comparatively many large-scale GWAS of behaviors related to cigarette smoking; the largest to date is, as for alcohol use, GSCAN (Liu et al. 2019), which considered up to 1.2 million subjects for "smoking initiation" and hundreds of thousands of subjects for several other smoking phenotypes, including cigarettes per day (in which the lead variant mapped to *CHRNA5* with $P = 1.2 \times 10^{-278}$) and smoking cessation. Other strongly implicated genes included *BDNF, REV3L,* and *BRWD1*. This study was well-powered for extensive and highly informative *in silico* follow-up analyses, showing a wide range of significant genetic correlations of smoking behaviors with outcomes related to mental and physical health, including psychiatric disorders and cardiovascular diseases (Liu et al. 2019). Additionally, pathway enrichment analyses highlighted dopaminergic and glutamatergic neurotransmission among several brain regions that may be involved in reward-based learning and drug-seeking behavior. Mendelian randomization studies based on GWAS data further explored the relation of smoking behaviors to psychiatric disorders and other behavioral traits, observing positive causal effects of smoking initiation and lifetime smoking on bipolar disorder (Vermeulen et al. 2019) and a causal association between low educational attainment and increased risk for smoking (Gage et al. 2018).

Two studies of cannabis dependence genetics so far have yielded genomewide significant results (Agrawal et al. 2018; Sherva et al. 2016), and one study of cannabis-related aggression mapped a risk locus to the serotonin type 2B receptor gene (*HTR2B*) (Montalvo-Ortiz et al. 2018). These studies can all be viewed as promising, but they lack sufficient power for extensive *in silico* follow-up analyses; they require replication. Larger consortium studies of cannabis use have greater power and more consistent findings (Pasman et al. 2018), but the relation of their findings to pathological cannabis use is less certain. Analyses based on the largest cannabis use GWAS (N=184,765 [Pasman et al. 2018]) showed positive genetic correlations with smoking and alcohol use and dependence and also with attention-deficit/hyperactivity disorder and schizophrenia. The GWAS data also were used to dissect the causal mechanisms linking cannabis use to schizophrenia. Mendelian randomization tests found stronger evidence for a positive causal influence of schizophrenia risk on lifetime cannabis use than for a causal influence in the opposite direction. Larger studies of cannabis dependence are sorely needed; the biobanks likely will be somewhat helpful with this issue.

Other SUDs (e.g., cocaine dependence [Gelernter et al. 2014c]) have been studied at the GWAS level, but generally with small to moderate sample sizes and with need of replication, notwithstanding statistically significant results.

Epigenetics

Epigenetics is the study of the gene expression changes resulting from molecular changes in the genomes that are not related to DNA base sequence changes. Epigenetic modifications, such as DNA methylation (at CpG sites) and histone modification, can be reversible, can differ across tissues and cell types, and can alter DNA accessibility and chromatin structure, regulating gene function across biological processes also in response to environmental stimuli. Similar to the genomewide microarrays that are used to acquire SNP data, high-throughput platforms have been developed to assay methylation changes in hundreds of thousands of CpG dinucleotides across the genomes. Currently, the MethylationEPIC BeadChip microarray from Illumina Inc. (San Diego, CA) can assess epigenetic modification in more than 850,000 CpG sites (Pidsley et al. 2016). This high-throughput technology has permitted investigators to conduct epigenomewide association studies (EWASs) of numerous complex traits, including some that are pertinent to the SUDs. Although sample sizes in SUD-related EWASs have so far been quite limited, EWASs appear to have greater statistical power in comparison with GWASs conducted in samples of the same size. This is because epigenetic changes, unlike genetic variation, can be related to causative mechanisms (i.e., epigenetic change is causal with respect to the trait of interest) or to downstream consequences (i.e., epigenetic change is induced by the trait), with a consistent overrepresentation of the latter with respect to the former, and accordingly often have higher effect sizes (Osório 2014). Additionally, epigenetic variability across tissues and cell types could reflect different aspects of the biology of the phenotypes investigated. For SUDs, as for other psychiatric traits, the tissue of greatest interest is that of the brain, which is inaccessible in living persons. Therefore, epigenetic studies of SUDs face the limitation of focusing on the desired target tissue in postmortem studies or using a proxy tissue, such as blood or saliva, accessible in living participants, which we would then hope reflects changes in brain. A recent study reported that there is a consistent correlation in the regulatory mechanisms of gene expression and methylation profile between brain and blood, confirming that it is possible to identify gene targets for brain-related traits by using methylomic data from blood (Qi et al. 2018). As mentioned earlier, the reason to use blood rather than brain for these studies is mostly a practical one, but this practicality extends to clinical translation as well: predicting risk based on epigenomic profiles would have little utility if the procedure had to be based on brain but great utility if based on blood.

Among the addictive substances, nicotine has received the most investigation in blood-based EWASs thus far. This is because smoking, like alcohol use, is legal—a large percentage of the general population is exposed to nicotine, mainly via tobacco smoking. The studies conducted have highlighted the pervasive effect of tobacco smoking on epigenetic changes across the genome, also identifying several CpG sites within the *AHRR* (aryl-hydrocarbon receptor repressor) gene as very strongly and consistently affected by smoking behavior (Joehanes et al. 2016). The epigenetic changes induced by tobacco smoking appear to be reversible in former smokers (McCartney et al. 2018). Smoking-induced epigenetic changes also have been observed with respect to several traits that co-occur with tobacco use, including other psychiatric disorders (Smith et al. 2019), cancer (Murphy et al. 2018), and cardiovascular diseases (Dogan et al. 2017).

Although the epigenetic changes were not as pervasive as those observed for tobacco smoking (McCartney et al. 2018), alcohol consumption and alcohol use disorder were associated with methylation changes in several loci, including *GABRD* (γ-aminobutyric acid A receptor delta), *GABBR1* (γ-aminobutyric acid B receptor subunit 1), and *NR3C1* (the gene encoding the glucocorticoid receptor) (Gatta et al. 2019; Liu et al. 2018). Beyond nicotine- and alcohol-related traits, very limited information is available about the epigenetic changes associated with illicit drug use and abuse. A recent study conducted in 220 European American women (140 case patients with opioid dependence; 80 opioid-exposed control subjects) identified three genomewide significant differentially methylated CpG sites mapping to *PARG, RERE,* and *CFAP77* (Montalvo-Ortiz et al. 2019). Because epigenetic changes can be used to assess the biological response to substance use and abuse, future epigenomewide studies are needed to target illicit substances in adequately powered cohorts.

Conclusion

Research on the genetics of complex traits—including psychiatric genetics—saw enormous progress in the latter half of the 2010s as a result of several trends that allowed for adequately powered studies and, consequently, locus discovery. The first of these trends was the use of large meta-analyses. Early successes for traits like schizophrenia demonstrated to investigators in the field the shared benefits of working together, with results that have transformed the field—first with locus discovery and biology based on *in silico* analyses (Schizophrenia Working Group of the Psychiatric Genomics Consortium 2014) and then with another wave of molecular biology (Sekar et al. 2016). As data from large biobank samples became available, investigators experienced another wave of remarkable progress. The pace of discovery has generally confirmed the hypothesis that for GWASs, it is common to see an "inflection point," depending on sample size; up to a certain point, different for each trait, few risk variants are identified, but after that point, a reliable number are seen for each participant added to the sample (Sullivan et al. 2018).

The degree of progress made in understanding the genetics of the SUDs has diverged greatly by substance, depending on the availability of applicable data in large biobanks. Studies of SUDs for which data are available—generally speaking, SUDs involving the legal substances—have seen enormous progress. Studies of SUDs for which data are not generally available—such as cocaine dependence, opioid dependence, and methamphetamine dependence—have been hampered in their progress by a lack of informative samples for analysis. From the vantage point of 2020, it is difficult to see how this situation can change substantially. Many psychiatric traits—for example, autism spectrum disorder—have strongly supportive public constituencies, but that is not the case for any illegal SUDs. Accordingly, all funding for studies in this area must come from public agencies like the National Institutes of Health. This current state has left the illegal SUDs far from their discovery inflection points and with no readily apparent way to reach the necessary sample sizes to achieve the power to discover many, not just a few, risk variants.

What does the future hold? This depends on many factors extrinsic to the science itself. Those in the field have made great progress in understanding the genetics of alcohol and tobacco use and are making progress on other fronts. Even for the former traits, however, we can still account for only a fraction of the genetic risk. That situation will improve as large biobanks (e.g., MVP, UKB, and AllofUS) continue to expand. GWASs alone will not be enough; substantial investments must be made to further the understanding of the epigenetics of these traits. Also, the relative contributions of common and rare variants to genetic risk are under active discussion. Such contributions surely vary by trait; however, a recent demonstration (Wainschtein et al. 2019) showed that for height, whole-genome sequencing recovered enough genetic variation to account for virtually all of the heritability of this complex trait. Whether a similar situation exists for any of the SUDs must be determined empirically.

References

Agrawal A, Chou YL, Carey CE, et al: Genome-wide association study identifies a novel locus for cannabis dependence. Mol Psychiatry 23(5):1293–1302, 2018 29112194

Border R, Johnson EC, Evans LM, et al: No support for historical candidate gene or candidate gene-by-interaction hypotheses for major depression across multiple large samples. Am J Psychiatry 176(5):376–387, 2019 30845820

Boyle EA, Li YI, Pritchard JK: An expanded view of complex traits: from polygenic to omnigenic. Cell 169(7):1177–1186, 2017 28622505

Bulik-Sullivan B, Finucane HK, Anttila V, et al: An atlas of genetic correlations across human diseases and traits. Nat Genet 47(11):1236–1241, 2015a 26414676

Bulik-Sullivan BK, Loh PR, Finucane HK, et al: LD score regression distinguishes confounding from polygenicity in genome-wide association studies. Nat Genet 47(3):291–295, 2015b 25642630

Check Hayden E: The rise and fall and rise again of 23andMe. Nature 550(7675):174–177, 2017 29022933

Cheng Z, Zhou H, Sherva R, et al: Genome-wide association study identifies a regulatory variant of RGMA associated with opioid dependence in European Americans. Biol Psychiatry 84(10):762–770, 2018 29478698

Collins R: What makes UK Biobank special? Lancet 379(9822):1173–1174, 2012 22463865

Davey Smith G, Hemani G: Mendelian randomization: genetic anchors for causal inference in epidemiological studies. Hum Mol Genet 23(R1):R89–R98, 2014 25064373

de Leeuw CA, Mooij JM, Heskes T, et al: MAGMA: generalized gene-set analysis of GWAS data. PLOS Comput Biol 11(4):e1004219, 2015 25885710

Dogan MV, Beach SRH, Philibert RA: Genetically contextual effects of smoking on genome wide DNA methylation. Am J Med Genet B Neuropsychiatr Genet 174(6):595–607, 2017 28686328

Duncan LE, Ostacher M, Ballon J: How genome-wide association studies (GWAS) made traditional candidate gene studies obsolete. Neuropsychopharmacology 44(9):1518–1523, 2019 30982060

Gage SH, Bowden J, Davey Smith G, et al: Investigating causality in associations between education and smoking: a two-sample Mendelian randomization study. Int J Epidemiol 47(4):1131–1140, 2018 29961807

Gatta E, Grayson DR, Auta J, et al: Genome-wide methylation in alcohol use disorder subjects: implications for an epigenetic regulation of the cortico-limbic glucocorticoid receptors (NR3C1). Mol Psychiatry June 25, 2019. [Epub ahead of print] 31239533

Gaziano JM, Concato J, Brophy M, et al: Million Veteran Program: a mega-biobank to study genetic influences on health and disease. J Clin Epidemiol 70:214–223, 2016 26441289

Gelernter J: Inviting in the exome for alcohol and smoking traits. Biol Psychiatry 85(11):889–890, 2019 31122339

Gelernter J, Gueorguieva R, Kranzler HR, et al; VA Cooperative Study #425 Study Group: Opioid receptor gene (OPRM1, OPRK1, and OPRD1) variants and response to naltrexone treatment for alcohol dependence: results from the VA Cooperative Study. Alcohol Clin Exp Res 31(4):555–563, 2007 17374034

Gelernter J, Kranzler HR, Sherva R, et al: Genome-wide association study of alcohol dependence: significant findings in African- and European-Americans including novel risk loci. Mol Psychiatry 19(1):41–49, 2014a 24166409

Gelernter J, Kranzler HR, Sherva R, et al: Genome-wide association study of opioid dependence: multiple associations mapped to calcium and potassium pathways. Biol Psychiatry 76(1):66–74, 2014b 24143882

Gelernter J, Sherva R, Koesterer R, et al: Genome-wide association study of cocaine dependence and related traits: FAM53B identified as a risk gene. Mol Psychiatry 19(6):717–723, 2014c 23958962

Gelernter J, Zhou H, Nuñez YZ, et al: Genomewide association study of alcohol dependence and related traits in a Thai population. Alcohol Clin Exp Res 42(5):861–868, 2018 29460428

Gelernter J, Sun N, Polimanti R, et al: Genome-wide association study of maximum habitual alcohol intake in >140,000 U.S. European and African American veterans yields novel risk loci. Biol Psychiatry 86(5):365–376, 2019 31151762

Joehanes R, Just AC, Marioni RE, et al: Epigenetic signatures of cigarette smoking. Circ Cardiovasc Genet 9(5):436–447, 2016 27651444

Kranzler HR, Zhou H, Kember RL, et al: Genome-wide association study of alcohol consumption and use disorder in 274,424 individuals from multiple populations. Nat Commun 10(1):1499, 2019 30940813

Li D, Zhao H, Kranzler HR, et al: Genome-wide association study of copy number variations (CNVs) with opioid dependence. Neuropsychopharmacology 40(4):1016–1026, 2015 25345593

Liu C, Marioni RE, Hedman AK, et al: A DNA methylation biomarker of alcohol consumption. Mol Psychiatry 23(2):422–433, 2018 27843151

Liu M, Jiang Y, Wedow R, et al: Association studies of up to 1.2 million individuals yield new insights into the genetic etiology of tobacco and alcohol use. Nat Genet 51(2):237–244, 2019 30643251

Mancuso N, Shi H, Goddard P, et al: Integrating gene expression with summary association statistics to identify genes associated with 30 complex traits. Am J Hum Genet 100(3):473–487, 2017 28238358

McCartney DL, Stevenson AJ, Hillary RF, et al: Epigenetic signatures of starting and stopping smoking. EBioMedicine 37:214–220, 2018 30389506

Montalvo-Ortiz JL, Zhou H, D'Andrea I, et al: Translational studies support a role for serotonin 2B receptor (HTR2B) gene in aggression-related cannabis response. Mol Psychiatry 23(12):2277–2286, 2018 30389506

Montalvo-Ortiz JL, Cheng Z, Kranzler HR, et al: Genomewide study of epigenetic biomarkers of opioid dependence in European-American women. Sci Rep 9(1):4660, 2019 30874594

Murphy SE, Park SL, Balbo S, et al: Tobacco biomarkers and genetic/epigenetic analysis to investigate ethnic/racial differences in lung cancer risk among smokers. NPJ Precis Oncol 2:17, 2018 30155522

Nelson EC, Agrawal A, Heath AC, et al: Evidence of CNIH3 involvement in opioid dependence. Mol Psychiatry 21(5):608–614, 2016 26239289

Oslin DW, Berrettini W, Kranzler HR, et al: A functional polymorphism of the mu-opioid receptor gene is associated with naltrexone response in alcohol-dependent patients. Neuropsychopharmacology 28(8):1546–1552, 2003 12813472

Oslin DW, Leong SH, Lynch KG, et al: Naltrexone vs placebo for the treatment of alcohol dependence: a randomized clinical trial. JAMA Psychiatry 72(5):430–437, 2015 25760804

Osório J: Obesity. Looking at the epigenetic link between obesity and its consequences—the promise of EWAS. Nat Rev Endocrinol 10(5):249, 2014 24686199

Pasman JA, Verweij KJH, Gerring Z, et al: GWAS of lifetime cannabis use reveals new risk loci, genetic overlap with psychiatric traits, and a causal influence of schizophrenia. Nat Neurosci 21(9):1161–1170, 2018 30150663

Pidsley R, Zotenko E, Peters TJ, et al: Critical evaluation of the Illumina MethylationEPIC BeadChip microarray for whole-genome DNA methylation profiling. Genome Biol 17(1):208, 2016 27717381

Polimanti R, Peterson RE, Ong JS, et al: Evidence of causal effect of major depression on alcohol dependence: findings from the psychiatric genomics consortium. Psychol Med 49(7):1218–1226, 2019 30929657

Qi T, Wu Y, Zeng J, et al: Identifying gene targets for brain-related traits using transcriptomic and methylomic data from blood. Nat Commun 9(1):2282, 2018 29891976

Quillen EE, Chen XD, Almasy L, et al: ALDH2 is associated to alcohol dependence and is the major genetic determinant of "daily maximum drinks" in a GWAS study of an isolated rural Chinese sample. Am J Med Genet B Neuropsychiatr Genet 165B(2):103–110, 2014 24277619

Saccone NL, Culverhouse RC, Schwantes-An TH, et al: Multiple independent loci at chromosome 15q25.1 affect smoking quantity: a meta-analysis and comparison with lung cancer and COPD. PLoS Genet 6(8):e1001053, 2010 20700436

Sanchez-Roige S, Palmer AA, Fontanillas P, et al: Genome-wide association study meta-analysis of the Alcohol Use Disorders Identification Test (AUDIT) in two population-based cohorts. Am J Psychiatry 176(2):107–118, 2019 30336701

Saunders JB, Aasland OG, Babor TF, et al: Development of the Alcohol Use Disorders Identification Test (AUDIT): WHO Collaborative Project on Early Detection of Persons With Harmful Alcohol Consumption—II. Addiction 88(6):791–804, 1993 8329970

Schizophrenia Working Group of the Psychiatric Genomics Consortium: Biological insights from 108 schizophrenia-associated genetic loci. Nature 511(7510):421–427, 2014 25056061

Sekar A, Bialas AR, de Rivera H, et al: Schizophrenia risk from complex variation of complement component 4. Nature 530(7589):177–183, 2016 26814963

Sherva R, Kranzler HR, Yu Y, et al: Variation in nicotinic acetylcholine receptor genes is associated with multiple substance dependence phenotypes. Neuropsychopharmacology 35(9):1921–1931, 2010 20485328

Sherva R, Wang Q, Kranzler H, et al: Genome-wide association study of cannabis dependence severity, novel risk variants, and shared genetic risks. JAMA Psychiatry 73(5):472–480, 2016 27028160

Smith AH, Jensen KP, Li J, et al: Genome-wide association study of therapeutic opioid dosing identifies a novel locus upstream of OPRM1. Mol Psychiatry 22(3):346–352, 2017 28115739

Smith AK, Ratanatharathorn A, Maihofer AX, et al: Epigenome-wide meta-analysis of PTSD across 10 military and civilian cohorts identifies novel methylation loci. bioRxiv, March 21, 2019. Available at: https://www.biorxiv.org/content/biorxiv/early/2019/03/21/585109.full.pdf. Accessed November 12, 2019.

Sullivan PF, Agrawal A, Bulik CM, et al: Psychiatric genomics: an update and an agenda. Am J Psychiatry 175(1):15–27, 2018 28969442

Thomasson HR, Edenberg HJ, Crabb DW, et al: Alcohol and aldehyde dehydrogenase genotypes and alcoholism in Chinese men. Am J Hum Genet 48(4):677–681, 1991 2014795

Tobacco and Genetics Consortium: Genome-wide meta-analyses identify multiple loci associated with smoking behavior. Nat Genet 42(5):441–447, 2010 20418890

Vermeulen J, Wootton R, Treur J, et al: Smoking and the risk for bipolar disorder: causal evidence from a bidirectional Mendelian randomization study. bioRxiv, January 17, 2019. Available at: https://www.biorxiv.org/content/biorxiv/early/2019/01/17/522268.full.pdf. Accessed November 12, 2019.

Wainschtein P, Jain DP, Yengo L, et al: Recovery of trait heritability from whole genome sequence data. bioRxiv, March 25, 2019. Available at: https://www.biorxiv.org/content/biorxiv/early/2019/03/25/588020.full.pdf. Accessed November 12, 2019.

Walters RK, Polimanti R, Johnson EC, et al: Transancestral GWAS of alcohol dependence reveals common genetic underpinnings with psychiatric disorders. Nat Neurosci 21(12):1656–1669, 2018b 30482948

Xu K, Kranzler HR, Sherva R, et al: Genomewide association study for maximum number of alcoholic drinks in European Americans and African Americans. Alcohol Clin Exp Res 39(7):1137–1147, 2015 26036284

Zhang Y, Qi G, Park JH, et al: Estimation of complex effect-size distributions using summary-level statistics from genome-wide association studies across 32 complex traits. Nat Genet 50(9):1318–1326, 2018 30104760

Zheutlin AB, Dennis J, Karlsson Linnér R, et al: Penetrance and pleiotropy of polygenic risk scores for schizophrenia in 106,160 patients across four health care systems. Am J Psychiatry 176(10):846–855, 2019 31416338

CHAPTER 3

Epidemiology of Addiction

Nathan D.L. Smith, A.L.M.

Linda B. Cottler, Ph.D., M.P.H., FACE

Addiction is a common mental health disorder with multiple complex features that has resisted simple definition and treatment. It is a ubiquitous subject in film, television, literature, and art. Nearly every person has been touched by addiction, and many have formed strong opinions on the disorder based on personal or family experiences, political beliefs, or moral philosophies. For all of these reasons, determining the epidemiology of addiction—the science of identifying how addiction is distributed in the population (Robins 1978)—is important and complicated. In this chapter, we present the historical framework of the epidemiology of addiction, where the field stands today, and thoughts on where the field is going and how it will get there.

The Past: The Three Eras and Landmark Studies

Those who study the epidemiology of addiction rely on the historical and pioneering work of the many psychiatrists, psychologists, and epidemiologists who have taken the field to where it is today. Modern addiction epidemiology was shaped by the methods used in three historical eras, with their landmark studies that have provided much of the commonly cited data on national prevalence of addictive disorders.

The Three Eras of Psychiatric Epidemiology

The history of psychiatric epidemiology can be divided into three broad eras (Regier et al. 1984), which we will identify by the way cases were distinguished from noncases. The first era relied on the self-selection of patients, the second on the direct expertise of clinical practitioners, and the third on carefully tested diagnostic protocols.

Relying on Patients (Before 1945)

The first era of psychiatric epidemiology relied on the reports of the patient and his or her family. To identify cases, researchers visited psychiatric institutions and surveyed individuals admitted—or, alternatively, they contacted psychiatric institutions and asked for a report on the number of cases of psychiatric disorders. This method was relatively simple and inexpensive but limited cases to people who had been admitted to a psychiatric institution and interviewed by a psychiatrist or another physician (Regier et al. 1984; Robins 1978). This method was capable of providing information on the number of individuals residing in hospitals and psychiatric facilities as well as basic demographic and geographic data for individuals with each mental disorder diagnosis. However, relying on the reports of patients to determine case status provided data on only the tip of the iceberg of mental disorders. This practice narrowed the numerator to only those who went to treatment, and the denominator was vaguely associated with all those at risk.

Counting individuals who are institutionalized is a measure of the population-level disorder only if the institutionalized individuals are representative of the population as a whole. Unfortunately, this was not the case, as noted by Dr. Edward Jarvis in his 1855 *Report on Insanity and Idiocy in Massachusetts,* which showed that the farther away a person lived from a psychiatric institution, the less likely he or she was to be found there (Hunter and Shannon 1985; Lincoln and Sumner 1855). Since then, other biases relating to who receives treatment and who does not have been identified, such as Berkson's bias. Berkson (1946) was the first to find that hospitalized people are sicker and have more comorbidities than nonhospitalized people, which can skew epidemiological findings on patients' diagnoses.

These kinds of persistent errors created the need for advancements in psychiatric epidemiology. Unfortunately, the tools required for this advancement were not developed until the end of World War II, which ushered in the second era of psychiatric epidemiology: reliance on the practitioner (Regier et al. 1984).

Relying on Practitioners (1945–1978)

To avoid the biases inherent in surveying only individuals in institutions, researchers had to broaden their pool of survey respondents to the population as a whole. To do this, either psychiatrists were sent into the field to interview participants directly, or a lay interviewer recorded participants' answers to predetermined questions, which were later reviewed by a psychiatrist (Regier et al. 1984). This type of study was capable of providing prevalence data for the relatively small geographic areas covered by the study, as well as considerably more accurate demographic and geographic data than were previously available. In addition, use of a general population survey produced information on individuals who had never received treatment, a group that had been left out of earlier studies.

Notable examples of survey studies from this era include the Midtown Manhattan and Stirling County studies. The Midtown Manhattan study included 1,660 individuals in the Midtown area of New York City interviewed between 1952 and 1960 (Kraines 1964), and the Stirling County study included 1,003 individuals in eastern Canada in 1952 (Hughes et al. 1960; Murphy et al. 2000). The studies used a structured interview administered by a trained interviewer and reviewed by a psychiatrist in order to obtain diagnoses (Hughes et al. 1960).

This research method had clear benefits, because cases were still determined by well-trained experts, and more representative samples could be procured than those found in mental institutions. However, relying on psychiatrists to evaluate every individual in a sample is expensive and time-consuming, and evidence indicates that psychiatrists may follow their own individualized line of thinking and overlook or discount certain diagnostic criteria that do not fit with their schemas (Cottler and Keating 1990). Relying on psychiatrists also made it nearly impossible to gather information on less-prevalent disorders, such as schizophrenia, which occurs in approximately 1% of the population. Including enough community members to achieve a reasonable sample of people with schizophrenia, say 100 cases, would require a random sample of about 10,000 people. Gathering a large enough sample to study rare disorders required the next major shift in psychiatric epidemiological methods, from relying on the practitioner to relying on a protocol.

Relying on Protocols (1979 to Present)

The shift from relying on the determinations of a professional to relying on a protocol was preceded by a major change in the way that psychiatric disorders were defined by the American Psychiatric Association. In the first edition of the *Diagnostic and Statistical Manual of Mental Disorders* (DSM), released in 1952 (American Psychiatric Association 1952), disorders were described generally, but responsibility for determining a case was left to the psychiatrist. For example, the diagnosis of "alcoholism" was to be used in "cases in which there is a well-established addiction to alcohol" (Hughes et al. 1960). DSM-III, released in 1980, represented a major advancement over the earlier DSM editions in the development of diagnoses; it provided specific criteria that had to be met in order to qualify for a diagnosis of alcohol abuse or alcohol dependence (American Psychiatric Association 1980). This shift in the specificity and clarity of definitions to a set of measurable criteria allowed for the creation of diagnostic assessment instruments that, if properly tested and used, could provide an accurate diagnosis for dozens of psychiatric conditions without requiring the services of a psychiatrist to verify each diagnosis. In this chapter, we use the term *protocol* to refer to all of the elements of a specific assessment measure or instrument—including the questions, probing techniques, and interviewer training—that make the assessment valid.

The first study to use this type of assessment instrument on a large scale was the Epidemiologic Catchment Area (ECA) study, which used the Diagnostic Interview Schedule (Eaton et al. 1981) to examine a wide range of mental disorders in the population. This program of research was a landmark community investigation of mental illness and was the first "modern" study to determine the prevalence of psychiatric conditions in the United States. The ECA project provided the blueprint for large-scale studies of psychiatric disorders, and all modern psychiatric epidemiology studies can trace their methodological lineages to this study (Regier et al. 1984; Smith and Cottler 2018).

The careful creation and testing of a psychiatric assessment instrument, such as the Diagnostic Interview Schedule, required that the assessment be capable of mimicking the diagnosis produced by an experienced psychiatrist. This allowed for the large-scale psychiatric prevalence surveys that are common today and are discussed in the next section (see "National Epidemiologic Survey on Alcohol and Related Conditions"). Relying on the protocol instead of on psychiatrists had several benefits, including cost-effectiveness and the ability to gather the large amounts of data needed to examine low-base-rate disorders in the community. The main problem in relying on a protocol was that creating a reliable and valid protocol was difficult and time-consuming, and any problems with the reliability or validity of the protocol affected the diagnoses of every participant in the survey. The protocol itself is what determines the difference between a case and a noncase. For this reason, the creation, testing, and verification of assessments used for this type of research are of paramount importance, because assessments with low reliability and validity will yield inferior and biased findings.

Modern Landmark Studies

Producing stable, representative prevalence data on national populations requires extremely large numbers of respondents from diverse backgrounds and living all across the United States, as well as enough trained interviewers to collect comprehensive information from each individual. For this reason, producing valid and reliable rates of psychiatric disorders in the general population is difficult, expensive, and time-consuming. Most of the widely quoted prevalence data for mental disorders in the United States were produced by a very few large-scale national surveys. In this section, we briefly review the major studies since the dawn of the third era of psychiatric epidemiology in 1979.

There is also a rich history of national surveys engaged in ongoing monitoring of psychoactive substance use in the population. These monitoring studies, the best known of which is probably the National Survey on Drug Use and Health (https://nsduhweb.rti.org/respweb/homepage.cfm), occupy a distinct parallel track with the studies of substance use disorders we discuss in this chapter.

Epidemiologic Catchment Area Study

In 1978, the National Institute of Mental Health (NIMH) concluded that the existing body of research could not answer two fundamental questions: 1) What is the prevalence of mental disorders in the United States? and 2) Are people with mental disorders receiving treatment? The project that came to be called the ECA study was designed to answer these two questions (Robins et al. 1981).

The ECA study sample came from five U.S. catchment areas in urban and rural areas: Baltimore, Maryland; St. Louis, Missouri; New Haven, Connecticut; Los Angeles, California; and Durham, North Carolina. The sample consisted of 18,571 persons who completed face-to-face interviews with the NIMH Diagnostic Interview Schedule (Robins et al. 1981), an interview protocol designed to be administered by lay interviewers that assessed psychiatric conditions as defined by DSM-III criteria. The data gathered by the ECA study allowed the field, for the first time, to evaluate the comorbidity of disorders, the temporal sequence of disorders, the duration of disorders, and the periods of risk for disorders. The Diagnostic Interview Schedule was the precursor to the Composite International Diagnostic Interview (CIDI), the Structured Clinical Interview for DSM-IV, the Psychiatric Research Interview for Substance and Mental Disorders (PRISM), the National Comorbidity Survey (NCS), the Alcohol Use Disorder and Associated Disabilities Interview Schedule, and other diagnostic interviews (Regier et al. 1988).

National Comorbidity Survey

The ECA study was able to provide reliable data on prevalence rates of mental disorder throughout the United States, but it was not designed to examine the very high rates of comorbidity that it uncovered. To address this issue, the Survey Research Center at the University of Michigan's Institute for Social Research conducted a national study of comorbidity—the National Comorbidity Survey—between 1990 and 1992 (Kessler et al. 1994). In this survey, trained lay interviewers administered a modified version of the World Health Organization's (WHO's) CIDI, which was based on the Diagnostic Interview Schedule, to 8,098 individuals representing the contiguous 48 states (Kessler et al. 1994). The CIDI provided lifetime and past-year (12-month) diagnoses based on DSM-III-R (American Psychiatric Association 1987) diagnostic criteria (Kessler et al. 1994).

National Epidemiologic Survey on Alcohol and Related Conditions

The National Epidemiologic Survey on Alcohol and Related Conditions (NESARC) was sponsored by the National Institute on Alcohol Abuse and Alcoholism to collect data on alcohol and drug use and disorders as well as associated psychiatric conditions. The sample was nationally representative of the U.S. population and included data from 43,093 completed face-to-face interviews conducted by trained lay interviewers. The original NESARC was conducted between 2000 and 2001 (Hasin and Grant 2015). Since then, two additional survey studies have been completed. The first, NESARC-II, followed up on the sample collected in the original NESARC (Grant and Kaplan 2005). The second, NESARC-III, tested the new DSM-5 (American Psychiatric Association 2013) diagnostic criteria in a national sample and is perhaps the best national source for current data on prevalence rates of mental disorders in the U.S. population (Grant et al. 2014).

World Mental Health Survey

The World Mental Health Survey (WMHS) was intended to yield estimates of the prevalence and severity of mental disorders that could be compared cross-nationally. The WMHS was conducted between 2001 and 2005 in 17 countries (Demyttenaere et al. 2004). The World Bank defined 7 countries as less developed (China, Colombia, Lebanon, Mexico, Nigeria, South Africa, and Ukraine) and the other 10 countries as developed (Belgium, France, Germany, Israel, Italy, Japan, Netherlands, New Zealand, Spain, and the United States) (Kessler et al. 2007). Sample sizes varied from 282 in Japan to 3,197 in the United States, and response rates varied from 50.6% in Belgium to 87.7% in Colombia. The WMHS interviewers completed the WHO CIDI in face-to-face interviews (Kessler et al. 2007). The WHO CIDI generates both ICD-10 (World Health Organization 1992) and DSM-IV (American Psychiatric Association 1994) diagnoses.

The Present: DSM-5 and Current Prevalence

The current state of addiction epidemiology has been primarily influenced by the definitional changes enacted in DSM-5, which was released in 2013 (American Psychiatric Association 2013). In this section, we review two common misunderstandings in addiction epidemiology, discuss some of the major changes to the substance-related disorders in DSM-5, and provide updated prevalence rates for a number of addictive disorders.

Common Errors: Conditional Diagnoses and "Substance Use Disorder"

Before addressing the changes made in DSM-5, it is worth clarifying two common errors encountered in addiction epidemiology: conditional diagnoses and "substance use disorder."

A conditional diagnosis occurs when a disorder can be diagnosed only in the presence of an underlying exposure. For example, posttraumatic stress disorder (PTSD) can be diagnosed only in people who have experienced a qualifying traumatic event. Therefore, the rate of the underlying exposure can make a significant difference in population rates of PTSD. Among the DSM-5 substance-related and addictive disorders, a use disorder involving a particular substance can be diagnosed only in an individual who has used that substance. For example, alcohol use disorder can be present only in individuals who have used alcohol. For this reason, the ambient level of substance use in a population can vastly increase the number of substance use disorders in the population, even if the same percentage of users have these disorders. Therefore, we recommend always reporting rates of substance use in populations along with rates of substance use disorders among substance users.

Another common error is reporting "substance use disorder" as a singular diagnosis. Although "Substance-Related and Addictive Disorders" is a category of conditions in DSM-5, this category is made up of specific disorders such as alcohol use disorder and opioid use disorder. The problem occurs when researchers aggregate symptoms experienced across a variety of specific use disorders and report this aggregated score as a blanket "substance use disorder." The category "substance use disorder" has no clinical or diagnostic meaning. It is, however, acceptable to report "*any* substance use disorder" as a category containing all individuals whose symptoms meet the criteria for a specific DSM-5 substance use disorder.

As an example, in a study sample in which 4% of subjects meet criteria for only alcohol use disorder, 3% meet criteria for only cannabis use disorder, and 3% meet criteria for both disorders, it would be acceptable to present a finding of 10% for "any substance use disorder" (i.e., alcohol use disorder + cannabis use disorder + both). However, one cannot lump together the symptoms of alcohol use disorder and cannabis use disorder and present people who meet two or more criteria as having a substance use disorder.

Major Changes in DSM-5

The publication of DSM-5 in 2013 brought significant changes to the diagnostic criteria for some substance use disorders. In this section, we highlight the changes from the previous edition (DSM-IV) in the removal of the "legal troubles" criterion and the broadening of the substance-related disorder category to include, for the first time, a non-substance-related addictive disorder—gambling disorder.

A Dimensional Approach to Substance Use Disorders

DSM-IV, published in 1994, separated substance use disorders into substance abuse and substance dependence (American Psychiatric Association 1994). As an example, alcohol abuse was diagnosed when a person reported one or more symptoms from a list of four harmful consequences of alcohol use: hazardous use, interpersonal problems, neglecting major roles because of use, and legal problems. Alcohol dependence was diagnosed when three or more of the following seven symptoms were reported: tolerance, withdrawal, repeated attempts to quit, using larger amounts than before, excessive time spent on using, physical or psychological problems related to use, and activities given up because of use (Hasin et al. 2013). DSM-IV also gave the two diagnoses a hierarchy, with alcohol dependence being the more severe of the two, and prohibited an alcohol abuse diagnosis when dependence was present (American Psychiatric Association 1994). The diagnoses of alcohol abuse and alcohol dependence were found to be highly reliable, but the system contained some other problems (Hasin et al. 2013). For example, under this system, a person who met one criterion for abuse would be diagnosed with abuse, but a person who met two criteria for dependence would not receive any diagnosis.

In DSM-5, the two categories of abuse and dependence were replaced with a single diagnosis—use disorder—which incorporates the criteria for DSM-IV abuse and dependence (American Psychiatric Association 2013). The DSM-5 diagnosis for alcohol use disorder now includes three severities: two to three symptoms indicate a mild alcohol use disorder, four to five indicate a moderate alcohol use disorder, and six or more symptoms indicate a severe alcohol use disorder. This relatively simple way of calculating severity was implemented because more complicated systems of weighting different criteria might not be universally applicable across subpopulations (Hasin et al. 2013).

Addition of Craving as a Criterion

Craving, the strong urge or desire to use a substance or engage in an activity, is strongly associated with the conceptualization of addiction in the popular psyche and has been included in discussions of addiction since at least 1906 (Kelynack 1906). However, craving was not included in the DSM-IV criteria for abuse or dependence (American Psychiatric Association 1994). For DSM-5, a craving item was tested and was found to be useful in identifying addiction to nicotine, alcohol, cannabis, and heroin, but not cocaine. Ultimately, craving was added to the listed criteria for all substance use disorders because it is a potential target for biological treatment (Hasin et al. 2013).

Elimination of Legal Troubles

Since at least 1980 (the publication date of DSM-III), there has been some mention of legal difficulties in the DSM definitions of addiction. As more research was done into substance use and criminology, it became clear that not all groups of people were equally likely to experience legal troubles related to their substance use. For example, marijuana use is much more common among white Americans than among African Americans, but many more African Americans are incarcerated for marijuana use than are white Americans (Smith et al. 1984). Using legal trouble as part of a diagnosis for a substance use disorder transfers the systemic racial bias into a psychiatric diagnosis.

The authors of DSM-5 extracted the societal bias from the diagnosis by removing the legal troubles criterion from each substance use disorder diagnosis. This change did not substantially affect the diagnosis of substance use disorders because 1) the legal troubles criterion was rarely endorsed, and 2) many people who endorsed the legal troubles criterion also endorsed several other criteria. This minimized the additional diagnostic information provided by the criterion (Hasin et al. 2012).

Addition of Gambling Disorder

DSM-5 also took a major step toward clarifying our understanding of behavioral addictions by renaming DSM-IV pathological gambling as gambling disorder and moving it from the "Impulse-Control Disorders Not Elsewhere Classified" section, which contained disorders such as kleptomania and pyromania, to the newly expanded "Substance-Related and Addictive Disorders" section (American Psychiatric Association 1994; Hasin et al. 2012). This change resolved some of the confusion associated with gambling disorder (which was defined by criteria that closely mirrored those defining addictive substance use disorders) by bringing these similar disorders together into the same category. This conceptual shift away from addiction requiring a substance also opens the door for other behavioral addictions to be added to this category in future DSM editions.

The Status of Video Games

Problematic video game playing, called Internet gaming disorder in DSM-5, will perhaps be the next behavioral addiction to become a future DSM diagnosis. In DSM-5, Internet gaming disorder is listed as a condition for further study (American Psychiatric Association 2013). However, in ICD-11, released in 2019, gaming disorder was included as a full-fledged disorder (World Health Organization 2019), even though this inclusion was strongly opposed by some in the field of addiction research (Aarseth et al. 2017). The next 10 years are likely to see a series of similar conflicts regarding potentially problematic behaviors such as social media use, Internet use, cell phone use, and other similar behaviors that may lead to negative health consequences.

Prevalence of Substance-Related and Addictive Disorders Reported in DSM-5

For each mental disorder diagnosis included, DSM-5 provides background information on diagnostic features, prevalence, development (including age at onset) and course, and other factors and issues useful for clinicians and researchers. Table 3–1 presents a summary of the 12-month prevalence rates of DSM-5 substance-related and addictive disorders, including rates for adolescents and adults and for men and women separately (American Psychiatric Association 2013).

Table 3–1 shows that the highest rates of substance-related disorders in adolescents (i.e., those ages 12–17 years) are for alcohol use disorder (4.6%) and cannabis use disorder (3.4%) (American Psychiatric Association 2013). Use disorder prevalences are lower among adults (i.e., those age 18 years or older) than among adolescents for all substances except alcohol and amphetamine-type stimulants, for which rates of use disorder are the same or higher in adults than in adolescents (alcohol use disorder:

TABLE 3–1.   **Twelve-month prevalence rates of DSM-5 substance-related and addictive disorders**

Disorder	12-Month prevalence (%)			
	Ages 12–17 y	Age ≥18 y	Men (≥18 y)	Women (≥18 y)
Alcohol use disorder	4.6	8.5	12.4	4.9
Amphetamine-type stimulant use disorder	0.2	0.2	0.2	0.2
Cannabis use disorder	3.4	1.5	2.2	0.8
Gambling disorder	NA	0.2–0.3	NA	NA
Inhalant use disorder	0.4	0.0	NA	NA
Tobacco use disorder (estimated via DSM-IV nicotine dependence)	NA	13.0	14.0	12.0
Opioid use disorder	1.0	0.4	0.5	0.3
Other hallucinogen use disorder	0.5	0.1	0.2	0.1
Sedative, hypnotic, or anxiolytic use disorder	0.3	0.2	NA	NA

Note. NA=not available.
Source. Data from "Prevalence" sections of respective DSM-5 substance use disorders (American Psychiatric Association 2013).

8.5% vs. 4.6%, respectively; amphetamine-type stimulant use disorder: 0.2% vs. 0.2%, respectively) (American Psychiatric Association 2013). Use disorder prevalence rates also are higher in men than in women for all substances except amphetamine-type stimulants (0.2% vs. 0.2% for men vs. women). It is worth noting that DSM-5 provides population rates, not conditional rates (see earlier subsection "Common Errors: Conditional Diagnoses and 'Substance Use Disorder'").

The Future: New Approaches to Overcoming Treatment Barriers and Measuring Substance Use

With the realities of the past and present states of addiction epidemiology in mind, we now turn our attention to issues that could dominate the next 10 years of research. In this section, we present ideas about two topics: 1) new approaches to address treatment barriers among individuals with SUDs, including reluctance to seek care and problems with treatment adherence; and 2) new technology allowing direct measurement of substance use, along with examples of notable studies.

Overcoming Barriers to Treatment: The Cascade of Care

Although treatment for substance use disorders has improved with recent advances in practice, such as medication-assisted treatment for opioid use disorder, dramatically improving the lives of people with substance use disorders, estimates of the proportion of individuals who seek treatment for their substance use disorders continue to hover between 10% and 15% (Substance Abuse and Mental Health Services Administration 2015). That means that of the 22.5 million individuals with a substance use disorder in the United States, about 20 million (or 88%) did not receive evidence-based treatment appropriate for their disease (Socías et al. 2016).

One way to combat low treatment seeking is to adopt a concept of treatment monitoring from the HIV/AIDS literature: the cascade of care. The cascade of care bridges the gap between having a disorder and attaining long-term recovery from that disorder by dividing the recovery process into discrete steps that build on one another. This sequential design allows for the monitoring of each individual step along the pathway and for identification of the points at which individuals prematurely exit the pathway (Socías et al. 2016). In one example of a cascade of care for opioid use disorders, the steps along the cascade would include 1) seeking treatment for severe opioid addiction, 2) receiving a diagnosis of opioid use disorder, 3) engaging in care, 4) initiating medication-assisted treatment, 5) remaining in medication-assisted treatment for at least 6 months, and 6) maintaining long-term abstinence. In theory, if 90% of patients who enter the cascade stay and complete each of the steps without dropping out (i.e., achieve a 90% retention goal), then 59% of persons with a severe opioid use disorder would achieve continuous abstinence (Williams et al. 2017). This relatively modest goal would represent a four- to sixfold improvement over current rates of treatment adherence.

Although promising, the cascade of care framework also has potential problems. First, agreement has not been reached on a set of validated criteria to assess the cascade of care in addiction. Considerable research and collaboration are will be needed to produce these criteria. Second, substance use disorders are often characterized by cycles of abstinence and relapse that may complicate the utility of a cascade of care (Socías et al. 2016). Finally, even exemplary treatment programs, such as medication-assisted treatment, have practical barriers to treatment, such as low rates of health insurance coverage, that hinder the achievement of retention goals; this situation is not likely to improve unless considerable structural changes are made to the U.S. health care system (Williams et al. 2017). These barriers must be overcome in order to build a cascade of care for substance use disorders that matches the effect on public health achieved by the model in HIV/AIDS.

Precise Measurement of Substances Ingested

Over the past 50 years, the technology for measuring the substances ingested by an individual has becoming cheaper, more accurate, and more available. It may not be long before a sensor the size of a Band-Aid can give an accurate reading of all the substances an individual has consumed over the past several weeks. This technology will allow scientists to directly measure the substances used by individuals in a way that has never before been possible. However, this technology will not address the harm experienced by an individual as a result of substance use. Although heavy use of a substance like alcohol may be dangerous for everyone, and the sensor can identify such use, the harm caused by alcohol is more complex and difficult to define. A well-calibrated sensor that can identify the substances used by an individual might be a starting point for determining exposure, but it will never replace an interview that gathers information on consequences or patterns of use, because an interview conducted by a qualified individual will always be a more sensitive detector of critical consequences of use.

New Initiatives in Addiction Epidemiology

As we have discussed, the history of the epidemiology of addiction is dominated by a small number of very important studies. We suspect that the future will be likewise guided by a few keystone studies. In this section, we discuss two studies that may guide the field forward over the next 10 years, and beyond.

Adolescent Brain Cognitive Development Study

Adolescence is an important period in the physiological, cognitive, psychological, and social development of an individual. The large longitudinal Adolescent Brain Cognitive Development (ABCD) investigation will follow children as they age and develop throughout adolescence (Volkow et al. 2018). The study uses a comprehensive protocol to collect data on physical health (e.g., height, weight, vision, medical history), mental health (e.g., mood, social relationships, impulsivity, resilience), substance use (knowledge and use of alcohol, tobacco, marijuana, and other substances), neurocognition (e.g., verbal IQ, attention, working memory, visuospatial processing), and culture and environment (e.g., parental supervision, cultural affiliation, acculturation, family dynamics), as well as data from brain imaging (e.g., functional magnetic resonance imaging, monetary delay task) and biospecimens (e.g., alcohol and drug screens, pubertal hormones, DNA, baby teeth) (Adolescent Brain Cognitive Development 2019). The ABCD study will enroll a large and diverse sample of more than 11,000 children age 9 or 10 years who will be followed for a decade. The findings will be generalizable to the general population and will provide valuable data to scientists for decades to come (Volkow et al. 2018).

Helping to End Addiction Long-term (HEAL)

In 2018, the National Institutes of Health (NIH) launched the Helping to End Addiction Long-term (HEAL) initiative to address the epidemic of opioid-related mortality in the United States (National Institutes of Health 2019a). The NIH has set aside more than $500 million that will be used in combating the problem of addiction from several directions (National Institutes of Health 2019b). Major areas of focus are improving treatment for addiction, including medicine-assisted treatment, and improving pain management, including testing nonaddictive treatments for chronic pain (National Institutes of Health 2019a). The initiative also provides resources for research that integrate a broader collection of stakeholders, including research on criminal justice issues and research in community-based settings (National Institutes of Health 2019b). The HEAL initiative is the largest funding source for studies of addiction in U.S. history.

Conclusion

For more than 100 years, researchers have tried to answer fundamental questions about addiction and society. How many people have addictive disorders? What factors are associated with the development of addictive disorders? How many people with addictive disorders get the treatment they need?

The history of research on the epidemiology of addiction shows a pattern of flattening power structures and broadening focus in terms of both who is included in research studies and what is considered an object of addiction. We suspect that the future of addiction epidemiology will continue this trend. Direct measures of substance use will allow more accurate data to be gathered from more people at more time points, and advances in tracking treatment progress will allow for the creation of better systems for providing all people with addictive disorders the treatment they need to live healthy lives.

References

Aarseth E, Bean AM, Boonen H, et al: Scholars' open debate paper on the World Health Organization ICD-11 Gaming Disorder proposal. J Behav Addict 6(3):267–270, 2017 28033714

Adolescent Brain Cognitive Development: Protocols. 2019. Available at: https://abcd-study.org/scientists/protocols. Accessed November 12, 2019.

American Psychiatric Association: Diagnostic and Statistical Manual: Mental Disorders. Washington, DC, American Psychiatric Association, 1952

American Psychiatric Association: Diagnostic and Statistical Manual of Mental Disorders, 3rd Edition. Washington, DC, American Psychiatric Association, 1980

American Psychiatric Association: Diagnostic and Statistical Manual of Mental Disorders, 3rd Edition, Revised. Washington, DC, American Psychiatric Association, 1987

American Psychiatric Association: Diagnostic and Statistical Manual of Mental Disorders, 4th Edition. Washington, DC, American Psychiatric Association, 1994

American Psychiatric Association: Diagnostic and Statistical Manual of Mental Disorders, 5th Edition. Arlington, VA, American Psychiatric Association, 2013

Berkson J: Limitations of the application of fourfold table analysis to hospital data. Biometrics 2(3):47–53, 1946 21001024

Cottler LB, Keating SK: Operationalization of alcohol and drug dependence criteria by means of a structured interview. Recent Dev Alcohol 8:69–83, 1990 2333396

Demyttenaere K, Bruffaerts R, Posada-Villa J, et al: Prevalence, severity, and unmet need for treatment of mental disorders in the World Health Organization World Mental Health Surveys. JAMA 291(21):2581–2590, 2004 15173149

Eaton WW, Regier DA, Locke BZ, et al: The Epidemiologic Catchment Area Program of the National Institute of Mental Health. Public Health Rep 96(4):319–325, 1981 6265966

Grant BF, Kaplan KD: Source and Accuracy Statement for the Wave 2 National Epidemiologic Survey on Alcohol and Related Conditions (NESARC). Rockville, MD, National Institute on Alcohol Abuse and Alcoholism, 2005

Grant BF, Amsbary M, Chu A, et al: Source and Accuracy Statement: National Epidemiologic Survey on Alcohol and Related Conditions-III (NESARC-III). Rockville, MD, National Institute on Alcohol Abuse and Alcoholism, 2014

Hasin DS, Grant BF: The National Epidemiologic Survey on Alcohol and Related Conditions (NESARC) Waves 1 and 2: review and summary of findings. Soc Psychiatry Psychiatr Epidemiol 50(11):1609–1640, 2015 26210739

Hasin DS, Fenton MC, Beseler C, et al: Analyses related to the development of DSM-5 criteria for substance use related disorders, 2: proposed DSM-5 criteria for alcohol, cannabis, cocaine and heroin disorders in 663 substance abuse patients. Drug Alcohol Depend 122(1–2):28–37, 2012 21963333

Hasin DS, O'Brien CP, Auriacombe M, et al: DSM-5 criteria for substance use disorders: recommendations and rationale. Am J Psychiatry 170(8):834–851, 2013 23903334

Hughes CC, Tremblay M-A, Rapoport RN, et al: People of Cove and Woodlot: Communities From the Viewpoint of Social Psychiatry. New York, Basic Books, 1960

Hunter JM, Shannon GW: Jarvis revisited: distance decay in service areas of mid-19th century asylums. Prof Geogr 37(3):296–302, 1985 11617962

Kelynack TN: The Alcohol Problem in Its Biological Aspect. London, Richard J. James, 1906

Kessler RC, McGonagle KA, Zhao S, et al: Lifetime and 12-month prevalence of DSM-III-R psychiatric disorders in the United States: results from the National Comorbidity Survey. Arch Gen Psychiatry 51(1):8–19, 1994 8279933

Kessler RC, Angermeyer M, Anthony JC, et al: Lifetime prevalence and age-of-onset distributions of mental disorders in the World Health Organization's World Mental Health Survey Initiative. World Psychiatry 6(3):168–176, 2007 18188442

Kraines SH: Life stress and mental health: the Midtown Manhattan Study (book review). JAMA 187(6):464, 1964

Lincoln L, Sumner I: Report on Insanity and Idiocy in Massachusetts. 1855. Available at: http://archive.org/details/reportoninsanity00mass. Accessed November 12, 2019.

Murphy JM, Laird NM, Monson RR, et al: A 40-year perspective on the prevalence of depression: the Stirling County Study. Arch Gen Psychiatry 57(3):209–215, 2000 10711905

National Institutes of Health: The Helping to End Addiction Long-term (HEAL) Initiative. 2019a. Available at: https://www.nih.gov/research-training/medical-research-initiatives/heal-initiative. Accessed November 12, 2019.

National Institutes of Health: NIH HEAL Initiative: Funding Opportunities. 2019b. Available at: https://www.nih.gov/research-training/medical-research-initiatives/heal-initiative/funding-opportunities. Accessed November 12, 2019.

Regier DA, Myers JK, Kramer M, et al: The NIMH Epidemiologic Catchment Area program: historical context, major objectives, and study population characteristics. Arch Gen Psychiatry 41(10):934–941, 1984 6089692

Regier DA, Boyd JH, Burke JD Jr, et al: One-month prevalence of mental disorders in the United States: based on five Epidemiologic Catchment Area sites. Arch Gen Psychiatry 45(11):977–986, 1988 3263101

Robins LN: Psychiatric epidemiology. Arch Gen Psychiatry 35(6):697–702, 1978 655768

Robins LN, Helzer JE, Croughan J, et al: National Institute of Mental Health Diagnostic Interview Schedule: its history, characteristics, and validity. Arch Gen Psychiatry 38(4):381–389, 1981 6260053

Smith DA, Visher CA, Davidson LA: Equity and discretionary justice: the influence of race on police arrest decisions. Journal of Criminal Law and Criminology 75(1):234–249, 1984. Available at: https://www.ncjrs.gov/App/Publications/abstract.aspx?ID=94870. Accessed February 10, 2020.

Smith NDL, Cottler LB: The epidemiology of post-traumatic stress disorder and alcohol use disorder. Alcohol Res 39(2):113–120, 2018 31198651

Socías ME, Volkow N, Wood E: Adopting the "cascade of care" framework: an opportunity to close the implementation gap in addiction care? Addiction 111(12):2079–2081, 2016 27412876

Substance Abuse and Mental Health Services Administration: Behavioral Health Barometer: United States, 2015. HHS Publication no. SMA–16–Baro–2015. Rockville, MD, Substance Abuse and Mental Health Services Administration, 2015. Available at: https://www.samhsa.gov/data/sites/default/files/2015_National_Barometer.pdf. Accessed July 22, 2020.

Volkow ND, Koob GF, Croyle RT, et al: The conception of the ABCD study: from substance use to a broad NIH collaboration. Dev Cogn Neurosci 32:4–7, 2018 29051027

Williams AR, Nunes E, Olfson M: To battle the opioid overdose epidemic, deploy the "cascade of care" model. Health Affairs Blog March 13, 2017. Available at: https://www.healthaffairs.org/do/10.1377/hblog20170313.059163/full. Accessed November 12, 2019.

World Health Organization: International Statistical Classification of Diseases and Related Health Problems, 10th Revision. Geneva, World Health Organization, 1992

World Health Organization: International Statistical Classification of Diseases and Related Health Problems, 11th Revision. Geneva, World Health Organization, 2019

CHAPTER 4

Substance Use Disorder Diagnoses in DSM-5

Deborah S. Hasin, Ph.D.

Farren R.R. Larson, M.A.

The *Diagnostic and Statistical* Manual of Mental Disorders (DSM), the standard classification of mental disorders published by the American Psychiatric Association (APA), is used for many clinical, research, policy, and reimbursement purposes. Since publication of the first edition in 1952 (American Psychiatric Association 1952), the manual has been revised six times. DSM-5 (American Psychiatric Association 2013), the current edition, included several changes to the criteria for and coverage of substance use disorders (SUDs). This chapter has two purposes: 1) to review some of the major changes made to SUDs in DSM-5, expanding on the background, methods, and rationales behind these changes (Hasin et al. 2013); and 2) to present new studies that have examined the reliability and validity of the DSM-5 SUD criteria since DSM-5 was published.

Updating the DSM-5 SUD criteria took several years. The APA convened experts to form the DSM-5 Substance-Related Disorders Work Group, which reviewed empirical studies of the strengths and weaknesses in the DSM-IV (American Psychiatric Association 1994) approach to SUDs, identified gaps in this literature, and published a series of literature reviews in the journal *Addiction* in 2006 (Saunders and Schuckit 2006). The work group then identified survey and clinical data sets to analyze to fill the gaps and investigate solutions to the problems identified. Work group members also monitored PubMed and other databases for new publications and formulated interim recommendations for changes to elicit feedback from others in the field (Hasin et al. 2013). This led to further analyses and adjustments before the final recommendations were made to the APA, reviewed, and incorporated into DSM-5.

Major Changes to Substance Use Disorders in DSM-5

Substance Abuse and Dependence Criteria Combined to Define a Single Substance Use Disorder

DSM-IV differentiated between substance abuse and substance dependence (Table 4–1) and created a hierarchy by stipulating that abuse should not be diagnosed if dependence was present. Studies showed that the DSM-IV criteria for substance dependence were highly reliable (Hasin et al. 2006a) and showed good validity with indicators such as treatment utilization, impaired functioning, consumption, and comorbidity (Compton et al. 2007; Dawson 2000; Grant et al. 2004; Hasin et al. 2007).

In contrast, the DSM-IV criteria for substance abuse were problematic. When DSM-IV abuse and dependence were diagnosed hierarchically, the reliability and validity of DSM-IV abuse were much lower than those for DSM-IV dependence; however, when the abuse criteria were analyzed without regard to dependence, their test–retest reliability improved (Hasin et al. 2006a), suggesting that the hierarchy, not the criteria, was responsible for the poor reliability of the DSM-IV abuse criteria. Problems with the DSM-IV hierarchy also included "diagnostic orphans" (Hasin and Paykin 1998, 1999a; McBride et al. 2009), defined as individuals who meet one or two dependence criteria and no abuse criteria. Cases involving dependence without abuse represented potentially more serious conditions than did cases involving abuse only but were ineligible for a diagnosis of dependence or abuse. Other common assumptions about the relation between abuse and dependence proved to be incorrect. Although abuse was often assumed to be milder than dependence, some abuse criteria pointed to clinically severe problems (e.g., failure to fulfill major responsibilities). Furthermore, the assumption that abuse was simply a prodromal condition that would eventually progress to dependence was not supported in prospective studies (Grant et al. 2001; Hasin et al. 1997; Schuckit et al. 2000). The assumption that all cases of dependence would also meet criteria for abuse was likewise not always supported, particularly among women and minority populations (Hasin and Grant 2004; Hasin et al. 2005). Additionally, a syndrome requires more than one symptom, but studies showed that about half of all abuse diagnoses were made on the basis of only one criterion—most often, hazardous use (e.g., driving while intoxicated) (Hasin and Paykin 1999b; Hasin et al. 1999). Finally, factor analyses of the DSM-IV dependence and abuse criteria showed that the criteria formed a single factor (Krueger et al. 2004) or two very highly correlated factors (Agrawal and Lynskey 2007; Blanco et al. 2007; Gillespie et al. 2007; Harford and Muthén 2001; Martin et al. 2006; Proudfoot et al. 2006; Teesson et al. 2002), suggesting that the criteria should be combined to define a single disorder.

Item Response Theory analysis was used to further investigate the relation between the DSM-IV abuse and dependence criteria. Two main findings emerged, with similar results across studies (Hasin et al. 2013). First, unidimensionality was found for all DSM-IV abuse and dependence criteria except legal problems, suggesting that dependence and the remaining abuse criteria indicated the same underlying condi-

TABLE 4–1.   **DSM-IV and DSM-5 criteria for substance use disorders**

Criteria	DSM-IV dependence[a] (historical)	DSM-IV abuse[b] (historical)	DSM-5 substance use disorder[c]
Withdrawal[d]	X	—	X
Tolerance	X	—	X
Used larger amounts/longer time	X	—	X
Repeated attempts to quit/control use	X	—	X
Much time spent using	X	—	X
Physical/psychological problems related to use	X	—	X
Activities given up to use	X	—	X
Hazardous use	—	X	X
Social/interpersonal problems related to use	—	X	X
Neglected major roles to use	—	X	X
Legal problems	—	X	—
Craving	—	—	X

[a]Three or more dependence criteria within a 12-month period.
[b]One or more abuse criteria within a 12-month period and no dependence diagnosis; applicable to all substances except nicotine.
[c]Two or more substance use disorder criteria within a 12-month period.
[d]Withdrawal not included for cannabis-, inhalant-, hallucinogen-, or phencyclidine-related disorders in DSM-IV; withdrawal added to criteria for cannabis use disorder in DSM-5.

tion. Second, the abuse and dependence criteria were always intermixed across the severity spectrum. DSM-IV abuse and dependence criteria were therefore combined into one SUD in DSM-5, as shown in Table 4–1.

Legal Problems Removed From DSM-5 Substance Use Disorder Diagnostic Criteria

Reasons to drop the criterion of legal problems included low prevalence (Hagman and Cohn 2011; Hasin et al. 2012; Mewton et al. 2011; Saha et al. 2006, 2007; Shmulewitz et al. 2010; Teesson et al. 2002), low discrimination (Hagman and Cohn 2011; Hasin et al. 2012; Lynskey and Agrawal 2007; Martin et al. 2006; Mewton et al. 2011; Saha et al. 2007), poor fit with other SUD criteria (Mewton et al. 2011; Saha et al. 2006; Teesson et al. 2002), and little added information in Item Response Theory analyses (Martin et al. 2006; Saha et al. 2012; Shmulewitz et al. 2010). Some clinicians were concerned that removing legal problems would leave patients with no diagnosis, an issue specifically addressed among heavy alcohol, cannabis, cocaine, and/or heroin users (Hasin et al. 2012). However, none of these patients reported substance-related legal problems as the only criterion met or "lost" a DSM-5 SUD diagnosis if this criterion was absent. Thus, the legal problems criterion was not found to be useful for SUD and was removed from the DSM-5 SUD criteria (see Table 4–1).

Craving Added to DSM-5 Substance Use Disorder Diagnostic Criteria

Craving was a substance dependence criterion in ICD-10 (World Health Organization 1993). Support for adding craving to the DSM-5 criteria came from behavioral (O'Brien et al. 1998; Waters et al. 2004), neurobiological (Heinz et al. 2009; Miller and Goldsmith 2001; Weiss 2005), pharmacological (O'Brien 2005), and genetics studies (Foroud et al. 2007). Item Response Theory analyses using general population and clinical samples (Casey et al. 2012; Cherpitel et al. 2010; Hasin et al. 2012; Keyes et al. 2011; Mewton et al. 2011; Shmulewitz et al. 2011) found that craving fit well with other SUD criteria and did not perturb their factor loadings, severity, or discrimination. Some studies suggested that craving was redundant with other criteria (Casey et al. 2012; Cherpitel et al. 2010; Mewton et al. 2011). When statistical tests were used to compare Item Response Theory results, the addition of craving to the dependence criteria did not significantly add information; however, when craving and the three abuse criteria were added to the dependence criteria, total information was increased for nicotine, alcohol, cannabis, and heroin use disorders (Hasin et al. 2012; Shmulewitz et al. 2011). Although the psychometric benefit of adding a craving criterion was equivocal, the view that craving could become a biological treatment target (a nonpsychometric perspective) prevailed. Craving was therefore added as a DSM-5 SUD criterion (see Table 4–1).

Diagnostic Threshold Set at Two or More Criteria

Studies have shown that the SUD criteria represent a dimensional condition with no natural threshold (Beseler and Hasin 2010; Hasin and Beseler 2009; Hasin et al. 2006b). However, a binary (yes/no) diagnostic decision is often needed in clinical practice. To avoid marked perturbations in prevalence, the work group sought a threshold for DSM-5 SUD that would yield the best agreement with the combined prevalence of DSM-IV substance abuse and dependence disorders. The work group used general population and clinical samples to calculate the prevalences of and the agreement (kappa) between the DSM-5 SUD criteria and the DSM-IV dependence and abuse criteria with thresholds of two or more to four or more DSM-5 criteria (Hasin et al. 2013). Prevalence was very similar across the thresholds, and agreement was maximized with the threshold of two or more criteria. Another large, independently conducted study further supported this threshold (Peer et al. 2013). Concerns that the threshold of two or more criteria was too low and would either produce overly heterogeneous groups or result in false-positive diagnoses (Martin et al. 2011) were weighed against the need to identify all cases meriting intervention, including milder cases (e.g., those in primary care). Concerns about the threshold can be further addressed by using the severity specifiers (see the following section), which clearly indicate that cases vary in severity.

An important exception to making a diagnosis of DSM-5 SUD on the basis of two criteria pertains to the supervised medical use of psychoactive substances (e.g., opioids when used to treat chronic pain). Regular use of opioids even for therapeutic purposes can produce tolerance and withdrawal as normal physiological adaptations, even when used appropriately. Under these conditions, the presence of tolerance and withdrawal in the absence of two or more additional criteria does not indicate an SUD and should not be diagnosed as such.

Severity Indicators (Determined Using a Criteria Count) for DSM-5 Substance Use Disorder Diagnoses

The DSM-5 Task Force asked work groups to provide severity indicators of mild, moderate, and severe for diagnoses. A count of the SUD criteria provided a simple, parsimonious approach, because the criteria are unidimensional, and as the count increases, so do SUD risk factors and consequences (Beseler and Hasin 2010; Dawson et al. 2010; Hasin and Beseler 2009; Hasin et al. 2006b). Mild SUDs are diagnosed when two to three criteria are met, moderate SUDs are diagnosed for four to five criteria, and severe SUDs are diagnosed for six or more criteria.

New Studies Since Publication of DSM-5

Since the publication of DSM-5, several studies within and outside the United States have examined the reliability and validity of the DSM-5 SUD criteria. These studies used a variety of measures and were conducted in community, clinical, and other unique samples (Table 4–2).

In a large U.S. sample, test–retest reliability for binary DSM-5 SUDs was fair to excellent (Grant et al. 2015), showing improved reliability when SUDs were assessed with dimensional scales, with most SUDs (e.g., alcohol, cannabis, opioids) in the good to excellent range. Similar results were obtained in a smaller study (Shankman et al. 2018); test–retest reliability was fair to excellent for DSM-5 SUDs and alcohol use disorder (AUD), and dimensional scales generally yielded better reliability than did categorical diagnoses. In a small Swedish sample (Gerdner and Wickström 2015), test–retest reliability for DSM-5 AUD, cannabis use disorder (CUD), and opioid use disorder was good to excellent and was comparable to that for DSM-IV abuse or dependence. In a genetics study (Denis et al. 2015), interobserver reliability was good to excellent for DSM-5 AUD, CUD, and opioid use disorder and was generally higher for DSM-5 SUDs than for DSM-IV diagnoses. Internal consistency for DSM-5 SUD criteria ranged from acceptable to good in a U.S. college student sample (Hagman 2017), a U.S.-based mixed community and clinical sample (Shankman et al. 2018), and a small Swedish clinical sample (Gerdner and Wickström 2015).

Agreement between two measures of DSM-5 SUDs was fair to good for most substances, including alcohol, cannabis, and opioids (Hasin et al. 2015). Concordance for dimensional measures was greater than that for binary diagnoses, ranging from good to excellent. Agreement between two measures of inhalant use disorder also was improved when counts of SUD criteria were used rather than categorical diagnoses and was better for the DSM-5 configuration of inhalant use disorder compared with that from DSM-IV (Ridenour et al. 2015). Regarding other convergent validators, DSM-5 AUD and SUD were significantly correlated with indicators of impaired functioning and distress in a mixed community and clinical sample (Shankman et al. 2018). In a study in a sample of college students, participants who met criteria for DSM-5 AUD had significantly higher levels of alcohol and drug use and of negative consequences related to drinking and drug use than did those who did not meet these criteria (Hagman 2017).

TABLE 4–2.   Reliability and validity studies of DSM-5 substance use disorders (SUDs)

Reference	Sample	Location	N	Measures	Main findings
Kelly et al. 2014	Community, adolescents	United States	525	CIDI-SAM	Strong agreement between DSM-5 SUDs and DSM-IV abuse/dependence (kappa=0.81 for alcohol; 0.84 for cannabis).
Murphy et al. 2014	Community	United States	104	SCID, PACS	Craving functioned similarly to other DSM-5 AUD criteria. It was endorsed at a similar rate to other AUD criteria and was significantly correlated with greater alcohol consumption, greater AUD severity, and more alcohol-related consequences. Factor analysis indicated good fit with other AUD criteria as part of a single latent syndrome.
Denis et al. 2015	Community and clinical	United States	173	SSADDA	Interobserver reliability was good to excellent (kappa=0.65–0.94). Reliability was generally higher for DSM-5 SUD than for DSM-IV abuse/dependence diagnoses.
Gerdner and Wickström 2015	Clinical	Sweden	30	ADDIS	Internal consistency for DSM-5 SUD criteria was satisfactory to excellent (α=0.87–0.96), comparable to criteria for DSM-IV dependence/abuse diagnoses. Test–retest reliability of DSM-5 SUDs ranged from moderate to almost perfect for most substances (kappa=0.67–0.85), comparable to DSM-IV diagnoses.
Grant et al. 2015	Community	United States	1,006	AUDADIS-5	Test–retest reliability was fair to excellent for past-year and prior-to-past-year binary DSM-5 SUDs (kappa=0.40–0.87). Dimensional scales showed better reliability than categorical diagnoses, with most SUDs in the good to excellent range (ICC=0.60–0.85). Reliability was comparable to DSM-IV diagnoses.
Hasin et al. 2015	Community	United States	712	AUDADIS-5, PRISM-5	Agreement between categorical past-year, prior-to-past-year, and lifetime SUD diagnoses was fair to good for most substances (kappa=0.40–0.68). Agreement for dimensional measures was good to excellent for most substances (ICC=0.68–0.92). Concordance levels were comparable to validity studies of DSM-IV measures.

TABLE 4–2. Reliability and validity studies of DSM-5 substance use disorders (SUDs) *(continued)*

Reference	Sample	Location	N	Measures	Main findings
Lundin et al. 2015	Community	Sweden	1,091	SCAN	Agreement between DSM-5 AUD and DSM-IV alcohol abuse/dependence was excellent (kappa=0.84). Agreement between DSM-5 AUD and ICD-10 harmful use/dependence was lower, although still good (kappa=0.62).
Ridenour et al. 2015	Community and clinical	United States	162	CIDI-SAM, SCAN	Assessment of inhalant use disorder was improved when treated as a continuous measure, with better agreement between measures for counts of criteria than for categorical diagnoses. Principal components analysis suggested that a single factor underlies all 4 inhalant types. Concordance and validity were better for, and more consistent with, DSM-5 inhalant use disorder than DSM-IV.
Lago et al. 2016	Community	Australia	5,552[a], 1,639[b]	WMH-CIDI	Factor analysis demonstrated a unifactorial model of AUD and CUD. Demographic and clinical correlates showed similar associations for alcohol and cannabis dependence in DSM-IV, ICD-10, and ICD-11; DSM-5 moderate/severe AUD was associated with a less persistent course of disorder, fewer mental/substance use comorbidities, lower likelihood of having received treatment, and lower level of social disadvantage. DSM-5 moderate/severe CUD followed a similar but less marked pattern of differences to cannabis dependence. Lifetime prevalence of any AUD and CUD was similar across DSM-IV, DSM-5, ICD-10, and ICD-11. For DSM-5, lifetime prevalence of moderate/severe SUD was higher than DSM-IV dependence for alcohol (13.1% vs. 6.2%) and cannabis (15.9% vs. 9.8%). Concordance for alcohol and cannabis dependence was excellent among DSM-IV, ICD-10, and ICD-11 (kappa=0.90–0.99). Agreement was lower between DSM-5 moderate/severe AUD and CUD and alcohol/cannabis dependence, although still fair to good (kappa=0.61–0.70).

TABLE 4–2. Reliability and validity studies of DSM-5 substance use disorders (SUDs) *(continued)*

Reference	Sample	Location	N	Measures	Main findings
Chung et al. 2017	Clinical, adolescents	United States	339	SCID[c]	Past-year prevalence of any AUD was similar between DSM-IV and DSM-5; these prevalences were significantly higher than ICD-10 and ICD-11. DSM-5 moderate/severe SUD had the highest level of agreement with ICD-11 dependence (kappa=0.73 for alcohol; 0.78 for cannabis), followed by ICD-10 (kappa=0.65 for alcohol; 0.71 for cannabis), and DSM-IV (kappa=0.54 for alcohol; 0.63 for cannabis).
Hagman 2017	College students	United States	923	Brief DSM-5 AUD Assessment	Internal consistency for DSM-5 AUD criteria was high (α=0.78). Participants with DSM-5 AUD had significantly higher levels of alcohol/drug use and negative consequences related to drinking/drug use compared with participants without AUD. Confirmatory factor analysis indicated a single factor underlying DSM-5 AUD criteria.
Degenhardt et al. 2019	Community	10 countries[d]	12,182[a], 1,788[b]	WMH-CIDI	Lifetime prevalence was similar among DSM-IV, DSM-5, ICD-10, and ICD-11 for AUDs and CUDs. Concordance among DSM-IV, ICD-10, and ICD-11 was excellent for all AUDs and CUDs (kappa=0.93–0.97). Concordance was lower between DSM-5 and the other diagnostic systems. For any AUDs and CUDs, agreement was good (kappa=0.65–0.71). For DSM-5 moderate/severe AUD and CUD, agreement with dependence was fair to good (kappa=0.61–0.70). For DSM-5 mild AUD and CUD, agreement with abuse/harmful use was poor to fair (kappa=0.39–0.42). Differences in demographic and clinical correlates were minimal for AUDs and CUDs across the diagnostic systems.

TABLE 4–2.	Reliability and validity studies of DSM-5 substance use disorders (SUDs) *(continued)*			
Reference	Sample	Location	N	Measures	Main findings
Serier et al. 2019	Clinical, Native Americans	United States	79	SCID	Confirmatory factor analysis indicated that DSM-5 AUD criteria reflect a single underlying construct. Previous findings regarding validity of DSM-5 AUD criteria were replicated in a treatment-seeking sample of Native Americans.
Shankman et al. 2018	Community and clinical	United States	234	SCID	Dimensional scales and categorical diagnoses were associated with significant concurrent validity for all validators. Internal consistency for dimensional assessment of current and lifetime AUD and SUD was in the moderate to substantial range (α=0.78–0.91) for dimensional scales (ICC=0.79–0.92 for lifetime; 0.38–0.76 for current) was generally better than for categorical diagnoses (kappa=0.84–0.87 for lifetime; 0.54–0.64 for current). Reliability for lifetime disorders (dimensional and categorical) was better than for current disorders, potentially because of small number of participants with current AUD or SUD.

Note. ADDIS=Alcohol Drog Diagnos InStrument (Swedish); AUD=alcohol use disorder; AUDADIS-5=Alcohol Use Disorder and Associated Disabilities Interview Schedule, DSM-5 Version; CIDI-SAM=Composite International Diagnostic Interview Substance Abuse Module; CUD=cannabis use disorder; ICC=intraclass correlation coefficient; PACS=Penn Alcohol Craving Scale; PRISM-5=Psychiatric Research Interview for Substance and Mental Disorders, DSM-5 Version; SCAN=Schedules for Clinical Assessment in Neuropsychiatry; SCID=Structured Clinical Interview for DSM; SSADDA=Semi-Structured Assessment for Drug Dependence and Alcoholism; WMH-CIDI=World Mental Health Survey Initiative version of the Composite International Diagnostic Interview.

[a] Alcohol users.

[b] Cannabis users.

[c] Adapted for use with adolescents.

[d] Argentina, Australia, Brazil, Colombia, Iraq, Northern Ireland, Poland, Portugal, Romania, and Spain.

Factor analyses indicated that DSM-5 AUD criteria were characterized by a single underlying factor in college students (Hagman 2017), a Native American sample (Serier et al. 2019), and a large Australian community sample (Lago et al. 2016) in which CUD criteria were also unidimensional. Factor analysis showed that craving fit well with other DSM-5 AUD criteria as part of the latent syndrome; functioned similarly to other AUD criteria; was endorsed at a similar rate; and was associated with greater alcohol consumption, greater AUD severity, and more alcohol-related consequences (Murphy et al. 2014).

As with the DSM-IV classification for SUDs, the ICD-10 classification system for SUDs included two separate, hierarchical diagnoses: harmful use and dependence (Saunders 2017). ICD-11 (World Health Organization 2019) retained the ICD-10 distinction between harmful substance use and substance dependence and most of the ICD-10 criteria but proposed combining individual criteria to form composite criteria to simplify diagnostic guidelines (Saunders 2017). Studies examining the agreement of DSM-5 SUDs with other diagnostic systems have generally shown good concordance—for example, in samples of adolescents, in which concordance for any AUD and CUD was good to excellent between DSM-5 and DSM-IV (Chung et al. 2017; Kelly et al. 2014), fair between DSM-5 and ICD-11, and poor between DSM-5 and ICD-10 (Chung et al. 2017). However, when severity was taken into account, moderate or severe DSM-5 AUD and CUD had the highest level of agreement with ICD-11 dependence (Chung et al. 2017).

In adult samples, good agreement also was found between DSM-5 AUD and DSM-IV alcohol abuse or dependence; agreement between DSM-5 AUD and ICD-10 harmful use of alcohol or alcohol dependence was lower but still good (Lundin et al. 2015). Lifetime prevalences of any AUD or CUD were similar across DSM-IV, DSM-5, ICD-10, and ICD-11 in two large international community studies (Degenhardt et al. 2019; Lago et al. 2016). Concordance among DSM-IV, ICD-10, and ICD-11 alcohol and cannabis dependence was excellent; concordance was lower, although still fair to good, between moderate or severe AUD and CUD in DSM-5 and alcohol and cannabis dependence in the other diagnostic systems (Degenhardt et al. 2019; Lago et al. 2016). Although the demographic and clinical correlates of alcohol and cannabis dependence as defined in DSM-IV, ICD-10, and ICD-11 showed a similar pattern of associations, the correlates of DSM-5 moderate or severe AUD and CUD exhibited a different pattern in one study (Lago et al. 2016). Compared with alcohol and cannabis dependence in the other diagnostic systems, moderate or severe AUD and CUD in DSM-5 were associated with a less persistent course of disorder, fewer mental and substance use disorder comorbidities, a lower likelihood of having received treatment, and less social disadvantage. However, differences in demographic and clinical correlates were not observed in another study (Degenhardt et al. 2019).

Conclusion

In summary, studies examining the reliability and validity of the DSM-5 SUD criteria have shown that these criteria demonstrated good internal consistency and reliability when a variety of measures were used. Factor analysis showed that DSM-5 SUD criteria are unidimensional. DSM-5 SUDs show good concurrent validity with indicators of problematic use and good agreement with other diagnostic classification systems. In general, the reliability and validity of the DSM-5 SUD criteria are comparable to the reliability and validity of their DSM-IV abuse or dependence counterparts. Importantly, DSM-5 SUDs are better conceptualized by using dimensional scales rather than binary diagnoses, because the dimensional DSM-5 SUD measures have better reliability and validity.

References

Agrawal A, Lynskey MT: Does gender contribute to heterogeneity in criteria for cannabis abuse and dependence? Results from the National Epidemiological Survey on Alcohol and Related Conditions. Drug Alcohol Depend 88(2–3):300–307, 2007 17084563

American Psychiatric Association: Diagnostic and Statistical Manual: Mental Disorders. Washington, DC, American Psychiatric Association, 1952

American Psychiatric Association: Diagnostic and Statistical Manual of Mental Disorders, 4th Edition. Washington, DC, American Psychiatric Association, 1994

American Psychiatric Association: Diagnostic and Statistical Manual of Mental Disorders, 5th Edition. Arlington, VA, American Psychiatric Association, 2013

Beseler CL, Hasin DS: Cannabis dimensionality: dependence, abuse and consumption. Addict Behav 35(11):961–969, 2010 20598807

Blanco C, Harford TC, Nunes E, et al: The latent structure of marijuana and cocaine use disorders: results from the National Longitudinal Alcohol Epidemiologic Survey (NLAES). Drug Alcohol Depend 91(1):91–96, 2007 17512682

Casey M, Adamson G, Shevlin M, et al: The role of craving in AUDs: dimensionality and differential functioning in the DSM-5. Drug Alcohol Depend 125(1–2):75–80, 2012 22516145

Cherpitel CJ, Borges G, Ye Y, et al: Performance of a craving criterion in DSM alcohol use disorders. J Stud Alcohol Drugs 71(5):674–684, 2010 20731972

Chung T, Cornelius J, Clark D, et al: Greater prevalence of proposed ICD-11 alcohol and cannabis dependence compared to ICD-10, DSM-IV, and DSM-5 in treated adolescents. Alcohol Clin Exp Res 41(9):1584–1592, 2017 28667763

Compton WM, Thomas YF, Stinson FS, et al: Prevalence, correlates, disability, and comorbidity of DSM-IV drug abuse and dependence in the United States: results from the National Epidemiologic Survey on Alcohol and Related Conditions. Arch Gen Psychiatry 64(5):566–576, 2007 17485608

Dawson DA: Drinking patterns among individuals with and without DSM-IV alcohol use disorders. J Stud Alcohol 61(1):111–120, 2000 10627104

Dawson DA, Saha TD, Grant BF: A multidimensional assessment of the validity and utility of alcohol use disorder severity as determined by item response theory models. Drug Alcohol Depend 107(1):31–38, 2010 19782481

Degenhardt L, Bharat C, Bruno R, et al: Concordance between the diagnostic guidelines for alcohol and cannabis use disorders in the draft ICD-11 and other classification systems: analysis of data from the WHO's World Mental Health Surveys. Addiction 114(3):534–552, 2019 30370636

Denis CM, Gelernter J, Hart AB, et al: Inter-observer reliability of DSM-5 substance use disorders. Drug Alcohol Depend 153:229–235, 2015 26048641

Foroud T, Wetherill LF, Liang T, et al: Association of alcohol craving with alpha-synuclein (SNCA). Alcohol Clin Exp Res 31(4):537–545, 2007 17374032

Gerdner A, Wickström L: Reliability of ADDIS for diagnoses of substance use disorders according to ICD-10, DSM-IV and DSM-5: test-retest and inter-item consistency. Subst Abuse Treat Prev Policy 10:14, 2015 25886630

Gillespie NA, Neale MC, Prescott CA, et al: Factor and item-response analysis DSM-IV criteria for abuse of and dependence on cannabis, cocaine, hallucinogens, sedatives, stimulants and opioids. Addiction 102(6):920–930, 2007 17523987

Grant BF, Stinson FS, Harford TC: Age at onset of alcohol use and DSM-IV alcohol abuse and dependence: a 12-year follow-up. J Subst Abuse 13(4):493–504, 2001 11775078

Grant BF, Stinson FS, Dawson DA, et al: Prevalence and co-occurrence of substance use disorders and independent mood and anxiety disorders: results from the National Epidemiologic Survey on Alcohol and Related Conditions. Arch Gen Psychiatry 61(8):807–816, 2004 15289279

Grant BF, Goldstein RB, Smith SM, et al: The Alcohol Use Disorder and Associated Disabilities Interview Schedule-5 (AUDADIS-5): reliability of substance use and psychiatric disorder modules in a general population sample. Drug Alcohol Depend 148:27–33, 2015 25595052

Hagman BT: Development and psychometric analysis of the Brief DSM-5 Alcohol Use Disorder Diagnostic Assessment: towards effective diagnosis in college students. Psychol Addict Behav 31(7):797–806, 2017 29144150

Hagman BT, Cohn AM: Toward DSM-V: mapping the alcohol use disorder continuum in college students. Drug Alcohol Depend 118(2–3):202–208, 2011 21514750

Harford TC, Muthén BO: The dimensionality of alcohol abuse and dependence: a multivariate analysis of DSM-IV symptom items in the National Longitudinal Survey of Youth. J Stud Alcohol 62(2):150–157, 2001 11327181

Hasin DS, Beseler CL: Dimensionality of lifetime alcohol abuse, dependence and binge drinking. Drug Alcohol Depend 101(1–2):53–61, 2009 19095379

Hasin DS, Grant BF: The co-occurrence of DSM-IV alcohol abuse in DSM-IV alcohol dependence: results of the National Epidemiologic Survey on Alcohol and Related Conditions on heterogeneity that differ by population subgroup. Arch Gen Psychiatry 61(9):891–896, 2004 15351767

Hasin D, Paykin A: Dependence symptoms but no diagnosis: diagnostic "orphans" in a community sample. Drug Alcohol Depend 50(1):19–26, 1998 9589269

Hasin D, Paykin A: Dependence symptoms but no diagnosis: diagnostic "orphans" in a 1992 national sample. Drug Alcohol Depend 53(3):215–222, 1999a 10080047

Hasin D, Paykin A: DSM-IV alcohol abuse: investigation in a sample of at-risk drinkers in the community. J Stud Alcohol 60(2):181–187, 1999b 10091956

Hasin DS, Van Rossem R, McCloud S, et al: Differentiating DSM-IV alcohol dependence and abuse by course: community heavy drinkers. J Subst Abuse 9:127–135, 1997 9494944

Hasin D, Paykin A, Endicott J, et al: The validity of DSM-IV alcohol abuse: drunk drivers versus all others. J Stud Alcohol 60(6):746–755, 1999 10606485

Hasin DS, Hatzenbuehler M, Smith S, et al: Co-occurring DSM-IV drug abuse in DSM-IV drug dependence: results from the National Epidemiologic Survey on Alcohol and Related Conditions. Drug Alcohol Depend 80(1):117–123, 2005 16157234

Hasin DS, Hatzenbuehler ML, Keyes K, et al: Substance use disorders: Diagnostic and Statistical Manual of Mental Disorders, Fourth Edition (DSM-IV) and International Classification of Diseases, Tenth Edition (ICD-10). Addiction 101 (suppl 1):59–75, 2006a 16930162

Hasin DS, Liu X, Alderson D, Grant BF: DSM-IV alcohol dependence: a categorical or dimensional phenotype? Psychol Med 36(12):1695–1705, 2006b 17038207

Hasin DS, Stinson FS, Ogburn E, et al: Prevalence, correlates, disability, and comorbidity of DSM-IV alcohol abuse and dependence in the United States: results from the National Epidemiologic Survey on Alcohol and Related Conditions. Arch Gen Psychiatry 64(7):830–842, 2007 17606817

Hasin DS, Fenton MC, Beseler C, et al: Analyses related to the development of DSM-5 criteria for substance use related disorders, 2: proposed DSM-5 criteria for alcohol, cannabis, cocaine and heroin disorders in 663 substance abuse patients. Drug Alcohol Depend 122(1–2):28–37, 2012 21963333

Hasin DS, O'Brien CP, Auriacombe M, et al: DSM-5 criteria for substance use disorders: recommendations and rationale. Am J Psychiatry 170(8):834–851, 2013 23903334

Hasin DS, Greenstein E, Aivadyan C, et al: The Alcohol Use Disorder and Associated Disabilities Interview Schedule-5 (AUDADIS-5): procedural validity of substance use disorders modules through clinical re-appraisal in a general population sample. Drug Alcohol Depend 148:40–46, 2015 25604321

Heinz A, Beck A, Grüsser SM, et al: Identifying the neural circuitry of alcohol craving and relapse vulnerability. Addict Biol 14(1):108–118, 2009 18855799

Kelly SM, Gryczynski J, Mitchell SG, et al: Concordance between DSM-5 and DSM-IV nicotine, alcohol, and cannabis use disorder diagnoses among pediatric patients. Drug Alcohol Depend 140:213–216, 2014 24793367

Keyes KM, Krueger RF, Grant BF, et al: Alcohol craving and the dimensionality of alcohol disorders. Psychol Med 41(3):629–640, 2011 20459881

Krueger RF, Nichol PE, Hicks BM, et al: Using latent trait modeling to conceptualize an alcohol problems continuum. Psychol Assess 16(2):107–119, 2004 15222807

Lago L, Bruno R, Degenhardt L: Concordance of ICD-11 and DSM-5 definitions of alcohol and cannabis use disorders: a population survey. Lancet Psychiatry 3(7):673–684, 2016 27371989

Lundin A, Hallgren M, Forsman M, et al: Comparison of DSM-5 classifications of alcohol use disorders with those of DSM-IV, DSM-III-R, and ICD-10 in a general population sample in Sweden. J Stud Alcohol Drugs 76(5):773–780, 2015 26402358

Lynskey MT, Agrawal A: Psychometric properties of DSM assessments of illicit drug abuse and dependence: results from the National Epidemiologic Survey on Alcohol and Related Conditions (NESARC). Psychol Med 37(9):1345–1355, 2007 17407621

Martin CS, Chung T, Kirisci L, et al: Item response theory analysis of diagnostic criteria for alcohol and cannabis use disorders in adolescents: implications for DSM-V. J Abnorm Psychol 115(4):807–814, 2006 17100538

Martin CS, Steinley DL, Vergés A, et al: The proposed 2/11 symptom algorithm for DSM-5 substance-use disorders is too lenient. Psychol Med 41(9):2008–2010, 2011 21557890

McBride O, Adamson G, Bunting BP, et al: Characteristics of DSM-IV alcohol diagnostic orphans: drinking patterns, physical illness, and negative life events. Drug Alcohol Depend 99(1–3):272–279, 2009 18848409

Mewton L, Slade T, McBride O, et al: An evaluation of the proposed DSM-5 alcohol use disorder criteria using Australian national data. Addiction 106(5):941–950, 2011 21205055

Miller NS, Goldsmith RJ: Craving for alcohol and drugs in animals and humans: biology and behavior. J Addict Dis 20(3):87–104, 2001 11681596

Murphy CM, Stojek MK, Few LR, et al: Craving as an alcohol use disorder symptom in DSM-5: an empirical examination in a treatment-seeking sample. Exp Clin Psychopharmacol 22(1):43–49, 2014 24490710

O'Brien CP: Anticraving medications for relapse prevention: a possible new class of psychoactive medications. Am J Psychiatry 162(8):1423–1431, 2005 16055763

O'Brien CP, Childress AR, Ehrman R, et al: Conditioning factors in drug abuse: can they explain compulsion? J Psychopharmacol 12(1):15–22, 1998 9584964

Peer K, Rennert L, Lynch KG, et al: Prevalence of DSM-IV and DSM-5 alcohol, cocaine, opioid, and cannabis use disorders in a largely substance dependent sample. Drug Alcohol Depend 127(1–3):215–219, 2013 22884164

Proudfoot H, Baillie AJ, Teesson M: The structure of alcohol dependence in the community. Drug Alcohol Depend 81(1):21–26, 2006 16005578

Ridenour TA, Halliburton AE, Bray BC: Does DSM-5 nomenclature for inhalant use disorder improve upon DSM-IV? Psychol Addict Behav 29(1):211–217, 2015 25134040

Saha TD, Chou SP, Grant BF: Toward an alcohol use disorder continuum using item response theory: results from the National Epidemiologic Survey on Alcohol and Related Conditions. Psychol Med 36(7):931–941, 2006 16563205

Saha TD, Stinson FS, Grant BF: The role of alcohol consumption in future classifications of alcohol use disorders. Drug Alcohol Depend 89(1):82–92, 2007 17240085

Saha TD, Compton WM, Chou SP, et al: Analyses related to the development of DSM-5 criteria for substance use related disorders, 1: toward amphetamine, cocaine and prescription drug use disorder continua using Item Response Theory. Drug Alcohol Depend 122(1–2):38–46, 2012 21963414

Saunders JB: Substance use and addictive disorders in DSM-5 and ICD 10 and the draft ICD 11. Curr Opin Psychiatry 30(4):227–237, 2017 28459730

Saunders JB, Schuckit MA: The development of a research agenda for substance use disorders diagnosis in the Diagnostic and Statistical Manual of Mental Disorders, Fifth Edition (DSM-V). Addiction 101 (suppl 1):1–5, 2006 16930155

Schuckit MA, Smith TL, Landi NA: The 5-year clinical course of high-functioning men with DSM-IV alcohol abuse or dependence. Am J Psychiatry 157(12):2028–2035, 2000 11097971

Serier KN, Venner KL, Sarafin RE: Evaluating the validity of the DSM-5 alcohol use disorder diagnostic criteria in a sample of treatment-seeking Native Americans. J Addict Med 13(1):35–40, 2019 30303888

Shankman SA, Funkhouser CJ, Klein DN, et al: Reliability and validity of severity dimensions of psychopathology assessed using the Structured Clinical Interview for DSM-5 (SCID). Int J Methods Psychiatr Res 27(1), 2018 29034525

Shmulewitz D, Keyes K, Beseler C, et al: The dimensionality of alcohol use disorders: results from Israel. Drug Alcohol Depend 111(1–2):146–154, 2010 20537809

Shmulewitz D, Keyes KM, Wall MM, et al: Nicotine dependence, abuse and craving: dimensionality in an Israeli sample. Addiction 106(9):1675–1686, 2011 21545668

Teesson M, Lynskey M, Manor B, et al: The structure of cannabis dependence in the community. Drug Alcohol Depend 68(3):255–262, 2002 12393220

Waters AJ, Shiffman S, Sayette MA, et al: Cue-provoked craving and nicotine replacement therapy in smoking cessation. J Consult Clin Psychol 72(6):1136–1143, 2004 15612859

Weiss F: Neurobiology of craving, conditioned reward and relapse. Curr Opin Pharmacol 5(1):9–19, 2005 15661620

World Health Organization: The ICD-10 Classification of Mental and Behavioural Disorders: Diagnostic Criteria for Research. Geneva, World Health Organization, 1993

World Health Organization: International Statistical Classification of Diseases and Related Health Problems, 11th Revision. Geneva, World Health Organization, 2019

PART II

Assessment and Treatment

CHAPTER 5

Assessment

Timothy Fong, M.D.

In the most recent *Practice Guidelines for the Psychiatric Evaluation of Adults*, the American Psychiatric Association (2016) recommends that the initial psychiatric evaluation of a patient include an assessment of the patient's use of tobacco, alcohol, psychoactive substances, prescribed medications, and any other supplements. In contrast to screening, which is designed to quickly identify risky patterns of substance use, a comprehensive assessment firmly establishes where on the continuum of substance use the patient falls—use, misuse, excessive use, or substance use disorder. This information will then add to the development of an appropriate and evidence-based treatment plan that fits the proper level of care.

In general, the basic components of a substance use assessment include 1) describing current and past patterns of substance use with an emphasis on characterizing use that may be excessive, harmful, or hazardous; 2) diagnosing any substance-related disorder that may be present currently; and 3) documenting the effect of substance use on an individual's mental and physical state. Understanding the patient's readiness to change, determining the presence of co-occurring psychiatric disorders, documenting medical history, performing a physical examination and laboratory tests, exploring the presence of substance use disorder in the patient's family, and conducting a review of social factors are also parts of the substance use assessment (Dugosh et al. 2017). In this chapter, I review techniques and strategies for conducting an efficient assessment of substance use and for synthesizing the substance use assessment with other parts of the psychiatric assessment.

Preparing for the Substance Use Assessment

A thorough substance use assessment starts with preparation before the first question is asked. Each interview setting, whether it be an office, emergency department, hospital unit, or residential treatment facility, has unique qualities and features that must be considered beforehand (Dugosh et al. 2017). For example, assessments in the emergency department will be shorter and more focused on the issue at hand while striving to maintain confidentiality in a chaotic environment. In an inpatient psychiatric hospital unit, patients may be less forthright and more likely to minimize their substance use, especially if they are admitted on an involuntary hold. Clinicians should keep in mind that patients who are presenting for care in a non–addiction treatment setting (such as an office visit for depression, insomnia, or anxiety) may not be expecting complex and vigorous questions about substance use; therefore, clinicians should describe to the patient, in clear terms, the purpose and intent of asking questions about substance use.

Maintaining the highest level of security and confidentiality in the interview room is fundamental to completing an accurate substance use assessment. Patients who feel uneasy or who do not trust that their medical records will be secure are unlikely to provide a frank and full disclosure of their use of substances and any consequences of such use (Vendetti et al. 2017). Conducting the interview in an open space (like those seen in emergency departments or hospital rooms) or in front of a large treatment team are examples of conditions that a patient may not perceive as safe and private and that would likely lead to minimization or denial of substance use (Schaper et al. 2016).

Electronic medical records have revolutionized the way that health care is practiced, and their use during the substance use assessment must be taken into consideration beforehand. The practice of typing and inputting information while interviewing (and thus making less eye contact) has drawn mixed reviews from clinicians and patients (Hollis et al. 2015; Papadakos 2013). Providers who first learned to document patient details in an electronic culture often will prefer to type while interviewing (Alkureishi et al. 2016). Because opportunities to engage in discussion around substances require finesse, empathy, and the ability to read patients' verbal and nonverbal cues, interviewers need to think about how their actions and behaviors will be perceived by patients before they begin the interview.

One final consideration in the substance use interview is to recognize the current physical and psychiatric state of the patient. Patients who use substances will present in a wide variety of states, ranging from intoxication to withdrawal. For obvious reasons, it is unlikely that a valid and reliable history would be obtainable from a patient in either of these states. If possible, an interview with an intoxicated patient should be limited to an assessment of the patient's physical and psychiatric safety (Simpson 2019). By the same token, it is unlikely that accurate information would be collected if the clinician fails to notice or to correctly identify the patient's current state; for example, a patient in withdrawal might easily be misperceived as being uncooperative or hostile or be misdiagnosed as having a personality disorder (Jansson and Nordgaard 2016).

In the following subsection, I describe the specific tasks that should be completed before the assessment.

Review the Medical Record Beforehand

Given the time constraints of clinical medicine today, it is critical before seeing any patient for the first time to review as much available information as possible. Electronic medical records will have many clues as to potential patterns of substance use and misuse—connections that previous providers may not have put together. For instance, patients records showing multiple emergency visits combined with frequent visits to primary care for symptoms such as headaches, insomnia, and back pain that result in prescription of controlled substances may provide clues to an unidentified substance use disorder. Some patients may have received a previous diagnosis of substance use disorder, which still may be active or may be in remission, but the problem list on the electronic record may not have been updated (Wright et al. 2015). Other potential clues in the electronic record include evidence of frequent physical injuries; laboratory findings of abnormalities in liver function, neuroimaging, or cardiac test results; infectious disease (e.g., HIV) test results; or even prior urine drug screening results.

Finally, clinicians should be aware that some health systems maintain records related to substance use disorder treatment behind electronic firewalls, in accordance with federal confidentiality law and regulations, which would limit the clinician's access to records and information (McCarty et al. 2017). The Confidentiality of Substance Use Disorder Patient Records (42 CFR Part 2) regulations serve to protect patient records by prohibiting law enforcement personnel from using the patient's records in criminal proceedings against the patient. Part 2 also restricts the disclosure of substance use disorder treatment records without patient consent, other than as statutorily authorized in the context of a bona fide medical emergency or an appropriate court order for good cause.

Check Prescription Drug Monitoring Program Database

Prescription drug monitoring programs (PDMPs) are highly effective tools used by government officials for reducing prescription drug abuse and diversion (Strickler et al. 2019). PDMPs collect, monitor, and analyze electronically transmitted prescribing and dispensing data submitted by pharmacies and dispensing practitioners. Conducting a PDMP review prior to—rather than after or during—the substance use assessment will yield valuable information that can be discussed during the assessment. Because each state has specific rules about when, how, and by whom PDMP databases can be checked, clinicians are urged to follow state-specific rules and guidelines around prescriptions for scheduled medications.

Administer and Review Substance Use Screening Forms in Advance

The challenges faced by clinicians who work in non–addiction treatment settings are different from those faced by providers who are identified as addiction treatment specialists. Because of denial, lack of education about symptoms of substance use disorder, resistance to treatment, stigma, and low motivation to seek treatment, patients with substance use disorder who present in non–addiction treatment settings may not easily volunteer information about their substance use and harmful consequences (Pickard 2016). Over the last 15 years, many screening instruments for a wide variety of substances have been validated, and use of these tools to collect information before the assessment can improve efficiency (Levy et al. 2016). Screening instruments can take time to complete but have been shown to yield accurate and valid information. Thus, health care providers in outpatient settings should encourage clients to arrive 30–40 minutes before their scheduled appointments to complete intake forms collecting baseline information.

Information gathered from questions during the initial psychiatric interview can be supplemented by administration of self-report rating scales, such as the DSM-5 Self-Rated Level 1 Cross-Cutting Symptom Measure, with administration of the DSM-5 Level 2 Measure—Substance Use if the patient gives a positive response on the Level 1 alcohol or substance use items (American Psychiatric Association 2013). These measures are available on the American Psychiatric Association website (www.psychiatry .org/psychiatrists/practice/dsm/educational-resources/assessment-measures).

Conducting the Substance Use Assessment

Interview Techniques

Patients are often reluctant to report behaviors related to substance use disorders, not only because the act of ingesting substances to alter one's mental state is associated with immorality and illegality but also because of shame related to harmful behaviors such as lying to or manipulating others or neglecting self-care (Zorland et al. 2018). At the time of the assessment, patients may be experiencing shame, embarrassment, or guilt or simply be in denial or lack awareness or understanding of the severity of their illness (Rahim and Patton 2015). With this in mind, interviewers should pay especially close attention to the patient's verbal and nonverbal clues, such as not listening to questions; minimizing use or consequences of use; changing the subject; discouraging inquiry by displaying irritation, anxiety, or other behaviors; and outright lying. Awareness of these clues will alert the interviewer to attempt to make a connection between the history of the details rather than passing a rapid and quick judgment.

Interviewing techniques to overcome these barriers include asking open-ended questions such as "Tell me about your relationship with alcohol" or "As a standard part of our interview today, I'd like to ask about your thoughts, feelings, and behaviors related to substances—I can assure you that what you tell me is protected by laws about confidentiality" (Rieckmann et al. 2016).

Too often, interviews are rushed because of time constraints, and interviewers often feel the need to push along the interview, which will result in closed-ended questions or preemptively judgmental questions such as "You wouldn't use illegal drugs, would you?" Providers are encouraged to review resources on motivational interviewing and guidelines on how to ask sensitive questions in a clear, concise manner (DiClemente et al. 2017). Being able to control the pace of the interview, especially in regard to reviewing all substances, is an important skill. If it appears that the time allotted for the interview is insufficient, the interviewer should consider scheduling additional visits as needed to obtain a full substance use assessment.

Interviewers should reserve some time (3–5 minutes) at the end of the interview to summarize the patient's history and to provide preliminary feedback about the findings—for example, "Our discussion suggests that you may have a moderate alcohol use disorder. Let me first tell you what that means, and then I'll talk about some options for the next steps" (DiClemente et al. 2017).

Structure of the Assessment

Substance Use History: Focus on Documenting Current Use

The first step in making an accurate substance use assessment is to document current substance use and connect those findings to the chief complaint and current symptoms (Dugosh et al. 2017). DSM-5 lists 10 separate classes of substances, and all of these classes need to be considered and reviewed during a comprehensive assessment. The clinician should inquire about the ingestion route, quantity, frequency, pattern, and setting of use, as well as about self-perceived risks and benefits of use.

The specific substances that the clinician inquires about may be licit or illicit and may include (but are not limited to) tobacco, alcohol, caffeine, marijuana, cocaine, methamphetamine, club drugs, inhalants, hallucinogens, and heroin (Wu et al. 2017). Questions about misuse of prescribed or over-the-counter medications or supplements often can be introduced while the clinician is taking a history of the patient's prescribed medications, including anabolic-androgenic steroids; benzodiazepines, barbiturates, and other sedative-hypnotics; muscle relaxants; and opioid medications. Over-the-counter medications or supplements that may be misused include dextromethorphan, diphenhydramine, chlorpheniramine, caffeine, nicotine replacement therapy, laxatives, and creatine. Newer substances of abuse are continuing to emerge and are frequently available over the counter, with names (e.g., "bath salts" or "spice") that can disguise their true nature as substances of abuse. This list is not exhaustive, and interviewers should not inquire about every single substance in a checklist fashion. The National Institute on Drug Abuse maintains an online database (www.drugabuse.gov/drugs-abuse) that provides current, scientifically accurate information about drugs of abuse.

To maximize the efficiency of the substance use interview, interviewers should continually work to increase their general knowledge about all of the major categories of addictive substances as well as their specialized knowledge about patterns of intoxication and withdrawal and diagnostic criteria for substance use disorders (Komaromy et al. 2016). Keeping this knowledge updated is essential for an accurate and timely substance use interview. One common clinician error is to ask patients about some but not all categories of substances, thereby leaving major omissions in the record. Another error is to make assumptions, such as asking a patient whether he or she uses any illegal drugs while inadvertently including cannabis in that category; in many states, cannabis use is actually legal and accepted as a conventionally used substance (Carliner et al. 2017).

If the patient exhibits obvious signs of intoxication or withdrawal during the course of the interview, scales such as the Clinical Institute Withdrawal Assessment for Alcohol—Revised (Higgins et al. 2019) or the Clinical Opiate Withdrawal Scale can be used to document signs and symptoms and to guide treatment plans (Wesson and Ling 2003). Copies of both of these withdrawal scales are readily available online, as they are not copyrighted.

To assist clinicians in keeping informed on current trends in how substances are used, several no-cost and scientifically credible resources are available. Most notably, the websites of the National Institute on Drug Abuse (DrugFacts: www.drugabuse .gov/publications/finder/t/160/drugfacts), the Substance Abuse and Mental Health Services Administration (SAMHSA) Treatment Improvement Protocols (known as the TIP Series; https://store.samhsa.gov/series/tip-series-treatment-improvement-pro- tocols-tips), the National Institute on Alcohol Abuse and Alcoholism (NIAAA; www .niaaa.nih.gov), and the Centers for Disease Control and Prevention (www.cdc.gov) are regularly updated and provide current information on each substance. In addition, the American Psychiatric Association's website (http://psychiatryonline.com) hosts freely accessible practice guidelines, newsletters, and resource sheets.

Ask About Non-Substance-Related Disorders (Behavioral Addictions)

In addition to inquiring about substances, clinicians should ask about other behaviors that lead to addictive disorders, such as gambling and Internet or video gaming. At this time, gambling disorder is classified in the DSM-5 chapter on substance-related and addictive disorders, and Internet gaming disorder is listed in the "Conditions for Further Study" chapter in DSM-5 Section III (American Psychiatric Association 2013; Fauth-Bleuer et al. 2017). A recommended opening question is "In addition to sub- stances, what are your experiences with gambling, video games, and time spent on the Internet?" (Himelhoch et al. 2015). Validated screening instruments for gambling and gaming are available, and two—the Brief Biosocial Gambling Screen (Brett et al. 2014) and the Internet Gaming Disorder Scale (Lemmens et al. 2015)—can be accessed free of charge online.

Distinguish Substance Use From Substance Use Disorder

One of the primary tasks of the substance use assessment is to distinguish substance use from substance use disorders. To make a diagnosis of substance use disorder in routine clinical practice, a clinical interview is generally used to identify which DSM-5 diagnostic criteria are or are not met. Structured diagnostic instruments (de- veloped to facilitate reliable and valid diagnoses for research) and semistructured tools are lengthy and require training to administer; nonetheless, these instruments can be used in clinical practice when a highly formalized and technical assessment is required (First 2014).

In DSM-5, substance-related disorders are divided into two groups—substance use disorders and substance-induced disorders; older terms such as *substance abuse* and *dependence* should be replaced by the more scientifically accurate *substance use dis- order,* which is defined globally as a maladaptive pattern of substance use leading to clinically significant impairment or distress, as manifested by persistent or recurrent social or interpersonal problems caused by substance use (American Psychiatric As- sociation 2013). A substance use disorder may include physical dependence (defined as brain changes that produce distressing symptoms of tolerance and withdrawal), but such dependence is not required for the diagnosis.

The first step to applying the diagnostic criteria is to inquire about the frequency of substance use as well as the amount of the substance used and the route of admin- istration (e.g., orally ingested, inhaled, insufflated or snorted, intravenously or subcutaneously injected). This information will help the interviewer understand the progression of substance use over time. Route of administration has value in suggesting risks of medical problems (e.g., perforated sinus from intranasal intake or infectious disease from injection) (Strang et al. 1998).

As the interview continues, the patient's answers to general questions about the consequences of substance use will be used to determine how much harm has occurred as a result of his or her substance use. The interview will focus on the concept of continuing use despite harmful consequences and will look for consequences of substance use—such as limitations, loss of functioning, or impairments in any life domains, including academic performance, occupational functioning, general life satisfaction, and interpersonal relationships—as well as medical or legal problems associated with substance use (Whiteford et al. 2015).

Once a substance use disorder diagnosis has been made, a specifier of severity is required. In DSM-5 (American Psychiatric Association 2013), severity is based on the number of diagnostic criteria met by the patient at the time of diagnosis of a substance use disorder: mild (two to three criteria), moderate (four to five criteria), or severe (six or more criteria). For a patient who previously met full criteria but currently meets no criteria (apart from craving) for a substance use disorder, DSM-5 provides two course specifiers: early remission and sustained remission (the DSM-5 work group eliminated the DSM-IV course specifier of partial remission). "In early remission" indicates that a period of at least 3 months but less than 12 months has elapsed since DSM-5 substance use disorder criteria (other than craving) were met, and "in sustained remission" denotes a period of 12 months or longer.

Substance Use Disorder Treatment History

The history of addiction treatment is an important component of the assessment that will help in developing a fuller understanding of how to best help the patient. It is critical that the interviewer closely examine the patient's experience with recovery and treatment and carefully document what has worked and what has not. The history of addiction treatment includes a review of hospital admissions for detoxification, as well as admissions to other controlled living situations (e.g., residential programs, halfway houses, sober houses) to support recovery. Outpatient programs such as partial hospital programs, as well as group, individual, and pharmacological therapies (e.g., disulfiram, naltrexone, buprenorphine-naloxone, methadone, nicotine replacement therapies), also may be a part of the patient's previous treatment. Information on which earlier treatments did or did not help the patient achieve and maintain abstinence can serve as a guide for treatment recommendations (Iqbal et al. 2019).

The interviewer also should ask the patient about involvement in mutual-help groups (e.g., Alcoholics Anonymous, Narcotics Anonymous, Self-Management and Recovery Training, Rational Recovery, Women for Sobriety). In particular, the interviewer should ask not just about attendance but also about whether the patient actively participated and showed commitment in meetings (e.g., setting up chairs, acting as treasurer, making coffee) in order to obtain a full picture. The interviewer should neither support nor discredit the patient's feelings about mutual-help groups but instead should seek to understand the patient's experiences, both to educate the patient about the effectiveness of mutual-help groups and to formulate a realistic treatment plan that will benefit the patient (Zemore et al. 2018).

Psychiatric History

Integrated treatment that addresses co-occurring psychiatric disorders and substance use disorders at the same time improves and enhances outcomes for both disorders (Grant et al. 2016). For this reason, the substance use assessment must include a complete and thorough psychiatric history with a focus on primary psychiatric conditions and substance-related disorders. Studies have shown that co-occurring substance-related and psychiatric disorders can each worsen the prognosis for the other disorder and are often misdiagnosed or not recognized (Lai et al. 2015). Traditionally, identifying psychiatric symptoms as being primary or secondary was considered a priority; however, work in the dual-diagnosis field over the last 20 years has changed this (McKetin et al. 2017). If a patient reports symptoms consistent with a psychiatric disorder, the interviewer should inquire about the temporal relation between substance use and the emergence, exacerbation, or remission of psychiatric symptoms. Reviewing the patient's history of psychiatric symptoms before the onset of substance use, during episodes of intoxication with or withdrawal from substances, and after cessation of substance use can help the interviewer distinguish between substance-induced mental disorders and co-occurring psychiatric and substance-related disorders. Often, this task is very difficult because of recall bias, poor recollection, or a lack of collateral information, and the interviewer is left with no option but to focus on documenting and treating the psychiatric symptoms that are currently leading to distress and loss of functioning (Compton et al. 2000).

Medical History

Conducting a complete medical history, including current and past medical problems, hospitalizations, surgical procedures, and medication allergies, is part of assessing the full effects of substance use. In addition, patients with substance use disorders often have neglected their health and routine medical care and are at risk for a wide variety of co-occurring medical disorders (Khalsa and Haber 2015). For each medical condition reported by the patient, the interviewer should try to determine whether the symptoms are related to or independent of substance use and should inquire about the temporal relation between the development of the medical condition and substance use.

Understanding the relation between the development and exacerbation of the patient's medical disorders and the patient's substance use provides the interviewer with information that may motivate the patient to change addictive behavior. The medical history also provides the information necessary to refer the patient to appropriate medical care, regardless of the origin of the medical disorder.

Family History

Substance use disorders have been shown to carry powerful genetic and familial risk, meaning that every assessment should include inquiry as to the presence or absence of substance use disorders in the patient's family (Hancock et al. 2018). Interviewers can educate patients about genetic vulnerability and family environmental factors associated with substance-related disorders. In addition to asking about genetic family history, providers should ask about family members' response to treatments for addictive disorders. For instance, a positive and therapeutic response to naltrexone on the part of a family member may predict improved outcome with this medication for the patient.

Social History

SAMHSA's principles of recovery focus on the domains of home, health, purpose, and community (Castillo et al. 2018). Using these domains to structure the social history will advance understanding of the true effect of substance use and of how to organize recovery activities and priorities. Questions about the home environment should focus on the stability and safety of the patient's living situation (always considering homelessness as a pivotal risk factor) as well as on what other people are present or absent in the home. A toxic and stressful home life is a major risk factor for ongoing substance use and risky behaviors.

A comprehensive social history will focus not only on assessing the patient's current living situation but also on identifying important people in the patient's current social network. Documenting both harmful and protective relationships is a major part of this assessment component, because that information will naturally lead to a discussion in the treatment plan about how to maintain or build this network and how to remove or reduce contributors to stress (Bradshaw et al. 2016).

Another important area of the social history that will be used in the treatment plan is the types of hobbies, pastimes, and activities the patient currently enjoys or previously engaged in before developing substance use problems. This information will be helpful in devising strategies for strengthening recovery treatment plans. For instance, restoring or redeveloping passions and connections can be crucial to successful recovery.

Importance of Collateral Information

Obtaining additional, objective information from sources other than the patient is a critical and valuable part of the substance use assessment (Petrik et al. 2015). Common sources of collateral information include family members, roommates, friends, employers, and other health care providers. Collateral informants may supply objective data and improve assessment, or they may advocate for a particular outcome and add to bias. Acquiring collateral information during the intake session can be both an enlightening and a difficult and emotional process. Addictive disorders and psychiatric disorders are often best managed with family support and education. However, the nature of substance use disorders also brings out lying, minimizing, and other behaviors that patients do not want their loved ones to know about. One way to manage collection of collateral information in an office-based setting is to ask the patient to allow 15–20 minutes of time toward the end of the interview to invite any family members or significant others who are present into the office for questions and feedback. Speaking with the patient's family or significant others at the first visit also allows the clinician to involve these individuals early in treatment planning and may help in establishing social networks that can potentially support the patient's recovery and help maintain abstinence.

Physical and Mental Status Examination

Physical and mental status examinations of patients are critical portions of the substance use assessment because of the high frequency of overlapping conditions between medical and psychiatric disorders found in this population. Substance use can disrupt the structure and functioning of virtually every organ system in the body, both acutely and chronically (Khalsa and Haber 2015). Findings from the mental status examination will vary considerably from case to case, which means that interviewers should complete each section of the mental status examination, including the cognitive and memory testing portion.

Laboratory Tests

When available, laboratory testing will provide additional information to consider in a substance use assessment. Examples of useful laboratory data include urine toxicology, blood alcohol levels, and measures of substance metabolites or the biological effects of substance use (e.g., abnormal liver function, mean corpuscular volume of erythrocytes [Volkow et al. 2015]). Routine urine drug screens typically are not part of outpatient office assessments, but the availability of office saliva testing makes that a viable option. Biological markers of alcohol use include phosphatidylethanol and ethyl glucuronide (covered in other chapters; see Chapter 9, "Treatment of Alcohol-Related Disorders," and Chapter 50, "Testing for Substances of Abuse"); however, biomarker testing is generally not used during the first visit (Bean et al. 2017). Currently, the use of neuroimaging tests such as magnetic resonance imaging (MRI), computed tomography (CT) scans, and positron emission tomography (PET) scans is not considered useful in the substance use assessment, unless such tests are used to rule out a neurological process that could potentially shed light on the patient's substance use (e.g., a brain tumor leading to disinhibited behavior) (Kwako et al. 2016).

Potential Adverse Events Related to the Substance Use Assessment

Of the potential adverse outcomes related to substance use assessment, failure to conduct a thorough assessment is likely the most serious. Missing the diagnosis and not putting together the clues indicating that a substance use disorder is present (i.e., a false-negative result) would lead to ongoing suffering, distress, and a high likelihood of misinterpretation of symptoms and exposure to unnecessary treatments (Zimmerman and Mattia 1999). Conversely, identifying a patient as having a substance use disorder when one is not present (i.e., a false-positive result) could result in unnecessary treatment for addiction and undertreatment of any psychiatric conditions that are present (Avery and Barnhill 2017).

Patients can become irritated or agitated during a substance use assessment, but this response is more likely to be related to the interviewer or the interview setting itself than to the nature and content of the questions. Clinicians who are not addiction specialists may be concerned about triggering urges or cravings to use simply by asking questions about substances. Much like the false notion that discussing suicide with patients will trigger suicidal ideation, discussion of substances and the manner and environment in which they are used is not likely to generate acute motivation or desire or to awaken uncontrolled urges to seek substances (DeCou and Schumann 2018).

Finally, substance use assessments can take time, especially with patients who have long histories of psychiatric conditions, substance use disorder treatment, and multiple medical conditions. Spending too much time on the substance use assessment may result in poorer outcomes by limiting the time available to address other issues of importance to the patient or of relevance to diagnosis and treatment planning. Clinicians are encouraged to think of substance use assessment as a process that begins at intake and continually evolves at each patient encounter.

Strategies to Improve Clinical Skills in Conducting a Substance Use Assessment

Despite the high prevalence of substance use disorders among patient populations in nearly every clinical setting in health care, many providers have not received specialty training in addiction psychiatry (Ruiz and Strain 2011). Providers with any background or level of experience can use the following practical tips to increase their clinical knowledge and skills related to conducting a more efficient and thorough substance use assessment:

- Attend the annual meeting of an addiction organization (e.g., American Academy of Addiction Psychiatry).
- Regularly review and refer to online addiction resources from SAMHSA, the National Institute on Drug Abuse, NIAAA, the American Academy of Addiction Psychiatry, and the American Psychiatric Association. Many of these organizations offer no-cost guides to screening, assessment, and enhancing clinical assessment skills. Examples of evidence-based guides for assessment include SAMHSA's TIP Series and NIAAA's *Helping Patients Who Drink Too Much: A Clinician's Guide* (Willenbring et al. 2009).
- Access the Provider's Clinical Support System (http://pcssnow.org). This online mentoring program offers a national network of trained clinicians with expertise in addiction medicine and pain management aimed at improving primary care providers' confidence and skills in preventing, identifying, and treating substance use disorders and chronic pain by using evidence-based practices.
- Visit local substance use disorder treatment programs to learn about available treatment options, effective treatment practices, and current trends in substance use.

Conclusion

A thorough substance use assessment includes a detailed inventory of the type, amount, frequency, and consequences of a patient's substance use; an evaluation of the patient's perceptions about the substance use and readiness to change; an assessment of co-occurring psychiatric disorders; a medical history, physical examination, and laboratory tests; a family history; and a review of social factors that may contribute to substance use or facilitate treatment. A careful and accurate assessment of the patient will provide the necessary information that will lead to the creation of an appropriate treatment plan.

References

Alkureishi MA, Lee WW, Lyons M, et al: Impact of electronic medical record use on the patient–doctor relationship and communication: a systematic review. J Gen Intern Med 31(5):548–560, 2016 26786877

American Psychiatric Association: Diagnostic and Statistical Manual of Mental Disorders, 5th Edition. Arlington, VA, American Psychiatric Association, 2013

American Psychiatric Association: The American Psychiatric Association Practice Guidelines for the Psychiatric Evaluation of Adults. Arlington, VA, American Psychiatric Association Publishing, 2016

Avery JD, Barnhill JW (eds): Co-Occurring Mental Illness and Substance Use Disorders: A Guide to Diagnosis and Treatment. Arlington, VA, American Psychiatric Association Publishing, 2017

Bean P, Brown G, Hallinan P, et al: Improved recovery of repeat intoxicated drivers using fingernails and blood spots to monitor alcohol and other substance abuse. Traffic Inj Prev 18(1):9–18, 2017 27285956

Bradshaw SD, Shumway ST, Wang EW, et al: Family functioning and readiness in family recovery from addiction. Journal of Groups in Addiction & Recovery 11(1):21–41, 2016. Available at: https://www.tandfonline.com/doi/full/10.1080/1556035X.2015.1104644. Accessed February 6, 2020.

Brett EI, Weinstock J, Burton S, et al: Do the DSM-5 diagnostic revisions affect the psychometric properties of the Brief Biosocial Gambling Screen? International Gambling Studies 14(3):447–456, 2014. Available at: https://www.tandfonline.com/doi/full/10.1080/14459795.2014.931449. Accessed February 6, 2020.

Carliner H, Brown QL, Sarvet AL, et al: Cannabis use, attitudes, and legal status in the U.S.: a review. Prev Med 104:13–23, 2017 28705601

Castillo EG, Chung B, Bromley E, et al: Community, public policy, and recovery from mental illness: emerging research and initiatives. Harv Rev Psychiatry 26(2):70–81, 2018 29381527

Compton WM 3rd, Cottler LB, Phelps DL, et al: Psychiatric disorders among drug dependent subjects: are they primary or secondary? Am J Addict 9(2):126–134, 2000 10934574

DeCou CR, Schumann ME: On the iatrogenic risk of assessing suicidality: a meta-analysis. Suicide Life Threat Behav 48(5):531–543, 2018 28678380

DiClemente CC, Corno CM, Graydon MM, et al: Motivational interviewing, enhancement, and brief interventions over the last decade: a review of reviews of efficacy and effectiveness. Psychol Addict Behav 31(8):862–887, 2017 29199843

Dugosh KL, Cacciola J, Saxon AJ: Clinical assessment of substance use disorders. UpToDate, April 18, 2017. Available at: https://www.uptodate.com/contents/clinical-assessment-of-substance-use-disorders. Accessed November 14, 2019.

Fauth-Bühler M, Mann K, Potenza MN: Pathological gambling: a review of the neurobiological evidence relevant for its classification as an addictive disorder. Addict Biol 22(4):885–897, 2017 26935000

First MB: Structured Clinical Interview for the DSM (SCID), in The Encyclopedia of Clinical Psychology. Edited by Cautin RL, Lilienfeld SO. New York, Wiley, 2014

Grant BF, Saha TD, Ruan WJ, et al: Epidemiology of DSM-5 drug use disorder: results from the National Epidemiologic Survey on Alcohol and Related Conditions-III. JAMA Psychiatry 73(1):39–47, 2016 26580136

Hancock DB, Markunas CA, Bierut LJ, et al: Human genetics of addiction: new insights and future directions. Curr Psychiatry Rep 20(2):8, 2018 29504045

Higgins J, Bugajski AA, Church D, et al: A psychometric analysis of CIWA-Ar in acutely ill and injured hospitalized patients. J Trauma Nurs 26(1):41–49, 2019 30624381

Himelhoch SS, Miles-McLean H, Medoff DR, et al: Evaluation of brief screens for gambling disorder in the substance use treatment setting. Am J Addict 24(5):460–466, 2015 25963048

Hollis C, Morriss R, Martin J, et al: Technological innovations in mental healthcare: harnessing the digital revolution. Br J Psychiatry 206(4):263–265, 2015 25833865

Iqbal MN, Levin CJ, Levin FR: Treatment for substance use disorder with co-occurring mental illness. FOCUS (Am Psychiatr Publ)17(2):88–97, 2019 31975963

Jansson L, Nordgaard J: The psychiatric interview: methodological and practical aspects, in The Psychiatric Interview for Differential Diagnosis. Cham, Switzerland, Springer, 2016, pp 27–51

Khalsa JH, Haber PS: Medical disorders and complications of alcohol and other drugs, pain, and addiction: an introduction, in Textbook of Addiction Treatment: International Perspectives. Edited by el-Guebaly N, Carrà G, Galanter M. New York, Springer, 2015, pp 1573–1576

Komaromy M, Duhigg D, Metcalf A, et al: Project ECHO (Extension for Community Healthcare Outcomes): a new model for educating primary care providers about treatment of substance use disorders. Subst Abus 37(1):20–24, 2016 26848803

Kwako LE, Momenan R, Litten RZ, et al: Addictions neuroclinical assessment: a neuroscience-based framework for addictive disorders. Biol Psychiatry 80(3):179–189, 2016 26772405

Lai HMX, Cleary M, Sitharthan T, et al: Prevalence of comorbid substance use, anxiety and mood disorders in epidemiological surveys, 1990–2014: a systematic review and meta-analysis. Drug Alcohol Depend 154:1–13, 2015 26072219

Lemmens JS, Valkenburg PM, Gentile DA: The Internet Gaming Disorder Scale. Psychol Assess 27(2):567–582, 2015 25558970

Levy SJ, Williams JF; Committee on Substance Use and Prevention: Substance use screening, brief intervention, and referral to treatment. Pediatrics 138(1):e20161211, 2016 27325634

McCarty D, Rieckmann T, Baker RL, et al: The perceived impact of 42 CFR Part 2 on coordination and integration of care: a qualitative analysis. Psychiatr Serv 68(3):245–249, 2017 27799017

McKetin R, Baker AL, Dawe S, et al: Differences in the symptom profile of methamphetamine-related psychosis and primary psychotic disorders. Psychiatry Res 251:349–354, 2017 28282630

Papadakos PJ: The rise of electronic distraction in health care: is addiction to devices contributing? Journal of Anesthesia & Clinical Research 4(3):e112, 2013. Available at: https://www.omicsonline.org/the-rise-of-electronic-distraction-in-health-care-is-addiction-to-devices-contributing-2155-6148.1000e112.php?aid=11833. Accessed February 6, 2020.

Petrik ML, Billera M, Kaplan Y, et al: Balancing patient care and confidentiality: considerations in obtaining collateral information. J Psychiatr Pract 21(3):220–224, 2015 25955265

Pickard H: Denial in addiction. Mind and Language 31(3):277–299, 2016. Available at: https://onlinelibrary.wiley.com/doi/abs/10.1111/mila.12106. Accessed February 7, 2020.

Rahim M, Patton R: The association between shame and substance use in young people: a systematic review. PeerJ 3:e737, 2015 25649509

Rieckmann TR, Abraham AJ, Bride BE: Implementation of motivational interviewing in substance use disorder treatment: research network participation and organizational compatibility. J Addict Med 10(6):402–407, 2016 27559847

Ruiz P, Strain EC (eds): Substance Abuse: A Comprehensive Textbook, 5th Edition. Philadelphia, PA, Lippincott Williams & Wilkins, 2011, pp 847–870

Schaper E, Padwa H, Urada D, et al: Substance use disorder patient privacy and comprehensive care in integrated health care settings. Psychol Serv 13(1):105–109, 2016 26845493

Simpson SA: A survey of clinical approaches to suicide risk assessment for patients intoxicated on alcohol. Psychosomatics 60(2):197–203, 2019 30093244

Strang J, Bearn J, Farrell M, et al: Route of drug use and its implications for drug effect, risk of dependence and health consequences. Drug Alcohol Rev 17(2):197–211, 1998 16203485

Strickler GK, Zhang K, Halpin JF, et al: Effects of mandatory prescription drug monitoring program (PDMP) use laws on prescriber registration and use and on risky prescribing. Drug Alcohol Depend 199:1–9, 2019 30954863

Vendetti J, Gmyrek A, Damon D, et al: Screening, brief intervention and referral to treatment (SBIRT): implementation barriers, facilitators and model migration. Addiction 112 (suppl 2):23–33, 2017 28074571

Volkow ND, Koob G, Baler R: Biomarkers in substance use disorders. ACS Chem Neurosci 6(4):522–525, 2015 25734247

Wesson DR, Ling W: The Clinical Opiate Withdrawal Scale (COWS). J Psychoactive Drugs 35(2):253–259, 2003 12924748

Whiteford HA, Ferrari AJ, Degenhardt L, et al: The global burden of mental, neurological and substance use disorders: an analysis from the Global Burden of Disease Study 2010. PLoS One 10(2):e0116820, 2015 25658103

Willenbring ML, Massey SH, Gardner MB: Helping patients who drink too much: an evidence-based guide for primary care clinicians. Am Fam Physician 80(1):44–50, 2009 19621845

Wright A, McCoy AB, Hickman TTT, et al: Problem list completeness in electronic health records: a multi-site study and assessment of success factors. Int J Med Inform 84(10):784–790, 2015 26228650

Wu LT, McNeely J, Subramaniam GA, et al: DSM-5 substance use disorders among adult primary care patients: results from a multisite study. Drug Alcohol Depend 179:42–46, 2017 28753480

Zemore SE, Lui C, Mericle A, et al: A longitudinal study of the comparative efficacy of Women for Sobriety, LifeRing, SMART Recovery, and 12-step groups for those with AUD. J Subst Abuse Treat 88:18–26, 2018 29606223

Zimmerman M, Mattia JI: Psychiatric diagnosis in clinical practice: is comorbidity being missed? Compr Psychiatry 40(3):182–191, 1999 10360612

Zorland JL, Gilmore D, Johnson JA, et al: Effects of substance use screening and brief intervention on health-related quality of life. Qual Life Res 27(9):2329–2336, 2018 29869747

CHAPTER 6

Screening and Brief Intervention

Richard Saitz, M.D., M.P.H., FACP, DFASAM

It has been more than 50 years since the first randomized trial found that a brief counseling intervention for patients with alcohol use disorder might lead to better outcomes. Screening and brief intervention (SBI) is now a well-established clinical practice supported by evidence from controlled clinical trials. However, in the same way that substance use disorders and their treatments represent a wide variety of conditions and effective management strategies, SBI also encompasses a wide variety of screening and intervention strategies with varying efficacy and degrees of supporting evidence. In this chapter I cover SBI for alcohol and other drugs, but not the specifics of SBI for tobacco. SBI simultaneously represents 1) a preventive intervention aimed at recurring behavioral risks and 2) an initial step in the management of moderate to severe substance use disorders. The best evidence supports the former aim—decreasing risk for people who use substances associated with future health harms but who have mild or no symptoms of a substance use disorder. Little evidence supports the latter aim. In addition, scant evidence supports the efficacy of SBI for substances other than alcohol. A systematic review of clinical trials (Glass et al. 2015) found no evidence to support the efficacy of referral to treatment as part of SBI; thus, the moniker "SBIRT" (SBI plus referral to treatment), mainly used by government programs, is a misnomer and is not used in this chapter.

Although screening can have goals other than reduction in substance use, clinicians need to be aware of substance use when diagnosing or managing health conditions and when prescribing any medications. The form of SBI with demonstrated efficacy—screening for risky alcohol use or a mild alcohol use disorder and conducting a brief intervention with those who screen positive—is among the most cost-effective preventive health services in existence and is recommended widely by professional organizations and quality assurance bodies. Nevertheless, SBI is also among the least implemented known-to-be-effective services in clinical practice.

SBI is a clinical preventive service and therefore is not geared primarily toward individuals with symptoms. Instead, it is intended to be implemented in settings in which the main purpose of the health care visit is not attention to substance use. SBI has been studied in hospitals, emergency departments, and primary care medical settings (as well as certain other locations, such as schools and pharmacies). In settings in which patients are seeking help or treatment for substance use and substance use disorders, or in which patients have symptoms or diagnoses for which substance use disorders rank high on the differential diagnosis, use of SBI alone makes no sense; in such settings (e.g., addiction treatment programs, psychiatric outpatient practices or hospitals), patients should have full expert assessments for substance use disorders. Some of the tools of SBI may be used as part of such expert assessments and subsequent management, but the concept of SBI simply does not apply.

Screening

Purpose of Screening

While this textbook is largely focused on addictive (i.e., substance use) disorders and their treatment, the target of screening is any unhealthy substance use (Saitz 2005). Unhealthy substance use is defined as any use of alcohol or other drugs that increases the risk for or has been related to health consequences. Thus, it includes use of any illicit drugs or misuse of prescription or nonprescription drugs known to cause risk or harm, and amounts of alcohol known to increase the risk for health consequences. Unhealthy use also includes use with consequences that do not yet meet criteria for a disorder, as well as use leading to a substance use disorder. Screening is aimed at detecting the entire spectrum of unhealthy use, from risky use to use with problems to a diagnosable disorder. Part of the rationale for this detection is not only to address the needs of people who are suffering from a chronic illness (e.g., severe substance use disorder) but also to identify and intervene with people who are at risk by either reducing their risk of consequences or preventing progression to a disorder (although the latter has never been a proven effect of SBI). The other reason to identify and intervene in unhealthy use is that the majority of health consequences on a population level do not accrue to those with severe substance use disorders, but instead occur in people who are simply drinking too much, with no severe disorder (Spurling and Vinson 2005). What constitutes an unhealthy amount of alcohol is determined by expert consensus, taking into consideration both individual and public health implications, and is based on conclusions drawn from numerous epidemiological studies. The National Institute on Alcohol Abuse and Alcoholism (NIAAA) defines "risky" amounts as more than 14 standard drinks per week on average or more than 4 drinks per day for men under age 65 years, and more than 7 drinks per week or 3 per day for women and for men age 65 years or older (National Institute on Alcohol Abuse and Alcoholism 2007). A standard drink is 12–14 grams of ethanol, which is the amount found in 12 ounces of regular-strength beer, 5 ounces of nonfortified wine, or 1.5 ounces of 80-proof liquors. Of note, because alcohol is an addictive carcinogen, any amount of exposure can be associated with serious health consequences, and low amounts have been associated with the development of cancers. Furthermore, recent high-quality methodological studies have raised serious questions regarding whether there are any health benefits of alcohol (for a review, see Stockwell et al. 2016). For other drugs, any use is generally thought to be unhealthy (e.g., a single use of cocaine can lead to dysrhythmia and sudden death, or if contaminated with fentanyl, death from overdose), although researchers are studying what levels of cannabis use substantially increase the risk for health consequences (e.g., cognitive limitations, psychosis, addiction). Screening does not simply mean "testing"; rather, screening is a clinical activity performed for patients without known symptoms of the target condition.

Screening Tools

Many screening tools have been validated for their accuracy. The key issues for selecting a tool for practice are brevity, wide applicability to populations, and validity for detecting the full spectrum of unhealthy use. The CAGE questions (Mayfield et al. 1974) and the Michigan Alcoholism Screening Test (MAST; Selzer 1971; Selzer et al. 1975) were among the first screening tools developed. (The acronym CAGE stands for four questions: Have you ever felt you should **C**ut down on your drinking? Have people **A**nnoyed you by criticizing your drinking? Have you ever felt bad or **G**uilty about your drinking? Have you ever taken a drink first thing in the morning [**E**ye-opener] to steady your nerves or to get rid of a hangover?) However, these tools are no longer recommended for screening because although they can identify alcohol use disorder, they are not sufficiently accurate for identifying the spectrum of unhealthy use, and the MAST is also too long. Laboratory testing (e.g., urine drug screening, carbohydrate-deficient transferrin) is also not recommended for screening; although such testing can identify use, it is insufficiently sensitive for identifying unhealthy use (particularly if use has been neither heavy nor very recent). However, a combination of screening and testing (e.g., CAGE, laboratory testing) might be useful for assessment or monitoring.

Single-item screening questions (SSQs) can be administered quickly and easily and have been validated in primary medical care settings. A single-question alcohol screening test is 82% sensitive and 79% specific for unhealthy alcohol use (Smith et al. 2009), and an SSQ about illicit drug use or nonmedical use of prescription drugs is 93% sensitive and 94% specific for any drug use (Smith et al. 2010). SSQs for alcohol use and drug use recommended by the NIAAA (National Institute on Alcohol Abuse and Alcoholism 2007) and the National Institute on Drug Abuse (2019), respectively, are presented in Table 6–1.

SSQs with different wording have been studied in emergency and primary care settings and have been found to be similarly accurate. Longer screening tools have two disadvantages: 1) they cannot be memorized and used as easily in medical interviews in busy settings, and 2) they are more difficult to score. Some longer screens (e.g., the Drug Abuse Screening Test [DAST; Skinner 1982]) have not been as extensively validated as SSQs in general health care settings. Nevertheless, if longer screening tools can be implemented (e.g., by patient self-administration, through administration by health care workers dedicated to the task, or by inclusion in an electronic

TABLE 6–1.	Recommended single-item screening questions for alcohol and drug use	
	Alcohol use	**Drug use**
Question	"How many times in the past year have you had five (four for women) or more drinks in a day?" **Note:** This question is often asked after first asking the question "Do you sometimes drink beer, wine, or other alcoholic beverages?"	"How many times in the past year have you used an illegal drug or used a prescription medication for nonmedical reasons?" **Note:** If asked by the patient to clarify the meaning of "nonmedical reasons," the interviewer can say, "For instance, you used it because of the experience or feeling it caused."
Scoring	A response greater than zero is considered a positive test result for unhealthy alcohol use.	A response greater than zero is considered a positive test result for unhealthy drug use.
Source	National Institute on Alcohol Abuse and Alcoholism 2007	National Institute on Drug Abuse 2019

medical record to prompt the clinician), they can provide more information about the severity of the risk identified, which is information required for an appropriate brief counseling intervention. Tools validated as part of controlled trials of SBI (e.g., the Alcohol Use Disorders Identification Test [AUDIT; Babor et al. 2001]) are therefore ideal.

The Alcohol Use Disorders Identification Test—Consumption (AUDIT-C) (Bradley et al. 2007) is a short screening version of the AUDIT with three alcohol consumption items (Table 6–2).

The AUDIT-C has been well validated. Its sensitivity is 73% and 86% for men and women, respectively (similar to that of the SSQ), and its specificity is 89% and 91%, respectively. A score of 7–10 or greater (maximum is 12) suggests a moderate to severe alcohol use disorder (Bradley et al. 2007; Rubinsky et al. 2010). The full 10-item AUDIT has been validated in many countries (Babor et al. 2001) and is available from the World Health Organization (www.who.int/substance_abuse/publications/alcohol/en/). The scoring range is 0 to 40. In primary care settings, a score of 4–7 (which is lower than the often-discussed cutoff of 8) provides optimal sensitivity and still reasonable specificity for unhealthy use (Bradley et al. 2007). A score of 20 or greater suggests a moderate to severe alcohol use disorder.

The Alcohol, Smoking, and Substance Involvement Screening Test (ASSIST) can have upwards of six dozen items, depending on how many substances the patient reports using (Humeniuk et al. 2008, 2010). It does not identify risky alcohol use amounts directly. Unless the ASSIST is administered with computerized skip patterns, it is unwieldy for screening. On the other hand, it provides risk-level information that is useful for brief intervention. For drugs other than tobacco and alcohol, a substance-specific ASSIST score of 4 or greater is considered risky. A score lower than 4 but greater than 0 means recent or past use (lower risk). A score of 27 or greater sug-

TABLE 6–2.	Alcohol Use Disorders Identification Test—Consumption questions (AUDIT-C)
AUDIT-C item	**Response (points)**
How often do you have a drink containing alcohol?	Never (0) Monthly or less (1) Two to four times a month (2) Two to three times a week (3) Four or more times a week (4)
How many drinks containing alcohol do you have on a typical day when you are drinking?	None, I do not drink (0) 1 or 2 (0) 3 or 4 (1) 5 or 6 (2) 7 to 9 (3) 10 or more (4)
How often do you have six (four for women)[a] or more drinks on one occasion?	Never (0) Less than monthly (1) Monthly (2) Weekly (3) Daily or almost daily (4)

Scoring: The total score is the sum of the scores from all items; 4 or more for men, and 3 or more for women, is considered a positive screening test for unhealthy alcohol use.
[a]Drink numbers should be altered to five for men and four for women when AUDIT-C is used in the United States, due to varying international drink sizes.

Source. Bradley et al. 2007. The AUDIT-C is available for use in the public domain.

gests a moderate to severe substance use disorder. An online version of the ASSIST modified for drugs is available free of charge (www.drugabuse.gov/nmassist/).

The 10-item version of the DAST is a longer option for screening for drugs that may provide additional information useful for discussion during a brief intervention (Yudko et al. 2007). A score of 3 or greater is considered positive. This version of the DAST is much less well validated for screening in primary care settings than the AUDIT for alcohol, and the results do not provide information on which drug might be a concern. Like the AUDIT, CAGE, MAST, and ASSIST, the 10-item version of the DAST may be useful as a tool to assess severity in people with a positive screening test.

Using different tools for different populations can be considered, but in general, any small advantages of this practice are outweighed by the added complexity that arises when trying to implement multiple tools. However, there are two specific populations—1) adolescents and 2) pregnant women or women aiming to conceive—for whom use of tailored screening tools is helpful, because for these patients, *any* use is unhealthy. For reasons similar to those discussed earlier regarding the CAGE and MAST, the CAGE and the CRAFFT (a brief questionnaire for youths [discussed in the following section, "Assessment"]) are not recommended as the sole tools for screening these two populations because the screening tools were validated to detect disorders, not unhealthy use.

The NIAAA has recommended use of the following two questions for adolescents (ages 14–18 years) (National Institute on Alcohol Abuse and Alcoholism 2011):

1. "In the past year, on how many days have you had more than a few sips of beer, wine, or any drink containing alcohol?" (Any number of days is a positive test.)
2. "If your friends drink, how many drinks do they usually drink on an occasion?" (More than three drinks for boys or more than two for girls is a positive test indicating the need for further assessment and brief counseling.)

Use of a screening test consisting of a single item only has not been validated for detecting unhealthy alcohol use among pregnant women. Nonetheless, in order to identify any alcohol use, all women who are pregnant or who are trying to conceive should be asked "Do you sometimes drink beer, wine, or other alcoholic beverages?" (or a similar question). The AUDIT-C (validated in women and in pregnancy) can be used. Many other brief screening tests have been validated in pregnancy (Burns et al. 2010). One of these, the T-ACE (Sokol et al. 1989), includes the C, A, and E questions from the CAGE (see list in first paragraph of this section) plus a question about tolerance: "How many drinks does it take to make you feel high?" (>2 drinks is a positive test for this question in the general population). For pregnant women, any positive response to any T-ACE question is a positive test. The rationale for using the T-ACE or similar questionnaires validated in pregnancy is that they do not ask directly about usual drinking amounts, questions that pregnant women may not answer directly because they may feel guilty. Another option, the 4Ps Plus (Chasnoff et al. 2007), has been validated for screening for alcohol and drug use in pregnancy. The instrument consists of five questions:

1. Did either of your parents ever have a problem with alcohol or drugs?
2. Does your partner have a problem with alcohol or drugs?
3. Have you ever drunk beer, wine, or liquor?
4. In the month before you knew you were pregnant, how many cigarettes did you smoke?
5. In the month before you knew you were pregnant, how many beers/how much wine/how much liquor did you drink?

Again, any use reported on the 4Ps Plus by a pregnant woman is considered positive (although many women who report substance use may not have engaged in such use during pregnancy).

Assessment

When a patient screens positive, the following three areas should be assessed before brief counseling interventions are started: 1) drinking amounts, drug used, and frequency; 2) substance use consequences, including substance use disorders; and 3) the patient's perception of his or her use and readiness to change. The reason for these brief assessments is to determine how to counsel the patient most effectively. Of note, although some of these recommended assessments have been validated, most have not, particularly not in the context of SBI. Assessments, as an extension of screening, can also be considered part of the intervention when done in the context of a therapeutic relationship. Reviewing use, consequences, and readiness to change can be the beginning of change.

Assessment of Use

To assess the quantity and frequency of alcohol use, the clinician can ask three questions:

1. On average, how many days per week do you drink alcohol?
2. On a typical day when you drink, how many drinks do you have?
3. What is the maximum number of drinks you had on any given occasion during the last month?

For drug use, the first item for each drug from the ASSIST could be asked, or the patient could simply be asked what drugs he or she uses, how many days in the past month the patient used those drugs or any drugs, and how many times per day (an approach taken from the Addiction Severity Index [ASI; McLellan et al. 1992], which is often used in treatment settings).

Assessment of Consequences

Although relatively brief validated tools are available to assess drug- and alcohol-related problems (e.g., the Short Inventory of Problems [SIP; Allensworth-Davies et al. 2012]), these instruments may not be as widely used as other ways of assessing consequences, either because they do not provide an indication (e.g., a specific cutoff value) of whether the disorder is moderate or severe or because they require (like the AUDIT) specific questions and response options to be available at the point of care. Clinicians may use AUDIT or AUDIT-C results from screening or may administer the ASSIST or CAGE as a brief structured assessment (using a cutoff score of ≥2 affirmative responses to the CAGE or the CAGE Adapted to Include Drugs [CAGE-AID]) items to indicate a higher likelihood of a disorder (Brown and Rounds 1995).

The CAGE-AID adds "or drug use" to items 1 through 3 and "or used drugs" to item 4, as follows:

1. Have you ever felt that you ought to **C**ut down on your drinking or drug use?
2. Have people **A**nnoyed you by criticizing your drinking or drug use?
3. Have you ever felt bad or **G**uilty about your drinking or drug use?
4. Have you ever had a drink or used drugs first thing in the morning (**E**ye-opener) to steady your nerves, e.g., get rid of a hangover, or get the day started?

Another alternative is a clinical interview (and physical examination) to identify medical, psychiatric, social, and legal consequences of use (details of which are beyond the scope of this chapter). In addition, a checklist of symptoms of substance use disorders from the fourth edition (DSM-IV) of the *Diagnostic and Statistical Manual of Mental Disorders* (American Psychiatric Association 1994), as suggested by the NIAAA publication "Helping Patients Who Drink Too Much: A Clinician's Guide" (National Institute on Alcohol Abuse and Alcoholism 2007), can help clinicians determine the presence or absence of a disorder using tools easily available online (such as at the NIAAA website http://rethinkingdrinking.niaaa.nih.gov/WhatsTheHarm/WhatAreSymptomsOfAnAlcoholUseDisorder.asp). Such checklists should be updated to capture the DSM-5 criteria (American Psychiatric Association 2013). For alcohol, Vinson et al. (2007) validated an assessment with two items (with a sensitivity of 77%–95% and a specificity of 62%–86% if either is positive):

1. In the past year, have you sometimes been under the influence of alcohol in situations where you could have caused an accident or gotten hurt?
2. Have there often been times when you had a lot more to drink than you intended to have?

For adolescents, the CRAFFT (which stands for **C**ar, **R**elax, **A**lone, **F**orget, **F**riends, and **T**rouble) can be used as a brief assessment to indicate the possible presence of a substance use disorder (Massachusetts Department of Public Health Bureau of Substance Abuse Services 2009):

- Have you ever ridden in a **C**AR driven by someone (including yourself) who was "high" or had been using alcohol or drugs?
- Do you ever use alcohol or drugs to **R**ELAX, feel better about yourself, or fit in?
- Do you ever use alcohol or drugs while you are by yourself, or **A**LONE?
- Do you ever **F**ORGET things you did while using alcohol or drugs?
- Do your family or **F**RIENDS ever tell you that you should cut down on your drinking or drug use?
- Have you ever gotten into **T**ROUBLE while you were using alcohol or drugs?

Two or more "yes" answers indicate a higher likelihood of a disorder. The reason for the focus on "disorder" is that many studies of treatments (e.g., pharmacotherapies, evidence-based psychosocial therapies, residential and intensive outpatient care) focus on and differentiate substance dependence as defined in DSM-IV (or earlier DSM editions) from substance use with less severe or fewer symptoms. Although DSM-IV substance dependence does not map directly or exactly onto DSM-5 moderate to severe substance use disorder, the two diagnoses are addressed in a similar manner clinically.

Assessment of the Patient's Perception and Readiness to Change

The simplest way to understand the patient's perception about his or her substance use is to ask something like "What do you think about your alcohol use?" or "Has your drug use caused you any trouble?" Readiness to change lies on a continuum and can be assessed by using simple visual analogue scale–type questions, such as "On a scale from 0 to 10, where 0 is not at all and 10 is the most, how ready are you to change your drinking?" Similarly, one can ask about the importance of changing and the patient's confidence in his or her ability to change should he or she decide to do so. An interviewer can also determine a patient's stage of change: precontemplation (patient is not considering making a change), contemplation (patient is thinking about change), determination (patient has decided to change), action (patient is making a change), maintenance (patient has made a change), or relapse (patient has returned to unhealthy use).

Brief Counseling Interventions

Performing a Brief Intervention

A brief intervention involves counseling to help the patient to abstain from or reduce substance use, or to reduce the risk of such use. Brief interventions consist of feedback, advice, and goal setting. The counseling is done based on the principles of motivational interviewing. The goal of a brief intervention depends on the level of severity of substance use and the patient's perception of the problem and readiness to change. In general, the best goal for individuals with moderate to severe substance use disorders is abstinence (and also initiation of or referral for treatment of the disorder); for others, the goal can be either abstinence or reduced use or reduced risks when using. Of note, most patients with a moderate to severe disorder identified by screening are not ready for treatment or referral, so these options should not be the only ones presented such patients. Another reason for not focusing on referral is that it lacks efficacy. Such options, however, should be included as "best medical advice" and also because patients with more severe disorders are more likely to recognize consequences during brief counseling that might motivate change. Furthermore, treatment can often be done in a primary care setting, an option that should be included in the discussion since it is often more acceptable to patients. To help individuals who are interested in obtaining specialty addiction treatment, the NIAAA provides directories of evidence-based treatment resources useful to patients and clinicians (https://alcoholtreatment.niaaa.nih.gov/), and the National Institute on Drug Abuse outlines principles of science-based treatment (www.drugabuse.gov/publications/principles-drug-addiction-treatment-research-based-guide-third-edition/principles-effective-treatment).

Abstinence is the best goal for youths, women who are pregnant or trying to conceive, people who are taking medications that interact with alcohol or who have medical conditions that are harmed by drinking, people who have tried and failed to cut down or quit, and people who are taking other drugs besides alcohol. Abstinence may also be best for individuals with a significant family history of addiction or for those with recurrent consequences of use. The goal for a brief intervention also depends on the patient's readiness to change. Goals can be wide ranging—for example, avoiding risky situations such as driving after drinking, or using a substance less frequently.

A brief intervention can be delivered as a single stand-alone session lasting from 5 to 45 minutes, or it might involve up to four sessions. Brief interventions include clinician feedback about the patient's risks and consequences of substance use (identified from the screening and assessment), specific advice (after asking permission to give it), and goal setting (which should consider a range or menu of options). A brief intervention can also include provision of information. The clinician has two initial concerns: 1) establishing a trusting and preferably ongoing relationship that includes follow-up and 2) determining how the brief intervention should be provided. The clinician should express concern about the patient's use and should use open-ended questions to find out what the patient thinks of the feedback or information given. In addition, patients should be reminded that only they can change and have responsibility for it. After giving advice, the clinician should ask what the patient thinks and assess what the patient's goals are and what the patient thinks might work to achieve them. A good way to do this is to, with permission, say something like "This is my best medical advice for most people in your situation, but I don't know how it will work for you or what you think of it. What do you think?" Telling patients to quit and how to do it is not likely to be effective. If the patient's goal is to abstain, and the patient has a plan, he or she is more likely to pursue that goal and achieve it. If the patient is unclear on a goal or plan, the clinician can provide options and alternatives— ways that others have succeeded in the past. In the end, the plan should arise from a balancing of patient desires, best medical advice, and readiness to change, with the idea that the plan can be reevaluated and changed in follow-up. Effective brief interventions require that the clinician use an empathic—as opposed to a directly confrontational—counseling style. When there is resistance or disagreement, it is best to agree to disagree or change the subject. Some patients will feel guilty about their substance use or feel that they cannot change their behavior. For them, reinforcement of self-efficacy (their confidence or belief that they can change) is important. The clinician can simply state his or her belief that the patient has the capacity to change, or remind the patient of other successes with substance use changes in the past or with other health behaviors. Reflective listening is a key skill of motivational interviewing that is helpful in brief behavior change counseling. Reflective listening involves repeating or paraphrasing what the patient has said (in the form of a statement, not a question). For example, if the patient says, "I missed my son's soccer game because I was hung over," the clinician could say, "You missed your son's game because you were hung over" or "You feel guilty that you missed a special time for your son because of your drinking." When the clinician uses reflective listening, patients feel that the clinician has heard or listened to them; even though what they hear is just a reflection of what they said, it can have a powerful impact.

Clinicians are often frustrated in brief interventions when patients are in the precontemplation stage. Success can be increased and frustration minimized if the clinician realizes that the goal should be to have the patient understand that there is a concern about his or her substance use. To do this, the clinician can express concern about the patient's use, say so nonjudgmentally, and agree to disagree if necessary. The best medical advice should still be shared with the patient, and sometimes a trial of changed use can be instructive. Patients should be invited to return even if they have not changed their substance use. For patients in the contemplation stage, it is useful to review the pros and cons of use from their perspective (by having the patient list them and then using reflective listening to encourage behavior change). A list can put into stark relief a discrepancy between the patient's values and actions, which can lead to change. Once a patient decides to make a change or has changed, working on motivation to change becomes less of a focus; instead, the goal will be to assist the patient in figuring out what to do and how to do it. This work involves negotiation and eliciting what the patient thinks of various options. During this time, reinforcement of self-efficacy becomes useful and a realistic discussion of the difficulty of change is helpful.

Evidence for Efficacy of Brief Intervention Among Patients Identified by Screening

An exhaustive review of the literature is beyond the scope of this chapter, but numerous systematic reviews have been published (e.g., Jonas et al. 2012; Kaner et al. 2011; O'Connor et al. 2018). One caution is that the literature on brief interventions among people not identified by screening cannot speak to the efficacy of brief interventions in people identified by screening. The reason that the general literature on brief interventions is not applicable is that the settings and context are quite different from those of SBI studies, and patients in brief intervention studies often have been seeking help. In SBI and in SBI studies, patients are undifferentiated with regard to motivation. There are no randomized efficacy trials of SBI versus no SBI to provide information regarding the impact of SBI; however, there are numerous randomized trials of brief interventions versus no brief interventions among people identified by screening. By far the best evidence of efficacy for brief interventions as part of SBI is for patients with nondependent (using DSM-IV criteria) unhealthy alcohol use (which would likely apply to those without moderate to severe alcohol use disorder in DSM-5) who were identified by screening in primary care settings (Jonas et al. 2012). Too little study has been done in adolescents, but studies are promising in terms of positive effects; it may be the case that SBI will have greater effects in youth because their behaviors are less well established.

The brief multicontact intervention was usually provided at least in part by the patient's primary care clinician (i.e., in a longitudinal relationship). The effect of brief interventions is to decrease risky drinking by about 10%–12% at 1 year and by about 3 drinks per week (Jonas et al. 2012). Although this is a small effect for an individual, it is large on a public health basis. However, there is some concern among SBI researchers that brief interventions offered as part of SBI may have no effect at all, given that studies are not blinded and are susceptible to social desirability bias (i.e., the likelihood that patients counseled to reduce drinking will report reduced drinking to please assessors to a greater extent than will comparison group patients not so counseled). Bolstering this concern is the observation that although some studies have found benefits for outcomes beyond drinking (e.g., reductions in motor vehicle crashes, less hospital or emergency department utilization, or even lower mortality), data at present are insufficient to draw firm conclusions about the impact of brief interventions on any of these outcomes.

Alcohol SBI has also been studied in hospitals and emergency department settings. Despite the fact that U.S. accreditation organizations encourage (for hospitals) or require (for trauma centers) SBI, the evidence for efficacy in these settings has been decidedly mixed. In hospitals, most studies have not found SBI to be beneficial for decreasing drinking or for increasing completion of referrals to treatment (McQueen et al. 2011). This may be in part because patients identified by screening in hospitals are more severely affected. There is very little evidence that SBI is efficacious for people with moderate to severe alcohol use disorder in any setting, in part because most SBI studies have excluded such patients. In emergency departments, many studies have found no benefit from brief interventions, other studies have found decreases in consequences of use, and still others have found decreases in drinking (Havard et al. 2008). Most studies in trauma centers have also been negative, finding no efficacy for brief interventions. In the most widely cited trauma SBI study (Gentilello et al. 1999), the primary outcome (recurrent injury) was not significantly affected by the brief intervention, and the self-report outcome of alcohol consumption (a decrease in drinking) was affected by the brief intervention, but about half the sample had been lost to follow-up. One implementation study found that in trauma centers in which staff were trained in SBI, injured patients had modestly lower AUDIT scores but no difference in heavy drinking (Zatzick et al. 2014). Although the results were encouraging, consideration of the results in the context of other negative studies raises concern that SBI is an insufficient response to the remarkably high co-occurrence of heavy drinking and serious trauma. The mixed results may be due to the fact that emergency and trauma clinicians often do not have a relationship with the patient and the intervention is a single session. In addition, although patients in these situations are often seen as being in a "teachable moment," it is also possible that such patients would be able to learn from these moments and change (e.g., stop drinking due to awareness that a serious crash was due to his or her intoxication, "a learnable moment") without receiving brief interventions. Although behavior change counseling can potentially have efficacy for any behavioral condition in any setting, it is becoming clear from studies that the context for these interventions (setting, patient experience, clinician) is likely a critical component that contributes to their success or failure. Another factor that may influence efficacy is comorbidity. One systematic review found that brief interventions were ineffective for individuals who had a co-occurring mental disorder or for those who used more than one substance (Kaner et al. 2011).

Far fewer studies have been done of SBI use with individuals taking drugs other than alcohol. One study in an urgent care setting found 5%–9% decreases in heroin and cocaine use as a result of brief interventions (Bernstein et al. 2005). Since then, a series of randomized trials for drug SBI in various settings have been published. The first was an international study in a variety of outpatient settings (one site was in the United States). It found that brief interventions for drugs were ineffective in the United States and that these interventions had a very small effect of questionable clinical significance when overall results were considered (Humeniuk et al. 2012). It stands to reason that a single brief counseling session with an individual identified by screening may be insufficient to change a chronic serious health behavior that is not socially sanctioned, such as heroin or cocaine use, or even cannabis use in an individual who is unconvinced of any health consequences. Consistent with this speculation, an authoritative systematic review found no effect of brief intervention on drug use or any other outcomes in primary care patients with drug use identified by screening (Patnode et al. 2020). In emergency departments, a large randomized multisite trial with high follow-up found that brief intervention had no effect on drug use or consequences (Bogenschutz et al. 2014). One smaller single-site study that examined in-person and computerized SBI found small effects on drug use (Blow et al. 2017). A study in a trauma center also had null results (Field et al. 2020). In summary, drug SBI lacks evidence of efficacy. The main justification for it is the value of knowing one's patients and what they are ingesting or using, because this information has value for prescribing and diagnosis and may open a long-term conversation about health behaviors.

Conclusion

SBI for unhealthy alcohol use is widely recommended on the basis of substantial evidence for efficacy in primary care settings (although its effects are largely limited to use and may not extend to other important health outcomes), yet that information has been poorly disseminated. Brief validated tools are available for screening, and it is important to identify the full spectrum of a patient's unhealthy use. Brief intervention is a clinical skill that can be learned and that is feasible to use in general health settings and is helpful for addressing health risk behaviors in general. Efforts should be made for widespread implementation, and electronic systems to prompt clinicians or even to provide the SBI itself may help. SBI has not yet shown efficacy for reducing drug use or consequences. The same is true for SBI for alcohol in settings outside of primary care. Future studies should move beyond SBI alone to address those risks in those settings. There are other reasons to identify alcohol and drug use in patients beyond identifying patients to undergo brief intervention with the expectation of a change in substance use. For example, clinicians should identify use when prescribing medications that might interact with substances of abuse, or when developing pain management plans, or when trying to make a diagnosis of symptoms that could arise from substance use. However, screening tools are generally not validated for those purposes (i.e., most tools identify risky use, not any use). Clearly, further research needs to be done in those areas where evidence is insufficient to determine whether SBI is effective and what else might be needed to address these serious problems when SBI is insufficient.

References

Allensworth-Davies D, Cheng DM, Smith PC, et al: The Short Inventory of Problems–Modified for Drug Use (SIP-DU): validity in a primary care sample. Am J Addict 21(3):257–262, 2012 22494228

American Psychiatric Association: Diagnostic and Statistical Manual of Mental Disorders, 4th Edition. Washington, DC, American Psychiatric Association, 1994

American Psychiatric Association: Diagnostic and Statistical Manual of Mental Disorders, 5th Edition. Arlington, VA, American Psychiatric Association, 2013

Babor TF, Higgins-Biddle JC, Saunders JB, et al: AUDIT: The Alcohol Use Disorders Identification Test: Guidelines for Use in Primary Health Care (WHO Publ No PSA/92.4). Geneva, Switzerland, World Health Organization, 2001

Bernstein J, Bernstein E, Tassiopoulos K, et al: Brief motivational intervention at a clinic visit reduces cocaine and heroin use. Drug Alcohol Depend 77(1):49–59, 2005 15607841

Blow FC, Walton MA, Bohnert ASB, et al: A randomized controlled trial of brief interventions to reduce drug use among adults in a low-income urban emergency department: the HealthiER You study. Addiction 112(8):1395–1405, 2017 28127808

Bogenschutz MP, Donovan DM, Mandler RN, et al: Brief intervention for patients with problematic drug use presenting in emergency departments: a randomized clinical trial. JAMA Intern Med 174(11):1736–1745, 2014 25179753

Bradley KA, DeBenedetti AF, Volk RJ, et al: AUDIT-C as a brief screen for alcohol misuse in primary care. Alcohol Clin Exp Res 31(7):1208–1217, 2007 17451397

Brown RL, Rounds LA: Conjoint screening questionnaires for alcohol and other drug abuse: criterion validity in a primary care practice. Wis Med J 94(3):135–140, 1995 7778330

Burns E, Gray R, Smith LA: Brief screening questionnaires to identify problem drinking during pregnancy: a systematic review. Addiction 105(4):601–614, 2010 20403013

Chasnoff IJ, Wells AM, McGourty RF, et al: Validation of the 4P's Plus screen for substance use in pregnancy validation of the 4P's Plus. J Perinatol 27(12):744–748, 2007 17805340

Field CA, Von Sternberg K, Velasquez MM: Randomized trial of screening and brief intervention to reduce injury and substance abuse in an urban Level I trauma center. Drug Alcohol Depend 208:107792, 2020 32028253

Gentilello LM, Rivara FP, Donovan DM, et al: Alcohol interventions in a trauma center as a means of reducing the risk of injury recurrence. Ann Surg 230(4):473–480, discussion 480–483, 1999 10522717

Glass JE, Hamilton AM, Powell BJ, et al: Specialty substance use disorder services following brief alcohol intervention: a meta-analysis of randomized controlled trials. Addiction 110(9):1404–1415, 2015 25913697

Havard A, Shakeshaft A, Sanson-Fisher R: Systematic review and meta-analyses of strategies targeting alcohol problems in emergency departments: interventions reduce alcohol-related injuries. Addiction 103(3):368–376, discussion 377–378, 2008 18190671

Humeniuk R, Ali R, Babor TF, et al: Validation of the Alcohol, Smoking and Substance Involvement Screening Test (ASSIST). Addiction 103(6):1039–1047, 2008 18373724

Humeniuk R, Henry-Edwards S, Ali R, et al: The Alcohol, Smoking and Substance Involvement Screening Test (ASSIST): Manual for Use in Primary Care. Geneva, World Health Organization, 2010. Available at: http://whqlibdoc.who.int/publications/2010/9789241599382_eng.pdf?ua=1. Accessed November 15, 2019.

Humeniuk R, Ali R, Babor T, et al: A randomized controlled trial of a brief intervention for illicit drugs linked to the Alcohol, Smoking and Substance Involvement Screening Test (ASSIST) in clients recruited from primary health-care settings in four countries. Addiction 107(5):957–966, 2012 22126102

Jonas DE, Garbutt JC, Amick HR, et al: Behavioral counseling after screening for alcohol misuse in primary care: a systematic review and meta-analysis for the U.S. Preventive Services Task Force. Ann Intern Med 157(9):645–654, 2012 23007881

Kaner EF, Brown N, Jackson K: A systematic review of the impact of brief interventions on substance use and co-morbid physical and mental health conditions. Mental Health and Substance Use 4(1):38–61, 2011. Available at: https://www.tandfonline.com/doi/abs/10.1080/17523281.2011.533449. Accessed December 12, 2019.

Kaner EFS, Beyer FR, Muirhead C, et al: Effectiveness of brief alcohol interventions in primary care populations. Cochrane Database Syst Rev (2):CD004148, 2018 29476653

Massachusetts Department of Public Health Bureau of Substance Abuse Services: Provider Guide: Adolescent Screening, Brief Intervention, and Referral to Treatment Using the CRAFFT Screening Tool. Boston, MA. Massachusetts Department of Public Health, 2009

Mayfield D, McLeod G, Hall P: The CAGE questionnaire: validation of a new alcoholism screening instrument. Am J Psychiatry 131(10):1121–1123, 1974 4416585

McLellan AT, Kushner H, Metzger D, et al: The fifth edition of the Addiction Severity Index. J Subst Abuse Treat 9(1–2):199–213, 1992 1334156

McQueen J, Howe TE, Allan L, et al: Brief interventions for heavy alcohol users admitted to general hospital wards. Cochrane Database Syst Rev (8):CD005191, 2011 21833953

National Institute on Alcohol Abuse and Alcoholism: Helping Patients Who Drink Too Much: A Clinician's Guide, Updated 2005 Edition (NIH Publ No 07-3769). Bethesda, MD, National Institutes of Health, reprinted May 2007. Available at: https://www.integration.samhsa.gov/clinical-practice/Helping_Patients_Who_Drink_Too_Much.pdf. Accessed March 3, 2020.

National Institute on Alcohol Abuse and Alcoholism: Alcohol Screening and Brief Intervention for Youth: A Practitioner's Guide (NIH Publ No 11-7805). Bethesda, MD, National Institutes of Health, 2011. Available at: www.niaaa.nih.gov/youthguide. Accessed November 15, 2019.

National Institute on Drug Abuse: NIDA Drug Screening Tool: Clinician's Screening Tool for Drug Use in General Medical Settings. 2019. Available at: http://www.drugabuse.gov/nmassist/. Accessed November 15, 2019.

O'Connor EA, Perdue LA, Senger CA, et al: Screening and behavioral counseling interventions to reduce unhealthy alcohol use in adolescents and adults: updated evidence report and systematic review for the US Preventive Services Task Force. JAMA 320(18):1910–1928, 2018 30422198

Patnode CD, Perdue LA, Rushkin M, et al: Screening for unhealthy drug use: updated evidence report and systematic review for the US Preventive Services Task Force. JAMA 323(22):2310–2328, 2020 32515820

Rubinsky AD, Kivlahan DR, Volk RJ, et al: Estimating risk of alcohol dependence using alcohol screening scores. Drug Alcohol Depend 108(1–2):29–36, 2010 20042299

Saitz R: Clinical practice. Unhealthy alcohol use. N Engl J Med 352(6):596–607, 2005 15703424

Selzer ML: The Michigan Alcoholism Screening Test: the quest for a new diagnostic instrument. Am J Psychiatry 127(12):1653–1658, 1971 5565851

Selzer ML, Vinokur A, van Rooijen L: A self-administered Short Michigan Alcoholism Screening Test (SMAST). J Stud Alcohol 36(1):117–126, 1975 238068

Skinner HA: The Drug Abuse Screening Test. Addict Behav 7(4):363–371, 1982 7183189

Smith PC, Schmidt SM, Allensworth-Davies D, et al: Primary care validation of a single-question alcohol screening test. J Gen Intern Med 24(7):783–788, 2009 19247718

Smith PC, Schmidt SM, Allensworth-Davies D, Saitz R: A single-question screening test for drug use in primary care. Arch Intern Med 170(13):1155–1160, 2010 20625025

Sokol RJ, Martier SS, Ager JW: The T-ACE questions: practical prenatal detection of risk-drinking. Am J Obstet Gynecol 160(4):863–868, discussion 868–870, 1989 2712118

Spurling MC, Vinson DC: Alcohol-related injuries: evidence for the prevention paradox. Ann Fam Med 3(1):47–52, 2005 15671190

Stockwell T, Zhao J, Panwar S, et al: Do "moderate" drinkers have reduced mortality risk? A systematic review and meta-analysis of alcohol consumption and all-cause mortality. J Stud Alcohol Drugs 77(2):185–198, 2016 26997174

Vinson DC, Kruse RL, Seale JP: Simplifying alcohol assessment: two questions to identify alcohol use disorders. Alcohol Clin Exp Res 31(8):1392–1398, 2007 17559544

Yudko E, Lozhkina O, Fouts A: A comprehensive review of the psychometric properties of the Drug Abuse Screening Test. J Subst Abuse Treat 32(2):189–198, 2007 17306727

Zatzick D, Donovan DM, Jurkovich G, et al: Disseminating alcohol screening and brief intervention at trauma centers: a policy-relevant cluster randomized effectiveness trial. Addiction 109(5):754–765, 2014 24450612

CHAPTER 7

Treating Addiction Like a Chronic Illness

A Practical Clinical Model

Jenna L. McCauley, Ph.D.

A. Thomas McLellan, Ph.D.

In this chapter we present a formative clinical model for the chronic care management of opioid use disorder in general medical settings. To facilitate development of this model, we draw on Chronic Care Model strategies and procedures currently in place for managing type 2 diabetes. Specifically, in keeping with the Chronic Care Model, this chapter argues for a proactive, team-based approach to the management of opioid use disorder that promotes patients' self-management of disease (i.e., recovery), modeled after the clinical management and monitoring protocols currently used in the treatment of adult-onset type 2 diabetes (Parchman et al. 2007). Through this effort, we hope to highlight critical but correctable discrepancies in our current approach to the management of opioid use disorder and other addictions, from prevention through screening and diagnosis, treatment, and ultimately patient self-management. For all major areas of discrepancy, we delineate key contributory factors and provide recommendations for achieving parity.

During the time of this work, Dr. McCauley received funding from the National Institute on Drug Abuse (K23 DA036566).

Substance Use Disorders Are Medical Illnesses

A diagnosis of a substance use disorder is based on evidence of impaired control, social impairment, risky use, and craving for the substance. The most serious and usually chronic form of a substance use disorder is commonly called an "addiction."

Substance use disorders are common. General population studies estimate the prevalence of substance use disorders as between 8% and 10%, or more than 21 million people age 12 years or older (Center for Behavioral Health Statistics and Quality 2015). Individuals with substance use disorders are overrepresented in health care settings, with prevalences estimated at 15%–20% in primary care settings, approximately 40% in hospital clinics, and greater than 70% in emergency departments and urgent care facilities (Mertens et al. 2003). In addition to being highly prevalent, substance use disorders are also costly to U.S. health care, accounting for more than $120 billion dollars annually in unnecessary or inappropriate health care procedures, avoidable hospital readmissions, and preventable injuries and infectious diseases (Centers for Disease Control and Prevention 2014a).

Research over the past three decades suggests that addictions are best considered as being acquired chronic illnesses (Volkow et al. 2016). These illnesses are considered to be acquired because the disease process begins with voluntary self-administration of intoxicants by the individual, usually starting in the adolescent years. Substance use disorders are considered to be chronic because repeated self-administration can produce gradual but progressive injury to specific brain circuits controlling inhibition, motivation, cognition, reward sensitivity, and stress tolerance (Volkow et al. 2016), and those brain changes are accompanied by characteristic behavioral symptoms of loss of control over use, emotional and motivational volatility, and reduced interest in previously rewarding social and vocational activities. The frequency/intensity/duration of substance use needed to produce these changes in brain function and disease onset differs appreciably across individuals and drug types/combinations. Similarly, the time required for these brain changes to resolve and return to "normal" during treatment also varies appreciably. Imaging studies of abstinent but previously addicted adults showed slow progress toward normalization of the affected brain circuits, yet those circuits still differed from those of "normal" control subjects even after 180 days of complete abstinence (Volkow et al. 2016). Thus, in common with other chronic illnesses such as diabetes, asthma, and hypertension, addictions can be effectively managed, but there is currently no treatment that will reliably produce a return to normal brain function and normal control of substance use— that is, there is presently no cure for addiction.

Legislative Calls for Parity in Treatment of Addiction

Despite estimates that approximately 20% of health care costs are spent treating conditions and complications resulting from addiction, only around 1% of U.S. health care dollars are spent treating addiction itself (Mark et al. 2015). Over time, scientific findings and legislative changes, like the Mental Health Equity and Addiction Parity Act and the Affordable Care Act, have provided a rationale and framework for operationalizing and rationalizing the financing of addiction treatment like treatments of other chronic illnesses (Roy and Miller 2010). Such a comparative clinical model would be beneficial for several reasons: 1) to provide the foundation on which medical and other health care professional training is based, 2) to promote integration of addiction treatment and mainstream health care information systems, 3) to develop practical quality assurance protocols, and 4) to enable payers to decide reimbursement schedules.

Clinical Model for Managing Chronic Illness

The Chronic Care Model (CCM) was developed as a framework for improving the quality of care delivered for the treatment of chronic medical conditions, namely diabetes (Stellefson et al. 2013). Virtually all chronic health conditions require initial clinical monitoring by a health care team to prepare the patient (and family) for ongoing self-management, with adjunctive monitoring and support provided by the health care system (Goodman et al. 2013). Currently within the American health care system, effective management of chronic health conditions is hindered by fragmented (and at times duplicative) service delivery and underdeveloped clinical information systems that prevent goal-directed coordination of care. The CCM provides a framework for addressing these and other systemic deficits and has been used as a model to guide contemporary diabetes care. The CCM framework has also been modified to support high-quality, patient-centered management of chronic diseases such as congestive heart failure, asthma, and depression. Table 7–1 outlines the core components of the CCM.

The Chronic Care Model and Opioid Use Disorder

While all substance use disorders are dangerous and costly, in this chapter we focus primarily on the treatment of opioid use disorder (OUD), particularly moderate-to-severe opioid use disorder. As of 2018, the United States was in its tenth year of an opioid epidemic that has resulted in more than 400,000 overdose deaths, has produced more than 6 million cases of opioid addiction during that period, and continues to escalate with respect to the morbidity and mortality toll (Seth et al. 2018). Most important, while there has been extensive basic and clinical research on the origins, course, and treatment of OUD, and that research has produced many effective, evidence-based prevention and treatment tools, very few physicians have received the minimum fundamental training necessary to screen for, diagnose, or treat OUD (Rosenblatt et al. 2015). Put simply, research findings combine to suggest that training in OUD can and should become part of general medical education, care, and insurance coverage, not only because these disorders are treatable illnesses in their own right, but also because they are so prevalent and so corrosive to the quality, costs, and outcomes of care for many other medical conditions that they may both cause and complicate.

TABLE 7–1.   **Components of the chronic care model intended to optimize patient-centered care**

Model component	Key characteristics
Delivery system design	Delivery system designed to be consistent with a proactive (rather than reactive) model of care delivery wherein planned visits are coordinated through a team-based approach that prioritizes determination of a plan of care and follow-up patient navigation to guide patients through the components of that plan
Self-management support	Support designed to empower and prepare patients to manage their health and health care through use of proven programs that foster self-efficacy and provide information, emotional support, and strategies for living with a chronic illness
Decision support	Support designed to promote implementation of evidence-based guidelines, appropriate integration of specialty care into treatment, and consideration of patient preferences in the determination of a plan of care
Clinical information systems	Systems designed to organize patient- and population-level data to facilitate efficient and effective health care
Community resources and policies	Programs and laws that promote and protect healthy lifestyle choices for patients with chronic illness
Health systems	Organizational/systemic mechanisms that promote safe, high-quality care—including provision of incentives for quality care and development of agreements facilitating care coordination within and across organizations

Source.   Tsai et al. 2005.

In the text that follows, we present a science-based, clinically practical model for screening, diagnosing, intervening, and (when necessary) treating and managing OUD. That model is informed by basic and clinical addiction science, but just as importantly by the practical clinical experience derived from screening, intervening in, and treating another chronic illness—type 2 adult-onset diabetes (T2D). Although every disease process is unique, as are the patients who experience those diseases, there are notable parallels in the onset, course, clinical management, and treatment goals between T2D and other chronic illnesses—including OUD. T2D can be characterized as the gradual loss of control of sugar metabolism brought on by progressive injury to pancreatic structures and function, usually through repeated inappropriate, unhealthy behaviors (diet, exercise, etc.), particularly among individuals with a genetic predisposition toward the illness. T2D is an apt clinical comparator for OUD for several key reasons. First, T2D and OUD have both been recognized as chronic health conditions that will typically require long-term management (American Diabetes Association 2018b; Bruneau et al. 2018). Second, both primary illnesses promote risk for additional, related diseases. Third, in both T2D and OUD, unhealthy behaviors are the primary trigger for onset of disease symptomatology. In recognition of these similarities, T2D was cited as a comparator case for parity in payment for addiction treatment in the aforementioned Affordable Care Act legislation.

Applying the Chronic Care Model to Disease Management: Comparing Type 2 Diabetes and Opioid Use Disorder

Delivery System Design

Primary care accounts for the majority of U.S. physician office visits. Thus, a key step toward implementing the CCM in T2D—and a key difference from the current approach to treating OUD—is integrating guideline-based OUD treatment (including screening, diagnosis, treatment, and monitoring) into all primary care settings, particularly in the context of pain management. Integration of addiction treatment into primary care could also have several advantages for health care in general, such as the following: increased ability to address comorbid physical illnesses, enhanced health and social function outcomes for patients, and decreased systemic costs of treatment (Substance Abuse and Mental Health Services Administration 2016). Table 7–2 provides a brief summary of key comparisons between mainstream approaches to the management of T2D and OUD in the United States.

The U.S. Preventive Services Task Force recommends regular (i.e., annually to every 3 years) T2D screening beginning in childhood for individuals at risk, use of objective measures (e.g., A1c), use of specific diagnostic cut points, early intervention, and immediate engagement in treatment when indicated (American Diabetes Association 2018b; Siu and U.S. Preventive Services Task Force 2015). Data indicate that there is much room for improvement in the implementation of guideline-concordant screening procedures (Mainous et al. 2016). Nonetheless, about 97% of primary care physicians ($N=1,256$) do screen for prediabetes by ordering one of the three recommended blood tests (Kaiser Permanente 2019) and using recommended diagnostic and treatment guidelines (e.g., American Diabetes Association 2018b; Kaiser Permanente 2019). Identification and diagnostic accuracy of T2D have been significantly improved by the emergence of laboratory-based criteria; among current cases ($N=34.2$ million), approximately 79% are appropriately diagnosed (Centers for Disease Control and Prevention 2020). Use of evidence-based laboratory criteria has also improved the management of diabetes, as indicated by substantial increases in the proportion of patients attaining recommended thresholds for hemoglobin A1c (HbA1c), blood pressure, and low-density lipoprotein (LDL) cholesterol (Ali et al. 2013).

First-line medication therapy for T2D usually consists of metformin, which may be combined or replaced with sulfonylureas, sodium-glucose cotransporter 2 (SGLT-2) inhibitors, or insulin if necessary (Kaiser Permanente 2019). More severe cases of T2D—those necessitating insulin therapies, as well as those involving multiple medical complexities—are more appropriately managed by or in consultation with specialist care, usually an endocrinologist (McCulloch et al. 2019). Many of these more complex patients need multiple agents and more intensive clinical interventions to achieve optimal disease management and to address common comorbidities and medical complexities (American Diabetes Association 2018b). Outcomes are best when there is stable adherence to medications for 2 years or longer (Nerat et al. 2016). However, appropriate use of prescribed medication is not the only focus of T2D management;

TABLE 7–2. Key comparisons between management of type 2 diabetes (TD2) and opioid use disorder (OUD) in the American health care system

	Type 2 diabetes	Opioid use disorder
Prevalence of preclinical symptoms	84.1 million adults meet criteria for prediabetes (Centers for Disease Control and Prevention 2017)	11.5 million adults report a history of opioid misuse (Davenport and Matthews 2018)
Diagnostic prevalence of condition	23.1 million diagnosed, 7.2 million (24%) undiagnosed (Centers for Disease Control and Prevention 2017)	1.5 million adults with public or private insurance diagnosed with opioid abuse, dependence, or poisoning; 1.9 million adults self-report being addicted to opioids (Davenport and Matthews 2018)
Association with mortality	Proportion of all deaths attributable to diabetes estimated at between 11.5% and 11.8% for time period spanning 1997–2011 (Stokes and Preston 2017)	Proportion of all deaths attributable to opioids increased by 292% from 2001 to 2016, accounting for 1.5% of deaths in 2016 (Gomes et al. 2018)
Average annual expenditures for health care	$3,560 in health care expenses (Agency for Healthcare Research and Quality 2016)	$6,552 for methadone treatment; $5,980 for buprenorphine treatment in OTP setting; $14,112 for naltrexone in OTP setting; costs vary, depending on treatment setting (National Institute on Drug Abuse 2018; Substance Abuse and Mental Health Services Administration 2016)
Cost of coverage for treatment	Majority (67%) covered by government insurance (including Medicare, Medicaid, and military); remainder covered by private insurance (~31%) and self-pay/uninsured (2%) (American Diabetes Association 2018a)	Largest share of substance use disorder treatment financing from state (non-Medicaid) and local governments (29%), often in the form of substance abuse prevention and treatment block grants (Substance Abuse and Mental Health Services Administration 2016)
Screening	Universal screening recommended for patients with identified risk factors (every 3 years for negative screen without complications; annually for patients with complicating conditions); screening conducted by primary care physicians	As of June 2020, screening recommendations were updated to support primary care screening of adults 18 years and older for unhealthy drug use when accurate diagnostics and effective treatment are available (U.S. Preventive Services Task Force et al. 2020); screening recommended for patients being treated with long-term opioid therapy for chronic pain

TABLE 7–2. Key comparisons between management of type 2 diabetes (TD2) and opioid use disorder (OUD) in the American health care system *(continued)*

	Type 2 diabetes	Opioid use disorder
Percentage of diagnosed patients entering treatment	Of patients diagnosed, 95.3% were linked to a usual care provider, and 91.7% reported two or more visits in the past year since diagnosis (Ali et al. 2014)	75% of patients with prescription OUD do not receive treatment within first decade after onset (Blanco et al. 2013)
Transition from diagnosis to treatment	Same physician/practice screening for T2D, so no "referral to treatment" necessary; upon diagnosis, care provider engages patient in treatment planning	If patient is diagnosed outside the specialty treatment setting, referral is needed; wait lists and limited availability of treatment options pervade most localities, particularly rural locations
Treatment components	Medication and self-management; referrals for comorbidities	Medication and psychosocial services to promote self-management; referrals for comorbidities
Medication use	Metformin, insulin, sulfonylureas, SGLT-2 inhibitors; evidence-based decision support to guide medication selection based on disease progression and treatment response	Methadone, naltrexone, buprenorphine (buprenorphine/naltrexone); no evidence-based clinical decision support to determine medication selection
Role of specialty care	Primary care provides majority of first-line care; diabetes team (endocrinology) referral for patients whose HbA1c is not controlled with trials of first-line medications	Specialty treatment facilities provide majority of first-line care for all levels of OUD; in 2014, only 40% of spending on substance abuse treatment went to outpatient treatment services, the majority of which were delivered at specialty facilities rather than in primary care settings (Substance Abuse and Mental Health Services Administration 2016)
Frequency of patient appointments	Patients visit primary care physician every 3 months for assessment of whether changes to therapy regimen are needed (barring complications); once HbA1c goal is attained, return for care annually	Daily (methadone), weekly (buprenorphine), or monthly (naltrexone) medication management appointments at outset of treatment; individual/group counseling sessions often required in addition to medication/medical management appointments; patients may progress to less-frequent appointments (monthly to biannually with buprenorphine and naltrexone) if meeting treatment goals

TABLE 7–2. Key comparisons between management of type 2 diabetes (TD2) and opioid use disorder (OUD) in the American health care system *(continued)*

	Type 2 diabetes	Opioid use disorder
Regulations around medication prescribing	No first-line medications are controlled/scheduled; all medications may be prescribed by any clinician credentialed to prescribe medications	Methadone available only in approved OTPs; buprenorphine requires additional controlled substance training and waiver; naltrexone is not controlled and can be prescribed by anyone credentialed to prescribe medications
Role of self-management and counseling	Critical—Self-monitoring of blood glucose is key to treatment monitoring and determining effectiveness of medication; lifestyle management is key to reducing risk for symptom development; discussion of management of "sick days" and guided planning for how to deal with them; patients continue to receive medication management even if nonadherent to self-management/counseling recommendations	Critical—Is usually a required psychosocial component (often individual or group counseling sessions) of MAT; the psychosocial component varies, but usually includes cognitive-behavioral approaches to promote lifestyle changes consistent with sobriety; most providers will not continue to prescribe medications if patient is nonadherent to counseling requirements
Treatment adherence	Recommended glycemic goals are achieved by fewer than 50% of patients (García-Pérez et al. 2013)	12-month adherence rates for patients engaged in MAT range from 30% to 40% (Ronquest et al. 2018)
Common additional clinical considerations	Depression; nutrition, vision care, foot care; atherosclerotic cardiovascular disease prevention	Other substances of abuse; depression, posttraumatic stress disorder, anxiety, infectious disease, chronic pain
Definition of recovery	HbA1c at goal and comorbidity risks managed/mitigated	Abstinence from illicit opioids and comorbidity risks managed/mitigated

Note.　HbA1c=hemoglobin A1c; MAT=medication-assisted treatment; OTP=opioid treatment program; SGLT-2=sodium-glucose cotransporter 2.

most T2D patients also require lifestyle management programming, often targeting nutrition and physical activity (Centers for Disease Control and Prevention 2012).

There are obvious parallels between T2D and OUD in onset, course, diagnosis, treatment, and management—but equally obvious differences in contemporary clinical methods. For example, OUD is not diagnosed with a biological test. Instead, diagnosis is typically based on an interview history provided by the patient, combined with a comprehensive physical examination (Kampman and Jarvis 2015). Whereas urine drug testing can be used to support a diagnostic decision, urine testing results are not in themselves definitive (Kampman and Jarvis 2015). Until June 2020, the U.S. Preventive Services Task Force noted that there was insufficient evidence to recommend universal screening for general drug use disorders in primary care settings (U.S. Preventive Services Task Force et al. 2020). Available estimates suggest that primary care physicians—particularly those seeing patients outside of chronic pain management—seldom screen for OUD (Venner et al. 2018).

The infrequency of OUD screening in primary care settings is particularly disheartening because early, accurate diagnosis could lead to treatment with any of the three U.S. Food and Drug Administration (FDA)–approved medications—naltrexone, methadone, and buprenorphine—to manage symptoms of OUD, in combination with additional counseling for lifestyle management. Methadone, an opioid agonist, is not approved for delivery in primary care settings and can only be delivered in federally certified opioid treatment programs. In contrast, naltrexone, an opioid antagonist, can be prescribed by any licensed health care provider. Buprenorphine, a partial opioid agonist with effectiveness equivalent to that of methadone, is available from any licensed prescriber who has passed an instructional course and received a specific waiver to prescribe (as set forth by the Drug Addiction Treatment Act of 2000 [DATA 2000]). Although the numbers of waivered prescribers have increased over the past decade (17.3 prescribers per 100,000 persons in 2019), the total number of waivered prescribers continues to represent fewer than 1 in 10 of all primary care providers (McBain et al. 2020). For this reason, the majority of OUD treatment continues to take place in specialty addiction treatment facilities that exist outside of mainstream medical practices and thus have limited medical staffing or even minimal functional interaction with mainstream health care settings. Thus, only about 1 in 10 individuals with OUD who enter specialty addiction care actually receives medication-assisted treatment (MAT) (Sandoe et al. 2018). In the context of the broader comparison of these two chronic illnesses, it is difficult to imagine the effects on the quality, outcomes, and costs if the majority of contemporary diabetes care were relegated to separate nonmedical centers that were largely unable to provide evidence-based medications.

As is true for patients with diabetes, patients with OUD do far better when they are stably adherent for a year or more in comprehensive, individualized care, with monitoring and appropriately prescribed medications (Ronquest et al. 2018). However 12-month MAT adherence rates hover between 30% and 40% in most insured populations (Ronquest et al. 2018). One exceptional program deserves comment: mandatory addiction treatment programs for physicians and airline pilots with substance use disorders (McLellan et al. 2008). These programs are compulsory (under threat of loss of license) and combine individualized care and supportive services with 4 years of clinical monitoring using unannounced drug screenings. Five-year outcome evaluations show that 78% or more of these patients ($N=802$) are stably in recovery and functioning well (McLellan et al. 2008), setting a recovery benchmark similar to that demonstrated by more widely available T2D care.

In light of the low uptake of MAT by either specialty addiction providers or the broader primary care system, the current U.S. opioid epidemic has spurred significant efforts to develop, evaluate, and disseminate models for integration of MAT into primary care (Chou et al. 2016). The current Screening, Treatment Initiation, and Referral approach initiated in emergency medicine and hospital settings is gaining empirical support for its feasibility, positive patient outcomes, and cost-effectiveness (Bernstein and D'Onofrio 2017). While such models show promise, additional work remains to be done to achieve levels of care availability and integration approaching those currently available for T2D treatment.

Lifestyle Change, "Disease Control," and "Recovery"

Self-management of disease control, the accepted clinical goal of T2D care, is operationally and conceptually very similar to the self-management of "recovery" in addiction care. Both require 1) reduction in the severity of the cardinal symptom of the illness to below problematic levels (e.g., in T2D, HbA1c levels below 6%); 2) improved health and function, which is important to both patients and payers and serves to maintain cardinal symptom improvement; and 3) training and motivation of the patient (and family) to maintain self-management of their care by continuing a healthier lifestyle and self-monitoring for signs of relapse.

Lifestyle management plays a significant role in the promotion of disease control in T2D. Lifestyle management includes diabetes education for patients and family, provision of social supports to enable lifestyle change, enhanced physical activity, smoking cessation counseling, and medical nutrition therapy. These lifestyle management interventions have generally strong evidence of improving key outcomes like self-care behaviors, HbA1c levels, and quality of life (American Diabetes Association 2018b). American Diabetes Association guideline recommendations identify four critical times to evaluate and respond to patients' need for self-management: at diagnosis, annually, when complications arise, and when transitions of care occur. Most costs associated with T2D lifestyle management programming are covered by public and private payers, although these services are often unavailable outside metropolitan areas (Rutledge et al. 2017).

In the case of OUD and other addictions, lifestyle management with the goal of recovery involves reduction of the cardinal symptom (substance use) through programmatic efforts to instill total abstinence and/or through implementation of MAT, as well as other positive lifestyle changes (Substance Abuse and Mental Health Services Administration 2016). Recovery support groups serve the important function of helping the patient to self-monitor and recognize signs of impending relapse and to take proactive action to prevent such relapse. Mutual aid groups such as Alcoholics Anonymous (AA) and Narcotics Anonymous (NA) constitute the best-known and most rigorously evaluated approach to recovery support. Whereas attitudinal barriers regarding MAT have traditionally existed in AA/NA groups and largely continue to persist, MAT-inclusive groups are becoming more prevalent. There is a need for well-controlled research examining the effectiveness of 12-step facilitation in conjunction with MAT.

Decision Support and Clinical Information Systems

Clear, evidence-based decision support for diabetes care has been developed and is accessible via electronic health records (EHRs) to guide physicians in diagnosing patients, prescribing medications, providing adjunctive support services, clinically monitoring patient progress, and interacting with other health care specialists and clinics (see, e.g., Kaiser Permanente 2019). Decision support paradigms engage patients through a combined reliance on patient self-monitoring of blood glucose and office-based measurement of HbA1c levels to assess the effectiveness and safety of glycemic control (American Diabetes Association 2018b). The major uptake of EHR, supported by the Affordable Care Act legislation, has provided enhanced opportunities to engage clinical information systems in the planning, delivery, and coordination of care for T2D. Clinical information systems, when combined with usual care interventions, are associated with improved glycemic control (Riazi et al. 2015).

Within the addiction treatment field, and despite the development of MAT guidelines (Kampman and Jarvis 2015), evidence-based clinical decision support remains in the early stages of development and evaluation. An additional challenge to developing clinical decision support systems in OUD care is the now-antiquated federal substance abuse confidentiality regulations (42 CFR Part 2—Confidentiality of Substance Use Disorder Patient Records) specific to addiction treatment, which restrict the sharing of even clinical information between an addiction treatment program and all other parts of the health care system. These restrictions impede clinical collaboration and even basic clinical interactions such as referral, consultation, and certain laboratory testing (see Substance Abuse and Mental Health Services Administration 2016).

Community Resources and Policies

The Centers for Disease Control and Prevention (CDC) disseminates many publicly available prevention resources for T2D, including the evidence-based Lifestyle Change Program (Knowler et al. 2009). Numerous additional community resources have been deployed to advocate for (e.g., American Diabetes Association, Diabetes Patient Advocacy Coalition) and to directly provide clinical and social supports and education (e.g., community health workers) for patients with diabetes.

Community-based resources that target the prevention and management of OUD have been more widely implemented and are more accessible than in the past, largely boosted by the federal response to the opioid crisis and infusions of funding provided through the 21st Century Cures Act Opioid State Targeted Response grants and the recently authorized State Opioid Response Grants (Johnson et al. 2018). Additionally, numerous federal, state, local, and private organizations have developed opioid-related prevention programming (e.g., Operation Prevention [www.operation-prevention.com]), although most of this programming focuses on prevention of prescription opioid abuse through public health education and prescription monitoring. Unfortunately, neither broad public health education nor prescription drug monitoring programs have demonstrated definitive empirical evidence of effectiveness (see, e.g., American Public Health Association 2015).

Broad reviews of health policy effects on access to and effectiveness of treatment for T2D and OUD are beyond the scope of this chapter. However, Medicaid expansion has emerged as a leading policy-level factor supporting access to care for—and identification and successful management of—OUD, as it has previously done for T2D (Meinhofer and Witman 2018). More specifically, increased ease of access to third-party reimbursement for OUD medications and specialty addiction care treatment has more than doubled utilization of these services (Meara and Frank 2005). Despite these advances, MAT coverage and benefits vary from state to state, with some states continuing to impose restrictions on length or type of treatment.

Health Systems: Population Health Measurement and Tracking Systems

Population health monitoring systems are critical for preventing new cases and for managing existing cases of all chronic illnesses, including evaluation of quality improvement initiatives. In the case of T2D, the Diabetes Quality Improvement Project was the first widely adopted comprehensive set of performance measures for any single disease, and was rapidly supported by organizations representing more than 80% of diabetic patients across the country (Fleming et al. 2001). The most recent Standards of Care in Diabetes, developed by the Agency for Healthcare Research and Quality, call for continued efforts toward quality improvement and patient-centered practice transformation in the treatment of T2D (Burstin and Johnson 2016).

No such clinical system of regular national reporting of new cases, or of treatment quality standards, exists in the addiction field. States vary widely in their approaches to measurement and reporting of substance use treatment quality indicators, and significant operational problems persist in the collection, analysis, interpretation, and use of these outcome measures. Recent efforts to address these problems in quality assessment have involved repurposing the "Cascade of Care" framework (Williams et al. 2017) introduced in the HIV/AIDS field as a model for closing gaps in access and quality of addiction care; however, these efforts are in the early stages of model development and have yet to be tested or implemented.

Barriers to Integrated Care for Opioid Use Disorder

In summary, to this point, there are sound clinical, practical, and commonsense reasons to extend current CCM methods, measures, and standards for preventing, intervening early in, and comprehensively treating T2D to the management of OUD. Thus far, we have emphasized many of the commonalities between these two chronic illnesses, but there are also some serious ideological and political differences in the public approach to these two illnesses that have contributed to notable discrepancies in their clinical management.

Stigma

Stigma exists toward diabetes and individuals with the illness—both in the general public and among health care professionals (Liu et al. 2017). However, stigma associated with addictive disorders is qualitatively different from that associated with diabetes. Because most addictions and overdoses have resulted from illegal acts, these conditions have traditionally been considered to be the purview of the justice system to be managed with social sanctions and punishments (Kopak 2015). Addiction has rarely been considered an illness or a public health problem to be dealt with by health care systems. For centuries, the public understanding of addiction was as a "character or personality disorder," an indicator of moral weakness expressed via wanton behaviors (Nathan et al. 2016). Only within the past three decades has neuropsychological and genetic research confirmed the biological foundation for the traditionally stigmatized addiction-related behaviors (Frank and Nagel 2017).

It was because of these now-outdated views that when addiction treatment was made available in the mid 1960s, it was purposely segregated from the rest of health care, including care delivery settings, insurance coverage, and medical education/ training (Roy and Miller 2010). Indeed, recent practitioner surveys indicate that stigma and criminalization remain key barriers to integrated care for OUD and a driver of disparities (Barnett et al. 2018). As with all other historical examples of segregation, this forced separation of services has delayed the application of public health prevention strategies and the chronic care model of treatment.

Access to Treatment

Evidence-based behavioral and medication-assisted treatments, when applied in a chronic care framework, have been shown to promote recovery, prevent relapse, and improve associated outcomes (e.g., increased employment, decreased criminal justice system involvement) that enhance overall quality of life (see Maglione et al. 2018). However, as previously discussed, rates of access to OUD care remain low, and treatment quality remains a significant concern. A major driver of poor access to treatment is lack of insurance reimbursement for continuing, comprehensive care management for addiction. As indicated previously, lack of insurance parity continues to exist despite federal legislation mandating such parity, and that disparity leads to many other issues impeding access to treatment. For example, lack of medical insurance coverage for the treatment of OUD has led to lack of motivation on the part of medical and nursing schools to teach and train health care workforces (Andrews et al. 2015); reluctance on the part of pharmaceutical firms and health care technology firms to develop and market new and better medications, monitoring systems, and decision support software products for addiction care; and unwillingness on the part of major health care organizations to include treatment for OUD or other addictions (Haffajee et al. 2018). These barriers to access are particularly problematic in rural, nonmetropolitan areas across the country, despite elevated demand for services in many of these areas (President's Commission on Combating Drug Addiction and the Opioid Crisis 2017). For OUD-diagnosed individuals with public or private insurance, prior-authorization requirements, treatment limits, and "fail first" insurance policies (which require that patients must fail to respond to nonmedication treatment alternatives prior to qualifying for MAT coverage) are among the major barriers faced. It is true that coverage for some T2D medications also requires initial "fail first" trials with inexpensive medications, but those policies are largely based on evidence-based, guideline-concordant care (American Diabetes Association 2018b).

Ineffective Institutionalized Treatment Approaches

Not only is evidence-based treatment for OUD inaccessible to many, but also the public understanding of addiction as a moral failure has historically led to ineffective, unappealing, short-term, and often punitive approaches to addiction treatment (Meara and Frank 2005). A prime example of such an approach is hospital-based detoxification without provision of aftercare, which continues to be the modal type of "treatment episode" year after year. This type of short-term care has never been shown to be effective in sustaining any of the goals of care or recovery, and it is quite expensive.

As indicated, addiction treatment services continue to be offered by separate legacy "programs" that typically offer only one part of the continuum of care (e.g., residential or intensive outpatient treatment). These piecemeal programs remain in practice because of long-standing, segregated, predominantly state-run licensing and funding regulations. The inherent design of these segmented programs prevents personalized care, impedes the movement of patients across the care continuum, and inhibits long-term monitoring of and support for recovery. Engagement in long-term treatment often requires patients to navigate transitions in care settings and providers, many involving significant delays and breaks in continuity, thereby contributing to treatment discontinuation and relapse (Williams et al. 2017). When patients do successfully transition to long-term treatment settings, their treatment durations are often significantly less than the 12 months recommended by clinical guidelines (Kampman and Jarvis 2015). Importantly, discontinuation of OUD treatment has the same consequences as discontinuation of T2D treatment—that is, rapid relapse of symptoms, resulting in the need for re-treatment, often in a hospital or emergency facility (Fiellin et al. 2008).

The segmented nature of "programmatic" addiction treatment virtually ensures that no single program has the full set of treatment options necessary to promote and sustain recovery. For example, among current opioid treatment programs, fewer than 20% offer injectable naltrexone, and only 25% offer buprenorphine (Substance Abuse and Mental Health Services Administration 2015). Finally, given that a nonphysician workforce delivers the majority of addiction treatment, few treatment programs have the capability to provide medical care for common physical comorbidities or psychiatric care for common mental health comorbidities (e.g., depression, posttraumatic stress disorder).

Recommendations for Improving the Chronic Care of Addiction

Our premise in this chapter is that *severe substance use disorders (i.e., addictions) should be treated and insured using the same methods; by the same clinical teams; and in the same general health care systems that now treat other chronic illnesses.* This is not a new concept. It has been discussed in over 30 years of replicated genetic, pharmacological, neurological, brain imaging, and clinical research papers. That research has been most effectively summarized in the Surgeon General's Report titled "Facing Addiction in America" (Substance Abuse and Mental Health Services Administration 2016).

Of course, problems of access and quality continue in the treatment of diabetes, but in that field there has been significant progress in translating basic and clinical research; most physicians and clinical teams have been trained, equipped, and incentivized to screen for and intervene with patients identified as having risk factors for diabetes. Because of this progress, patients with incipient cases of "pre-diabetes" are routinely helped to manage their health behaviors and to ultimately avoid the pancreatic injuries that are the cardinal marker of the illness. Moreover, even if the illness develops, there are well-developed and highly individualized clinical care regimens that combine one or more medications with during-treatment monitoring of patient symptoms and function, as well as continuing patient and family education and support for a healthier lifestyle. Although a cure is currently not possible, effective "disease control"—defined as normalization of sugar metabolism (HbA1c levels below 6%)—can be expected, as can improved health and functional status that are ultimately self-monitored and self-managed by the patient and family.

In comparison, there is also now a rich basic and clinical research literature on OUD and other addictions. There are research-proven but practical clinical protocols for comprehensive, individualized continuing care for OUD that are cost effective. But as described above and elsewhere (Substance Abuse and Mental Health Services Administration 2016), these research advances have generally not translated into available, accessible addiction care. The legacy system for the treatment of OUD and other addictions was designed in the mid-1960s based on the available, but scientifically inaccurate, conceptions about addiction and was quite purposely segregated from the rest of health care, clinically, administratively, financially, and culturally. Put simply, the system as currently structured simply cannot deliver evidence-based care and is incompatible with the concepts and methods used in the chronic care model of treatment used for other chronic illnesses. The remedy is full and immediate integration of prevention and treatment of OUD into the rest of mainstream health care, reserving specialty care for those individuals with severe cases that require additional care coordination.

Full integration of the continuum of services for substance use disorders into mainstream health care systems would likely significantly improve the quality, effectiveness, and safety of *all* health care. In regard to the treatment of patients with mild- to moderate-severity OUD, we recommend adaptation of the current CCM by existing care management teams within mainstream health care. Individuals with substance use disorders at all levels of severity can benefit from treatment, and research shows that integrating substance use disorder treatment into mainstream health care can improve the quality of treatment services. Using T2D as a benchmark, we make four key recommendations to promote integration of OUD treatment into mainstream health care systems.

Recommendation 1

Increase treatment capacity as well as availability of/access to care by treating the majority of OUD cases in primary care settings, reserving specialty care for individuals with severe cases needing additional structured management. The goals of substance use disorder treatment are very similar to the treatment goals for other chronic illnesses—to eliminate or reduce the primary symptoms (substance use), improve general health and functioning, and enhance the motivation and skills needed by patients and their families to manage threats of relapse. Even serious substance use disorders can be treated effectively, and can achieve reductions in recurrence rates equivalent to those achieved in other chronic illnesses such as diabetes, asthma, or hypertension. With comprehensive continuing care, recovery is an attainable outcome; more than 25 million individuals with a previous substance use disorder are estimated to be in remission (Substance Abuse and Mental Health Services Administration 2016).

However, the notable separation of substance use disorder treatment from the rest of health care has contributed to the lack of understanding of the medical nature of these conditions, lack of awareness among affected individuals that they have a significant health problem, and slow adoption of scientifically supported medical treatments by addiction treatment providers. Additionally, mainstream health care has been inadequately prepared to address the prevalent substance misuse–related problems of patients in many clinical settings. This has contributed to incorrect diagnoses, inappropriate treatment plans, poor adherence to treatment plans by patients, and high rates of emergency department and hospital admissions.

Recommendation 2

Enhance training, education, and workforce development to support capacity expansion across all health care disciplines, including physicians, nurse practitioners, psychologists, counselors, dentists, social workers, and peer recovery specialists. Integration of mental health and substance use disorder care into general health care will not be possible without a workforce that is competently cross-educated and trained in all of these areas. Only a minority of U.S. medical schools and residencies offer separate courses on addiction medicine or addiction medicine residencies. Similarly, a minority of training programs for other front-line health care professionals (e.g., physician assistant, nursing, pharmacy) require completion of separate addiction coursework or training (National Center on Addiction and Substance Abuse at Columbia University 2012). Federal education grants and low-cost loans for medical, nursing, and pharmacy students should require that the receiving educational institution have at least one required one-semester course on substance use disorders. Similarly, associations of clinical professionals should maintain their provision of continuing education and training courses—especially online courses—for those already in practice. Finally, practitioners' willingness and ability to prescribe medications for substance use disorders could be improved if there were a single, comprehensive prescriber module covering both controlled substances and all approved medications for treating substance use disorders. Ideally, this course module would include the current CDC guidelines for prescribing opioids, but its scope should be extended to also include training in other controlled substances and in the prescribing of all approved addiction treatment medications. Passing this standardized course module would serve to fulfill requirements for both a U.S. Drug Enforcement Administration authorization to prescribe all controlled substances and a current Substance Abuse and Mental Health Services Administration "waiver" to prescribe buprenorphine.

Recommendation 3

Implement and continue to evaluate evidence-based models to promote patient movement across the continuum of care and enhance collaboration between mainstream health care and specialty providers. This integration will not occur without robust policy changes at the federal and state levels. The federal government should immediately review the regulations governing clinical information exchange to harmonize those governing addiction treatment (i.e., 42 CFR Part 2) with those governing the rest of health care (i.e., the Health Insurance Portability and Accountability Act). This single act would markedly expand clinical interactions and create a broader market for improved clinical tracking and patient management software systems. States have substantial power to shape the nature of care within these programs. State licensing and financing policies should be designed to provide better financial incentives for addiction treatment programs that offer the following: 1) the full continuum of care (residential, outpatient, continuing monitoring, and recovery supports); 2) a full range of evidence-based behavioral treatments and medications; and 3) functional affiliations with general and mental health care professionals to integrate care. This is recommended to gradually move away from the existing set of state-licensed but unconnected and segmented standalone addiction treatment programs that simply cannot offer most evidence-based care.

Recommendation 4

Enforce parity in insurance coverage for services, reduce unnecessary payment barriers, and provide fiscal incentives for practices to integrate screening, early intervention, treatment, and recovery support services for addiction. Within general health care, federal and state educational, training, and clinical research grants to advance and further develop chronic care treatment models should explicitly require inclusion of substance use disorders as part of the eligibility requirements. Importantly, efforts at the federal level (Health and Human Services) and at the state level (state attorneys general; state insurance commissioners) should be undertaken to enforce the existing Parity Act legislation that will provide the financial incentives for this integration.

Conclusion

The goals of substance use disorder treatment are very similar to the treatment goals for other chronic illnesses: eliminate or reduce the primary symptoms (substance use), improve general health and function, and increase the motivation and skills of patients and their families to manage threats of relapse. Even serious substance use disorders can be treated effectively, achieving reductions in recurrence rates equivalent to those achieved in other chronic illnesses, such as diabetes, asthma, or hypertension. Integrated treatment can dramatically improve patient health and quality of life, reduce fatalities, address health disparities, and reduce societal costs that result from unrecognized and untreated substance use disorders among patients in the general health care system. However, most existing substance use disorder treatment programs lack the needed training, personnel, and infrastructure to provide treatment for co-occurring physical and mental illnesses. Similarly, most physicians, nurses, and other health care professionals working in general health care settings have not received training in screening, diagnosing, or treating substance use disorders, resulting in key gaps in parity between chronic care models for OUD compared with chronic care models for T2D. Increased legislative attention resulting from the current opioid epidemic crisis may provide a unique opportunity to bring OUD management and treatment paradigms into better alignment with management and treatment paradigms found to be effective for other chronic diseases.

References

Agency for Healthcare Research and Quality: Mean Expenses per Person with Care for Selected Conditions by Type of Service: United States, 2014. Medical Expenditure Panel Survey Household Component Data. 2016. Available at: https://meps.ahrq.gov/mepsweb/survey_comp/household.jsp. Accessed August 18, 2020.

Ali MK, Bullard KM, Gregg EW: Achievement of goals in U.S. Diabetes Care, 1999–2010. N Engl J Med 369(3):287–288, 2013 23863067

Ali MK, Bullard KM, Gregg EW, Del Rio C: A cascade of care for diabetes in the United States: visualizing the gaps. Ann Intern Med 161(10):681–689, 2014 25402511

American Diabetes Association: Economic costs of diabetes in the U.S. in 2017. Diabetes Care 41(5):917–928, 2018a 29567642

American Diabetes Association: Updates to the standards of medical care in diabetes—2018. Diabetes Care 41(9):2045–2047, 2018b 30135199

American Public Health Association: Prevention and Intervention Strategies to Decrease Misuse of Prescription Pain Medication. Policy Statements, No 20154, 2015. Available at: https://www.apha.org/policies-and-advocacy/public-health-policy-statements/policy-database/2015/12/08/15/11/prevention-and-intervention-strategies-to-decrease-misuse-of-prescription-pain-medication. Accessed November 10, 2019.

Andrews C, Abraham A, Grogan CM, et al: Despite resources from the ACA, most states do little to help addiction treatment programs implement health care reform. Health Aff (Millwood) 34(5):828–835, 2015 25941285

Barnett AI, Hall W, Fry CL, et al: Drug and alcohol treatment providers' views about the disease model of addiction and its impact on clinical practice: a systematic review. Drug Alcohol Rev 37(6):697–720, 2018 29239048

Bernstein SL, D'Onofrio G: Screening, treatment initiation, and referral for substance use disorders. Addict Sci Clin Pract 12(1):18, 2017 28780906

Blanco C, Iza M, Schwartz RP, et al: Probability and predictors of treatment-seeking for prescription opioid use disorders: a national study. Drug Alcohol Depend 131(1–2):143–148, 2013 23306097

Bruneau J, Ahamad K, Goyer ME, et al: Management of opioid use disorders: a national clinical practice guideline. CMAJ 190(9):E247–E257, 2018 29507156

Burstin H, Johnson K: Getting to better care and outcomes for diabetes through measurement. Am J Manag Care 22(4 Spec No.):SP145–SP146, 2016 29381308

Center for Behavioral Health and Statistics and Quality: Behavioral Trends in the United States: Results From the 2014 National Survey on Drug Use and Health (HHS Publ No SMA-15-4927, NSDUH Series H-50). Rockville, MD, Substance Abuse and Mental Health Services Administration, 2015

Centers for Disease Control and Prevention: Crude and Age-Adjusted Percentage of Adults With Diabetes Using Any Diabetes Medication, United States, 1997–2011. Diabetes Public Health Resource, 2012. Available at: https://www.cdc.gov/diabetes/statistics/meduse/fig3.htm. Accessed November 10, 2019.

Centers for Disease Control and Prevention: Excessive Drinking Costs US $249 Billion. 2014a. Available at: https://www.cdc.gov/features/costsofdrinking/index.html. Accessed July 7, 2020.

Centers for Disease Control and Prevention: National Diabetes Statistics Report: Estimates of Diabetes and Its Burden in the United States. U.S. Department of Health and Human Services, 2014b. Available at: https://www.cdc.gov/diabetes/pdfs/data/2014-report-estimates-of-diabetes-and-its-burden-in-the-united-states.pdf. Accessed November 10, 2019.

Centers for Disease Control and Prevention: New CDC report: More than 100 million Americans have diabetes or prediabetes. Press Release: July 18, 2017. Available at: https://www.cdc.gov/media/releases/2017/p0718-diabetes-report.html. Accessed July 6, 2020.

Centers for Disease Control and Prevention: National Diabetes Statistics Report, 2020: Estimates of Diabetes and Its Burden in the United States. Atlanta, GA, Centers for Disease Control and Prevention, U.S. Department of Health and Human Services, 2020. Available at: https://www.cdc.gov/diabetes/pdfs/data/statistics/national-diabetes-statistics-report.pdf. Accessed July 7, 2020.

Chou R, Korthuis PT, Weimer M, et al: Medication-Assisted Treatment Models of Care for Opioid Use Disorder in Primary Care Settings. Technical Brief No. 28. (Prepared by the Pacific Northwest Evidence-based Practice Center under Contract No. 290-2015-00009-I.) AHRQ Publ. No. 16(17)-EHC039-EF. Rockville, MD, Agency for Healthcare Research and Quality, December 2016. Available at: https://effectivehealthcare.ahrq.gov/sites/default/files/pdf/opioid-use-disorder_technical-brief.pdf. Accessed July 7, 2020.

Davenport S, Matthews K: Opioid use disorder in the United States: diagnosed prevalence by payer, age, sex, and state. Milliman White Paper, March 2018. Available at: https://www.milliman.com/-/media/Milliman/importedfiles/uploadedFiles/insight/2018/opioid_use_disorder_prevalence.ashx. Accessed July 6, 2020.

Fiellin DA, Moore BA, Sullivan LE, et al: Long-term treatment with buprenorphine/naloxone in primary care: results at 2–5 years. Am J Addict 17(2):116–120, 2008 18393054

Fleming BB, Greenfield S, Engelgau MM, et al: The Diabetes Quality Improvement Project: moving science into health policy to gain an edge on the diabetes epidemic. Diabetes Care 24(10):1815–1820, 2001 11574448

Frank LE, Nagel SK: Addiction and moralization: the role of the underlying model of addiction. Neuroethics 10(1):129–139, 2017 28725284

García-Pérez LE, Alvarez M, Dilla T, et al: Adherence to therapies in patients with type 2 diabetes. Diabetes Ther 4(2):175–194, 2013 23990497

Gomes T, Tadrous M, Mamdani MM, et al: The burden of opioid-related mortality in the United States. JAMA Netw Open 1(2):e180217, 2018 30646062

Goodman RA, Posner SF, Huang ES, et al: Defining and measuring chronic conditions: imperatives for research, policy, program, and practice. Prev Chronic Dis 10:E66, 2013 23618546

Haffajee RL, Bohnert ASB, Lagisetty PA: Policy pathways to address provider workforce barriers to buprenorphine treatment. Am J Prev Med 54 (6 suppl 3):S230–S242, 2018 29779547

Johnson K, Jones C, Compton W, et al: Federal response to the opioid crisis. Curr HIV/AIDS Rep 15(4):293–301, 2018 29968173

Kaiser Permanente: Type 2 Diabetes Screening and Treatment Guideline. Kaiser Permanente Clinical Guidelines, Washington State, April 2019. Available at: https://wa.kaiserpermanente.org/static/pdf/public/guidelines/diabetes2.pdf. Accessed November 10, 2019.

Kampman K, Jarvis M: American Society of Addiction Medicine (ASAM) National Practice Guideline for the Use of Medications in the Treatment of Addiction Involving Opioid Use. J Addict Med 9(5):358–367, 2015 26406300

Knowler WC, Fowler SE, Hamman RF, et al: 10-year follow-up of diabetes incidence and weight loss in the Diabetes Prevention Program Outcomes Study. Lancet 374(9702):1677–1686, 2009 19878986

Kopak AM: Breaking the addictive cycle of the system: improving US criminal justice practices to address substance use disorders. Int J Prison Health 11(1):4–16, 2015 25751703

Liu NF, Brown AS, Folias AE, et al: Stigma in people with type 1 or type 2 diabetes. Clin Diabetes 35(1):27–34, 2017 28144043

Maglione MA, Raaen L, Chen C, et al: Effects of medication assisted treatment (MAT) for opioid use disorder on functional outcomes: a systematic review. J Subst Abuse Treat 89:28–51, 2018 29706172

Mainous AG 3rd, Tanner RJ, Baker R: Prediabetes diagnosis and treatment in primary care. J Am Board Fam Med 29(2):283–285, 2016 26957387

Mark TL, Wier LM, Malone K, et al: National estimates of behavioral health conditions and their treatment among adults newly insured under the ACA. Psychiatr Serv 66(4):426–429, 2015 25555031

McBain RK, Dick A, Sorbero M, Stein BD: Growth and distribution of buprenorphine-waivered providers in the United States, 2007–2017. Ann Intern Med 172(7):504–506, 2020 31905379

McCulloch DK, Nathan DM, Mulder JE: Overview of medical care in adults with diabetes mellitus. UpToDate, October 20, 2019. Available at: https://www.uptodate.com/contents/overview-of-medical-care-in-adults-with-diabetes-mellitus. Accessed November 10, 2019.

McLellan AT, Skipper GS, Campbell M, et al: Five year outcomes in a cohort study of physicians treated for substance use disorders in the United States. BMJ 337:a2038, 2008 18984632

Meara E, Frank RG: Spending on substance abuse treatment: how much is enough? Addiction 100(9):1240–1248, 2005 16128713

Meinhofer A, Witman AE: The role of health insurance on treatment for opioid use disorders: evidence from the Affordable Care Act Medicaid expansion. J Health Econ 60:177–197, 2018 29990675

Mertens JR, Lu YW, Parthasarathy S, et al: Medical and psychiatric conditions of alcohol and drug treatment patients in an HMO: comparison with matched controls. Arch Intern Med 163(20):2511–2517, 2003 14609789

Nathan PE, Conrad M, Skinstad AH: History of the concept of addiction. Annu Rev Clin Psychol 12:29–51, 2016 26565120

National Center on Addiction and Substance Abuse at Columbia University: Addiction Medicine: Closing the Gap Between Science and Practice. June 2012. Available at: https://drugfree.org/reports/addiction-medicine-closing-the-gap-between-science-and-practice/. Accessed August 14, 2020.

National Institute on Drug Abuse: Medications to treat opioid use disorder: How much does opioid treatment cost? June 2018. Available at: https://www.drugabuse.gov/publications/research-reports/medications-to-treat-opioid-addiction/how-much-does-opioid-treatment-cost. Accessed July 6, 2020.

Nerat T, Locatelli I, Kos M: Type 2 diabetes: cost-effectiveness of medication adherence and lifestyle interventions. Patient Prefer Adherence 10:2039–2049, 2016 27757024

Parchman ML, Zeber JE, Romero RR, et al: Risk of coronary artery disease in type 2 diabetes and the delivery of care consistent with the chronic care model in primary care settings: a STARNet study. Med Care 45(12):1129–1134, 2007 18007162

President's Commission on Combating Drug Addiction and the Opioid Crisis: Final Report of the President's Commission on Combating Drug Addiction and the Opioid Crisis. 2017. Available at: https://www.whitehouse.gov/sites/whitehouse.gov/files/images/Final_Report_Draft_11-1-2017.pdf. Accessed November 10, 2019.

Riazi H, Larijani B, Langarizadeh M, et al: Managing diabetes mellitus using information technology: a systematic review. J Diabetes Metab Disord 14:49, 2015 26075190

Ronquest NA, Willson TM, Montejano LB, et al: Relationship between buprenorphine adherence and relapse, health care utilization and costs in privately and publicly insured patients with opioid use disorder. Subst Abuse Rehabil 9:59–78, 2018 30310349

Rosenblatt RA, Andrilla CH, Catlin M, et al: Geographic and specialty distribution of US physicians trained to treat opioid use disorder. Ann Fam Med 13(1):23–26, 2015 25583888

Roy K, Miller M: Parity and the medicalization of addiction treatment. J Psychoactive Drugs 42(2):115–120, 2010 20648906

Rutledge SA, Masalovich S, Blacher RJ, et al: Diabetes self-management education programs in nonmetropolitan counties—United States, 2016. MMWR Surveill Summ 66(10):1–6, 2017 28448482

Sandoe E, Fry CE, Frank RG: Policy Levers That States Can Use to Improve Opioid Addiction Treatment and Address the Opioid Epidemic. Health Affairs Blog, October 2, 2018. Accessed October 10, 2018. Available at: https://www.healthaffairs.org/do/10.1377/hblog20180927.51221/full/. Accessed November 10, 2019.

Seth P, Scholl L, Rudd RA, et al: Overdose deaths involving opioids, cocaine, and psychostimulants—United States, 2015–2016. MMWR Morb Mortal Wkly Rep 67(12):349–358, 2018 29596405

Siu AL; U.S. Preventive Services Task Force: Screening for abnormal blood glucose and type 2 diabetes mellitus: U.S. preventive services task force recommendation statement. Ann Intern Med 163(11):861–868, 2015 26501513

Stellefson M, Dipnarine K, Stopka C: The chronic care model and diabetes management in US primary care settings: a systematic review. Prev Chronic Dis 10:E26, 2013 23428085

Stokes A, Preston SH: Deaths attributable to diabetes in the United States: comparison of data sources and estimation approaches. PLoS One 12(1):e0170219, 2017 28121997

Substance Abuse and Mental Health Services Administration: National Survey of Substance Abuse Treatment Services (N-SSATS): 2015: Data on Substance Abuse Treatment Facilities. BHSIS Series S-88, HHS Publ No SMA-17-5031. 2015. Available at: https://www.samhsa.gov/data/sites/default/files/2015_National_Survey_of_Substance_Abuse_Treatment_Services.pdf. Accessed November 10, 2019.

Substance Abuse and Mental Health Services Administration: Reports of the Surgeon General Facing Addiction in America: The Surgeon General's Report on Alcohol, Drugs, and Health. Washington, DC, U.S. Department of Health and Human Services, 2016

Tsai AC, Morton SC, Mangione CM, Keeler EB: A meta-analysis of interventions to improve care for chronic illnesses. Am J Manag Care 11(8):478–488, 2005 16095434

U.S. Preventive Services Task Force, Krist AH, Davidson KW, et al: Screening for unhealthy drug use: US Preventive Services Task Force Recommendation Statement. JAMA 323(22):2301–2309, 2020 3251582

Venner KL, Sánchez V, Garcia J, et al: Moving away from the tip of the pyramid: screening and brief intervention for risky alcohol and opioid use in underserved patients. J Am Board Fam Med 31(2):243–251, 2018 29535241

Volkow ND, Koob GF, McLellan AT: Neurobiologic advances from the brain disease model of addiction. N Engl J Med 374(4):363–371, 2016 26816013

Williams AR, Nunes E, Olfson M: To Battle the Opioid Overdose Epidemic, Deploy the Cascade of Care Model. Health Affairs Blog, March 13, 2017. Available at: https://www.healthaffairs.org/do/10.1377/hblog20170313.059163/full/. Accessed November 10, 2019.

PART III

Specific Substances of Abuse:
Neurobiology and Pharmacotherapy

CHAPTER 8

Neurobiology of Alcohol

Markus Heilig, M.D., Ph.D.
Rainer Spanagel, Ph.D.

In this chapter we provide a summary of the molecular and neural mechanisms by which alcohol acts on the brain to promote the development of addiction in vulnerable individuals. We first define the terminology to be used, and then proceed to giving an account of interactions of alcohol with ligand-gated ion channels and G protein–coupled receptors, respectively. We next describe the complex effects of alcohol at the systems level that result from its multiple molecular effects, specifically focusing on the composite, biphasic nature of these systemic effects, with one phase being dominated by effects that are anxiolytic, sedative, and ataxic and the other being dominated by psychomotor stimulant–like and rewarding effects. We discuss individual vulnerability factors that interact with this composite profile of alcohol's actions and promote the development of addiction, in particular highlighting how genetics mediate low sedative/ataxic responses and prominent rewarding responses to alcohol, respectively. The subsequent section discusses neurobiological mechanisms underlying craving and relapse, with a focus on how alcohol-associated cues gain control over attention and reward seeking as addiction develops. We then discuss neuroadaptive changes in the brain that occur over the course of using alcohol, and how these neuroadaptations promote alcohol seeking and use to alleviate the stress and negative emotions that emerge with the progression of alcohol addiction. Finally, we highlight the role of impulsive decision making as both a risk factor for and a consequence of heavy alcohol use. In closing, we suggest that an improved understanding of the mechanisms summarized in this chapter may help identify targets for treatments for alcohol addiction, a devastating disease with large unmet medical needs.

Terminology

The active ingredient in "alcoholic" drinks, ethyl alcohol (or "ethanol" for short), is just one among the many organic chemicals called alcohols. Other alcohols are also present in our everyday lives. For instance, methanol and butanol are used as fuels or solvents, and the sugar alcohol xylitol is used in the food-processing industry (e.g., in "sugar free" chewing gum). It would therefore be useful if we could consistently refer to the form of alcohol used and abused by humans by its proper term, ethanol. But then, for consistency, we would perhaps also have to refer to the disorder as *ethanolism* rather than *alcoholism*. That is not a realistic proposition, given how firmly the latter term is established in the literature and in the public consciousness. For that reason, we will use the term *alcohol* throughout this chapter, although readers should bear in mind that unless stated otherwise, what we are referring to by that name is in fact ethanol.

There is broad agreement that a significant proportion—perhaps around 15%—of people who use alcohol develop a pathological relationship with the drug and continue to use it at the expense of healthy rewards, and despite knowledge of adverse consequences (Anthony et al. 1994). Yet the terms used to refer to this relationship keep changing. What was once referred to as *alcohol dependence* would in the DSM-5 era correspond to "alcohol use disorder, moderate to severe." That is not a very nimble term, and patients of course will continue to refer to their condition as "alcoholism." In the following sections, we will use the term *alcoholism* to denote alcohol addiction.

History

After humans settled down as farmers about 10,000 years ago, they learned how to use yeast to ferment sugars obtained from the crops. As early as 9,000 years ago, beer brewing was commonplace in the late Stone Age village of Jiahu in northern China. Hieroglyphic inscriptions from ancient Egypt of about 6,000 years ago describe production and consumption of wine. Recipes for making wine or beer are also found on clay tablets from Mesopotamia dated about a millennium later. In ancient Greece, fermented honey—mead—seems to have been the original alcoholic beverage, but wine-producing skills reached Greece in about 2000 B.C. Alcoholic beverages at that time were not necessarily consumed for their taste or intoxicating properties. Fermented beverages also provided a certain degree of protection against growth of microbes in drinking supplies. Because of this, fluid consumption in areas where fresh water was not readily available could to a large extent consist of beer or wine. Likewise, when ships went to sea, drinking supplies brought on board were often not in the form of water, but rather of beer. The alcohol content of these beverages was typically relatively low, probably not exceeding 4%. The protection afforded against the growth of bacteria was thus not optimal, given that alcohol is most effective as a disinfectant at concentrations around 70%.

Fermented beverages typically do not reach an alcohol content beyond approximately 15%. At higher concentrations, the yeast that produce alcohol from sugar die or become unable to maintain production. The concentration of alcohol in alcoholic beverages is an important factor, because a general principle of drug reward is that the rate at which drug concentrations rise in the brain in part determines the intensity of the "high"—and therefore the addictive potential—of the drug. It is difficult to work up a rapid rise of blood alcohol concentrations using beverages with low alcohol content. Acquiring the knowledge to make distilled spirits was therefore a landmark in the relationship between humans and alcohol. It is thought that the process of distillation was picked up from Arab chemists by the Salerno School of Medicine in southern Italy and was initially applied to produce alcohol quantities useful for human consumption in the twelfth century. By the thirteenth century, this expertise had spread to the rest of Europe. By the fourteenth century, the use of distilled spirits as medicinal elixirs was widespread, for instance, to provide protection or cure from the Black Death.

Basic Mechanisms of Action

Alcohol is unique among addictive drugs in the way it produces its brain actions. In contrast to opioids or stimulants, for example, alcohol does not have a unique molecular target in the central nervous system (CNS)—that is, it does not bind with high affinity to any specific neurotransmitter receptor or transporter. This fundamental difference is the reason why alcohol is psychoactive only at brain levels that are much higher than those required for other addictive substances. For instance, opioids are active at nanomolar concentrations. In contrast, the legal limit for alcohol intoxication in most states, 80 mg/dL, corresponds to a concentration of more than 17 mmol/L, whereas anesthetic effects are reached at concentrations of as much as 190 mmol/L. The lack of very specific high-affinity targets helps explain why the actions of alcohol are so complex and widely variable among individuals, much more so than the effects of most other addictive drugs. Also, because the amounts of alcohol that are typically consumed are, on a molar basis, about three orders of magnitude greater than the amounts consumed for other addictive drugs, the enzymes that metabolize alcohol become saturated. This results in elimination that follows zero-order (linear) kinetics, as opposed to the first-order kinetics seen for drugs acting at high affinities, and therefore in small amounts.

Because no high-affinity target for alcohol could be identified, it was once thought that the actions of alcohol in the brain were caused through effects on nerve cell membranes. As an organic solvent, alcohol was thought to enter these lipid bilayers and alter their properties. This in turn was thought to influence neurotransmitter receptors and transporters embedded in the membranes. In fact, although the very first steps in the actions of alcohol are still not entirely clear, proteins rather than lipids appear to be the primary targets. Current evidence supports the notion that alcohol enters pockets encoded by a conserved amino acid motif that is found in numerous transmembrane proteins (Kruse et al. 2003). A prototype for these pockets, called LUSH, is an odorant receptor in *Drosophila*. When the crystal structure of this protein was resolved, it was found that a group of three amino acids forms a network of hydrogen bonds between the protein and alcohol, providing the structural motif for alcohol binding. This motif seems to have been conserved in a number of mammalian ligand-gated ion channels that are directly implicated in the pharmacological effects of alcohol (Kruse et al. 2003). A similar motif is also found in a particularly alcohol-sensitive isoform (AC7) of the signal transduction enzyme adenylyl cyclase (Harris et al. 2008).

Among ligand-gated ion channels, glutamatergic, γ-aminobutyric acid (GABA)–ergic, and glycine-binding receptors are key mediators of alcohol's acute effects. Through concerted actions on these systems, alcohol intake results for the most part in CNS suppression. Alcohol acutely dampens glutamatergic transmission by de-

creasing the ion flux through the *N*-methyl-D-aspartate (NMDA) receptor upon its activation. Alcohol also potentiates GABA transmission by increasing the chloride flux
through $GABA_A$ receptors when these are activated, and probably also by increasing
presynaptic GABA release.

Because glutamate and GABA systems are so fundamental for the millisecond-to-
millisecond communication between nerve cells throughout the brain, the "first hit"
of alcohol on these primary targets results in an unusually broad range of secondary
effects. Among these effects are actions on systems that play a key role in reward from
addictive drugs, importantly including the dopamine, endorphin, and endocannabinoid systems (Spanagel 2009). In experimental animal studies, genetic deletion of
either μ-opioid or cannabinoid type 1 (CB_1) receptors decreases both alcohol consumption and measures of alcohol reward. Animal studies further indicate that endorphins are released by alcohol in several brain structures, including the ventral tegmental area, the origin of the classic dopamine projection thought to make up a final
common reward pathway. Endorphin release triggered by alcohol in this area is
thought to remove inhibitory tone from the dopamine cells, leading to their disinhibition and resulting in increased dopamine release in their terminal areas in the nucleus accumbens. Alcohol intake also results in endorphin release in the nucleus
accumbens itself. Although the ventral tegmental area is not easily visualized with
positron emission tomography (PET), alcohol-induced endorphin release in the nucleus accumbens and in regions of the prefrontal cortex has been confirmed in the
human brain through use of this methodology (Mitchell et al. 2012). Alcohol-induced
dopamine release in the nucleus accumbens had previously been demonstrated
through use of PET (Boileau et al. 2003). In agreement with these data, functional
magnetic resonance imaging (fMRI) studies have shown that alcohol triggers activation of the human nucleus accumbens and that this activation correlates strongly with
the subjective feeling of intoxication (Gilman et al. 2008).

Alcohol-associated stimuli appear to induce cravings in part by activating the same
circuitry as that involved in mediating reward from alcohol. A meta-analysis of functional brain imaging studies showed that the nucleus accumbens/ventral striatum is
activated by alcohol-associated cues. This activation is correlated with subjective cravings, overlaps with activations seen in response to natural rewards (Noori et al. 2016),
and is attenuated by successful treatment (Schacht et al. 2013). Endogenous opioids
also appear to play a role in alcohol craving through actions exerted locally in the nucleus accumbens, but the exact mechanism is unclear. An original PET study reported
that abstinent alcohol-dependent patients displayed an increase in μ-opioid receptors
in the ventral striatum, including the nucleus accumbens, and that this correlated with
the severity of patients' alcohol craving (Heinz et al. 2005). More recently, however, an
analysis of postmortem brain tissue from alcohol-dependent individuals showed
markedly lower, rather than higher, μ-opioid receptor densities (Hermann et al. 2017).

Complex Actions of Alcohol: A Composite of Stimulant and Sedative/Ataxic Effects

By acting on multiple targets, alcohol has the potential to produce a wide range of
effects. In general, limited quantities of alcohol dampen anxiety, cause behavioral dis-

inhibition, and produce varying degrees of psychomotor stimulation. Higher alcohol levels instead tend to produce more pronounced CNS depressant actions, resulting in ataxia, progressive cognitive impairment, and transient anterograde amnesia ("blackouts," or, if incomplete, "grayouts"). With consumption of still higher amounts of alcohol, the broadly depressant effects become dominant, producing sleep, unconsciousness, and ultimately death due to respiratory depression. These multifaceted effects of alcohol are classically described as a biphasic progression, in which the first phase is dominated by the anxiolytic, rewarding, and stimulant-like actions, which then become overshadowed by the depressant effects at higher doses. This biphasic nature of the dose-response relationship is useful for didactic purposes, but it is important to recognize that it represents an idealization. Because so many different actions combine to produce the net effect of alcohol on the brain, there is great potential for individual variation, and that is indeed what is observed. Genetic factors, early life experience, prior drug exposure history, and current environmental influences are all able to shape the response to alcohol in important ways.

The aspect of individual variation in sensitivity to alcohol that has received perhaps the most attention is the differential sensitivity people show to alcohol's sedative and ataxic actions. The heritability of alcoholism is in the range of 50%–60% (Goldman et al. 2005). When sons of alcoholic parents and sons of parents without alcohol problems were followed before subjects in either group had developed any alcohol problems of their own, a low level of sedative/ataxic response to alcohol—measured, for example, as magnitude of body sway—was found among the sons of alcoholic parents. Because this study design eliminated the potential confounds of tolerance and other consequences of alcohol consumption, the results showed that the low sedative/ataxic response to alcohol is a phenotypic marker of genetic alcoholism risk (Schuckit 1994). On the basis of these findings, it was hypothesized that this trait may place people at higher risk in part because they lack the protection against heavy drinking afforded by sensitivity to alcohol-induced sedation. In this scenario, the rewarding and stimulant-like actions of alcohol would remain unopposed and thus would continue to dominate the drinking experience, even after high levels of alcohol intake.

In fact, the role of "low alcohol response" in humans seems to be somewhat more complex. A phenomenon called "acute functional tolerance" refers to the observation that a given blood alcohol level (BAL) produces a greater degree of sedative/ataxic effects on the ascending limb of the BAL curve than when BALs decline. According to a proposed "differentiator" model, an important aspect of individual variation in sensitivity to alcohol is the extent to which an individual develops acute functional tolerance (Newlin and Thomson 1990). More recently, King et al. (2016) showed that while heavy drinkers indeed exhibit lower sensitivity to the sedative and cortisol release–inducing effects of alcohol, they also show higher reactivity to alcohol's stimulating and rewarding effects. This ambitious effort followed a cohort of heavy and light drinkers over time, and also showed that in heavy drinkers with symptom trajectories leading to alcohol dependence, heightened alcohol stimulation and reward persisted over time (King et al. 2016). In contrast, heavy drinkers with trajectories associated with no (or only low levels of) dependence symptoms showed reduced alcohol stimulation over time and lower reward throughout the follow-up.

Whatever the mechanism, people with low sensitivity to alcohol's depressant actions are clearly able to consume larger amounts of the drug with predominantly rewarding and stimulant-like consequences. At the other end of the spectrum, in people with high sensitivity to alcohol's CNS depressant effects, an initial reduction of tension and anxiety at low alcohol doses may be followed by sedation as doses increase, thereby limiting intake. Importantly, this "brake" on consumption may still be removed if the individual engages in frequent consumption over long periods, resulting in tolerance. An important implication is that if a preexisting anxiety disorder provides an incentive for regular use of alcohol for its anxiolytic properties, an individual might be able to develop enough tolerance to ultimately escalate the amounts consumed to levels otherwise achieved by people with an inborn low response to alcohol's sedative/ataxic effects.

Biological Substrates of Individual Variation in Alcohol Reward

Urban et al. (2010) reported that individuals vary widely in their response both to alcohol's sedative/ataxic actions and to its rewarding and psychomotor stimulant–like effects. Perhaps the most fundamental aspect of this variation is its sex dependence; human PET data have shown that the nucleus accumbens dopamine response to alcohol is markedly more pronounced in men than in women. This finding led these authors to hypothesize that a corresponding higher alcohol reward may contribute to the well-established difference in alcoholism risk between men and women, reflected in the approximately 2:1 male:female prevalence ratio for this disorder (Urban et al. 2010).

Furthermore, individuals who have a family history positive for alcoholism show a more pronounced response to the rewarding and stimulant-like effects of alcohol. This enhanced response may be related to differences in opioid signaling, given that these individuals are also preferentially sensitive to blockade of alcohol's stimulant-like actions by the μ-preferring opioid antagonist naltrexone, and also given that male sex and family history of alcoholism are predictors of a clinical response to naltrexone (Garbutt et al. 2014). Collectively, these observations indicate that μ-opioid receptors are critically involved in the rewarding and stimulant-like effects of alcohol.

Given the importance of opioid signaling in alcohol reward, genetic variation within this system could potentially contribute to differential sensitivity to the rewarding effects of alcohol. Functional genetic variation is present at the gene locus that encodes the μ-opioid receptor. This *OPRM1* A118G single nucleotide polymorphism (SNP) encodes an amino acid exchange in the receptor protein (Bond et al. 1998). Among healthy social drinkers, carriers of the minor 118G allele at this locus show a more vigorous nucleus accumbens dopamine response to alcohol, a finding also replicated in humanized mice carrying the respective human receptor variants (Ramchandani et al. 2011). Direct evaluation of naltrexone in these mouse lines showed an enhanced ability of this medication to suppress alcohol intake in 118G allele carriers (Bilbao et al. 2015). These findings suggest that *OPRM1* A118G variation may serve as a predictor of clinical naltrexone response, thereby offering a potential strategy for personalizing this treatment. Meta-analyses of clinical naltrexone studies seemed to support this conclusion but were based on retrospective secondary analyses (Garbutt et al. 2014). A subsequent attempt to prospectively evaluate *OPRM1* A118G variation as a predictor of naltrexone response did not detect this effect, but this result was not informative, since the study also did not detect an overall naltrexone effect, irrespective of genotype (Oslin et al. 2015). Thus, this issue remains unresolved.

Of note, the observations of alcohol's effects on brain reward circuitry reviewed above were obtained in healthy, moderate social drinkers. As we have already mentioned (see section "Complex Actions of Alcohol"), drug use history is another critical factor that contributes to individual differences in alcohol response. Accordingly, nucleus accumbens activation in response to alcohol is much attenuated in heavy compared with light drinkers (Gilman et al. 2012). It has been suggested that alcoholic individuals have a decreased availability of dopamine type 2 (D_2) receptors in the nucleus accumbens (Volkow et al. 1996), and animal studies suggest that high D_2 availability may be protective against escalation of alcohol intake (Volkow et al. 2006). It is unclear whether the decreased availability of D_2 receptors in alcohol-dependent persons reflects a preexisting vulnerability, a consequence of heavy alcohol use, or both. Regardless, it has been hypothesized that these changes reflect a hypodopaminergic tone in the reward system and result in a "reward deficit syndrome" in relation to natural reinforcers (Volkow et al. 2019). In combination with a vigorous reward response to alcohol, low sensitivity to alcohol's sedative/ataxic actions as a "brake," or both, this reward deficit state is likely to drive a progression into alcohol addiction. Although this framework is appealing, one investigation has suggested the possibility of a more complex process, in which a hypodopaminergic state would be followed by a reversal into a state of elevated dopamine activity (Hirth et al. 2016).

Craving and Brain Activation in Response to Alcohol-Associated Stimuli

Alcohol-dependent patients commonly experience cravings in response to alcohol-associated stimuli, an observation that is replicated in the laboratory (Monti et al. 1993). Cravings triggered by alcohol-associated stimuli are a powerful predictor of relapse to heavy drinking (Sinha et al. 2011a), a finding consistent with observations that these stimuli trigger alcohol-seeking behavior in experimental animals (Bossert et al. 2013). Cravings and drug seeking arise as a consequence of associative learning that occurs as stimuli are repeatedly paired with the subjective experience of consuming alcohol. Laboratory procedures, both in rodents and in humans, commonly utilize discrete cues such as the smell of alcohol to elicit behavioral responses. In clinical practice, complex contextual stimuli—in particular, those that are of a social nature—are the most powerful triggers of craving and relapse.

Because cravings triggered by alcohol-associated stimuli precede and predict relapse, it was hypothesized that extinguishing these responses would result in clinical benefits. This hypothesis resulted in the development of Cue Exposure Therapy (CET) by Monti and colleagues (Monti 2002). In a meta-analysis of seven available studies, however, only modest evidence in support of CET being effective was found (Mellentin et al. 2017). CET showed only a moderate effect on the latency to relapse, and the overall quality of evidence was graded as low. Similar conclusions have been reached for other substance use disorders (Conklin and Tiffany 2002). The context dependency of extinction learning and the spontaneous renewal of extinguished re-sponses over time pose challenges to this strategy. Nevertheless, naltrexone's clinical efficacy is associated with its ability to attenuate cue-induced cravings (O'Malley et al. 2002).

Patterns of brain activation induced by exposure to alcohol-associated stimuli can be captured by fMRI studies and can provide important insights into the nature of cravings. Schacht et al. (2013) used activation likelihood estimation, a quantitative, coordinate-based meta-analytic method, to analyze the pattern of brain areas acti-vated by alcohol-associated stimuli and to examine whether these neural signatures differed between cases and controls. They also examined potential correlations be-tween self-reported measures of craving and patterns of brain activation. Finally, Schacht and colleagues assessed treatment effects on brain activations induced by alco-hol-associated stimuli. In alcohol-dependent patients, but not in healthy control sub-jects, alcohol-associated stimuli cues elicited robust activation of a limbic-prefrontal network that included the ventral striatum, the anterior cingulate, and the ventro-medial prefrontal cortex (Schacht et al. 2013). This network shows considerable over-lap with structures activated by natural rewards (Noori et al. 2016). Activation in the ventral striatum was correlated with self-reported cravings and was reduced with treatment.

Collectively, these observations suggest that associative learning allows alcohol-associated stimuli to gain control over the activity of reward networks otherwise ac-tivated by alcohol itself, becoming a relapse trigger similar to that of a priming drink. Interventions that effectively suppress brain responses to alcohol-associated stimuli in a context-independent manner are likely to possess therapeutic potential.

Alcohol Dependence–Induced Neuroadaptations

Heavy alcohol consumption over an extended period of time leads to the develop-ment of tolerance, after which cessation of intake results in the emergence of with-drawal (Heilig et al. 2010). The acute alcohol withdrawal syndrome is characterized by a general nervous system hyperexcitability that is largely a mirror image of alco-hols' depressant actions. This hyperexcitability is mainly driven by a rebound hyper-activity of glutamatergic transmission and results in increased anxiety, tremor, and autonomic dysfunction, as well as an increased potential for seizures. After a single heavy-consumption episode, CNS excitability typically normalizes within 3–5 days. Following prolonged exposure of the brain to cycles of intoxication and withdrawal, however, more persistent neuroadaptations begin to emerge and contribute to a pro-gression into addiction.

Escalated alcohol consumption and relapse are among the behavioral hallmarks of this progression. These behaviors are, however, typically accompanied by additional psychopathological manifestations, such as low mood and elevated anxiety in re-sponse to a wide range of stressors, often referred to collectively as a negative emo-tional state. Baseline anxiety, which is elevated during acute withdrawal, declines to normal levels over the course of 3–6 weeks following cessation of heavy alcohol use; however, an increased reactivity to stressors persists for much longer and heightens relapse risk. As patients discover, these manifestations of negative emotionality can be temporarily normalized by resumption of alcohol use, but that solution comes at the expense of further progression of the process that leads to addiction. Along the way, the motivation for alcohol seeking and relapse undergoes a fundamental shift. From initially being driven by positive reinforcement (i.e., "reward"), alcohol use becomes increasingly driven by negative reinforcement (i.e., "relief") (Heilig and Koob 2007) (see next section, "Stress Systems and Progression Into Negatively Reinforced Alcohol Use").

A persistent hyperglutamatergic state is an important element of neuroadaptations that result from a prolonged history of alcohol dependence and contribute to escalation of voluntary alcohol intake (Spanagel et al. 2005). Animal studies have shown that transiently elevated CNS glutamate levels initially observed during acute alcohol withdrawal become more persistent following repeated cycles of alcohol intoxication and withdrawal. A hyperglutamatergic state also contributes to augmented excitatory synaptic plasticity within the reward system. In particular, postsynaptic α-amino-3-hydroxy-5-methyl-4-isoxazolepropionic acid (AMPA) receptor function shows enhanced activation after alcohol self-administration, making reward-mediating neurons more sensitive to alcohol and alcohol-conditioned cues. In sum, enhanced excitatory synaptic plasticity and a hyperglutamatergic state contribute to excessive alcohol consumption, and human magnetic resonance spectroscopy studies support the notion that these observations translate to the human condition (Hermann et al. 2012; Umhau et al. 2010). The functional glutamate antagonist acamprosate is able to normalize elevated CNS glutamate levels both in experimental animals and in alcohol-dependent individuals. Meanwhile, work in mice (Spanagel et al. 2005) has shown that elevation of extracellular glutamate levels achieved through a genetic modification is sufficient to mimic the escalation of voluntary alcohol intake otherwise observed following a history of dependence. This research demonstrated that the ability of acamprosate to normalize glutamate levels is associated with an ability to reverse escalated voluntary consumption (Spanagel et al. 2005).

Together, these data provide a neurobiological basis for the hypothesis that acamprosate—and perhaps other medications targeting glutamatergic neuroadaptations—may be preferentially (or even exclusively) active in individuals in whom dependence-induced neuroadaptations have reached a certain level. Indeed, animal experiments provide support for this notion, because acamprosate decreased alcohol consumption only after a prolonged history of dependence and left basal levels of consumption in nondependent animals unaffected (Rimondini et al. 2002). These findings suggest the possibility that a personalized medicine approach may be required when using medications targeting glutamatergic neuroadaptations. Discrepancies among clinical studies in their findings regarding the effects of acamprosate as an alcoholism medication, which will be discussed in Chapter 9 ("Treatment of Alcohol-Related Disorders"), may in fact be accounted for by this neurobiological mechanism.

Stress Systems and Progression Into Negatively Reinforced Alcohol Use

Beyond glutamatergic neuroadaptations, multiple stress-related systems become dysregulated as people progress into fully developed alcohol addiction (Heilig et al.

2010). Both clinical and experimental studies have documented disturbances in endocrine stress responses involving the hypothalamic-pituitary-adrenal (HPA) axis following chronic alcohol exposure. For example, acute alcohol withdrawal is associated with heightened HPA axis activation. This activation usually resolves within a few days and is followed by a blunted HPA axis responsiveness to stress challenges that persists for a prolonged period of time. However, animal studies show that behavioral phenomena observed in later stages of alcohol addiction, such as increased vulnerability to stress-induced relapse, are not directly driven by changes in HPA axis function. Instead, expression of these addictive behaviors is largely mediated by extrahypothalamic stress systems. The activity of the HPA axis and the resulting glucocorticoid receptor activation are thought to promote neuroadaptations that confer increased sensitivity to stress and vulnerability to stress-induced relapse (Vendruscolo et al. 2012).

The hypothalamic release factor that activates the HPA axis, corticotropin-releasing hormone (CRH; also referred to as corticotropin-releasing factor [CRF]), is also expressed in extrahypothalamic structures that mediate behavioral, rather than endocrine, stress responses, such as the amygdala complex and the bed nucleus of the stria terminalis (BNST). CRH in these structures mediates its pro-stress actions predominantly through the CRH_1 receptor subtype. Numerous animal studies have shown that extrahypothalamic CRH activity plays a key role in mediating anxiety and dysphoria during both acute alcohol withdrawal and protracted abstinence. Upregulated CRH and CRH_1 receptor expression within the amygdala underlies the increased behavioral sensitivity to stress following development of alcohol dependence in laboratory animals (Heilig and Koob 2007). Animal studies have also suggested that CRH activity plays a major role in mediating relapse provoked by stressors, as well as escalation of drinking following a prolonged history of dependence.

These findings led to the expectation that brain-penetrant CRH_1 receptor antagonists would block stress-induced craving and relapse in people with alcohol addiction (Zorrilla et al. 2013). However, studies to date have not supported this prediction (Kwako et al. 2015; Schwandt et al. 2016). Although these studies have by no means been definitive, CRH_1 receptor antagonists have also failed to show utility in other stress-related psychiatric conditions, such as depression, anxiety, and posttraumatic stress disorder (PTSD), for which they were expected to confer clinical benefits. In one study, the CRH_1 receptor antagonist verucerfont was found to exacerbate, rather than alleviate, fear symptoms (Grillon et al. 2015). The reason for these failures is presently unknown. However, CRH_1 receptor development programs in the pharmaceutical industry have been discontinued, leaving little hope that medications targeting this system will become therapeutics for negatively reinforced alcohol seeking.

Modulation of noradrenergic transmission has been suggested as another strategy for targeting stress-induced relapse and escalation of alcohol consumption. Prevention of postsynaptic consequences of noradrenergic activity may be possible through use of antagonists of α_1-adrenergic receptors, while agonists of α_2-adrenergic receptors have the ability to suppress the activity of noradrenergic (e.g., locus coeruleus) neurons themselves. Medications that target α_1- and α_2-adrenergic receptors, such as prazosin and guanfacine, respectively, have long been available as blood pressure medications and have received renewed interest as potential relapse-preventive medications in alcoholism (Sinha et al. 2011b). However, despite promising pilot results, an ambitious clinical trial in patients with comorbid alcohol use disorder and PTSD did not support the efficacy of prazosin (Petrakis et al. 2016).

Other stress-related systems have also been implicated in alcohol consumption and relapse (Schank et al. 2012). For instance, the κ-opioid receptor and its endogenous ligand dynorphin contribute to the behavioral effects of stress and have been shown to block escalated alcohol self-administration as well as stress-induced relapse in preclinical models (Domi et al. 2018). Evaluation of this mechanism in humans has not yet been accomplished.

Impulsivity: Action Without Forethought

Cravings for the rewarding properties of alcohol or for its ability to relieve negative emotional states are important in alcoholism but are insufficient to fully explain relapse, the core phenomenon of any addictive disorder. People with alcoholism frequently make disastrous behavioral choices in ways that people without addictive disorders simply are unlikely to do. When faced with seemingly trivial choices that determine whether they will be able to keep a job, hold together a family, or simply survive, alcoholic individuals frequently choose against what is in their own best interest. Afterward, the patients themselves and the people around them appear to find these choices equally difficult to comprehend. Maladaptive decisions of this nature represent a breakdown of some of the most sophisticated cognitive functions of which the human brain is capable. Supported by several areas of the prefrontal cortex, these functions have evolved further in humans than in any other species and normally allow people to successfully navigate highly complex and ever-changing environments. However, these functions break down at several levels in alcoholism.

For choices to be guided by their consequences, the different future scenarios that can be expected to follow a set of decisions must be represented in the brain. Outcomes associated with such "memories of the future" then need to be assigned different values, and choices made on the basis of hunches sensed in real time (Jentsch and Taylor 1999). When deciding among different options, people take into account not only the absolute value of the associated outcome but also how far into the future that outcome can be expected. A certain degree of what is called "temporal discounting" is often rational, given that outcomes that are distant in time, no matter how appealing, may in fact never materialize. But when cohorts with addictive disorders, including alcoholism, are evaluated under laboratory conditions, most studies find that these patients apply steeper temporal discounting than do healthy control subjects (Reynolds 2006). This finding presumably reflects these patients' increased susceptibility, in real life, to choose the reward from a drink now over the reward from a paycheck 2 weeks from today. Alcohol-dependent individuals also discount risk to a higher degree than do healthy control subjects. Once a choice is made, pursuing it often requires inhibiting ongoing activity and switching tasks. Both of these functions are also impaired in people with alcoholism, frequently resulting in rigid, maladaptive behaviors. Collectively, these traits make up facets of what is frequently called "impulsivity," a construct that is in fact quite complex (Dick et al. 2010).

Although increased impulsivity is well established in alcoholism, a key question is whether this is a consequence of prolonged heavy alcohol use, a preexisting susceptibility factor, or both. Both human data and findings from experimental studies in nonhuman primates indicate that innate elevated impulsivity, associated with low activity of CNS serotonin transmission, indeed confers an increased risk for heavy alcohol consumption and, in humans, alcoholism. In a study involving a large sample of almost 2,000 14-year-olds, Whelan et al. (2012) found that hypofunctioning of the lateral orbitofrontal cortex was associated with a greater likelihood of initiating alcohol use in early adolescence. This finding showed that preexisting alterations in prefrontal connectivity not only drive different dimensions of impulsivity but also confer susceptibility to excessive alcohol consumption. It is, however, also clear that alcohol use ultimately results in structural damage to the brain, with loss of gray matter, leading to further impairment of cognitive function and impulse control.

Conclusion

Alcohol has a potential for producing addiction and adverse consequences that is comparable to that of "hard" drugs such as cocaine or heroin (Nutt et al. 2010). Multiple neurobiological systems contribute to alcohol's actions. Systems mediating both the positively reinforcing and the negatively reinforcing properties of alcohol offer multiple targets for treatment. Impulsivity and impaired decision making in alcoholism may offer an additional category of treatment targets. An understanding of the neurobiological mechanisms underlying alcoholism is important not only because it offers the promise of mechanism-based therapies. Understanding the neurobiological mechanisms of alcohol addiction is one of the most important paths toward removing the stigma of this disease.

References

Anthony JC, Warner LA, Kessler RC: Comparative epidemiology of dependence on tobacco, alcohol, controlled substances, and inhalants: basic findings from the National Comorbidity Survey. Experimental and Clinical Psychopharmacology 2(3):244–268, 1994. Available at: https://www.hcp.med.harvard.edu/publications/comparative-epidemiology-dependence-tobacco-alcohol-controlled-substances-and-inhalants. Accessed December 12, 2019.

Bilbao A, Robinson JE, Heilig M, et al: A pharmacogenetic determinant of mu-opioid receptor antagonist effects on alcohol reward and consumption: evidence from humanized mice. Biol Psychiatry 77(10):850–858, 2015 25442002

Boileau I, Assaad JM, Pihl RO, et al: Alcohol promotes dopamine release in the human nucleus accumbens. Synapse 49(4):226–231, 2003 12827641

Bond C, LaForge KS, Tian M, et al: Single-nucleotide polymorphism in the human mu opioid receptor gene alters beta-endorphin binding and activity: possible implications for opiate addiction. Proc Natl Acad Sci USA 95(16):9608–9613, 1998 9689128

Bossert JM, Marchant NJ, Calu DJ, et al: The reinstatement model of drug relapse: recent neurobiological findings, emerging research topics, and translational research. Psychopharmacology (Berl) 229(3):453–476, 2013 23685858

Conklin CA, Tiffany ST: Applying extinction research and theory to cue-exposure addiction treatments. Addiction 97(2):155–167, 2002 11860387

Dick DM, Smith G, Olausson P, et al: Understanding the construct of impulsivity and its relationship to alcohol use disorders. Addict Biol 15(2):217–226, 2010 20148781

Domi E, Barbier E, Augier E, et al: Preclinical evaluation of the kappa-opioid receptor antagonist CERC-501 as a candidate therapeutic for alcohol use disorders. Neuropsychopharmacology 43(9):1805–1812, 2018 29463912

Garbutt JC, Greenblatt AM, West SL, et al: Clinical and biological moderators of response to naltrexone in alcohol dependence: a systematic review of the evidence. Addiction 109(8):1274–1284, 2014 24661324

Gilman JM, Ramchandani VA, Davis MB, et al: Why we like to drink: a functional magnetic resonance imaging study of the rewarding and anxiolytic effects of alcohol. J Neurosci 28(18):4583–4591, 2008 18448634

Gilman JM, Ramchandani VA, Crouss T, et al: Subjective and neural responses to intravenous alcohol in young adults with light and heavy drinking patterns. Neuropsychopharmacology 37(2):467–477, 2012 21956438

Goldman D, Oroszi G, Ducci F: The genetics of addictions: uncovering the genes. Nat Rev Genet 6(7):521–532, 2005 15995696

Grillon C, Hale E, Lieberman L, et al: The CRH1 antagonist GSK561679 increases human fear but not anxiety as assessed by startle. Neuropsychopharmacology 40(5):1064–1071, 2015 25430779

Harris RA, Trudell JR, Mihic SJ: Ethanol's molecular targets. Sci Signal 1(28):re7, 2008 18632551

Heilig M, Koob GF: A key role for corticotropin-releasing factor in alcohol dependence. Trends Neurosci 30(8):399–406, 2007 17629579

Heilig M, Egli M, Crabbe JC, et al: Acute withdrawal, protracted abstinence and negative affect in alcoholism: are they linked? Addict Biol 15(2):169–184, 2010 20148778

Heinz A, Reimold M, Wrase J, et al: Correlation of stable elevations in striatal mu-opioid receptor availability in detoxified alcoholic patients with alcohol craving: a positron emission tomography study using carbon 11-labeled carfentanil. Arch Gen Psychiatry 62(1):57–64, 2005 15630073

Hermann D, Weber-Fahr W, Sartorius A, et al: Translational magnetic resonance spectroscopy reveals excessive central glutamate levels during alcohol withdrawal in humans and rats. Biol Psychiatry 71(11):1015–1021, 2012 21907974

Hermann D, Hirth N, Reimold M, et al: Low μ-opioid receptor status in alcohol dependence identified by combined positron emission tomography and post-mortem brain analysis. Neuropsychopharmacology 42(3):606–614, 2017 27510425

Hirth N, Meinhardt MW, Noori HR, et al: Convergent evidence from alcohol-dependent humans and rats for a hyperdopaminergic state in protracted abstinence. Proc Natl Acad Sci USA 113(11):3024–3029, 2016 26903621

Jentsch JD, Taylor JR: Impulsivity resulting from frontostriatal dysfunction in drug abuse: implications for the control of behavior by reward-related stimuli. Psychopharmacology (Berl) 146(4):373–390, 1999 10550488

King AC, Hasin D, O'Connor SJ, et al: A prospective 5-year re-examination of alcohol response in heavy drinkers progressing in alcohol use disorder. Biol Psychiatry 79(6):489–498, 2016 26117308

Kruse SW, Zhao R, Smith DP, Jones DN: Structure of a specific alcohol-binding site defined by the odorant binding protein LUSH from Drosophila melanogaster. Nat Struct Biol 10(9):694–700, 2003 12881720

Kwako LE, Spagnolo PA, Schwandt ML, et al: The corticotropin releasing hormone-1 (CRH1) receptor antagonist pexacerfont in alcohol dependence: a randomized controlled experimental medicine study. Neuropsychopharmacology 40(5):1053–1063, 2015 25409596

Mellentin AI, Skøt L, Nielsen B, et al: Cue exposure therapy for the treatment of alcohol use disorders: a meta-analytic review. Clin Psychol Rev 57:195–207, 2017 28781153

Mitchell JM, O'Neil JP, Janabi M, et al: Alcohol consumption induces endogenous opioid release in the human orbitofrontal cortex and nucleus accumbens. Sci Transl Med 4(116):116ra6, 2012 22238334

Monti PM: Treating Alcohol Dependence: A Coping Skills Training Guide, 2nd Edition. New York, Guilford, 2002, pp xii, 196

Monti PM, Rohsenow DJ, Rubonis AV, et al: Alcohol cue reactivity: effects of detoxification and extended exposure. J Stud Alcohol 54(2):235–245, 1993 8384678

Newlin DB, Thomson JB: Alcohol challenge with sons of alcoholics: a critical review and analysis. Psychol Bull 108(3):383–402, 1990 2270234

Noori HR, Cosa Linan A, Spanagel R: Largely overlapping neuronal substrates of reactivity to drug, gambling, food and sexual cues: a comprehensive meta-analysis. Eur Neuropsychopharmacol 26(9):1419–1430, 2016 27397863

Nutt DJ, King LA, Phillips LD, et al: Drug harms in the UK: a multicriteria decision analysis. Lancet 376(9752):1558–1565, 2010 21036393

O'Malley SS, Krishnan-Sarin S, Farren C, et al: Naltrexone decreases craving and alcohol self-administration in alcohol-dependent subjects and activates the hypothalamo-pituitary-adrenocortical axis. Psychopharmacology (Berl) 160(1):19–29, 2002 11862370

Oslin DW, Leong SH, Lynch KG, et al: Naltrexone vs placebo for the treatment of alcohol dependence: a randomized clinical trial. JAMA Psychiatry 72(5):430–437, 2015 25760804

Petrakis IL, Desai N, Gueorguieva R, et al: Prazosin for veterans with posttraumatic stress disorder and comorbid alcohol dependence: a clinical trial. Alcohol Clin Exp Res 40(1):178–186, 2016 26683790

Ramchandani VA, Umhau J, Pavon FJ, et al: A genetic determinant of the striatal dopamine response to alcohol in men. Mol Psychiatry 16(8):809–817, 2011 20479755

Reynolds B: A review of delay-discounting research with humans: relations to drug use and gambling. Behav Pharmacol 17(8):651–667, 2006 17110792

Rimondini R, Arlinde C, Sommer W, et al: Long-lasting increase in voluntary ethanol consumption and transcriptional regulation in the rat brain after intermittent exposure to alcohol. FASEB J 16(1):27–35, 2002 11772933

Schacht JP, Anton RF, Myrick H: Functional neuroimaging studies of alcohol cue reactivity: a quantitative meta-analysis and systematic review. Addict Biol 18(1):121–133, 2013 22574861

Schank JR, Ryabinin AE, Giardino WJ, et al: Stress-related neuropeptides and addictive behaviors: beyond the usual suspects. Neuron 76(1):192–208, 2012 23040815

Schuckit MA: Low level of response to alcohol as a predictor of future alcoholism. Am J Psychiatry 151(2):184–189, 1994 8296886

Schwandt ML, Cortes CR, Kwako LE, et al: The CRF1 antagonist verucerfont in anxious alcohol-dependent women: translation of neuroendocrine, but not of anti-craving effects. Neuropsychopharmacology 41(12):2818–2829, 2016 27109623

Sinha R, Fox HC, Hong KI, et al: Effects of adrenal sensitivity, stress- and cue-induced craving, and anxiety on subsequent alcohol relapse and treatment outcomes. Arch Gen Psychiatry 68(9):942–952, 2011a 21536969

Sinha R, Shaham Y, Heilig M: Translational and reverse translational research on the role of stress in drug craving and relapse. Psychopharmacology (Berl) 218(1):69–82, 2011b 21494792

Spanagel R: Alcoholism: a systems approach from molecular physiology to addictive behavior. Physiol Rev 89(2):649–705, 2009 19342616

Spanagel R, Pendyala G, Abarca C, et al: The clock gene Per2 influences the glutamatergic system and modulates alcohol consumption. Nat Med 11(1):35–42, 2005 15608650

Umhau JC, Momenan R, Schwandt ML, et al: Effect of acamprosate on magnetic resonance spectroscopy measures of central glutamate in detoxified alcohol-dependent individuals: a randomized controlled experimental medicine study. Arch Gen Psychiatry 67(10):1069–1077, 2010 20921123

Urban NB, Kegeles LS, Slifstein M, et al: Sex differences in striatal dopamine release in young adults after oral alcohol challenge: a positron emission tomography imaging study with [11C]raclopride. Biol Psychiatry 68(8):689–696, 2010 20678752

Vendruscolo LF, Barbier E, Schlosburg JE, et al: Corticosteroid-dependent plasticity mediates compulsive alcohol drinking in rats. J Neurosci 32(22):7563–7571, 2012 22649234

Volkow ND, Wang GJ, Fowler JS, et al: Decreases in dopamine receptors but not in dopamine transporters in alcoholics. Alcohol Clin Exp Res 20(9):1594–1598, 1996 8986209

Volkow ND, Wang GJ, Begleiter H, et al: High levels of dopamine D2 receptors in unaffected members of alcoholic families: possible protective factors. Arch Gen Psychiatry 63(9):999–1008, 2006 16953002

Volkow ND, Michaelides M, Baler R: The neuroscience of drug reward and addiction. Physiol Rev 99(4):2115–2140, 2019 31507244

Whelan R, Conrod PJ, Poline JB, et al: Adolescent impulsivity phenotypes characterized by distinct brain networks. Nat Neurosci 15(6):920–925, 2012 22544311

Zorrilla EP, Heilig M, de Wit H, et al: Behavioral, biological, and chemical perspectives on targeting CRF(1) receptor antagonists to treat alcoholism. Drug Alcohol Depend 128(3):175–186, 2013 23294766

CHAPTER 9

Treatment of Alcohol-Related Disorders

Alyssa Braxton, M.D.

Tara M. Wright, M.D.

Hugh Myrick, M.D.

Excessive alcohol use led to roughly 88,000 deaths and 2.5 million years of potential life lost each year in the United States from 2006 to 2010 (Centers for Disease Control and Prevention 2020; Stahre et al. 2014). Unfortunately, alcohol use disorder (AUD) is underdiagnosed and difficult to treat. Clinical management of AUD begins with identification and management of withdrawal states. In this chapter we focus on various relapse-prevention strategies, including both pharmacological and social interventions.

General Management

In nonemergent situations, questionnaires can be helpful in detecting problematic drinking. The four-question CAGE (Mayfield et al. 1974) screening tool can prompt further investigation into problem drinking with the patient (Ewing 1984). Longer questionnaires such as the 10-item Alcohol Use Disorder Identification Test (AUDIT) and the 25-item Michigan Alcohol Screening Test (MAST) can also indicate problems with alcohol use (Conley 2001; Saunders et al. 1993).

In addition to self-report screening questionnaires, various biomarkers can be utilized in the clinical setting to screen for alcohol use. Alcohol can be detectable for several hours after consumption via a breathalyzer, blood, or urine. Other laboratory studies measure chronic alcohol use through its effects on liver enzymes such as gamma-glutamyl transpeptidase (GGT), aspartate aminotransferase (AST), and alanine aminotransferase (ALT). An AST-to-ALT ratio of 2:1 or greater is suggestive of excessive alcohol use, especially in combination with an elevated GGT. GGT has a sensitivity of 40%–60% and a specificity of 80% for heavy alcohol use; however, it is limited in its ability to identify recent relapse or intoxication.

Several newer tests, including measurement of percentage carbohydrate-deficient transferrin (%CDT), ethyl glucuronide (EtG), ethyl sulfate (EtS), and phosphatidylethanol (PEth), can also be useful in monitoring alcohol intake. EtG and EtS remain detectable in the urine for several hours to days, depending on the amount of alcohol consumed (Dahl et al. 2011). %CDT, which measures the transient change in glycosylation pattern of transferrin, has a diagnostic specificity of approximately 70% in patients with non-alcohol-induced liver cirrhosis, 88.2% in hepatitis patients, and 93.5% in patients with elevated GGT (Hock et al. 2005). Therefore, the combination of measuring GGT and %CDT enhances a provider's ability to detect heavy drinking. Another direct alcohol biomarker, known as Peth, is formed on the phospholipid membrane of blood cells in the presence of alcohol, and can be particularly helpful in identifying alcohol misuse in people who have severe liver dysfunction or who are awaiting liver transplantation (Gnann et al. 2012).

Alcohol Withdrawal

Signs and Symptoms

Cessation of or reduction in prolonged and heavy alcohol consumption may result in a characteristic withdrawal syndrome. Alcohol withdrawal symptoms typically begin between 6 and 48 hours after reduction or cessation of alcohol use and can last between 2 and 7 days. It is important to remember that symptoms of alcohol withdrawal can emerge before the blood alcohol level reaches zero.

Symptoms of alcohol withdrawal can include autonomic hyperactivity (sweating or tachycardia); tremor; insomnia; nausea or vomiting; transient visual, tactile, or auditory hallucinations; motor arousal (agitation); anxiety; irritability; and seizures. If symptoms are left untreated or are undertreated, progression to the most severe syndrome, delirium tremens, can occur. Delirium tremens (DTs) is characterized by decreased attention and awareness, with fluctuating disturbances in consciousness, memory, orientation, and perception. It also is commonly associated with autonomic instability and hyperpyrexia. Onset of DTs typically occurs around the third day of abstinence from alcohol, and the syndrome lasts on average from 1 to 8 days. Most literature estimates that 3%–5% of patients admitted for alcohol withdrawal will develop DTs (Mirijello et al. 2015). DTs must be considered a medical emergency, because without treatment, the mortality rate can be as high as 20% for patients who progress to this stage (Mayo-Smith et al. 2004). Death typically occurs as a result of hyperthermia, cardiac arrhythmias, withdrawal seizure complications, or comorbid medical disorders.

Alcohol withdrawal seizures are another major complication that can occur during the withdrawal period. These seizures are typically generalized tonic-clonic in type and are estimated to occur in 5%–15% of patients. Withdrawal seizures typically occur within the first 24 hours after cessation of alcohol use, but they can occur up to 5 days later (Victor 1990). An important risk factor for alcohol withdrawal seizures is a past history of alcohol withdrawal seizures, referred to as the "kindling" phenomenon (Brown et al. 1988).

In addition to experiencing the initial symptoms of alcohol withdrawal, many patients report longer-lasting symptoms referred to as *protracted withdrawal syndrome.* Symptoms can include restlessness, anxiety, insomnia, dysphoria, cravings, fatigue, anorexia, and low energy. Because of the lack of literature support and unclear delineation between acute and protracted withdrawal, this syndrome has not been included in DSM-5 (American Psychiatric Association 2013).

Inpatient Versus Outpatient Treatment

Inpatient Treatment

Inpatient treatment provides the safest setting for the treatment of alcohol withdrawal because it allows the patient to be closely monitored. Inpatient treatment may also allow for separation from environmental triggers of alcohol or other drug use and enable patients to engage in the start of the rehabilitative process. For certain patient populations, such as individuals with a history of significant past episodes of alcohol withdrawal, recent drinking at very high levels, or a history of withdrawal seizures or DTs, treatment in an inpatient setting would be advisable. Inpatient treatment would also be recommended for individuals with serious comorbid medical or psychiatric illness. In addition, patients with multiple past detoxifications may be at an increased risk of complications due to the kindling effect of withdrawal and therefore should be considered for inpatient detoxification (Brown et al. 1988).

Outpatient Treatment

Over the past two decades, there has been a major shift from the inpatient to the outpatient setting for the treatment of alcohol withdrawal. In a review of the literature on ambulatory detoxification, Abbott et al. (1995) found that only 10%–20% of patients required admission. In the studies reviewed, the completion rates for ambulatory detoxification ranged from 35% to 95%, with most studies reporting completion rates above 70% (Abbott et al. 1995). In the majority of studies reviewed, approximately half of patients continued in alcohol rehabilitation, including group and individual therapy, after detoxification. Most important, this literature review found no reports of mortality or serious medical complications, with the exception of one program reporting a patient who had a seizure after starting detoxification (Abbott et al. 1995).

Although no specific criteria exist for determining which patients can be safely treated in an outpatient setting, practical considerations would dictate exclusion of patients with severe withdrawal symptoms, comorbid severe medical or psychiatric illness, a past history of seizures or delirium tremens, or lack of a reliable support system.

Assessment of Withdrawal

Quantitative scales have been developed in order to assess the severity of alcohol withdrawal symptoms. These scales are based on a combination of subjective and behavioral variables. The assessment tool most often cited in current alcohol withdrawal literature is the Clinical Institute Withdrawal Assessment for Alcohol, revised (CIWA-Ar) (Sullivan et al. 1991). This clinician-rated checklist is a 10-item scale used to monitor the clinical course of withdrawal symptoms, such as nausea/vomiting; headache; tremor; sweating; anxiety; agitation; tactile, auditory, and visual disturbances; and clouding of sensorium. For each of the 10 symptom items, a severity number (0 to 7) can be assigned; thus, the higher the score, the more severe the alcohol withdrawal symptoms.

General Management

The general management of individuals presenting for alcohol detoxification includes adjunctive management of a variety of medical conditions. A physical examination should be performed with particular emphasis on assessing for cardiac conditions, liver disease, pancreatic disease, gastrointestinal bleeding, infections, and neurological impairment. If the patient has unstable vital signs, stabilization should be a top priority.

Individuals with AUD may also have electrolyte abnormalities such as hypomagnesemia, hypophosphatemia, and hypokalemia. Oral multivitamins containing folic acid should be given for several weeks to correct any nutritional deficits resulting from either dietary insufficiencies or alcohol-related changes in the digestive tract. The treatment of thiamine deficiency is particularly important, given thiamine's role in Wernicke's encephalopathy. It is imperative that thiamine be replaced prior to glucose administration in order to prevent exacerbation of Wernicke's encephalopathy.

Medication Management of Detoxification

Benzodiazepines have historically been viewed as the gold standard in the treatment of alcohol withdrawal, given the depth of the evidence supporting their efficacy (Anton and Becker 1995). However, there is increasing evidence supporting the use of anticonvulsants in the management of alcohol withdrawal. Both classes of agents will be discussed in this section.

Benzodiazepines

Benzodiazepines are the first-line treatment for alcohol withdrawal due to their efficacy and safety profile. Benzodiazepines enhance γ-aminobutyric acid (GABA) transmission, balancing the surge of glutamate responsible for many alcohol withdrawal symptoms. Choice of specific benzodiazepines should be determined on the basis of individual clinical factors such as age, liver function, and history of seizures. Based on meta-analyses, no specific benzodiazepine appears to be superior in the treatment of alcohol withdrawal (Mayo-Smith and American Society of Addiction Medicine Working Group on Pharmacological Management of Alcohol Withdrawal 1997). Agents with longer half-lives, such as chlordiazepoxide and diazepam, can provide a smoother withdrawal due to the "auto-taper" provided by gradual excretion of active metabolites; however, such agents have the potential to cause oversedation, coordination difficulties, and confusion in elderly persons or those with liver dysfunction. Therefore, shorter-acting agents such as oxazepam and lorazepam may be preferred in this population.

The three most commonly used dosing strategies in the treatment of alcohol withdrawal are fixed dosing, loading dosing, and symptom-triggered treatment. *Fixed dosing* involves dosing at regular intervals, independent of the patient's symptoms, over 4–7 days; this strategy is typically used in inpatients with a heightened risk of alcohol withdrawal. *Loading dosing* involves initial administration of a higher single dose of a long-acting benzodiazepine in order to produce sedation, with tapering occurring via drug metabolism. Because this method carries a higher risk of benzodiazepine toxicity at the beginning of treatment, it requires close clinical monitoring. More recently, clinicians have used *symptom-triggered treatment* guided by CIWA-Ar scores to determine the need for benzodiazepines (Saitz et al. 1994). Trials comparing different dosing strategies have not found clear evidence of the superiority of one strategy over another. Studies have shown that symptom-triggered dosing requires lower total benzodiazepine doses in low-risk patients, which could produce less sedation and thus allow patients to more readily engage in other treatment activities (Saitz et al. 1994). For moderate to severe withdrawal symptoms, intravenous administration should be the preferred route of administration because it provides a rapid onset of action.

Anticonvulsants

Although not approved by the U.S. Food and Drug Administration (FDA) for the treatment of alcohol withdrawal, nonbenzodiazepine anticonvulsants have increasingly been shown to be as efficacious as benzodiazepines for the medical management of alcohol withdrawal. Advantages of anticonvulsants over benzodiazepines include their lack of abuse potential, lack of sedation, and lack of increased central nervous system depression if used concomitantly with alcohol (Book and Myrick 2005). These advantages can be especially important in the management of alcohol withdrawal in the outpatient setting.

Both clinical and basic science data strongly suggest that detoxified individuals are likely to experience incremental symptoms over multiple detoxification episodes akin to a sensitization or kindling phenomenon (Becker 1999). Because anticonvulsants have shown anti-kindling properties, that effect would be another reason to consider their use in the treatment of alcohol withdrawal. Several research studies evaluating adjunctive anticonvulsant use during acute withdrawal and postwithdrawal support this suggestion (Anton et al. 2009, 2011). Therefore, anticonvulsants not only may help ameliorate alcohol withdrawal symptoms but also may have a positive effect on return to drinking.

Several anticonvulsant agents have been evaluated in the treatment of alcohol withdrawal. These include older agents (e.g., valproic acid, carbamazepine) as well as new agents (e.g., gabapentin, pregabalin, levetiracetam). In most studies, the anticonvulsant was found to have efficacy similar to a benzodiazepine. Although it is beyond the scope of this chapter to discuss all of the studies using anticonvulsants, a few are worth mentioning. Malcolm et al. (2002) compared carbamazepine and lorazepam in the treatment of alcohol withdrawal in outpatients. The drugs appeared to be equally effective in acutely reducing the symptoms of alcohol withdrawal. However, carbamazepine was found to be superior to lorazepam in postwithdrawal treatment, significantly reducing the number of drinks per drinking day and significantly increasing the probability of not drinking at all. Whereas these effects were evident in the overall sample, they were most pronounced in the subgroup of individuals who had undergone two or more prior alcohol detoxifications, supporting the hypothesis that the "antikindling" effects of anticonvulsants may be important to their efficacy in the treatment of alcohol withdrawal.

Another agent that has received particular interest in the treatment of alcohol withdrawal is gabapentin. Gabapentin has multiple advantages over the older anticonvulsants: it lacks hepatic metabolism, does not bind to plasma proteins or induce hepatic enzymes, has no bone marrow toxicity, is not a scheduled drug, and is eliminated by renal excretion as an unchanged drug. In addition, gabapentin has a very benign side-effect profile. Myrick et al. (2009) compared gabapentin and lorazepam in the treatment of outpatient alcohol withdrawal. Gabapentin was well tolerated and was at least as effective as lorazepam in reducing the symptoms of alcohol withdrawal. Of note, as found with carbamazepine, there was less drinking in the immediate postwithdrawal period when gabapentin was utilized instead of lorazepam (Myrick et al. 2009).

Treatment of Complicated Withdrawal

Alcohol withdrawal seizures and DTs represent the most severe complications of alcohol withdrawal. Primary alcohol withdrawal seizures are self-limited and typically require supportive treatment and benzodiazepines. The treatment of DTs is somewhat less straightforward. Benzodiazepines are used to decrease autonomic hyperactivity, decrease risk of alcohol withdrawal seizures, and control agitation. Despite these beneficial effects, benzodiazepines may iatrogenically contribute to the behavioral disinhibition and confusion that are components of DTs. Treatment of DTs may include fluid repletion, nutritional supplementation, and correction of electrolyte abnormalities. If intravenous rehydration is needed, thiamine should be administered prior to giving glucose to avoid precipitating Wernicke's encephalopathy. Low doses of dopamine antagonists such as haloperidol can be given to help with the behavioral agitation resulting from psychosis or hallucinations, although these medications should be used judiciously because they can lower the seizure threshold (Mayo-Smith et al. 2004).

Emerging treatments for DTs in the intensive care unit setting include the use of alpha$_2$-agonists (e.g., dexmedetomidine and clonidine), which can be helpful in alleviating autonomic hyperactivity (e.g., hypertension, tachycardia) and (as an adjuvant with benzodiazepines) in potentially reducing the total benzodiazepine requirement and improving patient communication. One notable disadvantage of these medications is their potential to induce bradycardia. Another medication being implemented in patients with severe DTs with poor response to high doses of benzodiazepines is propofol. With its short duration of effect, propofol allows for quick assessment of a patient's mental status upon discontinuation. A drawback is that administration of propofol requires endotracheal intubation, mechanical ventilation, and close clinical monitoring.

Relapse Prevention

Four medications have been approved by the FDA for the treatment of AUD: disulfiram, naltrexone (both oral and long-acting injectable formulations), and acamprosate. However, medications for treating AUD are both underutilized and underprescribed.

Disulfiram

Disulfiram is an alcohol-deterrent drug that has been FDA approved since 1949. It interferes with the metabolism of alcohol by irreversibly inhibiting aldehyde dehydrogenase, thereby blocking the breakdown of acetaldehyde to acetate. Inhibiting this enzyme rapidly increases the serum concentration of acetaldehyde, producing a reaction characterized by facial flushing, nausea and vomiting, headache, hypotension, and palpitations. The patient's fear of this disulfiram-alcohol reaction, particularly after experiencing it, is presumed to serve as a strong reinforcement for abstinence. Due to the potentially dangerous effects of the disulfiram–ethanol interaction, it is inadvisable to prescribe disulfiram for the purpose of reducing alcohol consumption (as opposed to its indicated use for maintenance of abstinence).

A large placebo-controlled trial of disulfiram found no significant between-group differences in rates of abstinence or time to first drinking day (Fuller et al. 1986). Patient nonadherence was likely a main contributor to the negative finding, as only 20% of the 577 patients who completed the study were adherent to the disulfiram regimen. However, among patients who drank and had a complete set of assessment interviews, those in the 250-mg disulfiram group reported significantly fewer drinking days than those in the 1-mg or the no-disulfiram group. A significant relationship between adherence to the drug regimen and complete abstinence was found in all groups. Fuller et al. (1986) concluded that disulfiram may help reduce drinking frequency after relapse but did not enhance the effects of nonpharmacological treatments such as cognitive-behavioral therapy or 12-step facilitation in helping alcohol-dependent patients to sustain continuous abstinence or delay resumption of drinking. Fuller et al. (1986) also suggested that older, more motivated men seemed to be more adherent to treatment and to have better outcomes with disulfiram.

Adherence is a limitation in determining the generalization of disulfiram's effectiveness. Some authors have shown that supervised disulfiram treatment and incentive-driven interventions are associated with decreased alcohol consumption and increased rates of abstinence (Wright and Moore 1990). A detailed meta-analysis found that evidence for the efficacy of disulfiram was lacking overall, but the authors also pointed out that some evidence suggested that disulfiram could be effective when given under supervision (Berglund et al. 2003).

Naltrexone (Oral Formulation)

Naltrexone is a nonselective antagonist of the mu (μ), kappa (κ), and gamma (γ) opioid receptors; it is hypothesized to reduce the mesolimbic reward of alcohol consumption via blocking the release of dopamine induced by the consumption of alcohol. After it was shown to reduce drinking frequency and the likelihood of relapse to heavy drinking, naltrexone was approved by the FDA for the treatment of alcohol dependence in 1994 (O'Malley et al. 1992; Volpicelli et al. 1992). Naltrexone is believed to reduce alcohol craving and loss of control by reducing the rewarding effects of alcohol. It is relatively well tolerated, with the most common side effects being somnolence, nausea, vomiting, decreased appetite, and abdominal pain.

A large meta-analysis involving 27 randomized controlled trials (RCTs) of naltrexone found that short-term treatment with naltrexone decreased relapse risk, with a risk ratio of 0.64 and a number needed to treat (NNT) of 7 (Srisurapanont and Jarusuraisin 2005). The meta-analysis also found that in comparison with placebo, naltrexone lowed the risk of treatment dropout in alcohol-dependent patients by 28% (NNT=13) (Srisurapanont and Jarusuraisin 2005). A crucial consideration for the clinician and patient is that naltrexone is an opioid antagonist and can therefore induce withdrawal in an opioid-dependent individual. Special consideration must also be given to pain control, as naltrexone will block the effects of opioid analgesics. In a supervised hospital setting, the antagonist properties of naltrexone can be overridden by increased doses of opioid analgesics.

The efficacy of naltrexone was supported by the COMBINE (Combined Pharmacotherapies and Behavioral Interventions for Alcohol Dependence) study, a large double-blind RCT of relapse prevention medications (Anton et al. 2006). The COMBINE study evaluated the efficacy of naltrexone, acamprosate, or both, in comparison with each other and with placebo, with health care provider–delivered medical management, and with or without a specialized combined behavioral intervention (CBI). It included 1,383 recently abstinent volunteers with a diagnosis of alcohol dependence recruited from 11 U.S. academic sites (Anton et al. 2006). Individuals receiving naltrexone plus medical management or naltrexone plus medical management and CBI had a higher percentage of days abstinent compared with those receiving placebo plus medical management. Naltrexone also reduced the risk of heavy drinking days over time. Acamprosate had no impact on alcohol outcomes in this study.

The fact that not all studies of naltrexone have been positive suggests that there may be subgroups of individuals who are more likely to respond to naltrexone. King et al. (1997) found a differential response to naltrexone based on paternal history of alcoholism and level of stimulation experienced during alcohol drinking.

Evidence exists that there are variants in the gene encoding the μ-opioid receptor (OPRM1) that may alter the affinity of the receptor for endogenous ligands, resulting in variations in response to naltrexone. In a post hoc study that combined three previously collected datasets, subjects of European descent with one or two copies of the 118G variant allele treated with naltrexone had significantly lower rates of relapse and a longer time to return to heavy drinking than those homozygous for this allele (Oslin et al. 2003). These differences were not found among subjects assigned to placebo.

Naltrexone (Long-Acting Formulation)

Because patient adherence is clearly critical to the success of naltrexone, a long-acting injectable formulation of naltrexone (NTX-XR) was FDA approved in 2006. Garbutt et al. (2005) conducted a double-blind RCT of extended-release injectable naltrexone in 624 actively drinking alcohol-dependent adults. Participants were randomly assigned to one of three conditions: 1) a monthly intramuscular injection of 380 mg of NTX-XR, 2) a monthly intramuscular injection of 190 mg of NTX-XR, or 3) a matching volume of placebo combined with 12 sessions of a low-intensity psychosocial intervention (Garbutt et al. 2005). Compared with subjects assigned to the placebo group, those receiving 380 mg of NTX-XR showed a 25% decrease in the event rate of heavy drinking days, and those receiving 190 mg of NTX-XR showed a 17% decrease. The study also found that men (as compared with women) and individuals with lead-in abstinence exhibited greater treatment effects (Garbutt et al. 2005). NTX-XR has adverse effects similar to those of the oral formulation with the addition of injection site reactions.

Acamprosate

Acamprosate was approved by the FDA for the treatment of alcohol dependence in 2004. Acamprosate is structurally similar to GABA and is thought to exert its therapeutic effect by modulating the excitatory glutamate amino acid system (N-methyl-D-aspartate [NMDA] receptor) in the brain. Because acamprosate is poorly absorbed, it is generally given in high doses of about 2 g/day, in TID dosing. Acamprosate has been found to be generally well tolerated in all of the clinical trials to date. Diarrhea is the most common side effect, but headache, dizziness, and pruritus have also been reported, although to a much lesser degree. By functioning to increase GABAergic activity and/or to inhibit glutamatergic activity via modulation of the NMDA receptor, acamprosate may ameliorate alcohol withdrawal symptoms (Boeijinga et al. 2004).

Multiple trials conducted in Europe and elsewhere support the efficacy and safety of acamprosate. In a meta-analysis of 17 RCTs, Mann et al. (2004) found that continuous abstinence rates at 6 months were significantly higher in the acamprosate-treated patients. However, not all studies of acamprosate have shown its efficacy in comparison with placebo. As reported earlier in chapter, the COMBINE study (Anton et al. 2006) did not support the efficacy of acamprosate in intent-to-treat analyses. There has been much speculation as to the reasons for this finding, including differences in study populations and design. In the COMBINE study, patients were initiated on study drugs as outpatients, after a minimum of 4 days of abstinence (Anton et al. 2006). However, more than 50% of participants reported more than 4 days of abstinence prior to randomization. In summary, at present it is unclear which alcohol-dependent individuals are most likely to respond to acamprosate, although the weight of the data does suggest that individuals with a strong commitment to abstinence who take the medication for several weeks while abstaining might have better outcomes in the long run.

Combination Therapy

Whereas studies have shown that naltrexone and acamprosate are safe and well tolerated in combination, findings supporting superior efficacy for combination therapy over naltrexone monotherapy have been mixed. Although some trials have shown superior efficacy (Feeney et al. 2006; Kiefer and Wiedemann 2004), the COMBINE trial did not show a superior effect of naltrexone and acamprosate over naltrexone alone (Anton et al. 2006).

Non-FDA-Approved Medications

Gabapentin

The proposed mechanism of action of gabapentin is blockade of a subunit of the voltage-gated calcium channel, indirectly modulating GABA neurotransmission. Preclinical research has shown that gabapentin reverses the stress-induced GABA activation in the amygdala associated with AUD (Roberto et al. 2008). In a 12-week RCT comparing gabapentin dosages of 900 mg/day and 1,800 mg/day in 150 adults with AUD, participants receiving gabapentin showed higher rates of abstinence (11% and 17% for the 900 mg/day and the 1,800 mg/day group, respectively) in comparison with participants receiving placebo (4%) (Mason et al. 2014). One major drawback of this study was the high (43%) dropout rate. The most common adverse effects were dizziness, somnolence, ataxia, and peripheral edema.

Topiramate

Topiramate is postulated to reduce cravings for alcohol by targeting the glutamate pathways in the brain. Dosing in AUD trials has ranged from 75 mg/day to 300 mg/day. A meta-analysis (Blodgett et al. 2014) involving seven randomized clinical trials found that topiramate had a small effect in increasing the number of abstinent days and in lowering the frequency of binge drinking in comparison with placebo. Side effects of topiramate included paresthesias, anorexia, difficulty with concentration and attention, and cognitive slowing. Use of topiramate is contraindicated in patients with renal calculi, secondary angle glaucoma, or metabolic acidosis.

Nonpharmacological Treatment Options

Psychodynamic psychotherapy, cognitive-behavioral therapy (CBT), motivational enhancement therapy (MET), 12-step facilitation (TSF), contingency management, network therapy, group therapy, and family therapy have all been used in the treatment of AUD.

Project MATCH (Matching Alcoholism Treatments to Client Heterogeneity) was a multisite clinical trial that investigated whether matching of treatments to patients resulted in improved treatment outcomes (Project MATCH Research Group 1997). Subjects ($N=1,726$) were randomly assigned to TSF, CBT, or MET over a 12-week period. Overall, study subjects showed significant and sustained improvement, with increased percentages of abstinent days and decreased numbers of drinks per drinking day, and with few clinically significant outcome differences among the three treatments. There was no difference in sustained abstinence among treatments. However, outpatients who received TSF were more likely than those who received the other treatments to remain completely abstinent in the year following treatment. The overarching conclusion appears to be that once patients have reached the point at which they are willing to consider abstinence, their motivation and individual characteristics are likely to be better predictors of outcome than is any specific aspect of the treatment program (Project MATCH Research Group 1997, 1998).

Conclusion

Alcoholism is a devastating illness that leads to huge societal losses. Despite the fact that alcoholism is underdiagnosed, effective identification strategies are available and need to be more widely used in medical settings. In particular, there have been developments in both the treatment strategies for alcohol withdrawal and the locations in which detoxification may occur. There have been many new developments in the prevention of relapse to alcohol use. Despite these advances, there is a need for more effective interventions for individuals with AUD. An increased understanding of the neurobiological underpinnings of AUD, including the role of pharmacogenetics, may lead to enhanced effectiveness of future treatment strategies.

References

Abbott PJ, Quinn D, Knox L: Ambulatory medical detoxification for alcohol. Am J Drug Alcohol Abuse 21(4):549–563, 1995 8561102

American Psychiatric Association: Diagnostic and Statistical Manual of Mental Disorders, 5th Edition. Arlington, VA, American Psychiatric Association, 2013

Anton RF, Becker HC: Pharmacology and pathophysiology of alcohol withdrawal, in The Pharmacology of Alcohol Abuse (Handbook of Experimental Pharmacology Series, Vol 114). Edited by Kranzler HR. Springer-Verlag, 1995, pp 315–367

Anton RF, O'Malley SS, Ciraulo DA, et al: Combined pharmacotherapies and behavioral interventions for alcohol dependence: the COMBINE study: a randomized controlled trial. JAMA 295(17):2003–2017, 2006 16670409

Anton RF, Myrick H, Baros AM, et al: Efficacy of a combination of flumazenil and gabapentin in the treatment of alcohol dependence: relationship to alcohol withdrawal symptoms. J Clin Psychopharmacol 29(4):334–342, 2009 19593171

Anton RF, Myrick H, Wright TM, et al: Gabapentin combined with naltrexone for the treatment of alcohol dependence. Am J Psychiatry 168(7):709–717, 2011 21454917

Becker HC: Alcohol withdrawal: neuroadaption and sensitization. CNS Spectr 4(1):38–65, 1999. Available at: https://www.cambridge.org/core/journals/cns-spectrums/article/alcohol-withdrawal-neuroadaptation-and-sensitization/800C80335B7B9-FA55460DEB035BB7208. Accessed December 14, 2019.

Berglund M, Thelander S, Salaspuro M, et al: Treatment of alcohol abuse: an evidence-based review. Alcohol Clin Exp Res 27(10):1645–1656, 2003 14574236

Blodgett JC, Del Re AC, Maisel NC, et al: A meta-analysis of topiramate's effects for individuals with alcohol use disorders. Alcohol Clin Exp Res 38(6):1481–1488, 2014 24796492

Boeijinga PH, Parot P, Soufflet L, et al: Pharmacodynamic effects of acamprosate on markers of cerebral function in alcohol-dependent subjects administered as pretreatment and during alcohol abstinence. Neuropsychobiology 50(1):71–77, 2004 15179024

Book SW, Myrick H: Novel anticonvulsants in the treatment of alcoholism. Expert Opin Invest Drugs 14(4):371–376, 2005 15882114

Brown ME, Anton RF, Malcolm R, et al: Alcohol detoxification and withdrawal seizures: clinical support for a kindling hypothesis. Biol Psychiatry 23(5):507–514, 1988 3345323

Centers for Disease Control and Prevention: Alcohol and Public Health: Alcohol-Related Disease Impact (ARDI) Application (web page). July 30, 2020. Centers for Disease Control and Prevention, National Center for Chronic Disease Prevention and Health Promotion, Division of Population Health. Available at: https://nccd.cdc.gov/DPH_ARDI/Default/Default.aspx. Accessed August 10, 2020.

Conley TB: Construct validity of the MAST and AUDIT with multiple offender drunk drivers. J Subst Abuse Treat 20(4):287–295, 2001 11672645

Dahl H, Voltaire Carlsson A, Hillgren K, et al: Urinary ethyl glucuronide and ethyl sulfate testing for detection of recent drinking in an outpatient treatment program for alcohol and drug dependence. Alcohol Alcohol 46(3):278–282, 2011 21339184

Ewing JA: Detecting alcoholism. The CAGE questionnaire. JAMA 252(14):1905–1907, 1984 6471323

Feeney GF, Connor JP, Young RM, et al: Combined acamprosate and naltrexone, with cognitive behavioural therapy is superior to either medication alone for alcohol abstinence: a single centres' experience with pharmacotherapy. Alcohol Alcohol 41(3):321–327, 2006 16467406

Fuller RK, Branchey L, Brightwell DR, et al: Disulfiram treatment of alcoholism. A Veterans Administration cooperative study. JAMA 256(11):1449–1455, 1986 3528541

Garbutt JC, Kranzler HR, O'Malley SS, et al: Efficacy and tolerability of long-acting injectable naltrexone for alcohol dependence: a randomized controlled trial. JAMA 293(13):1617–1625, 2005 15811981

Gnann H, Weinmann W, Thierauf A: Formation of phosphatidylethanol and its subsequent elimination during an extensive drinking experiment over 5 days. Alcohol Clin Exp Res 36(9):1507–1511, 2012 22458353

Hock B, Schwarz M, Domke I, et al: Validity of carbohydrate-deficient transferrin (%CDT), gamma-glutamyltransferase (gamma-GT) and mean corpuscular erythrocyte volume (MCV) as biomarkers for chronic alcohol abuse: a study in patients with alcohol dependence and liver disorders of non-alcoholic and alcoholic origin. Addiction 100(10):1477–1486, 2005 16185209

Kiefer F, Wiedemann K: Combined therapy: what does acamprosate and naltrexone combination tell us? Alcohol Alcohol 39(6):542–547, 2004 15456690

King AC, Volpicelli JR, Frazer A, et al: Effect of naltrexone on subjective alcohol response in subjects at high and low risk for future alcohol dependence. Psychopharmacology (Berl) 129(1):15–22, 1997 9122358

Malcolm R, Myrick H, Roberts J, et al: The effects of carbamazepine and lorazepam on single versus multiple previous alcohol withdrawals in an outpatient randomized trial. J Gen Intern Med 17(5):349–355, 2002 12047731

Mann K, Lehert P, Morgan MY: The efficacy of acamprosate in the maintenance of abstinence in alcohol-dependent individuals: results of a meta-analysis. Alcohol Clin Exp Res 28(1):51–63, 2004 14745302

Mason BJ, Quello S, Goodell V, et al: Gabapentin treatment for alcohol dependence: a randomized clinical trial. JAMA Intern Med 174(1):70–77, 2014 24190578

Mayfield D, McLeod G, Hall P: The CAGE questionnaire: validation of a new alcoholism screening instrument. Am J Psychiatry 131(10):1121–1123, 1974 4416585

Mayo-Smith MF; American Society of Addiction Medicine Working Group on Pharmacological Management of Alcohol Withdrawal: Pharmacological management of alcohol withdrawal. A meta-analysis and evidence-based practice guideline. JAMA 278(2):144–151, 1997 9214531

Mayo-Smith MF, Beecher LH, Fischer TL, et al: Management of alcohol withdrawal delirium. An evidence-based practice guideline. Arch Intern Med 164(13):1405–1412, 2004 15249349

Mirijello A, D'Angelo C, Ferrulli A, et al: Identification and management of alcohol withdrawal syndrome. Drugs 75(4):353–365, 2015 25666543

Myrick H, Malcolm R, Randall PK, et al: A double-blind trial of gabapentin versus lorazepam in the treatment of alcohol withdrawal. Alcohol Clin Exp Res 33(9):1582–1588, 2009 19485969

O'Malley SS, Jaffe AJ, Chang G, et al: Naltrexone and coping skills therapy for alcohol dependence. A controlled study. Arch Gen Psychiatry 49(11):881–887, 1992 1444726

Oslin DW, Berrettini W, Kranzler HR, et al: A functional polymorphism of the mu-opioid receptor gene is associated with naltrexone response in alcohol-dependent patients. Neuropsychopharmacology 28(8):1546–1552, 2003 12813472

Project MATCH Research Group: Project MATCH secondary a priori hypotheses. Addiction 92(12):1671–1698, 1997 9581001

Project MATCH Research Group: Matching alcoholism treatments to client heterogeneity: treatment main effects and matching effects on drinking during treatment. J Stud Alcohol 59(6):631–639, 1998 9811084

Roberto M, Gilpin NW, O'Dell LE, et al: Cellular and behavioral interactions of gabapentin with alcohol dependence. Version 2. J Neurosci 28(22):5762–5771, 2008 18509038

Saitz R, Mayo-Smith MF, Roberts MS, et al: Individualized treatment for alcohol withdrawal. A randomized double-blind controlled trial. JAMA 272(7):519–523, 1994 8046805

Saunders JB, Aasland OG, Babor TF, et al: Development of the Alcohol Use Disorders Identification Test (AUDIT): WHO collaborative project on early detection of persons with harmful alcohol consumption—II. Addiction 88(6):791–804, 1993 8329970

Srisurapanont M, Jarusuraisin N: Opioid antagonists for alcohol dependence. Cochrane Database Syst Rev (1):CD001867, 2005 15674887

Stahre M, Roeber J, Kanny D, et al: Contribution of excessive alcohol consumption to deaths and years of potential life lost in the United States. Prev Chronic Dis 11:E109, 2014 24967831

Sullivan JT, Swift RM, Lewis DC: Benzodiazepine requirements during alcohol withdrawal syndrome: clinical implications of using a standardized withdrawal scale. J Clin Psychopharmacol 11(5):291–295, 1991 1684974

Victor M: Alcohol withdrawal seizures: an overview, in Alcohol and Seizures. Edited by Porter R. New York, FA Davis, 1990

Volpicelli JR, Alterman AI, Hayashida M, et al: Naltrexone in the treatment of alcohol dependence. Arch Gen Psychiatry 49(11):876–880, 1992 1345133

Wright C, Moore RD: Disulfiram treatment of alcoholism. Am J Med 88(6):647–655, 1990 2189310

CHAPTER 10

Neurobiology of Stimulants

Mehmet Sofuoglu, M.D., Ph.D.

Elise E. DeVito, Ph.D.

Thomas R. Kosten, M.D.

Stimulants, also called psychostimulants, activate the central nervous system (CNS) and induce euphoria. As prescription medicines (e.g., lisdexamfetamine, methylphenidate, amphetamine), they treat attention-deficit/hyperactivity disorder (ADHD) or narcolepsy. Stimulants, especially cocaine, methamphetamine, or 3,4-methylenedioxymethamphetamine (MDMA, ecstasy), are also widely misused for their performance-enhancing effects. In this chapter on the neurobiology of stimulants, we focus on cocaine and methamphetamine because of their worldwide prevalence.

Pharmacology of Stimulants

Cocaine is commonly used intranasally (snorted), inhaled by smoking (in its freebase form, crack), or administered intravenously. Methamphetamine is commonly used orally, intravenously, or by inhalation ("ice," "crank") (Courtney and Ray 2014). The route of administration influences the reinforcing effects of stimulants, because faster drug delivery is more reinforcing. In comparison with oral or intranasal routes, intravenous or inhalation routes produce a more rapid onset of effects (less than 5 minutes vs. longer than 15–30 minutes) and more intense euphoria. Methamphetamine has a longer duration of action than cocaine (8–12 hours vs. 20–30 minutes) following intravenous delivery or inhalation.

Stimulants increase synaptic levels of monoamines (dopamine, serotonin, and norepinephrine) by blocking the dopamine, serotonin, and norepinephrine transporters (e.g., cocaine, methylphenidate) or releasing monoamines by inhibition of the vesicular monoamine transporter 2 (VMAT-2) (e.g., methamphetamine) (Moszczynska and Callan 2017). The reinforcing effects of stimulants are attributed to increased dopamine levels in the mesolimbic dopamine pathway (Haber 2014). This pathway originates from the ventral tegmental area (VTA) of the midbrain and has projections to several limbic and cortical areas, including the nucleus accumbens, the amygdala, and the prefrontal cortex (Haber 2014). Both stimulatory (type 1 [D_1]) and inhibitory (type 2 [D_2]) dopamine receptors are activated as a result of stimulant exposure. Activation of D_1 receptors is necessary for the rewarding effects of stimulants. Norepinephrine mediates the stimulant effects of increased arousal and cardiovascular and stress pathway activation. Activation of the serotonergic system mediates stimulant effects on mood (Müller and Homberg 2015).

Stimulants also interact with other neurotransmitters, including glutamate, γ-aminobutyric acid (GABA), acetylcholine, oxytocin, corticotropin-releasing factor (CRF), and other stress hormones (Koob and Volkow 2016). Glutamate and GABA are the main excitatory and inhibitory neurotransmitters in the brain, respectively. Glutamate release is thought to play a crucial role in facilitating the development of sensitization and craving in response to stimulants. In contrast, GABA attenuates reinforcement from stimulants and response to drug cues. Stimulant-induced acetylcholine release in the prefrontal cortex improves sustained attention. Oxytocin release has been linked to increased sociability following stimulant use. CRF release following stimulant exposure activates stress pathways that facilitate drug seeking and relapse.

Neuroimmune system activation, especially of microglia, has more recently been recognized to modulate the reinforcing effects of stimulants (Bachtell et al. 2017). Activation of Toll-like receptor 4 (TLR4), located on microglia, seems to be an essential step for the reinforcing effects of cocaine. TLR4 participates in immune surveillance of pathogens (e.g., bacteria, viruses), endogenous danger signals (i.e., substances released by cellular injury), and exogenous small molecules (e.g., cocaine, methamphetamine, opioids). In humans, the medication minocycline, which inhibits microglia activation, attenuates the subjective rewarding effects from amphetamine use (Sofuoglu et al. 2011). Thus, the neuroimmune system may be a novel treatment target for stimulant use disorder.

Acute Effects of Stimulants in Humans

Acute effects of stimulants include euphoria, grandiosity, enhanced energy, alertness, suppression of appetite, sexual stimulation, and sociability. In addition, dysphoria, anxiety, restlessness, stereotypic behavior, psychomotor agitation, and impaired judgment are also commonly observed (Courtney and Ray 2014). Heavy stimulant use can produce psychosis (hallucinations and delusions), vomiting, seizures, and stimulant delirium, which is characterized by a state of confusion and excitement. Physiological effects of stimulants include increased blood pressure and heart rate, dilated pupils, hyperthermia, perspiration, and chills.

In positron emission tomography (PET) imaging studies, acute administration of a euphoria-inducing (40 mg) cocaine dose occupied 80%–90% of the dopamine transporter (DAT), whereas a 5-mg cocaine dose, which produces perceptible effects but no euphoria, occupied about 40% of the DAT (Gatley et al. 1997). Functional magnetic resonance imaging (fMRI) studies have shown that acute cocaine administration activates many brain regions, including the nucleus accumbens, basal ganglia, thalamus, insula, cingulate, hippocampus, and cortical regions. Subjective ratings of cocaine "rush" were associated with activity in regions showing rapid activity increases following cocaine administration but with a short duration (e.g., VTA, pons, basal forebrain, caudate, cingulate, lateral prefrontal cortex), whereas "craving" ratings were associated with activity in regions showing sustained increases (nucleus accumbens, parahippocampal gyrus, regions of lateral prefrontal cortex) or decreases (amygdala) in blood-oxygen-level-dependent (BOLD) signals of blood flow and assumed neural activity (Risinger et al. 2005).

Stimulant Addiction

Development of Addiction

Development of addiction is a complex process influenced by the unique pharmacological properties of drugs, individual vulnerability factors (e.g., sex/gender, age, race, genetic makeup, psychiatric comorbidities), and environmental and social factors (e.g., drug availability, stress, poverty). Animal models of addiction have traditionally focused on the pharmacological properties of drugs, producing a wealth of information regarding underlying mechanisms of addiction. However, drug exposure and availability are necessary but not sufficient for development of addiction. For example, among individuals who have used cocaine, it is estimated that approximately 15%–16% will develop an addiction within 10 years (Wagner and Anthony 2002). Incorporation of individual vulnerability factors, which this relatively low rate of progression to addiction indicates, into animal models of addiction may improve their direct translation to clinical populations (Müller 2018).

Several addiction models for stimulants have been proposed, mostly based on animal models of addiction. An influential theory of drug addiction, the *incentive sensitization theory,* emphasizes the long-lasting sensitization of dopamine and glutamate neurons in the mesolimbic system following prolonged drug use, resulting in hyperreactivity of the mesolimbic system to drug-related cues and contexts (Berridge and Robinson 2016). This hyperreactivity of the system produces an automatic appetitive process, or incentive salience, that invokes a conditioned response of "wanting" a drug. Accordingly, drug cues become so salient that they induce "wanting" craving independent of any pleasure they yield (Berridge and Robinson 2016). Thus, the incentive sensitization theory predicts an increase in craving over time even if the euphoric effects of the drug are diminished. Clinical studies have provided partial support for the incentive sensitization theory, although whether and how long craving increases over time remains unclear (Small et al. 2009). A similar theory, *psychomotor sensitization,* emphasizes gradual increases in locomotor activity following repeated exposure to stimulants. The neural adaptations for development of incentive sensitization may not be similar to those for development of psychomotor sensitization, and this clearly needs testing. Stimulant-induced psychomotor sensitization also is not well demonstrated in humans, only in rodents (Vanderschuren and Pierce 2010).

Cellular and Molecular Mechanisms of Stimulant Addiction

Neuroadaptations or neuroplastic changes associated with the development of addiction affect a wide range of neurotransmitter systems in the CNS, including dopamine, norepinephrine, serotonin, glutamate, GABA, acetylcholine, opioid peptides, oxytocin, CRF, and orexin (Koob and Volkow 2016). These neuroadaptations include changes in synaptic transmission, in the strength of synaptic connections, and in the larger-scale neurocircuitry. A growing body of preclinical and clinical literature has described the neuroadaptations associated with development of stimulant addiction (Korpi et al. 2015).

Prolonged exposure to stimulants induces neuroplastic changes in the VTA, nucleus accumbens, hippocampus, amygdala, and prefrontal cortex (Korpi et al. 2015). The neuroplastic changes in the VTA are especially significant, given that the VTA is mainly responsible for assigning salience to environmental stimuli. A single dose of cocaine can induce potentiation of the excitatory input to the VTA dopamine cells (Kauer and Malenka 2007). This increased excitatory input is likely due to changes in glutamate transmission, and two possible mechanisms have been proposed: 1) increased permeability of the NMDA (N-methyl-D-aspartate) receptor to calcium, with a resultant increase in CaMKII (Ca2+/calmodulin-dependent protein kinase II) signaling; and 2) increased ratio of AMPA (α-amino-3-hydroxy-5-methyl-4-isoxazole-propionic acid) to NMDA receptor signaling to the VTA dopamine cells (Kauer and Malenka 2007). The end result of these neuroadaptations is increased dopamine transmission in the mesolimbic reward circuitry, which presumably represents a critical step in development of addiction to stimulants.

In comparison with the VTA, the nucleus accumbens is less sensitive to stimulant-induced synaptic neuroplasticity, a finding that supports the primary role of the VTA in inducing such changes in the nucleus accumbens. The medium spiny neurons (MSNs) are GABA projection neurons and represent more than 95% of the neurons in the nucleus accumbens. The MSNs are subdivided on the basis of whether they express the stimulatory D_1 or the inhibitory D_2 type of dopamine receptor. D_1 receptors are closely linked to reward signaling in the CNS and show low affinity to dopamine (Keeler et al. 2014). In rodents, activation of D_1 receptors facilitates cocaine self-administration, and blockage of these receptors inhibits cocaine self-administration. In contrast, activation of D_2 receptors, which have a high affinity for dopamine, may prevent reward and induce punishment-related signals (Kravitz et al. 2012). Importantly, repeated exposure to stimulants upregulates the excitatory D_1 dopamine receptors and downregulates the inhibitory D_2 receptors, resulting in enhanced dopamine transmission.

Short-term (i.e., 5 days) exposure to stimulants also induces expression of many genes in the striatum, including those involved in transcription, angiogenesis, cell adhesion, apoptosis, and neuronal development (Korpi et al. 2015). Among these genes, ongoing research has focused on transcription factors such as ΔFosB (delta FBJ murine osteosarcoma viral oncogene homolog B), CREB (cAMP [cyclic adenosine monophosphate] response element binding), NF-κB (nuclear factor kappa-B), and MEF2 (myocyte enhancer factor-2) (Nestler 2005). Induction of ΔFosB in the nucleus accumbens increases the rewarding effects of stimulants, whereas induction of CREB has the opposite effects. Stimulant-induced increases in NF-kB enhance the rewarding effects of stimulants and increase the dendritic spines in the nucleus accumbens. Similarly, MEF2 modulates increases in spine density induced by cocaine. These transcription factors may serve as potential targets for the development of novel medications for stimulant addiction.

Functional Neuroimaging Studies

Neuroimaging studies have provided insight into the neuroadaptations associated with chronic stimulant use and development of addiction in humans. Single-photon emission computerized tomography (SPECT) and PET imaging studies have been valuable in quantifying the changes in dopamine receptor and DAT density associated with stimulant use and addiction. A meta-analysis of neuroimaging studies found reductions in amphetamine- or methylphenidate-induced striatal dopamine release and D_2/D_3 receptor availability in cocaine or methamphetamine users compared with healthy control subjects (Ashok et al. 2017). DAT availability was significantly reduced in methamphetamine users, but results from cocaine users were inconclusive. Importantly, the reduced D_2/D_3 receptor density and striatal dopamine release were found to persist even after 9 months of abstinence, suggesting the long-term or irreversible nature of these changes (Ashok et al. 2017). Alternatively, these findings may simply be due to preexisting downregulation of the dopamine system that renders the individual vulnerable to stimulant addiction. We need longitudinal studies to tease apart these possibilities.

Functional connectivity can be measured with several fMRI techniques, which allow assessment of connections within and between functional brain networks in the absence of external stimuli (e.g., resting-state functional connectivity) or during in-scanner task performance, including in functional networks that subserve functions such as inhibitory control, attention, and emotional regulation, which are thought to contribute to addiction. In comparison with healthy control subjects, cocaine-dependent individuals exhibit altered resting-state and task-based functional connectivity in a range of networks, including corticostriatal networks and the default mode network (Ma et al. 2015). Given the associations between these functional connectivity measures and clinical outcomes, and the effect of pharmaceutical stimulants (e.g., methylphenidate) on functional connectivity measures, connectivity in these circuits may be a meaningful target for treatment of cocaine dependence (Ma et al. 2015).

Prolonged stimulant use has also been tied to changes in striatal activation patterns associated with development of stimulant addiction. One popular hypothesis is that escalation of stimulant addiction coincides with relative shifts in activity from the ventral to the dorsal striatum in parallel with a shift from substance use being impulsive to such use being more compulsive (Everitt and Robbins 2016). In an fMRI study, increased ventral striatal activity was found during anticipation of a nondrug reward among patients with moderate to severe cocaine use disorder (Jia et al. 2011), a finding that may suggest hypersensitivity of this region to reward anticipation. In abstinent cocaine users, dopamine release in the dorsal striatum was found to be increased in response to cocaine cues versus neutral cues (Volkow et al. 2006). Furthermore, greater cue-induced dorsal striatal dopamine release was positively associated with cocaine craving, withdrawal, and addiction severity, suggesting that diminished dorsal striatum activation may be a reasonable treatment target in stimulant-addicted individuals (Volkow et al. 2006).

Relapse to Stimulant Use

Stimulant addiction, like other addictions, is a chronic disorder with high rates of relapse during abstinence. Exposure to stimulant drugs ("priming"), stimulant-associated cues or contexts ("people, places, and things"), stress, and withdrawal or withdrawal-associated cues all can trigger relapse.

Laboratory animals have been used to model relapse using extinction-reinstatement paradigms. In these models, laboratory animals in which stimulant self-administration has been extinguished are exposed to various stimuli (e.g., a priming dose of stimulants, stimulant-associated cues or context, withdrawal states, or stress) designed to induce nonreinforced stimulant seeking (Koob and Volkow 2016). These studies led to significant advances in identifying the neurocircuitry of reinstatement induced by different methods (e.g., a priming dose of stimulants, cues, stress). For drug-induced reinstatement (i.e., reinstatement induced by a priming dose of stimulants), the neurocircuitry includes glutamatergic projections from the prefrontal cortex to the nucleus accumbens (Koob and Volkow 2016). Both D_1 and D_2 receptors in the prefrontal cortex modulate these glutamatergic projections. For cue-induced reinstatement, the neurocircuitry includes glutamatergic projections from the prefrontal cortex, basolateral amygdala, and ventral subiculum that modulate dopamine transmission to the nucleus accumbens. Stress-induced reinstatement of drug-related responding in animal models appears to depend on the activation of both CRF and norepinephrine in elements of the extended amygdala (i.e., central medial amygdala, sublenticular substantia innominata, the nucleus accumbens shell, and the bed nucleus of the stria terminalis) and the VTA. These findings further highlight the complexity of relapse and provide potential targets for novel treatments.

Functional neuroimaging studies in cocaine users show that greater drug cue or stress cue reactivity is associated with a higher likelihood of relapse (Courtney et al. 2016). In PET imaging studies, cue-induced craving for cocaine is associated with increased dopamine release in the striatum, amygdala, and prefrontal cortex and with increased opioid peptide release in the anterior cingulate and frontal cortex. These changes in reward circuitry activation in humans are consistent with those observed in rodent studies during drug consumption and drug seeking.

Incubation of cocaine craving means that cue-induced craving may increase in magnitude with prolonged abstinence. For example, in rats trained to press a lever to obtain cocaine, the ability of cocaine-related cues to induce lever pressing (i.e., induce "drug seeking") progressively increased across a 2-month cocaine abstinence period, despite the fact that lever-pressing was not reinforced by cocaine delivery during these 2 months (Grimm et al. 2001). Incubation of craving also has been extended to humans (Li et al. 2015). Methamphetamine-dependent humans similarly showed a progressive increase in cocaine cue–induced craving during 3 months of abstinence, and then a decrease at 6 months and 1 year of abstinence (Wang et al. 2013). The neurobiological mechanism of cocaine craving incubation seems to involve enhanced responsiveness of the nucleus accumbens to glutamatergic input, possibly due to greater conductance of the calcium-permeable AMPA receptors compared with calcium-impermeable AMPA receptors. This neuroadaptation is observed after 30 days of abstinence, coinciding with increased response to cocaine cues (Dong et al. 2017). Incubation of craving emphasizes the need to not only monitor patients for increases in craving but also provide long-term relapse-prevention treatments that address this increase in cue-induced craving.

Stimulant Withdrawal

Abstinence from stimulants can induce withdrawal symptoms, which manifest as depressive symptoms such as dysphoric mood, anhedonia, irritability, increased sleep and fatigue, and loss of motivation for nondrug rewards. However, only a subgroup of cocaine users experience withdrawal symptoms, and those with a past history of depression are more likely to experience withdrawal after use (Sofuoglu et al. 2003). Animal studies have consistently demonstrated that stimulant withdrawal is associated with reward deficits (as indicated by elevations of the reward threshold in intracranial self-stimulation procedures) and reduced dopamine transmission in the nucleus accumbens (D'Souza and Markou 2010). Consistent with these findings, a PET imaging study of cocaine users found that striatal dopamine release induced by amphetamine or methylphenidate was 50% lower in detoxified users and 80% lower in ongoing users compared with healthy control subjects (Ashok et al. 2017). Although cocaine withdrawal symptoms include diminished response to natural rewards, in a human laboratory study, cocaine users who reported experiencing withdrawal symptoms during abstinence rated cocaine delivery as more rewarding ("high," "feel effects") than did cocaine users who reported not experiencing withdrawal during abstinence. This combination of negative affect and anhedonia during abstinence paired with enhanced drug reward may contribute to maintenance of stimulant use (Sofuoglu et al. 2003).

Stimulant Tolerance

Although tolerance to the positive subjective effects of cocaine (e.g., high) is well known clinically, the magnitude of this tolerance is less prominent compared with the tolerance that occurs in users of alcohol and opioids. In PET imaging studies, cocaine-addicted individuals show less striatal dopamine release and euphoria (i.e., self-reported "high") in response to methylphenidate than do healthy control subjects (Volkow et al. 1997), a finding that possibly reflects tolerance development as a result of regular cocaine use. In preclinical studies using an extended-access cocaine self-administration model, escalation of cocaine intake coincided with development of tolerance to cocaine-induced dopamine release and reduced maximal rates of dopamine uptake by the DAT (Calipari et al. 2014). Thus, tolerance to the rewarding effects of stimulants may trigger craving as a means of compensating for the reduction in actual versus expected stimulant-induced euphoria.

Stimulant-Induced Psychosis

Transient psychotic symptoms are commonly experienced by both cocaine and methamphetamine users, with rates ranging from 50% to 75% (Arunogiri et al. 2020). Symptoms can include paranoia, auditory hallucinations, increased activity, and stereotyped compulsive behavior (McKetin 2018). More persistent psychosis is less common (i.e., an estimated prevalence of 15%–25% among dependent stimulant users), and is most often observed in men with heavy intravenous or smoked stimulant use, persons with a history of psychotic disorder or other psychiatric comorbidities (e.g., bipolar disorder, depression, antisocial personality disorder), and persons who also use cannabis (McKetin et al. 2006). Methamphetamine users have more severe positive symptoms (e.g., delusions, suspiciousness, unusual thought content, hallucinations, grandiosity) than do cocaine users (Alexander et al. 2017). The lag period between the initial stimulant use and the onset of psychotic disorder is about 5 years.

Although the pathophysiology of stimulant-induced psychosis has not been well characterized, exposure to repeated doses of stimulant results in greater sensitivity to increased dopamine release in the mesocorticolimbic areas and sensitization to the development of psychotic symptoms (Hsieh et al. 2014). Stimulant-induced psychosis is associated with high rates of developing schizophrenia, suicidal behavior, and high utilization of health services (Callaghan et al. 2012). Consistent with these findings, in fMRI studies, individuals with stimulant-induced psychotic disorder show reduced frontotemporal cortical thickness and smaller volumes of hippocampus and thalamus (Uhlmann et al. 2016). These findings are consistent with previous reports in schizophrenic patients (Wright et al. 2000) and may represent common neural changes associated with psychosis in general.

Stimulant Neurotoxicity and Neurocognitive Effects of Stimulants

Stimulant Neurotoxicity

Animal studies have demonstrated that chronic methamphetamine exposure has direct neurotoxic effects on dopamine neurons, including those in the nigrostriatal pathway (Moszczynska and Callan 2017). The underlying mechanism for this neurotoxicity is thought to involve elevations in dopamine levels in the cytosol of neurons due to inhibition of VMAT-2, rather than increases in synaptic dopamine levels. Stimulants differentially affect VMAT-2 function; whereas methamphetamine inhibits VMAT-2 activity, cocaine stimulates VMAT-2 function. In the cytoplasm, excess dopamine can produce reactive oxygen and nitrogen species, with subsequent induction of oxidative stress. In addition, methamphetamine-induced increases in extracellular glutamate can induce neurotoxicity by increasing reactive nitrogen species and activating calcium-dependent proteases, resulting in cytoskeletal damage (Moszczynska and Callan 2017). Furthermore, methamphetamine exposure can activate a neuroimmune response, resulting in the release of cytokines, chemokines, and adhesion molecules, which may contribute to neurotoxicity in different brain regions. In contrast to the dose-dependent damage inflicted by methamphetamine on dopamine neurons in animals, findings from human studies are less clear. For example, recreational methamphetamine use does not seem to cause damage to dopamine neurons in humans (Kish et al. 2017). Although many methamphetamine users show persistent CNS deficits consistent with damage to dopamine neurons, these deficits do not seem to be correlated with the total amount of methamphetamine consumed (Kish et al. 2017).

Neurocognitive Effects

Comparisons of cocaine or methamphetamine users with healthy control subjects show similar cognitive deficits in the stimulant users (Sofuoglu et al. 2016), although cocaine is more often associated with working memory impairments (which are typically linked with prefrontal cortex dysfunction), whereas methamphetamine is more often associated with memory impairments that are linked with temporal and parietal lobe dysfunction (Hall et al. 2018). These cognitive deficits may persist for months and/or may reflect preexisting cognitive deficits (e.g., response inhibition) that make individuals more vulnerable to initiating drug use and/or becoming drug-dependent.

Structural neuroimaging studies in cocaine and methamphetamine users have found a broad range of abnormalities, including diminished cortical gray matter volume and reduced white matter integrity. Reductions in white matter myelination and axon caliber and associated fiber density and organization are reflected in reduced fractional anisotropy (Ersche et al. 2013; London et al. 2015). These structural abnormalities may contribute to the cognitive deficits associated with chronic stimulant use, such as those affecting the executive functions of response inhibition, cognitive control, decision making, and cognitive flexibility (London et al. 2015). Diminished gray matter volume in the inferior and middle frontal gyri is associated with longer durations of stimulant use (Ersche et al. 2013). However, more importantly, recovery is possible, and longer durations of abstinence are positively correlated with greater increases in gray matter volume (London et al. 2015). Some structural brain differences in stimulant-dependent individuals may represent heritable traits predating drug use, given findings that these patients' non-drug-using siblings also differed from healthy control subjects in some of these same white matter and subcortical gray matter brain abnormalities (Ersche et al. 2013). Diminished frontal gray matter volume was present only in the stimulant-dependent individuals, and not their siblings (Ersche et al. 2013). Furthermore, better white matter integrity was associated with longer periods of cocaine abstinence (Xu et al. 2010). Together, these findings suggest the clinical relevance and potential reversal of structural brain abnormalities in stimulant users.

Comorbidity

Although most of the preclinical research and human clinical trials focus on stimulant addiction in isolation, the majority of individuals with stimulant addiction have psychiatric comorbidities, most commonly other substance use and mood disorders (MacLean and Sofuoglu 2018). A recent meta-analysis estimated that cocaine is frequently used concurrently (i.e., within 30 days) with other substances, including alcohol (77%) and cannabis (64%) (Liu et al. 2018). Human studies have shown that both alcohol and cannabis may enhance cocaine's acute subjective effects. Evidence also suggests that concurrent alcohol use may worsen the neurocognitive deficits associated with stimulant use and may negatively influence treatment outcomes. However, only a few preclinical studies have focused on stimulant use with other drugs of abuse (Liu et al. 2018).

A possible common link between stimulant use disorder and depression is the mesocorticolimbic reward pathway. In addition to its key role in mediating the rewarding effects of drugs and natural rewards, the mesocorticolimbic pathway has also been linked to depressive symptoms, especially to anhedonia (i.e., reduced ability to experience pleasure), a core symptom of major depressive disorder as well as of stimulant withdrawal (D'Souza and Markou 2010). Anhedonia or depressive symptoms may enhance the rewarding effects of stimulants, including cocaine in cocaine users and amphetamines in non-drug-using individuals (MacLean and Sofuoglu 2018). These findings provide a possible mechanism by which depression or anhedonia may facilitate stimulant use.

Impact of Sex and Sex Hormones

Women account for about one-third of stimulant users in the United States (Substance Abuse and Mental Health Services Administration 2018). Important sex differences in stimulant addiction include greater vulnerability in women for development of substance use disorder and more harmful consequences from substance use disorder than in men (McRae-Clark et al. 2017). Women with stimulant addiction also experience more frequent comorbid anxiety and mood disorders and have more severe medical and psychosocial problems than men with stimulant addiction. Preclinical studies suggest that females are more sensitive than males to stress-induced reinstatement, mediated by CRF and noradrenergic activation (McRae-Clark et al. 2017). In human studies, cocaine-dependent women showed greater sensitivity to stressful stimuli and noradrenergic stimulation than did men. Consistent with these findings, in a neuroimaging study using guided imagery of stressful or drug-related events, cocaine-dependent women showed greater activation to stressful imagery than did non-substance-using women, whereas cocaine-dependent men showed greater activation to drug-related imagery than did non-substance-using men (Potenza et al. 2012). Thus, treatments targeting the CRF and noradrenergic systems may be particularly effective in women with stimulant use disorders.

Preclinical and clinical studies have shown that the female sex hormones estradiol and progesterone modulate the rewarding effects of stimulant drugs (Andersen et al. 2012). Whereas estradiol enhances the rewarding effects of stimulants and dopamine release in the nucleus accumbens, progesterone attenuates stimulants' rewarding effects. In comparison with women who were in the follicular phase (high estradiol, low progesterone) of the menstrual cycle, women who were in the luteal phase (high progesterone) showed attenuated responses to the positive subjective effects of cocaine or amphetamine (Peltier and Sofuoglu 2018). The sudden drop in progesterone levels following childbirth may also contribute to high rates of relapse to drug use, including to stimulants, during the postpartum period. A double-blind, randomized, placebo-controlled study using progesterone showed promising results with progesterone in preventing relapse to cocaine use among postpartum women with a history of cocaine use (Yonkers et al. 2014).

Conclusion

Stimulant addiction is a chronic disorder of compulsive drug use that has high rates of relapse. Characteristic withdrawal, tolerance, psychotic symptoms, and neurotoxicity occur especially with methamphetamine use, and use of animal models of addiction has allowed us to gain a better understanding of the neuroadaptations and molecular mechanisms underlying these characteristics. Further refinement of these models by incorporating both individual and environmental factors may improve their application to humans. Commonly encountered comorbidities of stimulant addiction, including other addictions and psychiatric disorders, are rarely addressed in preclinical and clinical studies and warrant future investigation.

References

Alexander PD, Gicas KM, Willi TS, et al: A comparison of psychotic symptoms in subjects with methamphetamine versus cocaine dependence. Psychopharmacology (Berl) 234(9–10):1535–1547, 2017 28190084

Andersen ML, Sawyer EK, Howell LL: Contributions of neuroimaging to understanding sex differences in cocaine abuse. Exp Clin Psychopharmacol 20(1):2–15, 2012 21875225

Arunogiri S, McKetin R, Verdejo-Garcia A, et al: The methamphetamine-associated psychosis spectrum: a clinically focused review. International Journal of Mental Health and Addiction 18:54–65, 2020. Available at: https://doi.org/10.1007/s11469-018-9934-4. Accessed June 25, 2020.

Ashok AH, Mizuno Y, Volkow ND, et al: Association of stimulant use with dopaminergic alterations in users of cocaine, amphetamine, or methamphetamine: a systematic review and meta-analysis. JAMA Psychiatry 74(5):511–519, 2017 28297025

Bachtell RK, Jones JD, Heinzerling KG, et al: Glial and neuroinflammatory targets for treating substance use disorders. Drug Alcohol Depend 180:156–170, 2017 28892721

Berridge KC, Robinson TE: Liking, wanting, and the incentive-sensitization theory of addiction. Am Psychol 71(8):670–679, 2016 27977239

Calipari ES, Ferris MJ, Jones SR: Extended access of cocaine self-administration results in tolerance to the dopamine-elevating and locomotor-stimulating effects of cocaine. J Neurochem 128(2):224–232, 2014 24102293

Callaghan RC, Cunningham JK, Allebeck P, et al: Methamphetamine use and schizophrenia: a population-based cohort study in California. Am J Psychiatry 169(4):389–396, 2012 22193527

Courtney KE, Ray LA: Methamphetamine: an update on epidemiology, pharmacology, clinical phenomenology, and treatment literature. Drug Alcohol Depend 143:11–21, 2014 25176528

Courtney KE, Schacht JP, Hutchison K, et al: Neural substrates of cue reactivity: association with treatment outcomes and relapse. Addict Biol 21(1):3–22, 2016 26435524

D'Souza MS, Markou A: Neural substrates of psychostimulant withdrawal-induced anhedonia, in Behavioral Neuroscience of Drug Addiction. Edited by Self DW, Staley JK. New York, Springer, 2010, pp 119–178

Dong Y, Taylor JR, Wolf ME, et al: Circuit and synaptic plasticity mechanisms of drug relapse. J Neurosci 37(45):10867–10876, 2017 29118216

Ersche KD, Williams GB, Robbins TW, et al: Meta-analysis of structural brain abnormalities associated with stimulant drug dependence and neuroimaging of addiction vulnerability and resilience. Curr Opin Neurobiol 23(4):615–624, 2013 23523373

Everitt BJ, Robbins TW: Drug addiction: updating actions to habits to compulsions ten years on. Annu Rev Psychol 67:23–50, 2016 26253543

Gatley SJ, Volkow ND, Gifford AN, et al: Model for estimating dopamine transporter occupancy and subsequent increases in synaptic dopamine using positron emission tomography and carbon-11-labeled cocaine. Biochem Pharmacol 53(1):43–52, 1997 8960062

Grimm JW, Hope BT, Wise RA, et al: Neuroadaptation. Incubation of cocaine craving after withdrawal. Nature 412(6843):141–142, 2001 11449260

Haber SN: The place of dopamine in the cortico-basal ganglia circuit. Neuroscience 282:248–257, 2014 25445194

Hall MG, Hauson AO, Wollman SC, et al: Neuropsychological comparisons of cocaine versus methamphetamine users: a research synthesis and meta-analysis. Am J Drug Alcohol Abuse 44(3):277–293, 2018 28825847

Hsieh JH, Stein DJ, Howells FM: The neurobiology of methamphetamine induced psychosis. Front Hum Neurosci 8:537, 2014 25100979

Jia Z, Worhunsky PD, Carroll KM, et al: An initial study of neural responses to monetary incentives as related to treatment outcome in cocaine dependence. Biol Psychiatry 70(6):553–560, 2011 21704307

Kauer JA, Malenka RC: Synaptic plasticity and addiction. Nat Rev Neurosci 8(11):844–858, 2007 17948030

Keeler JF, Pretsell DO, Robbins TW: Functional implications of dopamine D1 vs. D2 receptors: a "prepare and select" model of the striatal direct vs. indirect pathways. Neuroscience 282:156–175, 2014 25062777

Kish SJ, Boileau I, Callaghan RC, et al: Brain dopamine neurone "damage": methamphetamine users vs. Parkinson's disease—a critical assessment of the evidence. Eur J Neurosci 45(1):58–66, 2017 27519465

Koob GF, Volkow ND: Neurobiology of addiction: a neurocircuitry analysis. Lancet Psychiatry 3(8):760–773, 2016 27475769

Korpi ER, den Hollander B, Farooq U, et al: Mechanisms of action and persistent neuroplasticity by drugs of abuse. Pharmacol Rev 67(4):872–1004, 2015 26403687

Kravitz AV, Tye LD, Kreitzer AC: Distinct roles for direct and indirect pathway striatal neurons in reinforcement. Nat Neurosci 15(6):816–818, 2012 22544310

Li X, Caprioli D, Marchant NJ: Recent updates on incubation of drug craving: a mini-review. Addict Biol 20(5):872–876, 2015 25440081

Liu Y, Williamson V, Setlow B, et al: The importance of considering polysubstance use: lessons from cocaine research. Drug Alcohol Depend 192:16–28, 2018 30195242

London ED, Kohno M, Morales AM, et al: Chronic methamphetamine abuse and corticostriatal deficits revealed by neuroimaging. Brain Res 1628(Pt A):174–185, 2015 25451127

Ma L, Steinberg JL, Moeller FG, et al: Effect of cocaine dependence on brain connections: clinical implications. Expert Rev Neurother 15(11):1307–1319, 2015 26512421

MacLean RR, Sofuoglu M: Stimulants and mood disorders. Current Addiction Reports 5:323–329, 2018. Available at: https://link.springer.com/article/10.1007%2Fs40429-018-0212-0. Accessed December 22, 2019.

McKetin R: Methamphetamine psychosis: insights from the past. Addiction 113(8):1522–1527, 2018 29516555

McKetin R, McLaren J, Lubman DI, Hides L: The prevalence of psychotic symptoms among methamphetamine users. Addiction 101(10):1473–1478, 2006 16968349

McRae-Clark AL, Cason AM, Kohtz AS, et al: Impact of gender on corticotropin-releasing factor and noradrenergic sensitivity in cocaine use disorder. J Neurosci Res 95(1–2):320–327, 2017 27870396

Moszczynska A, Callan SP: Molecular, behavioral, and physiological consequences of methamphetamine neurotoxicity: implications for treatment. J Pharmacol Exp Ther 362(3):474–488, 2017 28630283

Müller CP: Animal models of psychoactive drug use and addiction—present problems and future needs for translational approaches. Behav Brain Res 352:109–115, 2018 28641965

Müller CP, Homberg JR: The role of serotonin in drug use and addiction. Behav Brain Res 277:146–192, 2015 24769172

Nestler EJ: Is there a common molecular pathway for addiction? Nat Neurosci 8(11):1445–1449, 2005 16251986

Peltier MR, Sofuoglu M: Role of exogenous progesterone in the treatment of men and women with substance use disorders: a narrative review. CNS Drugs 32(5):421–435, 2018 29761343

Potenza MN, Hong KI, Lacadie CM, et al: Neural correlates of stress-induced and cue-induced drug craving: influences of sex and cocaine dependence. Am J Psychiatry 169(4):406–414, 2012 22294257

Risinger RC, Salmeron BJ, Ross TJ, et al: Neural correlates of high and craving during cocaine self-administration using BOLD fMRI. Neuroimage 26(4):1097–1108, 2005 15886020

Small AC, Kampman KM, Plebani J, et al: Tolerance and sensitization to the effects of cocaine use in humans: a retrospective study of long-term cocaine users in Philadelphia. Subst Use Misuse 44(13):1888–1898, 2009 20001286

Sofuoglu M, Dudish-Poulsen S, Brown SB, et al: Association of cocaine withdrawal symptoms with more severe dependence and enhanced subjective response to cocaine. Drug Alcohol Depend 69(3):273–282, 2003 12633913

Sofuoglu M, Mooney M, Kosten T, et al: Minocycline attenuates subjective rewarding effects of dextroamphetamine in humans. Psychopharmacology (Berl) 213(1):61–68, 2011 20838775

Sofuoglu M, DeVito EE, Waters AJ, et al: Cognitive function as a transdiagnostic treatment target in stimulant use disorders. J Dual Diagn 12(1):90–106, 2016 26828702

Substance Abuse and Mental Health Services Administration: Key substance use and mental health indicators in the United States: results from the 2017 National Survey on Drug Use and Health (HHS Publ. No. SMA 18-5068, NSDUH Series H-53). Rockville, MD, Center for Behavioral Health Statistics and Quality, SAMHSA, 2018. Available at: https://www.samhsa.gov/data/sites/default/files/cbhsq-reports/NSDUHFFR2017/NSDUHFFR2017.pdf. Accessed June 25, 2020.

Uhlmann A, Fouche JP, Koen N, et al: Fronto-temporal alterations and affect regulation in methamphetamine dependence with and without a history of psychosis. Psychiatry Res Neuroimaging 248:30–38, 2016 26792587

Vanderschuren LJ, Pierce RC: Sensitization processes in drug addiction. Curr Top Behav Neurosci 3:179–195, 2010 21161753

Volkow ND, Wang GJ, Fowler JS, et al: Decreased striatal dopaminergic responsiveness in detoxified cocaine-dependent subjects. Nature 386(6627):830–833, 1997 9126741

Volkow ND, Wang GJ, Telang F, et al: Cocaine cues and dopamine in dorsal striatum: mechanism of craving in cocaine addiction. J Neurosci 26(24):6583–6588, 2006 16775146

Wagner FA, Anthony JC: From first drug use to drug dependence; developmental periods of risk for dependence upon marijuana, cocaine, and alcohol. Neuropsychopharmacology 26(4):479–488, 2002 11927172

Wang G, Shi J, Chen N, et al: Effects of length of abstinence on decision-making and craving in methamphetamine abusers. PLoS One 8(7):e68791, 2013 23894345

Wright IC, Rabe-Hesketh S, Woodruff PW, et al: Meta-analysis of regional brain volumes in schizophrenia. Am J Psychiatry 157(1):16–25, 2000 10618008

Xu J, DeVito EE, Worhunsky PD, et al: White matter integrity is associated with treatment outcome measures in cocaine dependence. Neuropsychopharmacology 35(7):1541–1549, 2010 20393459

Yonkers KA, Forray A, Nich C, et al: Progesterone reduces cocaine use in postpartum women with a cocaine use disorder: a randomized, double-blind study. Lancet Psychiatry 1(5):360–367, 2014 25328863

CHAPTER 11

Treatment of Stimulant-Related Disorders

Richard A. Rawson, Ph.D.

Kristen Schmidt, M.D.

Larissa J. Mooney, M.D.

The category of "stimulant" drugs encompasses the amphetamine-type stimulants as well as the various forms of cocaine-derived products (e.g., powder cocaine, crack). Amphetamine-type stimulants include methamphetamine as well as prescription medications primarily used for the treatment of attention-deficit/hyperactivity disorder (ADHD), such as amphetamine, methylphenidate, and dextroamphetamine. In the Middle East, fenethylline, a stimulant sold in tablet form (Captagon), is widely used and is the leading reason for treatment admissions in Saudi Arabia and other countries in the region. Khat, a naturally occurring herb with stimulant properties, also poses a significant public health problem in Yemen and East Africa. In the United States, the most commonly used amphetamine-type stimulant is methamphetamine ("crystal," "crank," "speed") or "ice," its smokable form. Methamphetamine is mass-produced and trafficked by Mexican cartels and can also be domestically produced in smaller quantities; such production typically occurs in home-based "mom and pop" labs most often located throughout the western and midwestern United States. Cocaine (and "crack," its smokable freebase form) is a derivative of the coca plant and is imported into the United States from Central and South America.

Methamphetamine and cocaine have the intoxicating properties of euphoria, hyperactivity, restlessness, alertness, and sympathomimetic hyperarousal, as delineated in the *Diagnostic and Statistical Manual of Mental Disorders,* 5th Edition (DSM-5; American Psychiatric Association 2013). They can be injected, smoked, snorted, or ingested orally. Stimulants may be procured illicitly as street drugs or legally through a physician's prescription, or they can be naturally harvested, as in the case of khat.

Epidemiology

Prevalence statistics from the Substance Abuse and Mental Health Services Administration indicate that in 2017, 2.2 million people ages 12 years and older (1%) reported use of cocaine/crack during the previous month, and 774,000 used methamphetamine, whereas 1.8 million misused prescription stimulants (Substance Abuse and Mental Health Services Administration 2018). This represented a 10% increase from 2014 levels for cocaine/crack and an approximately 14% increase for methamphetamine; there was a 6% rise in prescription stimulant misuse. Based on data from the Centers for Disease Control and Prevention (CDC), deaths from "drug poisonings" involving stimulants have also escalated rapidly in recent years (Ahmad et al. 2019). According to the CDC, annual drug poisoning deaths reported as being due to "psychostimulants with abuse potential" (excluding cocaine) increased from 5,716 to 10,333 between 2015 and 2017 (U.S. Department of Justice Drug Enforcement Administration 2019), as illustrated in Figure 11–1. Deaths due to cocaine increased at an even higher rate, from 6,784 to 13,942, over the same period, as illustrated in Figure 11–2.

A number of other indicators reflect the increasing use of stimulants in the United States. For example, in parts of the United States that have successfully expanded the use of medications for opioid use disorder, there are reports of substantial increases in stimulant use among this patient population. In the eastern United States, cocaine appears to be the most widely used stimulant, while in the West and the Midwest, methamphetamine is used at an increasing rate among this patient population (Ellis et al. 2018; Seth et al. 2018).

The neurobiological differences between amphetamine-type stimulants and cocaine are important to note. Whereas cocaine inhibits dopamine reuptake by binding to presynaptic dopamine reuptake transporters, amphetamine-type stimulants have additional effects. For example, methamphetamine increases dopamine efflux by binding to both vesicular monoamine transporters and reuptake inhibitor transporters. The half-life of methamphetamine (11–12 hours) is significantly longer than that of cocaine (90 minutes) (Romanelli and Smith 2006); as a result, methamphetamine's physiological and subjective effects are far more durable than those of cocaine and have a far greater potential for toxicity (Newton et al. 2005).

Clinical Management of Stimulant-Related Disorders

Intoxication

Ingestion of cocaine and methamphetamine causes a surge in catecholamines in the central nervous system. A potent release of dopamine and norepinephrine leads to euphoria, hyperexcitability, hypersexuality, increased locomotor activity, agitation, and psychotic symptoms, including paranoia and hallucinations. Objective findings of hypertension, tachycardia, and arrhythmias on electrocardiograms (ECGs) of users reflect sympathetic overdrive.

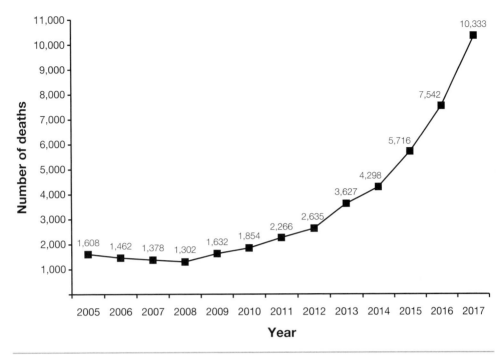

FIGURE 11–1. Drug poisoning deaths involving psychostimulants, 2005–2017.

Source. U.S. Department of Justice Drug Enforcement Administration 2019.

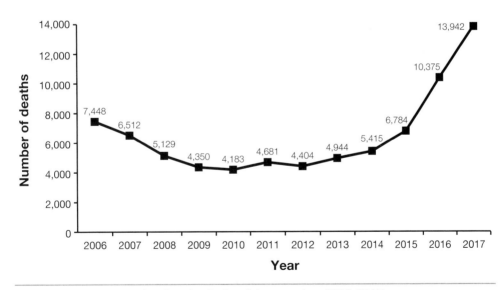

FIGURE 11–2. Drug poisoning deaths involving cocaine, 2006–2017.

Source. U.S. Department of Justice Drug Enforcement Administration 2019.

Acute agitation from cocaine/methamphetamine intoxication is most often the condition that leads users to seek medical attention, and "talking down" the patient in a calm environment is the first course of action. Addressing possible cocaine/

methamphetamine toxicity may involve emetics or lavage to remove methamphet-amine pills, but toxicity from IV or smoked routes of administration may necessitate the use of charcoal and medications such as ammonium chloride to hasten clearance from the gastrointestinal tract and the circulatory system. No medications are avail-able to reverse methamphetamine overdose.

Benzodiazepines may be especially effective in acute management of agitation and distress and may reduce seizure potential in patients, particularly with cocaine toxic-ity. In order to avoid hypertensive crises, blood pressure medication may prove help-ful, although it is important to avoid beta antagonists such as propranolol, which can exacerbate matters through unopposed alpha receptor stimulation. Due to cocaine's shorter duration of action, cocaine intoxication generally resolves more rapidly (2–4 hours) than methamphetamine intoxication, which can last up to 12 hours or longer.

Acute Stimulant Psychosis

The presentations of cocaine and methamphetamine psychosis are similar; however, psychosis is more common among methamphetamine users, and its severity and du-ration are often greater due to the longer half-life of methamphetamine. As sensiti-zation to stimulants develops, psychosis can be triggered with even small doses of cocaine or methamphetamine. The psychotic symptoms frequently include auditory hallucinations and visual (flashing lights, peripheral artifacts), olfactory, and tactile sensations. In addition, powerful paranoia and persecutory delusions are extremely common, along with ideas of reference, stereotypy and compulsive acts, blunted af-fect, poverty of speech, delirium, and violence.

Management of stimulant-induced psychosis, which generally is transient, may re-quire use of either a benzodiazepine or an antipsychotic, both of which should be dis-continued when acute symptoms have resolved. Antipsychotics such as risperidone and olanzapine are less likely to cause extrapyramidal symptoms compared with first-generation agents, and their sedative properties may ameliorate psychomotor agitation. It is, however, important to monitor for hyperthermia and dehydration when antipsychotics are used in patients with acute stimulant intoxication.

Chronic Methamphetamine Psychosis

Persistent symptoms of psychosis are rarely reported among cocaine users in the ab-sence of other comorbid psychiatric disorders. However, symptoms of persistent or chronic methamphetamine psychosis are often so similar to those of schizophrenia that some clinicians may regard them as clinically equivalent conditions, although it has been argued that methamphetamine *produces* a persistent psychosis that resembles schizophrenia (O'Daly et al. 2005). Regardless of the causal direction or association, the symptoms of schizophrenia and those of persistent methamphetamine psychosis are not readily distinguishable; therefore, the treatment for the two conditions is ba-sically the same.

Stimulant Withdrawal

Stimulant withdrawal symptoms consist of severe fatigue, cognitive impairment, feelings of depression and anxiety, anergia, confusion, and paranoia. For the majority of patients experiencing acute withdrawal or early-phase abstinence, most symptoms will resolve within 2–10 days. Rest, exercise, and a healthy diet may be the best management approach for most people experiencing withdrawal. Individuals with heightened agitation and sleep disturbance may respond to benzodiazepines, but acute depression and anhedonia associated with early abstinence generally resolve without intervention. Again, clinicians should be aware of the potential for dehydration and hyperthermia.

Stimulant Use Disorder

Stimulant use disorder, like other substance use disorders, is marked by loss of control over stimulant use despite adverse consequences caused by such use. To qualify for a DSM-5 (American Psychiatric Association 2013) diagnosis of substance use disorder, an individual must have experienced at least 2 of the following 11 symptoms within the past year: 1) difficulty cutting down or stopping use; 2) excessive time spent obtaining, using, or recovering from use; 3) use in excess of what was intended; 4) cravings; 5) tolerance; 6) withdrawal; 7) failure to meet important role obligations; 8) recurrent use in physically hazardous situations; 9) important activities given up because of use, 10) use despite social or interpersonal problems; and 11) use despite psychological or medical consequences. The severity of the use disorder is coded according to the number of symptom criteria met over the past 12 months: mild (2–3 symptoms), moderate (4–5 symptoms), or severe (6 or more symptoms). Common comorbidities observed in stimulant users include depression and anxiety disorders; stimulant use is also associated with an elevated risk of suicidal ideation or behaviors.

Certain clinical challenges are commonly encountered by clinicians who treat stimulant users. Although this response is not unique to users of stimulants, persons who use cocaine and methamphetamine can develop a powerful Pavlovian craving response that is "triggered" when they come into contact with cues previously associated with stimulant use. These cues or "triggers" can include objects (e.g., cash), people (e.g., drug user friends), other substances (e.g., alcohol), places (e.g., areas where stimulants are sold or used), time periods (e.g., weekends, after work), and emotional states (e.g., depression, boredom). This powerful craving response frequently plays a key role in relapse during the initial months of abstinence. A related aspect of this Pavlovian response concerns the relationship between stimulant use and sexual behavior. Research has demonstrated that users of cocaine and methamphetamine frequently combine their drug use with sexual activity (Rawson et al. 2002). During treatment, hypersexuality may continue and can be associated with relapse.

Similarly, there has been extensive research on the impact of stimulants (especially methamphetamine) on cognition. A variety of cognitive deficits, including attention and memory problems, have been documented during early weeks and months of abstinence and can be severe enough to interfere with functioning (Simon et al. 2010). Symptoms of depression are very common during withdrawal from stimulants and typically abate over the first few weeks of abstinence. However, feelings of anhedonia often persist longer, into the first several months of abstinence. Finally, poor engagement and retention of stimulant users in treatment is a frequent challenge, and since an extended period of involvement in treatment is associated with better outcomes, this difficulty in retaining patients in treatment is an important challenge.

Vulnerable Populations

There are a number of stimulant user categories and characteristics that are noteworthy from a treatment perspective. Women who use stimulants are more likely than men to use stimulants for weight loss and should be screened and treated for eating disorders in order to prevent relapse when normal weight is achieved. Stimulant-using men who have sex with men, particularly methamphetamine users, are at elevated risk of HIV transmission due to high-risk sexual behavior associated with their stimulant use. Treatment of stimulant use disorder in this population should be delivered in conjunction with HIV education and HIV harm-reduction strategies. Individuals who use stimulants heavily (daily) or via injection require more intensive treatment (frequently inpatient/residential level care). Patients receiving medication-assisted treatment (methadone or buprenorphine) for opioid use disorder (OUD) are at very high risk for stimulant use disorder, and failure to treat the stimulant use disorder can lead to deterioration of the treatment progress for OUD.

Pharmacotherapeutic Treatment of Stimulant-Related Disorders

Long-term stimulant use has deleterious effects on neurobiological homeostasis. Changes in norepinephrine, serotonin, γ-aminobutyric acid (GABA), glutamate, and dopamine systems occur. In addition, there is disruption of the neuroendocrine machinery and the hypothalamic-pituitary-adrenal axis. After 30 years of intensive effort, no medications have been approved by the U.S. Food and Drug Administration (FDA) for use in the treatment of stimulant use disorder. There are, however, a number of compounds that have supportive research evidence, making them promising candidates, as well as a large number of other possible targets involving all of the systems above for potential treatment of cocaine and methamphetamine users.

Promising Candidate Medications

Topiramate

Topiramate is an anticonvulsant, GABA-enhancing medication that is also used to prevent migraines. GABAergic neurons inhibit dopamine release and activation of the reward system. A number of double-blind, placebo-controlled studies have demonstrated positive results for topiramate in curbing cocaine use, but others have yielded negative results; however, combining topiramate with long-acting stimulants has shown promise (Kampman 2019). Topiramate may be especially beneficial as an adjunct to behavioral approaches, such as group therapy and motivational interviewing (Baldaçara et al. 2016).

Topiramate has also accrued some consistent supportive evidence for its utility in methamphetamine treatment. In a 13-week multicenter randomized double-blind, placebo-controlled multicenter study, 30 of 69 methamphetamine-dependent subjects were identified as showing a favorable response to topiramate in the form of either abstinence or reduced methamphetamine use over time (Ma et al. 2013). Topiramate's beneficial effects may be due not only to GABA activation but also to glutamate inhibition via α-amino-3-hydroxy-5-methyl-4-isoxazolepropionic acid (AMPA) receptor antagonism.

Bupropion

Studies involving bupropion, an antidepressant with dopamine and norepinephrine reuptake inhibition, have suggested its utility in cocaine use disorder. Randomized controlled trials have demonstrated improved rates of cocaine abstinence associated with bupropion compared with placebo, according to a Cochrane review (Castellis et al. 2016).

Other research evidence suggests that bupropion may also be helpful in reducing relapse to methamphetamine use. However, the severity of the methamphetamine use may play a role in determining the benefit received from bupropion, with light users (but not heavy users) showing reduced use (Shoptaw et al. 2008).

Naltrexone

The opioid antagonist naltrexone has demonstrated benefit in reducing cocaine use, both when used alone (Schmitz et al. 2001) and when used in combination with the partial opioid agonist buprenorphine (Gerra et al. 2006). This beneficial effect may be due to the kappa antagonism action of buprenorphine.

Several studies have suggested a potential role for naltrexone in reducing methamphetamine use. In regard to the efficacy of extended-release injectable formulations, the data have been mixed (Mooney and McCance-Katz 2016; Pal et al. 2015).

Amphetamine/Methylphenidate

Amphetamine-type stimulants, including D-amphetamine, methamphetamine, and methylphenidate, increase dopamine release in the synapse by blocking dopamine transporters. A three-arm placebo-controlled trial found that for patients with comorbid ADHD and cocaine use, extended-release mixed amphetamine salts and cognitive-behavioral therapy (CBT) ameliorated the ADHD symptoms and reduced cocaine use (Levin et al. 2015).

Studies have demonstrated that agonist therapy with stimulants used for ADHD have also shown reduced cravings for methamphetamine, although this was not necessarily accompanied by reduced methamphetamine use (Galloway et al. 2011). Because of the potential for misuse of these medications, the risk–benefit ratio requires careful consideration in treating stimulant use disorder.

Modafinil

Modafinil, a weak inhibitor of dopamine and norepinephrine transporters that is FDA approved for use in the treatment of narcolepsy, obstructive sleep apnea, and shift work disorder, has been explored for cocaine use disorder, with mixed results. In some studies, modafinil appeared to be useful in reducing cocaine craving and use (Kampman et al. 2015); however, other trials failed to demonstrate a benefit (Dackis et al. 2012).

Disulfiram

Disulfiram, a medication originally utilized for alcohol use disorder because of its acetyl aldehyde dehydrogenase inhibition, has shown limited efficacy in the treatment of cocaine use disorder (Pani et al. 2010). Disulfiram increases dopamine levels by inhibiting the enzyme dopamine beta-hydroxylase, which converts dopamine into norepinephrine. In a placebo-controlled study of cocaine-dependent, alcohol-using individuals, participants receiving disulfiram showed significant reductions in cocaine and alcohol use compared with those receiving placebo, with sustained effects that were independent from alcohol consumption (Carroll et al. 2004). Disulfiram may delay cocaine metabolism and should be used with caution in individuals with preexisting cardiovascular risk factors (Mooney and McCance-Katz 2016).

Mirtazapine

Mirtazapine is an antidepressant that increases serotonin indirectly through antagonism of serotonin (5-hydroxytryptamine [5-HT]) type 2 (5-HT$_2$) and type 3 (5-HT$_3$) receptors. It has shown some utility in reducing methamphetamine use and high-risk sexual behaviors in methamphetamine users independently of its effects on depression (Coffin et al. 2019; Colfax et al. 2011).

Other Pharmacotherapy Research

Cocaine vaccines have been developed through use of a cholera-toxin protein conjugated to a cocaine structure in order to produce an immune response to the drug. Antibody levels in subjects have varied, as have findings regarding the vaccine's efficacy (Kosten et al. 2014; Shen et al. 2011).

Summary of Best Evidence

The use of any pharmacotherapy to target stimulant use disorder is considered off-label at this time. Limitations of the aforementioned trials include limited power, methodological deficiencies, and high attrition rates. Low-strength evidence does exist for topiramate, bupropion, modafinil, sustained-release mixed amphetamine salts, disulfiram, and naltrexone/buprenorphine for targeting cocaine use (Chan et al. 2018). Topiramate, mirtazapine, bupropion, naltrexone, and sustained-release methylphenidate may be indicated for targeting methamphetamine use disorder (Chan et al. 2018).

There are many important clinical issues to consider before prescribing experimental medications to patients with stimulant use disorder, such as medical and psychiatric comorbidities, whether or not a patient has a history of prescription stimulant use disorder, and the ability of providers to monitor patients closely for adverse medication effects or relapse potential.

Behavioral Approaches to Treatment of Stimulant-Related Disorders

Behavioral interventions are the mainstay of stimulant use disorder treatment. There are a number of studies in which cocaine users and methamphetamine users have been treated in the same research trials, and those treatments were applied clinically to both groups using the same protocols, personnel, and measures. In all of these studies, treatment response in cocaine users and methamphetamine users has been comparable (e.g., Petry et al. 2005; Rawson et al. 2004). For this reason, unlike the previous review of medications, we will review the evidence for the following behavioral strategies with the assumption that results from cocaine users will generalize to methamphetamine user populations and vice versa. The approaches with the most substantial empirical support will be reviewed in some detail, followed by those with less evidence but some supportive evidence.

During the past decade, there have been a number of systematic reviews of treatments for stimulant use disorder, including two Cochrane reviews (Knapp et al. 2007; Minozzi et al. 2016), a review by the World Health Organization for its mental health guidelines document (Mental Health Gap Action Programme [mhGAP; https://www.who.int/mental_health/mhgap/en/), and a meta-analysis by De Crescenzo et al. (2018). In all of these analyses, contingency management was recognized as having the strongest evidence base. For example, in the Knapp et al. (2007) review, the following conclusion was reached from the analysis: "The comparisons between different types of behavioral interventions showed results in favor of treatments with some form of contingency management in respect to both reducing dropouts and lowering cocaine use" (p. 1). Furthermore, the 2018 meta-analysis (De Crescenzo et al. 2018) also concluded that contingency management (together with the community reinforcement approach) produced the best evidence of effectiveness for generating a variety of positive outcomes.

Behavioral Approaches With Robust Empirical Support

Contingency Management

Contingency management (CM; also known as motivational incentives) applies the principles of positive reinforcement to promote performance of desired behaviors consistent with abstinence from cocaine or methamphetamine. CM involves the contingent delivery of an incentive for behaviors such as attendance at treatment sessions, a drug-negative urine specimen, or documented completion of a homework assignment. Incentives include desired items or privileges, such as vouchers. There are a variety of ways to structure and individualize CM, and a variable schedule of reinforcement can be applied with the "fishbowl approach," which uses low-cost incentives (Petry 2000). This relatively simple positive-reinforcement intervention has been shown to produce and sustain substantial and clinically meaningful reductions in stimulant use.

Specific research findings supporting CM for the treatment of stimulant use disorder include the landmark paper by Higgins et al. (1991) that documented highly significant reductions in cocaine use and very large and significant increases in extended periods of cocaine abstinence using CM. Roll et al. (2006) extended these findings to methamphetamine users and reported that CM produced significantly greater retention in treatment and significantly more methamphetamine-negative urine samples. Rawson et al. (2002) found that among individuals in methadone treatment who also used cocaine, CM produced significantly more cocaine-free urine samples than did no treatment (other than methadone) or CBT. Furthermore, the addition of CBT did not produce additional benefits over and above CM alone.

Although there is strong empirical support for CM, its application in real-world treatment settings has been limited, even though the National Institute on Drug Abuse (NIDA) and the Substance Abuse and Mental Health Services Administration

(SAMHSA) have collaborated to produce a set of "Blending" manuals and materials to support the use of CM (www.drugabuse.gov/nidasamhsa-blending-initiative). Roll et al. (2009) described some of the obstacles that interfere with broad-scale application of CM in community treatments. One effort that has shown promise is a large implementation trial promoting the use of CM as a routine treatment approach within the U.S. Department of Veterans Affairs (VA). The effectiveness of this implementation project has been documented by DePhilippis et al. (2018), who reported that CM is being successfully implemented across a large number of VA sites and that patient outcomes were significantly improved by the addition of CM within these treatment settings.

Community Reinforcement Approach

The Community Reinforcement Approach (CRA) involves a combination of behavioral strategies that target the role of environmental contingencies in encouraging or discouraging drug use and attempt to rearrange these contingencies so that a non-drug-using lifestyle is more rewarding than a drug-using one. CRA components include behavioral skills training, social and recreational counseling, marital therapy, motivational enhancement, job counseling, and relapse prevention. In a number of CRA trials for cocaine use disorder, a voucher-based CM reinforcement program was added. Higgins et al. (1991) established the efficacy of CRA and vouchers (CM) for the treatment of cocaine dependence. In order to isolate the effects of CRA, Higgins et al. (2003) replicated this study, comparing CRA plus vouchers versus vouchers only. Study results demonstrated that while both conditions produced significant reductions in cocaine use, participants in the CRA-plus-vouchers condition were better retained in treatment and had fewer days of cocaine or alcohol use. Furthermore, participants treated with CRA plus vouchers had more employed days, fewer hospital admissions and legal problems, and reduced depression symptoms. A systematic review of CRA (Roozen et al. 2004) concluded that CRA has evidence of support for reducing cocaine use, and CRA together with CM produced higher rates of abstinence than CRA alone. To promote the dissemination of CRA plus CM, NIDA has produced a manual describing the approach in detail (Budney and Higgins 1998).

Cognitive-Behavioral Therapy

CBT is a form of "talk therapy" based on principles of social learning theory that is used to teach, encourage, and support individuals in reducing or stopping their harmful drug use (Carroll et al. 1998). CBT provides skills that are valuable in assisting people in gaining initial abstinence from drugs (or in reducing their drug use) and provides skills to help people sustain abstinence. CBT addresses negative thought patterns and teaches individuals how to cope with distress in order to prevent relapse. A systematic review of randomized controlled trials using CBT as an intervention for methamphetamine users concluded that CBT was associated with reductions in stimulant use and improvements in mood and other areas of functioning (Lee and Rawson 2008), and a review of CBT for a variety of substance use disorders likewise concluded that it is an effective approach (Dutra et al. 2008). Carroll and colleagues conducted studies establishing the efficacy of CBT for the treatment of cocaine use disorder (Carroll et al. 1994a, 1994b). These studies demonstrated that the use of their CBT manual reduced cocaine use over a 1-year period. In fact, their report suggests that CBT produces especially efficacious results at follow-up points. In a meta-analysis of behavioral treatments for cocaine or methamphetamine use disorder (De Crescenzo et al. 2018), studies evaluating the efficacy of CBT consistently showed positive findings. However, data in this meta-analysis indicated that in numerous trials in which CBT was compared with CM, CM strategies consistently resulted in greater reductions in stimulant use.

CBT has become more accessible with the advent of computerized delivery (Carroll et al. 2008). A randomized trial among cocaine-using individuals in methadone maintenance treatment showed that participants receiving computer-based training for CBT ("CBT4CBT") were significantly more likely than control subjects receiving standard treatment to achieve three or more consecutive weeks of abstinence from cocaine (Carroll et al. 2014).

Behavioral Approaches With Some Supportive Evidence

The following behavioral strategies have been the subject of at least one randomized clinical trial demonstrating superior outcomes in comparison with control procedures.

Exercise Therapy

Exercise is a simple and effective intervention for substance use disorders. By increasing endogenous opioid release, exercise helps potentiate dopamine efflux and improves mood and cognition and can help prevent relapse (Abel et al. 2019; Meeusen 2005). An 8-week trial showed that methamphetamine-using participants randomly assigned to a supervised, progressive endurance and resistance training three times per week demonstrated improved dopamine receptor binding compared with individuals receiving health education only (Robertson et al. 2016). In addition, the participants who received the exercise intervention had lower anxiety and depression scores (as measured with the Beck Anxiety Inventory and the Beck Depression Inventory) over the study period (Rawson et al. 2015a), and individuals with lower-severity methamphetamine use at baseline had significantly lower relapse rates after discharge from residential care (Rawson et al. 2015b). A large randomized controlled trial funded by NIDA also explored the relationship between stimulant use and exercise in residential treatment programs (Trivedi et al. 2017). This study found a modestly higher (but significant) percentage of days abstinent for participants receiving exercise who were adherent to their regimens compared with participants receiving only health education.

Mindfulness

Mindfulness is a practice derived from Buddhist teachings that centers on a conscious presence in the here and now with focused attention and nonjudgmental monitoring (Garland and Howard 2018). Positive effects with regard to stress and cue reactivity in individuals with alcohol and/or cocaine use disorder receiving mindfulness compared with CBT have been reported (Brewer et al. 2009). A systematic review of the literature concluded that mindfulness behavioral interventions could reduce consumption of cocaine and amphetamines to a greater extent than control conditions (e.g., waitlist controls, nonspecific educational support groups) (Chiesa and Serretti 2014). A small pilot trial of a 10-week mindfulness therapy found that abstinence rates in cocaine-using participants who received mindfulness therapy were greater than abstinence rates in historical comparison groups (Dakwar and Levin 2013).

Transcranial Magnetic Stimulation

Transcranial magnetic stimulation (TMS) is FDA approved for treatment-resistant depression and has demonstrated preliminary evidence of potential efficacy for stimulant use disorder. A pilot trial that randomly assigned participants with cocaine use disorder to receive repetitive TMS (rTMS) delivered to the left dorsolateral prefrontal cortex (DLPFC) found significant reductions in craving and in numbers of cocaine-positive urine tests in the rTMS group compared with the control group (Terraneo et al. 2016). Similarly, five sessions of rTMS delivered to the left DLPFC significantly reduced cravings in patients with methamphetamine use disorder while also improving cognitive function (Su et al. 2017). A subsequent study confirmed that cue-induced cravings for methamphetamine were diminished by rTMS of the DLPFC, irrespective of delivery side or frequency (Liu et al. 2017). This noninvasive treatment modality has few side effects and may provide a unique way to target disordered stimulant use.

Matrix Model

The Matrix Model of Intensive Outpatient Treatment (Obert et al. 2000) is a combination of therapeutic strategies—CBT, motivational interviewing, family involvement, and psychoeducation—delivered in a manner to produce an integrated outpatient treatment experience. In a large randomized multisite trial comparing the Matrix Model with treatment as usual, methamphetamine users who received Matrix treatment stayed in treatment longer, provided higher numbers of methamphetamine-negative urines, and had longer periods of abstinence compared with those who received treatment as usual (Rawson et al. 2004). The Matrix counselor's treatment manual is available from SAMHSA (Substance Abuse and Mental Health Services Administration 2013).

Motivational Interviewing

Motivational interviewing (MI) is a technique that aims to help individuals resolve their ambivalence about enacting positive change. In a randomized clinical trial, MI demonstrated positive effects, with decreased methamphetamine use and lower cravings in participants receiving MI, regardless of treatment intensity (Polcin et al. 2014). Of note, intensive MI lasting 9 weeks was found to be especially helpful for women with methamphetamine use disorder and comorbid alcohol use (Korcha et al. 2014). Another randomized trial examining MI for cocaine use found that individuals who used cocaine on 15 or more of the 30 days prior to baseline showed significantly higher mean reductions in days of cocaine use following MI in comparison with those assigned to the control group (Stein et al. 2009).

Twelve-Step Facilitation

Twelve-step facilitation is a therapy founded on the principles of Alcoholics Anonymous and traditionally involves nondirected participation in meetings, engagement in social support (fellowship), and acquisition of a sponsor for guidance in recovery from substance use. A large randomized multisite trial sponsored by NIDA found evidence that participation in 12-step therapy resulted in significant reductions in reported stimulant use and cravings and led to prosocial service engagement (Donovan et al. 2013). A secondary analysis suggested that having a sponsor was associated with a higher likelihood of sustained abstinence from stimulants at follow-up (Wendt et al. 2017).

Conclusion

Stimulant use disorder involving cocaine and amphetamine-type substances has profound effects on the monoamine neurotransmitters and the sympathetic nervous system. Although the FDA has not approved any pharmacotherapy to treat stimulant use disorder, research targeting neural pathways involved in reward function is under way. Behavioral interventions such as contingency management in particular, and including the community reinforcement approach and cognitive-behavioral therapy, have robust evidence supporting their efficacy in the treatment of stimulant use disorder. Other behavioral approaches have more limited evidence. Populations with stimulant use disorder have unique vulnerabilities and clinical challenges and should be screened for comorbid psychiatric and medical disorders.

To summarize the current state of treatment for stimulant-related disorders, we provide the following three key points:

- Although some medications show limited benefit in reducing cravings and stimulant use, there are currently no FDA-approved medications to treat stimulant use disorder.
- Behavioral therapies including contingency management, community reinforcement approach, and cognitive-behavioral therapy are evidence-based approaches with strong empirical support for efficacy in the treatment of stimulant use disorder.
- Special screening and treatment considerations should be given to women, men who have sex with men, and stimulant-injecting individuals.

References

Abel JM, Nesil T, Bakhti-Suroosh A, et al: Mechanisms underlying the efficacy of exercise as an intervention for cocaine relapse: a focus on mGlu5 in the dorsal medial prefrontal cortex. Psychopharmacology (Berl) 236(7):2155–2171, 2019 31161451

Ahmad FB, Rossen LM, Spencer MR, et al: Provisional Drug Overdose Death Counts. National Center for Health Statistics, 2019. Available at: https://www.cdc.gov/nchs/nvss/vsrr/drug-overdose-data.htm. Accessed November 19, 2019.

American Psychiatric Association: Diagnostic and Statistical Manual of Mental Disorders, 5th Edition. Arlington, VA, American Psychiatric Association, 2013

Baldaçara L, Cogo-Moreira H, Parreira BL, et al: Efficacy of topiramate in the treatment of crack cocaine dependence: a double-blind, randomized, placebo-controlled trial. J Clin Psychiatry 77(3):398–406, 2016 27046312

Brewer JA, Sinha R, Chen JA, et al: Mindfulness training and stress reactivity in substance abuse: results from a randomized, controlled stage I pilot study. Subst Abus 30(4):306–317, 2009 19904666

Budney AJ, Higgins ST: Therapy Manual for Drug Addiction Manual 2—A Community Rein-
    forcement Plus Vouchers Approach: Treating Cocaine Addiction. National Institute on Drug
    Abuse, 1998. Available at: https://www.ncjrs.gov/App/Publications/abstract.aspx?ID=
    180293. Accessed November 19, 2019.
Carroll KM, Rounsaville BJ, Gordon LT, et al: Psychotherapy and pharmacotherapy for ambu-
    latory cocaine abusers. Arch Gen Psychiatry 51(3):177–187, 1994a 8122955
Carroll KM, Rounsaville BJ, Nich C, et al: One-year follow-up of psychotherapy and pharma-
    cotherapy for cocaine dependence. Delayed emergence of psychotherapy effects. Arch
    Gen Psychiatry 51(12):989–997, 1994b 7979888
Carroll KM, Nich C, Ball SA, et al: Treatment of cocaine and alcohol dependence with psycho-
    therapy and disulfiram. Addiction 93(5):713–727, 1998 9692270
Carroll KM, Fenton LR, Ball SA, et al: Efficacy of disulfiram and cognitive behavior therapy in
    cocaine-dependent outpatients: a randomized placebo-controlled trial. Arch Gen Psychia-
    try 61(3):264–272, 2004 14993114
Carroll KM, Ball SA, Martino S, et al: Computer-assisted delivery of cognitive-behavioral ther-
    apy for addiction: a randomized trial of CBT4CBT. Am J Psychiatry 165(7):881–888, 2008
    18450927
Carroll KM, Kiluk BD, Nich C, et al: Computer-assisted delivery of cognitive-behavioral ther-
    apy: efficacy and durability of CBT4CBT among cocaine-dependent individuals main-
    tained on methadone. Am J Psychiatry 171(4):436–444, 2014 24577287
Castellis X, Cunill R, Pérez-Mañá C, et al: Psychostimulant drugs for cocaine dependence. Co-
    chrane Database Syst Rev (9):CD007380, 2016 27670244
Chan B, Kondo K, Ayers C, et al: Pharmacotherapy for Stimulant Use Disorders: A Systematic
    Review of the Evidence. Washington, DC, Department of Veterans Affairs, 2018
Chiesa A, Serretti A: Are mindfulness-based interventions effective for substance use disor-
    ders? A systematic review of the evidence. Subst Use Misuse 49(5):492–512, 2014 23461667
Coffin PO, Santos GM, Hern J, et al: Effects of mirtazapine for methamphetamine use disorder
    among cisgender men and transgender women who have sex with men: a placebo-con-
    trolled randomized clinical trial. JAMA Psychiatry 77(3):246–255, 2019 31825466
Colfax GN, Santos GM, Das M, et al: Mirtazapine to reduce methamphetamine use: a random-
    ized controlled trial. Arch Gen Psychiatry 68(11):1168–1175, 2011 22065532
Dackis CA, Kampman KM, Lynch KG, et al: A double-blind, placebo-controlled trial of moda-
    finil for cocaine dependence. J Subst Abuse Treat 43(3):303–312, 2012 22377391
Dakwar E, Levin FR: Individual mindfulness-based psychotherapy for cannabis or cocaine de-
    pendence: a pilot feasibility trial. Am J Addict 22(6):521–526, 2013 24131158
De Crescenzo F, Ciabattini M, D'Alò GL, et al: Comparative efficacy and acceptability of psy-
    chosocial interventions for individuals with cocaine and amphetamine addiction: a sys-
    tematic review and network meta-analysis. PLoS Med 15(12):e1002715, 2018 30586362
DePhilippis D, Petry NM, Bonn-Miller MO, et al: The national implementation of contingency
    management (CM) in the Department of Veterans Affairs: attendance at CM sessions and
    substance use outcomes. Drug Alcohol Depend 185:367–373, 2018 29524874
Donovan DM, Daley DC, Brigham GS, et al: Stimulant abuser groups to engage in 12-step: a
    multisite trial in the National Institute on Drug Abuse Clinical Trials Network. J Subst
    Abuse Treat 44(1):103–114, 2013 22657748
Dutra L, Stathopoulou G, Basden SL, et al: A meta-analytic review of psychosocial interven-
    tions for substance use disorders. Am J Psychiatry 165(2):179–187, 2008 18198270
Ellis MS, Kasper ZA, Cicero TJ: Twin epidemics: the surging rise of methamphetamine use in
    chronic opioid users. Drug Alcohol Depend 193:14–20, 2018 30326396
Galloway GP, Buscemi R, Coyle JR, et al: A randomized, placebo-controlled trial of sustained-
    release dextroamphetamine for treatment of methamphetamine addiction. Clin Pharmacol
    Ther 89(2):276–282, 2011 21178989
Garland EL, Howard MO: Mindfulness-based treatment of addiction: current state of the field
    and envisioning the next wave of research. Addict Sci Clin Pract 13(1):14, 2018 29669599
Gerra G, Fantoma A, Zaimovic A: Naltrexone and buprenorphine combination in the treatment
    of opioid dependence. J Psychopharmacol 20(6):806–814, 2006 16401652

Higgins ST, Delaney DD, Budney AJ, et al: A behavioral approach to achieving initial cocaine abstinence. Am J Psychiatry 148(9):1218–1224, 1991 1883001

Higgins ST, Sigmon SC, Wong CJ, et al: Community reinforcement therapy for cocaine-dependent outpatients. Arch Gen Psychiatry 60(10):1043–1052, 2003 14557150

Kampman KM: The treatment of cocaine use disorder. Sci Adv 5(10):eaax1532, 2019 31663022

Kampman KM, Lynch KG, Pettinati HM, et al: A double blind, placebo controlled trial of modafinil for the treatment of cocaine dependence without co-morbid alcohol dependence. Drug Alcohol Depend 155:105–110, 2015 26320827

Knapp WP, Soares B, Farrell M, et al: Psychosocial interventions for cocaine and psychostimulant amphetamines related disorders. Cochrane Database Syst Rev (3):CD003023, 2007 17636713

Korcha RA, Polcin DL, Evans K, et al: Intensive motivational interviewing for women with concurrent alcohol problems and methamphetamine dependence. J Subst Abuse Treat 46(2):113–119, 2014 24074649

Kosten TR, Domingo CB, Shorter D, et al: Vaccine for cocaine dependence: a randomized double-blind placebo-controlled efficacy trial. Drug Alcohol Depend 140:42–47, 2014 24793366

Lee NK, Rawson RA: A systematic review of cognitive and behavioural therapies for methamphetamine dependence. Drug Alcohol Rev 27(3):309–317, 2008 18368613

Levin FR, Mariani JJ, Specker S, et al: Extended-release mixed amphetamine salts vs placebo for comorbid adult attention-deficit/hyperactivity disorder and cocaine use disorder: a randomized clinical trial. JAMA Psychiatry 72(6):593–602, 2015 25887096

Liu Q, Shen Y, Cao X, et al: Either at left or right, both high and low frequency rTMS of dorsolateral prefrontal cortex decreases cue induced craving for methamphetamine. Am J Addict 26(8):776–779, 2017 29134789

Ma JZ, Johnson BA, Yu E, et al: Fine-grain analysis of the treatment effect of topiramate on methamphetamine addiction with latent variable analysis. Drug Alcohol Depend 130(1–3):45–51, 2013 23142494

Meeusen R: Exercise and the brain: insight in new therapeutic modalities. Ann Transplant 10(4):49–51, 2005 17037089

Minozzi S, Saulle R, De Crescenzo F, et al: Psychosocial interventions for psychostimulant misuse. Cochrane Database Syst Rev (9):CD011866, 2016 27684277

Mooney L, McCance-Katz E: Psychopharmacological treatments for substance use disorders, in Clinical Textbook of Addictive Disorders, 4th Edition. Edited by Mack A, Brady K, Miller S, et al. New York, Guilford, 2016, pp 666–704

Newton TF, De La Garza R 2nd, Kalechstein AD, et al: Cocaine and methamphetamine produce different patterns of subjective and cardiovascular effects. Pharmacol Biochem Behav 82(1):90–97, 2005 16112720

Obert JL, McCann MJ, Marinelli-Casey P, et al: The matrix model of outpatient stimulant abuse treatment: history and description. J Psychoactive Drugs 32(2):157–164, 2000 10908003

O'Daly OG, Guillin O, Tsapakis E-M, et al: Schizophrenia and substance abuse co-morbidity: a role for dopamine sensitization? Journal of Dual Diagnosis 1(2):11–40, 2005. Available at: https://www.tandfonline.com/doi/abs/10.1300/J374v01n02_03. Accessed December 12, 2019.

Pal R, Mendelson JE, Flower K, et al: Impact of prospectively determined A118G polymorphism on treatment response to injectable naltrexone among methamphetamine-dependent patients: an open-label, pilot study. J Addict Med 9(2):130–135, 2015 25622123

Pani PP, Troqu E, Vacca R, et al: Disulfiram for the treatment of cocaine dependence. Cochrane Database Syst Rev (1):CD007024, 2010 20091613

Petry NM: A comprehensive guide to the application of contingency management procedures in clinical settings. Drug Alcohol Depend 58(1–2):9–25, 2000 10669051

Petry NM, Peirce JM, Stitzer ML, et al: Effect of prize-based incentives on outcomes in stimulant abusers in outpatient psychosocial treatment programs: a national drug abuse treatment clinical trials network study. Arch Gen Psychiatry 62(10):1148–1156, 2005 16203960

Polcin DL, Bond J, Korcha R, et al: Randomized trial of intensive motivational interviewing for methamphetamine dependence. J Addict Dis 33(3):253–265, 2014 25115166

Rawson RA, Huber A, McCann M, et al: A comparison of contingency management and cognitive-behavioral approaches during methadone maintenance treatment for cocaine dependence. Arch Gen Psychiatry 59(9):817–824, 2002 12215081

Rawson RA, Marinelli-Casey P, Anglin MD, et al: A multi-site comparison of psychosocial approaches for the treatment of methamphetamine dependence. Addiction 99(6):708–717, 2004 15139869

Rawson RA, Chudzynski J, Gonzales R, et al: The impact of exercise on depression and anxiety symptoms among abstinent methamphetamine-dependent individuals in a residential treatment setting. J Subst Abuse Treat 57:36–40, 2015a 25934458

Rawson RA, Chudzynski J, Mooney L, et al: Impact of an exercise intervention on methamphetamine use outcomes post-residential treatment care. Drug Alcohol Depend 156:21–28, 2015b 26371404

Robertson CL, Ishibashi K, Chudzynski J, et al: Effect of exercise training on striatal dopamine D2/D3 receptors in methamphetamine users during behavioral treatment. Neuropsychopharmacology 41(6):1629–1636, 2016 26503310

Roll JM, Petry NM, Stitzer ML, et al: Contingency management for the treatment of methamphetamine use disorders. Am J Psychiatry 163(11):1993–1999, 2006 17074952

Roll JM, Madden GJ, Rawson R, et al: Facilitating the adoption of contingency management for the treatment of substance use disorders. Behav Anal Pract 2(1):4–13, 2009 22477692

Romanelli F, Smith KM: Clinical effects and management of methamphetamine abuse. Pharmacotherapy 26(8):1148–1156, 2006 16863490

Roozen HG, Boulogne JJ, van Tulder MW, et al: A systematic review of the effectiveness of the community reinforcement approach in alcohol, cocaine and opioid addiction. Drug Alcohol Depend 74(1):1–13, 2004 15072802

Schmitz JM, Stotts AL, Rhoades HM, et al: Naltrexone and relapse prevention treatment for cocaine-dependent patients. Addict Behav 26(2):167–180, 2001 11316375

Seth P, Scholl L, Rudd RA, et al: Overdose deaths involving opioids, cocaine, and psychostimulants—United States, 2015–2016. MMWR Morb Mortal Wkly Rep 67(12):349–358, 2018 29596405

Shen X, Orson FM, Kosten TR: Anti-addiction vaccines. F1000 Med Rep 3:20, 2011 22003367

Shoptaw S, Heinzerling KG, Rotheram-Fuller E, et al: Randomized, placebo-controlled trial of bupropion for the treatment of methamphetamine dependence. Drug Alcohol Depend 96(3):222–232, 2008 18468815

Simon SL, Dean AC, Cordova X, et al: Methamphetamine dependence and neuropsychological functioning: evaluating change during early abstinence. J Stud Alcohol Drugs 71(3):335–344, 2010 20409426

Stein MD, Herman DS, Anderson BJ: A motivational intervention trial to reduce cocaine use. J Subst Abuse Treat 36(1):118–125, 2009 18657938

Su H, Zhong N, Gan H, et al: High frequency repetitive transcranial magnetic stimulation of the left dorsolateral prefrontal cortex for methamphetamine use disorders: a randomised clinical trial. Drug Alcohol Depend 175:84–91, 2017 28410525

Substance Abuse and Mental Health Services Administration: Matrix Intensive Outpatient Treatment for People With Stimulant Use Disorders: Counselor's Treatment Manual (HHS Publ No SMA13-4152). Rockville, MD, Center for Substance Abuse Treatment, 2013. Available at: https://store.samhsa.gov/product/Matrix-Intensive-Outpatient-Treatment-for-People-With-Stimulant-Use-Disorders-Counselor-s-Treatment-Manual/SMA13-4152. Accessed May 19, 2020.

Substance Abuse and Mental Health Services Administration: Key Substance Use and Mental Health Indicators in the United States: Results From the 2017 National Survey on Drug Use and Health (HHS Publ. No. SMA 18-5068, NSDUH Series H-53). Rockville, MD, Center for Behavioral Health Statistics and Quality, SAMHSA, 2018. Available at: https://www.samhsa.gov/data/sites/default/files/cbhsq-reports/NSDUHFFR2017/NSDUHFFR2017.pdf. Accessed June 25, 2020.

Terraneo A, Leggio L, Saladini M, et al: Transcranial magnetic stimulation of dorsolateral pre-frontal cortex reduces cocaine use: a pilot study. Eur Neuropsychopharmacol 26(1):37–44, 2016 26655188

Trivedi MH, Greer TL, Rethorst CD, et al: Randomized controlled trial comparing exercise to health education for stimulant use disorder: results from the CTN-0037 STimulant Reduction Intervention Using Dosed Exercise (STRIDE) study. J Clin Psychiatry 78(8):1075–1082, 2017 28199070

U.S. Department of Justice Drug Enforcement Administration: 2019 National Drug Threat Assessment (DEA-DCT-DIR-007-20). December 2019. Available at: https://www.dea.gov/sites/default/files/2020-01/2019-NDTA-final-01-14-2020_Low_Web-DIR-007-20_2019.pdf. Accessed October 8, 2020.

Wendt DC, Hallgren KA, Daley DC, et al: Predictors and outcomes of twelve-step sponsorship of stimulant users: secondary analyses of a multisite randomized clinical trial. J Stud Alcohol Drugs 78(2):287–295, 2017 28317510

CHAPTER 12

Neurobiology of Opioids

Jermaine D. Jones, Ph.D.

Charles J. Levin, B.A.

Mudassir Mumtaz, B.S.

Sandra D. Comer, Ph.D.

Within the context of substance use disorders, the endogenous opioid system has been described as a chief mediator of "pain and pleasure." This characterization results from the important role that endogenous and exogenous opioids play in pain perception and hedonic states. However, the physiology of this system is multifaceted, both in itself and in its interactions with other neurobiological components. Thus, the endogenous opioid system may be critical to the etiology and treatment of several disease states. This chapter reviews what we know about the neurobiology of opioids. The authors attempt to detail how opioid neurobiology modulates physiology and behavior, and how this knowledge is being translated into the development of novel therapeutics and treatment strategies.

Naturally Occurring Opioids and Their Interactions With Opioid Receptors

Opioid receptors are present throughout the body, both centrally (e.g., in the brain and spinal cord) and peripherally (e.g., in the heart and gut). The primary opioid receptors that have been identified are the mu (μ), kappa (κ), and delta (δ) subtypes (Corder et al. 2018). Endogenous peptides that activate these subtypes are endorphins for μ, dynorphins for κ, and enkephalins for δ receptors, and these are derived from other endogenous substances, including proopiomelanocortin, prodynorphin, and preproenkephalin. More recently, nociception receptors were identified, which are activated by the endogenous peptide nociceptin/orphanin FQ (Corder et al. 2018). All of the opioid receptor subtypes are seven-transmembrane G protein–coupled receptors (GPCRs) that can exist in both active and inactive conformations. It has been known for some time that opioid agonists bind to inhibitory G proteins, which ultimately activate various effectors and signaling cascades. When opioid receptors are activated, release of the neurotransmitter γ-aminobutyric acid (GABA) is reduced. GABA normally produces a tonic inhibition of dopamine release, so opioid-induced inhibition of GABA produces an increase in dopamine release. In the past few years, several important advances have occurred in our understanding of opioid receptor functioning, including biased signaling, allosteric regulation, and heteromerization. Each of these advances will be reviewed briefly in the following subsections. For more comprehensive reviews of this literature, readers are referred to Corder et al. (2018) and Valentino and Volkow (2018).

G Protein and Beta-Arrestin Signaling

As noted above, both endogenous and exogenous opioid agonists bind to inhibitory GPCRs, specifically $G_{\alpha i/0}$, which leads to uncoupling of the G_α and $G_{\beta\gamma}$ subunits, inhibition of adenylate cyclase, reduction in cyclic adenosine monophosphate production, and modulation of calcium and potassium ion channels (Al-Hasani and Bruchas 2011). Recent research has suggested that, in addition to interacting with G proteins, opioid receptors interact with β-arrestins, which also regulate signaling (Schmid et al. 2017). Of particular interest is the notion that an opioid molecule binding to an opioid receptor can simultaneously activate $G_{\alpha i/0}$ and β-arrestin pathways. Activation of G protein pathways is thought to mediate the analgesic and antipruritic effects of opioids, while activation of β-arrestin pathways may mediate respiratory depression and constipation. The extent to which the two pathways are activated depends on the agonist, with some agonists, such as morphine, having a greater propensity to activate the G protein pathway and others, such as fentanyl and sufentanil, having a greater propensity to activate the β-arrestin pathway (Schmid et al. 2017). The relative effects of an agonist on the two pathways are termed *biased agonism*, or *functional selectivity* (Schmid et al. 2017). Drug development is now targeting biased agonists, such as TRV130 and PMZ21, that preferentially activate the G protein pathway and that therefore, in theory, may be safer and have fewer unwanted side effects (Schmid et al. 2017).

Allosteric Regulation

Another important line of research suggests that substances that bind to allosteric sites on opioid receptors can affect the potency, efficacy, and affinity of substances that bind to orthosteric sites on opioid receptors (Livingston and Traynor 2018). By definition, orthosteric sites are those that bind to endogenous opioid peptides, including the endorphins, dynorphins, and enkephalins, while allosteric sites are those that are spatially distinct from the orthosteric sites. Substances that bind to the allosteric sites typically do not directly activate or inhibit the receptor, but they can enhance the effects of an orthosteric ligand (i.e., a positive allosteric modulator [PAM]), inhibit the effects of an orthosteric ligand (i.e., a negative allosteric modulator [NAM]), or occupy the allosteric site without affecting the orthosteric ligand (i.e., a silent allosteric modulator [SAM]). PAMs at μ-opioid receptors potentially can enhance the effects of currently used opioid medications, such as morphine or oxycodone, so that lower dosages of these medications can be used, which could decrease their unwanted side effects (e.g., constipation and respiratory depression). Perhaps even more intriguing is the possibility that PAMs could be used to enhance the effects of endogenous opioids that may be released in response to stress and/or pain (Livingston and Traynor 2018). This latter approach is appealing because it also would avoid the unwanted side effects of exogenous opioids and be temporally limited to the duration of the stress or pain. At present, the clinical utility of NAMs and SAMs is unclear. Although in vitro techniques have been used to characterize selective allosteric modulators for the μ- and δ-opioid receptor subtypes (Livingston et al. 2018), in vivo studies are needed to support this research. Furthermore, no selective allosteric modulators have been identified for κ-opioid and nociceptin receptors. For a more comprehensive review of this literature, readers are referred to Livingston and Traynor (2018).

Receptor Heteromers

Opioid agonists can bind to opioid receptors in their monomeric forms to produce their cascade of effects on G proteins and β-arrestins, as described above, but this does not prevent the receptors from forming heterodimers (Derouiche and Massotte 2019). Research suggests that opioid receptors may form heteromers with other opioid receptors, such as μ–δ, μ–κ, δ–κ, and μ–nociceptin, or with non-opioid receptors, such as δ–cannabinoid and μ–galanin (Valentino and Volkow 2018). For validation of heteromer formation in GPCRs, there must be evidence of at least two of the following (Derouiche and Massotte 2019):

1. A physical association between the different monomers
2. A specific function of the heteromer that differs from each individual monomer
3. Alteration of the functioning of the heteromer when the physical association is disrupted

Perhaps the most well-studied heterodimer has been the μ–δ combination. Multiple assays, including double fluorescent knock-in mice, μ–δ–selective antibodies, μ–δ coimmunoprecipitation, and administration of a bivalent μ agonist–δ antagonist ligand (MDAN-21), support the existence of μ–δ heterodimers in the brain (Derouiche and Massotte 2019; Valentino and Volkow 2018). Although the functional significance of these opioid heteromers has been more difficult to ascertain, the ability to synthesize bivalent compounds is intriguing and may represent a novel target for development. These advances and others, as described below, have been important for the development of compounds capable of retaining the therapeutic benefits of opioids while minimizing their adverse effects.

Opioid Interactions With Other Endogenous Systems

Glia

Glia (or immunocompetent cells) are non-neuronal cells that are estimated to constitute up to 90% of the cells in the central nervous system (CNS; Herculano-Houzel 2014). The mature CNS contains three types of glial cells: astrocytes, oligodendrocytes, and microglial cells. The term "glia," meaning "glue," reflects what was once thought to be their passive function as physical support for neurons. However, we now know that glia play key roles in many neuronal processes and disease states. Researchers have been studying the interaction between opioids and glia for almost 40 years. This area of investigation has shown that glia express opioid receptors and the messenger RNA (mRNA) needed to produce them. Although it is now recognized that opioid peptides are synthesized in glia, little is known about neuropeptide storage and release from glia.

Exogenous opioid administration typically increases vulnerability to infection, suggesting that opioids are immunosuppressive. However, recent research indicates that opioids may have both activating and inhibitory effects. Investigations into how opioids interact with glia typically examine the effects of the classical μ-receptor agonist morphine. Both acute and chronic administration of morphine increases the expression of cellular markers associated with glial cell activation, such as microglial CD11b and astrocytic glial fibrillary acidic protein (GFAP [Beitner-Johnson et al. 1993; Hutchinson et al. 2010a]). This effect of morphine on GFAP can be antagonized by the nonselective opioid receptor antagonist naltrexone (Beitner-Johnson et al. 1993). Administration of morphine can also lead to increased expression of glial cell–signaling proteins, such as cytokines (interleukin 1β [IL-1β] and tumor necrosis factor α [TNFα]) and chemokines (C-C motif chemokine ligand-5 [CCL5] and monocyte chemoattractant protein 1 [MCP-1]) (Sawaya et al. 2009). Evidence also suggests that morphine enhances microglial migration (Horvath and DeLeo 2009). This area of research has identified several potential mechanisms by which opioids modify glial cell activity.

Several studies have demonstrated that opioids directly activate glial cells in a nonclassical opioid receptor manner (He et al. 2011; Hutchinson et al. 2010b; Wang et al. 2012). Opioid drugs interact with glia through the pattern-recognition receptor Toll-like receptor 4 (TLR4), which is widely expressed in all glia types. In binding to the TLR4 co-receptor myeloid differentiation factor 2 (MD-2), morphine induces TLR4 oligomerization that results in glial activation (i.e., proinflammation [Hutchinson et al. 2010a]). Mice with genetic knockout of TLR4/MD-2 exhibited suppression of the morphine-induced neuroinflammatory response and potentiation of the analgesic effects of morphine (Hutchinson et al. 2012). In addition to supporting the proposed mechanism by which opioids interact with glia, these findings demonstrated that opioid effects on glia may modulate their analgesic actions. Growing evidence suggests that opioid receptors expressed on glia are causally involved in the development of opioid analgesic tolerance, opioid physiological dependence, and opioid-induced hyperalgesia (Watkins et al. 2009).

Opioid-induced increases in proinflammatory cytokine release are thought to oppose opioid analgesic effects. This hypothesis is supported by research showing that the development of hyperalgesia and spinal analgesic tolerance to morphine is correlated (using real-time reverse transcription polymerase chain reaction) with glial activation and cytokine release (Raghavendra et al. 2002). Morphine-induced inflammatory signaling via TLR4 has also been shown to contribute to deficits in glutamate transmission. Opioid-induced changes in glutamate transmission are thought to be related to the development of opioid tolerance and dependence. In rats, pharmacological blockade of TLR4 attenuates morphine tolerance and potentiates the analgesic effects of morphine (Eidson and Murphy 2013).

Opioid interactions with glial cells may also contribute to opioid actions within the brain's reward center (i.e., the mesolimbic dopamine pathway), thereby mediating the drug's potential to be abused. As noted above, morphine increases GFAP levels in the ventral tegmental area, nucleus accumbens, striatum, and frontal cortex—areas hypothesized to contribute to the positive reinforcing effects of stimuli (Koob and Volkow 2016). Administration of astrocyte-related proinflammatory cytokines and chemokines potentiates the preference for morphine-associated cues (Narita et al. 2006). Furthermore, TLR4 knockout mice show impaired development of morphine conditioned place preference, an animal model used to study the rewarding and aversive effects of drugs (Hutchinson et al. 2012).

Taken together, there is a strong body of preclinical evidence suggesting that opioid effects on glia contribute to both analgesia and the behavioral effects associated with opioid misuse and dependence. Consistent with this literature, preclinical studies have demonstrated that pharmacological modulation of opioid–glia interactions may improve the clinical utility of opioid drugs (for a review, see Jones 2020). The TNFα inhibitor ibudilast was found to shift the dose–response curve for morphine-induced analgesia leftward, decreasing the minimum effective analgesic dose (Hutchinson et al. 2009). Ibudilast also delayed the development of morphine tolerance and hyperalgesia (Johnson et al. 2014). Minocycline, a microglia inhibitor, has been shown to enhance morphine-induced antinociception (Kosarmadar et al. 2015).

Minocycline also attenuated the development of opioid-induced hyperalgesia and potentiated the analgesic effects of morphine (Mika et al. 2007). Similar results have been shown with propentofylline, which inhibits GFAP, CD11b, IL-1β, IL-6, and TNFα (Raghavendra et al. 2003). When fluorocitrate, an inhibitor of glial metabolism, was administered in combination with chronic morphine, it attenuated the development of tolerance to the analgesic effects of morphine (Song and Zhao 2001). Finally, statins are potent inhibitors of various glial pathways and products and have been shown to exert significant protective effects against tolerance to the antinociceptive effects of morphine and the development of physiological dependence in mice and rats (Pajohanfar et al. 2017). This area of research has also led to the development of promising single-molecular-entity compounds that simultaneously inhibit glia and stimulate the μ-opioid receptor as treatments for chronic pain without tolerance (Akgün et al. 2019).

Glia-modulating drugs have also been shown to decrease the rewarding effects of opioids. Ibudilast significantly reduced the magnitude of morphine-induced dopamine transmission within the reward pathway and morphine-induced conditioned place preference (Bland et al. 2009). Minocycline and propentofylline also antagonized the rewarding effects of morphine, as demonstrated in the conditioned place preference paradigm (Narita et al. 2006). Finally, pioglitazone, which inhibits the expression of cytokines by monocytes/macrophages and microglia, attenuated the development of morphine tolerance, opioid withdrawal, and heroin self-administration and dopamine release (de Guglielmo et al. 2017; Ghavimi et al. 2014). These preclinical data strongly support the therapeutic potential of glia modulators for the treatment of several aspects of opioid use disorder.

Clinical research is only beginning to replicate the promising preclinical findings concerning the treatment potential of glia-modulating drugs. Cooper et al. (2016) found that ibudilast reduced subjective ratings of abstinence-induced opioid withdrawal among opioid-dependent participants. Metz et al. (2017) extended these findings by testing the effects of ibudilast on the subjective, reinforcing, and analgesic effects of oral oxycodone. While under active ibudilast maintenance, subjects' ratings of oxycodone "liking" were significantly decreased, along with oxycodone self-administration. Mogali et al. (2014) also found that minocycline attenuated the positive subjective effects of oral oxycodone, along with opioid craving. Finally, Jones et al. (2018) assessed the effects of pioglitazone on the abuse potential of heroin and found that pioglitazone maintenance significantly reduced opioid craving.

Despite this extensive body of work, the full extent of opioid and glial interactions is not fully understood. However, our understanding of their association continues to grow. The current body of literature suggests that manipulation of the interaction between opioids and glia may be a means of both improving the clinical utility of opioids and reducing nonmedical use of opioids.

Hypothalamic-Pituitary-Adrenal Axis

The hypothalamic-pituitary-adrenal (HPA) axis refers to the three neuroendocrine glands that function in tandem to help regulate metabolic and immunological processes throughout the body. This system of glands also plays a major role in the regulation of stress. When an individual is exposed to a stressor (defined as any real or perceived threat to one's well-being), the hypothalamus—or, more specifically, the medial parvocellular subdivision—releases corticotropin-releasing factor (CRF) (Smith and Vale 2006). CRF binding causes the pituitary to release adrenocorticotropic hormone (ACTH), which binds to the adrenal gland, resulting in the release of glucocorticoids—more specifically, cortisol in humans (Smith and Vale 2006). Cortisol release increases blood sugar and available glucose to the brain, as well as reparative metabolic processes, and slows digestion (Nesse et al. 2016). While HPA axis activation in response to an immediate threat is adaptive, chronic activation of the HPA axis has been implicated in the development or worsening of obesity, depression, abnormal sleep patterns, and memory deficits (Buckley and Schatzberg 2005).

The HPA axis also is affected by opioids and thus may play a role in opioid use disorder. In primates, self-administration of high doses of the potent µ-opioid agonist fentanyl decreased plasma cortisol and ACTH (Broadbear et al. 2004). In contrast, the µ-receptor-selective antagonist naltrexone, but not the δ-selective antagonist naltrindole, increased ACTH and plasma cortisol levels (Williams et al. 2003, 2004). However, the µ-receptor-selective antagonist clocinnamox failed to increase ACTH. The long-lasting κ-selective antagonist norbinaltorphimine increased ACTH on the day of injection but not at later time points (24 hour) when its κ-antagonist effects were still evident (Williams et al. 2003).

Clinical studies in humans typically report an opioid-induced suppression of HPA axis function. In one study, six healthy male volunteers were administered five different µ-opioid-receptor-selective agonists (morphine, methadone, pentazocine, nalorphine, and D-Ala$_2$,MePhe$_4$Met[O]$_5$-ol enkephalin). For all five drugs, acute administration produced a significant decrease in serum cortisol relative to placebo (Delitala et al. 1983). The prototypical µ-opioid receptor agonist morphine has also been shown to suppress the release of ACTH, a finding that helps to explain the accompanying decrease in serum cortisol (Allolio et al. 1987). Other studies also have shown that long-term users of heroin have lower serum cortisol levels compared with healthy control subjects (Kreek and Koob 1998). However, among opioid-dependent individuals, cortisol levels vary as a function of opioid withdrawal state. In a study by Zhang et al. (2008), individuals seeking treatment for opioid use disorder were treated with either non-opioid medications (i.e., benzodiazepines and clonidine) or methadone. In comparison with healthy control participants, opioid-using participants who were not maintained on an opioid agonist medication had significantly higher cortisol levels during acute withdrawal. Meanwhile, cortisol levels were lower (versus healthy controls) among participants maintained on methadone.

The specific pathways by which the opioid receptor system modulates HPA axis activity are not completely understood. However, there is some evidence to suggest that κ-opioid receptor binding in the hypothalamus may mediate the effects of opioids on the HPA axis (Pfeiffer et al. 1986). Individuals with Cushing's disease also appear to be resistant to the opioid-induced ACTH- and cortisol-suppressing effects seen in healthy control subjects (Yanovski 1993). Cushing's disease is a condition in which either tumors or hyperplasia of the pituitary gland causes excess ACTH release and therefore cortisol production. Thus, the findings of Yanovski (1993) implicate action at the pituitary as a factor in the HPA axis–suppressing effects of opioids. Ultimately, the current body of evidence supports the claim that opioids may exert their influence over the HPA axis by directly binding to the hypothalamus and pituitary gland.

Gonadal Hormones

The endogenous opioid system is one of numerous neuroendocrine modulators of the hypothalamic-pituitary-gonadal (HPG) axis. Opioids exert an inhibitory effect on the pulsatile secretion of gonadotropin-releasing hormone (GnRH) from the hypothalamus, which subsequently inhibits secretion of follicle-stimulating hormone (FSH) and luteinizing hormone (LH) from the anterior pituitary gland. The end result of this opioid-induced cascade is an inhibition of sex hormone release from reproductive organs. Administration of the opioid antagonist naloxone to healthy individuals has been shown to increase GnRH levels, suggesting tonic inhibition of gonadotropin release by endogenous opioids (Seyfried and Hester 2012).

In women, the endogenous opioid system is tightly coupled to the menstrual cycle (Leyendecker et al. 1990). The early follicular phase of the menstrual cycle is marked by low opioid tone and thus uninhibited, pulsatile GnRH secretion from the hypothalamus. A rise in estrogen levels follows, with an accompanying rise in endogenous opioid tone, leading to a slowing of GnRH release. Increased progesterone during the luteal phase of the cycle maintains a high opioid tone, resulting in the onset of menstruation, during which estrogen, progesterone, and opioid levels fall and pulsatile GnRH secretion resumes uninhibited (Leyendecker et al. 1990).

GnRH levels decrease in response to administration of exogenous opioids, which contributes to the sexual and menstrual dysfunction seen with long-term opioid use (Colameco and Coren 2009). Opioids additionally reduce testosterone and estrogen production by decreasing adrenal androgen production, which is dependent on serum cortisol levels (Colameco and Coren 2009). Continuous exposure to exogenous opioids leads to hypogonadism, with symptoms such as decreased libido and erectile dysfunction in men and amenorrhea in women. Administration of μ-opioid receptor antagonists, such as naltrexone, leads to resumption of normal GnRH secretion and restoration of menstrual cycles and sexual function in these individuals, however (Böttcher et al. 2017). Opioid receptors are also found on cells throughout the male and female reproductive systems, and opioids have been suggested to play a role in the regulation of numerous reproductive functions, including proliferation of testicular cells, sperm motility, and uterine contractions. Disruptions to these functions likely contribute to the sexual and endocrine dysfunction associated with repeated administration of exogenous opioids. However, the precise role of opioids in the pathogenesis of disorders of the endocrine system remains incompletely understood (Böttcher et al. 2017).

Therapeutic Uses of Exogenous Opioids

Exogenous administration of opioids is used therapeutically for multiple indications. One of the most common uses of opioids is for pain control. In addition, opioids reduce cough and diarrhea and induce loss of consciousness, which is useful for anesthesia in surgical settings.

Pain

Opioids are commonly prescribed to treat acute pain after surgery or trauma, as well as to manage chronic pain. Although there are numerous types of opioid drugs, with varying pharmacodynamic and pharmacokinetic profiles, all opioids function by binding to and activating one or more of the opioid receptor subtypes. The μ-opioid receptor has been suggested to play a central role in analgesia, given that all current opioid analgesics exert their effects, at least in part, through μ-opioid receptor activation (Al-Hasani and Bruchas 2011).

The opioid receptors mediating pain control are primarily located in the dorsal horn of the spinal cord (which relays nociceptive input from the periphery to the brain via the spinothalamic tract) and are also located in subcortical brain regions from which pain-modulating pathways emerge, including the thalamus, periaqueductal gray area, rostral ventromedial medulla, and locus coeruleus (Trang et al. 2015). In the spinal dorsal horn, opioids produce analgesia through effects on both presynaptic afferent neurons and postsynaptic projection neurons of the spinothalamic tract. Activation of opioid receptors in presynaptic neurons results in activation of receptor-associated inhibitory G proteins, producing a decrease in cytosolic cyclic adenosine monophosphate (cAMP) and inhibition of voltage-gated calcium channels that are required for release of nociceptive neurotransmitters (e.g., substance P). On postsynaptic neurons of the spinal cord, activation of the receptor-associated G protein leads to an increase in potassium conductance and hyperpolarization of the cell, which decreases activity. An alternate mechanism by which opioids achieve pain control is by indirect stimulation of descending inhibitory pain pathways from the midbrain (Williams 2008). Opioid receptor activation in this region produces disinhibition of inhibitory GABAergic pathways acting on the periaqueductal gray area (PAG) and rostral ventromedial medulla (RVM). The net result of this process is the activation of descending inhibitory pathways from the PAG and RVM that suppress nociceptive transmission in the spinal cord.

Management of chronic pain with opioids may be difficult due to the development of analgesic tolerance, which is defined as the need for increasing amounts of a drug in order to achieve the same effect. Opioid receptor internalization and phosphorylation by downstream signaling molecules likely play key roles in the development of tolerance (Raehal and Bohn 2014). A major downstream consequence of μ-opioid receptor activation is the activation of receptor tyrosine kinases, such as platelet-derived growth factor receptor–β (PDGFR-β) (Wang et al. 2012). Activation of PDGFR-β can lead to phosphorylation of the μ-opioid receptor, which facilitates binding of β-arrestin to the receptor. The opioid receptor is thus prevented from associating with another G protein and is instead targeted for internalization. This process contributes to the development of tolerance because the target cell now expresses fewer opioid receptors and would be less responsive to subsequent opioid stimulation.

In contrast to tolerance, dependence is defined as the appearance of specific physiological and psychological symptoms upon cessation of a drug or administration of an opioid antagonist. Physiological opioid dependence is characterized by the emergence—usually within 12 hours of abstinence from opioids or sooner, depending on the opioid agonist—of withdrawal symptoms such as restlessness, yawning, lacrimation, rhinorrhea, chills, hyperhidrosis, nausea, vomiting, diarrhea, and myalgias. Although physical dependence on a drug usually accompanies tolerance to the drug, the two processes do not necessarily occur by the same mechanism. β-Arrestin knockout mice do not become tolerant to opioid effects, for example, but still become physiologically dependent (Raehal and Bohn 2014). These data suggest that opioid dependence is dissociable from opioid tolerance and may develop through a separate mechanism.

The precise mechanisms of opioid dependence and withdrawal are not completely understood, but the neuronal hyperexcitability that characterizes withdrawal states indicates a role of the autonomic nervous system in this process. This enhanced neuronal excitability is thought to arise from a compensatory increase in expression of proteins and effector molecules downstream from the opioid receptor secondary to the inhibitory effects of opioid stimulation (Burma et al. 2017). For example, opioids inhibit norepinephrine (noradrenaline) release from the locus coeruleus (LC), contributing to the reduction in respiratory rate seen during opioid intoxication. Tonic suppression of norepinephrine release from the LC results in compensatory upregulation of this pathway in order to preserve normal physiological function in the presence of opioids. Abrupt cessation of opioid stimulation, therefore, results in increased norepinephrine release due to loss of inhibition of this upregulated pathway. Other features of opioid dependence and withdrawal, such as CNS pain sensitization and negative affective states, may arise from similar mechanisms.

Anesthesia

Opioids are routinely used in surgical procedures (along with other anesthetic agents) due to their analgesic properties and ability to suppress the HPA axis. Opioids commonly used as anesthetic agents include morphine, fentanyl, and other fentanyl analogs such as alfentanil and remifentanil. These agents are typically administered intravenously or intrathecally, and the dose is adjusted until the desired effect is achieved.

The primary benefit of using opioids in anesthetic procedures is their ability to produce analgesia while maintaining cardiac stability (Bovill et al. 1984). These functions arise primarily from the actions of these drugs on μ-opioid receptors (as discussed earlier), including inhibition of ascending and descending pain pathways and suppression of the HPA axis. The inhibitory effects of opioids on the release of adrenal hormones (including cortisol and aldosterone) are especially important during intraoperative anesthesia, because surgery is often associated with extreme increases in blood pressure and heart rate, which may otherwise contribute to morbidity and mortality.

Cough

Opioids are among the most commonly used and potent antitussive agents. In particular, codeine (a prodrug that is metabolized to morphine) and hydrocodone have long been considered to be the "gold standard" narcotic (opioid) antitussives. Although the exact mechanism by which these agents produce their effects is unclear, cough suppression likely arises from inhibitory effects on the medullary cough center and the vagal afferent and efferent nerves in the airways (Takahama and Shirasaki 2007). These effects are likely mediated primarily by the μ-opioid receptor, and, to a lesser extent, the κ-opioid receptor.

Diarrhea

One of the more common side effects seen with opioids is constipation (Ahmedzai and Boland 2010). For this reason, coprescription of a laxative is quite common, particularly when opioids are prescribed for extended periods of time, such as in chronic pain or terminal illness. The binding of opioids—specifically μ agonists—to peripheral receptors located in the gastrointestinal tract inhibits gastrointestinal mobility, ultimately leading to constipation (Murphy et al. 1997). However, under certain circumstances, this outcome can be desirable. For example, the peripheral opioid receptor agonist loperamide decreases peristalsis and fluid secretion (Baker 2007). These effects, combined with loperamide's minimal action in the CNS, make it an effective treatment for diarrhea without the risk of dependence associated with many centrally acting opioid agonists (Baker 2007). The constipation observed with long-term opioid use can be rapidly reversed with selective peripherally acting μ-opioid antagonists such as methylnaltrexone (Rosow 1997). Interestingly, diarrhea is a symptom of opioid withdrawal (Wesson and Ling 2003) and likely results from a rebound increase in intestinal motility after extended periods of constipation associated with long-term opioid use.

Off-Label Uses: Depression

Pharmacotherapy has become the primary treatment approach for depression, which is estimated to affect just over 4% of the global population, or approximately 339 million individuals (World Health Organization 2017). Pharmacotherapy for depression includes medications such as selective serotonin reuptake inhibitors (SSRIs) and tricyclic antidepressants (TCAs). Unfortunately, only approximately 40% of individuals treated with SSRIs—the more effective of the two medication classes—show a response (Khan and Brown 2015). These medications also have a slow onset of therapeutic action, with symptom relief typically requiring weeks to take effect.

In response to the need for improved pharmacotherapies for depression, researchers have explored the utility of agents that act on the opioid receptor system. Some studies have linked the severity of depressive symptoms to deficiencies in μ-opioid receptor density and binding potential in cortical brain regions associated with emotional processing (e.g., anterior cingulate cortex [Kennedy et al. 2006]). The opioid receptor system has also been shown, through extensive research, to interact with the HPA axis (as detailed in the section "Hypothalamic-Pituitary-Adrenal Axis"). Postmortem examination of suicide victims' brains has also shown an increased density of μ-opioid receptors in the frontal cortex and caudate (Gross-Isseroff et al. 1990). Others have shown, however, that prefrontal cortex μ-opioid receptor binding affinity is significantly lower among suicide victims than in healthy control subjects (Zalsman et al. 2005). The combination of receptor site insensitivity and deficiency in the total number of opioid receptor sites suggests that unresponsiveness to endogenous opioids may be linked to suicidal tendencies.

Although the exact nature of the relationship between the endogenous opioid system and depression is unknown, researchers are investigating opioids such as tianeptine, which is approved in Europe for the treatment of depression. Despite having a chemical structure similar to that of other TCAs, tianeptine differs significantly from other TCAs and even SSRIs in that it increases serotonin reuptake as opposed to inhibiting it (Wagstaff et al. 2001). Research from the past decade strongly implicates the opioid receptor system in the effects of tianeptine as well. An in vitro study by Gassaway et al. (2014) demonstrated that tianeptine has a high affinity for the human μ-opioid receptor, ultimately acting as a μ-opioid receptor agonist, with negligible binding affinity for either δ or κ receptors. This study also found that tianeptine had virtually no agonist or antagonist effects on metabotropic glutamate receptors, a finding suggesting that direct modulation of the glutamate system, which researchers have put forth as an alternative theory to explain tianeptine's effects, is unlikely.

Recent research has also examined the efficacy of a mixture containing samidorphan and buprenorphine as a treatment for depression in individuals who fail to respond to first-line medications. Buprenorphine is a well-established medication used primarily for the treatment of opioid use disorder. It is a partial μ-opioid receptor agonist, a κ-opioid receptor antagonist, and a weak δ-opioid receptor antagonist (Walsh and Middleton 2013). Samidorphan, on the other hand, functions as a μ-opioid receptor antagonist (Fava et al. 2016). Delivering the two drugs in combination theoretically increases the κ receptor antagonist effects of buprenorphine while attenuating its μ receptor partial-agonist effects, which should decrease its potential for nonmedical use (Ragguett et al. 2018). Although some clinical studies of buprenorphine plus samidorphan in the treatment of depression appeared to show its promise (Fava et al. 2016; Ragguett et al. 2018), an advisory panel of the U.S. Food and Drug Administration recently voted 20–3 that the pharmaceutical company had not provided sufficient evidence that the combination formulation was effective in treating depression. In addition to buprenorphine plus samidorphan, other κ-opioid-receptor-selective medications are also in various stages of clinical development for this indication.

Abuse Potential of Opioids

Although opioids are among the most commonly used drugs for treating pain, their clinical utility as analgesics is tempered by their potential to be misused. It is now widely recognized that the misuse of opioid analgesics is a substantial contributor to the development of opioid use disorder and a pathway to heroin use (Cicero et al. 2014). The role of the various opioid receptor subtypes in opioid misuse has been investigated extensively. Opioid-induced euphoria is thought to be the initiating factor in the development of opioid use disorder (Koob and Volkow 2016). Repeated drug exposure produces changes in multiple brain circuits, resulting in increases in the threshold at which euphoria is experienced (i.e., tolerance) and emergence of withdrawal symptoms in the absence of the drug (i.e., dependence). Because tolerance and dependence were discussed earlier in this chapter, this section will focus on the factors that contribute to the initiation stage in the development of opioid use disorder. The euphoric effects of opioids increase the probability of repeated opioid use through either positive or negative reinforcement. Positive reinforcement is typically thought of as increased behavior in order to obtain the pleasurable hedonic feeling produced by a drug. Negative reinforcement refers to increased behavior in order to remove an unpleasant stimulus or state. Both of these processes contribute to continued opioid use.

The reinforcing effects of opioids have been attributed to their actions at μ-opioid receptors. In the preclinical conditioned place preference (CPP) model, a drug is first paired with a distinct environment and then the amount of time the animal subsequently spends in the drug-paired environment relative to the placebo-paired environment is used as a measure of the rewarding effects of the drug. Morphine produces a CPP, but this effect is not observed in μ-opioid-receptor-deficient mice (Becker et al. 2000). Pharmacological antagonism of μ-opioid receptors has also been shown to block the rewarding and reinforcing effects of opioids (Rowlett and Woolverton 1997). Research has further established that μ-opioid receptor activation within the ventral tegmental area (VTA) of the mesolimbic dopamine pathway is the critical site for opioid-mediated reward (Fields and Margolis 2015). Opioid-induced CPP can be blocked by intra-VTA μ-opioid-receptor-selective antagonists (Olmstead and Franklin 1997). Similar results have been observed with VTA site-specific genetic manipulation of μ-opioid-receptor levels (Zhang et al. 2009). Opioids are also self-administered directly into the VTA, but not in other sites in the brain. Similarly, morphine-induced CPP is also site-specific for the VTA (Bals-Kubick et al. 1993).

In the canonical model of the neurobiology of drug reward, dopamine is the neurotransmitter associated with the reinforcing effects of all drugs of abuse. As noted previously, when opioids activate μ receptors, they reduce the tonic inhibition of dopaminergic neurons by GABAergic interneurons, resulting in increased mesolimbic dopamine release (Jalabert et al. 2011). Although a considerable portion of the rewarding effects of opioids may be related to their indirect activation of dopamine transmission, such activation is not an essential component of opioid reward. Dopamine-depleted mice still acquire morphine CPP (Hnasko et al. 2005), although these findings can be dependent on specific testing parameters.

The role that δ-opioid receptors play in the rewarding effects of opioids has only recently been elucidated using genetic techniques. The rewarding and reinforcing effects of morphine are retained in δ-opioid receptor knockout mice, suggesting minimal δ-opioid receptor modulation of reward processes (Le Merrer et al. 2011). Nonetheless, opioid effects on δ-opioid receptors may reinforce drug taking in other ways. δ-Opioid receptor activation produces anxiolytic and antidepressant effects (Pradhan et al. 2011). The effects of opioids on stress systems were detailed earlier in the chapter (see section "Hypothalamic-Pituitary-Adrenal Axis"). Opioids may also be negatively reinforcing in other ways. μ-Opioid receptor activation has been implicated in the modulation of prosocial behavior, anhedonia, and attachment (Der-Avakian and Markou 2012). As a result, "social pain" (e.g., social dysfunction and isolation) may motivate opioid use. The negatively reinforcing effects of opioids may be a separate or complementary contributor to their abuse potential. The role that negative reinforcement plays in the initiation of opioid misuse deserves further study because nonmedical opioid use resulting from positive and negative reinforcement may constitute two distinct phenotypes of the behavior and subsequent development of opioid use disorder. In conclusion, the pleasurable effects of opioids are primarily the result of their activation of the μ-opioid receptor and facilitation of mesolimbic dopamine transmission.

Opioid use disorder stems from the progressive adaptation of the brain to repeated opioid exposure, resulting in tolerance, physiological dependence, and a shift from drug taking being pleasurable (positively reinforcing) to drug taking being necessary in order to feel "normal" (negatively reinforcing). However, substantial individual variability exists in subjective response to opioids and in what initiates nonmedical opioid use. A better understanding of the factors that motivate nonmedical opioid use could significantly improve our ability to identify individuals at risk and may lead to more targeted treatment approaches.

Conclusion

Endogenous opioid peptides (endorphins, enkephalins, dynorphins, and nociceptin) exert their effects through activity at four G protein–coupled receptor subtypes: μ, δ, κ, and nociceptin. Opioid peptides and their receptors are distributed throughout the CNS and the peripheral nervous system and are important mediators of stress response, autonomic activity, pain, and reward. Opioid-induced suppression of HPA axis function mediates responses to stressors. Endogenous opioids, along with exogenous μ-opioid receptor agonists, typically have antistress or anxiolytic effects, suggesting that altered activity in the endogenous opioid system may be involved in anxiety, depression, and suicidality. Currently, opioid medications are being investigated for the treatment of depression. Exogenous opioids are among the most effective and widely used medications for treating pain. However, μ-opioid receptor agonists produce pleasurable effects that lead to nonmedical use and abuse. Universal features of prolonged opioid use such as tolerance and dependence help to maintain opioid use that can ultimately lead to the development of opioid use disorder. We are just beginning to understand the extent and nature of the interaction between opioids and glia. A growing body of literature suggests that opioid–glia interactions contribute to the development of opioid-related tolerance, dependence, and abuse potential. Targeting medications that alter glial functioning may lead to the development of novel, non-opioid pharmacotherapies to treat opioid use disorder. In summary, endogenous and exogenous opioids influence many neurobiological systems. For this reason, these interactions are important topics of investigation as they relate to the clinical utility and abuse potential of opioids as well as to the development of novel pharmacotherapies for treating opioid use disorder.

References

Ahmedzai SH, Boland J: Constipation in people prescribed opioids. BMJ Clin Evid 2010:2407, 2010 21718572

Akgün E, Lunzer MM, Portoghese PS: Combined glia inhibition and opioid receptor agonism afford highly potent analgesics without tolerance. ACS Chem Neurosci 10(4):2004–2011, 2019 30110531

Al-Hasani R, Bruchas MR: Molecular mechanisms of opioid receptor-dependent signaling and behavior. Anesthesiology 115(6):1363–1381, 2011 22020140

Allolio B, Schulte HM, Deuss U, et al: Effect of oral morphine and naloxone on pituitary-adrenal response in man induced by human corticotropin-releasing hormone. Acta Endocrinol (Copenh) 114(4):509–514, 1987 3033966

Baker DE: Loperamide: a pharmacological review. Rev Gastroenterol Disord 7 (suppl 3):S11–S18, 2007 18192961

Bals-Kubik R, Ableitner A, Herz A, Shippenberg TS: Neuroanatomical sites mediating the motivational effects of opioids as mapped by the conditioned place preference paradigm in rats. J Pharmacol Exp Ther 264(1):489–495, 1993 8093731

Becker A, Grecksch G, Brödemann R, et al: Morphine self-administration in mu-opioid receptor-deficient mice. Naunyn Schmiedebergs Arch Pharmacol 361(6):584–589, 2000 10882032

Beitner-Johnson D, Guitart X, Nestler EJ: Glial fibrillary acidic protein and the mesolimbic dopamine system: regulation by chronic morphine and Lewis-Fischer strain differences in the rat ventral tegmental area. J Neurochem 61(5):1766–1773, 1993 8228992

Bland ST, Hutchinson MR, Maier SF, et al: The glial activation inhibitor AV411 reduces morphine-induced nucleus accumbens dopamine release. Brain Behav Immun 23(4):492–497, 2009 19486648

Böttcher B, Seeber B, Leyendecker G, Wildt L: Impact of the opioid system on the reproductive axis. Fertil Steril 108(2):207–213, 2017 28669481

Bovill JG, Sebel PS, Stanley TH: Opioid analgesics in anesthesia: with special reference to their use in cardiovascular anesthesia. Anesthesiology 61(6):731–755, 1984 6150663

Broadbear JH, Winger G, Woods JH: Self-administration of fentanyl, cocaine and ketamine: effects on the pituitary-adrenal axis in rhesus monkeys. Psychopharmacology (Berl) 176(3–4):398–406, 2004 15114434

Buckley TM, Schatzberg AF: On the interactions of the hypothalamic-pituitary-adrenal (HPA) axis and sleep: normal HPA axis activity and circadian rhythm, exemplary sleep disorders. J Clin Endocrinol Metab 90(5):3106–3114, 2005 15728214

Burma NE, Kwok CH, Trang T: Therapies and mechanisms of opioid withdrawal. Pain Manag 7(6):455–459, 2017 29125396

Cicero TJ, Ellis MS, Surratt HL, Kurtz SP: The changing face of heroin use in the United States: a retrospective analysis of the past 50 years. JAMA Psychiatry 71(7):821–826, 2014 24871348

Colameco S, Coren JS: Opioid-induced endocrinopathy. J Am Osteopath Assoc 109(1):20–25, 2009 19193821

Cooper ZD, Johnson KW, Pavlicova M, et al: The effects of ibudilast, a glial activation inhibitor, on opioid withdrawal symptoms in opioid-dependent volunteers. Addict Biol 21(4):895–903, 2016 25975386

Corder G, Castro DC, Bruchas MR, Scherrer G: Endogenous and exogenous opioids in pain. Annu Rev Neurosci 41:453–473, 2018 29852083 de Guglielmo G, Kallupi M, Scuppa G, et al: Pioglitazone attenuates the opioid withdrawal and vulnerability to relapse to heroin seeking in rodents. Psychopharmacology (Berl) 234(2):223–234, 2017 27714428

Delitala G, Grossman A, Besser M: Differential effects of opiate peptides and alkaloids on anterior pituitary hormone secretion. Neuroendocrinology 37(4):275–279, 1983 6633817

Der-Avakian A, Markou A: The neurobiology of anhedonia and other reward-related deficits. Trends Neurosci 35(1):68–77, 2012 22177980

Derouiche L, Massotte D: G protein-coupled receptor heteromers are key players in substance use disorder. Neurosci Biobehav Rev 106:73–90, 2019 30278192

Eidson LN, Murphy AZ: Blockade of Toll-like receptor 4 attenuates morphine tolerance and facilitates the pain relieving properties of morphine. J Neurosci 33(40):15952–15963, 2013 24089500

Fava M, Memisoglu A, Thase ME, et al: Opioid modulation with buprenorphine/samidorphan as adjunctive treatment for inadequate response to antidepressants: a randomized double-blind placebo-controlled trial. Am J Psychiatry 173(5):499–508, 2016 26869247

Fields HL, Margolis EB: Understanding opioid reward. Trends Neurosci 38(4):217–225, 2015 25637939

Gassaway MM, Rives ML, Kruegel AC, et al: The atypical antidepressant and neurorestorative agent tianeptine is a μ-opioid receptor agonist. Transl Psychiatry 4:e411, 2014 25026323

Ghavimi H, Hassanzadeh K, Maleki-Dizaji N, et al: Pioglitazone prevents morphine antinociception tolerance and withdrawal symptoms in rats. Naunyn Schmiedebergs Arch Pharmacol 387(9):811–821, 2014 24899385

Gross-Isseroff R, Dillon KA, Israeli M, Biegon A: Regionally selective increases in mu opioid receptor density in the brains of suicide victims. Brain Res 530(2):312–316, 1990 2176118

He L, Li H, Chen L, et al: Toll-like receptor 9 is required for opioid-induced microglia apoptosis. PLoS One 6(4):e18190, 2011 21559519

Herculano-Houzel S: The glia/neuron ratio: how it varies uniformly across brain structures and species and what that means for brain physiology and evolution. Glia 62(9):1377–1391, 2014 24807023

Hnasko TS, Sotak BN, Palmiter RD: Morphine reward in dopamine-deficient mice. Nature 438(7069):854–857, 2005 16341013

Horvath RJ, DeLeo JA: Morphine enhances microglial migration through modulation of P2X4 receptor signaling. J Neurosci 29(4):998–1005, 2009 19176808

Hutchinson MR, Lewis SS, Coats BD, et al: Reduction of opioid withdrawal and potentiation of acute opioid analgesia by systemic AV411 (ibudilast). Brain Behav Immun 23(2):240–250, 2009 18938237

Hutchinson MR, Lewis SS, Coats BD, et al: Possible involvement of toll-like receptor 4/myeloid differentiation factor-2 activity of opioid inactive isomers causes spinal proinflammation and related behavioral consequences. Neuroscience 167(3):880–893, 2010a 20178837

Hutchinson MR, Zhang Y, Shridhar M, et al: Evidence that opioids may have toll-like receptor 4 and MD-2 effects. Brain Behav Immun 24(1):83–95, 2010b 19679181

Hutchinson MR, Northcutt AL, Hiranita T, et al: Opioid activation of toll-like receptor 4 contributes to drug reinforcement. J Neurosci 32(33):11187–11200, 2012 22895704

Jalabert M, Bourdy R, Courtin J, et al: Neuronal circuits underlying acute morphine action on dopamine neurons. Proc Natl Acad Sci USA 108(39):16446–16450, 2011 21930931

Johnson JL, Rolan PE, Johnson ME, et al: Codeine-induced hyperalgesia and allodynia: investigating the role of glial activation. Transl Psychiatry 4:e482, 2014 25386959

Jones JD: Potential of glial cell modulators in the management of substance use disorders. CNS Drugs 34(7):697–722, 2020 32246400

Jones JD, Bisaga A, Metz VE, et al: The PPARgamma agonist pioglitazone fails to alter the abuse potential of heroin, but does reduce heroin craving and anxiety. J Psychoactive Drugs 50(5):390–401, 2018 30204554

Kennedy SE, Koeppe RA, Young EA, Zubieta JK: Dysregulation of endogenous opioid emotion regulation circuitry in major depression in women. Arch Gen Psychiatry 63(11):1199–1208, 2006 17088500

Khan A, Brown WA: Antidepressants versus placebo in major depression: an overview. World Psychiatry 14(3):294–300, 2015 26407778

Koob GF, Volkow ND: Neurobiology of addiction: a neurocircuitry analysis. Lancet Psychiatry 3(8):760–773, 2016 27475769

Kosarmadar N, Ghasemzadeh Z, Rezayof A: Inhibition of microglia in the basolateral amygdala enhanced morphine-induced antinociception: possible role of GABAA receptors. Eur J Pharmacol 765:157–163, 2015 26297974

Kreek MJ, Koob GF: Drug dependence: stress and dysregulation of brain reward pathways. Drug Alcohol Depend 51(1–2):23–47, 1998 9716928

Le Merrer J, Plaza-Zabala A, Del Boca C, et al: Deletion of the delta opioid receptor gene impairs place conditioning but preserves morphine reinforcement. Biol Psychiatry 69(7):700–703, 2011 21168121

Leyendecker G, Waibeltreber S, Wildt L: The central control of follicular maturation and ovulation in the human. Oxf Rev Reprod Biol 12:93–146, 1990 2075005

Livingston KE, Traynor JR: Allostery at opioid receptors: modulation with small molecule ligands. Br J Pharmacol 175(14):2846–2856, 2018 28419415

Livingston KE, Stanczyk MA, Burford NT, et al: Pharmacologic evidence for a putative conserved allosteric site on opioid receptors. Mol Pharmacol 93(2):157–167, 2018 29233847

Metz VE, Jones JD, Manubay J, et al: Effects of ibudilast on the subjective, reinforcing, and analgesic effects of oxycodone in recently detoxified adults with opioid dependence. Neuropsychopharmacology 42(9):1825–1832, 2017 28393896

Mika J, Osikowicz M, Makuch W, Przewlocka B: Minocycline and pentoxifylline attenuate allodynia and hyperalgesia and potentiate the effects of morphine in rat and mouse models of neuropathic pain. Eur J Pharmacol 560(2–3):142–149, 2007 17307159

Mogali S, Jones JD, Manubay J, et al: Effects of minocycline on oxycodone-induced responses in humans. Drug and Alcohol Dependence 140:e153, 2014. Available at: https://www.sciencedirect.com/science/article/abs/pii/S0376871614004888?via%3Dihub. Accessed April 26, 2020.

Murphy DB, Sutton JA, Prescott LF, Murphy MB: Opioid-induced delay in gastric emptying: a peripheral mechanism in humans. Anesthesiology 87(4):765–770, 1997 9357876

Narita M, Miyatake M, Narita M, et al: Direct evidence of astrocytic modulation in the development of rewarding effects induced by drugs of abuse. Neuropsychopharmacology 31(11):2476–2488, 2006 16407899

Nesse RM, Bhatnagar S, Ellis B: Evolutionary origins and functions of the stress response system, in Stress: Concepts, Cognition, Emotion, and Behavior (Handbook of Stress Series, Vol 1). Edited by Fink G. Cambridge, MA, Academic Press, 2016, pp 95–101. Available at: https://www.sciencedirect.com/science/article/pii/B978012800951200011X. Accessed April 26, 2020.

Olmstead MC, Franklin KB: The development of a conditioned place preference to morphine: effects of microinjections into various CNS sites. Behav Neurosci 111(6):1324–1334, 1997 9438801

Pajohanfar NS, Mohebbi E, Rad A, et al: Protective effects of atorvastatin against morphine-induced tolerance and dependence in mice. Brain Res 1657:333–339, 2017 28062186

Pfeiffer A, Knepel W, Braun S, et al: Effects of a kappa-opioid agonist on adrenocorticotropic and diuretic function in man. Horm Metab Res 18(12):842–848, 1986 3028922

Pradhan AA, Befort K, Nozaki C, et al: The delta opioid receptor: an evolving target for the treatment of brain disorders. Trends Pharmacol Sci 32(10):581–590, 2011 21925742

Raehal KM, Bohn LM: Beta-arrestins: regulatory role and therapeutic potential in opioid and cannabinoid receptor-mediated analgesia. Handb Exp Pharmacol 219:427–443, 2014 24292843

Ragguett RM, Rong C, Rosenblat JD, et al: Pharmacodynamic and pharmacokinetic evaluation of buprenorphine + samidorphan for the treatment of major depressive disorder. Expert Opin Drug Metab Toxicol 14(4):475–482, 2018 29621905

Raghavendra V, Rutkowski MD, DeLeo JA: The role of spinal neuroimmune activation in morphine tolerance/hyperalgesia in neuropathic and sham-operated rats. J Neurosci 22(22):9980–9989, 2002 12427855

Raghavendra V, Tanga F, Rutkowski MD, DeLeo JA: Anti-hyperalgesic and morphine-sparing actions of propentofylline following peripheral nerve injury in rats: mechanistic implications of spinal glia and proinflammatory cytokines. Pain 104(3):655–664, 2003 12927638

Rosow CE: Methylnaltrexone: reversing the gastrointestinal effects of opioids. Anesthesiology 87(4):736–737, 1997 9357871

Rowlett JK, Woolverton WL: Self-administration of cocaine and heroin combinations by rhesus monkeys responding under a progressive-ratio schedule. Psychopharmacology (Berl) 133(4):363–371, 1997 9372536

Sawaya BE, Deshmane SL, Mukerjee R, et al: TNF alpha production in morphine-treated human neural cells is NF-kappaB-dependent. J Neuroimmune Pharmacol 4(1):140–149, 2009 19023660

Schmid CL, Kennedy NM, Ross NC, et al: Bias factor and therapeutic window correlate to predict safer opioid analgesics. Cell 171(5):1165–1175.e13, 2017 29149605

Seyfried O, Hester J: Opioids and endocrine dysfunction. Br J Pain 6(1):17–24, 2012 26516462

Smith SM, Vale WW: The role of the hypothalamic-pituitary-adrenal axis in neuroendocrine responses to stress. Dialogues Clin Neurosci 8(4):383–395, 2006 17290797

Song P, Zhao ZQ: The involvement of glial cells in the development of morphine tolerance. Neurosci Res 39(3):281–286, 2001 11248367

Takahama K, Shirasaki T: Central and peripheral mechanisms of narcotic antitussives: codeine-sensitive and -resistant coughs. Cough 3:8, 2007 17620111

Trang T, Al-Hasani R, Salvemini D, et al: Pain and poppies: the good, the bad, and the ugly of opioid analgesics. J Neurosci 35(41):13879–13888, 2015 26468188

Valentino RJ, Volkow ND: Untangling the complexity of opioid receptor function. Neuropsychopharmacology 43(13):2514–2520, 2018 30250308

Wagstaff AJ, Ormrod D, Spencer CM: Tianeptine: a review of its use in depressive disorders. CNS Drugs 15(3):231–259, 2001 11463130

Walsh S, Middleton L: Buprenorphine pharmacodynamics and pharmacokinetics, in Handbook of Methadone Prescribing and Buprenorphine Therapy. Edited by Cruciani R, Knotkova H. New York, Springer, 2013, pp 163–181

Wang X, Loram LC, Ramos K, et al: Morphine activates neuroinflammation in a manner parallel to endotoxin. Proc Natl Acad Sci USA 109(16):6325–6330, 2012 22474354

Watkins LR, Hutchinson MR, Rice KC, Maier SF: The "toll" of opioid-induced glial activation: improving the clinical efficacy of opioids by targeting glia. Trends Pharmacol Sci 30(11):581–591, 2009 19762094

Wesson DR, Ling W: The Clinical Opiate Withdrawal Scale (COWS). J Psychoactive Drugs 35(2):253–259, 2003 12924748

Williams J: Basic opioid pharmacology. Rev Pain 1(2):2–5, 2008 26524987

Williams KL, Ko MC, Rice KC, Woods JH: Effect of opioid receptor antagonists on hypothalamic-pituitary-adrenal activity in rhesus monkeys. Psychoneuroendocrinology 28(4):513–528, 2003 12689609

Williams KL, Broadbear JH, Woods JH: Noncontingent and response-contingent intravenous ethanol attenuates the effect of naltrexone on hypothalamic-pituitary-adrenal activity in rhesus monkeys. Alcohol Clin Exp Res 28(4):566–571, 2004 15100607

World Health Organization: Depression and Other Common Mental Disorders: Global Health Estimates (p. 8). Geneva, World Health Organization, 2017. Available at: https://www.who.int/mental_health/management/depression/prevalence_global_health_estimates/en/. Accessed April 25, 2020.

Yanovski J: Loperamide to diagnose Cushing's syndrome—Reply. JAMA 270(19):2302, 1993. Available at: https://jamanetwork.com/journals/jama/article-abstract/409239. Accessed April 25, 2020.

Zalsman G, Molcho A, Huang Y, et al: Postmortem mu-opioid receptor binding in suicide victims and controls. J Neural Transm (Vienna) 112(7):949–954, 2005 15937639

Zhang GF, Ren YP, Sheng LX, et al: Dysfunction of the hypothalamic-pituitary-adrenal axis in opioid dependent subjects: effects of acute and protracted abstinence. Am J Drug Alcohol Abuse 34(6):760–768, 2008 19016181

Zhang Y, Landthaler M, Schlussman SD, et al: Mu opioid receptor knockdown in the substantia nigra/ventral tegmental area by synthetic small interfering RNA blocks the rewarding and locomotor effects of heroin. Neuroscience 158(2):474–483, 2009 18938225

CHAPTER 13

Methadone and Buprenorphine Maintenance Treatment of Opioid-Related Disorders

Eric C. Strain, M.D.

Kenneth B. Stoller, M.D.

In this chapter we review the use of methadone and buprenorphine for the treatment of opioid-related disorders. Both of these medications are effective and safe and are widely used throughout the world.

Methadone has been in use since the 1960s. In the early years of its use, methadone demonstrated that opioid use disorder, previously seen as having a poor prognosis, could be effectively treated. In the United States as well as other parts of the world, methadone treatment is often delivered through a special clinic system. While for many years methadone clinics existed on the fringes of the health care system, recent years have seen these clinics and the clinic system become more integrated into mainstream medical care. Today, standards of treatment for opioid use disorder follow approaches used in other health care settings.

Buprenorphine likewise has made a substantial impact on the treatment of patients with opioid use disorder. Buprenorphine has been used for this indication for more than 20 years, and in the United States it can be prescribed in office-based practices, providing improved access to treatment for patients who do not have methadone clinics (now called *opioid treatment programs* in the United States) located near them.

Methadone and buprenorphine are effective, but the complexities of treating patients with opioid use disorder often require nonpharmacological treatments as well, such as counseling and contingency management strategies. While not the focus of this chapter, those treatments combined with these medications can exert powerful positive impacts on patients. Through integrated medication and nonmedication treatments, patients can be assisted in addressing the direct and indirect consequences of their use of opioids, and grow and thrive in their lives.

Methadone Treatment

Methadone was originally developed in the mid-1960s for the treatment of opioid dependence. Work conducted by Vincent Dole, Marie Nyswander, and Mary Jeanne Kreek at Rockefeller University demonstrated its efficacy and safety (Dole et al. 1966). Although methadone was not the first medication used to treat an addictive disorder (disulfiram was available to treat alcoholism years before methadone was developed), methadone's dramatic efficacy for what had been a significant problem unresponsive to other treatments made it a lifesaving intervention for countless persons with opioid use disorder. Methadone continues to be one of the primary pharmacotherapies for a substance use disorder, with extensive use throughout the world.

Pharmacology of Methadone

Methadone's primary therapeutic effect is mediated by its action as a μ-opioid receptor agonist. However, it also has activity at the N-methyl-D-aspartate (NMDA) receptor, where it acts as a weak antagonist. Methadone has good oral bioavailability, and while there is considerable variability in studies that have looked at its absorption, it is generally considered to have 70%–80% bioavailability when swallowed (Walsh and Strain 2006). Peak effects vary depending on whether the person is physically dependent on opioids; in a nondependent person, the peak effects are generally reached at around 2–3 hours, while in a dependent person, it may take somewhat longer. Methadone's half-life is somewhat complex, as it can vary considerably between individuals as a function of factors such as genetic differences in enzymatic activity, the duration of treatment, co-prescribed medications, and the pH of the urine (Eap et al. 2002). In addition to these sorts of factors, as a person stabilizes on methadone, there can be some increase in metabolism (autoinduction) with a resultant decrease in the half-life. Studies in humans of the half-life of methadone usually find it to be between 15 and 36 hours (about an average of 24 hours), which permits methadone to be dosed once per day in most patients. Methadone is metabolized in the liver, and a small percentage (about 10%) is excreted unchanged in the urine.

Methadone produces several physiological effects. It is a very effective analgesic, and it was initially developed for this indication. Methadone is still used for this purpose, although less so recently due to recognition of the risk of toxicity from accumulation effects of the medication when higher-than-advisable doses are ingested. Methadone can be administered orally, rectally, or by injection. The duration of methadone's analgesic effects is shorter than its pharmacokinetic half-life would suggest, necessitating dosing 2–4 times per day when used for pain control. Methadone can also function as a respiratory depressant, an effect that reflects its agonism at the μ-opioid receptor. Such respiratory effects are more likely to be seen in a nondependent person who receives a relatively high dose of methadone. Other effects include miosis (especially notable in a nondependent person), nausea and vomiting (again, more likely in a nondependent person), histaminic effects (itching, flushing, sweating), and constipation. Evidence suggests that methadone is associated with prolongation of the QTc interval and ventricular arrhythmias (Chou et al. 2014a, 2014b). Although routine electrocardiogram (ECG) screening is recommended for patients with risk factors for QTc prolongation, there is limited evidence supporting ECG screening for individuals without such risk (Cruciani et al. 2005).

Even at low doses, methadone can effectively suppress spontaneous withdrawal in a person with opioid physical dependence who stops their usual use of opioid. At moderate doses, methadone reduces craving for opioids. In a person who takes methadone daily (and thus has developed tolerance to its effects), an adequate dosage of methadone produces cross-blockade of the other effects of a µ-opioid agonist (i.e., the person who takes an opioid while on an adequate dose of methadone will not experience a "high" from that opioid). These are the three critical pharmacological effects of methadone—withdrawal suppression, craving reduction, and cross-blockade—that help to exert its therapeutic effect for opioid use disorder.

Finally, it is important to briefly address methadone's psychological and cognitive/performance effects. Acute doses of methadone can produce positive subjective effects, and methadone is mildly reinforcing. Nondependent persons can also experience sedation with acute doses of methadone. Higher doses of acute methadone can produce lethargy and may produce fewer desirable effects in a nondependent person. While acute doses of methadone in a nondependent person can produce impairments on performance tasks, methadone use under chronic dosing conditions appears to produce no substantial or gross problems in psychomotor performance or cognitive functioning.

Treatment of Opioid Use Disorder With Methadone

Methadone treatment for opioid use disorder (also known as opioid dependence) in the United States is provided at special clinics devoted to this modality of care (i.e., an opioid treatment program [OTP]). Such clinics are health care sites that provide both pharmacotherapy (almost always methadone, and, increasingly, buprenorphine and/or naltrexone) and other services such as counseling, urine toxicology testing, mental health assessment, case management, peer support, and vocational assistance. OTPs have a physician medical director, additional medical providers (depending on clinic size), counseling staff (with a patient-to-counselor ratio sometimes determined by local regulations), nursing staff, and other support staff. Patients initially attend the clinic either 6 or 7 days per week (some clinics are routinely closed on Saturdays or Sundays). For days that the patient is not required to attend the clinic, a "take home" or "takeaway" dose of medication is provided. The maximum number of methadone take-home doses allowed per week is clearly specified in federal regulations and is tied to the patient's response to and time in treatment. As a patient progresses in treatment and achieves stability, more take-home doses can be provided. In the United States, it is possible for patients to receive up to a month's worth of take-home doses of medication, although an individual must have spent at least 2 years in treatment for that number of take-home doses to be considered.

When at the clinic, the patient receives a supervised dose of methadone (or buprenorphine) provided by a nurse at the clinic dispensary. The methadone dose is typically delivered in a flavored liquid form, diluted with juice or water (e.g., 30–60 mL). While in the clinic setting, the patient may be asked to provide a urine sample for drug testing, to have medical or mental health issues addressed with staff, and/ or to attend an individual or group counseling session.

Two different approaches are used in methadone treatment: supervised withdrawal (i.e., detoxification) and methadone maintenance. Supervised withdrawal involves a period of initial stabilization on a dose of methadone, followed by a gradual dosage reduction process. Longer and more gradual withdrawal regimens are more effective than shorter ones (Senay et al. 1977), although outcomes from opioid withdrawal (however long the duration) can be poor. Methadone maintenance treatment, on the other hand, consists of an induction period followed by stable dosing of daily methadone; patients in maintenance treatment may remain on methadone for many years. Outcomes of methadone maintenance treatment can be excellent, as discussed below (see section "Efficacy and Safety of Methadone").

Counseling provided during methadone treatment can vary, depending on the indicators of the patient's clinical stability, such as concurrent drug or alcohol use, level of social needs, effectiveness of coping skills, and vocational/legal status. Early in treatment, there is usually an emphasis on engaging the patient in treatment, stopping drug use, educating the patient regarding risk behaviors, and assisting the patient in obtaining other needed services (e.g., stable housing, medical care, social services, other psychiatric services). These elements of care can be addressed in individual counseling sessions, and strategies are often reinforced in group treatment. Peer recovery advocates are increasingly used in programs to provide encouragement and support (often brokering recovery services), activities that can improve early treatment retention and response. As the patient stabilizes in treatment and shows evidence of sustained abstinence from all illicit drug use and from problematic alcohol use, counseling may decrease in frequency and intensity and shift to addressing the consequences of use (e.g., repairing damaged familial relationships, resuming productive work and educational pursuits) and focusing on relapse prevention.

Various counseling approaches (e.g., motivational enhancement, cognitive-behavioral therapy) may be used in conjunction with pharmacological treatment of opioid use disorder; these modalities are addressed in Part IV ("Nonpharmacotherapeutic Treatment Modalities") in this volume (see Chapters 22–30). Notably, contingency management is particularly useful in the context of methadone treatment, in which the availability of methadone take-home doses can serve as a very powerful incentive for desired behavioral changes (e.g., cessation of non-opioid drug use, regular attendance of counseling sessions) (Dutra et al. 2008). Adaptive stepped-care models, which adjust the scope and intensity of counseling services based on objective indicators of treatment response, have been shown to be particularly effective in conjunction with contingencies that encourage treatment adherence (Brooner and Kidorf 2002).

Methadone Dosing

Dosing with methadone can be broadly conceptualized as consisting of four phases: induction, stabilization, maintenance, and withdrawal (the last not being relevant in cases of maintenance treatment). The *induction* phase can be viewed as covering up to the first 2 weeks of dosing—the period during which methadone dosing is initiated. Induction typically begins with a first-day dose of 10–30 mg, with a possible additional 5- to 10-mg dose if there is an indication for such (e.g., the patient shows evidence of opioid withdrawal 2–3 hours after the first dose). It is generally recommended that the total first-day dose not exceed 40 mg. In general, it is helpful to monitor the patient for several hours on the first day of dosing to ensure that the first dose is neither too high (leading to signs of sedation) nor too low (leading to significant withdrawal). Dosage increases of methadone during this period should be in increments of 5–10 mg and are typically timed to occur 3–5 days apart (but should be no more frequent than 3 days apart). A balance between the goal of achieving an effective dosage to minimize ongoing opioid use and the goal of ensuring safety is critical during this period. Due to the long half-life of methadone, serum levels may accumulate for up to 5–7 days following dosage increases, placing the patient at risk of excessive opioid agonist effects (including rare cases of overdose). It is important that patients be carefully educated to understand that even though they may not be "held" for a full 24 hours during this period (withdrawal symptoms may still emerge before the next day's dose), illicit opioid use on top of methadone may result in overdose. The *stabilization* phase is the period during which the patient's optimal dosage is determined and the patient is engaged in treatment and is beginning to achieve functional stability. Some illicit opioid use may still occur during stabilization, but there should be an overall trend of decreasing illicit use. The *maintenance* phase is the period during which a stable dosage of methadone is provided, no illicit opioid use occurs, and other issues in treatment (e.g., other drug use, psychosocial issues) are being well addressed (Chou et al. 2014a).

Efficacy and Safety of Methadone

Methadone is a very effective medication for the treatment of opioid use disorder, especially when used properly (i.e., an appropriate dose for the patient, concurrent nonpharmacological services). Outcomes with methadone medication are dose related; lower dosages (20–40 mg/day) are effective in suppressing opioid withdrawal but may not be sufficient to decrease craving or to block the effects of other opioids (Strain et al. 1993a, 1993b). There is great variability in the effective dosage of methadone for different patients, but maintenance dosages are generally in the range of 80–120 mg/day (although some patients respond well to dosages lower than 80 mg/day and some patients may require dosages higher than 120 mg/day). The blood level of methadone does not correspond well to dosage, and there is considerable variability among patients in the effective dosage. In part, this variability may reflect differences in the isomeric forms of methadone, which are not typically assessed when obtaining a methadone blood level. However, there may be value in checking peak (2–3 hours postdose) and trough (24 hours postdose) blood levels in patients who report that their dose is not holding them, especially if these patients are on a dosage of 120 mg/day or higher or are taking other medications known to alter the serum methadone level. Peak-to-trough level ratios greater than 2 can be seen in rapid metabolizers, who may benefit from having their total daily dosage split into 2–3 doses rather than continuing to increase a once-daily dose. It is important to note that in the United States, providing these doses as take-homes may require special "exception" requests to the Substance Abuse and Mental Health Services Administration (SAMHSA) and to the state opioid treatment authority if the patient has been in treatment for less than 1 year.

Although methadone medication can be very useful for suppressing withdrawal and blocking the effects of other opioids, methadone treatment also provides a context in which several other prosocial activities and other health issues can be addressed. A number of studies have shown that methadone treatment can be highly effective, as assessed by outcomes such as reduced risk of drug overdose and improved treatment retention and rates of abstinence from illicit opioid use (e.g., as measured by urine testing) (Larochelle et al. 2018; Ling et al. 1996; Mattick et al. 2009; Sees et al. 2000; Strain et al. 1993a, 1999). In addition, methadone treatment is associated with reductions in criminal activity, illegal income-generating pursuits, and non-opioid illicit drug use. Greater amounts of nonpharmacological treatment in the context of methadone treatment are generally thought to be associated with better outcomes (McLellan et al. 1993), although a review of specific structured psychosocial treatments (vs. usual counseling) failed to show significantly better results for the structured treatments across a variety of outcomes (Amato et al. 2011). A stepped-care approach that tailors the amount of services to the needs of the patient has been shown to be a practical and effective strategy for treating patients in an opioid treatment program (Brooner and Kidorf 2002), and such individualized and tailored treatment may be a more appropriate approach for the allocation of nonpharmacological resources.

Methadone medication is also a safe treatment (Center for Substance Abuse Treatment 2005; Kreek 1973). There can be side effects associated with methadone (e.g., increased sweating, constipation); however, as noted above (see earlier section "Pharmacology of Methadone"), for persons maintained on a steady dose of methadone, there do not appear to be problems with performance or clinically significant cognitive impairment. There has been some controversy regarding the extent to which methadone can induce prolongation of the QTc interval, but studies to date have lacked consistency in their ECG findings on this matter, and professional organizations have issued variable recommendations on screening and monitoring with an ECG (Chou et al. 2014a, 2014b). For patients who have other risk factors for QTc prolongation (e.g., co-occurring use of other medications that can prolong the QTc interval, preexisting cardiac conditions, electrolyte abnormalities) or who are on dosages greater than 120 mg/day, monitoring of the QTc interval appears to be warranted.

Summary of Methadone Treatment

Methadone treatment is a widely used and well-established pharmacological treatment approach for opioid use disorder that has been shown in numerous studies to be effective and safe. For many patients, optimal outcomes appear to be achieved when medication is combined with nonpharmacological services, and the efficacy of both medication and nonpharmacological treatments is dose related. In the United States, methadone for opioid use disorder is limited to use in specialized clinics (OTPs), and because such clinics may not be near people in need of treatment and may have long wait times for treatment admission, access to methadone-based treatment often does not meet the demand.

Buprenorphine Treatment

Buprenorphine was initially developed as an analgesic and was marketed for this purpose for decades before it was approved as a treatment for opioid dependence. However, in the 1970s it was also identified as having a pharmacological profile suggestive of its potential usefulness as a treatment for opioid dependence (Jasinski et al. 1978). The studies used to reach approval for this indication were conducted and supported by the somewhat unusual combination of the company that developed it, the U.S. National Institute on Drug Abuse (NIDA), and several academic medical centers. Buprenorphine was approved by the U.S. Food and Drug Administration (FDA) in 2002 for the treatment of opioid dependence, but the United States was not the first country to use this medication for opioid use disorder treatment—it had been approved for this indication in France 6 years earlier, and quickly became the standard pharmacological approach for the treatment of opioid dependence in that country (where there was very limited methadone treatment available). In the United States, as well as in other parts of the world, buprenorphine has become a widely used medication for opioid dependence treatment, and its availability either within or outside the traditional opioid treatment program system has served to transform the treatment of opioid use disorder in the United States. Buprenorphine is best viewed as a complement to methadone (and naltrexone treatment), given that it has a different pharmacological profile of effects and a unique set of legal stipulations governing the context in which it can be used.

Pharmacology of Buprenorphine

Buprenorphine is one of a number of analgesic medications that have been classified as "mixed agonist–antagonist opioids" (others include butorphanol, nalbuphine, and pentazocine). For many years, the profile of pharmacological effects for buprenorphine was thought to be accounted for by its actions as a partial μ-opioid receptor agonist combined with antagonist effects at the κ-opioid receptor. However, it has become apparent that buprenorphine's partial agonist effects at the opioid receptor–like (ORL)-1 receptor are probably the feature that accounts for its unusual profile of effects. The dose–response curve for buprenorphine is bell-shaped—that is, as the buprenorphine dosage increases, a corresponding increase is seen in specific measured effects of the drug (e.g., analgesia, decreased gastrointestinal motility, respiratory depression), typical of what would be expected with μ-opioid receptor agonist effects. However, with further increases beyond a certain dosage of the drug, the response curve begins to flatten and then descend, so that increasing the dosage beyond this point produces less of an effect (producing the downward portion of the bell-shaped curve). This profile has been demonstrated in several animal models (Bryant et al. 1983; Doxey et al. 1982; Lizasoain et al. 1991), although it has not yet been clearly demonstrated in a human study. However, this bell-shaped dose–response curve suggests that there should be increased safety with buprenorphine (i.e., there would be less respiratory depression with very high doses of the medication), in comparison with a full μ-opioid receptor agonist such as methadone. There is some evidence to suggest that the descending portion of the curve may be due to the ORL-1 effects of buprenorphine, given that studies using knockout rodent models that have no ORL-1 receptors have shown that buprenorphine appears to behave as a full μ-opioid receptor agonist (Lutfy et al. 2003; Marquez et al. 2008). Buprenorphine has a high affinity for and slow dissociation from the μ-opioid receptor.

Buprenorphine was initially approved as a parenteral analgesic in the United States; it was also approved as a sublingual analgesic in other parts of the world, such as New Zealand. In the treatment of opioid use disorder, buprenorphine is most often ingested via the transmucosal (XMCL) route—which provides slightly better bioavailability than ingestion via the gastrointestinal (oral swallowing) route—and can be administered as a long-acting injectable/implantable formulation. Buprenorphine also has reasonable bioavailability when taken intranasally, although it is not marketed in such a form. (A transdermal patch is also marketed for the treatment of pain, but not opioid use disorder; this product is not addressed in this chapter.)

Buprenorphine has a long duration of action, which allows once-daily dosing when the drug is taken transmucosally. Several studies have shown that it can be dosed less frequently than daily (e.g., every 48–72 hours, and perhaps even at longer intervals), although the most common practice appears to be having patients take it daily. Buprenorphine is metabolized by cytochrome P450 (CYP) 3A4, with a primary metabolite (norbuprenorphine) that has some bioactivity. Buprenorphine (and norbuprenorphine) is primarily excreted in bile. As with methadone, bioavailability studies indicate that patients can show wide variability in the blood levels of buprenorphine produced by a given dose (Strain et al. 2004).

Buprenorphine for the treatment of opioid use disorder is marketed as a XMCL tablet, a XMCL soluble film, a long-acting (6-month) implant, and a long-acting (once-monthly) subcutaneous injection formulation. XMCL formulations typically contain naloxone, an opioid receptor antagonist that will precipitate opioid withdrawal if administered by injection to a person who is physically dependent on typical μ-opioid receptor agonist opioids (e.g., heroin, oxycodone). The inclusion of naloxone in buprenorphine tablets and soluble films is not for therapeutic purposes, but rather is a pharmacological strategy to discourage parenteral misuse of buprenorphine tablets and film strips. Doses of up to 2 mg of naloxone have been shown to have poor sublingual bioactivity (compared with buprenorphine's fairly good sublingual bioavailability) (Preston et al. 1990). However, injected naloxone has good bioavailability. The logic of the addition of naloxone to sublingual buprenorphine is that there will be no naloxone effect if the buprenorphine/naloxone is taken as indicated (i.e., transmucosally); however, if the buprenorphine/naloxone is misused—for example, by being dissolved and injected—by a person who is physically dependent on opioids, it will likely precipitate opioid withdrawal in that person (Stoller et al. 2001). Buprenorphine/naloxone tablets and soluble films are marketed in a dose ratio of 4 to 1 (e.g., 12/3 mg, 8/2 mg, 4/1 mg), and some marketed forms have doses (e.g., 5.7/1.4 mg) that provide bioequivalence to the originally approved formulations (i.e., 8/2 mg). (In the remainder of this chapter, reference will be made to buprenorphine XMCL doses without the naloxone dose, but the preferred XMCL formulation is the combination dose that contains naloxone. Parenteral forms of buprenorphine do not contain naloxone.)

There are currently two long-acting formulations of buprenorphine, marketed under the trade names Probuphine and Sublocade. Probuphine consists of rods (consisting of a polymeric matrix composed of ethylene vinyl acetate and buprenorphine) that are placed in the upper arm and that provide continuous exposure to a 6-month dose of buprenorphine. Insertion and removal of the rods are minor office-based surgical procedures that require training, and the total time of use is 12 months (i.e., they can be used once in each arm). Because of the limited amount of buprenorphine delivered by Probuphine, this formulation is intended for use by individuals who have attained clinical stability on low to moderate dosages (≤8 mg/day) of XMCL buprenorphine. Sublocade is a once-monthly subcutaneous injection of buprenorphine into the abdomen; no removal is necessary at the end of the month, as the product is absorbed over this period. The injection site is rotated monthly around the four quadrants of the abdomen, and there is no limit on the duration of the use. Both Probuphine and Sublocade require initial XMCL stabilization on buprenorphine, both have demonstrated efficacy, and both may be useful as strategies to address problems with adherence and diversion of the XMCL product. (Another injectable formulation of buprenorphine that is absorbed over time [and is similar to Sublocade in this respect] is under development by Braeburn Pharmaceuticals but as of August 2020 is not yet FDA approved. This product, which is to be marketed under the trade name Brixadi, includes a once-weekly and a once-monthly form, and unlike the two other products described here, it does not require prestabilization on XMCL buprenorphine.)

A final note on buprenorphine's pharmacology is that its actions as a partial μ-opioid receptor agonist confer another potential effect. A partial-agonist opioid can occupy a receptor but will produce less activation at that receptor relative to a full-agonist opioid. This means that administration of a dose of buprenorphine to a person who is physically dependent on a full-agonist opioid such as heroin could produce a net decrease in receptor effect, resulting in precipitation of opioid withdrawal. Indeed, this effect has been demonstrated in opioid-dependent persons under laboratory conditions (Rosado et al. 2007; Strain et al. 1995) and has been anecdotally reported by some clinicians. In order to minimize the risk of buprenorphine-precipitated withdrawal, it is best that the first XMCL dose be low (e.g., 2–4 mg) and that it be given well after the last dose of the opioid agonist (i.e., at least 4 hours, depending on the half-life of the opioid being used). Ideally, the patient would be in early opioid withdrawal (e.g., a Clinical Opiate Withdrawal Scale [COWS; Wesson and Ling 2003] score of 5 or higher). In addition, special care should be taken if the person has a higher level of opioid physical dependence (i.e., daily doses of an opioid agonist that are equivalent to 40–50 mg or more of methadone). This cautionary guidance has unfortunately become more important given the increased penetration of illicit, highly potent, and lipophilic fentanyl and related analogs into the drug supply.

Treatment of Opioid Use Disorder With Buprenorphine

In the United States, buprenorphine can be prescribed for the treatment of opioid dependence (opioid use disorder) by a physician in an office-based setting (in contrast to methadone, which is only available through OTPs). In addition, buprenorphine can be provided at an OTP; all of the regulations for methadone treatment apply to OTP-based buprenorphine treatment, except that the limitations on take-home doses based on treatment duration do not apply in the case of buprenorphine. The legal capability to prescribe buprenorphine outside the context of an OTP is derived from the

Drug Addiction Treatment Act of 2000 (DATA 2000), a federal law that set up the stipulations under which physicians could prescribe an opioid medication for the maintenance treatment of opioid addiction in an office setting (Substance Abuse and Mental Health Services Administration 2020). Notably, DATA 2000 does not limit such practice to buprenorphine (and in fact never mentions buprenorphine); rather, it sets up a set of conditions for use of an FDA-approved opioid, and buprenorphine is the only medication that has fulfilled those conditions at this time. However, it is possible that other scheduled medications may be developed that could also be used under the parameters of DATA 2000. Although DATA 2000 limited prescribing to physicians, subsequent legislation—the Comprehensive Addiction and Recovery Act (CARA), signed into law in 2016 (Substance Abuse and Mental Health Services Administration 2020)—expanded the provider group to include nurse practitioners (NPs) and physician assistants (PAs). The physician who prescribes buprenorphine must complete a special 8-hour training course (or can achieve the qualification through some other mechanisms, such as being board-certified in addiction psychiatry) and then must apply for a special U.S. Department of Justice Drug Enforcement Administration (DEA) number (often called an "X number," as the letter X always precedes the number) before prescribing buprenorphine. NPs and PAs must take 24 hours of special training, and other state-level requirements may also apply to their prescribing of buprenorphine. There is a limit on the number of patients a physician can concurrently treat with buprenorphine (30 in the first year, then the physician can apply to treat up to 100, followed by another request to treat up to 275 patients). An NP or PA can have a case load of up to 30 patients being treated with buprenorphine.

Patients started on XMCL buprenorphine should begin with a relatively low dose (either 2 or 4 mg/day) and ideally should be experiencing slight opioid withdrawal prior to the first dose. A second dose can be given the same day after 1–2 hours if the first dose is tolerated without problems. If the person is not physically dependent on opioids (e.g., a person who was on buprenorphine previously, was then incarcerated, and now has returned to restart buprenorphine), a low dose (2 mg) should be given to start, and stabilization should be slowed. Typical maintenance doses of buprenorphine are in the range of 8–16 mg/day, although some patients have required higher doses (e.g., 24 mg/day). If a patient seems to require high doses (e.g., 24–32 mg/day), it would be prudent to consider whether there is any risk of diversion or misuse of the medication.

Probuphine and Sublocade are used at 6- and 1-month intervals, respectively. Induction to these formulations typically occurs after initial treatment with XMCL formulations. Under no circumstances should either formulation be self-administered; both are implantations/injections administered by a trained practitioner in an office setting.

As is the case with methadone, buprenorphine can be used for medically supervised withdrawal as well as maintenance treatment. When tapering buprenorphine, 2-mg increments are typically used. Tablets are not intended to be broken, and the soluble films are not designed to be cut (although some clinicians do cut them, and it is a convenient mechanism to produce doses that contain less than 2 mg of buprenorphine). Gradual rather than rapid withdrawal regimens are probably more effective, although there is limited research on buprenorphine tapers. Maintenance on buprenorphine can extend for years (similar to methadone). Physicians can prescribe a month's worth of the medication with up to five refills (although early in treatment, it is probably better to prescribe a reduced number of days of medication, and not provide refills). The long-acting implantable or injectable formulations may be useful options for patients who are stable, for patients with whom diversion and misuse of XMCL forms is a concern, or for patients who have a tendency to skip doses or stop taking the medication prematurely and then relapse. Because its sequestration in fat stores (i.e., its lipophilicity) causes fentanyl to remain in the body for a prolonged period, patients maintained on buprenorphine who relapse to illegal fentanyl use are at risk of discontinuing their buprenorphine to avoid the risk of precipitated withdrawal. Hence, the utility of long-acting buprenorphine formulations may grow as fentanyl becomes increasingly commonplace in the drug supply.

Providing nonpharmacological treatment along with buprenorphine is recommended for most patients (especially early in treatment).

Efficacy and Safety of Buprenorphine

Beginning in the late 1980s and continuing throughout the 1990s, numerous clinical trials investigated the efficacy of buprenorphine in comparison with placebo and methadone. In general, these studies showed that buprenorphine produced outcomes that were superior to the outcomes seen with placebo or placebo-like doses of medication (i.e., very low doses of buprenorphine) (Johnson et al. 1995; Ling et al. 1998) and were similar to the outcomes seen with methadone at dosages of about 50–60 mg/day. However, the magnitude of response seen with higher dosages of methadone (i.e., 80 mg/day or greater) was generally not seen with daily buprenorphine in these controlled trials (Hser et al. 2014; Ling et al. 1996). These findings that higher doses of methadone (80+ mg/day) were more effective than the doses of buprenorphine used were somewhat surprising, given that clinical pharmacology studies suggest that buprenorphine has a plateau of effects at higher dosages (Walsh et al. 1994, 1995). However, the important point is that several clinical trials have shown that buprenorphine is effective, as assessed by outcomes such as treatment retention and decreases in opioid use (measured both by self-report and through urine testing) (Mattick et al. 2014).

Buprenorphine has also been shown to be a safe medication. Despite initial concerns that it might cause a slight increase in liver function tests in persons with a history of hepatitis (Petry et al. 2000), a large multicenter trial did not find such problems with buprenorphine or with methadone (the comparison condition) over the first 6 months of treatment (Saxon et al. 2013). During the early years of buprenorphine's use in France, there were fatalities in individuals who injected high doses of buprenorphine in conjunction with an injectable form of a benzodiazepine. This problem has not been seen in the United States, and it is notable that a number of early clinical trials found that concurrent use of benzodiazepines by buprenorphine-treated patients did not result in any reports of adverse events. As is the case with other μ-opioid drugs, buprenorphine can cause constipation and increased sweating. There do not appear to be significant cognition- or performance-impairing effects associated with buprenorphine treatment for opioid use disorder, and there is no evidence of QTc interval prolongation with its use.

Summary of Buprenorphine Treatment

Buprenorphine has expanded the capacity for opioid use disorder treatment in the United States as well as many other parts of the world, and its use has concurrently expanded the treatment of an illicit drug use disorder into mainstream medical practice. Despite this success, it is notable that only a small percentage of physicians have obtained the waiver to use the medication (somewhere on the order of 5% of physicians in the United States), and those who do prescribe often do so for relatively few patients. However, even with the relatively small number of prescribing physicians, there appear to be a substantial number of patients who receive the medication (Mark et al. 2009; Pashmineh Azar et al. 2020). Buprenorphine is effective and safe, and has the advantage of being able to be prescribed by a physician, an NP, or a PA in an office setting—a difference from methadone that is legal in nature but that also reflects what is believed to be an overall safer profile for this medication. Providers who are interested in learning more about buprenorphine should consider taking a course on its use and can also consult other resources available through professional organizations and government agencies (e.g., the Providers Clinical Support System [https://pcssnow.org]).

Conclusion

Methadone and buprenorphine are first-line treatments for opioid use disorder. Their use has been extensively studied, and clinical trials have shown that both are effective and safe treatments that can be have a direct impact on improving patients' lives, and that can also provide a context for comprehensive treatment that is often needed for this patient population. Key take-away points from this chapter include the following:

- Methadone and buprenorphine are safe and effective medications, especially when used in the context of other services (e.g., group and individual counseling, case management, urine testing, contingency management); and each is associated with a broad array of positive treatment outcomes.
- In the United States, methadone treatment for opioid use disorder is primarily available through a specialized clinic system (i.e., opioid treatment programs [OTPs]). OTPs are required to deliver a combination of methadone medication and nonpharmacological services, both of which have dose-related efficacy.
- In the United States, buprenorphine treatment for opioid use disorder can be prescribed in office settings by physicians, nurse practitioners, and physician assistants who have obtained the necessary U.S. Drug Enforcement Administration (DEA) permission ("X number"). Buprenorphine is also available through the specialized OTP clinic system. Effective buprenorphine treatment should also include nonpharmacological services.
- Providers should be familiar with both of these medications. A provider should consider obtaining DEA authorization to prescribe buprenorphine. Even if a provider chooses not to obtain a waiver to prescribe buprenorphine, familiarity with methadone and buprenorphine is important, given the increasing use of these medications and the extent of opioid-related problems.

References

Amato L, Minozzi S, Davoli M, et al: Psychosocial combined with agonist maintenance treatments versus agonist maintenance treatments alone for treatment of opioid dependence. Cochrane Database Syst Rev (10):CD004147, 2011 21975742

Brooner RK, Kidorf M: Using behavioral reinforcement to improve methadone treatment participation. Sci Pract Perspect 1(1):38–47, 2002 18567965

Bryant RM, Olley JE, Tyers MB: Antinociceptive actions of morphine and buprenorphine given intrathecally in the conscious rat. Br J Pharmacol 78(4):659–663, 1983 6687818

Center for Substance Abuse Treatment: Medication-Assisted Treatment for Opioid Addiction in Opioid Treatment Programs. Rockville, MD, Substance Abuse and Mental Health Services Administration, 2005

Chou R, Cruciani RA, Fiellin DA, et al: Methadone safety: a clinical practice guideline from the American Pain Society and College on Problems of Drug Dependence, in collaboration with the Heart Rhythm Society. J Pain 15(4):321–337, 2014a 24685458

Chou R, Weimer MB, Dana T: Methadone overdose and cardiac arrhythmia potential: findings from a review of the evidence for an American Pain Society and College on Problems of Drug Dependence clinical practice guideline. J Pain 15(4):338–365, 2014b 24685459

Cruciani RA, Sekine R, Homel P, et al: Measurement of QTc in patients receiving chronic methadone therapy. J Pain Symptom Manage 29(4):385–391, 2005 15857742

Dole VP, Nyswander ME, Kreek MJ: Narcotic blockade. Arch Intern Med 118(4):304–309, 1966 4162686

Doxey JC, Everitt JE, Frank LW, et al: A comparison of the effects of buprenorphine and morphine on the blood gases of conscious rats. British Journal of Pharmacology 75 (suppl 1):118P, 1982. Available at: https://bpspubs.onlinelibrary.wiley.com/doi/epdf/10.1111/j.1476-5381.1982.tb17346.x. Accessed December 22, 2019.

Dutra L, Stathopoulou G, Basden SL, et al: A meta-analytic review of psychosocial interventions for substance use disorders. Am J Psychiatry 165(2):179–187, 2008 18198270

Eap CB, Buclin T, Baumann P: Interindividual variability of the clinical pharmacokinetics of methadone: implications for the treatment of opioid dependence. Clin Pharmacokinet 41(14):1153–1193, 2002 12405865

Hser YI, Saxon AJ, Huang D, et al: Treatment retention among patients randomized to buprenorphine/naloxone compared to methadone in a multi-site trial. Addiction 109(1):79–87, 2014 23961726

Jasinski DR, Pevnick JS, Griffith JD: Human pharmacology and abuse potential of the analgesic buprenorphine: a potential agent for treating narcotic addiction. Arch Gen Psychiatry 35(4):501–516, 1978 215096

Johnson RE, Eissenberg T, Stitzer ML, et al: A placebo controlled clinical trial of buprenorphine as a treatment for opioid dependence. Drug Alcohol Depend 40(1):17–25, 1995 8746920

Kreek MJ: Medical safety and side effects of methadone in tolerant individuals. JAMA 223(6):665–668, 1973 4739193

Larochelle MR, Bernson D, Land T, et al: Medication for opioid use disorder after nonfatal opioid overdose and association with mortality: a cohort study. Ann Intern Med 169(3):137–145, 2018 29913516

Ling W, Wesson DR, Charuvastra C, et al: A controlled trial comparing buprenorphine and methadone maintenance in opioid dependence. Arch Gen Psychiatry 53(5):401–407, 1996 8624183

Ling W, Charuvastra C, Collins JF, et al: Buprenorphine maintenance treatment of opiate dependence: a multicenter, randomized clinical trial. Addiction 93(4):475–486, 1998 9684386

Lizasoain I, Leza JC, Lorenzo P: Buprenorphine: bell-shaped dose-response curve for its antagonist effects. Gen Pharmacol 22(2):297–300, 1991 2055424

Lutfy K, Eitan S, Bryant CD, et al: Buprenorphine-induced antinociception is mediated by mu-opioid receptors and compromised by concomitant activation of opioid receptor-like receptors. J Neurosci 23(32):10331–10337, 2003 14614092

Mark TL, Kassed CA, Vandivort-Warren R, et al: Alcohol and opioid dependence medications: prescription trends, overall and by physician specialty. Drug Alcohol Depend 99(1–3):345–349, 2009 18819759

Marquez P, Borse J, Nguyen AT, et al: The role of the opioid receptor-like (ORL1) receptor in motor stimulatory and rewarding actions of buprenorphine and morphine. Neuroscience 155(3):597–602, 2008 18634857

Mattick RP, Breen C, Kimber J, et al: Methadone maintenance therapy versus no opioid replacement therapy for opioid dependence. Cochrane Database Syst Rev (3):CD002209, 2009 19588333

Mattick RP, Breen C, Kimber J, et al: Buprenorphine maintenance versus placebo or methadone maintenance for opioid dependence. Cochrane Database Syst Rev (2):CD002207, 2014 24500948

McLellan AT, Arndt IO, Metzger DS, et al: The effects of psychosocial services in substance abuse treatment. JAMA 269(15):1953–1959, 1993 8385230

Pashmineh Azar AR, Cruz-Mullane A, Podd JC, et al: Rise and regional disparities in buprenorphine utilization in the United States. Pharmacoepidemiol Drug Saf 29(6):708–715, 2020 32173955

Petry NM, Bickel WK, Piasecki D, et al: Elevated liver enzyme levels in opioid-dependent patients with hepatitis treated with buprenorphine. Am J Addict 9(3):265–269, 2000 11000922

Preston KL, Bigelow GE, Liebson IA: Effects of sublingually given naloxone in opioid-dependent human volunteers. Drug Alcohol Depend 25(1):27–34, 1990 2323306

Rosado J, Walsh SL, Bigelow GE, et al: Sublingual buprenorphine/naloxone precipitated withdrawal in subjects maintained on 100 mg of daily methadone. Drug Alcohol Depend 90(2–3):261–269, 2007 17517480

Saxon AJ, Ling W, Hillhouse M, et al: Buprenorphine/naloxone and methadone effects on laboratory indices of liver health: a randomized trial. Drug Alcohol Depend 128(1–2):71–76, 2013 22921476

Sees KL, Delucchi KL, Masson C, et al: Methadone maintenance vs 180-day psychosocially enriched detoxification for treatment of opioid dependence: a randomized controlled trial. JAMA 283(10):1303–1310, 2000 10714729

Senay EC, Dorus W, Goldberg F, Thornton W: Withdrawal from methadone maintenance. Rate of withdrawal and expectation. Arch Gen Psychiatry 34(3):361–367, 1977 843188

Stoller KB, Bigelow GE, Walsh SL, et al: Effects of buprenorphine/naloxone in opioid-dependent humans. Psychopharmacology (Berl) 154(3):230–242, 2001 11351930

Strain EC, Stitzer ML, Liebson IA, et al: Dose-response effects of methadone in the treatment of opioid dependence. Ann Intern Med 119(1):23–27, 1993a 8498759

Strain EC, Stitzer ML, Liebson IA, et al: Methadone dose and treatment outcome. Drug Alcohol Depend 33(2):105–117, 1993b 8261875

Strain EC, Stitzer ML, Liebson IA, et al: Comparison of buprenorphine and methadone in the treatment of opioid dependence. Am J Psychiatry 151(7):1025–1030, 1994 8010359

Strain EC, Preston KL, Liebson IA, et al: Buprenorphine effects in methadone-maintained volunteers: effects at two hours after methadone. J Pharmacol Exp Ther 272(2):628–638, 1995 7853176

Strain EC, Bigelow GE, Liebson IA, et al: Moderate- vs high-dose methadone in the treatment of opioid dependence: a randomized trial. JAMA 281(11):1000–1005, 1999 10086434

Strain EC, Moody DE, Stoller KB, et al: Relative bioavailability of different buprenorphine formulations under chronic dosing conditions. Drug Alcohol Depend 74(1):37–43, 2004 15072805

Substance Abuse and Mental Health Services Administration: Statutes, Regulations, and Guidelines (web page). Last Updated: August 20, 2020. Available at: https://www.samhsa.gov/medication-assisted-treatment/statutes-regulations-guidelines. Accessed August 29, 2020.

Walsh SL, Strain EC: Pharmacology of methadone, in The Treatment of Opioid Dependence. Edited by Strain EC, Stitzer ML. Baltimore, MD, Johns Hopkins University Press, 2006, pp 60–76

Walsh SL, Preston KL, Stitzer ML, et al: Clinical pharmacology of buprenorphine: ceiling effects at high doses. Clin Pharmacol Ther 55(5):569–580, 1994 8181201

Walsh SL, Preston KL, Bigelow GE, et al: Acute administration of buprenorphine in humans: partial agonist and blockade effects. J Pharmacol Exp Ther 274(1):361–372, 1995 7542336

Wesson DR, Ling W: The Clinical Opiate Withdrawal Scale (COWS). J Psychoactive Drugs 35(2):253–259, 2003 12924748

CHAPTER 14

Opioid Antagonist Treatment of Opioid-Related Disorders

Michael Capata, M.D.

Karen J. Hartwell, M.D.

Opioid antagonists have an important role in the treatment of opioid use disorder (OUD), including reversing an opioid overdose and reducing the risk of relapse. Opioid antagonists block or diminish the reinforcing effects of opioids and decrease the risk of overdose with resumption of opioid use. Research suggests that injectable extended-release naltrexone may attenuate craving (Lee et al. 2018; Tanum et al. 2017). In this chapter we focus on opioid antagonists—specifically, the use of oral and injectable extended-release naltrexone to treat OUD, as well as the use of naloxone to reverse opioid overdose. Topics that will be addressed include indications, antagonist pharmacology, routes of administration, adverse effects, effectiveness, and treatment choice considerations.

Clinical experience and research repeatedly find that in the treatment of OUD, addressing withdrawal alone is inadequate to ensure continued abstinence. Ongoing treatment is essential to prevent relapse, and this thought process led to the use of opioid agonist treatment in the 1970s. The first clinical trial of an opioid antagonist involved the compound cyclazocine (Schecter 1980). Naltrexone (*N*-cyclopropylmethylnoroxymorphone), a synthetic analog of oxymorphone with no opioid agonist properties, was initially developed to block the euphoric effects of morphine and was approved by the U.S. Food and Drug Administration (FDA) in 1984 for the blockade of exogenously administered opioids. Naltrexone was FDA approved for relapse prevention in alcohol use disorders in 1994. Problems with adherence to oral naltrexone followed by treatment dropout and relapse limited its effectiveness, which led to the development of extended-release formulations (Sudakin 2016). The injectable extended-release formulation of naltrexone (XR-NTX), branded as Vivitrol, was FDA approved in 2006 for the treatment of alcohol dependence and in 2010 for the treatment of OUD. In recent years, an implantable formulation of naltrexone has been developed and is primarily used in Australia and Russia. No implantable formulations have been FDA approved in the United States (Bisaga et al. 2018a). Nalmefene, a 6-methylene analog of naltrexone, is an opioid antagonist used primarily to treat alcohol dependence outside the United States, as it lacks FDA approval. Both oral naltrexone and XR-NTX are indicated for the prevention of relapse in OUD, following opioid detoxification.

Naltrexone

Clinical Pharmacology

Naltrexone acts a competitive μ-opioid receptor antagonist with a high receptor affinity and, to a lesser extent, an antagonist at the κ- and δ-opioid receptors. The recommended dosing for oral naltrexone is an initial 25-mg dose followed by 50 mg daily if no withdrawal symptoms occur. An alternative strategy with three-times-per-week dosing of 100 mg, 100 mg, and 150 mg is also generally sufficient to block the subjective and physiological effects of opioids (Kampman and Jarvis 2015). Naltrexone is readily absorbed by the gastrointestinal tract, with peak serum concentrations of 15 ng/mL at 2 hours following a 100-mg dose (Verebey et al. 1976). Oral naltrexone, at 50 mg daily dosing, has been shown to occupy 95% of brain μ-opioid receptors. After a single 50-mg dose of naltrexone, 91% of the receptors are still occupied after 2 days and 30% after 7 days (Lee et al. 1988). XR-NXT is administered in a monthly 380-mg intramuscular injection that continuously releases biodegradable polymer microspheres, resulting in naltrexone levels of greater than 1–2 ng/mL, the critical concentration for opioid blockade (Bigelow et al. 2012). Naltrexone undergoes first-pass metabolism in the liver by dihydrodiol dehydrogenase to 6β-naltrexol, a less-potent μ-opioid receptor antagonist with a longer duration of action (a half-life of approximately 13 hours) compared with naltrexone (a half-life of approximately 4 hours), followed primarily by renal excretion (Meyer et al. 1984). The half-lives of XR-NXT and 6β-naltrexol vary from 5 to 10 days, depending on the erosion of the polymer. The duration of action is about 1–2 days for oral naltrexone and about 5–6 weeks for the extended-release form, after which patients are at a higher risk for relapse. The duration of treatment is dependent on clinical judgment, as there is no recommended length of treatment in current guidelines.

Clinical laboratory studies have demonstrated the ability of naltrexone to attenuate the subjective and physiological effects of acute opioid administration. One of the earliest laboratory studies found that an oral dose of naltrexone 30 mg completely blocked the subjective and attenuated the pupillary response of a 50-mg dose of morphine and reduced the effects of a 100-mg morphine challenge (Martin et al. 1973). In a similar study, oral naltrexone (20–200 mg) produced a dose-dependent reduction in the direct effects of heroin 25 mg administered intravenously (Resnick et al. 1974). Likewise, a clinical laboratory study of XR-NXT found a dose-dependent blockade or reduction of the subjective and physiological effects of escalating doses of hydromorphone (3–6 mg), with an almost complete blockade of feeling any drug effect for a month following administration of a single intramuscular dose of 300 mg (Bigelow et al. 2012). Injectable and depot formulations have the advantage of bypassing the first-pass metabolism in the liver, resulting in a higher plasma ratio of naltrexone to 6β-naltrexol with minimization of the peaks and troughs that occur with oral dosing.

Tanum et al. (2017) found comparable treatment retention rates and reduction of opioid use between patients who were able to successfully initiate treatment with either buprenorphine or XR-NTX. However, because of the need for total opioid abstinence for 6–10 days prior to induction, initiation of OUD individuals on XR-NTX can be more challenging than initiating buprenorphine. For example, in a recent study, 72% of participants were successfully inducted to XR-NTX, compared with 94% of those who started buprenorphine. After induction, the relapse rates were comparable: 52% for the XR-NTX group and 56% for the buprenorphine group (Lee et al. 2018). According to estimates by Jarvis et al. (2018), approximately 47% of patients opted to continue XR-NTX 6 months after starting the monthly injections.

Adverse Effects

Naltrexone can result in severe withdrawal in patients who are physiologically dependent on opioids. Before initiating naltrexone, it is important to determine whether the patient is adequately detoxified and is no longer dependent, or the use of naltrexone can result in precipitated withdrawal. Precipitated withdrawal can be prolonged and severe due to the long half-life of naltrexone and its high affinity for the μ-opioid receptor. A complete history, a physical examination, evidence of opioid detoxification, documented abstinence in a drug-free environment, and an opioid-negative toxicology screen are recommended prior to initiating treatment. In order to avoid precipitated withdrawal, patients should be abstinent from short-acting opioids for approximately 6 days and from long-acting opioids (e.g., methadone, buprenorphine) for 7–10 days (Kampman and Jarvis 2015). Naloxone is a short-acting opioid antagonist (half-life of 30–120 minutes, depending on the route) utilized to reverse opioid overdose (discussed later in chapter in the "Naloxone" section). A naloxone challenge or a test of low-dose oral naltrexone can be administered to ensure that the patient can tolerate the medication without going into withdrawal. Because of naloxone's short half-life, precipitated withdrawal following its administration is not as protracted as NTX-precipitated withdrawal. XR-NTX can be administered immediately following a successful challenge. Once initiated on XR-NTX, patients may still experience prolonged withdrawal symptoms of anxiety, irritability, insomnia, and decreased energy. Methylphenidate and quetiapine have been used to target these protracted withdrawal symptoms (Bisaga et al. 2018a).

Safety and tolerability with naltrexone has generally been good. In patients who received 380 mg of long-acting injectable naltrexone (N=205), the most common adverse events were nausea (33%), headache (22%), and fatigue (20%), with 12% reporting pain, bruising, swelling, or tenderness at the injection site for XR-NTX (Garbutt et al. 2005). Severe injection site reactions such as cellulitis, abscess, necrosis, or hematoma have been observed, some requiring surgical debridement. Rare cases of hypersensitivity and eosinophilic pneumonia have been reported. It is commonly recommended that liver function tests (i.e., aspartate aminotransferase [AST], alanine aminotransferase [ALT], γ-glutamyl transferase [GGT], and bilirubin) be monitored at baseline and periodically during naltrexone treatment; however, hepatotoxicity has typically only been seen at oral doses closer to 300 mg/day (Mitchell et al. 2012). Hepatic toxicity has not been problematic with daily oral naltrexone 50 mg or with XR-NTX, and naltrexone has been safely used in patients with liver disease, hepatitis C, or HIV (Mitchell et al. 2012; Tetrault et al. 2012). However, naltrexone should be used with caution in patients with acute liver failure or hepatitis.

A small proportion of patients (approximately 5%) experience depression, anxiety, suicidal thoughts, suicidal behavior, dysphoria, or generalized malaise early in treatment, resulting in discontinuation. The anxiogenic effect of naltrexone may be related to its antagonism of the opioid receptors. Opioid antagonists increase activity in the hypothalamic-pituitary-adrenal (HPA) axis and alter the hypothalamic-pituitary-gonadal (HPG) system by blocking the tonic, inhibitory effects of β-endorphin on the hypothalamus (Vuong et al. 2010). Naltrexone's blockade of endogenous opioids could potentially alter the normal hedonic response or result in depression. However, in both clinical practice and clinical trials, this has not been problematic. In a recent study by Latif et al. (2019), XR-NTX was just as effective as agonist therapy in reducing rates of anxiety and depression, and was superior to agonist therapy in reducing symptoms of insomnia. It was also found that average opioid craving was initially less for XR-NTX compared with buprenorphine-naloxone ($P=0.0012$) at week 7; however, findings for the two groups had converged by 6 months ($P=0.20$) (Lee et al. 2018).

Treatment Considerations

Patients who are most likely to be successful on naltrexone are those who are highly motivated to change, who have a lower level of dependence on opioids, and who do not need opioids for pain management (Sigmon et al. 2012). In general, oral naltrexone is not recommended due to poor adherence and should be reserved for highly motivated patients who are willing to comply with strategies to improve adherence, such as observed dosing (Kampman and Jarvis 2015). As an example, a previous Cochrane review of 13 randomized trials involving more than 1,100 opioid-dependent participants treated with naltrexone with and without psychotherapy determined that oral naltrexone was not superior to placebo in either treatment retention or reduction in illicit opioid use, supporting the use of XR-NTX (Minozzi et al. 2011). Individuals with high tolerance would likely benefit from agonist therapy, because they may not be able to maintain sobriety and, if using more than 60 mg (or 6 bags) of heroin per day, would likely receive more benefit from methadone treatment (Sigmon et al. 2012).

XR-NTX may be beneficial for patients failed to respond or adhere to treatment with buprenorphine or methadone, who are living in a drug-free environment (e.g., a rehabilitation program, a prison, a community without access to agonist therapies), or who do not want to take opioid agonists. XR-NTX is often the preferred option for individuals who must demonstrate a low risk of opioid use to professional licensing boards or criminal justice officials. A third preparation used internationally is an implantable device that maintains therapeutic naltrexone levels in patients for up to 6 months. In a randomized controlled trial of oral versus implanted naltrexone, patients treated with oral naltrexone were more likely than those treated with the implant to relapse early in treatment, to return to regular heroin use ($P=0.03$) at 6 months, and to have low blood naltrexone levels (Hulse et al. 2009). Barriers to use of XR-NTX include the capacity to administer intramuscular medications, patient acceptance, and high cost due to the lack of a generic formulation.

Naltrexone is contraindicated in individuals who have severe hepatic impairment, who are allergic to naltrexone, or who have a history of sensitivity to polylactide-co-glycolide, carboxycellulose, or any other components of the diluent. XR-NTX should not be given to patients whose body mass precludes the use of the provided 2-inch needle, as inadvertent subcutaneous injection can precipitate a severe injection-site reaction.

Induction Strategies

There is no single best detoxification strategy for naltrexone induction; rather, there exist a set of pharmacological approaches that can be adapted to the treatment setting and the needs of the individual patient. In the absence of physiological dependence, such as following treatment in a controlled environment without access to opioids, extended-release naltrexone can be administered immediately (Bisaga et al. 2018a). Patients who present to treatment during active opioid use represent a bigger challenge in the initiation of XR-NTX. The simplest induction strategy involves using only supportive medications (alpha-agonists, benzodiazepines, and antiemetics) to allow the patient to completely withdraw from opioids, and then administering XR-NTX. However, a recent systematic review found that across multiple studies, roughly 40% of patients intending to start XR-NTX were unable to go through the detoxification process (Jarvis et al. 2018).

Substitution and gradual taper with a longer-acting opioid or buprenorphine facilitates a more measured recovery from the underlying neuroadaptation from chronic opioid use. The use of buprenorphine to manage withdrawal in combination with low doses of oral naltrexone to facilitate the accelerated introduction of XR-NTX has shown promise in preclinical research, with findings indicating that exposure to the opioid antagonist naloxone reversed the μ-opioid receptor internalization secondary to opioid administration and upregulated the surface receptors from the downregulated state (Zaki et al. 2000).

In a review of induction strategies, Sigmon et al. (2012) recommended a short taper of buprenorphine if needed, a titration of oral naltrexone, and use of ancillary medications (e.g., clonidine, hydroxyzine, cyclobenzaprine, promethazine, loperamide) to manage withdrawal symptoms, followed by extended-release naltrexone on days 1–7 or 4–7 days after titration, depending on the level of opioid dependence and the clinical setting. These investigators compared two different outpatient detoxification regimens: 1) a 7-day buprenorphine taper followed by the first XR-NTX injection on day 15, and 2) a single day of buprenorphine followed by ascending doses of naltrexone 1 mg, 3 mg, 12 mg, and 25 mg on days 4, 5, and 7, respectively, with XR-NTX on day 8. Ancillary medications to manage withdrawal were available in both groups (Sullivan et al. 2017). Of the 150 participants, 56% of the naltrexone-assisted detoxification group were successfully inducted to XR-NTX, compared with only 33% of the buprenorphine-assisted detoxification group, with the naltrexone-assisted group being 2.78 times more likely to receive a second XR-NTX injection. Of note, the severity of withdrawal symptoms during days 8–15 was about the same in the two groups. The additional 7-day wait in the buprenorphine-assisted detox group contributed to the lower success rate, with a 29% relapse rate during the waiting period (Sullivan et al. 2017). A follow-up study compared the effectiveness of three regimens for detoxification and induction to XR-NTX: 1) low-dose oral naltrexone with a brief 3-day buprenorphine taper; 2) low-dose naltrexone and placebo buprenorphine; or 3) both placebo naltrexone and buprenorphine with ancillary medications as needed to manage withdrawal (Bisaga et al. 2018b). Participants randomly assigned to one of the naltrexone groups received two doses of naltrexone on a titration schedule during each study visit: 0.25 mg, 0.5 mg, 1.5 mg, 4 mg, 7.5 mg, and 15 mg on days 1–7, respectively, with the second dose held if withdrawal symptoms did not sufficiently abate after 2 hours. The buprenorphine taper consisted of 2 mg administered twice during the first study visit, with an additional 2-mg dose for take-home treatment if needed, followed by 2 mg on days 2 and 3. Participants passing a naloxone challenge test on day 8 received a dose of XR-NTX. Similar rates of induction (~44%) and mild withdrawal symptoms were found across the groups, with prescription opioid users more likely to initiate XR-NTX treatment (Bisaga et al. 2018b). This was comparable to findings in other studies (Bisaga et al. 2015; Lee et al. 2018; Sullivan et al. 2017) showing that induction to XR-NTX with similar strategies had success rates of 55%–72% when done on an inpatient basis and of 33%–56% when done on an outpatient basis. Results from this study suggest that ancillary medications are sufficient in an outpatient setting for patients transitioning from prescription opioids to XR-NTX (Bisaga et al. 2018b). However, Bisaga and colleagues currently recommend inpatient detoxification for patients transitioning from heroin to XR-NTX. Additional research is needed before these methods can be accepted as the standard of care.

The need for a compounding pharmacy is a barrier to expanding low-dose naltrexone inductions beyond research. However, dermatologists are using low-dose naltrexone to treat a variety of disorders, and a recent study reported that crushing commercially available 50-mg naltrexone tablets (e.g., ten 50-mg tablets) into 500 mL of orange juice results in a 1 mg/mL solution with 3 months of stability (Bronfenbrener 2019). This strategy for compounding low-dose naltrexone could be adapted to XR-NTX induction as described by Bisaga et al. (2018b).

Naloxone and naltrexone have been utilized in anesthesia-assisted ultrarapid opioid detoxification. This methodology has not been demonstrated to improve subjective withdrawal scores or short-term or 12-month abstinence rates (Sigmon et al. 2012). Due to the high risk of serious adverse events associated with this detoxification strategy, governmental agencies and professional associations such as the American Society for Addiction Medicine (Centers for Disease Control and Prevention 2013) do not recommend use of anesthesia-assisted ultrarapid opioid detoxification in clinical settings.

Adjunctive Treatments to Enhance Adherence

Current treatment guidelines recommend the use of psychosocial treatments in conjunction with any form of pharmacotherapy for OUD, including oral and extended-release naltrexone, with a psychosocial needs assessment, referral to community services, provision of links to existing family supports, and supportive counseling (Kampman and Jarvis 2015). A variety of interventions have been utilized in the treatment of OUD, including contingency management, motivational interviewing, cognitive-behavioral therapy (CBT), acceptance and commitment therapy, behavioral drug and HIV risk reduction counseling, community reinforcement, family training for treatment retention, and general supportive counseling (Dugosh et al. 2016). Contingency management and CBT are the two most widely studied psychosocial interventions provided in conjunction with pharmacotherapy for opioid dependence, with methadone being the pharmacotherapy most commonly used in these studies. There are a limited number of studies with naltrexone. Trials of behavioral therapies (e.g., contingency management, CBT) consistently demonstrate improvement in treatment retention with oral naltrexone, with most reporting reductions in the number of opioid-positive urines; however, limitations of these trials include small to medium effect sizes (0.24–0.60) and substantial dropout across studies (Nunes et al. 2006). These results suggest that there may be a limit to the efficacy of psychosocial interventions in overcoming poor adherence to oral naltrexone.

The effectiveness of XR-NTX as monotherapy without accompanying psychosocial treatment has not been established, as most of the research to date included some form of psychosocial support. In a study among unemployed opioid-dependent adults ($N=38$), a contingency intervention involving employment-based reinforcement significantly improved the number of XR-NTX injections, with 74% of participants in the XR-NTX plus contingency group receiving all injections over the 6-month study ($P=0.02$), compared with 26% of participants who were prescribed XR-NTX alone (DeFulio et al. 2012). Another study examining the utility of adding weekly behavioral therapy (to promote adherence and support treatment) to medication treatment with either oral naltrexone or XR-NTX found that the XR-NTX plus therapy group had twice the retention in treatment at 6 months compared with the oral naltrexone plus therapy group, with the two groups showing similar rates of opioid-positive toxicology, suggesting that most patients remain abstinent when adherent to naltrexone and engaged in treatment (Sullivan et al. 2019). These findings support the use of behavioral therapy in combination with XR-NTX as an efficacious treatment for individuals who prefer non-agonist therapy for relapse prevention.

Current treatment guidelines do not consider mutual-help programs as standalone treatments (Kampman and Jarvis 2015). Many providers recommend these programs to their patients, as mutual self-help groups are ancillary services that promote long-term recovery and are valuable community resources. Narcotics Anonymous (NA) was founded in 1953. It is an adaptation of the Alcoholics Anonymous 12-step format for narcotic (i.e., opioid) dependence. Other mutual-help programs include Moderation Management and Self-Management and Recovery Therapy (SMART). NA does not express a specific opinion regarding medication-assisted treatment for OUD and instead focuses on providing a recovery environment where attendees can share their recovery stories with each other. Methadone Anonymous and Medication-Assisted Recovery Anonymous meetings are held in some communities as a result of anecdotal reports that some 12-step groups are less accepting of patients receiving medication-assisted treatment.

Mortality Following Treatment Discontinuation

Opioid overdose is the leading cause of premature death from opioid-related causes. During sustained treatment with opioid agonists and naltrexone, the risk of opioid overdose is decreased compared with untreated opioid dependence. Previous research has indicated that the risk of return to opioid use and overdose increases rapidly following discontinuation of oral naltrexone. For example, in an analysis of multiple trials in Australia, participants who discontinued oral naltrexone experienced eight times the rate of heroin overdose (44% within the first 2 weeks after discontinuation) compared with those who discontinued agonist therapy (Digiusto et al. 2004). Concerns regarding the efficacy of oral naltrexone and the high risk of overdose following discontinuation combined with substantially lower mortality risk with agonist therapy reinforce recommendations to avoid oral naltrexone. In a review of case reports of fatal overdoses associated with XR-NTX, Saucier et al. (2018) found that approximately 85% of the deaths occurred within 2 months of the last injection, indicating that this is a high-risk period for overdose. In an open-label randomized controlled multisite trial, participants assigned to receive XR-NTX experienced more relapse events than participants assigned to receive sublingual buprenorphine/naloxone (hazard ratio 1.36), with the majority of events occurring early in treatment and no differences in overdoses between the two groups (Lee et al. 2018). A retrospective study of 46,846 commercially insured individuals diagnosed with OUD examined the risk of opioid overdose associated with different medication treatments. Patients were prescribed XR-NTX (median filled prescriptions: 9 months), oral naltrexone (5 months), or buprenorphine (19 months) at least once during the 6-year period (Morgan et al. 2019). Buprenorphine, unlike oral naltrexone or XR-NTX, was associated with a significant reduction in the risk of opioid overdose compared with no treatment. In sum, the research indicates that considerable risk of opioid overdose and death is associated with discontinuation of either form of naltrexone compared with discontinuation of agonist therapy, and that extended-release formulations are preferable to oral naltrexone.

Special Considerations

Pregnancy

Naltrexone is currently classified by the FDA as pregnancy category C, meaning that animal studies have demonstrated adverse fetal effects and there are no well-controlled studies in humans to guide its use during pregnancy. Data from a case series using a formulation of XR-NTX not available in the United States suggested a possible increased risk of early pregnancy loss, with no identifiable increased risk of other adverse obstetric or neonatal outcomes, including anomaly risk, with the exception of possible rare urogenital abnormalities found in a retrospective study examining exposure to a naltrexone implant (Jones and Terplan 2018). The data to date do not support the initiation of naltrexone during pregnancy. Careful assessment of the potential benefits of continuing naltrexone and maintaining abstinence weighed against the potential risks to the mother (postpartum pain management) and the fetus may warrant continued use with informed consent. If a patient is highly motivated to remain sober while pregnant, she should discuss with her physician coming off of naltrexone. However, if a patient were to relapse while pregnant, it is not recommended to restart naltrexone. The most serious risk to a fetus is opioid withdrawal. Therefore, if a pregnant patient were to relapse, buprenorphine or methadone would usually be the recommended treatment (Kampman and Jarvis 2015; Tran et al. 2017).

Naltrexone and the 6-beta-naltrexol metabolite can be found in breast milk. One case report found that the total relative infant dose with both compounds (as naltrexone equivalents) was only 0.86% to 1.06% of the maternal 50-mg daily dose in a healthy infant who achieved anticipated milestones while breastfeeding (Chan et al. 2004). Given the lack of additional information, the use of naltrexone during breastfeeding should always be part of an informed consent and individual risk-benefit discussion.

Pain Management and Surgery

The management of pain during treatment with naltrexone can be challenging. Oral naltrexone should be stopped 2–3 days prior to surgery, and XR-NTX should ideally be stopped 1 month prior to surgery (Kampman and Jarvis 2015). Most pain can be treated with non-opioid analgesics (e.g., nonsteroidal anti-inflammatory drugs) and regional anesthesia. In the event of an acute emergency, naltrexone opioid receptor blockade can be overridden with the use of high-affinity opioids. Due to the risk of respiratory depression, this procedure should be performed only when necessary and only in a hospital setting capable of managing acute opioid overdose.

Youth

First-line treatment for youth with OUD should be buprenorphine/naloxone, with methadone as an alternative when the disorder cannot be managed with optimal doses of buprenorphine/naloxone. Additional research is needed to assess the effectiveness of naltrexone in youth, as some patients and families prefer naltrexone over opioid agonist treatment. The safe use of naltrexone in youth younger than 18 years of age has not been well established. The use of oral naltrexone is not recommended, because of low adherence rates and the risk of fatal overdose from the loss of tolerance. The literature on the use of XR-NTX in adolescent patients has been limited to case series reports. A chart review in a convenience sample of 16 youths (mean age 18.5 years) found that treatment with XR-NTX was well tolerated and accepted, with 63% retained in treatment for at least 4 months and 56% substantially reducing opioid use and improving in at least one psychosocial domain, with no new problems related to substance use (Fishman et al. 2010). Future studies are needed to look at the effectiveness of buprenorphine and methadone compared with XR-NTX in youth.

Naloxone

On October 26, 2017, the U.S. Department of Health and Human Services declared the opioid crisis a public health emergency. More people are now dying from opioid overdoses than from motor vehicle accidents. In 2017, there were more than 47,000 overdose deaths involving opioids, with increases across racial/ethnic groups, age groups, and county urbanization levels (Scholl et al. 2018). Synthetic opioids such as fentanyl were responsible for a 45.2% increase in opioid-related deaths in 2017 compared with the previous year. Opioid antagonists have an obvious therapeutic role in the treatment of opioid overdoses. Tolerance to the respiratory depressant effects of opioids develops more slowly than does tolerance to opioid analgesic or euphoric effects, leading to a heightened risk of overdose when users increase their dosage to maintain the same effects (White and Irvine 1999). Tolerance also rapidly decreases with abstinence, leading to an increased risk of overdose if the abstinent person resumes use.

Pharmacology

Naloxone was first approved for the treatment of opioid overdose by the FDA in 1971. Naloxone is a safe and effective reversal antidote that has saved countless lives and has become a key component in the prevention of opioid-related overdose deaths. Naloxone (N-allylnoroxymorphone) is a competitive antagonist with no intrinsic opioid agonist properties. Naloxone readily crosses the blood-brain barrier and binds to µ-opioid receptors with a high affinity; it has a lower affinity for the κ- and δ-opioid receptors (Peng et al. 2007). The onset of action in the central nervous system occurs within 2 minutes with intravenous use and takes slightly longer with intranasal or intramuscular administration. The duration of action is 20–120 minutes, depending on the route of administration. Naloxone is metabolized primarily by glucuronidation in the liver, with half-life of 30–120 minutes, depending on the route of administration.

There are three FDA-approved forms of naloxone: intranasal spray, injection (for intravenous or intramuscular use), and auto-injection. There are no oral formulations on the market, given naloxone's poor oral bioavailability and extensive first-pass metabolism in the liver. In the community setting, naloxone nasal spray has been the easiest method to train people to use (Ashrafioun et al. 2016). A 4-mg dose delivered in a single device (0.1 mL) can be used by both first responders and the lay public, providing a critical and potentially life-saving intervention (Krieter et al. 2016). In hospital settings, naloxone dosing is empirical and dependent on formulation availability and clinical response. Typically, the initial dose of naloxone is 0.4 mg (intravenously or intramuscularly), with the dose increased every 2–3 minutes (to 0.5 mg, 2 mg, 4 mg, 10 mg, 15 mg) until respiratory function is restored (Boyer 2012). A low dose may be adequate in some patients without precipitating withdrawal; however, for larger overdoses, repeated dosing or continuous infusion may be necessary due to the short half-life of naloxone (20–90 minutes, which is much shorter than the half-life of many opioids). Naloxone-precipitated withdrawal typically lasts for 30–60 minutes.

Use for Acute Emergent Treatment of Opioid Overdose

Opioids are potent depressants of respiratory function. Opioid overdose is characterized by pinpoint pupils (miosis), hypopnea (fewer than 12 breaths/minute), and apnea, leading to cerebral hypoxia and impaired consciousness, with cardiac arrest occurring as a later complication. Miosis is an inconsistent finding and may be absent in overdoses involving meperidine, propoxyphene, tramadol, or multiple drugs (Boyer 2012).

Emergency opioid overdose management involves maintaining an airway, restoring adequate ventilation, and administering naloxone (intravenously, intramuscularly, or intranasally, depending on availability and setting). Assessment and treatment of commonly associated complications, such as rhabdomyolysis, pulmonary edema, compartment syndrome (from compression in muscle groups resulting in disruption in blood flow), and hepatic damage (from acetaminophen-containing analgesics), are also critical to successful treatment outcomes. Because of naloxone's short half-life, multiple doses are often needed to revive a patient before the patient can receive more advanced interventions in an emergency care setting. Likewise, in a health care setting, continuous infusion may be necessary to support respiratory function until higher-potency opioids (e.g., fentanyl) or longer-acting opioids have been sufficiently metabolized and cleared. Close monitoring for the return of respiratory function after the initial administration of naloxone is recommended. Some patients will respond to low-dose naloxone without experiencing precipitated opioid withdrawal. In a prospective observational study of 1,192 opioid overdoses, 33% of patients treated with naloxone by emergency medical services experienced opioid withdrawal symptoms, 32% were confused or restless, 22% complained of headaches, and 4% had seizures (Buajordet et al. 2004). The high rate of headaches and seizures was thought to be related to cerebral hypoxia, given that the majority of patients were severely cyanotic prior to naloxone administration.

Because of its safety and efficacy, naloxone can be used by trained laypersons in the community. Family and friends are often the first to witness the symptoms of an opioid overdose. The provision of naloxone rescue kits and the accompanying instructions is a cost-effective and critical strategy to reduce overdose deaths.

Special Considerations: Pregnancy

Naloxone is not recommended in pregnancy apart from life-threatening overdoses. However, naloxone should obviously not be withheld from a pregnant woman who needs it to reverse a life-threatening opioid overdose (Kampman and Jarvis 2015). The administration of naloxone may be critical to reverse the overdose and may benefit the fetus by reversing maternal hypoxia. Naloxone crosses the placenta and can precipitate withdrawal in the fetus in addition to the mother. Acute withdrawal could potentially cause maternal seizures and death in a vulnerable fetus and should be avoided if possible. To avoid precipitated withdrawal, the smallest effective dose should be administered, and an ambulance should be called regardless of the gestational age of the fetus. The FDA classifies naloxone as a pregnancy category B drug, indicating that there have been no reports of teratogenicity in humans or animals.

Availability and Legal Protection

In an effort to stem the rise in opioid overdose deaths, the majority of the states in the United States have enacted legislation to improve access to naloxone for both first responders and the lay public (Davis and Carr 2017). It is imperative to administer naloxone as soon as possible, as the risk of death and permanent injury increases with the duration of respiratory depression. Access to naloxone and Good Samaritan laws have been associated with about a 25% reduction in overdose deaths (McClellan et al. 2018). Good Samaritan laws provide legal protection for individuals who report an overdose for the purpose of requesting emergency medical assistance. Naloxone is available over the counter in many states and by prescription throughout the United States. Cost varies by formulation. Overdose Education and Naloxone Distribution (ONED) programs provide access to naloxone. They also provide training to opioid-using individuals and their family members and peers, who may be the first to witness an overdose. Evidence has demonstrated that naloxone administration by bystanders is associated with increased odds of recovery, and that overdose education programs such as ONED result in improved recognition and management of overdoses in nonclinical settings (Giglio et al. 2015).

The number of naloxone prescriptions dispensed in retail pharmacies increased substantially between 2012 and 2018, with an 106% increase from 2017 to 2018; however, rates of naloxone prescriptions per high-dose opioid prescriptions remain low

(Guy et al. 2019). Efforts to improve access to and distribution of naloxone are critical to reducing and preventing deaths related to opioid overdose.

Conclusion

Opioid antagonists have an important role in the treatment of opioid use disorders. The significant take-home points for this chapter are as follows:

- Injectable extended-release naltrexone is preferable to oral naltrexone due to the latter's poor adherence, elevated dropout rates, high relapse rates, and risk of overdose on oral preparations.
- Oral naltrexone should be avoided except in very select patients who accept the risks, agree to observed dosing and close monitoring, and have adequate support.
- Introduction of low-dose naltrexone during detoxification, with a tapering course of buprenorphine in conjunction with ancillary medications to manage withdrawal, shows promise in facilitating induction of extended-release naltrexone.
- Naloxone is a life-saving treatment for opioid overdoses. Naloxone rescue kits should be prescribed to all individuals with opioid use disorder, ideally in association with training for family and significant others who may be the first to witness an overdose.

References

Ashrafioun L, Gamble S, Herrmann M, et al: Evaluation of knowledge and confidence following opioid overdose prevention training: a comparison of types of training participants and naloxone administration methods. Subst Abus 37(1):76–81, 2016 26514071

Bigelow GE, Preston KL, Schmittner J, et al: Opioid challenge evaluation of blockade by extended-release naltrexone in opioid-abusing adults: dose-effects and time-course. Drug Alcohol Depend 123(1–3):57–65, 2012 22079773

Bisaga A, Sullivan MA, Glass A, et al: The effects of dronabinol during detoxification and the initiation of treatment with extended release naltrexone. Drug Alcohol Depend 154:38–45, 2015 26187456

Bisaga A, Mannelli P, Sullivan MA, et al: Antagonists in the medical management of opioid use disorders: historical and existing treatment strategies. Am J Addict 27(3):177–187, 2018a 29596725

Bisaga A, Mannelli P, Yu M, et al: Outpatient transition to extended-release injectable naltrexone for patients with opioid use disorder: a phase 3 randomized trial. Drug Alcohol Depend 187:171–178, 2018b 29674251

Boyer EW: Management of opioid analgesic overdose. N Engl J Med 367(2):146–155, 2012 22784117

Bronfenbrener R: Inexpensive compounding of low dose naltrexone (LDN) with orange juice. J Am Acad Dermatol March 28, 2019 [Epub ahead of print] 30930087

Buajordet I, Naess AC, Jacobsen D, et al: Adverse events after naloxone treatment of episodes of suspected acute opioid overdose. Eur J Emerg Med 11(1):19–23, 2004 15167188

Centers for Disease Control and Prevention: Deaths and severe adverse events associated with anesthesia-assisted rapid opioid detoxification—New York City, 2012. MMWR Morb Mortal Wkly Rep 62(38):777–780, 2013 24067581

Chan CF, Page-Sharp M, Kristensen JH, et al: Transfer of naltrexone and its metabolite 6,beta-naltrexol into human milk. J Hum Lact 20(3):322–326, 2004 15296587

Davis C, Carr D: State legal innovations to encourage naloxone dispensing. J Am Pharm Assoc 57(2, suppl):S180–S184, 2017 28073688

DeFulio A, Everly JJ, Leoutsakos JM, et al: Employment-based reinforcement of adherence to an FDA approved extended release formulation of naltrexone in opioid-dependent adults: a randomized controlled trial. Drug Alcohol Depend 120(1–3):48–54, 2012 21782353

Digiusto E, Shakeshaft A, Ritter A, et al: Serious adverse events in the Australian National Evaluation of Pharmacotherapies for Opioid Dependence (NEPOD). Addiction 99(4):450–460, 2004 15049745

Dugosh K, Abraham A, Seymour B, et al: A systematic review on the use of psychosocial interventions in conjunction with medications for the treatment of opioid addiction. J Addict Med 10(2):93–103, 2016 26808307

Fishman MJ, Winstanley EL, Curran E, et al: Treatment of opioid dependence in adolescents and young adults with extended release naltrexone: preliminary case-series and feasibility. Addiction 105(9):1669–1676, 2010 20626723

Garbutt JC, Kranzler HR, O'Malley SS, et al: Efficacy and tolerability of long-acting injectable naltrexone for alcohol dependence: a randomized controlled trial. JAMA 293(13):1617–1625, 2005 15811981

Giglio RE, Li G, DiMaggio CJ: Effectiveness of bystander naloxone administration and overdose education programs: a meta-analysis. Inj Epidemiol 2(1):10, 2015 27747742

Guy GP Jr, Haegerich TM, Evans ME, et al: Vital signs: pharmacy-based naloxone dispensing—United States 2012–2018. MMWR Morb Mortal Wkly Rep 68(31):679–686, 2019 31393863

Hulse GK, Morris N, Arnold-Reed D, et al: Improving clinical outcomes in treating heroin dependence: randomized, controlled trial of oral or implant naltrexone. Arch Gen Psychiatry 66(10):1108–1115, 2009 19805701

Jarvis BP, Holtyn AF, Subramaniam S, et al: Extended-release injectable naltrexone for opioid use disorder: a systematic review. Addiction 113(7):1188–1209, 2018 29396985

Jones CW, Terplan M: Pregnancy and naltrexone pharmacotherapy. Obstet Gynecol 132(4):923–925, 2018 30204703

Kampman K, Jarvis M: American Society of Addiction Medicine (ASAM) national practice guideline for the use of medications in the treatment of addiction involving opioid use. J Addict Med 9(5):358–367, 2015 26406300

Krieter P, Chiang N, Gyaw S, et al: Pharmacokinetic properties and human use characteristics of an FDA-approved intranasal naloxone product for the treatment of opioid overdose. J Clin Pharmacol 56(10):1243–1253, 2016 27145977

Latif ZE, Šaltyte Benth J, Solli KK, et al: Anxiety, depression, and insomnia among adults with opioid dependence treated with extended-release naltrexone vs buprenorphine-naloxone: a randomized clinical trial and follow-up study. JAMA Psychiatry 76(2):127–134, 2019 30566177

Lee MC, Wagner HN Jr, Tanada S, et al: Duration of occupancy of opiate receptors by naltrexone. J Nucl Med 29(7):1207–1211, 1988 2839637

Lee JD, Nunes EV Jr, Novo P, et al: Comparative effectiveness of extended-release naltrexone versus buprenorphine-naloxone for opioid relapse prevention (X:BOT): a multicentre, open-label, randomised controlled trial. Lancet 391(10118):309–318, 2018 29150198

Martin WR, Jasinski DR, Mansky PA: Naltrexone, an antagonist for the treatment of heroin dependence. Effects in man. Arch Gen Psychiatry 28(6):784–791, 1973 4707988

McClellan C, Lambdin BH, Ali MM, et al: Opioid-overdose laws association with opioid use and overdose mortality. Addict Behav 86:90–95, 2018 29610001

Meyer MC, Straughn AB, Lo MW, et al: Bioequivalence, dose-proportionality, and pharmacokinetics of naltrexone after oral administration. J Clin Psychiatry 45(9 Pt 2):15–19, 1984 6469932

Minozzi S, Amato L, Vecchi S, et al: Oral naltrexone maintenance treatment for opioid dependence. Cochrane Database Syst Rev (4):CD001333, 2011 21491383

Mitchell MC, Memisoglu A, Silverman BL: Hepatic safety of injectable extended-release naltrexone in patients with chronic hepatitis C and HIV infection. J Stud Alcohol Drugs 73(6):991–997, 2012 23036218

Morgan JR, Schackman BR, Weinstein ZM, et al: Overdose following initiation of naltrexone and buprenorphine medication treatment for opioid use disorder in a United States commercially insured cohort. Drug Alcohol Depend 200:34–39, 2019 31082666

Nunes EV, Rothenberg JL, Sullivan MA, et al: Behavioral therapy to augment oral naltrexone for opioid dependence: a ceiling on effectiveness? Am J Drug Alcohol Abuse 32(4):503–517, 2006 17127538

Peng X, Knapp BI, Bidlack JM, et al: Pharmacological properties of bivalent ligands containing butorphan linked to nalbuphine, naltrexone, and naloxone at mu, delta, and kappa opioid receptors. J Med Chem 50(9):2254–2258, 2007 17407276

Resnick RB, Volavka J, Freedman AM, et al: Studies of EN-1639A (naltrexone): a new narcotic antagonist. Am J Psychiatry 131(6):646–650, 1974 4827793

Saucier R, Wolfe D, Dasgupta N: Review of case narratives from fatal overdoses associated with injectable naltrexone for opioid dependence. Drug Saf 41(10):981–988, 2018 29560596

Schecter A: The role of narcotic antagonists in the rehabilitation of opiate addicts: a review of naltrexone. Am J Drug Alcohol Abuse 7(1):1–18, 1980 6254356

Scholl L, Seth P, Kariisa M, et al: Drug and opioid-involved overdose deaths—United States, 2013–2017. MMWR Morb Mortal Wkly Rep 67(5152):1419–1427, 2018 30605448

Sigmon SC, Bisaga A, Nunes EV, et al: Opioid detoxification and naltrexone induction strategies: recommendations for clinical practice. Am J Drug Alcohol Abuse 38(3):187–199, 2012 22404717

Sudakin D: Naltrexone: not just for opioids anymore. J Med Toxicol 12(1):71–75, 2016 26546222

Sullivan M, Bisaga A, Pavlicova M, et al: Long-acting injectable naltrexone induction: a randomized trial of outpatient opioid detoxification with naltrexone versus buprenorphine. Am J Psychiatry 174(5):459–467, 2017 28068780

Sullivan MA, Bisaga A, Pavlicova M, et al: A randomized trial comparing extended-release injectable suspension and oral naltrexone, both combined with behavioral therapy, for the treatment of opioid use disorder. Am J Psychiatry 176(2):129–137, 2019 30336703

Tanum L, Solli KK, Latif ZE, et al: Effectiveness of injectable extended-release naltrexone vs daily buprenorphine-naloxone for opioid dependence: a randomized clinical noninferiority trial. JAMA Psychiatry 74(12):1197–1205, 2017 29049469

Tetrault JM, Tate JP, McGinnis KA, et al: Hepatic safety and antiretroviral effectiveness in HIV-infected patients receiving naltrexone. Alcohol Clin Exp Res 36(2):318–324, 2012 21797892

Tran TH, Griffin BL, Stone RH, et al: Methadone, buprenorphine, and naltrexone for the treatment of opioid use disorder in pregnant women. Pharmacotherapy 37(7):824–839, 2017 28543191

U.S. Department of Health & Human Services: HHS Acting Secretary Declares Public Health Emergency to Address National Opioid Crisis (press release). October 26, 2017. Available at: https://www.hhs.gov/about/news/2017/10/26/hhs-acting-secretary-declares-public-health-emergency-address-national-opioid-crisis.html. Accessed July 10, 2020.

Verebey K, Kogan MJ, DePace A, et al: Quantitative determination of naltrexone and beta-naltrexol in human plasma using electron capture detection. J Chromatogr A 118(3):331–335, 1976 1254668

Vuong C, Van Uum SHM, O'Dell LE, et al: The effects of opioids and opioid analogs on animal and human endocrine systems. Endocr Rev 31(1):98–132, 2010 19903933

White JM, Irvine RJ: Mechanisms of fatal opioid overdose. Addiction 94(7):961–972, 1999 10707430

Zaki PA, Keith DE Jr, Brine GA, et al: Ligand-induced changes in surface mu-opioid receptor number: relationship to G protein activation? J Pharmacol Exp Ther 292(3):1127–1134, 2000 10688632

CHAPTER 15

Neurobiology and Treatment of Hallucinogen Use Disorder

Elias Dakwar, M.D.

Fame is finally the sum of all the misunderstandings that surround a new name.

—Rainer Maria Rilke

On October 4, 1969, Diane Linkletter, a 20-year-old aspiring actor, jumped from her apartment window and fell several stories. Within hours of her death, her father, the popular radio and television host Art Linkletter, proposed that the most probable cause of death was the serotonergic hallucinogen lysergic acid diethylamide (LSD), which he alleged had led to a "bum trip" and nervous breakdown 6 months earlier. Mr. Linkletter further speculated that she had likely been intoxicated with LSD when she jumped to her death, because she was "not herself" at the time (even though toxicology reports and a personal account of her behavior prior to the fall indicated that no drugs were in her system) (Bleeker 2016). This event, following on the heels of the horrific Manson Family murders earlier that year, which had also been reputed to implicate repeated LSD use, shook the nation.

Mr. Linkletter would go on to become a prominent campaigner for drug criminalization, with a focus on the dangers of LSD, which had been emerging as a popular drug with the counterculture. Young people who were otherwise healthy, he said, were falling into madness, violence, and antisocial behavior; and there were also indications that these drugs might lead to chromosomal damage, cognitive impairments, and irrevocable personality changes (Kornheiser 1981). In less than 5 years,

227

and in the wake of a proliferation of comparable headlines depicting young people gone mad, LSD and most other so-called hallucinogens—once touted as wonder drugs for the treatment of depression, anxiety, criminal behavior, and addiction—were criminalized, with any research into their medical value also aborted.

The rapid fall from grace of hallucinogens represents a case study of how drugs come to be demonized. Reasoned argument or even evidence are rarely involved. Instead, scapegoating, facile moralizing, fear, and other irrational forces often have the upper hand. It has become clear, decades later, that cultural issues, sensationalistic news reports, generational tensions, and the confusions brought on by rapidly shifting societal norms and values were crucial factors in the criminalization of LSD and other hallucinogens (DiPaolo 2018). Furthermore, some reports of risk were either overblown or entirely spurious (Bakalar and Grinspoon 1997; Hofmann 2009; Marlan 2019). It remains difficult, even today, to delineate what is real and what is not when it comes to hallucinogens.

The story of hallucinogens presents an opportunity to more lucidly and empirically understand how and why psychoactive substances can be dangerous. One major problem with unreasonably denigrating a substance is that this works to obscure what its real dangers might be and how one might approach it responsibly. Accordingly, more rigorous investigation of the risks of hallucinogens by first examining the facts and carefully sifting through the distortions and myths is preferable. Therefore, this chapter on hallucinogens begins by clarifying their actions, psychoactive effects, historical uses, potential therapeutic benefits, and neural mechanisms. When appropriate, this chapter calls attention to, and dispels, the misconceptions that have continued to surround them. The chapter concludes with a survey of their risks, as well as a discussion of the various settings in which these adverse effects might be either worsened or minimized.

Names, Categories, Biological Effects

It does not take long to stumble into misconceptions; they begin with the name. "Hallucinogens" is the accepted medical term for this class of substances, even though they do not typically engender hallucinations (sensations perceived as real without an actual referent). Instead, these substances might be more properly characterized as engendering nonordinary states of consciousness comparable to meditation, trance, dreaming, or mystical experience, as well as to certain features of psychosis, such as overvalued ideas, distortions, and idiosyncratic thought processes. Other names given to these substances include "psychedelics" and "entheogens"; however, these terms carry bias because they overemphasize the "mystical" and "revelatory" effects of these substances, just as the term *hallucinogen* is biased because it confers a negative valence on these effects, conflating them with psychopathology. Despite these problems with *hallucinogen,* that term will be employed throughout this chapter, in deference to the accepted medical-scientific lexicon.

Hallucinogens encompass many distinct substances, some with widely varying neurobiological and psychoactive effects (Bakalar and Grinspoon 1997). These various agents can be organized either by their immediate neurobiological effects or by their molecular structure. The two broadest molecular subgroups are the indoleamines and the phenethylamines (Figure 15–1). The indoleamines include LSD, dimethyltrypta-mine (DMT), psilocybin, ibogaine, and harmaline. The phenethylamines include nat-urally occurring compounds such as mescaline as well as an ever-expanding number of synthetic compounds, such as 2,5-dimethoxy-4-bromophenethylamine (2-CB), 3,4-methylenedioxymethamphetamine (MDMA), 3,4-methylenedioxyamphetamine (MDA), and 2,5-dimethoxy-4-methylamphetamine (DOM).

Classical hallucinogens are widely believed to exert their psychoactive effects by di-rect agonism of the serotonin (5-hydroxytryptamine [5-HT]) type 2A (5-HT$_{2A}$) recep-tor, though other serotonin receptors may also be involved. Classical hallucinogens include psilocybin, LSD, mescaline, and DMT. These compounds, despite sharing neurobiological activity, are derived from quite diverse sources; for example, psilocy-bin can be isolated from a mushroom, and mescaline can be obtained from cacti (pey-ote and San Pedro).

Hallucinogens may also exert their psychoactive effects by *nonclassical* mecha-nisms. These mechanisms include serotonin release or nonspecific serotonin receptor activation, as in the case of MDMA ("Ecstasy" or "Molly") and some phenethyl-amines; N-methyl-D-aspartate receptor (NMDAr) or glutamatergic modulation, as with ketamine and phencyclidine; cannabinoid receptor activation; and κ-opioid re-ceptor agonism, as with *Salvia divinorum*. These mechanisms are by no means exhaus-tive; there are other compounds (e.g., nitrous oxide, the fly agaric mushroom) that work by quite different mechanisms (Bakalar and Grinspoon 1997; Glennon 2008; Malleson 1971). Interestingly, research suggests that classical hallucinogens and dis-sociative anesthetics, despite their apparent differences in acute neurobiological ac-tivity, exert their effects through a common final pathway of prefrontal glutamatergic modulation (Vollenweider and Kometer 2010).

The effects of classical hallucinogens on cerebral blood flow (CBF) and brain activ-ity remain a subject of active study. Whereas psilocybin had been demonstrated to in-crease blood flow to and activity in the prefrontal brain areas when administered orally (Gouzoulis-Mayfrank et al. 1999; Schreckenberger et al. 1998; Vollenweider and Kometer 2010), more recent functional magnetic resonance imaging (fMRI) research by a single group (Carhart-Harris et al. 2012) has suggested that psilocybin adminis-tered as a bolus dose by the intravenous route may *decrease* CBF to certain prefrontal areas, as well as reduce prefrontal activity. These changes in CBF and brain activity appear to correlate with certain psychoactive effects. Furthermore, intravenous psilo-cybin has been shown by the same group (Carhart-Harris et al. 2012, 2013) to attenu-ate functional connectivity, synchronize anti-correlated networks, and reduce resting-state activity of the default mode network (DMN), which is thought to correspond to self-referential processing and the structuring of experience. These latter effects on functional connectivity and the DMN are consistent with brain activity associated with other altered states, such as meditation and psychosis, as well as with the effects of subanesthetic infusions of ketamine (Scheidegger et al. 2012).

Psychoactive Effects

The psychoactive effects of hallucinogens can be markedly different, depending on the type of drug and its route of administration. Even agents from the same subgroup

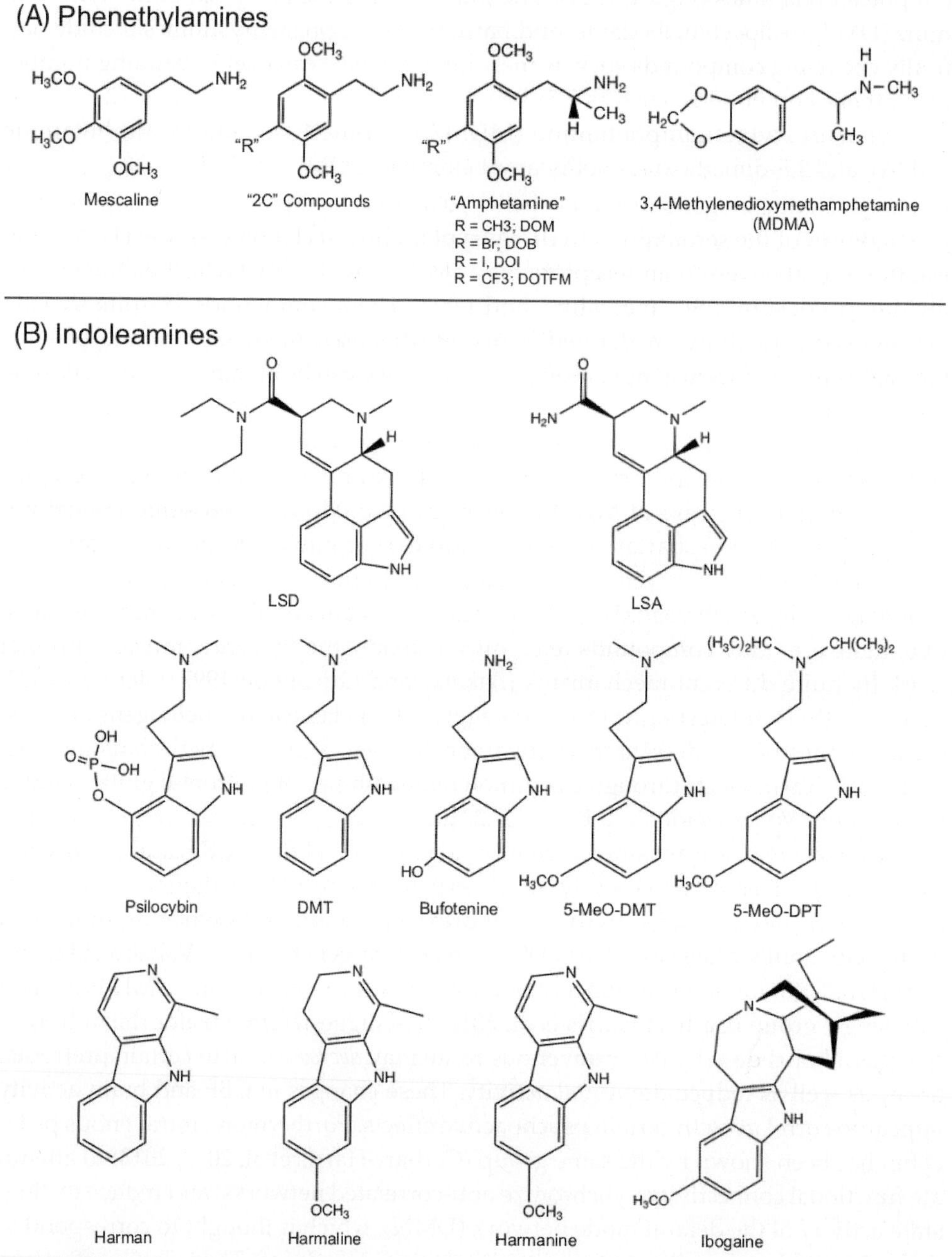

(A) Phenethylamines

Mescaline

"2C" Compounds

"Amphetamine"
R = CH3; DOM
R = Br; DOB
R = I, DOI
R = CF3; DOTFM

3,4-Methylenedioxymethamphetamine
(MDMA)

(B) Indoleamines

LSD

LSA

Psilocybin

DMT

Bufotenine

5-MeO-DMT

5-MeO-DPT

Harman

Harmaline

Harmanine

Ibogaine

FIGURE 15–1. Hallucinogens by molecular group.

(A) Phenethylamines: "2C" compounds–family of phenethylamines containing methoxy groups on the 2 and 5 positions of a benzene ring; DOB=dimethoxybromoamphetamine; DOI=2,5-dimethoxy-4-iodo-amphetamine; DOM=2,5-dimethoxy-4-methylamphetamine; DOTFM=2,5-dimethoxy-4-trifluoromethyl-amphetamine; MDA=3,4-methylenedioxyamphetamine; MDMA=3,4-methylenedioxymethamphetamine; "R"=R group. (B) Indoleamines: 5-MeO-DIPT=5-methoxy-N,N-diisopropyltryptamine; 5-MeO-DMT= 5-methoxy-N,N-dimethyltryptamine; DMT=dimethyltryptamine; LSA=lysergic acid amide; LSD=lysergic acid diethylamide.

(e.g., mescaline and MDMA) can have quite dissimilar effects. In this section, the aim is to describe all *potential* hallucinogenic effects involving alterations of consciousness. Classical hallucinogens are the subgroup that typically exhibits the widest range of these alterations (Bakalar and Grinspoon 1997; Glennon 2008; Malleson 1971; Vollenweider and Kometer 2010).

These alterations of consciousness can be grouped into several categories, all of which can be experienced concurrently (Figure 15–2) (Bakalar and Grinspoon 1997; Studerus et al. 2011; Vollenweider and Kometer 2010). The first and most basic category of alterations is *perceptual changes.* These include an intensification of sensory phenomena; greater sensitivity to latent phenomena (e.g., patterns or textures that are ordinarily overlooked); changes in the perception of time or space; conflation of sensory modalities, as in synesthesia; the production of eidetic imagery, such as spirals, shapes, and arabesques; heightened aesthetic appreciation; illusions; pseudo-hallucinations (with intact reality testing); and an altered sense of the body.

The second category of alterations is *experiential changes.* These changes include alterations in mood (euphoria, hilarity, terror, or anxiety); altered relatedness to others or to objects (empathy, alienation, connectedness, or merging); greater philosophical/ existential concerns; increased insight; dissociation; emergence of pseudo-delusional or overvalued ideas (e.g., the world will end in the near future); suggestibility; and a reliving of past memories or a resurgence of apparently resolved conflicts.

Mystical-type or transpersonal experiences constitute the third category. These are experiences characterized by heightened spirituality or mysticism, similar in nature to those described by mystics, philosophers, or religious figures in historical accounts. Such experiences can include a struggle or conflict of archetypal dimensions; a sense of life's absurdity or lack of purpose; an experience of complete oneness with all that is; near-death or birthlike experiences; immersion in a total void; ego diffusion, as in so-called oceanic boundlessness; ego dissolution; a sense of the sacred; spiritual ecstasy; spatiotemporal transcendence; nondiscursive or ineffable understanding (e.g., knowledge beyond the reach of language); an overwhelming sense of finiteness or sinfulness; identification with the divine; reincarnation; reevaluation of values; redemption; and metaphysical/cosmological speculation. Research with psilocybin suggests that the personal significance of such experiences can be enduring, with some individuals continuing to report 1 year later that the experience was among the most important in their lives (Griffiths et al. 2006, 2008).

Cultural Uses

As is the case with many psychoactive substances, hallucinogens have been accorded an important, and sometimes sacramental, place in various cultural traditions and groups. The use of the hallucinogen might be ritualized or ceremonialized, symbolically integrated into the group's beliefs and traditions, or invested with supernatural importance (Figure 15–3). Indeed, the unique psychoactive profile of hallucinogens, and particularly their capacity to engender mystical-type experiences, has made them especially well-suited for use in religious, initiation, or healing ceremonies (Bakalar and Grinspoon 1997; Hofmann and Schultes 1979).

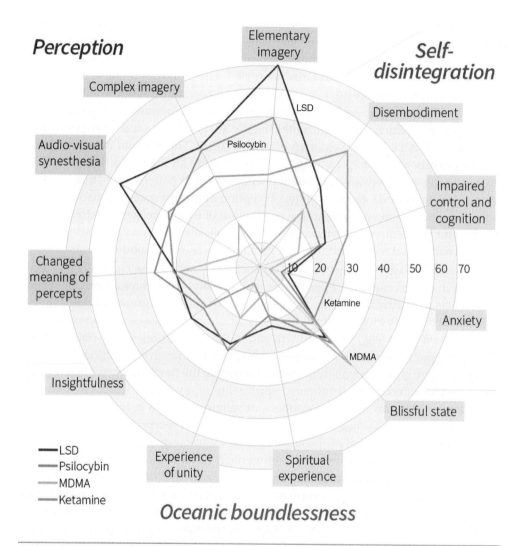

FIGURE 15–2.   Psychoactive effects of common hallucinogens according to the Five Dimensions of Altered States of Consciousness (5D-ASC) scale.

To view this figure in color, see Plate 4 in Color Gallery in middle of book.

Data mapped in the figure were compiled from separate trials, each administering a single psychoactive substance. The 5D-ASC dimensions of psychoactive effects studied—oceanic boundlessness, ego disintegration, and perception—each contain elements of the perceptual, experiential, and mystical-type/transpersonal effects discussed in chapter text. LSD=lysergic acid diethylamide; MDMA=3,4-methylenedioxymethamphetamine.

Source.   Reprinted from "The Psychedelic Experience According to the 5D-ASC Scale" (chart) in Marlene Rupp, "The Psychedelic Experience," *Sapiensoup Blog*, June 27, 2017. Available at: https://sapiensoup.com/psychedelic-experience. Accessed June 19, 2020. Used with permission.

Indigenous groups in the Americas have a robust and diverse history of incorporating hallucinogens into their rituals and ceremonies, likely because of the wealth of naturally occurring psychoactive substances in these continents. The Aztecs ritualized the use of psilocybin-containing mushrooms for millennia; peyote (mescaline) and salvia are used by indigenous groups in Mexico; and harmalines and DMT, in the form of ayahuasca or yage, are central to shamanic or religious rituals in various indigenous

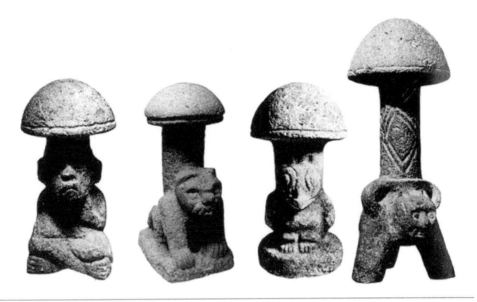

FIGURE 15–3. Various mushroom stones.

These stones, dating from 1000 B.C. to 500 A.D., are approximately 1 foot in height. They suggest the religious and cultural importance accorded to psychoactive mushrooms by the cultural/ethnic groups that consume them sacramentally, ritually, or ceremonially.

Source. Reprinted from *Plants of the Gods*, by Richard Evans Schultes, Albert Hofmann, and Christian Rätsch; copyright © 2001. Used with permission of Inner Traditions International and Bear & Company (www.innertraditions.com).

and syncretic Amazonian traditions. Despite the fact that DMT and mescaline are illegal in the United States, they can be licitly used in their naturally occurring forms by members of certain religions that are recognized by the U.S. government as requiring these substances for proper worship. Of note, both DMT (as ayahuasca) and mescaline (as peyote) are used by their respective communities to promote health and to address certain ailments, such as addiction. The spiritually oriented framework encompassing the ritualistic use of hallucinogens has led some researchers to propose that psychospiritual mechanisms account for their putative benefits. Researchers have accordingly proposed hallucinogen-based treatment models that aim to elicit mystical states similar to those cultivated in hallucinogen-oriented rituals (Bakalar and Grinspoon 1997; Hoffer 1970; Hofmann and Schultes 1979).

The widespread use of hallucinogens in the United States and Europe among the young during the 1960s is also worth discussing, not least because it contributed to the criminalization campaign mentioned earlier. In addition to being valued for their profound ability to alter and enhance sensory experience, hallucinogens (and primarily LSD) were celebrated by the counterculture as potent tools for self-discovery, direct mystical experience, and transcendence beyond ordinary consensus reality. This attitude toward hallucinogens, fueled by such popular figures as Aldous Huxley, Timothy Leary, and Alan Watts, among many others, gained particular momentum in the context of the social problems and generational conflicts that characterized the late 1950s and 1960s, with many people, and particularly the young, having become disillusioned with the belligerent imperialism, consumerism, materialism, and conformity that had come to shape their societies. In this troubled time, hallucinogens came to represent, much as in some indigenous cultures, a means by which to access deeper truths and to initiate communal renewal. Unlike these indigenous cultures, however, the United States and other Western countries lacked the cultural framework to effectively incorporate hallucinogen use, to support individuals who sought to use these substances, and to respond creatively to the powerful experiences occasioned by them. Instead, unsupervised and irresponsible use proliferated, traumatic or sensational adverse events made headlines, and the substances were condemned as dangerous and bereft of benefit. The importance of a supportive and guided framework that adequately screens and prepares individuals before hallucinogen administration cannot be overstated; such a framework should guide both the clinical and the cultural use of these compounds so as to minimize their potential risks and optimize their benefits (Bakalar and Grinspoon 1997; Leuner 1994).

Adverse Effects

The paradox of hallucinogens, and one of the reasons they constitute such an intriguing class of agents, is that the very same effects that might be therapeutic are also those associated with risk. This is of course the case with most drugs and medications; the stimulation elicited by amphetamines, for example, leads to both improvements in concentration and difficulties with appetite and sleep. But hallucinogens call our attention, quite clearly, to the different variables distinguishing harmful from therapeutic use. These same variables are also relevant to other drugs, even if they may seem less conspicuous.

The psychoactive effects of hallucinogens represent the most common cause of risk. Research suggests that the behavioral and psychoactive risks associated with hallucinogens may be effectively minimized and managed by the context in which the agents are administered. It has been recognized that hallucinogen-occasioned alterations in consciousness are shaped, to an extent, by the past experiences, expectations/intentions, preparation, and attributes of the user (the *set*), as well as by the context (including presence of other individuals, medical staff, or a guide) in which the experience occurs (the *setting*) (Bakalar and Grinspoon 1997; Imperi et al. 1968; Malleson 1971; Studerus et al. 2012; Vollenweider and Kometer 2010). The set and setting may play primary roles in whether the hallucinogen experience is pleasant and enriching or dysphoric and upsetting. Most importantly, the set and setting also constitute the most salient modifiable variables affecting whether or not hallucinogen-related toxicity occurs. Many reports from the heyday of hallucinogen research—the 1950s and 1960s—have consistently shown that with appropriate patient selection, preparation, guidance, and follow-up care, hallucinogens can be safely administered in medical settings, with minimal reports of behavioral toxicity or persistent adverse effects (Bakalar and Grinspoon 1997; Malleson 1971; Studerus et al. 2011; Vollenweider and Kometer 2010). Most accounts of behavioral toxicity or persistent distress in fact occur outside of medical settings, when these substances are used irresponsibly. These findings are now being replicated by more recent investigations as human-oriented hallucinogen research carefully resumes (Johnson et al. 2008).

Hallucinogens are most likely to cause harm, therefore, when they are consumed by unprepared or unstable individuals or in the absence of a supportive, responsive framework. In such circumstances, hallucinogens may lead to acute behavioral disturbances or persistent distress that may require emergency treatment. Common adverse effects of hallucinogens include anxiety or dysphoria, generally limited to the period of intoxication; loss of behavioral control (manifesting as passivity, disorganization, indecision, and suboptimal functioning) during acute intoxication; and, more rarely, the emergence of persistent anxiety or of affective or psychotic disturbances in vulnerable individuals (Bakalar and Grinspoon 1997; Imperi et al. 1968; Johnson et al. 2008; Vollenweider and Kometer 2010). It should be noted that in some treatment models, the emergence of anxiety or dysphoria during a session may be a valuable component of the therapeutic process and may represent an abreaction of previously repressed or suppressed psychic content (Hoffer 1970).

The most common—and sometimes the most dangerous—source of hallucinogen-related acute distress is simple intoxication. In unprepared or unguided individuals, hallucinogens can occasionally lead to such high levels of distress that individuals may seek medical help in the midst of the experience out of fear that they are about to die, become insane, or undergo some catastrophe. The acutely distressed individual will present to an acute setting, by ambulance or otherwise, and health care workers will be confronted by a terrified, possibly incoherent, and behaviorally disorganized person who may not be able to properly recount what happened, including whether a hallucinogen was taken. Physiological signs of intoxication, such as dilated pupils, diaphoresis, and altered psychomotor status, may serve as clues in the absence of a clear history.

Hallucinogen-related distress can constitute a psychiatric emergency, and may involve many of the usual features of acute decompensation, including poor engagement with health care workers, agitation, aggression, elopement risk, or suicidality. A one-on-one sitter should therefore be assigned. Caution should of course be exercised, and if the patient does not respond to supportive therapy, relaxation exercises, and redirection, a low dose of a fast-acting benzodiazepine, such as lorazepam, should be sufficient to ameliorate distress. The medication should initially be offered by mouth; if the medication is refused and pharmacological restraint is deemed necessary, the medication should be provided intramuscularly.

The persistent effects of hallucinogens can include the precipitation of psychosis, depression, or anxiety in vulnerable individuals, or the exacerbation of psychiatric distress in patients with unstable mental illness. A rare consequence of hallucinogen use is hallucinogen persisting perception disorder (HPPD), more colloquially referred to as "flashbacks." HPPD differs from psychosis in that the effects are purely perceptual rather than involving cognition, behavior, or ideation. Unfortunately, there are no known treatments for this seldom-encountered but distressing condition.

Psychiatric distress should be managed as it would be in other circumstances; worsening psychosis merits the initiation of higher doses of an antipsychotic, mania requires mood stabilization, and worsening anxiety or depressive symptoms require proper pharmacotherapy and psychotherapy. Clear cases of acute hallucinogen-induced depression or anxiety, however, should not be treated with pharmacotherapy immediately; instead, watchful waiting, along with psychotherapy, is advised. If the depression or anxiety persists for more than 4 weeks after the hallucinogen use, or if symptoms are so severe that they require immediate clinical attention, then pharmacotherapy may be necessary.

The management of hallucinogen-induced psychosis is less clear-cut, as this effect has not been properly studied. Furthermore, cases may be time-limited and may resolve on their own without pharmacotherapy. However, it is currently impossible at the onset of the disturbance to discriminate between time-limited cases and those that might persist for some time. Expert opinion encourages the judicious use of antipsychotics for hallucinogen-induced psychosis, although the role of maintenance pharmacotherapy remains unclear.

Although these terms are now obsolete in the current DSM-5 (American Psychiatric Association 2013) conceptualization of substance use disorders, the distinctions between *abuse* and *dependence* offer a valuable way to understand disordered patterns of hallucinogen use. Although hallucinogens may be used irresponsibly or abused (e.g., repeatedly ingested despite the emergence of behavioral distress or other adverse effects), findings from animal models indicate that classical hallucinogens do not present a risk for dependence; these agents are not self-administered, do not create conditioned place preference or physiological dependence, and do not lead to dopamine release from reward pathways (Fantegrossi et al. 2008). Results from recent U.S. population surveys of adolescents and adults parallel these findings and strongly suggest that hallucinogens are infrequently used. According to data from the 2018 National Survey on Drug Use and Health (NSDUH), hallucinogens are most commonly used in late adolescence and young adulthood, with up to 17% of respondents between the ages of 18 and 25 years reporting having used a hallucinogen at least once in their lifetime (Substance Abuse and Mental Health Services Administration 2019). Hallucinogen use is generally sporadic, clustered, or infrequent, as evidenced by the finding that only 7% of respondents in the 18- to 25-year age group reported such use over the past year. It is uncommon for hallucinogen use to persist beyond young adulthood; only 1.3% of respondents older than 25 years reported past-year use of hallucinogens (Substance Abuse and Mental Health Services Administration 2019).

Barring atypical substances that might be grouped with hallucinogens—such as ketamine, nitrous oxide, certain phenethylamines (i.e., MDMA), or cannabis—hallucinogens do not create physiological dependence or tolerance, and dependence phenomena, such as an inability to stop using, are rarely seen (Fantegrossi et al. 2008; Glennon 2008; Passie et al. 2002). Hallucinogen abuse occurs when an individual continues to use hallucinogens despite repeatedly incurring any of the above adverse effects to the point of medical or psychosocial impairment. Thus, a hallucinogen use disorder (American Psychiatric Association 2013), especially if it involves classical hallucinogens, is unlikely to qualify for a "severe" specification (based on the number of DSM-5 criteria met), given the absence of dependence phenomena.

The criminalization of hallucinogens in 1966 was predicated on various claims of risk that are now recognized as false but that have nonetheless managed to persist despite a lack of supportive evidence (Bakalar and Grinspoon 1997). These unsubstantiated claims include concerns that classical hallucinogens cause chromosomal damage (Cohen and Shiloh 1977–1978); that they lead to suicide, murder, or debauchery, even when used in appropriate clinical settings (Malleson 1971; Studerus et al. 2011); or that they engender schizotypal personality changes or lasting psychotic disturbances in individuals without a pre-existing vulnerability (Malleson 1971; Studerus et al. 2011; Vardy and Kay 1983).

Conclusion

In the United States, classical hallucinogens are classified as Schedule I substances; this classification is reserved for substances of high abuse liability with no known medical benefits. Inasmuch as hallucinogens can be associated with substantial risks and are not established to be effective for any medical conditions, this classification is appropriate. However, the classification is problematic because it a priori dismisses agents with hallucinogenic effects as being without medical benefit. This blanket dismissal has led to difficult cultural, legal, and financial obstacles being placed in the way of investigators who seek to obtain a better understanding of the clinical utility, or lack thereof, of these compounds.

Despite such challenges, hallucinogen research has resumed in various academic centers around the world, and there is widespread interest in examining these compounds' clinical efficacy. Pharmaceutical companies have even emerged with an interest in taking certain hallucinogens, primarily psilocybin, to market. There is therefore greater attention being given to the therapeutic frameworks in which—and the clinical guidelines under which—these substances might be provided to optimal effect. This increased attention has allowed for a more sensitive appraisal of the risks and benefits of this substance class, and of how those risks and benefits might be balanced appropriately.

The story of hallucinogens awaits its next chapter. It is not yet clear whether these compounds are as helpful or as clinically effective as preliminary research suggests. Nevertheless, there are important lessons we can draw from these compounds thus far—lessons that we may generalize to even cocaine and heroin. The most important lesson is that most drugs are only as dangerous as how they are used. For many drugs, helpfulness overlaps with harmfulness—that is, the same properties that might be beneficial may also present risk. Hallucinogens reveal this paradox to us quite clearly and thus underscore the importance of a responsible and knowledgeable approach to psychoactive compounds.

Hallucinogens are only as dangerous, in other words, as we are—in all our carelessness, irresponsibility, and insensitivity. Perhaps the psychedelic (mind-manifesting) quality attributed to hallucinogens extends beyond psychological revelation. The mirror might reveal much else. We look into the reflection these substances provide, and find, for better or worse, ourselves.

References

American Psychiatric Association: Diagnostic and Statistical Manual of Mental Disorders, 5th Edition. Arlington, VA, American Psychiatric Association, 2013

Bakalar J, Grinspoon L: Psychedelic Drugs Reconsidered, 3rd Edition. New York, The Lindemith Center, 1997

Bleeker T: Diane Linkletter: A Princess Wrongly Accused. Scotts Valley, CA, CreateSpace Independent Publishing Platform, 2016

Carhart-Harris RL, Erritzoe D, Williams T, et al: Neural correlates of the psychedelic state as determined by fMRI studies with psilocybin. Proc Natl Acad Sci USA 109(6):2138–2143, 2012 22308440

Carhart-Harris RL, Leech R, Erritzoe D, et al: Functional connectivity measures after psilocybin inform a novel hypothesis of early psychosis. Schizophr Bull 39(6):1343–1351, 2013 23044373

Cohen MM, Shiloh Y: Genetic toxicology of lysergic acid diethylamide (LSD-25). Mutat Res 47(3–4):183–209, 1977–1978 99650

DiPaolo M: LSD and the hippies: a focused analysis of criminalization and persecution in the sixties. The People, Ideas, and Things (PIT) Journal, Social Science category, Cycle 9, 2018. Available at: http://pitjournal.unc.edu/content/lsd-and-hippies-focused-analysis-criminalization-and-persecution-sixties. Accessed August 18, 2020.

Fantegrossi WE, Murnane KS, Reissig CJ: The behavioral pharmacology of hallucinogens. Biochem Pharmacol 75(1):17–33, 2008 17977517

Glennon RA: Neurobiology of hallucinogens, in The American Psychiatric Publishing Textbook of Substance Abuse Treatment, 4th Edition. Washington, DC, American Psychiatric Publishing, 2008, pp 181–189

Gouzoulis-Mayfrank E, Schreckenberger M, Sabri O, et al: Neurometabolic effects of psilocybin, 3,4-methylenedioxyethylamphetamine (MDE) and d-methamphetamine in healthy volunteers. A double-blind, placebo-controlled PET study with [18F]FDG. Neuropsychopharmacology 20(6):565–581, 1999 10327426

Griffiths RR, Richards WA, McCann U, et al: Psilocybin can occasion mystical-type experiences having substantial and sustained personal meaning and spiritual significance. Psychopharmacology (Berl) 187(3):268–283; discussion 284–292, 2006 16826400

Griffiths R, Richards W, Johnson M, et al: Mystical-type experiences occasioned by psilocybin mediate the attribution of personal meaning and spiritual significance 14 months later. J Psychopharmacol 22(6):621–632, 2008 18593735

Hoffer A: Treatment of alcoholism with psychedelic therapy, in The Uses and Implications of Hallucinogenic Drugs. Edited by Aaronson B, Osmond H. London, Hogarth Press, 1970, pp 357–366

Hofmann A: LSD—My Problem Child: Reflections on Sacred Drugs, Mysticism and Science, 4th Edition. Santa Cruz, CA, Multidisciplinary Association for Psychedelic Studies, 2009

Hofmann A, Schultes RE: Plants of the Gods: Their Sacred, Healing, and Hallucinogenic Powers. New York, McGraw-Hill, 1979

Imperi LL, Kleber HD, Davie JS: Use of hallucinogenic drugs on campus. JAMA 204(12):1021–1024, 1968 5694746

Johnson M, Richards W, Griffiths R: Human hallucinogen research: guidelines for safety. J Psychopharmacol 22(6):603–620, 2008 18593734

Kornheiser T: Art Linkletter: He Stooped To Conquer. The Washington Post, October 11, 1981. Available at: https://www.washingtonpost.com/archive/lifestyle/style/1981/10/11/art-linkletter-he-stooped-to-conquer/18b1dd82-3c36-4eb8-ba81-31b2374e3214/. Accessed August 18, 2020.

Leuner H: Hallucinogens as an aid in psychotherapy: basic principles and results, in 50 Years of LSD: Current Status and Perspectives of Hallucinogen Research. Edited by Pletscher A, Ladewig D. New York, Parthenon, 1994, pp 175–190

Malleson N: Acute adverse reactions to LSD in clinical and experimental use in the United Kingdom. Br J Psychiatry 118(543):229–230, 1971 4995932

Marlan D: Beyond cannabis: psychedelic decriminalization and social justice. Lewis & Clark Law Review 23(3):851–892, 2019. Available at: https://law.lclark.edu/live/files/28626-lcb233article3marlanwebsitepdf. Accessed August 18, 2020.

Passie T, Seifert J, Schneider U, et al: The pharmacology of psilocybin. Addict Biol 7(4):357–364, 2002 14578010

Scheidegger M, Walter M, Lehmann M, et al: Ketamine decreases resting state functional network connectivity in healthy subjects: implications for antidepressant drug action. PLoS One 7(9):e44799, 2012 23049758

Schreckenberger M, Gouzoulis-Mayfrank E, Sabri O, et al: The psilocybin psychosis as a model psychosis paradigm for acute schizophrenia: a PET study with 18-FDG. European Journal of Nuclear Medicine 25(8):877, 1998. Available at: https://link.springer.com/article/10.1007/BF02793931. Accessed December 22, 2019.

Studerus E, Kometer M, Hasler F, et al: Acute, subacute and long-term subjective effects of psilocybin in healthy humans: a pooled analysis of experimental studies. J Psychopharmacol 25(11):1434–1452, 2011 20855349

Studerus E, Gamma A, Kometer M, et al: Prediction of psilocybin response in healthy volunteers. PLoS One 7(2):e30800, 2012 22363492

Substance Abuse and Mental Health Services Administration: Key substance use and mental health indicators in the United States: results from the 2018 National Survey on Drug Use and Health (HHS Publication No. PEP19-5068, NSDUH Series H-54). Rockville, MD, Center for Behavioral Health Statistics and Quality, Substance Abuse and Mental Health Services Administration, August 2019. Available at: https://www.samhsa.gov/data/sites/default/files/cbhsq-reports/NSDUHNationalFindingsReport2018/NSDUHNationalFindingsReport2018.pdf. Accessed August 18, 2020.

Vardy MM, Kay SR: LSD psychosis or LSD-induced schizophrenia? A multimethod inquiry. Arch Gen Psychiatry 40(8):877–883, 1983 6870484

Vollenweider FX, Kometer M: The neurobiology of psychedelic drugs: implications for the treatment of mood disorders. Nat Rev Neurosci 11(9):642–651, 2010 20717121

CHAPTER 16

Neurobiology of Marijuana

Gregory Sahlem, M.D.

Brian Sherman, Ph.D.

Aimee McRae-Clark, Pharm.D.

Though often thought of as a singular substance, marijuana—or, more accurately, cannabis—consists of at least 100 phytochemicals with distinct chemical structures. The behavioral effects of cannabis have been well described for centuries, but the endogenous system that cannabis works upon was only discovered in the early 1990s. Since that time, much research has been done to uncover the substrates and neural systems associated with the endocannabinoid system.

In this chapter we review the structure of the endocannabinoid system, the endogenous ligands and metabolic pathways that regulate it, and the most well described exogenous cannabinoids that activate it. We also look at the current state of the literature in reference to the neurobiology of several of the oft-described behavioral effects of cannabis—namely, its cognitive, analgesic, soporific, and sedative effects.

The Endocannabinoid System

In 1964, the main active cannabinoid substance of the cannabis plant, Δ^9-tetrahydrocannabinol (THC), was isolated. This advance was followed by the discovery of the G protein–coupled cannabinoid type 1 (CB_1) brain receptor, through which THC exerts its psychoactive effects. Given that other brain receptors, such as opioid receptors, have endogenous ligands, subsequent research focused on identification of endogenous cannabinoids. Anandamide, the first endogenous cannabinoid, was found in 1992, followed by 2-arachidonoylglycerol (2-AG) in 1993, along with the discovery of a second cannabinoid receptor (CB_2); other endogenous cannabinoid ligands have since been identified. The term "endocannabinoid (eCB) system" is often used to refer to these endogenous ligands along with the cannabinoid receptors and enzymes responsible for ligand biosynthesis and deactivation (Di Marzo et al. 2004).

The eCB system is involved in a myriad of physiological processes. CB_1 receptors are concentrated primarily in the central nervous system. The highest densities of CB_1 receptors are found in the basal ganglia and cerebellum, which likely accounts for the well-described impact of cannabis and cannabinoids on movement and coordination. Memory impairments associated with cannabis are likely related to the presence of CB_1 receptors in the hippocampal region and cortex. CB_1 receptors are also found in ascending and descending pain pathways, as well as in brain regions associated with reward, such as the nucleus accumbens. In contrast, the CB_2 receptor is largely restricted to immune tissues and cells and may be implicated in inflammatory and chronic pain processes.

The marijuana plant, *Cannabis sativa*, contains at least 100 phytocannabinoids that interact with the natural eCB system. The two most widely studied phytocannabinoids are THC and cannabidiol (CBD). THC is a partial CB_1 agonist with a strong affinity for CB_1 receptors (Di Marzo and Piscitelli 2015); CBD has low affinity for CB_1 receptors, but it can provide functional antagonism at CB_1 receptors at low concentrations (Pertwee 2008). Plant-based cannabis contains varying levels of THC, CBD, and other cannabinoids. Currently, there are also commercially available purified preparations of THC (dronabinol) and CBD, as well as a synthetic THC analog (nabilone). In addition, there is a commercially available oromucosal spray that combines purified THC and CBD in a 1:1 ratio.

Functional Significance of Endocannabinoid System and Impacts of Cannabis Use

Cognition and Brain Development

The eCB system plays a critical role in neurodevelopment and cognition (for reviews, see Curran et al. 2016, Dow-Edwards and Silva 2017, and Sagar and Gruber 2018). The eCB system is heavily involved in the neurogenesis and synaptic pruning that occur during critical stages of cortical development. Exogenous cannabinoid exposure during these developmental periods is thought to affect this process. THC, the primary intoxicating component of cannabis, has been shown to disrupt the natural eCB system, including the neuroplastic processes of long-term potentiation and long-term depression, and to alter brain structure and function. In contrast, growing evidence suggests that CBD exerts opposing effects on neural function and may ameliorate cognitive decrements associated with THC exposure (Lorenzetti et al. 2016). Furthermore, a preclinical study indicated that THC exposure may actually enhance cognitive performance in older adulthood by stimulating the aging eCB system (Bilkei-Gorzo et al. 2017), suggesting potential differential impacts of THC exposure based on age and stage of brain development.

Extensive literature documents the effects of cannabis on cognitive functioning across various domains. There is a general consensus that cannabis use is associated with decrements in certain aspects of memory and executive function (for a review, see Broyd et al. 2016), although other findings are equivocal. Acute effects of cannabis include decrements in working and episodic memory; however, evidence on the non-acute effects of cannabis on working memory is mixed. Robust evidence supports the association between cannabis use and deficits in verbal learning and memory, particularly on measures of encoding, recall, and recognition. Aspects of executive functioning such as response inhibition, planning, and decision making have shown consistent impairment in both current and recent cannabis users. The association between cannabis use and other aspects of memory such as visuospatial and associative memory is less clear. Fewer studies have examined processing speed, but some evidence suggests reduced processing speed in cannabis users compared with nonusers. This heterogeneity of findings on the cognitive effects of cannabis may be due to several moderating factors, including frequency and quantity of use, periods of abstinence, and age at onset of use. Although further research is needed to account for these factors, converging evidence largely suggests the reversal of cognitive decrements within 4 weeks of abstinence.

Evidence on whether cannabis affects overall IQ is also equivocal. An initial large prospective cohort study found up to a six-point decline in IQ from ages 7–13 years to age 38 years among individuals with persistent cannabis dependence (Meier et al. 2012). However, two prospective cohort studies with larger samples did not find an association with cannabis use and IQ between users and nonusing control subjects (Mokrysz et al. 2016) or among twin pairs that were discordant on use (Jackson et al. 2016). All three studies had limitations, including retrospective self-report of cannabis use and inability to adjust for variations in cannabis potency or delivery method. For this reason, the relationship between cannabis use and IQ remains inconclusive.

Brain imaging studies have led to a better understanding of the neural substrates associated with cannabis-related functional impairment (for reviews, see Curran et al. 2016 and Sagar and Gruber 2018). Numerous studies of executive function in cannabis users (Gruber and Yurgelun-Todd 2005; Kober et al. 2014; Sagar et al. 2015) have found altered activation in the frontal cortex (including the anterior cingulate and dorsolateral prefrontal cortex), a region typically associated with impulse control, problem solving, and judgment, among other functions. In functional magnetic resonance imaging (fMRI) studies examining working memory (Kanayama et al. 2004; Padula et al. 2007; Smith et al. 2010), cannabis users demonstrate significantly increased neural activation compared with healthy nonusing control subjects, yet perform similarly on spatial working memory tasks. Similar task performance despite increased activation may reflect inefficient use of neural resources among cannabis users (i.e., cannabis users expend greater neural resources to achieve the same outcome). Cannabis use may also result in sensitization of the incentive-motivational reward pathway, as evidenced by hyperactivation of the striatum during monetary incentive delay tasks (Jager et al. 2013; Nestor et al. 2010).

Alterations in brain structure have been found in cannabis users, particularly in brain regions high in CB_1 receptor density (Lorenzetti et al. 2016; Sagar and Gruber 2018). However, evidence shows bidirectional volumetric changes in gray matter. For example, among cannabis users, studies show larger gray matter volume in the cerebellum and striatum but smaller gray matter volume in the hippocampus (Batalla et al. 2013). White matter integrity has also been investigated with diffusion tensor imaging. Adult and adolescent cannabis users show reduced white matter fiber tract integrity in prefrontal, limbic, parietal, and cerebellar tracts (Batalla et al. 2013; Sagar and Gruber 2018). Notably, there is evidence to suggest that CBD may mitigate structural alterations (Lorenzetti et al. 2016; Yücel et al. 2016), and because most studies do not account for cannabis composition (THC:CBD ratio), individual variation in total CBD vs. THC exposure could explain some of the discordant findings regarding brain alterations. Likewise, early onset of cannabis use is associated with structural changes in both gray and white matter (Clark et al. 2012; Filbey et al. 2015; Gruber et al. 2014).

In summary, the eCB system is intimately involved in neurodevelopment, homeostasis, and cognition. Existing evidence suggests that exogenous cannabis exposure disrupts the body's natural eCB system, resulting in cognitive impairment and alterations in brain structure and function. These effects may be heightened during adolescence, which is a particularly vulnerable period of cortical development. However, evidence is not sufficient to infer causality, as there are several potential moderating factors, including age at onset of use, frequency and quantity of use, length of abstinence, cannabis composition (THC:CBD ratio), and premorbid intellectual functioning. Future research should account for these factors.

Pain

Pain relief is one of the most commonly reported medicinal uses of cannabis (Ilgen et al. 2013). The term *pain,* however, is a catchall term used to describe a variety of conditions, each with different etiologies, characteristics, and courses. Furthermore, the experience of pain is divided into sensory aspects (the signal itself) and emotional aspects (the reaction to the signal), and the term *pain* describes both acute pain (the sensory and emotional experience directly linked to an ongoing injury) and chronic pain (a sensory and emotional experience that is the result of a remote injury or an occult etiology, as is the case in fibromyalgia).

As discussed above, CB_1 receptors are located diffusely throughout both the central and peripheral nervous systems, and they have a high density throughout several brain regions with known importance in the pain system (e.g., peripheral pain pathways, the ascending pain portion of the spinal cord, and higher central pain-related regions such as the medial prefrontal cortex). CB_2 receptors are also found in the central nervous system; however, they are predominately found peripherally in immune cells involved in the inflammatory response system. The eCB system thus has a direct input into several pathways important in the conduction and modulation of pain. Several preclinical studies have demonstrated that activation of the eCB system via a variety of means (orthosterically, allosterically, and through blockade of degradation enzymes) results in an analgesic effect in a diverse series of animal models and pain paradigms (Woodhams et al. 2017). Despite promising preclinical work, clinical trials activating the eCB system have largely been disappointing; however, utilizing this system remains an active area of study.

A number of trials have directly tested the administration of cannabinoids (both plant-based and synthetically derived preparations) for analgesia. Analgesia is commonly measured experimentally using objective laboratory-based paradigms (often termed quantitative sensory testing [QST]). In QST, a painful experimental stimulus is applied at either a fixed or an escalating intensity. *Pain threshold* (defined as the minimum stimulus experienced as painful) and *pain tolerance* (i.e., the maximum bearable stimulus) are measured objectively, and the associated subjective experience is measured by participant report and separated into sensory (intensity) and affective (unpleasantness) experiences. In a recent meta-analysis, De Vita et al. (2018) reviewed data from studies that used QST to investigate the acute analgesic effects of cannabinoid administration. Some of the studies reviewed demonstrated that cannabinoids had a positive effect in QST testing (primarily in the domains of pain threshold, pain tolerance, and the affective component of pain), although cannabinoids did not appear to confer any benefit in pain intensity or hyperalgesia paradigms. The pooled effect sizes were small to medium overall, and cannabinoids appeared to be most robust in reducing the affective component of pain. Generally, plant-based cannabis had a larger effect than isolated THC (dronabinol) or synthetic THC (nabilone), and higher doses had a larger effect than lower doses. To date, there have been no studies exploring the utility of isolated CBD in the reduction of laboratory-induced pain. Although interesting, the existing literature is limited by studies strictly using psychoactive cannabinoids (with the resultant feeling of being high) and not exploring pain paradigms inducing neuropathic pain.

There have also been a multitude of studies testing the utility of cannabinoid administration in various pain conditions (see Stockings et al. 2018 for a comprehensive review and meta-analysis of chronic noncancer pain, and Davis 2016 for a review of cancer pain); however, with the exception of studies examining pain related to multiple sclerosis, to date, there have been only a few studies performed that would be considered highly rigorous (e.g., including well-defined populations and outcomes, using a double-blind design, and having a placebo control condition). In chronic noncancer pain, the majority of trials have studied the utility of various cannabinoids in neuropathic pain. Although less well investigated, there are also studies evaluating the efficacy of cannabinoids in other mixed pain conditions such as rheumatoid arthritis and fibromyalgia. When all of these trials are considered together, there appears to be a consistent but small analgesic effect; however, it should be noted that the literature in this area is heterogeneous, and some trials have reported larger beneficial effects. Two recent trials evaluated the use of combined THC and CBD in cancer pain, with one suggesting a benefit (Johnson et al. 2010) and the other failing to achieve an effect in the planned analysis (Portenoy et al. 2012), further suggesting that the use of cannabinoids for clinical pain disorders is complex.

The majority of published studies have been short in duration, and only a few trials have included a placebo condition that mimics the psychoactive effects of cannabis. Areas in need of further study include the determination of which cannabinoid preparation is most efficacious for pain and the optimal frequency, route of administration, and dose of cannabinoid. In addition, beneficial effects must be weighed against the potential consequences of cannabinoid use (Volkow et al. 2014).

Sleep

Sleep disruption is a common complaint among adults worldwide, with clinically relevant sleep disruption described by 10%–15% of the population (Morin and Jarrin 2013). Given the often-described sedative-hypnotic properties of cannabis, it is unsurprising that users of medicinal cannabis cite insomnia as a common therapeutic reason for its use (Ilgen et al. 2013). Sleep is colloquially thought to be a static process; however, sleep itself is divided into physiologically distinct stages, often referred to as the architecture of sleep. The main architectural components of sleep include rapid eye movement (REM) sleep, which is important in certain types of memory consolidation and emotion regulation, and non-REM (NREM) sleep, which is important in other types of memory consolidation and the maintenance of daytime vigilance and wakefulness. Furthermore, sleep is more appropriately thought of as one pole in the interdependent sleep-wake cycle. The sleep-wake cycle is dependent on both behavioral factors and intrinsic physiological factors governed by the intrinsic rhythmic pacemaker of the body, the suprachiasmatic nucleus.

The eCB system appears to play a role in the sleep-wake cycle and vice versa (Prospéro-García et al. 2016). Work with animals has demonstrated that there are diurnal variations in CB_1 receptor density, the concentration of both of the endocannabinoid ligands (2-AG and anandamide), and the degradative enzymes involved in the eCB system (monoacylglycerol lipase [MAGL] and fatty acid amide hydrolase [FAAH]). Furthermore, CB_1 receptors have been found on the suprachiasmatic nucleus, and activation of the eCB system may alter processes involved in circadian shifts in the sleep-wake system. Early human data are consistent with preclinical studies, with a variation of 2-AG levels that is similar between humans and animals. Consistent with behavioral reports of a sedative-hypnotic effect of cannabis, administration of anandamide and 2-AG increases sleep in animal models and reduces wakefulness, and the eCB system appears to have a higher level of activation during sleep compared with wakefulness. A noteworthy exception to the increased activity of the eCB system during sleep is that there are higher plasma levels of 2-AG during the daytime in humans, which may be related to a U-shaped dose-response curve.

Studies examining the effect of cannabinoid administration in general, and especially administration prior to sleep, have suggested a more complicated picture than the intuitive and commonly made assertion that cannabinoids have hypnotic effects (Babson et al. 2017). Of note, the majority of trials on this topic would not be considered to be of high scientific rigor, and most commonly report the effect of various cannabinoids on the sleep of healthy volunteers or chronic users of cannabis. Despite these limitations, several studies have reported that cannabinoids improve subjective sleep quality; however, findings from studies looking at sleep architecture have been notably mixed. In general terms, cannabinoids acutely administered to nonchronic cannabis smokers prior to sleep have resulted in improved measures of sleep architecture, although there have been both positive and negative reports. Sleep studies in more chronic users of cannabis have yielded results suggestive of sleep disruption, although these types of studies are methodologically challenging, and definitive conclusions are difficult to draw. One of the more consistently reported effects of cannabis on sleep is the clear and substantial sleep disruption that accompanies the withdrawal syndrome (Budney et al. 2008; Vandrey et al. 2011). Sleep disruption during withdrawal can be long-lasting and is predictive of relapse during quit attempts (Babson et al. 2013). The data in this regard thus suggest that the sedative effects of cannabinoids are most pronounced with acute administration, and that there is an accommodation to this effect (similar to that with benzodiazepines). To date, there have not been any rigorous trials testing the effects of cannabinoids in the treatment of insomnia disorder; however, studies looking at the sleep disruption accompanying posttraumatic stress disorder (PTSD) (Jetly et al. 2015) and fibromyalgia (Ware et al. 2010) have reported sleep improvements in both conditions with cannabinoid administration.

Despite the common assertion that cannabinoids are useful as hypnotics, the existing literature is unclear in this regard, especially in the case of using cannabinoids therapeutically. As is the case with other potential clinical uses for cannabinoids, further research in this area that employs rigorous study designs is needed.

Stress Response

Among chronic users of cannabis, stress has been shown to be a significant factor in maintenance of use (for a review, see Hyman and Sinha 2009). In treatment-seeking samples, stress relief is a commonly reported benefit from and reason for continuing cannabis use. Studies have also shown that coping motives are associated with levels of cannabis use and cannabis-related problems (Bonn-Miller et al. 2007; Simons et al. 2005). Additionally, stress-related factors such as negative life events and traumatic stress have demonstrated associations with cannabis use.

In response to acute stress, the hypothalamic-pituitary-adrenal (HPA) axis releases corticotropin-releasing hormone (CRH) from the hypothalamus, which in turn promotes the release of adrenocorticotropic hormone (ACTH) from the anterior pituitary gland and cortisol from the adrenal cortex. Additional neuropeptides, such as oxytocin and vasopressin, act synergistically with CRH to stimulate ACTH release from the pituitary. Stress response is terminated through glucocorticoid-mediated negative feedback, primarily at the level of the paraventricular nucleus (PVN) and the pituitary. Of note, CB_1 receptors are highly expressed in multiple brain regions involved in HPA axis response, such as the hippocampus, amygdala, prefrontal cortex, and PVN, and stress produces rapid changes in eCB signaling in stress-responsive brain pathways (Micale and Drago 2018). Furthermore, the eCB system is also involved in rapid negative-feedback control of the HPA axis system during stress.

Both chronic stress and substance use have been shown to disrupt normal HPA axis functioning (Koob and Kreek 2007). Several, but not all, laboratory-based studies have found an increased cortisol response following acute cannabis administration (for a review, see Cservenka et al. 2018). Some work suggests that abstinent individuals with cannabis use disorder have a blunted cortisol response compared with nonusers after THC administration (D'Souza et al. 2008; Ranganathan et al. 2009), which may suggest development of tolerance to the impact of cannabis on HPA axis reactivity. Acute stress exposure has been associated with reduced cortisol activity in heavy cannabis users compared with healthy control subjects (Cuttler et al. 2017; Nusbaum et al. 2017). More longitudinal research is needed to determine the impact of chronic cannabis use on HPA axis functioning and to determine whether cannabis-related HPA axis dysregulation contributes to continued cannabis use.

Given the role of the eCB system in stress responsivity, as well as clinical reports from patients that cannabis use alleviates stress-related symptoms, significant recent research has focused on a potential role for cannabinoids in the treatment of PTSD. Preclinical studies have shown that administration of a CB_1/CB_2 agonist after exposure to a stress model of PTSD prevents development of behavioral and neuroendocrine sequelae of the trauma (Ganon-Elazar and Akirav 2012, 2013). Furthermore, CB_1 activation in rodents impairs retrieval of aversive memories and facilitates their extinction, a finding that may have clinical relevance for PTSD-related flashbacks, intrusive memories, and nightmares (Marsicano et al. 2002; Niyuhire et al. 2007). However, clinical treatment trials to date have been limited and (like the studies in pain and sleep discussed in previous subsections) lacking in methodological rigor. A small preliminary trial of nabilone, an oral synthetic cannabinoid agonist, in male military personnel with PTSD-related nightmares reported reductions in nightmares and improvement in functioning (Jetly et al. 2015); positive findings were also reported in a small open-label trial of adjunctive dronabinol (oral Δ^9-tetrahydrocannabinol) in outpatients with PTSD (Roitman et al. 2014). A placebo-controlled trial of smoked cannabis for PTSD among veterans was recently conducted; results are not yet available.

Conclusion

The eCB system is critical for numerous physiological processes related to both normal and pathological functioning and may hold significant promise for novel therapeutic avenues. A growing body of preclinical research has elucidated the role of the eCB system in cognitive processes, pain, the response to stress, and sleep. However, more clinical research into the physiological, as well as potentially pathophysiological, roles of eCB activation and manipulation is needed.

References

Babson KA, Boden MT, Harris AH, et al: Poor sleep quality as a risk factor for lapse following a cannabis quit attempt. J Subst Abuse Treat 44(4):438–443, 2013 23098380

Babson KA, Sottile J, Morabito D: Cannabis, cannabinoids, and sleep: a review of the literature. Curr Psychiatry Rep 19(4):23, 2017 28349316

Batalla A, Bhattacharyya S, Yücel M, et al: Structural and functional imaging studies in chronic cannabis users: a systematic review of adolescent and adult findings (review). PLoS One 8(2):e55821, 2013 23390554

Bilkei-Gorzo A, Albayram O, Draffehn A, et al: A chronic low dose of delta9-tetrahydrocannabinol (THC) restores cognitive function in old mice. Nat Med 23(6):782–787, 2017 28481360

Bonn-Miller MO, Vujanovic AA, Feldner MT, et al: Posttraumatic stress symptom severity predicts marijuana use coping motives among traumatic event-exposed marijuana users. J Trauma Stress 20(4):577–586, 2007 17721963

Broyd SJ, van Hell HH, Beale C, et al: Acute and chronic effects of cannabinoids on human cognition—a systematic review. Biol Psychiatry 79(7):557–567, 2016 26858214

Budney AJ, Vandrey RG, Hughes JR, et al: Comparison of cannabis and tobacco withdrawal: severity and contribution to relapse. J Subst Abuse Treat 35(4):362–368, 2008 18342479

Clark DB, Chung T, Thatcher DL, et al: Psychological dysregulation, white matter disorganization and substance use disorders in adolescence. Addiction 107(1):206–214, 2012 21752141

Cservenka A, Lahanas S, Dotson-Bossert J: Marijuana use and hypothalamic-pituitary-adrenal axis functioning in humans. Front Psychiatry 9:472, 2018 30327619

Curran HV, Freeman TP, Mokrysz C, et al: Keep off the grass? Cannabis, cognition and addiction. Nat Rev Neurosci 17(5):293–306, 2016 27052382

Cuttler C, Spradlin A, Nusbaum AT, et al: Blunted stress reactivity in chronic cannabis users. Psychopharmacology (Berl) 234(15):2299–2309, 2017 28567696

Davis MP: Cannabinoids for symptom management and cancer therapy: the evidence. J Natl Compr Canc Netw 14(7):915–922, 2016 27407130

De Vita MM, Moskal D, Maisto SA, et al: Association of cannabinoid administration with experimental pain in healthy adults: a systematic review and meta-analysis. JAMA Psychiatry 75(11):1118–1127, 2018 30422266

Di Marzo V, Piscitelli F: The endocannabinoid system and its modulation by phytocannabinoids. Neurotherapeutics 12(4):692–698, 2015 26271952

Di Marzo V, Bifulco M, De Petrocellis L: The endocannabinoid system and its therapeutic exploitation. Nat Rev Drug Discov 3(9):771–784, 2004 15340387

Dow-Edwards D, Silva L: Endocannabinoids in brain plasticity: Cortical maturation, HPA axis function and behavior. Brain Res 1654(Pt B):157–164, 2017 27569586

D'Souza DC, Ranganathan M, Braley G, et al: Blunted psychotomimetic and amnestic effects of delta-9-tetrahydrocannabinol in frequent users of cannabis. Neuropsychopharmacology 33(10):2505–2516, 2008 18185500

Filbey FM, McQueeny T, DeWitt SJ, Mishra V: Preliminary findings demonstrating latent effects of early adolescent marijuana use onset on cortical architecture. Dev Cogn Neurosci 16:16–22, 2015 26507433

Ganon-Elazar E, Akirav I: Cannabinoids prevent the development of behavioral and endocrine alterations in a rat model of intense stress. Neuropsychopharmacology 37(2):456–466, 2012 21918506

Ganon-Elazar E, Akirav I: Cannabinoids and traumatic stress modulation of contextual fear extinction and GR expression in the amygdala-hippocampal-prefrontal circuit. Psychoneuroendocrinology 38(9):1675–1687, 2013 23433741

Gruber SA, Yurgelun-Todd DA: Neuroimaging of marijuana smokers during inhibitory processing: a pilot investigation. Brain Res Cogn Brain Res 23(1):107–118, 2005 15795138

Gruber SA, Dahlgren MK, Sagar KA, et al: Worth the wait: effects of age of onset of marijuana use on white matter and impulsivity. Psychopharmacology (Berl) 231(8):1455–1465, 2014 24190588

Hyman SM, Sinha R: Stress-related factors in cannabis use and misuse: implications for prevention and treatment. J Subst Abuse Treat 36(4):400–413, 2009 19004601

Ilgen MA, Bohnert K, Kleinberg F, et al: Characteristics of adults seeking medical marijuana certification. Drug Alcohol Depend 132(3):654–659, 2013 23683791

Jackson NJ, Isen JD, Khoddam R, et al: Impact of adolescent marijuana use on intelligence: results from two longitudinal twin studies. Proc Natl Acad Sci USA 113(5):E500–E508, 2016 26787878

Jager G, Block RI, Luijten M, Ramsey NF: Tentative evidence for striatal hyperactivity in adolescent cannabis-using boys: a cross-sectional multicenter fMRI study. J Psychoactive Drugs 45(2):156–167, 2013 23909003

Jetly R, Heber A, Fraser G, et al: The efficacy of nabilone, a synthetic cannabinoid, in the treatment of PTSD-associated nightmares: a preliminary randomized, double-blind, placebo-controlled cross-over design study. Psychoneuroendocrinology 51:585–588, 2015 25467221

Johnson JR, Burnell-Nugent M, Lossignol D, et al: Multicenter, double-blind, randomized, placebo-controlled, parallel-group study of the efficacy, safety, and tolerability of THC:CBD extract and THC extract in patients with intractable cancer-related pain. J Pain Symptom Manage 39(2):167–179, 2010 19896326

Kanayama G, Rogowska J, Pope HG, et al: Spatial working memory in heavy cannabis users: a functional magnetic resonance imaging study. Psychopharmacology (Berl) 176(3–4):239–247, 2004 15205869

Kober H, DeVito EE, DeLeone CM, et al: Cannabis abstinence during treatment and one-year follow-up: relationship to neural activity in men. Neuropsychopharmacology 39(10):2288–2298, 2014 24705568

Koob G, Kreek MJ: Stress, dysregulation of drug reward pathways, and the transition to drug dependence. Am J Psychiatry 164(8):1149–1159, 2007 17671276

Lorenzetti V, Solowij N, Yücel M: The role of cannabinoids in neuroanatomic alterations in cannabis users. Biol Psychiatry 79(7):e17–e31, 2016 26858212

Marsicano G, Wotjak CT, Azad SC, et al: The endogenous cannabinoid system controls extinction of aversive memories. Nature 418(6897):530–534, 2002 12152079

Meier MH, Caspi A, Ambler A, et al: Persistent cannabis users show neuropsychological decline from childhood to midlife. Proc Natl Acad Sci USA 109(40):E2657–E2664, 2012 22927402

Micale V, Drago F: Endocannabinoid system, stress and HPA axis. Eur J Pharmacol 834:230–239, 2018 30036537

Mokrysz C, Landy R, Gage SH, et al: Are IQ and educational outcomes in teenagers related to their cannabis use? A prospective cohort study. J Psychopharmacol 30(2):159–168, 2016 26739345

Morin CM, Jarrin DC: Epidemiology of insomnia: prevalence, course, risk factors, and public health burden. Sleep Medicine Clinics 8(3):281–297, 2013. Available at: https://www.sleep .theclinics.com/article/S1556-407X(13)00054-4/fulltext. Accessed August 17, 2020.

Nestor L, Hester R, Garavan H: Increased ventral striatal BOLD activity during non-drug reward anticipation in cannabis users. Neuroimage 49(1):1133–1143, 2010 19631753

Niyuhire F, Varvel SA, Martin BR, et al: Exposure to marijuana smoke impairs memory retrieval in mice. J Pharmacol Exp Ther 322(3):1067–1075, 2007 17586723

Nusbaum AT, Whitney P, Cuttler C, et al: Altered attentional control strategies but spared executive functioning in chronic cannabis users. Drug Alcohol Depend 181:116–123, 2017 29045919

Padula CB, Schweinsburg AD, Tapert SF: Spatial working memory performance and fMRI activation interaction in abstinent adolescent marijuana users. Psychol Addict Behav 21(4):478–487, 2007 18072830

Pertwee RG: Ligands that target cannabinoid receptors in the brain: from THC to anandamide and beyond. Addict Biol 13(2):147–159, 2008 18482430

Portenoy RK, Ganae-Motan ED, Allende S, et al: Nabiximols for opioid-treated cancer patients with poorly-controlled chronic pain: a randomized, placebo-controlled, graded-dose trial. J Pain 13(5):438–449, 2012 22483680

Prospéro-García O, Amancio-Belmont O, Becerril Meléndez AL, et al: Endocannabinoids and sleep. Neurosci Biobehav Rev 71:671–679, 2016 27756691

Ranganathan M, Braley G, Pittman B, et al: The effects of cannabinoids on serum cortisol and prolactin in humans. Psychopharmacology (Berl) 203(4):737–744, 2009 19083209

Roitman P, Mechoulam R, Cooper-Kazaz R, et al: Preliminary, open-label, pilot study of add-on oral delta9-tetrahydrocannabinol in chronic post-traumatic stress disorder. Clin Drug Investig 34(8):587–591, 2014 24935052

Sagar KA, Gruber SA: Marijuana matters: reviewing the impact of marijuana on cognition, brain structure and function, & exploring policy implications and barriers to research. Int Rev Psychiatry 30(3):251–267, 2018 29966459

Sagar KA, Dahlgren MK, Gönenç A, et al: The impact of initiation: early onset marijuana smokers demonstrate altered Stroop performance and brain activation. Dev Cogn Neurosci 16:84–92, 2015 25936584

Simons JS, Gaher RM, Correia CJ, et al: An affective-motivational model of marijuana and alcohol problems among college students. Psychol Addict Behav 19(3):326–334, 2005 16187813

Smith AM, Longo CA, Fried PA, et al: Effects of marijuana on visuospatial working memory: an fMRI study in young adults. Psychopharmacology (Berl) 210(3):429–438, 2010 20401748

Stockings E, Campbell G, Hall WD, et al: Cannabis and cannabinoids for the treatment of people with chronic noncancer pain conditions: a systematic review and meta-analysis of controlled and observational studies. Pain 159(10):1932–1954, 2018 29847469

Vandrey R, Smith MT, McCann UD, et al: Sleep disturbance and the effects of extended-release zolpidem during cannabis withdrawal. Drug Alcohol Depend 117(1):38–44, 2011 21296508

Volkow ND, Baler RD, Compton WM, et al: Adverse health effects of marijuana use. N Engl J Med 370(23):2219–2227, 2014 24897085

Ware MA, Fitzcharles MA, Joseph L, et al: The effects of nabilone on sleep in fibromyalgia: results of a randomized controlled trial. Anesth Analg 110(2):604–610, 2010 20007734

Woodhams SG, Chapman V, Finn DP, et al: The cannabinoid system and pain. Neuropharmacology 124:105–120, 2017 28625720

Yücel M, Lorenzetti V, Suo C, et al: Hippocampal harms, protection and recovery following regular cannabis use. Transl Psychiatry 6:e710, 2016 26756903

CHAPTER 17

Treatment of Cannabis-Related Disorders

Christina Brezing, M.D.

Souparno Mitra, M.D.

Frances R. Levin, M.D.

Cannabis is the third most common psychoactive substance used worldwide, after alcohol and tobacco (United Nations Office on Drugs and Crime 2015). In the United States alone, 4.2 million people report past-year cannabis use disorder (CUD) (Substance Abuse and Mental Health Services Administration 2017), which is associated with significant impairment and disability (Degenhardt et al. 2013), psychiatric and medical comorbidity, poor performance, and legal consequences. In 2014, 15% of all substance abuse treatment admissions (representing almost 300,000 people) had cannabis use as the primary presenting problem (Substance Abuse and Mental Health Services Administration 2016). There is clearly a need for treatment development in this area.

With the legalization of medical and recreational use of marijuana in the United States, the prevalence of marijuana use has increased (Washington State Institute for Public Policy 2017), accompanied by a decrease in perceived risk (Substance Abuse and Mental Health Services Administration 2017).

Modes of Use

Cannabis has been used since 4,000 B.C., and has traditionally been ingested by smoking the dried leaves (e.g., marijuana, Mary Jane) or the resin derived from cannabis (hashish). Marijuana is smoked (in pipes or bongs or as joints, blunts, or spliffs [mixed with nicotine]) or is inhaled in aerosol form via small handheld vaporizing devices (e.g., Juul)—referred to as "vaping." Resins and dried leaves are also mixed with milk and food products and consumed in the form of "edibles" such as gummy candy or baked goods.

Spice/K2 is a synthetic cannabinoid that has gained popularity among the college student population as well as marginalized populations (e.g., people with past drug-related charges) (Seely et al. 2012).

Neurobiology of Cannabis

Mechanism of Action

The two known cannabinoid receptor subtypes are CB_1 and CB_2, although recent evidence suggests the existence of additional receptors (Morales and Reggio 2017). Endogenous ligands of cannabinoid receptors include anandamide and 2-arachidonoyl-glycerol (2-AG), as well as several lesser-known endocannabinoids and related compounds. CB_1 receptors are found in high concentrations in the hippocampus, neocortex, basal ganglia, and cerebellum (Glass et al. 1997). This receptor distribution helps to explain the modulation of pain and the mediation of motivation, mood, and cognition by the endocannabinoid system. CB_2 receptors are present in peripheral tissues and are believed to modulate immune and inflammatory response. More recently, CB_2 receptors have been found on microglial cells in the brain and spinal cord, where they exist in increased quantities during injury (Ashton and Glass 2007). Phytocannabinoids (derived from plants) include Δ^9-tetrahydrocannabinol (THC), a CB_1 and CB_2 receptor partial agonist; cannabidiol (CBD), a CB_1 and CB_2 antagonist; and Δ^9-tetrahydrocannabivarin (THCV), a CB_1 and CB_2 antagonist in vivo and a partial agonist in vitro.

Neurochemical Actions Mediating Reward

The potency of marijuana is typically measured on the basis of the amount of THC present. However, marijuana's psychoactive and addictive properties may depend on the activity of endocannabinoids, other cannabinoids in the smoked marijuana, or interactions with other cannabinoids at receptors. High-dose CBD potentiates the effects of THC via a CB_1 receptor–dependent mechanism (Hayakawa et al. 2008). Cannabis use also corresponds to dopamine release in the ventral striatum, increased extracellular dopamine in the nucleus accumbens, and increased activity of dopamine neurons in the ventral tegmental area, and THC blocks synaptic plasticity in the nucleus accumbens (Bossong et al. 2009).

Neurobiological Aspects of Chronic Use

Chronic THC administration in rats results in downregulation and desensitization of CB_1 receptors (Breivogel et al. 2003), suggesting that the withdrawal is driven by a compensatory downregulation of the endocannabinoid system. THC decreases sensitivity to cannabinoids at GABA (γ-aminobutyric acid)–ergic and glutamatergic synapses, and CB_1 is coexpressed with serotonin and dopamine receptors such that a compensatory downregulation of the endocannabinoid system would interact with other neurotransmitters (Best and Regehr 2008; Melis et al. 2004).

Clinical Features

Acute Symptoms

The acute symptoms of cannabis use include dry mouth, increased appetite, euphoria, slurred speech, conjunctival injection, slowed reaction time, tachycardia, and elevated blood pressure. Users may experience anxiety, dysphoria, and panic as well as social withdrawal (Ashton 2001).

Chronic Use

Individuals with chronic (i.e., heavy and prolonged) use of cannabis have higher risks of bronchitis, cognitive impairment, and psychotic disorders (especially if they have a personal or family history of psychotic symptoms or disorders). Among adolescents, there may be impaired educational attainment. The most important effect seen is the development of CUD (Hall and Degenhardt 2014).

Withdrawal

In the fifth edition or the *Diagnostic and Statistical Manual of Mental Disorders* (DSM-5; American Psychiatric Association 2013), cannabis withdrawal is defined as having three or more of the following signs and symptoms that develop within 1 week after the abrupt reduction or cessation of heavy and prolonged cannabis use: 1) irritability, anger, or aggression; 2) nervousness or anxiety; 3) sleep difficulty (e.g., insomnia, disturbing dreams); 4) decreased appetite or weight loss; 5) restlessness; 6) depressed mood; and 7) at least one of the following physical symptoms that causes significant discomfort: abdominal pain, shakiness/tremors, sweating, fever, chills, or headache (American Psychiatric Association 2013, p. 518).

Treatment

Psychotherapy

Psychotherapy for substance use disorders was one of the first modalities used to treat CUD. The most effective modalities found so far include cognitive-behavioral therapy (CBT), motivational enhancement therapy (MET), contingency management (CM), a combination of the above, and some newer tested modalities (see subsection "Other Therapeutic Modalities").

Cognitive-Behavioral Therapy

CBT focuses on the learning processes involved in behavior. It employs strategies to prevent relapse, such as exploring positive and negative consequences of continued use, self-monitoring to recognize cravings and high-risk situations, and developing coping strategies for high-risk situations. Research has shown the efficacy of CBT in reducing the frequency of cannabis use and the severity of cannabis dependence (Gates et al. 2016). CBT is more effective than MET in maintaining abstinence; however, the combination of CBT plus MET is more efficacious than either used alone.

Motivational Enhancement Therapy

Motivational interviewing is a nonconfrontational counseling style that focuses on exploring and resolving ambivalence about drug use behaviors and on strengthening the motivation to change these behaviors. MET, an adaptation of motivational interviewing that is delivered in four sessions, has been shown to be effective in reducing the frequency of use and the severity of dependence (Gates et al. 2016). As mentioned above, the combination of MET and CBT has shown even greater efficacy than either modality alone.

Contingency Management

CM involves the utilization of monetary incentives such as vouchers for abstinence (confirmed by drug-negative urine tests). It has shown benefit in helping adolescents to achieve and maintain abstinence in clinical trials (Stanger et al. 2009). CM has also been shown to boost the effects of CBT/MET.

Other Therapeutic Modalities

For adolescents with substance use disorders, interventions may include family-based approaches or components. The Cannabis Youth Treatment Study (Dennis et al. 2004) compared five different short-term interventions for adolescents with cannabis use disorder ($N=600$): 1) a 5-session regimen of MET/CBT (MET/CBT5); 2) a 12-session regimen of MET/CBT (MET/CBT12); 3) family support network (FSN) therapy, consisting of MET/CBT plus six parent education classes; 4) the adolescent community reinforcement approach (ACRA), a blend of CBT, MET, family therapy, and systems-based approaches; and 5) multidimensional family therapy (MDFT), consisting of case management added to individual and family therapy. Across all treatments, adolescents increased their number of days abstinent by 24% (an average of 13 out of 54 days), with no significant differences between treatments (Dennis et al. 2004). However, the most cost-effective approaches were CBT/MET5 and ACRA.

Technology has also been incorporated into the delivery of therapy in innovative ways. The Peer Network Counseling Text services (Mason et al. 2018) divided participants into the treatment group who received text messages and an assessment-only control group. The study sent 112 texts over 4 weeks. The study found reduction of cannabis use in less severe CUD at 3 months of assessment. Sherman et al. (2018) used Approach Biased Modification Protocol. This protocol utilized four sessions based on the push-versus-pull model of CBT. The study used the Cannabis Approach Avoidance Task, a computerized task that aims to modify the approach bias or the impulse to approach rather than avoid a substance cue (Jacobus et al. 2018). In this task, participants were presented with cannabis-related and neutral images and asked to push (zoom out: avoidance) or pull (zoom in: approach) in response to a non-content-related stimulus feature. The intervention consisted of four sessions wherein the participants were trained to push when presented with cannabis-related stimuli. The study showed decreased sessions of cannabis use in men when compared with women in the active-use arm at the end of the trial, as well as decreased cue reactivity to cannabis-related images in the active-use arm (Sherman et al. 2018). Budney et al. (2015) evaluated the efficacy of a computer-delivered MET/CBT/CM intervention in

promoting abstinence from cannabis use. In the study, which involved 75 participants, the computer-based modality produced longer durations of abstinence than
MET alone during treatment. The computer-based interventions was just as effective
as the therapist-delivered version in maintaining abstinence rates and reductions in
days of use, while costing an average of $130 less (Budney et al. 2015).

Adherence-focused, guidance-enhanced, web-based self-help intervention with
social presence (Amann et al. 2018) is a new therapy protocol currently being tested in
a three-arm randomized controlled trial for its efficacy in reducing cannabis use in frequent users. The trial uses *CANreduce,* a web-based self-help intervention developed
by the Swiss Research Institute of Public Health and Addiction. This tool consists of a
dashboard, a consumption diary, and eight modules based on the principles of motivational interviewing and CBT that are administered over a period of 6 weeks. One of
the two treatment arms also includes social presence in the form of an eCoach, who
communicates with and helps motivate participants as they complete the modules.

Pharmacotherapy

Noncannabinoid Medications

Adrenergic agents.   The initial research investigating pharmacotherapy for CUD
was based on a study by Budney et al. (2008) that showed overlap in the phenotypes
of cannabis and nicotine withdrawal. The similarities between the phenotypes of
nicotine and cannabis withdrawal led to trials of sustained-release bupropion (Zyban), which inhibits the reuptake of norepinephrine and dopamine. However, in a
double-blind trial of bupropion for CUD, Haney et al. (2001) found that this drug exacerbated symptoms of cannabis withdrawal.

Participants with DSM-IV (American Psychiatric Association 1994) cannabis dependence ($N=13$) treated with atomoxetine in an open-label trial (Tirado et al. 2008)
showed a trend toward reduction of cannabis use. However, 80% of the subjects experienced gastrointestinal side effects (e.g., nausea, vomiting, loose stools) and could
not tolerate the medication.

In a placebo-controlled study of extended-release venlafaxine, both groups showed
improvement in mood; however, abstinence rates were low and were worse in the
group taking venlafaxine compared with the group receiving placebo (Levin et al.
2013). A secondary analysis (Kelly et al. 2014) demonstrated that individuals in the
venlafaxine group had more severe withdrawal symptoms than did those in the placebo group, despite not changing their cannabis use.

Mirtazapine is an antidepressant that enhances noradrenergic and serotonergic
transmission by blocking presynaptic inhibitory α_2 autoreceptors, resulting in sedation and increased appetite. A study from a human laboratory model of relapse prevention showed that although mirtazapine improved appetite and sleep symptoms,
it did not lead to any reductions in relapse. Mirtazapine may help with certain symptoms but has not shown efficacy as monotherapy (Haney et al. 2010).

Data from literature show that noradrenergic agents are not promising agents for
CUD. At best, they can help mitigate certain symptoms of cannabis withdrawal, and
at worst, these agents can cause severe side effects or exacerbate cannabis use.

Serotonergic agents.   Buspirone, a serotonin type 1A active agent, has been considered for treatment of CUD. A pilot placebo-controlled trial (McRae-Clark et al. 2009) found reductions in rates of cannabinoid-positive urine tests in treatment completers. However, the same group (McRae-Clark et al. 2015) completed a fully powered randomized controlled trial that did not replicate the pilot study findings. This study had a greater than 50% dropout rate and also demonstrated statistically significant negative urine tests in women in the placebo group and men in the treatment group, suggesting that gender may be an important independent variable in the development and evaluation of new treatments for CUD (McRae-Clark et al. 2015).

Studies have also been conducted with fluoxetine, vilazodone, and escitalopram (Cornelius et al. 2010; McRae-Clark et al. 2016; Weinstein et al. 2014), with limited evidence of benefit in CUD. Thus, serotonergic agents are not considered to be useful in the treatment of CUD other than for treatment of comorbid conditions or for targeting of specific symptoms such as food intake or sleep. Also, medication selection may depend on specific patient characteristics such as gender.

GABAergic agents.   Another approach to pharmacotherapy involves mitigation of additional symptoms of cannabis withdrawal such as irritability, mood lability, insomnia, and anxiety. A double-blind, placebo-controlled pilot study in a clinical setting (Levin et al. 2004) examined the efficacy of divalproex sodium in the treatment of CUD. Although both treatment and control groups showed reduced cannabis use with a decrease in irritability, divalproex had no added benefit. Participants were also found to be poorly adherent to divalproex sodium based on blood levels. The study concluded that the drug had no utility in the treatment of CUD.

Baclofen, a GABA class B (GABA$_B$) receptor agonist, was explored for the treatment of CUD, based on previous research (Haney et al. 2006) that showed its efficacy in reducing self-administration and mood symptoms in the context of other drugs of abuse (cocaine, heroin). Although baclofen was found to reduce craving for cannabis dose-dependently, it did not reduce relapse or have an effect on mood (Haney et al. 2010). Baclofen worsened one measure of sleep (i.e., early awakening) and one measure of cognitive performance (i.e., tracking on the Divided Attention Task).

Investigation of agents that target the GABA class A (GABA$_A$) receptor has been more promising. Sleep difficulty during abstinence may be an important factor in relapse. Vandrey et al. (2011) postulated that the use of extended-release zolpidem for treating sleep difficulty associated with abstinence from cannabis could be effective in preventing relapse. Using polysomnography, they found that zolpidem attenuated the effect of abstinence on sleep architecture and also improved subjective measures of sleep quality without any effects on next-day cognitive performance. Vandrey et al. (2011) concluded that the drug could be useful adjunctively as part of treatment. However, zolpidem is a benzodiazepine receptor–like drug and has been found to have abuse potential, dangerous withdrawal symptoms when dependence is established, and problematic side effects, including parasomnias (Keuroghlian et al. 2012). These risks must be kept in mind if the use of zolpidem for CUD is being considered.

Gabapentin indirectly modulates the GABAergic mechanism by blocking the α_{2d} subunit of voltage-gated calcium channels at selective presynaptic sites. It has been seen to increase extrahypothalamic corticotropin-releasing factor, thus modulating an anxiogenic-like state and restoring brain homeostasis in the context of stress (Roberto et al. 2008). A proof-of-concept pilot study by Mason et al. (2012) investigated the efficacy of gabapentin in CUD and found significant reductions in urine cannabinoids, cannabis use via self-report, withdrawal symptoms including craving, and problems secondary to marijuana use. Gabapentin also improved executive functioning in the study, although a cause-effect relationship could not be established. A larger, fully powered controlled trial was completed, and although publication is pending, preliminary results available on clinicaltrials.gov suggest a negative trial (NCT00974376).

Another GABAergic medication studied by Miranda et al. (2017) was topiramate. Topiramate blocks voltage-sensitive sodium and calcium channels, which results in potentiation of GABA with enhancement of $GABA_A$ receptor function in addition to antagonist activity at AMPA (α-amino-3-hydroxy-5-methyl-4-isoxazolepropionic acid)/kainate glutamate receptors. It was thought that this activity would be helpful in reducing the reinforcing effects of cannabis. The study found that youth taking topiramate reduced their use significantly in terms of grams per day; however, they experienced notable side effects, and many dropped out (Miranda et al. 2017). The clinician should bear in mind that slower titration and lower doses of medication, in addition to a good working alliance with the patient and close follow-up, may mitigate the risk of patient dropout from treatment and may achieve reductions in cannabis use. Also, adults may respond differently than youth to topiramate.

$GABA_A$ agonist sleep agents and other medications with $GABA_A$ activity, such as gabapentin and topiramate, show promise in the treatment of CUD to target difficulties with sleep as a result of withdrawal and/or maintenance treatment of CUD by decreasing cannabis use, respectively (Brezing and Levin 2018). Larger, fully powered placebo-controlled trials need to be completed.

Naltrexone. The μ-opioid receptor antagonist naltrexone has demonstrated some positive results in the treatment of CUD. Although one study demonstrated that acute treatments with different doses of naltrexone prior to smoking increased the positive subjective effects of cannabis in non-treatment-seeking heavy users (Cooper and Haney 2010), a second placebo-controlled human laboratory study with chronic naltrexone administration demonstrated a significant reduction in both active cannabis self-administration and self-report of positive effects as compared with placebo (Haney et al. 2015). The effect continued outside the laboratory. A follow-up open-label trial of injectable intramuscular naltrexone, consistent with long-term naltrexone dosing, not only demonstrated good overall tolerance of the medication and feasibility of its use in the outpatient treatment of CUD, but also showed a significant reduction in the number of cannabis use days per week (Notzon et al. 2018). Maintenance administration of naltrexone more accurately represents the use of this medication in the clinical setting. Given that long-term administration of naltrexone has been shown to reduce self-administration and days of cannabis use, further investigation of this medication is warranted.

Other agents. *N*-acetylcysteine (NAC) is a prodrug of the amino acid cysteine, which is a main component in the cysteine-glutamate exchanger, which controls glutamate levels. Gray et al. (2012) demonstrated that NAC treatment resulted in more than twice the odds of having a negative urine cannabinoid test compared with placebo in adolescents; however, this finding was not replicated in adults (Gray et al. 2017), a result suggesting that benefits from NAC may depend on patient age or CUD severity.

Lofexidine is an α_{2A}-adrenergic receptor agonist that has been tried in the treatment of CUD. A randomized, placebo-controlled study (Levin et al. 2016) with dronabinol 20 mg three times a day and lofexidine 0.6 mg three times a day showed a correlation between baseline amount of marijuana use and 21-day abstinence and a withdrawal score decrease in the treatment arm. However, participants experienced notable side effects, and there was no significant impact on cannabis use.

Guanfacine is a selective α_{2A} receptor agonist that has also been postulated to help in the treatment of CUD. In one study, 1 mg guanfacine was administered for 6 days followed by 1.5 mg for 4 days (Haney et al. 2018). The medication group demonstrated reductions in irritability and sleep latency and improvements in sleep efficiency, but guanfacine had no effect on relapse.

A novel agent that inhibits fatty acid amide hydrolase (FAAH), the enzyme responsible for breakdown of the endocannabinoids anandamide and 2-AG, has been studied for its potential utility in the treatment of CUD and cannabis withdrawal. In a double-blind randomized controlled trial in which men with cannabis dependence were randomly assigned to receive either the FAAH inhibitor (4 mg/day) or placebo, D'Souza et al. (2019) found reduced symptoms of cannabis withdrawal and diminished use of cannabis at week 4 in the group treated with the FAAH inhibitor.

Cannabinoid Medications

The use of CB_1 receptor agonists was considered because of the success seen with the use of agonist medications in the treatment of other substance use disorders. Generally, an ideal agonist substitute in the treatment of substance abuse has the properties of low abuse potential and less hazardous route of administration; it acts to reduce withdrawal symptoms and craving and decreases the reinforcing effects of the target drug, in this case, cannabis and its most psychoactive component, THC, and leads to an improvement in functioning (Balter et al. 2014).

Dronabinol.   Dronabinol (oral THC) has been approved by the U.S. Food and Drug Administration (FDA) to treat AIDS-associated anorexia. Haney et al. (2004) found that dronabinol 40 mg/day alleviated some symptoms of marijuana withdrawal, such as craving and decreased food intake, physical symptoms, and mood disturbance, without producing intoxication, but it failed to prevent relapse. This finding was replicated in further human laboratory studies (Vandrey et al. 2013). In a well-powered placebo-controlled trial (Levin et al. 2011), it was found that dronabinol had no effect on abstinence but did decrease withdrawal symptoms.

The mostly negative results of dronabinol in the treatment of CUD likely have to do with its poor bioavailability (Bedi et al. 2013), in conjunction with the differences in study designs. Dronabinol's slow onset and long duration of action can decrease craving and symptoms of withdrawal at doses that should produce minimal intoxication and thereby give dronabinol a role in this specific component of treatment. However, dronabinol's mixed effects on attenuating subjective effects and inability to impact reductions or abstinence rates in the clinical setting suggest that it is not sufficient as a monotherapy or in combination with lofexidine in the treatment of CUD.

Nabilone.   Nabilone, classified as a Schedule II drug by the U.S. Drug Enforcement Administration, is a potent synthetic cannabinoid that is currently FDA approved at dosages up to 6 mg/day for the second-line treatment of nausea and vomiting related to cancer chemotherapy. In comparison with dronabinol, nabilone has better oral bio-availability, improved efficacy, and a more linear dose effect (Bedi et al. 2013). Because nabilone (unlike the naturally derived oral THC dronabinol) is a synthetic cannabinoid, it has distinct urinary metabolites, allowing for monitoring with urine cannabinoid testing as usual.

Nabilone has been found to significantly decrease cannabis self-administration as a model of relapse, in addition to reducing ratings of irritability and "bad effect" during precipitated abstinence (Haney et al. 2013). High-dose nabilone also decreased craving. Nabilone reversed abstinence-induced sleep disturbances and changes in food intake. Nabilone also significantly reversed characteristic and problematic symptoms of cannabis withdrawal, in addition to decreasing a model of relapse, by not only decreasing cannabis self-administration but also reducing the use of cannabis in individuals who had relapsed from their baseline use (Haney et al. 2013). Although there is a theoretical risk of abuse that is greater with nabilone than with oral THC, human laboratory studies showed that participants reported few subjective effects from nabilone. It is likely that nabilone's properties as a long-acting and slow-onset-of-action agonist may make it less likely to have the abuse liability of smoked cannabis.

A clinical trial using nabilone (Hill et al. 2017) found a decrease in compulsivity, emotionality, and total scores on the Marijuana Craving Questionnaire (Heishman et al. 2001), but there was no difference in number of cannabis use sessions, percentage of use days at end of treatment, and number of inhalations at end of treatment between nabilone and placebo. However, the study results were restricted because the study was underpowered ($N=12$) and the dosages used were below the maximum prescribed limit of 6 mg/day (initial dosage of 0.5 mg/day with weekly increments to 2 mg/day).

Nabiximols.   Nabiximols contains extracts from the *Cannabis sativa* plant. These extracts include THC, which provides the agonist action, and CBD, a cannabinoid with proposed benefit in attenuating paranoia, euphoria, anxiety, and depression. A nabiximols buccal spray containing THC and CBD in a 1:1 ratio provides a more rapid onset of action and more favorable pharmacokinetics than oral THC.

In one study, nabiximols (113.4 mg THC/105 mg CBD) was administered as needed daily for 12 weeks with MET/CBT. Although there was a significant effect on time to relapse, there was no difference in abstinence rates between the nabiximols and placebo groups (Trigo et al. 2018). Cannabis use showed a 70.5% decrease in the nabiximols group versus 42.6% in the placebo group. Nabiximols also had a significant positive effect on craving and duration of withdrawal.

Cannabidiol.   Cannabidiol has minimal direct effect at cannabinoid receptors but has pharmacological actions such as inhibiting the hydrolysis and reuptake of endocannabinoids (Freeman et al. 2020). Freeman and colleagues conducted a randomized controlled trial to study the impact of cannabidiol (400 mg or 800 mg) on reduction of cannabis use. The study found that both 400 mg and 800 mg of cannabidiol decreased use (Freeman et al. 2020). However, the findings warrant a larger trial and replication of the findings.

Rimonabant.   Rimonabant is a high-affinity CB_1 receptor antagonist. Human laboratory studies of both a single high dose (90 mg) of rimonabant and repeated lower doses (40 mg) demonstrated reduced physiological and subjective effects of smoked cannabis (Huestis et al. 2007). However, the serious adverse psychiatric effects of rimonabant, which include anxiety, depression, and suicidality, led to discontinuation of its use in clinical trials (Roberfroid et al. 2010).

Treatment of Comorbid Psychiatric Conditions

Providers must be cognizant of comorbid psychiatric disorders when treating individuals with CUDs. Studies have suggested that receiving treatment for comorbid psychiatric disorders increases the likelihood that an individual will abstain from or reduce cannabis use. Two useful questions to consider in this context are 1) "If this patient were less depressed, would he or she be more likely to adhere to CBT treatment for relapse prevention?" and 2) "Among the different medications available to treat this patient's psychiatric disorder, would some be more likely than others to have a beneficial impact on the patient's substance use?"

A study in patients with co-occurring schizophrenia and CUD by Machielsen et al. (2018) found that clozapine was associated with greater decreases in marijuana craving and in positive and negative symptoms of schizophrenia than was risperidone. Similarly, another study in individuals with co-occurring attention-deficit/hyperactivity disorder (ADHD), cocaine use disorder, and CUD found that mixed amphetamine salts were associated with greater abstinence rates among patients receiving medication compared with those receiving placebo (Notzon et al. 2016). Thoughtful consideration and treatment of both the CUD and the co-occurring psychiatric disorders should be the primary approach taken by clinicians who care for patients with dual diagnoses.

Conclusion

A number of factors need to be considered in the treatment of CUD, including patient-centric factors such as severity of use, comorbid conditions, gender, and age. At present, there are no FDA-approved medications for treatment of CUD; however, there are various effective treatment modalities that show promise. Psychotherapies such as CBT, MET, CM, or a combination of these have been shown to be effective. In regard to pharmacotherapy, certain off-label noncannabinoid medications such as gabapentin, naltrexone, and NAC have shown efficacy. Also, cannabinoid medications such as nabilone, nabiximols, and cannabidiol, as well as a new FAAH-inhibiting agent capable of modulating endocannabinoid function, have shown promise in the treatment of CUD and cannabis withdrawal.

Finally, although many studies set their sights on abstinence as the primary outcome, few participants achieve this. It is more usual for studies to find reductions in use, although often not at higher rates than in the placebo-treated group. Reduction in use has been considered a reasonable outcome in medication treatment studies of other substance use disorders and is likely a reasonable goal in the treatment of CUD as well. However, at present, there is no consensus about what constitutes clinically meaningful reductions in cannabis use. Future research should explore functional outcomes that correlate with changes in cannabis use to better inform our conclusions about promising medications and other treatments for CUD.

References

Amann M, Haug S, Wenger A, et al: The effects of social presence on adherence-focused guidance in problematic cannabis users: protocol for the CANreduce 2.0 randomized controlled trial. JMIR Res Protoc 7(1):e30, 2018 29386176

American Psychiatric Association: Diagnostic and Statistical Manual of Mental Disorders, 4th Edition. Washington, DC, American Psychiatric Association, 1994

American Psychiatric Association: Diagnostic and Statistical Manual of Mental Disorders, 5th Edition. Arlington, VA, American Psychiatric Association, 2013

Ashton CH: Pharmacology and effects of cannabis: a brief review. Br J Psychiatry 178:101–106, 2001 11157422

Ashton JC, Glass M: The cannabinoid CB2 receptor as a target for inflammation-dependent neurodegeneration. Curr Neuropharmacol 5(2):73–80, 2007 18615177

Balter RE, Cooper ZD, Haney M: Novel pharmacologic approaches to treating cannabis use disorder. Curr Addict Rep 1(2):137–143, 2014 24955304

Bedi G, Cooper ZD, Haney M: Subjective, cognitive and cardiovascular dose-effect profile of nabilone and dronabinol in marijuana smokers. Addict Biol 18(5):872–881, 2013 22260337

Best AR, Regehr WG: Serotonin evokes endocannabinoid release and retrogradely suppresses excitatory synapses. J Neurosci 28(25):6508–6515, 2008 18562622

Bossong MG, van Berckel BN, Boellaard R, et al: Delta 9-tetrahydrocannabinol induces dopamine release in the human striatum. Neuropsychopharmacology 34(3):759–766, 2009 18754005

Breivogel CS, Scates SM, Beletskaya IO, et al: The effects of delta9-tetrahydrocannabinol physical dependence on brain cannabinoid receptors. Eur J Pharmacol 459(2–3):139–150, 2003 12524139

Brezing CA, Levin FR: The current state of pharmacological treatments for cannabis use disorder and withdrawal. Neuropsychopharmacology 43(1):173–194, 2018 28875989

Budney AJ, Vandrey RG, Hughes JR, et al: Comparison of cannabis and tobacco withdrawal: severity and contribution to relapse. J Subst Abuse Treat 35(4):362–368, 2008 18342479

Budney AJ, Stanger C, Tilford JM, et al: Computer-assisted behavioral therapy and contingency management for cannabis use disorder. Psychol Addict Behav 29(3):501–511, 2015 25938629

Cooper ZD, Haney M: Opioid antagonism enhances marijuana's effects in heavy marijuana smokers. Psychopharmacology (Berl) 211(2):141–148, 2010 20490465

Cornelius JR, Bukstein OG, Douaihy AB, et al: Double-blind fluoxetine trial in comorbid MDD-CUD youth and young adults. Drug Alcohol Depend 112(1–2):39–45, 2010 20576364

Degenhardt L, Ferrari AJ, Calabria B, et al: The global epidemiology and contribution of cannabis use and dependence to the global burden of disease: results from the GBD 2010 study. PLoS One 8(10):e76635, 2013 24204649

Dennis M, Godley SH, Diamond G, et al: The Cannabis Youth Treatment (CYT) study: main findings from two randomized trials. J Subst Abuse Treat 27(3):197–213, 2004 15501373

D'Souza DC, Cortes-Briones J, Creatura G, et al: Efficacy and safety of a fatty acid amide hydrolase inhibitor (PF-04457845) in the treatment of cannabis withdrawal and dependence in men: a double-blind, placebo-controlled, parallel group, phase 2a single-site randomised controlled trial. Lancet Psychiatry 6(1):35–45, 2019 30528676

Freeman TP, Hindocha C, Baio G, et al: Cannabidiol for the treatment of cannabis use disorder: a phase 2a, double-blind, placebo-controlled, randomised, adaptive Bayesian trial. Lancet Psychiatry July 28, 2020 [Online ahead of print] 32735782

Gates PJ, Sabioni P, Copeland J, et al: Psychosocial interventions for cannabis use disorder. Cochrane Database Syst Rev (5):CD005336, 2016 27149547

Glass M, Dragunow M, Faull RL: Cannabinoid receptors in the human brain: a detailed anatomical and quantitative autoradiographic study in the fetal, neonatal and adult human brain. Neuroscience 77(2):299–318, 1997 9472392

Gray KM, Carpenter MJ, Baker NL, et al: A double-blind randomized controlled trial of N-acetylcysteine in cannabis-dependent adolescents. Am J Psychiatry 169(8):805–812, 2012 22706327

Gray KM, Sonne SC, McClure EA, et al: A randomized placebo-controlled trial of N-acetylcysteine for cannabis use disorder in adults. Drug Alcohol Depend 177:249–257, 2017 28623823

Hall W, Degenhardt L: The adverse health effects of chronic cannabis use. Drug Test Anal 6(1–2):39–45, 2014 23836598

Haney M, Ward AS, Comer SD, et al: Bupropion SR worsens mood during marijuana withdrawal in humans. Psychopharmacology (Berl) 155(2):171–179, 2001 11401006

Haney M, Hart CL, Vosburg SK, et al: Marijuana withdrawal in humans: effects of oral THC or divalproex. Neuropsychopharmacology 29(1):158–170, 2004 14560320

Haney M, Hart CL, Foltin RW: Effects of baclofen on cocaine self-administration: opioid- and non-opioid-dependent volunteers. Neuropsychopharmacology 31(8):1814–1821, 2006 16407903

Haney M, Hart CL, Vosburg SK, et al: Effects of baclofen and mirtazapine on a laboratory model of marijuana withdrawal and relapse. Psychopharmacology (Berl) 211(2):233–244, 2010 20521030

Haney M, Cooper ZD, Bedi G, et al: Nabilone decreases marijuana withdrawal and a laboratory measure of marijuana relapse. Neuropsychopharmacology 38(8):1557–1565, 2013 23443718

Haney M, Ramesh D, Glass A, et al: Naltrexone maintenance decreases cannabis self-administration and subjective effects in daily cannabis smokers. Neuropsychopharmacology 40(11):2489–2498, 2015 25881117

Haney M, Cooper ZD, Bedi G, et al: Guanfacine decreases symptoms of cannabis withdrawal in daily cannabis smokers. Addict Biol 24(4):707–716, 2018 29659126

Hayakawa K, Mishima K, Hazekawa M, et al: Cannabidiol potentiates pharmacological effects of Delta(9)-tetrahydrocannabinol via CB(1) receptor-dependent mechanism. Brain Res 1188:157–164, 2008 18021759

Heishman SJ, Singleton EG, Liguori A: Marijuana Craving Questionnaire: development and initial validation of a self-report instrument. Addiction 96(7):1023–1034, 2001 11440613

Hill KP, Palastro MD, Gruber SA, et al: Nabilone pharmacotherapy for cannabis dependence: a randomized, controlled pilot study. Am J Addict 26(8):795–801, 2017 28921814

Huestis MA, Boyd SJ, Heishman SJ, et al: Single and multiple doses of rimonabant antagonize acute effects of smoked cannabis in male cannabis users. Psychopharmacology (Berl) 194(4):505–515, 2007 17619859

Jacobus J, Taylor CT, Gray KM, et al: A multi-site proof-of-concept investigation of computerized approach-avoidance training in adolescent cannabis users. Drug Alcohol Depend 187:195–204, 2018 29679914

Kelly MA, Pavlicova M, Glass A, et al: Do withdrawal-like symptoms mediate increased marijuana smoking in individuals treated with venlafaxine-XR? Drug Alcohol Depend 144:42–46, 2014 25283697

Keuroghlian AS, Barry AS, Weiss RD: Circadian dysregulation, zolpidem dependence, and withdrawal seizure in a resident physician performing shift work. Am J Addict 21(6):576–577, 2012 23082842

Levin FR, McDowell D, Evans SM, et al: Pharmacotherapy for marijuana dependence: a double-blind, placebo-controlled pilot study of divalproex sodium. Am J Addict 13(1):21–32, 2004 14766435

Levin FR, Mariani JJ, Brooks DJ, et al: Dronabinol for the treatment of cannabis dependence: a randomized, double-blind, placebo-controlled trial. Drug Alcohol Depend 116(1–3):142–150, 2011 21310551

Levin FR, Mariani J, Brooks DJ, et al: A randomized double-blind, placebo-controlled trial of venlafaxine-extended release for co-occurring cannabis dependence and depressive disorders. Addiction 108(6):1084–1094, 2013 23297841

Levin FR, Mariani JJ, Pavlicova M, et al: Dronabinol and lofexidine for cannabis use disorder: a randomized, double-blind, placebo-controlled trial. Drug Alcohol Depend 159:53–60, 2016 26711160

Machielsen MWJ, Veltman DJ, van den Brink W, et al: Comparing the effect of clozapine and risperidone on cue reactivity in male patients with schizophrenia and a cannabis use disorder: a randomized fMRI study. Schizophr Res 194:32–38, 2018 28351544

Mason BJ, Crean R, Goodell V, et al: A proof-of-concept randomized controlled study of gabapentin: effects on cannabis use, withdrawal and executive function deficits in cannabis-dependent adults. Neuropsychopharmacology 37(7):1689–1698, 2012 22373942

Mason MJ, Zaharakis NM, Moore M, et al: Who responds best to text-delivered cannabis use disorder treatment? A randomized clinical trial with young adults. Psychol Addict Behav 32(7):699–709, 2018 30265057

McRae-Clark AL, Carter RE, Killeen TK, et al: A placebo-controlled trial of buspirone for the treatment of marijuana dependence. Drug Alcohol Depend 105(1–2):132–138, 2009 19699593

McRae-Clark AL, Baker NL, Gray KM, et al: Buspirone treatment of cannabis dependence: a randomized, placebo-controlled trial. Drug Alcohol Depend 156:29–37, 2015 26386827

McRae-Clark AL, Baker NL, Gray KM, et al: Vilazodone for cannabis dependence: a randomized, controlled pilot trial. Am J Addict 25(1):69–75, 2016 26685701

Melis M, Pistis M, Perra S, et al: Endocannabinoids mediate presynaptic inhibition of glutamatergic transmission in rat ventral tegmental area dopamine neurons through activation of CB1 receptors. J Neurosci 24(1):53–62, 2004 14715937

Miranda R Jr, Treloar H, Blanchard A, et al: Topiramate and motivational enhancement therapy for cannabis use among youth: a randomized placebo-controlled pilot study. Addict Biol 22(3):779–790, 2017 26752416

Morales P, Reggio PH: An update on non-CB1, non-CB2 cannabinoid related G-protein-coupled receptors. Cannabis Cannabinoid Res 2(1):265–273, 2017 29098189

Notzon DP, Mariani JJ, Pavlicova M, et al: Mixed-amphetamine salts increase abstinence from marijuana in patients with co-occurring attention-deficit/hyperactivity disorder and cocaine dependence. Am J Addict 25(8):666–672, 2016 28051838

Notzon DP, Kelly MA, Choi CJ, et al: Open-label pilot study of injectable naltrexone for cannabis dependence. Am J Drug Alcohol Abuse 44(6):619–627, 2018 29420073

Roberfroid D, Lachat C, Lucet C: Termination of the CRESCENDO trial. Lancet 376(9757):1983–1984, author reply 1984–1985, 2010 21146095

Roberto M, Gilpin NW, O'Dell LE, et al: Cellular and behavioral interactions of gabapentin with alcohol dependence. J Neurosci 28(22):5762–5771, 2008 18509038

Seely KA, Lapoint J, Moran JH, Fattore L: Spice drugs are more than harmless herbal blends: a review of the pharmacology and toxicology of synthetic cannabinoids. Prog Neuropsychopharmacol Biol Psychiatry 39(2):234–243, 2012 22561602

Sherman BJ, Baker NL, Squeglia LM, et al: Approach bias modification for cannabis use disorder: a proof-of-principle study. J Subst Abuse Treat 87:16–22, 2018 29471922

Stanger C, Budney AJ, Kamon JL, et al: A randomized trial of contingency management for adolescent marijuana abuse and dependence. Drug Alcohol Depend 105(3):240–247, 2009 19717250

Substance Abuse and Mental Health Services Administration: Treatment Episode Data Set (TEDS): 2004–2014. Rockville, MD, Center for Behavioral Health Statistics and Quality, 2016

Substance Abuse and Mental Health Services Administration: Behavioral Health Trends in the United States: Results From the 2014 National Survey on Drug Use and Health (NSDUH Series H-50). Rockville, MD, Center for Behavioral Health Statistics and Quality, 2017

Tirado CF, Goldman M, Lynch K, et al: Atomoxetine for treatment of marijuana dependence: a report on the efficacy and high incidence of gastrointestinal adverse events in a pilot study. Drug Alcohol Depend 94(1–3):254–257, 2008 18182254

Trigo JM, Soliman A, Quilty LC, et al: Nabiximols combined with motivational enhancement/cognitive behavioral therapy for the treatment of cannabis dependence: a pilot randomized clinical trial. PLoS One 13(1):e0190768, 2018 29385147

United Nations Office on Drugs and Crime: World Drug Report 2015, Sales no E.15.XI.6 2015. United Nations, 2015. Available at: http://www.wsipp.wa.gov/ReportFile/1670/Wsipp_I-502-Evaluation-and-Benefit Cost-Analysis-Second-Required-Report_Report.pdf. Accessed November 22, 2019.

Vandrey R, Smith MT, McCann UD, et al: Sleep disturbance and the effects of extended-release zolpidem during cannabis withdrawal. Drug Alcohol Depend 117(1):38–44, 2011 21296508

Vandrey R, Stitzer ML, Mintzer MZ, et al: The dose effects of short-term dronabinol (oral THC) maintenance in daily cannabis users. Drug Alcohol Depend 128(1–2):64–70, 2013 22921474

Washington State Institute for Public Policy: I-502 Evaluation and Benefit-Cost Analysis: Second Required Report, 14. September 2017. Available at: http://www.wsipp.wa.gov/ReportFile/1670/Wsipp_I-502-Evaluation-and-Benefit-Cost-Analysis-Second-Required-Report_Report.pdf. Accessed November 22, 2019.

Weinstein AM, Miller H, Bluvstein I, et al: Treatment of cannabis dependence using escitalopram in combination with cognitive-behavior therapy: a double-blind placebo-controlled study. Am J Drug Alcohol Abuse 40(1):16–22, 2014 24359507

CHAPTER 18

Neurobiology of Nicotine and Tobacco

Noah R. Gubner, Ph.D.

Neal L. Benowitz, M.D.

Nicotine is found in the leaves of plants in the *Solanaceae* family and acts as a natural insecticide. Among plants in this family, the tobacco plant (*Nicotiana tabacum*) contains the highest concentrations of nicotine; however, significantly lower levels of nicotine are also found in other members of the *Solanaceae* family, including tomatoes, potatoes, and eggplants. Use of tobacco by humans dates back at least 2,500 years to the Mayans, with its introduction to Europe occurring in the early 1500s. Snuff and pipe tobacco were the most prevalent early forms used, followed by cigars in the 1800s. The first commercially available cigarettes were produced in the mid-1800s, and they became the most prevalent form used. There are currently an estimated 1 billion smokers worldwide. Smoking remains one of the leading preventable causes of death in the world.

There are over 7,000 different compounds found in tobacco smoke, some of which (in addition to nicotine) are psychoactive (Margolis et al. 2017). These include compounds such as minor tobacco alkaloids, monoamine oxidase (MAO) inhibitors, and acetaldehyde. Nicotine accounts for approximately 95% of the alkaloid content found in tobacco, with the primary minor alkaloids being anatabine, anabasine, and norcotinine (von Weymarn et al. 2016).

The pharmacological actions of nicotine have the largest role in contributing to tobacco addiction (Figure 18–1). Nicotine can exist in two *stereoisomeric forms* (the same atoms arranged in differing spatial arrangements): R-nicotine and S-nicotine. In the tobacco plant, nicotine is produced primarily (~90%) in the S (versus the R) isomeric form, whereas synthesized formulations of nicotine contain similar proportions of both stereoisomers. The stereoisomers of nicotine differ in their receptor-binding properties and psychoactive effects; the S isomer is more biologically active, and the R form is a weaker agonist.

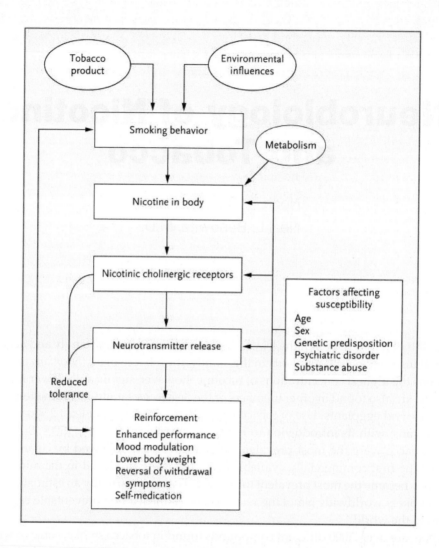

FIGURE 18–1.   Biobehavioral model showing factors and processes that contribute to nicotine/tobacco dependence.

Nicotine acts on nicotinic cholinergic receptors, triggering the release of neurotransmitters that produce psychoactive effects that are rewarding. With repeated exposure, tolerance develops to many of the effects of nicotine, thereby reducing its primary reinforcing effects and inducing physical dependence (i.e., withdrawal symptoms in the absence of nicotine). Smoking behavior is influenced by pharmacological feedback and by environmental factors such as smoking cues, friends who smoke, stress, and product advertising. Levels of nicotine in the body in relation to a particular level of nicotine intake from smoking are modulated by the rate of nicotine metabolism, which occurs in the liver largely by means of the enzyme CYP2A6. Other factors that influence smoking behavior include age, sex, genetics, mental illness, and substance abuse.

Source.   Reprinted from Figure 1 ("The Biology of Nicotine Addiction") in Benowitz NL: "Nicotine Addiction." *New England Journal of Medicine* 362(24):2295–2303, 2010. Copyright 2010, Massachusetts Medical Society. Used with permission.

As a tertiary amine, nicotine can exist in both a charged and an uncharged form (i.e., ionized and un-ionized). The ratio of ionized to un-ionized nicotine is altered by pH, with the majority of nicotine molecules being ionized in more acidic conditions (e.g., a pH of ≤5.5) and un-ionized in more alkaline conditions (e.g., a pH of ≥6.5). Charged and uncharged nicotine molecules differ in their membrane permeability. Un-ionized nicotine is lipophilic and can be absorbed through the skin and buccal membrane, whereas ionized nicotine cannot (Benowitz et al. 2009). The pH of tobacco smoke influences nicotine absorption and behavior among users. Cigarette smoke and cigar smoke differ in pH, with smoke from cigars being alkaline and smoke from most cigarettes being acidic. These differences between cigars and cigarettes are due to the type of tobacco used, the method for curing after harvesting, and the addition of chemicals during processing and formulation. In cigar smoke, a higher proportion of the nicotine molecules are un-ionized and can be absorbed in the mouth through the buccal membrane, allowing for nicotine absorption without inhalation. In contrast, cigarette smoke has a higher proportion of ionized nicotine molecules, which are lipophobic and not readily absorbed through the buccal membrane, resulting in limited absorption in the mouth without inhalation. In smokeless tobacco, the pH is adjusted to be more alkaline, resulting in a high proportion of un-ionized nicotine and more rapid buccal absorption of nicotine.

Tobacco can be smoked or chewed, and nicotine can be ingested in the form of gum, a lozenge, or spray; applied as a dermal patch; or inhaled as an aerosol through an electronic cigarette device or inhaler. Electronic cigarette devices heat a solution of nicotine and flavorant mixed with propylene glycol and/or glycerin into an aerosol, which is inhaled by the user. There are multiple types of electronic cigarette devices, which differ in design, formulations dispensed, and efficacy of nicotine delivery.

Nicotine from cigarette smoke is rapidly absorbed in the small airways and alveoli of the lung. Smoking one cigarette results in absorption of approximately 1–1.5 mg of nicotine systemically, depending on the smoking pattern and nicotine concentration in the cigarette (Benowitz and Jacob 1984). Nicotine from cigarette smoke is rapidly delivered to the brain within 15 seconds after inhalation (Berridge et al. 2010). The swift delivery of nicotine to the brain from smoking a cigarette contributes to the increased abuse liability of cigarettes compared with other routes of nicotine administration (Benowitz 2010; Benowitz et al. 1988). Nicotine has a half-life of approximately 2 hours in humans, although genetic and other factors (e.g., medications, diet, sex, estrogen, use of menthol cigarettes, compounds in tobacco smoke) contribute to individual differences in the rate of nicotine metabolism (Benowitz et al. 2009). With regular smoking, nicotine levels build up throughout the day, plateauing at 4–6 hours and then decreasing slowly overnight, but with significant levels still present first thing in the morning. Thus, nicotine is present in the brain 24 hours a day, facilitating the development of tolerance and dependence, as discussed in the section "Individual Vulnerability to Nicotine Dependence." Tolerance also develops throughout each day, with the greatest effects being experienced from the first cigarette of the day and subsequent cigarette craving and smoking being triggered at least in part by the need to relieve or avoid withdrawal symptoms.

Basic Mechanism of Action

Nicotine crosses the blood-brain barrier and acts as an agonist at nicotinic acetylcholine receptors (nAChRs), which are widely distributed in the central nervous system (CNS). There are multiple different nAChR subtypes, composed of different combinations of nAChR subunits (five subunits combined per nAChR). Sixteen known nicotinic receptor subunits exist; however, only 11 of these (α_2–α_7, α_9, α_{10}, and β_2–β_4) are expressed in the mammalian brain (Dani 2015). Heteromeric nAChRs are formed by the combination of α and β nAChR subunits to form multiple pentameric combinations (primarily with two α subunits combined with three β subunits). The only homomeric combination (composed of a single subunit type) is the α_7 nAChR. The most common nAChR subtypes found in the CNS are $\alpha_4\beta_2$ (most abundant) and α_7 nAChRs, both of which are widely expressed throughout the brain. The $\alpha_4\beta_2$ nAChR can occur in two different assemblies: three α_4 with two β_2 subunits or two α_4 with three β_2 subunits. These assemblies have different properties; the $\alpha_4\beta_2$ nAChRs consisting of two α_4 and three β_2 subunits have approximately a 100-fold higher affinity for nicotine (Morales-Perez et al. 2016). The α_5 and α_6 nAChR subunits can combine with $\alpha_4\beta_2$ subunits in various configurations to form different nAChRs. The $\alpha_3\beta_4$ nAChRs are highly expressed in the medial habenula and can combine with α_5 nAChR subunits.

The pharmacodynamic effects of nicotine are complex, with initial nAChR activation followed by receptor desensitization. There are three conformational states of nAChRs: 1) closed, at the resting state; 2) open, allowing for the translocation of ions across the cell membrane, causing membrane depolarization, and initiation of intercellular signaling; and 3) desensitized, during which the receptor is unresponsive to nAChR agonists such as nicotine or acetylcholine. The kinetic properties of nAChRs are dynamic, and the length of time the nAChR stays in the desensitized state can vary based on the subunit composition and dose/pattern of nicotine exposure (Dani 2015).

Neuronal nAChRs are present in presynaptic, postsynaptic, and nonsynaptic locations. In the CNS, nAChR subunits form a channel, which when activated allows the passage of ions including sodium, potassium, and calcium. Activation of presynaptic nAChRs causes an efflux of intracellular calcium, resulting in increased neurotransmitter release. Activation of postsynaptic nAChRs can also modulate postsynaptic processes such as depolarization and calcium signaling (Dani and Balfour 2011), although these actions of nAChRs have been less well characterized compared with the actions of presynaptic nAChRs.

Nicotine can affect multiple neurotransmitter systems, including acetylcholine, γ-aminobutyric acid (GABA), serotonin, glutamate, dopamine, and norepinephrine. Of particular importance, nicotine affects the mesolimbic dopamine pathway, which plays a central role in signaling pleasure and in the neurobiology of addiction. The mesolimbic dopamine pathway consists of dopamine neurons that project from the ventral tegmental area (VTA) to the nucleus accumbens. These dopamine neurons fire action potentials at low frequencies (tonic firing) but can also fire rapid bursts of action potentials (phasic or burst firing). Drugs of abuse or novel stimuli can cause burst firing of these dopamine neurons, resulting in increased dopamine efflux in the nucleus accumbens, a process thought to play an important role in addiction. Activation of nAChRs on dopamine cell bodies modulates the likelihood for cell depolarization and subsequent dopamine efflux at the synapse (Livingstone and Wonnacott 2009; Nisell et al. 1994). These actions of nicotine contribute to the reinforcing and cognition-enhancing effects of nicotine. Positive reinforcement likely plays a larger role in smoking behavior among new users or light/nondaily smokers. Nicotine has also been found to enhance reinforcement from nondrug rewards (Perkins et al. 2017).

GABAergic and glutamatergic neurons modulate burst firing of dopamine neurons projecting from the VTA to the nucleus accumbens. Activation of glutamatergic neurons increases, whereas activation of GABAergic neurons decreases, the likelihood of burst firing of these dopamine neurons. In the mesolimbic dopamine system, $\alpha_4\beta_2$ nAChRs, which have the highest affinity for nicotine, are predominantly located on inhibitory presynaptic GABAergic neurons. Nicotine initially activates and subsequently desensitizes $\alpha_4\beta_2$ nAChRs on inhibitory GABAergic neurons, which initially induces short-term activation of inhibitory GABAergic transmission (lasting several minutes), followed by more prolonged inhibition of GABAergic transmission (lasting for more than an hour) (Mansvelder and McGehee 2000; Mansvelder et al. 2002). The desensitization (sustained inactivation) of GABAergic neurons is thought to "remove the brake" on the mesolimbic dopamine system (i.e., inhibit the inhibitory GABAergic system). In comparison, nicotine more weakly activates α_7 nAChRs, which have a lower affinity for nicotine and are predominantly located on excitatory presynaptic glutamatergic afferent neurons. The α_7 nAChRs are more resistant to desensitization (Koukouli and Maskos 2015; Picciotto et al. 2008). Nicotine may decrease inhibitory GABAergic transmission (i.e., disinhibition), resulting in a shift to greater excitatory activation of dopamine neurons. Thus, nicotine may directly activate dopaminergic neurons while also decreasing inhibitory modulation by GABAergic signaling, leading to greater net excitation (Li et al. 2014; Zickler 2003). The abovementioned disinhibition mechanism may play a key role in the rewarding effects of nicotine. Disinhibition of GABAergic neurons by nicotine may contribute to the co-use of tobacco with many other drugs of abuse, including alcohol, cocaine, and opiates (Klenowski and Tapper 2018; Kohut 2017), which can induce dopamine efflux through other signaling pathways. This means that nicotine may decrease the "brake" on the mesolimbic dopamine system, allowing for greater activation to be induced by other drugs of abuse.

The opioid system is involved in drug reward and dependence. Endogenous opioids released in the brain, along with drugs such as morphine and heroin, act on opioid receptors. Nicotine has known analgesic effects and can induce the release of endogenous opioids (Berrendero et al. 2010). Nicotine-induced endogenous opioid release may play an important role in the reinforcing effects of nicotine and contribute to tobacco use disorder. Studies indicate that the α_7 nAChRs play a large role in nicotine's effects on the endogenous opioid system (Kishioka et al. 2014).

Genetically engineered mice with inactivated genes (also known as "knockout" mice) have helped to shed light on the roles of the various nAChR subunits. It is important to note that because nAChRs are widely distributed in the brain, it is difficult to predict how systemic activation or inhibition of nAChRs, which are involved in multiple different systems, will affect neurochemical and behavioral responses. Knockout studies have found that the β_2 nAChR subunit (along with the α_4 nAChR subunit with which it is often assembled) is necessary for nicotine-related reward and for addiction-related behaviors, whereas the α_7 nAChRs may have a more limited role (Mineur and Picciotto 2008). The α_6 nAChR subunit, which often combines with β_2 subunits, is highly expressed in the mesolimbic dopamine pathway. Knockout studies indicate an important role for α_6-containing nAChRs in nicotine-induced activation of dopamine neurons (Champtiaux et al. 2002). Knockout studies in mice indicate that α_5 nAChRs modulate the aversive effects of nicotine, with α_5 knockout mice showing fewer somatic signs of nicotine withdrawal (Salas et al. 2009). The β_4-containing nAChRs also appear to have a role in mediating nicotine withdrawal symptoms, with β_4 knockout mice showing reduced nicotine withdrawal symptoms (such as excessive grooming, chewing, scratching, shaking, leg tremors, and cage scratching) (Salas et al. 2004).

Upregulation of Nicotinic Acetylcholine Receptors

Smokers have a higher density of nAChRs in multiple brain areas compared with nonsmokers (Perry et al. 1999). Upregulation of nAChRs is thought to contribute to the development of dependence and withdrawal symptoms experienced by smokers during nicotine abstinence. When a chronic smoker is abstinent from nicotine, a higher proportion of nAChRs are open (i.e., not in a desensitized conformation), which may increase the inhibitory activity of GABAergic neurons in the VTA, leading to decreased tonic activity (i.e., inhibition) of dopamine terminals in the nucleus accumbens (Mansvelder and McGehee 2000; Mansvelder et al. 2002).

Different nAChR subtypes show different levels of upregulation in response to nicotine exposure, with the largest effects found for $\alpha_4\beta_2$ nAChRs located on GABAergic versus dopaminergic neurons in the VTA (Nashmi et al. 2007). In animal models, after chronic nicotine treatment, messenger ribonucleic acid (mRNA) levels of nAChR subunits are not affected (i.e., mRNA production of protein subunits is not increased). This implies that nicotine-induced upregulation of nAChRs is mediated by a posttranslational mechanism (Govind et al. 2009). Upregulation of nAChRs from chronic nicotine exposure was originally thought to occur because of nAChR desensitization; however, recent research suggests that such desensitization most likely does not play a primary role in nicotine-induced upregulation of nAChRs (Henderson and Lester 2015). Upregulation of nAChRs by nicotine likely occurs via a "chaperoning" mechanism in which nicotine enters the endoplasmic reticulum, binds to trapped nAChRs, and facilitates the assembly and escorted delivery of nAChRs to the cell membrane (Srinivasan et al. 2011), although this process is not fully understood (for a review, see Henderson and Lester 2015).

Psychoactive Effects of Nicotine

Nicotine's psychoactive and subjective effects are influenced by the dose, route of administration, speed of drug delivery, and concentration and length of time at nAChRs (for a review, see Benowitz et al. 2009). The rapid uptake of nicotine in the blood and brain from cigarettes smoked has been implicated in the greater abuse liability of cigarettes compared with other routes of nicotine administration. The psychoactive effects of nicotine are influenced by prior exposure to nicotine, which can induce neuroadaptations and tolerance.

Subjective effects of nicotine in smokers include arousal, increased attention, enhanced mood, and reduced anxiety or stress reactivity. However, some or most of the positive subjective effects reported by regular smokers are due to attenuation of withdrawal symptoms that accrue during periods of nicotine abstinence. For this reason, the perceived benefits of nicotine among smokers are in part mediated through *negative reinforcement* (i.e., the removal of adverse subjective effects). This distinction has important implications for the treatment and management of nicotine withdrawal during tobacco cessation.

Neuroadaptation

Individuals who are chronically exposed to nicotine rapidly develop tolerance to its dysphoric effects, including headache, nausea, and dizziness, as well as to some of its positive rewarding effects (Figure 18–1). Smokers are able to control the dose of nicotine that reaches the brain by altering the puff volume and frequency when smoking, as well as the duration between cigarettes, to maintain a desired level of nicotine in the brain. This pattern of regular smoking often leads to compulsive smoking behavior and dependence. Both the positive reinforcing effects (e.g., enhanced mood, increased attention, reduced anxiety) and the negative reinforcing effects (e.g., avoidance of withdrawal) contribute to the development and maintenance of addiction.

Regular smoking results in repeated exposure to smoking-related cues (e.g., sight/ taste/smell of smoke, tobacco packaging), which become conditioned over time. These conditioned stimuli, along with environmental cues, contribute to cigarette dependence. Nicotine also influences behavioral conditioning through activation of memory processes in the hippocampus linked to the mesolimbic pathway. Over time, smoking leads to reinforcement of conditioned environmental cues, which play an important role in tobacco use disorder. Cues associated with smoking can trigger craving and relapse, and particular cues can continue to trigger craving responses for prolonged periods of time after complete cessation—and in some cases may never fully extinguish.

Withdrawal

Nicotine withdrawal symptoms include irritability, anger, impatience, anxiety, dysphoria, anhedonia, impairment of cognitive function and performance, weight gain, and craving. The neural processes and nAChR subtypes that mediate nicotine withdrawal symptoms are different from the processes and subtypes that mediate nicotine reward and reinforcement. The medial habenula, located above the thalamus, and its primary output, the interpeduncular nucleus, are thought to play an important role in mediating nicotine withdrawal (for a review, see Baldwin et al. 2011). These brain regions have a high expression of α_2, α_3, α_5, and β_4 nAChRs, and antagonism of these receptors has been shown to block nicotine withdrawal symptoms in mice (Salas et al. 2004, 2009). Because distinct systems have been identified as mediating nicotine reward and withdrawal, both systems are thought to contribute to tobacco use disorder.

Nicotine also activates the hypothalamic-pituitary-adrenal (HPA) axis, the central stress response system, through a hypothalamus-mediated mechanism (Rohleder and Kirschbaum 2006). Chronic nicotine exposure results in a blunted HPA axis response to stress, which likely contributes to the reported stress/anxiety response among smokers when in withdrawal from nicotine.

Corticotropin-releasing hormone receptor 1 (CRF_1) is a peptide hormone that contributes to the HPA axis stress response. Increases in CRF–CRF_1 signaling are associated with negative mood states. It is well established that nicotine withdrawal is associated with increases in anxiety and negative mood states, and the CRF system has been found to contribute to nicotine withdrawal symptoms. Rodent studies have found that nicotine withdrawal can induce overactivation of the CRF–CRF_1 signaling system (George et al. 2007). Nicotine-induced withdrawal can drive nicotine intake through *negative reinforcement* (a behavior strengthened by stopping/removing a negative outcome). Administration of MPZP (*N,N*-bis[2-methoxyethyl]-3-[4-methoxy-2-methylphenyl]-2,5-dimethyl-pyrazolo[1,5α]pyrimidin-7-amine), a specific CRF_1 antagonist (i.e., an agent that blocks the CRF_1 system), was found to attenuate nicotine self-administration induced by nicotine withdrawal in mice (George et al. 2007).

The orexin/hypocretin neuropeptide system contributes to both sleep and arousal states and also has been found to play a role in drug-induced reinforcement. The insular cortex has dense populations of neurons containing hypocretin 1, also known as orexin A (Kenny 2011). Neurons in the insular cortex innervate the mesolimbic dopamine system. Individuals with strokes that cause lesions to the insular cortex have been found to have reduced craving and withdrawal symptoms during tobacco abstinence (Abdolahi et al. 2015, 2017). One explanation for this phenomenon is that hypocretin 1–containing neurons in the insular cortex modulate the responsiveness of the mesolimbic dopamine system to cue-induced craving (Kenny 2011). This could provide an additional biological mechanism contributing to nicotine dependence and withdrawal.

Chronic desensitization of nAChRs induced by prolonged smoking results in upregulation in the number of receptors in the CNS. In smokers during abstinence, there are a greater number of nAChRs in open conformation (i.e., not desensitized), which may contribute to nicotine withdrawal symptoms. In smokers during a period of nicotine abstinence, levels of nAChRs eventually return to levels similar to those seen in nonsmokers; however, this process takes time. Higher levels of nAChRs in the brain are found up to 1 month after smoking cessation in humans, but levels appear to normalize to nonsmoker levels after approximately 6–12 weeks of abstinence (Cosgrove et al. 2009). Nicotine can induce upregulation of nAChRs through multiple routes of administration in animal models. Because nicotine replacement therapy (NRT) attenuates the rewarding effects of smoking, it has been hypothesized that use of NRT may maintain upregulation of nAChRs in the brain (Brody et al. 2013). Mice exposed to the smoking cessation medication varenicline for 10–14 days were found to have upregulation of nAChRs in the brain (Marks et al. 2015; Turner et al. 2011). This suggests that both varenicline and NRT may maintain upregulation of nAChRs in the brains of smokers, which could contribute to relapse when patients stop taking these smoking cessation pharmacotherapies.

The two smoking behavior variables that are the most predictive of severity of cigarette dependence are 1) number of cigarettes smoked per day and 2) time to first cigarette after waking. The number of cigarettes smoked per day reflects both dose of nicotine and frequency of self-administration behaviors, whereas time to first cigarette is thought to reflect degree of physical dependence—that is, a need to take nicotine to relieve withdrawal symptoms after overnight abstinence. Cigarette dependence among smokers can be assessed through use of a combination of these two measures, called the Heaviness of Smoking Index, a subset of the Fagerström Test for Nicotine Dependence (Heatherton et al. 1989). These scales have also been adapted to assess electronic cigarette dependence (Foulds et al. 2015).

Individual Vulnerability to Nicotine Dependence

Genetic factors are known to contribute to individual differences in risk for the development of nicotine addiction. The rs16969968 single nucleotide polymorphism (SNP) on chromosome 15 is associated with increased susceptibility to nicotine dependence (Bierut et al. 2008). This SNP is also associated with a lower likelihood of successful smoking cessation, an increased risk for lung cancer, and an earlier age at lung cancer diagnosis (Chen et al. 2015; Xu et al. 2015). The relationship with the SNP is thought to be causally associated with smoking. The rs16969968 SNP is located within the *CHRNA5* gene, which encodes for the α_5 nAChR subunit. As previously discussed, α_5 nAChRs appear to play an important role in mediating the aversive effects of nicotine (Salas et al. 2009). The rs16969968 SNP is associated with loss of function of the α_5 nAChR, which is hypothesized to increase the tolerability—and therefore the daily dosing—of nicotine, which would increase risk for tobacco use disorder.

Genetic and other factors influence the rate of nicotine metabolism (Benowitz et al. 2009). Nicotine is metabolized primarily by the hepatic enzyme cytochrome P450 (CYP) 2A6, which exhibits considerable population polymorphism. Asians and African Americans have a higher prevalence of CYP2A6 gene variants associated with reduced nicotine metabolism (Tanner and Tyndale 2017). Individuals with a faster rate of nicotine metabolism experience withdrawal symptoms more quickly (Liakoni et al. 2019). Among smokers with a faster rate of nicotine metabolism, smoking cigarettes to attenuate nicotine withdrawal symptoms may play a large role in maintaining dependence. Individuals with a faster rate of nicotine metabolism have a more difficult time quitting. Differences in the rate of nicotine metabolism have been associated with differences in the efficacy of smoking cessation pharmacotherapies, with faster metabolizers showing greater benefit from varenicline versus NRT (Lerman et al. 2015).

The prevalence of cigarette smoking is higher among individuals with co-occurring drug or alcohol use disorders (Guydish et al. 2016; McKee and Weinberger 2013). In one study, daily smokers were three times more likely to meet criteria for hazardous drinking and alcohol use disorder (McKee et al. 2007). Alcohol use and tobacco use are not just associated with one another but also occur during the same episodes. In a survey of college students who were nondaily smokers ($N=217$), 74% of all reported smoking episodes occurred while drinking alcohol (McKee et al. 2004). Multiple mechanisms are thought to contribute to the concurrent use of tobacco and alcohol or other drugs of abuse: 1) shared genetic susceptibility; 2) one drug reducing the negative effects (e.g., craving, cognitive impairment, withdrawal, side effects) of the other drug; and 3) greater rewarding effects when drugs are used in combination versus either drug alone. It is important to note that most studies have found that quitting smoking has either a positive impact or no impact on treatment outcomes for other substance use disorders (see reviews by McKelvey et al. 2017 and Thurgood et al. 2016).

In comparison with the general population, individuals with mental illness smoke at higher rates and are heavier smokers. Smoking rates are particularly high among individuals with depressive disorders, bipolar disorder, posttraumatic stress disorder, or schizophrenia (Prochaska et al. 2017). Several mechanisms have been hypothesized to explain the high comorbidity of smoking and mental illness: 1) smoking is used as self-medication to reduce impairment in cognitive function and to suppress psychotic symptoms; 2) the association between smoking and mental disorders may reflect a shared genetic vulnerability; and 3) smoking constitutes a risk factor for the development of mental illness (Chen et al. 2016). All of these proposed mechanisms may contribute to tobacco use among individuals with mental illness, and they are not mutually exclusive. The higher rates of smoking among individuals with schizophrenia and other mental illnesses may also be due to the use of cigarette smoking to minimize the adverse effects (e.g., cognitive impairment) of conventional antipsychotic medications. Tobacco cessation has been associated with improvements in depression and anxiety symptoms (Prochaska et al. 2017), a finding that highlights the importance of treating tobacco use among individuals with mental illness. Cigarette smoke is a known inducer of CYP1A2 and therefore can increase the rate of clearance of certain conventional and atypical antipsychotic medications (e.g., chlorpromazine, clozapine) (Desai et al. 2001), resulting in reduced plasma concentrations of these drugs, which can diminish the efficacy or require the use of higher dosages of these medications.

Other Compounds in Tobacco With Psychoactive Effects

Cigarette smoking is associated with reduced MAO activity. MAOs are a family of enzymes that catalyze the oxidation of monoamines such as dopamine, serotonin, and norepinephrine. Inhibition of MAO activity reduces the breakdown and clearance of monoamine neurotransmitters from the synapse, increasing their availability for postsynaptic binding, which can have antidepressant effects. The inhibitory effect of tobacco smoke on MAO activity is not caused by nicotine but instead occurs through exposure to other constituents of tobacco smoke (Talhout et al. 2007). Acetaldehyde, which is present in high concentrations in cigarette smoke and which has been found to increase nicotine self-administration in rodent models, can combine with biogenic amines to form harman and salsolinol (Lewis et al. 2007). These compounds can inhibit MAO enzyme activity. The inhibitory effect of tobacco smoke on MAO activity may contribute to the rewarding effects of cigarettes and thus to dependence. Rodent models have shown that MAO inhibitors increase nicotine self-administration and enhance the reinforcing effects of nicotine (Guillem et al. 2005; Smith et al. 2016). Acetaldehyde, at levels found in tobacco smoke, was found to increase nicotine self-administration in adolescent rats (Belluzzi et al. 2005). This suggests that acetaldehyde may increase the reinforcing effects of nicotine and may contribute to tobacco dependence. As noted earlier, cigarette smoking is highly prevalent among individuals with mental illness (Prochaska et al. 2017). MAO inhibition from tobacco smoke may be one factor contributing to this correlation.

Conclusion

Dependence on tobacco is maintained by the positive reinforcing effects of nicotine, the conditioned stimuli associated with smoking, and the negative reinforcing effects of nicotine withdrawal. The pharmacological actions of nicotine are complex and involve multiple brain pathways and different nAChR types. Nicotine's effects are influenced by both genetic and environmental factors, as well as by prior nicotine exposure. The $\alpha_4\beta_2$ nAChRs (on GABA neurons) and the α_7 nAChRs (on glutamate neurons) play a key role in the pharmacological actions of nicotine in the mesolimbic dopamine pathway. The α_5 nAChRs, through a separate mechanism, have a role in mediating nicotine-induced aversion and withdrawal, and variants of the α_5 nAChR gene with reduced function are associated with an increased risk of nicotine dependence and tobacco-induced disease. Nicotine interacts with a number of other neurotransmitter systems, and this interaction contributes to nicotine's psychopharmacological effects. Chronic exposure to nicotine induces neuroadaptation (e.g., upregulation of $\alpha_4\beta_2$ nAChRs) and tolerance through desensitization of nAChRs. Tobacco smoke can inhibit MAO activity, and MAO inhibition may contribute to tobacco use disorder, particularly among individuals with mental illness. The rate of nicotine metabolism is also related to nicotine dependence; faster nicotine metabolizers have higher levels of dependence (as evidenced by smoking more cigarettes per day), more severe withdrawal symptoms during abstinence, and greater difficulty in quitting smoking with some interventions. Cigarette smoking is highly comorbid with mental illness as well as with other substance use disorders, a finding that highlights the importance of treating tobacco use disorder among populations with these disorders.

References

Abdolahi A, Williams GC, Benesch CG, et al: Damage to the insula leads to decreased nicotine withdrawal during abstinence. Addiction 110(12):1994–2003, 2015 26347067

Abdolahi A, Williams GC, Benesch CG, et al: Immediate and sustained decrease in smoking urges after acute insular cortex damage. Nicotine Tob Res 19(6):756–762, 2017 28199722

Baldwin PR, Alanis R, Salas R: The role of the habenula in nicotine addiction. J Addict Res Ther S1(2):002, 2011 22493758

Belluzzi JD, Wang R, Leslie FM: Acetaldehyde enhances acquisition of nicotine self-administration in adolescent rats. Neuropsychopharmacology 30(4):705–712, 2005 15496937

Benowitz NL: Nicotine addiction. N Engl J Med 362(24):2295–2303, 2010 20554984

Benowitz NL, Jacob P 3rd: Daily intake of nicotine during cigarette smoking. Clin Pharmacol Ther 35(4):499–504, 1984 6705448

Benowitz NL, Porchet H, Sheiner L, et al: Nicotine absorption and cardiovascular effects with smokeless tobacco use: comparison with cigarettes and nicotine gum. Clin Pharmacol Ther 44(1):23–28, 1988 3391001

Benowitz NL, Hukkanen J, Jacob P 3rd: Nicotine chemistry, metabolism, kinetics and biomarkers. Handb Exp Pharmacol 192(192):29–60, 2009 19184645

Berrendero F, Robledo P, Trigo JM, et al: Neurobiological mechanisms involved in nicotine dependence and reward: participation of the endogenous opioid system. Neurosci Biobehav Rev 35(2):220–231, 2010 20170672

Berridge MS, Apana SM, Nagano KK, et al: Smoking produces rapid rise of [11C]nicotine in human brain. Psychopharmacology (Berl) 209(4):383–394, 2010 20232056

Bierut LJ, Stitzel JA, Wang JC, et al: Variants in nicotinic receptors and risk for nicotine dependence. Am J Psychiatry 165(9):1163–1171, 2008 18519524

Brody AL, Mukhin AG, Shulenberger S, et al: Treatment for tobacco dependence: effect on brain nicotinic acetylcholine receptor density. Neuropsychopharmacology 38(8):1548–1556, 2013 23429692

Champtiaux N, Han ZY, Bessis A, et al: Distribution and pharmacology of alpha 6-containing nicotinic acetylcholine receptors analyzed with mutant mice. J Neurosci 22(4):1208–1217, 2002 11850448

Chen J, Bacanu SA, Yu H, et al: Genetic relationship between schizophrenia and nicotine dependence. Sci Rep 6:25671, 2016 27164557

Chen LS, Hung RJ, Baker T, et al: CHRNA5 risk variant predicts delayed smoking cessation and earlier lung cancer diagnosis—a meta-analysis. J Natl Cancer Inst 107(5):djv100, 2015 25873736

Cosgrove KP, Batis J, Bois F, et al: beta2-Nicotinic acetylcholine receptor availability during acute and prolonged abstinence from tobacco smoking. Arch Gen Psychiatry 66(6):666–676, 2009 19487632

Dani JA: Neuronal nicotinic acetylcholine receptor structure and function and response to nicotine. Int Rev Neurobiol 124:3–19, 2015 26472524

Dani JA, Balfour DJ: Historical and current perspective on tobacco use and nicotine addiction. Trends Neurosci 34(7):383–392, 2011 21696833

Desai HD, Seabolt J, Jann MW: Smoking in patients receiving psychotropic medications: a pharmacokinetic perspective. CNS Drugs 15(6):469–494, 2001 11524025

Foulds J, Veldheer S, Yingst J, et al: Development of a questionnaire for assessing dependence on electronic cigarettes among a large sample of ex-smoking e-cigarette users. Nicotine Tob Res 17(2):186–192, 2015 25332459

George O, Ghozland S, Azar MR, et al: CRF-CRF1 system activation mediates withdrawal-induced increases in nicotine self-administration in nicotine-dependent rats. Proc Natl Acad Sci USA 104(43):17198–17203, 2007 17921249

Govind AP, Vezina P, Green WN: Nicotine-induced upregulation of nicotinic receptors: underlying mechanisms and relevance to nicotine addiction. Biochem Pharmacol 78(7):756–765, 2009 19540212

Guillem K, Vouillac C, Azar MR, et al: Monoamine oxidase inhibition dramatically increases the motivation to self-administer nicotine in rats. J Neurosci 25(38):8593–8600, 2005 16177026

Guydish J, Tajima B, Pramod S, et al: Use of multiple tobacco products in a national sample of persons enrolled in addiction treatment. Drug Alcohol Depend 166:93–99, 2016 27449271

Heatherton TF, Kozlowski LT, Frecker RC, et al: Measuring the heaviness of smoking: using self-reported time to the first cigarette of the day and number of cigarettes smoked per day. Br J Addict 84(7):791–799, 1989 2758152

Henderson BJ, Lester HA: Inside-out neuropharmacology of nicotinic drugs. Neuropharmacology 96(Pt B):178–193, 2015 25660637

Kenny PJ: Tobacco dependence, the insular cortex and the hypocretin connection. Pharmacol Biochem Behav 97(4):700–707, 2011 20816891

Kishioka S, Kiguchi N, Kobayashi Y, et al: Nicotine effects and the endogenous opioid system. J Pharmacol Sci 125(2):117–124, 2014 24882143

Klenowski PM, Tapper AR: Molecular, neuronal, and behavioral effects of ethanol and nicotine interactions. Handb Exp Pharmacol 248:187–212, 2018 29423839

Kohut SJ: Interactions between nicotine and drugs of abuse: a review of preclinical findings. Am J Drug Alcohol Abuse 43(2):155–170, 2017 27589579

Koukouli F, Maskos U: The multiple roles of the alpha7 nicotinic acetylcholine receptor in modulating glutamatergic systems in the normal and diseased nervous system. Biochem Pharmacol 97(4):378–387, 2015 26206184

Lerman C, Schnoll RA, Hawk LW Jr, et al: Use of the nicotine metabolite ratio as a genetically informed biomarker of response to nicotine patch or varenicline for smoking cessation: a randomised, double-blind placebo-controlled trial. Lancet Respir Med 3(2):131–138, 2015 25588294

Lewis A, Miller JH, Lea RA: Monoamine oxidase and tobacco dependence. Neurotoxicology 28(1):182–195, 2007 16859748

Li X, Semenova S, D'Souza MS, et al: Involvement of glutamatergic and GABAergic systems in nicotine dependence: implications for novel pharmacotherapies for smoking cessation. Neuropharmacology 76(Pt B):182–195, 2014 16859748

Liakoni E, Edwards KC, St Helen G, et al: Effects of nicotine metabolic rate on withdrawal symptoms and response to cigarette smoking after abstinence. Clin Pharmacol Ther 105(3):641–651, 2019 30242831

Livingstone PD, Wonnacott S: Nicotinic acetylcholine receptors and the ascending dopamine pathways. Biochem Pharmacol 78(7):744–755, 2009 19523928

Mansvelder HD, McGehee DS: Long-term potentiation of excitatory inputs to brain reward areas by nicotine. Neuron 27(2):349–357, 2000 10985354

Mansvelder HD, Keath JR, McGehee DS: Synaptic mechanisms underlie nicotine-induced excitability of brain reward areas. Neuron 33(6):905–919, 2002 11906697

Margolis KA, Bernat JK, Keely O'Brien E, et al: Online information about harmful tobacco constituents: a content analysis. Nicotine Tob Res 19(10):1209–1215, 2017 27613931

Marks MJ, O'Neill HC, Wynalda-Camozzi KM, et al: Chronic treatment with varenicline changes expression of four nAChR binding sites in mice. Neuropharmacology 99:142–155, 2015 26192545

McKee SA, Weinberger AH: How can we use our knowledge of alcohol-tobacco interactions to reduce alcohol use? Annu Rev Clin Psychol 9:649–674, 2013 23157448

McKee SA, Hinson R, Rounsaville D, et al: Survey of subjective effects of smoking while drinking among college students. Nicotine Tob Res 6(1):111–117, 2004 14982695

McKee SA, Falba T, O'Malley SS, et al: Smoking status as a clinical indicator for alcohol misuse in US adults. Arch Intern Med 167(7):716–721, 2007 17420431

McKelvey K, Thrul J, Ramo D: Impact of quitting smoking and smoking cessation treatment on substance use outcomes: an updated and narrative review. Addict Behav 65:161–170, 2017 27816663

Mineur YS, Picciotto MR: Genetics of nicotinic acetylcholine receptors: relevance to nicotine addiction. Biochem Pharmacol 75(1):323–333, 2008 17632086

Morales-Perez CL, Noviello CM, Hibbs RE: X-ray structure of the human alpha4beta2 nicotinic receptor. Nature 538(7625):411–415, 2016 27698419

Nashmi R, Xiao C, Deshpande P, et al: Chronic nicotine cell specifically upregulates functional alpha 4* nicotinic receptors: basis for both tolerance in midbrain and enhanced long-term potentiation in perforant path. J Neurosci 27(31):8202–8218, 2007 17670967

Nisell M, Nomikos GG, Svensson TH: Systemic nicotine-induced dopamine release in the rat nucleus accumbens is regulated by nicotinic receptors in the ventral tegmental area. Synapse 16(1):36–44, 1994 8134899

Perkins KA, Karelitz JL, Boldry MC: Nicotine acutely enhances reinforcement from non-drug rewards in humans. Front Psychiatry 8:65, 2017 28507522

Perry DC, Dávila-García MI, Stockmeier CA, et al: Increased nicotinic receptors in brains from smokers: membrane binding and autoradiography studies. J Pharmacol Exp Ther 289(3):1545–1552, 1999 10336551

Picciotto MR, Addy NA, Mineur YS, et al: It is not "either/or": activation and desensitization of nicotinic acetylcholine receptors both contribute to behaviors related to nicotine addiction and mood. Prog Neurobiol 84(4):329–342, 2008 18242816

Prochaska JJ, Das S, Young-Wolff KC: Smoking, mental illness, and public health. Annu Rev Public Health 38:165–185, 2017 27992725

Rohleder N, Kirschbaum C: The hypothalamic-pituitary-adrenal (HPA) axis in habitual smokers. Int J Psychophysiol 59(3):236–243, 2006 16325948

Salas R, Pieri F, De Biasi M: Decreased signs of nicotine withdrawal in mice null for the beta4 nicotinic acetylcholine receptor subunit. J Neurosci 24(45):10035–10039, 2004 15537871

Salas R, Sturm R, Boulter J, et al: Nicotinic receptors in the habenulo-interpeduncular system are necessary for nicotine withdrawal in mice. J Neurosci 29(10):3014–3018, 2009 19279237

Smith TT, Rupprecht LE, Cwalina SN, et al: Effects of monoamine oxidase inhibition on the reinforcing properties of low-dose nicotine. Neuropsychopharmacology 41(9):2335–2343, 2016 26955970

Srinivasan R, Pantoja R, Moss FJ, et al: Nicotine up-regulates alpha4beta2 nicotinic receptors and ER exit sites via stoichiometry-dependent chaperoning. J Gen Physiol 137(1):59–79, 2011 21187334

Talhout R, Opperhuizen A, van Amsterdam JG: Role of acetaldehyde in tobacco smoke addiction. Eur Neuropsychopharmacol 17(10):627–636, 2007 17382522

Tanner JA, Tyndale RF: Variation in CYP2A6 activity and personalized medicine. J Pers Med 7(4):E18, 2017 29194389

Thurgood SL, McNeill A, Clark-Carter D, et al: A systematic review of smoking cessation interventions for adults in substance abuse treatment or recovery. Nicotine Tob Res 18(5):993–1001, 2016 26069036

Turner JR, Castellano LM, Blendy JA: Parallel anxiolytic-like effects and upregulation of neuronal nicotinic acetylcholine receptors following chronic nicotine and varenicline. Nicotine Tob Res 13(1):41–46, 2011 21097981

von Weymarn LB, Thomson NM, Donny EC, et al: Quantitation of the minor tobacco alkaloids nornicotine, anatabine, and anabasine in smokers' urine by high throughput liquid chromatography-mass spectrometry. Chem Res Toxicol 29(3):390–397, 2016 26825008

Xu ZW, Wang GN, Dong ZZ, et al: CHRNA5 rs16969968 polymorphism association with risk of lung cancer—evidence from 17,962 lung cancer cases and 77,216 control subjects. Asian Pac J Cancer Prev 16(15):6685–6690, 2015 26434895

Zickler P: Nicotine's multiple effects on the brain's reward system drive addiction. NIDA Notes 17(6):1–2, 2003. Available at: https://archives.drugabuse.gov/news-events/nida-notes/2003/03/nicotines-multiple-effects-brains-reward-system-drive-addiction. Accessed December 26, 2019.

CHAPTER 19

Treatment of Tobacco-Related Disorders

Jill M. Williams, M.D.

Nina Cooperman, Psy.D.

Vamsee Chaguturu, M.D.

Although tobacco use has declined in the past 50 years, it remains one of the main causes of preventable death in the United States. More than 480,000 deaths annually are attributable to tobacco use (U.S. Department of Health and Human Services 2014). Policy and public health efforts to educate the public, restrict smoking, and change social norms pertaining to tobacco have been very successful in driving down smoking rates. Even in more recent years, the proportion of U.S. adults who smoke cigarettes has continued to decline (from 20.9% in 2005 to 13.7% in 2018; U.S. Department of Health and Human Services 2020). However, important disparities in cigarette smoking persist. Cigarette smoking rates are higher among males, Native Americans, people with lower levels of education or income, and people who lack health insurance or who are insured through Medicaid (Jamal et al. 2018). Much higher tobacco use rates are also seen in military veterans, people with a disability, and people who identify as lesbian, gay, or bisexual (Odani et al. 2018). Some of the highest rates of smoking are reported among individuals who have a mental illness or another substance use disorder (SUD); smoking rates among these individuals are at least double the rates reported for the general population (Centers for Disease Control and Prevention 2013). There is also evidence that smoking rates are not declining as rapidly in these groups as they are in the population as a whole, suggesting that smoking will become increasingly concentrated among these subsets of the population if more is not done.

The burden of smoking morbidity and mortality remains high and costly. Tobacco use is a major contributor to heart disease, chronic obstructive pulmonary disease (COPD), and cancer. The annual cost of direct medical care attributable to cigarette smoking is now estimated at more than $130 billion (Xu et al. 2015). The disease risks from smoking for women have risen sharply over the past 50 years and are now equal to those for men. Research continues to identify new diseases caused by smoking, including diabetes mellitus, rheumatoid arthritis, and colorectal cancer (U.S. Department of Health and Human Services 2014). In addition to causing multiple diseases, cigarette smoking affects the body adversely in many other ways, such as triggering inflammation and impairing immune function. On average, smokers die 10 years earlier than nonsmokers (U.S. Department of Health and Human Services 2014).

The smoke from burning cigarettes is estimated to contain thousands of different chemical components, more than 65 of which are known to be carcinogenic. Acetaldehyde, benzene, ammonia, formaldehyde, and nitrosamines are just a few of the many toxins in cigarette smoke. The negative effects of the products of combustion, including carbon monoxide, on cardiovascular health are well documented. Although nicotine is responsible for the addiction to tobacco, it is not in itself the cause of the numerous cancers and other chronic diseases that are attributed to smoking; rather, these diseases are caused by the other chemicals found in tobacco and cigarette smoke.

Smoke is toxic to others in the environment; secondhand smoke is designated as a known human carcinogen. In adults, secondhand smoke has immediate adverse effects on the cardiovascular system and causes coronary heart disease and lung cancer. Children exposed to secondhand smoke are at an increased risk for sudden infant death syndrome, acute respiratory infections, ear problems, and more severe asthma. There is no risk-free level of exposure to secondhand smoke; therefore, eliminating smoking in indoor spaces is the only way to fully protect nonsmokers from exposure to secondhand smoke. In 2017, the U.S. Department of Housing and Urban Development issued a national ruling mandating that public housing be smoke-free in order to protect the health of residents, visitors, and staff. An estimated 10% of U.S. women smokers continue to smoke during pregnancy (U.S. Department of Health and Human Services 2014), and the risks of negative outcomes for mother and baby are quite high and include low birth weight, preterm birth, placental abnormalities, and birth defects.

At the same time that use of cigarettes is declining, use of other cigarette products remains stable or is increasing, requiring surveillance of a widening variety of products whose safety has not been determined. Switching one tobacco product for another is not felt to be an effective alternative to quitting and can still result in significant exposure to toxins (i.e., carcinogenic nitrosamines are still present in oral tobacco). The increase in products that heat nicotine but do not burn it (i.e., electronic cigarettes [e-cigarettes]) raises the potential for a product that could result in reduced harm, but this has not yet been proven. The rapid rise in e-cigarette use and vaping among teenagers and young adults is cause for concern. Recently reported increases in nicotine vaping among high school students represent the largest single-year change ever recorded for any substance in the 44 years of the Monitoring the Future study (Johnston et al. 2019).

Quitting smoking saves lives and is beneficial at any age. Predictors of successful quitting include a variety of biopsychosocial factors.Sociodemographic factors such as age, educational attainment, and income predict greater success in quitting. Having fewer smokers in one's social network and using smoking cessation treatments are also associated with higher abstinence rates (U.S. Department of Health and Human Services 2020). Having a behavioral health condition or a higher level of nicotine dependence generally makes it harder to quit. Gender is emerging as an important factor, with women having more difficulty quitting smoking on a given quit attempt than men (Smith et al. 2016).

Effective treatments for tobacco use disorder include medications and behavioral counseling; in addition, clinical practice guidelines have been implemented to broadly integrate tobacco treatment into the health care system (Fiore et al. 2008). There is a dose–response relationship between the amount of time spent counseling a patient about tobacco use and the patient's success in quitting smoking, with more counseling time resulting in better outcomes; many people still attempt to quit on their own, and treatments have a high rate of relapse, measured as return to smoking at 1 year. Although a majority of cigarette smokers make a quit attempt each year, fewer than one-third use cessation medications approved by the U.S. Food and Drug Administration (FDA) or behavioral counseling to support quit attempts (U.S. Department of Health and Human Services 2020). In this chapter, we review the evidence for effective approaches to the treatment of tobacco use disorder.

Assessment of Tobacco Use Disorder

Assessment of tobacco use disorder is important, as higher levels of addiction severity are associated with more severe withdrawal symptoms and greater difficulty in quitting. Unsuccessful attempts to stop smoking, difficulty in controlling use, and previous experiences of withdrawal symptoms during a period of abstinence are criteria for tobacco use disorder in both DSM-5 (American Psychiatric Association 2013) and ICD-10 (World Health Organization 1992). Addiction to tobacco may be best characterized as a dimensional rather than a categorical phenomenon, which makes assessments such as the Fagerström Test for Nicotine Dependence (FTND; Heatherton et al. 1991) useful in defining levels of severity and predicting outcomes.

Nicotine Pharmacology

Nicotine has a short half-life (2 hours), and levels can fluctuate throughout the day, resulting in periods of withdrawal. Smoking or inhaling a drug into the lungs is an extremely effective way to deliver a high dose rapidly to the brain, making the nicotine from cigarettes highly addictive (U.S. Department of Health and Human Services 2014). Cigarettes are often trivialized (being a legal substance) or considered "not a real drug," yet it is well documented that nicotine activates the brain reward pathways similarly to other addicting substances.

Although nicotine does not usually have intoxicating effects, there are significant withdrawal symptoms that occur with abrupt cessation or periods of abstinence, including the following: frustration, irritability/anger, anxiety, sad or depressed mood, impaired concentration, insomnia, restlessness, and increased appetite. Nicotine/tobacco withdrawal symptoms can interfere with daily functioning and result in relapsing back to tobacco use, although there is wide symptom heterogeneity. Because withdrawal symptoms can emerge hours after the last cigarette, they may be mistaken for other symptoms of mental illness or substance withdrawal. Affective or mood symptoms, which play a prominent part in this withdrawal syndrome, may be more important than physical symptoms of withdrawal in the maintenance of addiction (Koob and Le Moal 2005). As with other SUDs, it is important that patients receive proper treatment in order to diminish withdrawal, which can undermine attempts at abstinence.

Clinical Assessment Tools

Assessment is an important first step in the treatment of any SUD, and there are several easy measures of tobacco use that are clinically relevant. The FTND is a six-item scale that has been shown to predict withdrawal symptom and craving severity, and it is the most widely used questionnaire measure of tobacco use severity. The abbreviated two-item version of the FTND, which consists of simply asking about 1) the number of cigarettes smoked per day and 2) the minutes to first cigarette smoked upon awakening (two queries known as the Heaviness of Smoking Index), performs as well as the full-length FTND in assessing tobacco use severity and predicting cessation (Heatherton et al. 1991). The time in the morning until someone smokes his or her first cigarette is a good indicator of tobacco use severity and is an assessment of morning withdrawal. Individuals who smoke at least 10 cigarettes per day (or who smoke within 30 minutes of waking) are considered to be moderately nicotine dependent, and those smoking more than 20 cigarettes per day (or within 5 minutes of waking) are highly nicotine dependent. More recent studies of the development of tobacco use severity among young people have suggested that loss of control over one's smoking (as a central criterion for dependence) can develop with much lower levels of consumption, including less than one cigarette per day (DiFranza et al. 2002).

Biochemical Measures of Nicotine Dependence

Despite the usefulness of biochemical measures of nicotine, or of its main metabolite cotinine, in blood or saliva, such measures are often not available in clinical settings. The most commonly used biochemical measurement is expired breath carbon monoxide (CO), which can be taken with a handheld digital monitor. Afternoon concentrations of expired CO are typically in the range of 8–40 parts per million in smokers and drop down to 0–4 parts per million (i.e., nonsmoker levels) in ex-smokers within 2–3 days of quitting (U.S. Department of Health and Human Services 2014). The CO measurement reflects the last 3 days of smoking behavior but can be less accurate for very low levels of smoking. In addition to documenting the level of smoke exposure and verifying abstinence, CO measurement can also be used as a motivational tool. Smokers may be unaware that combustible tobacco products generate deadly carbon monoxide, which reduces body oxygen levels and is a major risk factor for cardiovascular disease. This effect is reversible, and the level returns to normal within only a few days of stopping smoking. The follow-up CO measurement serves as feedback that stopping smoking results in both immediate and long-term health benefits.

Patient Motivation/Engagement and Brief Approaches

In surveys, most smokers report that they want to quit, and more than half report having made a quit attempt during the past year (Fiore et al. 2008). For smokers who are not ready to quit immediately, interventions such as motivational interviewing can help to engage these individuals and encourage them to start thinking about and taking initial steps toward quitting (Miller and Rollnick 2013). According to the Stages of Change model of behavior change (Prochaska and DiClemente 1992), interventions targeting behavior change should be tailored to an individual's stage of change (i.e., precontemplation, contemplation, preparation, action, or maintenance stage). Resolving ambivalence about making changes in one's behavior is a key focus of motivational interviewing. Framing tobacco dependence as an SUD requiring "treatment" (as opposed to using action-oriented language like "quitting" or "stopping") is consistent with motivational approaches and may be more engaging to clients and lead to less resistance to pursuing behavior change.

Individuals who receive even brief advice to quit smoking from their physicians are 30% more likely to try to quit than those who do not receive this advice (Fiore et al. 2008). The 2008 Clinical Practice Guidelines (Fiore et al. 2008) from the U.S. Department of Health and Human Services recommended that in clinical settings, tobacco users should, at a minimum, be identified and advised to quit. The "five A's" were developed as a model for addressing tobacco use by health care providers. This model recommends the following: *Ask* a patient if they smoke. *Assess* tobacco use and desire to quit. *Advise* the patient to quit. *Assist* the patient with a quit plan. *Arrange* follow-up. To enhance motivation, the five A's can be implemented in the spirit of motivational interviewing (e.g., asking permission before giving advice and tailoring plans and recommendations based on the change readiness of and ideas provided by the patient). The five A's take less than 10 minutes to administer, and this intervention may also be replaced with even briefer strategies, such as "two A's and an R" (i.e., ask, advise, and refer [Fiore et al. 2008]).

To incentivize physicians to provide screening, brief intervention, and referral for tobacco use disorder, the Centers for Medicare and Medicaid Services developed Current Procedural Terminology (CPT) codes for reimbursement of these services. The codes are based on the time spent on smoking cessation counseling (CPT 99406 for between 3 and 10 minutes and CPT 99407 for more than 10 minutes). Current Medicare reimbursement rates for physicians and other recognized providers are low, and reimbursement codes have strict limitations on how they can be used, such as that counseling/treatment must be provided as an adjunctive and not a primary service. One of the ongoing challenges in treating patients with tobacco use disorder is that there are very few options to bill for intensive counseling or treatment for this condition as a primary disorder, as most insurance plans will not allow such billing.

Counseling Approaches

The Clinical Practice Guidelines (Fiore et al. 2008) recommended interventions that include support, encouragement, and practical counseling. These interventions often focus on helping individuals designate a date on which they plan to stop using tobacco, enlist support from their social network, and anticipate challenges they might encounter and develop a plan for dealing with them. Counseling may include cognitive-behavioral strategies that enable individuals to observe their smoking patterns, increase their awareness of situations that are associated with smoking, and break the links between smoking-associated situations and their smoking behavior. Interventions teach people to understand tobacco withdrawal, to become familiar with pharmacotherapy options, and to learn strategies for coping with cravings and triggers. These interventions can also help people replace maladaptive habits with healthy coping skills. Counseling is traditionally provided in a face-to-face individual or group format and is more effective than briefer interventions (Fiore et al. 2008).

Other emerging psychosocial interventions such as mindfulness meditation and acceptance and commitment therapy (ACT) have shown promise in the treatment of tobacco use disorder (Maglione et al. 2017). Methods for increasing mindfulness include meditation and yoga, which can help tobacco users in several ways. Mindfulness meditation increases awareness, reduces automatic behaviors, and helps individuals choose more adaptive responses, thus impacting relapse. Mindfulness practice also teaches individuals to simply observe negative experiences, without judgment or behavioral reaction, in order to disconnect and dismantle the negative reinforcement cycle. Mindfulness training helps individuals to tolerate cravings without immediately satisfying them, by "sitting with" or "riding out" their cravings. ACT helps people to develop core skills to increase cognitive flexibility, practice mindfulness, and promote overall success. These skills include being in and experiencing the present moment without judgment, developing insight into one's own values and then committing to actions that are consistent with those values, and learning to observe oneself in a way that is separate from one's emotions, thoughts, and memories (Dindo et al. 2017).

Psychosocial interventions delivered or accessed through telephone, Internet, or mobile technology have been developed, and studies have found these interventions to show promise for smoking cessation (Taylor et al. 2017; Whittaker et al. 2016). Telephone-based "quit line" services provide effective counseling; key advantages include accessibility, ease of use, and low cost. Most patients receive an average of three or fewer counseling calls, although in general, more sessions are associated with greater success (Stead et al. 2013). Every state has a state and/or federally funded quit line that offers free or low-cost services. Internet and mobile phone interventions enable individuals who would otherwise not have access to traditional counseling to obtain information and support. These interventions may send individuals tailored and supportive text messages or emails and provide education through written materials, videos, or interactive exercises.

Pharmacotherapy for Tobacco Use Disorder

Pharmacological treatments for tobacco use disorder have a strong evidence base for increasing the likelihood of a successful quit attempt. These medications reduce tobacco withdrawal symptoms and block the pleasurable effects of nicotine in the brain. They are associated with twofold to threefold increased success in quitting. Medications are most effective in combination with counseling, although they are also effective when used alone. The FDA has approved three different types of medications for use as an aid to smoking cessation: nicotine replacement therapies (NRTs), bupropion SR, and varenicline. Choice of treatment depends on the patient's preference, his or her experience during previous quit attempts, the presence of any comorbid medical or psychiatric disorders, and the severity of the patient's tobacco use disorder. Vareni-cline has demonstrated superior efficacy in comparison with NRT or bupropion (Ca-hill et al. 2013). Combining a long-acting nicotine patch with a short-acting nicotine replacement agent (e.g., gum, lozenge) is also an effective strategy that improves out-comes in comparison with use of a single type of NRT or bupropion monotherapy (Carpenter et al. 2013; Fiore et al. 2008). Better outcomes are associated with longer durations of treatment of around 6 months (Schnoll et al. 2015).

Nicotine Replacement Therapies

Six different NRT formulations are available: patch, gum, lozenge, inhaler, nasal spray, and the new oral spray. It is helpful to remind the patient that it is always safer to use NRT instead of smoking tobacco, because these products contain only nicotine and not the thousands of toxins and carcinogens found in tobacco smoke. About 25% of users of NRT are able to stay away from smoking at 6 months (Fiore et al. 2008). Nicotine poses little risk to a tobacco user who has developed physiological tolerance to nicotine. Decades of research on nicotine have demonstrated that it has little to no cardiotoxicity and does not cause cancer; furthermore, nicotine has no clinically sig-nificant drug–drug interactions. Estrogen-containing oral contraceptives speed the metabolism of nicotine, which can lead to reduced serum levels—and perhaps re-duced effectiveness—of NRT in women (Allen et al. 2019).

The patch, gum, and lozenge formulations are available over the counter (OTC) in the United States. However, because the cost of the OTC preparations can be a barrier to their use by low-income populations, many state Medicaid programs now cover these medications with a prescription (American Lung Association 2019).

Psychoeducation can help patients to maximize the effectiveness of NRT, because most patients take it at too low a dose or for too short a period of time. NRTs generally produce blood nicotine levels that are lower than those produced by smoking, and taking two NRT products simultaneously provides better withdrawal and craving re-lief (Carpenter et al. 2013). Dosing nicotine all day long produces better outcomes than using it only as needed for cravings, because this provides a steady level of nico-tine in the blood that helps to minimize withdrawal symptoms. Oral absorption of nicotine is reduced in an acidic environment; therefore, the patient should be advised not to use nicotine gum, lozenge, or inhaler products with beverages like coffee or soda. An advantage of the immediate-acting forms of NRT such as the gum or loz-enge is that they provide immediate relief from cravings and can be used as a rescue medication to supplement the longer-acting patch. In 2013, the FDA revised the guidelines for NRTs so that they are less restrictive than the previous recommenda-tions and reflect current evidence for safety and efficacy. Labeling on NRT products now states that there are no significant safety concerns associated with 1) using more than one NRT, 2) using NRT at the same time as a cigarette, and 3) using NRT for lon-ger than 12 weeks (U.S. Food and Drug Administration 2013).

Nicotine patches provide slow, transdermal delivery of nicotine, with peak con-centrations achieved 2–6 hours after application. There is no strict timeline for taper-ing the dose (from 21 mg to 14 mg and then to 7 mg); however, patients should be mostly free from cravings before dose reductions are considered. The patch can be as-sociated with local skin irritation, which can be minimized by rotating the patch site every day. Some patients develop insomnia or unpleasant dreams while wearing the patch overnight; otherwise, it is generally recommended that the patch be worn for 24 hours to deliver the full dose and reduce the risk for early-morning relapse.

Both nicotine gum and nicotine lozenges are available in 2-mg and 4-mg doses. These NRTs work best as scheduled medications taken every 1–2 hours, with additional doses taken as needed for cravings. Nicotine gum must be chewed slowly and held in the cheek for about 20 minutes. Poor adherence to the recommended usage technique can result in low nicotine blood levels and dyspepsia if too much nicotine is swallowed. Nicotine gum is not recommended for patients with poor dentition or temporomandibular joint problems. The nicotine lozenge is not chewed but instead is held in the mouth until it dissolves. Only about 50% of the nicotine contained in the gum or lozenge is absorbed, making them low-dose delivery products.

A nicotine inhaler requires a prescription but provides a dose that is pharmacologically similar to that provided by the gum or lozenge. The inhaler is an oral puffer consisting of a mouthpiece and a replaceable nicotine cartridge. The patient can puff for 20–30 minutes to allow the nicotine to be absorbed through the oral mucosa. Recommended usage is 6–16 cartridges per day. The nicotine nasal spray also requires a prescription; however, this product is rarely used. Although it delivers a high dose of nicotine, the nasal spray has an 80% discontinuation rate due to adverse effects such as nasal irritation, rhinitis, coughing, and watering eyes. There is some dependence liability with the nicotine nasal spray due to the more rapid absorption of nicotine through the nasal mucosa in comparison with absorption through the skin or oral mucosa.

A nicotine oral spray was FDA approved for OTC use in September 2019. Each spray to the mouth delivers about 1 mg of nicotine, and the spray can be used up to 4 times per hour and 64 times per day. Because of the smaller nicotine droplet size, the oral spray offers faster absorption of nicotine through the oral mucosa compared with other forms of NRT, which may provide more rapid relief of craving (Kraiczi et al. 2011). As with other oral forms of nicotine, the spray can cause gastrointestinal side effects—including hiccups and nausea as well as mild throat irritation—if too much nicotine is swallowed. The nicotine oral spray has been available for several years in Europe, Canada, and other countries, where it has not been associated with product abuse. It has demonstrated efficacy similar to that of other NRT products. One potential concern is that the oral spray contains a tiny amount of ethanol (<100 mg per spray). At the maximum dose of 64 sprays per day, the user would ingest about the same amount of ethanol contained in 5 mL (<1 teaspoon) of wine with 12% alcohol content (GlaxoSmithKline 2019).

Bupropion

Bupropion SR is a nonsedating antidepressant classified as a norepinephrine and dopamine reuptake inhibitor (NDRI). It was later discovered to be a noncompetitive nicotinic receptor antagonist (Slemmer et al. 2000). This may explain its efficacy as a smoking cessation aid, an effect not observed with most other antidepressants. For tobacco cessation, bupropion SR at a daily dosage of 150 mg or 300 mg can be effective, and its overall effectiveness is similar to that of NRT. Although bupropion can be an excellent choice for a smoker who experiences depression, its ability to help people quit smoking is independent of its effect on depression.

Adverse effects commonly reported with bupropion include dry mouth, headache, and insomnia. Because bupropion can lower the seizure threshold, its use is contraindicated in patients with history of seizures or bulimia. Bupropion is a strong cytochrome P450 (CYP) 2D6 inhibitor, which means that drug–drug interactions are possible. Bupropion at a daily dosage of 300 mg is associated with the lowest reported weight gain linked to stopping smoking. Although the FDA reviewed data on the sustained-release formulation when the medication was first approved for smoking cessation, the extended-release once-daily dosing formulation (bupropion XL) is likely bioequivalent and is often preferred in clinical practice, as it may enhance treatment adherence and reduce side effects.

Varenicline

Varenicline is a partial agonist at $\alpha_4\beta_2$ nicotinic acetylcholine receptors, which are found in the ventral tegmental area, an area involved in the biology of addiction in the brain. Varenicline promotes the release of small amounts of dopamine at the nucleus accumbens and helps to prevent tobacco withdrawal by maintaining tone in the mesolimbic pathway. Varenicline has a higher affinity than nicotine at the receptor, blocking the effects of nicotine when an individual uses tobacco (Cahill et al. 2016). In this way, varenicline diminishes the reward experienced from tobacco use.

Varenicline is titrated to a dose of 1 mg twice a day in the first week. The medication should be taken with food to reduce the main side effect of nausea. Other possible side effects of varenicline include constipation, insomnia, and abnormal dreams. A meta-analysis showed greater efficacy for varenicline among women smokers compared with men smokers for short- and immediate-term outcomes (McKee et al. 2016). This advantage of varenicline over bupropion and the nicotine patch is greater for women than for men, and clinicians should consider varenicline as the first-option treatment for women (Smith et al. 2017).

The EAGLES (Evaluating Adverse Events in a Global Smoking Cessation Study) trial was a large multisite study of more than 8,000 smokers with and without mental illness. In addition to confirming the superiority of varenicline over placebo, nicotine patch, and bupropion, the study confirmed the absence of severe neuropsychiatric side effects from varenicline, with no differences between medication groups (Anthenelli et al. 2016). This and other studies have validated varenicline's efficacy in smokers with mental illnesses, including major depressive disorder and schizophrenia (Anthenelli et al. 2013; Williams et al. 2012). In 2016, as a result of considerable evidence, the FDA removed the black box warning for severe neuropsychiatric symptoms (U.S. Food and Drug Administration 2016). The EAGLES trial further confirmed the lack of major adverse cardiovascular events (cardiovascular death, nonfatal myocardial infarction, and nonfatal stroke) associated with the nicotine patch, bupropion, or varenicline (Benowitz et al. 2018). Policies restricting or banning varenicline use, especially among those with behavioral health conditions, should be revisited, because the risk of tobacco far outweighs the potential risk from medications, and tobacco users should be given access to every available FDA-approved treatment. Combinations of varenicline with nicotine are generally not recommended, although combinations of varenicline and bupropion are safe and may enhance outcomes (Rose and Behm 2017).

Harm-Reduction Strategies for Tobacco Use Disorder

Smoking Reduction

Pharmacotherapy can also be effective in helping smokers who are not immediately ready to stop smoking. Several trials have tested NRT as an intervention to assist with smoking reduction. Use of NRT is associated with significant reductions in smoking as well as an increased likelihood of quitting among smokers who have been unable or unwilling to quit (Lindson-Hawley et al. 2016). Varenicline is also effective for smoking reduction. A large 24-week trial of varenicline versus placebo in smokers not willing or able to immediately quit demonstrated that varenicline was associated with much higher rates of abstinence from smoking at 6 and 12 months than was placebo (Ebbert et al. 2015). Varenicline reduction strategies have been so successful that they are part of the on-label FDA-approved usage recommendations. Recommendations are to start varenicline and encourage the patient to reduce smoking by 50% within the first 4 weeks and then by 50% again in the next 4 weeks, with the goal of reaching complete abstinence by 12 weeks. There is less evidence to support the use of behavioral interventions alone (without medication) for smoking reduction. In reduction studies, quantifying smoking reduction with biomarkers such as carbon monoxide or nicotine metabolite levels is more reliable than measures of cigarettes per day. In sum, these studies (Ebbert et al. 2015; Lindson-Hawley et al. 2016) suggest that treatments for smokers not yet ready to quit, but willing to reduce their cigarette consumption, are viable strategies for working with tobacco users.

Electronic Cigarettes

Alternative products that deliver heated nicotine but do not burn have been developed, and there is controversy in the field as to whether these products represent viable harm reduction alternatives for tobacco users. Electronic cigarettes (or e-cigarettes) are tobacco products that deliver nicotine. In addition to containing nicotine, e-cigarettes often include solvents, flavoring agents, and low levels of carcinogens (U.S. Department of Health and Human Services 2016). These products heat nicotine but do not produce the same products of combustion that are in cigarette smoke. The "vape" (i.e., heated nicotine vapor) generated from an e-cigarette is estimated to contain about 1% of the toxins present in a combustible cigarette, suggesting that e-cigarettes could represent a reduced-risk alternative for smokers who are unable or unwilling to quit. Studies have yielded mixed evidence as to whether e-cigarettes are effective in helping smokers to quit (Malas et al. 2016; McRobbie et al. 2014), and at best, they are felt to be about as effective as NRT. Because these products are so new and are rapidly changing, gaps exist in the knowledge base; therefore, a cautious approach is recommended.

One of the biggest concerns about e-cigarettes is their rapid uptake among young people. As usage rates of traditional cigarettes fall, new tobacco products that can appeal to a younger market are continually being developed. The newly expanding tobacco market also includes flavored and filtered cigars, new forms of chewing tobacco, and hookah, in addition to e-cigarettes (which can be easily modified to administer illicit substances). There is often the misperception that these products represent a risk-free alternative to cigarettes. Because these products contain nicotine, they carry a risk for dependence, and there is emerging evidence among teens that e-cigarettes are associated with greater use of cigarettes and marijuana (Leventhal et al. 2016). New nicotine vaporizers are discreetly sized and have the appearance of a computer flash drive. They employ a new nicotine salt preparation that delivers a very high nicotine dose to the user (Goniewicz et al. 2019). These vaporizers have become extremely popular among high school students, with 30% of U.S. twelfth graders reporting nicotine vaping in 2018 (Johnston et al. 2019). Action should be taken at the federal, state, and local levels to limit young people's access to tobacco products, including e-cigarettes. Bans on the use of flavoring agents in e-cigarettes may be a useful step in reducing their appeal among young people. Increased vigilance is warranted, because this represents an intentional effort by the tobacco industry to engage new populations in tobacco use as the popularity of traditional cigarettes declines.

Tobacco Use in Populations With Mental Illness or With Other Substance Use Disorders

Among individuals with mental illness, the prevalence of all types of SUDs, including tobacco use disorder, is much higher, and is associated with worse treatment outcomes. People with current mental illness or SUD make up at least one-third of current smokers in the United States, and they purchase at least one-third of all tobacco products (Centers for Disease Control and Prevention 2013; Lawrence et al. 2009). Among both people with mental disorders (Callaghan et al. 2014) and people with substance use disorders, tobacco is the number one cause of death, even surpassing rates for deaths due to alcohol or other drugs (Hurt et al. 1996; Veldhuizen and Callaghan 2014). Tobacco use also threatens recovery for these individuals by negatively impacting finances, employability, and housing. Tobacco smoke is a potent inducer of the CYP1A2 isoenzyme, reducing serum levels of several psychiatric medications.

Several studies have now linked tobacco use to worse mental health or other substance use outcomes (Hagman et al. 2008; Poorolajal and Darvishi 2016; Weinberger et al. 2017). Although many individuals report using tobacco to reduce anxiety, there are abundant human and animal data showing the opposite—that tobacco or nicotine exposure *increases* anxiety (Morissette et al. 2007). Because anxiety is also part of the withdrawal syndrome, it is likely that it is tobacco users' temporary relief from withdrawal that is mistaken for an anxiolytic effect. A meta-analysis of 26 longitudinal studies that assessed mental health in adult participants before and after smoking cessation found that anxiety, depression, and stress significantly decreased in quitters compared with individuals who continued to smoke (Taylor et al. 2014). In addition, both psychological quality of life and positive affect significantly improved in quitters during the same period. Among individuals with other SUDs, continuing or initiating smoking is associated with greater odds of SUD relapse (Weinberger et al. 2017).

People with mental illness have an increased vulnerability to tobacco use disorder and experience more difficulty in quitting tobacco use, which warrants a specialized or more intensive treatment approach. Tobacco users with psychiatric comorbidity have higher levels of nicotine dependence and tobacco use severity (Hagman et al. 2008; Pratt and Brody 2010). There is also evidence that these individuals experience higher levels of tobacco withdrawal symptoms, making it more challenging for them to quit and supporting the need for intensive treatments and more pharmacotherapies (Weinberger et al. 2010).

Given these challenges, an approach to integrating tobacco use disorder treatment into usual treatment could borrow from strategies for other co-occurring substance use disorders. Matching interventions to patient motivational level, and taking a long-term perspective, as is done with other co-occurring disorders, would be beneficial (Williams et al. 2014). Despite recommendations that smoking cessation treatment be integrated into behavioral health care programs, change has been slow, as evidenced by a recent Centers for Disease Control and Prevention review that found that fewer than half of U.S. mental health treatment facilities screen patients for tobacco use or have a smoke-free campus (Marynak et al. 2018). Rates of implementation for specific treatment interventions are even lower. Full integration of tobacco cessation interventions into behavioral health treatment, coupled with implementation of tobacco-free campus policies in behavioral health treatment settings, could decrease tobacco use and could improve health outcomes substantially among persons with mental disorders and SUDs.

Conclusion

The burden of tobacco use morbidity and mortality remains high and costly, and more efforts should be directed toward helping tobacco users to quit, particularly in the behavioral health treatment setting. Quitting smoking saves lives and is beneficial at any age. When asked, roughly a quarter of tobacco users say that they are ready to try to quit in the next 30 days. Evidence-based treatments are associated with better outcomes, and all tobacco users should be offered counseling and medication approaches. Tobacco users with higher levels of dependence will have greater difficulty quitting and may benefit from more intensive approaches. Motivational approaches are helpful to specifically engage individuals who are not ready to change, to resolve ambivalence about change, and to plan initial steps toward change. Nicotine replacement therapies, bupropion, and varenicline are all effective for quitting smoking, but better outcomes are associated with varenicline monotherapy or combinations of NRT products (long-acting plus short-acting). Practical tobacco use counseling may include cognitive-behavioral strategies that enable individuals to observe and change their smoking patterns, practice strategies for coping with cravings, and education about nicotine/tobacco withdrawal and options for pharmacotherapy. The rapid rise in e-cigarette use among teens and young adults is cause for concern; in addition, the widening variety of new tobacco products should be approached with caution, because their safety has not been determined.

References

Allen AM, Weinberger AH, Wetherill RR, et al: Oral contraceptives and cigarette smoking: a review of the literature and future directions. Nicotine Tob Res 21(5):592–601, 2019 29165663

American Lung Association: State Tobacco Cessation Coverage. 2019. Available at: http://www.lungusa2.org/cessation2/. Accessed November 25, 2019.

American Psychiatric Association: Diagnostic and Statistical Manual of Mental Disorders, 5th Edition. Arlington, VA, American Psychiatric Association, 2013

Anthenelli RM, Morris C, Ramey TS, et al: Effects of varenicline on smoking cessation in adults with stably treated current or past major depression: a randomized trial. Ann Intern Med 159(6):390–400, 2013 24042367

Anthenelli RM, Benowitz NL, West R, et al: Neuropsychiatric safety and efficacy of varenicline, bupropion, and nicotine patch in smokers with and without psychiatric disorders (EAGLES): a double-blind, randomised, placebo-controlled clinical trial. Lancet 387(10037):2507–2520, 2016 27116918

Benowitz NL, Pipe A, West R, et al: Cardiovascular safety of varenicline, bupropion, and nicotine patch in smokers: a randomized clinical trial. JAMA Intern Med 178(5):622–631, 2018 29630702

Cahill K, Stevens S, Perera R, et al: Pharmacological interventions for smoking cessation: an overview and network meta-analysis. Cochrane Database Syst Rev (5):CD009329, 2013 23728690

Cahill K, Lindson-Hawley N, Thomas KH, et al: Nicotine receptor partial agonists for smoking cessation. Cochrane Database Syst Rev (5):CD006103, 2016 27158893

Callaghan RC, Veldhuizen S, Jeysingh T, et al: Patterns of tobacco-related mortality among individuals diagnosed with schizophrenia, bipolar disorder, or depression. J Psychiatr Res 48(1):102–110, 2014 24139811

Carpenter MJ, Jardin BF, Burris JL, et al: Clinical strategies to enhance the efficacy of nicotine replacement therapy for smoking cessation: a review of the literature. Drugs 73(5):407–426, 2013 23572407

Centers for Disease Control and Prevention: Vital signs: current cigarette smoking among adults aged ≥18 years with mental illness—United States, 2009–2011. MMWR Morb Mortal Wkly Rep 62(5):81–87, 2013 23388551

Centers for Medicare and Medicaid Services: Counseling to Prevent Tobacco Use. MLN Matters, December 10, 2012. Available at: https://www.cms.gov/Outreach-and-Education/Medicare-Learning-Network-MLN/MLNMattersArticles/downloads/MM7133.pdf. Accessed November 25, 2019.

DiFranza JR, Savageau JA, Fletcher K, et al: Measuring the loss of autonomy over nicotine use in adolescents: the DANDY (Development and Assessment of Nicotine Dependence in Youths) study. Arch Pediatr Adolesc Med 156(4):397–403, 2002 11929376

Dindo L, Van Liew JR, Arch JJ: Acceptance and commitment therapy: a transdiagnostic behavioral intervention for mental health and medical conditions. Neurotherapeutics 14(3):546–553, 2017 28271287

Ebbert JO, Hughes JR, West RJ, et al: Effect of varenicline on smoking cessation through smoking reduction: a randomized clinical trial. JAMA 313(7):687–694, 2015 25688780

Fiore M, Jaén C, Baker TB, et al: Treating Tobacco Use and Dependence: 2008 Update. Clinical Practice Guideline. Rockville, MD, U.S. Department of Health and Human Services, Public Health Service, 2008

GlaxoSmithKline: Nicotine Oral Spray, Nonprescription Drugs Advisory Committee of the U.S. Food and Drug Administration, September 18, 2019. Available at: https://www.fda.gov/media/131058/download. Accessed July 9, 2020.

Goniewicz ML, Boykan R, Messina CR, et al: High exposure to nicotine among adolescents who use Juul and other vape pod systems ("pods"). Tob Control 28(6):676–677, 2019 18158218

Hagman BT, Delnevo CD, Hrywna M, et al: Tobacco use among those with serious psychological distress: results from the national survey of drug use and health, 2002. Addict Behav 33(4):582–592, 2008 18158218

Heatherton TF, Kozlowski LT, Frecker RC, et al: The Fagerström test for nicotine dependence: a revision of the Fagerström Tolerance Questionnaire. Br J Addict 86(9):1119–1127, 1991 1932883

Hurt R, Offord KP, Croghan IT, et al: Mortality following inpatient addictions treatment. Role of tobacco use in a community-based cohort. JAMA 275(14):1097–1103, 1996 8601929

Jamal A, Phillips E, Gentzke AS, et al: Current cigarette smoking among adults—United States, 2016. MMWR Morb Mortal Wkly Rep 67(2):53–59, 2018 29346338

Johnston LD, Miech RA, O'Malley PM, et al: Monitoring the Future: National Survey Results on Drug Use 1975–2018: Overview, Key Findings on Adolescent Drug Use. Ann Arbor, MI, Institute for Social Research, University of Michigan, 2019

Koob GF, Le Moal M: Plasticity of reward neurocircuitry and the "dark side" of drug addiction. Nat Neurosci 8(11):1442–1444, 2005 16251985

Kraiczi H, Hansson A, Perfekt R: Single-dose pharmacokinetics of nicotine when given with a novel mouth spray for nicotine replacement therapy. Nicotine Tob Res 13(12):1176–1182, 2011 21849415

Lawrence D, Mitrou F, Zubrick SR: Smoking and mental illness: results from population surveys in Australia and the United States. BMC Public Health 9:285, 2009 19664203

Leventhal AM, Stone MD, Andrabi N, et al: Association of e-cigarette vaping and progression to heavier patterns of cigarette smoking. JAMA 316(18):1918–1920, 2016 27825000

Lindson-Hawley N, Hartmann-Boyce J, Fanshawe TR, et al: Interventions to reduce harm from continued tobacco use. Cochrane Database Syst Rev (10):CD005231, 2016 27734465

Maglione MA, Maher AR, Ewing B, et al: Efficacy of mindfulness meditation for smoking cessation: a systematic review and meta-analysis. Addict Behav 69:27–34, 2017 28126511

Malas M, van der Tempel J, Schwartz R, et al: Electronic cigarettes for smoking cessation: a systematic review. Nicotine Tob Res 18(10):1926–1936, 2016 27113014

Marynak K, VanFrank B, Tetlow S, et al: Tobacco cessation interventions and smoke-free policies in mental health and substance abuse treatment facilities—United States, 2016. MMWR Morb Mortal Wkly Rep 67(18):519–523, 2018 29746451

McKee SA, Smith PH, Kaufman M, et al: Sex differences in varenicline efficacy for smoking cessation: a meta-analysis. Nicotine Tob Res 18(5):1002–1011, 2016 26446070

McRobbie H, Bullen C, Hartmann-Boyce J, et al: Electronic cigarettes for smoking cessation and reduction. Cochrane Database Syst Rev (12):CD010216, 2014 25515689

Miller WR, Rollnick S (eds): Motivational Interviewing: Helping People Change, 3rd Edition. New York, Guilford, 2013

Morissette SB, Tull MT, Gulliver SB, et al: Anxiety, anxiety disorders, tobacco use, and nicotine: a critical review of interrelationships. Psychol Bull 133(2):245–272, 2007 17338599

Odani S, Agaku IT, Graffunder CM, et al: Tobacco product use among military veterans— United States, 2010–2015. MMWR Morb Mortal Wkly Rep 67(1):7–12, 2018 29324732

Poorolajal J, Darvishi N: Smoking and suicide: a meta-analysis. PLoS One 11(7):e0156348, 2016 2739133

Pratt LA, Brody DJ: Depression and Smoking in the U.S. Household Population Aged 20 and Over, 2005–2008. NCHS Data Brief, Vol 34. Hyattsville, MD, National Center for Health Statistics, 2010

Prochaska JO, DiClemente CC: Stages of change in the modification of problem behaviors. Prog Behav Modif 28:183–218, 1992 1620663

Rose JE, Behm FM: Combination varenicline/bupropion treatment benefits highly dependent smokers in an adaptive smoking cessation paradigm. Nicotine Tob Res 19(8):999–1002, 2017 29054128

Schnoll RA, Goelz PM, Veluz-Wilkins A, et al: Long-term nicotine replacement therapy: a randomized clinical trial. JAMA Intern Med 175(4):504–511, 2015 25705872

Slemmer JE, Martin BR, Damaj MI: Bupropion is a nicotinic antagonist. J Pharmacol Exp Ther 295(1):321–327, 2000 10991997

Smith PH, Bessette AJ, Weinberger AH, et al: Sex/gender differences in smoking cessation: a review. Prev Med 92:135–140, 2016 27471021

Smith PH, Weinberger AH, Zhang J, et al: Sex differences in smoking cessation pharmacotherapy comparative efficacy: a network meta-analysis. Nicotine Tob Res 19(3):273–281, 2017 27613893

Stead LF, Hartmann-Boyce J, Perera R, et al: Telephone counselling for smoking cessation. Cochrane Database Syst Rev (8):CD002850, 2013 23934971

Taylor G, McNeill A, Girling A, et al: Change in mental health after smoking cessation: systematic review and meta-analysis. BMJ 348:g1151, 2014 24524926

Taylor GMJ, Dalili MN, Semwal M, et al: Internet-based interventions for smoking cessation. Cochrane Database Syst Rev (9):CD007078, 2017 28869775

U.S. Department of Health and Human Services: The Health Consequences of Smoking—50 Years of Progress: A Report of the Surgeon General. Atlanta, GA, U.S. Department of Health and Human Services, Centers for Disease Control and Prevention, National Center for Chronic Disease Prevention and Health Promotion, Office on Smoking and Health, 2014

U.S. Department of Health and Human Services: E-Cigarette Use Among Youth and Young Adults: A Report of the Surgeon General—Executive Summary. Atlanta, GA, U.S. Department of Health and Human Services, Centers for Disease Control and Prevention, National Center for Chronic Disease Prevention and Health Promotion, Office on Smoking and Health, 2016

U.S. Department of Health and Human Services: Smoking Cessation: A Report of the Surgeon General—Executive Summary. Atlanta, GA, U.S. Department of Health and Human Services, Centers for Disease Control and Prevention, National Center for Chronic Disease Prevention and Health Promotion, Office on Smoking and Health, 2020. Available at: https://www.hhs.gov/sites/default/files/2020-cessation-sgr-executive-summary.pdf. Accessed July 13, 2020.

U.S. Department of Housing and Urban Development: Instituting Smoke-Free Public Housing. A Rule by the Housing and Urban Development Department on 12/05/2016. Effective date February 3, 2017. Available at: https://www.federalregister.gov/documents/2016/12/05/2016-28986/instituting-smoke-free-public-housing. Accessed July 9, 2020.

U.S. Food and Drug Administration: Modifications to Labeling of Nicotine Replacement Therapy Products for Over-the-Counter Human Use. Federal Register, April 2, 2013. Available at: www.federalregister.gov/documents/2013/04/02/2013–07528/modifications-to-labeling-of-nicotine-replacement-therapy-products-for-over-the-counter-human-use. Accessed November 25, 2019.

U.S. Food and Drug Administration: FDA Drug Safety Communication: FDA Revises Description of Mental Health Side Effects of the Stop-Smoking Medicines Chantix (Varenicline) and Zyban (Bupropion) to Reflect Clinical Trial Findings. Center for Drug Evaluation and Research, December 16, 2016. Available at: www.fda.gov/Drugs/DrugSafety/ucm532221.htm. Accessed November 25, 2019.

Veldhuizen S, Callaghan RC: Cause-specific mortality among people previously hospitalized with opioid-related conditions: a retrospective cohort study. Ann Epidemiol 24(8):620–624, 2014 25084705

Weinberger AH, Desai RA, McKee SA: Nicotine withdrawal in U.S. smokers with current mood, anxiety, alcohol use, and substance use disorders. Drug Alcohol Depend 108(1–2):7–12, 2010 20006451

Weinberger AH, Platt J, Esan H, et al: Cigarette smoking is associated with increased risk of substance use disorder relapse: a nationally representative, prospective longitudinal investigation. J Clin Psychiatry 78(2):e152–e160, 2017 28234432

Whittaker R, McRobbie H, Bullen C, et al: Mobile phone-based interventions for smoking cessation. Cochrane Database Syst Rev (4):CD006611, 2016 27060875

Williams JM, Anthenelli RM, Morris CD, et al: A randomized, double-blind, placebo-controlled study evaluating the safety and efficacy of varenicline for smoking cessation in patients with schizophrenia or schizoaffective disorder. J Clin Psychiatry 73(5):654–660, 2012 22697191

Williams JM, Stroup TS, Brunette MF, et al: Tobacco use and mental illness: a wake-up call for psychiatrists. Psychiatr Serv 65(12):1406–1408, 2014 25270381

World Health Organization: International Statistical Classification of Diseases and Related Health Problems, 10th Revision. Geneva, World Health Organization, 1992

Xu X, Bishop EE, Kennedy SM, et al: Annual healthcare spending attributable to cigarette smoking: an update. Am J Prev Med 48(3):326–333, 2015 25498551

CHAPTER 20

Neurobiology and Treatment of Sedative-, Hypnotic-, and Anxiolytic-Related Disorders

Jennifer L. Jones, M.D.

Amy VandenBerg, Pharm.D., BCPP

Robert Malcolm, M.D.

Throughout history, numerous compounds have been utilized to restore tranquility and promote sleep. These therapeutic agents have gone by various names, including tranquilizers, sedatives, hypnotics, and anxiolytics. Consumption of alcohol and opium alkaloids derived from the poppy plant for their sedative-hypnotic properties predates written history. In the late nineteenth and early twentieth centuries, other compounds such as chloral hydrate, paraldehyde, and the bromide salts were also utilized in medicine for their sedative properties, although they have never been approved by the U.S. Food and Drug Administration (FDA). In modern times, compounds with these intended effects have been characterized as sedative-hypnotic agents. Although alcohol and opium possess sedative-hypnotic properties, they are considered separately in this textbook because of their unique pharmacology and abuse liability. Sedative-hypnotic agents are commonly categorized according to their chemical structure as barbiturates, benzodiazepines, and nonbenzodiazepine hypnotics (colloquially referred to as "Z-drugs" because their generic names typically start with the letter "z").

Treatment Applications

Historical Uses

Barbituric acid, the first of the modern sedative-hypnotics (Figure 20–1), was synthesized in 1864 by Adolf von Baeyer, who went on to found the Bayer Chemical Company. It was not until 1904, however, when diethylbarbituric acid (more commonly known as barbital) was developed and brought to market by Bayer, that barbiturates became used clinically (López-Muñoz et al. 2005). During the First and Second World Wars, barbital and its many subsequent analogs were widely used for induction of anesthesia and for their effects on many refractory psychiatric and neurological conditions of the time, including severe emotional repression, neuroses, psychoses, insomnia, and epilepsy (López-Muñoz et al. 2005). Barbiturates achieved their greatest clinical popularity in the 1940s and 1950s for the treatment of anxiety and insomnia (López-Muñoz et al. 2005). With this rising popularity, however, came a gradual increased awareness of the high rates of physiological dependence, the addictive potential, and the risk of respiratory depression associated with these agents. By the late 1960s, the overdose potential of barbiturates had become well known in American society following the fatal barbiturate overdoses of several celebrities, including Marilyn Monroe and Judy Garland.

In light of the abuse liability, physical dependence risks, and withdrawal severity of the barbiturates, novel agents were sought to replace these agents. In 1955, Hoffmann-La Roche chemist Leo Sternbach identified chlordiazepoxide (Librium), the first benzodiazepine (Wick 2013). This compound showed promise as a safer alternative to the barbiturate family, while retaining anxiolytic, hypnotic, and muscle-relaxant properties. Chlordiazepoxide was soon followed by diazepam (Valium). These agents appeared to be less toxic than the barbiturates and to carry a lower risk of respiratory depression; they were subsequently widely adopted by clinicians. By the mid-1970s, benzodiazepines were in widespread use for the management of daily stressors, nervousness, and insomnia. Valium prescribing peaked in the late 1970s, with Americans receiving more than 2.3 billion Valium tablets annually (Ainsworth 2013).

With escalating prescribing, however, came an awareness of the darker side of benzodiazepines and a push for legislative controls. Flunitrazepam (Rohypnol) was increasingly implicated in date rapes, leading to the Drug-Induced Rape Prevention and Punishment Act of 1996 (Wick 2013). The overdose potential, particularly when taken in combination with other respiratory depressants, was more broadly identified. Clinicians also began to recognize the unique risks of benzodiazepine use in the elderly, who seemed to be less sensitive to the therapeutic effects while being more sensitive to the adverse effects, such as delirium, falls, and cognitive impairment. Although benzodiazepines remained on the World Health Organization's list of essential drugs, they were excluded from coverage in Medicare Part D plans under the 2003 Medicare Modernization Act (Wick 2013). The benzodiazepine coverage exclusion was reversed by the 2010 Affordable Care Act (Wick 2013), but benzodiazepines remained on the recommended avoidance list of the 2012 Beers Criteria produced by the American Geriatric Society. Despite these cautionary measures, benzodiazepine

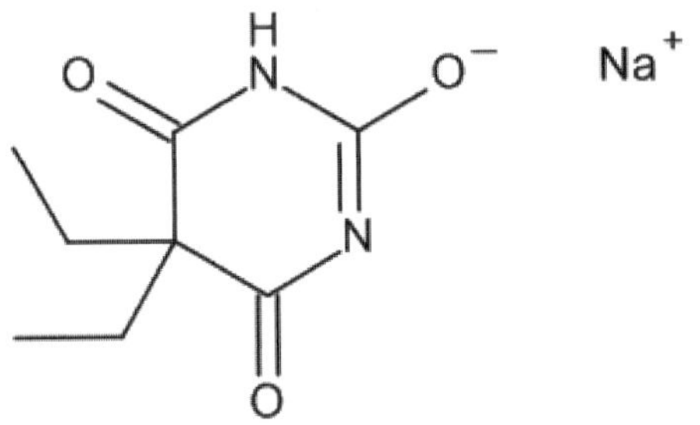

FIGURE 20–1. Barbital—the first of the modern sedative-hypnotics.

Barbital is the flagship compound from which more than 2,500 analogs were ultimately developed.

prescriptions have risen steadily over the past 25 years, increasing by 67% from 1996 to 2013, and the rates of overdose involving a benzodiazepine rose precipitously over this time period, from 0.58 per 100,000 in 1996 to 3.07 per 100,000 in 2013 (Bachhuber et al. 2016). Some studies estimate that 75% of opioid overdoses involve a benzodiazepine (Jones and McAninch 2015).

Nonbenzodiazepine alternatives with sedative and anxiolytic properties have been pursued over the past 30 years. This has led to the development of the "Z-drug" class of agents for the treatment of insomnia, the first of which were zopiclone, zolpidem, and zaleplon. These agents are associated with a risk (albeit low) of abuse and physical dependence, and consequently are recommended for short-term use only.

Current Medical Uses

Medical indications for use of these compounds are treatment of anxiety disorders (including perioperative anxiety), sleep disorders, seizure disorders, and muscle spasticity and movement disorders. Benzodiazepines are clinically useful in the management of acute intoxication of some substances (notably, stimulants such as cocaine and amphetamines), as well as in the management of acute withdrawal syndromes (particularly alcohol withdrawal). Barbiturates are still in use for the treatment of seizures (e.g., phenobarbital, primidone), for general anesthesia (e.g., sodium thiopental), and for animal euthanasia. Sedative-hypnotics are also used off-label for adjunctive treatment of mood and psychotic spectrum disorders (including catatonia), as well as for irritable bowel syndrome, physician-assisted suicide, and capital punishment.

Diagnosis of Problematic Use

In the fifth edition of the *Diagnostic and Statistical Manual of Mental Disorders* (DSM-5; American Psychiatric Association 2013), the substance-related and addictive disorders category comprises 10 separate classes of drugs. Although alcohol and opioids have sedative-hypnotic properties, they are grouped separately from their modern counterparts, which include barbiturates, benzodiazepines, and selective nonbenzodiazepine hypnotics. This diagnostic class is now labeled "sedative-, hypnotic-, or anxiolytic-related disorders" and includes the following: sedative, hypnotic, or anxiolytic use disorder; sedative, hypnotic, or anxiolytic intoxication; sedative, hypnotic, or anxiolytic withdrawal; other sedative-, hypnotic-, or anxiolytic-induced disorders; and unspecified sedative-, hypnotic-, or anxiolytic-related disorder.

In DSM-IV (American Psychiatric Association 1994), diagnostic distinctions were made between *abuse* and *dependence* with respect to substance use. These distinctions were intended to separate the psychosocial problems that accompany *abuse* (i.e., problematic use) of a substance from the physiological changes that accompany *chronic use* of that substance. However, in DSM-5, as the result of emerging recognition that the biopsychosocial problems associated with substance use occur on a spectrum, abuse and dependence were combined to form a single category, substance use disorder, defined by criteria encompassing 11 key biopsychosocial problem areas. Specifiers to denote severity and remission status are also provided with the DSM-5 diagnostic criteria for sedative, hypnotic, or anxiolytic (SHA) use disorder, as shown in Table 20–1.

Epidemiology

Prevalence of Use and Misuse

The Substance Abuse and Mental Health Services Administration (SAMHSA) publishes prevalence estimates from data collected annually in the National Survey on Drug Use and Health (NSDUH) on the use of different substances of abuse. In the NSDUH, benzodiazepines are classified under the monikers of *prescription tranquilizers*—a category including medications prescribed for the treatment of anxiety or muscle spasms (primarily benzodiazepines) and skeletal muscle relaxants (i.e., cyclobenzaprine and carisoprodol)—and *prescription sedatives*—a category including the barbiturates, the Z-drugs, and benzodiazepine agents commonly prescribed for insomnia (e.g., temazepam, triazolam, flurazepam). According to data from the 2017 NSDUH (collected from 68,032 individuals who completed the interview survey), an estimated 15% of U.S. adults ages 18 years and older reported use of prescription tranquilizers in the previous year, and an estimated 6.5% reported use of prescription sedatives (Substance Abuse and Mental Health Services Administration 2018). Among those adult respondents who reported use, 14.8% reported misuse (defined in the survey as use in any way not directed by a doctor) of tranquilizers, and 7.9% reported misuse of sedatives (Substance Abuse and Mental Health Services Administration 2018). Interestingly, whereas overall rates of prescription tranquilizer use among youth ages 12–17 years were lower than those in the general adult population (4.6% of youth respondents vs. 15% of adults), rates of past-year misuse among youth were considerably higher than those in adults (40.3% vs. 14.8%) (Substance Abuse and Mental Health Services Administration 2018). Similarly, overall rates of prescription sedative use among youth were lower than those among adults (2.3% vs. 6.5%); however, 13.1% of adolescent users reported misuse during the previous year, compared with 7.9% of adult users (Substance Abuse and Mental Health Services Administration 2018).

TABLE 20–1. **DSM-5 diagnostic criteria for sedative, hypnotic, or anxiolytic use disorder**

A. A problematic pattern of sedative, hypnotic, or anxiolytic use leading to clinically significant impairment or distress, as manifested by at least two of the following, occurring within a 12-month period:

   1. Sedatives, hypnotics, or anxiolytics are often taken in larger amounts or over a longer period than was intended.

   2. There is a persistent desire or unsuccessful efforts to cut down or control sedative, hypnotic, or anxiolytic use.

   3. A great deal of time is spent in activities necessary to obtain the sedative, hypnotic, or anxiolytic; use the sedative, hypnotic, or anxiolytic; or recover from its effects.

   4. Craving, or a strong desire or urge to use the sedative, hypnotic, or anxiolytic.

   5. Recurrent sedative, hypnotic, or anxiolytic use resulting in a failure to fulfill major role obligations at work, school, or home (e.g., repeated absences from work or poor work performance related to sedative, hypnotic, or anxiolytic use; sedative-, hypnotic-, or anxiolytic-related absences, suspensions, or expulsions from school; neglect of children or household).

   6. Continued sedative, hypnotic, or anxiolytic use despite having persistent or recurrent social or interpersonal problems caused or exacerbated by the effects of sedatives, hypnotics, or anxiolytics (e.g., arguments with a spouse about consequences of intoxication; physical fights).

   7. Important social, occupational, or recreational activities are given up or reduced because of sedative, hypnotic, or anxiolytic use.

   8. Recurrent sedative, hypnotic, or anxiolytic use in situations in which it is physically hazardous (e.g., driving an automobile or operating a machine when impaired by sedative, hypnotic, or anxiolytic use).

   9. Sedative, hypnotic, or anxiolytic use is continued despite knowledge of having a persistent or recurrent physical or psychological problem that is likely to have been caused or exacerbated by the sedative, hypnotic, or anxiolytic.

   10. Tolerance, as defined by either of the following:

       a. A need for markedly increased amounts of the sedative, hypnotic, or anxiolytic to achieve intoxication or desired effect.

       b. A markedly diminished effect with continued use of the same amount of the sedative, hypnotic, or anxiolytic.

       Note: This criterion is not considered to be met for individuals taking sedatives, hypnotics, or anxiolytics under medical supervision.

   11. Withdrawal, as manifested by either of the following:

       a. The characteristic withdrawal syndrome for sedatives, hypnotics, or anxiolytics (refer to Criteria A and B of the criteria set for sedative, hypnotic, or anxiolytic withdrawal, DSM-5 pp. 557–558).

       b. Sedatives, hypnotics, or anxiolytics (or a closely related substance, such as alcohol) are taken to relieve or avoid withdrawal symptoms.

       Note: This criterion is not considered to be met for individuals taking sedatives, hypnotics, or anxiolytics under medical supervision.

TABLE 20–1.   **DSM-5 diagnostic criteria for sedative, hypnotic, or anxiolytic use disorder *(continued)***

Specify if:

In early remission: After full criteria for sedative, hypnotic, or anxiolytic use disorder were previously met, none of the criteria for sedative, hypnotic, or anxiolytic use disorder have been met for at least 3 months but for less than 12 months (with the exception that Criterion A4, "Craving, or a strong desire or urge to use the sedative, hypnotic, or anxiolytic," may be met).

In sustained remission: After full criteria for sedative, hypnotic, or anxiolytic use disorder were previously met, none of the criteria for sedative, hypnotic, or anxiolytic use disorder have been met at any time during a period of 12 months or longer (with the exception that Criterion A4, "Craving, or a strong desire or urge to use the sedative, hypnotic, or anxiolytic," may be met).

In a controlled environment: This additional specifier is used if the individual is in an environment where access to sedatives, hypnotics, or anxiolytics is restricted.

Specify current severity:

Mild: Presence of 2–3 symptoms.

Moderate: Presence of 4–5 symptoms.

Severe: Presence of 6 or more symptoms.

Source.   Reprinted from American Psychiatric Association: *Diagnostic and Statistical Manual of Mental Disorders,* 5th Edition, Arlington, VA, American Psychiatric Association, 2013, pp. 550–552. Copyright © 2013, American Psychiatric Association. Used with permission.

Characteristics of Misuse

In an analysis of data on benzodiazepine use patterns from the 2015 and 2016 NSDUH, misuse of benzodiazepines (i.e., taking drugs other than as prescribed) accounted for 17.2% of total benzodiazepine use, and rates of misuse in younger adults (ages 18–25 years) were as high as rates of use as prescribed (Maust et al. 2019). Maust et al. (2019) further noted that coprescription of other controlled substances (e.g., stimulants, opioids) was strongly associated with risk for benzodiazepine misuse (Maust et al. 2019). The highest rates of overall benzodiazepine use were among adults ages 50–64 years, which is troubling, because this age cohort had previously been characterized as having higher rates of at-risk and binge use of alcohol and other substances compared with earlier generations of this age cohort (Maust et al. 2019).

Among responders to the 2017 NSDUH who reported misuse of sedatives, the sedatives were obtained from a health care provider (or more than one health care provider) 42.6% of the time and were acquired from a friend or relative (given for free, taken without asking, or purchased) 50.9% of the time (Center for Behavioral Health Statistics and Quality 2018). Similarly, tranquilizers were obtained from health care providers 82.5% of the time and from relatives or friends 12.7% of the time (Center for Behavioral Health Statistics and Quality 2018). Of particular concern, patients with a current prescription for benzodiazepines were 1.8 times more likely than those without a current prescription to be given a new prescription for an opioid during an ambulatory care visit, although naltrexone is coprescribed in fewer than 1% of all visits (Ladapo et al. 2018; Paulozzi et al. 2015). Enrollment in multiple health care systems (e.g., concurrent enrollment in Medicare and in the U.S. Department of Veterans Affairs system) is also associated with increased rates of benzodiazepine/opioid coprescription (Carico et al. 2018; Gellad et al. 2017). Taken together, these data strongly suggest that clinicians can play an important role in preventing the development of SHA use disorder through conscientious prescribing habits.

Neurobiology and Pharmacology

GABA Receptors

γ-Aminobutyric acid (GABA), the predominant inhibitory receptor in the central nervous system (CNS), was discovered more than 50 years ago; however, research is still ongoing to improve our understanding of activity in this system. The GABA class A (GABA$_A$) receptor complex is a ligand-gated ion channel consisting of five subunits with a multitude of binding sites. When GABA binds to receptors, the channel opens to allow chloride influx, which hyperpolarizes the postsynaptic neuron, preventing activation. Hence, GABA acts as an inhibitory neurotransmitter by blocking excitatory transmission. The channels are composed of different combinations of 19 known subunits: six of α, three of β, three of γ, three of ρ, and one each of δ, ε, π, and θ subunits. Although there are nearly a million potential subunit combinations, only certain combinations respond to medications, and fewer than 50 combinations are thought to occur naturally (Stephens et al. 2017). More than half of the GABA$_A$ receptors are composed of either $\alpha_1\beta_2\gamma_2$ or $\alpha_2\beta_2/3\gamma_2$. The full implications of specific receptor subtype combinations are still not known; however, differential expression of α_1 and α_2 subunits has been associated with different levels of addiction risk (Jembrek and Vlainić 2015).

In addition to containing binding sites for GABA, the receptor complex includes binding sites for anesthetics, anticonvulsants, barbiturates, benzodiazepines, ethanol, and neurosteroids (e.g., allopregnanolone), which cause different conformational changes to enhance the inhibitory effect of GABA. Some neurosteroids, anesthetics, and high-dose barbiturates may also directly activate the GABA$_A$ receptor in the absence of GABA.

Barbiturates

Barbiturates have fallen out of favor for the treatment of anxiety and insomnia with the increased use of benzodiazepines. When barbiturates bind to the GABA$_A$ complex, they increase the duration rather than the frequency of channel opening. Additionally, because barbiturates are capable of activating the GABA$_A$ complex in the absence of GABA, their use increases the risk of CNS depression, making these agents more toxic in overdose. The most commonly used barbiturates are phenobarbital, the phenobarbital prodrug primidone, and butalbital (typically used in combination with an analgesic and caffeine for migraine headaches). Phenobarbital is a potent inducer of oxidative hepatic metabolism as well as of P-glycoprotein, which may decrease the effectiveness of many medications if taken concurrently. It also has a very long half-life, making it prone to accumulation with long-term use (Jembrek and Vlainić 2015; Mihic et al. 2018).

Traditional Benzodiazepines

Benzodiazepines are thought to bind to GABA$_A$ receptors at the interface between the α and γ subunits. Receptors without γ subunits do not respond to benzodiazepines, and different α subunits confer varying response to pharmacological agents (Jembrek and Vlainić 2015; Stephens et al. 2017). When benzodiazepines bind to the GABA$_A$ receptor, they cause allosteric conformational changes to the receptor that increase the frequency of channel opening and hyperpolarization. Although dichotomously classified as either anxiolytics or sedative-hypnotics, all benzodiazepines have both anxiolytic and sedative-hypnotic effects (Mihic et al. 2018). Benzodiazepines vary in their pharmacokinetic parameters, resulting in different onsets and durations of action. In general, benzodiazepine drugs with a *faster onset* of action and a *shorter duration* of action are considered to have greater potential for misuse (see Table 20–2 in "Benzodiazepine Dose Equivalency" section below). Benzodiazepine drugs without active metabolites (e.g., lorazepam, oxazepam, temazepam) are safer for use in elderly patients and those with compromised hepatic function.

Benzodiazepine Dose Equivalency

The notion of equivalent dosing was first proposed in a 1984 study of 12 patients undergoing benzodiazepine withdrawal in which every 1 mg of lorazepam was initially converted to 10 mg of diazepam (Ashton 1984). Subsequently, approximate equivalent doses were assigned to other benzodiazepines available at the time. Many equivalence tables have since been published, with fairly consistent agreement about dosing equivalencies (Table 20–2).

Z-Drugs

The Z-drugs—zaleplon, zolpidem, zopiclone, and eszopiclone—were developed as sedative-hypnotic alternatives to benzodiazepines. Although they are structurally dissimilar to benzodiazepines, Z-drugs selectively bind at the benzodiazepine receptor site on specific subtypes of GABA$_A$ receptors that possess an α$_1$ subunit. Because of their more specific hypnotic activity (vs. anxiolytic, anticonvulsant, or muscle-relaxant activity), the Z-drugs were believed to have a better safety profile; however, postmarketing data contradicted this notion (Brandt and Leong 2017). Tolerance, physical dependence, abuse potential, and CNS side effects have been reported for the Z-drugs at rates similar to those reported for traditional benzodiazepines (Brandt and Leong 2017).

Safety and Toxicity

All benzodiazepines, Z-drugs, and barbiturates are controlled substances and have the potential to be misused and to cause dependence, tolerance, and withdrawal. For all three classes, use is associated with increased motor vehicle accidents, falls, and fractures, likely due to psychomotor impairments. Driving impairment (based on driving simulator studies, monitored driving studies, and epidemiological studies of actual accidents) is dose related and is more common soon after treatment initiation and with agents with a longer half-life. The Z-drugs have also been associated with

TABLE 20–2.   **Benzodiazepine equivalency**

Benzodiazepine	Approximately equivalent oral dose (mg)[a]	Elimination half-life (hours) (active metabolite)	Metabolism[c]
Alprazolam	0.5	6–12	CYP3A4
Chlordiazepoxide	10,[b,d] 25[c]	5–10 (36–200)	CYP3A4
Clonazepam	0.25,[b] 0.5,[c] 0.25–0.5[d]	18–50	Glucuronide and sulfate conjugation
Clorazepate	7.5[b,d]		CYP3A4
Diazepam	5,[b,d] 10[c]	20–100 (36–200)	CYP3A4, 2C19
Flurazepam	30,[b] 15–30,[c] 5[d]	40–250	CYP3A4
Lorazepam	1	10–20	Hepatic
Oxazepam	15,[b] 20,[c] 15–30[d]	4–15	Glucuronide conjugation
Temazepam	30,[b] 20,[c] 5[d]	8–22	CYP2B6, 2C8/9, 2C19, 3A4
Triazolam	0.25,[b] 0.1[d]		CYP3A4

Note.   CYP=cytochrome 450.
[a]Agreement among references b–d unless otherwise noted.
[b]Chouinard 2004.
[c]Ashton 2005.
[d]Lexi-Drugs 2018.

parasomnia behaviors (e.g., sleep driving), which increases the risk for accidents (Brandt and Leong 2017). Any new prescriptions for these agents should involve a discussion of driving safety and the recommendation to avoid driving after initial doses. As with driving, fall risk (and associated fractures) appears to correlate with higher doses and initial weeks of treatment. Older age, use of interacting medications, and variant expression of the cytochrome P450 (CYP) 2C9 allele also confer increased risk (Brandt and Leong 2017).

In 2008, the FDA issued an alert regarding increased risk of suicidality with all antiepileptic drugs (AEDs). The warning was based on a meta-analysis of 11 AEDs that did not include any benzodiazepines; however, the alert and subsequent labeling changes applied to many benzodiazepines, including clonazepam (Hersdorffer et al. 2010). A review of published studies revealed a twofold to fourfold increased risk of suicidality and self-injurious behavior across various patient populations and study designs (Dodds 2017). Because of the potential for benzodiazepines to increase fatality risk in a multidrug overdose, the risk of suicidality and assessment of suicide risk should be discussed with all patients prior to prescribing a benzodiazepine.

Because benzodiazepines are dependent on GABA release for their activity, they are relatively safe in monotherapy overdose. As synaptic GABA is depleted, the effects of benzodiazepines plateau. In multidrug overdose, however, benzodiazepines can contribute to respiratory depression and death. Overdose deaths involving benzodiazepines have increased since 2002, with the majority involving concurrent opioid overdose. The prescribing rate for benzodiazepines tripled between 1996 and 2013. Alprazolam appears to pose a higher risk of overdose compared with other benzodiazepines, with an increased rate of high-level clinical interventions such as intensive care unit admission, ventilation, and flumazenil reversal (Brandt and Leong 2017).

Flumazenil for Benzodiazepine Toxicity

Benzodiazepines have an additional measure of safety over barbiturates: the antidote flumazenil. Flumazenil is an imidazobenzodiazepine derivative that binds to the $GABA_A$ complex, competitively inhibits binding of benzodiazepines, and rapidly reverses their effects. It can only be administered intravenously and requires careful monitoring. Peak reversal occurs within 30 minutes and wears off within 60 minutes. Flumazenil must be used with great caution in patients with chronic use of benzodiazepines or a history of seizures because of the risk of inducing acute withdrawal seizures. Additionally, patients with severe benzodiazepine toxicity, especially from long-half-life agents, may require multiple doses because of the short half-life of flumazenil (Lexi-Drugs 2018; Mihic et al. 2018).

Adverse Effects

Benzodiazepines have been in use for about six decades, and they represent psychopharmacological anachronisms in that they were developed and marketed prior to the regulatory requirements mandated for current psychiatric medication clinical trial development. Postmarketing surveillance of adverse events was not required, because the Medical Dictionary for Regulatory Activities (MedDRA; developed to standardize reporting of adverse events) was not implemented until 2016 (International Council for Harmonization 2016). Consequently, conclusions on the acute and chronic health consequences of benzodiazepine use are primarily based on postmarketing case series and epidemiological examinations of databases. Despite the limitations of these sources, several worrisome patient and public health adverse events have repeatedly emerged.

The clinical phase III studies for FDA approval of alprazolam provide a quantitative overview of the incidence of adverse effects (Xanax [alprazolam] package insert 2016). Over the 4-week study period in the clinical trial of alprazolam for approval for the treatment of generalized anxiety disorder, the most common adverse events were drowsiness 41% (vs. 22% in the placebo group); lightheadedness 21% (vs. 19%); depression 14% (vs. 18%); headache 13% (vs. 20%); confusion 10% (vs. 10%), and insomnia 9% (vs. 18%). Adverse events associated with alprazolam in the clinical trial for its approval for the treatment of panic disorder were similar during a 3-month study window (Xanax [alprazolam] package insert 2016). The 2016 revision of the alprazolam package insert emphasized the hazards of taking alprazolam with opioids, alcohol, street drugs, or other CNS depressants. In addition to the previously mentioned common adverse events, the revised insert noted the risk of slowed mentation and cautioned against driving and operating heavy machinery while using alprazolam. This revision of the package insert also emphasized that use of alprazolam had not been studied for longer than 4 months for generalized anxiety disorder and 10 weeks for panic disorder (Xanax [alprazolam] package insert 2016). In general, the prevalence and severity of benzodiazepine side effects depend on dosage, duration of use, pharmacokinetic profile, and patient age. Clinical evaluation of side effects can be complicated by the use of long-half-life benzodiazepines, which often produce rising serum levels over several days, resulting in an insidious onset of adverse events.

Risk of Suicide

In the past two decades, the incidence of suicides involving benzodiazepines and the number of benzodiazepine prescriptions in the United States have both risen, suggesting a theoretical association (Dodds 2017). A review of 17 studies evaluated the relationship between benzodiazepine overdose and suicide; 16 studies found a statistically significant relationship between benzodiazepines and suicide attempts, with odds ratios varying between 2.5 and 6.2 (Dodds 2017). Additional risk factors for suicide attempts associated with benzodiazepine use include presence of severe mental illness, presence of borderline personality disorder, and veteran status (Dodds 2017). The Z-drugs (zolpidem, zaleplon, and eszopiclone) are likewise associated with an increased risk of suicidal ideation and suicide attempts, with an adjusted significant odds ratio approximately twice that of matched control subjects (Brandt and Leong 2017; Brower et al. 2011). This relationship between suicidality and benzodiazepine use has held true in both inpatient and outpatient settings (including office-based practices of primary care physicians and mental health specialists), and there appears to be a dose–response effect for longer-half-life, high-potency benzodiazepines (Brower et al. 2011; Dodds 2017). FDA requirements for clinical trials of psychotropic medications now include prospective assessment of suicidal ideation, suicide attempts, and completed suicides using a standardized instrument (Posner et al. 2011).

Cognitive Impairment

As a consequence of impaired psychomotor control, driving impairment and falls may result from taking benzodiazepines. The data regarding automobile accidents associated with benzodiazepines are primarily derived from emergency department visits in which serum benzodiazepine levels have been obtained, double-blind prospective automobile driving simulator experiments, and epidemiological databases. The risk of having an automobile accident for an individual who drives while taking benzodiazepines is far greater (adjusted odds ratio 1.6–3.75) than that for an otherwise comparable driver who is not taking benzodiazepines (Brandt and Leong 2017).

The relationship between long-term benzodiazepine use and falls (both those that result in fractures and those that do not) is somewhat more complicated (Stone et al. 2008). Sleep disorders, benzodiazepine or Z-drug use, pharmacokinetic differences, age, gender, and comorbid illnesses with medication treatments all contribute to fall risk. There is conservatively a 13%–30% increase in fall risk when taking benzodiazepines or Z-drugs (Brandt and Leong 2017).

In addition to the short-term risks conferred by psychomotor impairment, long-term use of benzodiazepines may also be associated with dementia. A recent meta-analysis of 10 studies (mean subject age=70 years) found that taking benzodiazepines was associated with a significantly increased risk (relative risk [RR]=1.51; 95% confidence interval [CI]=1.17–1.95) of developing dementia (He et al. 2019). Longer duration of use (>3 years) and use of a benzodiazepine with a longer-half-life (>20 hours) were associated with higher risks. He et al. (2019) noted that causality could not be established and suggested that anxiety and insomnia were among several independent risk factors for dementia. However, based on current scientific understanding, counseling appropriate patients about benzodiazepine use as a possible risk for dementia seems prudent.

Additional Risks With Concurrent Opioid Use

Another major risk factor contributing to suicide and accidental death involving benzodiazepines is the concurrent use of opioid analgesics. In a study using a case cohort epidemiological design, Park et al. (2015) evaluated approximately 400,000 veterans over 5 years. There were 2,400 opioid-related overdose deaths, about half of which were associated with a prescription for concurrent benzodiazepines. The adjusted odds ratio of death by overdose for patients taking opioids and having an active prescription for a benzodiazepine was 3.86 (95% CI=3.49–4.26), and that for patients taking opioids and having had a benzodiazepine prescription in the past was 2.33 (95% CI=2.05–2.64) (Park et al. 2015). With one exception, for all benzodiazepines prescribed, there was an almost fourfold increase in the risk of death by opioid overdose. Temazepam, prescribed as a hypnotic in the United States, inexplicably was associated with a 50% *lower* risk of death by overdose, although intentional versus accidental overdose could not be determined from the authors' data (Park et al. 2015). Collectively, these findings underscore the danger of opioid and benzodiazepine coprescription.

Evaluation and Management Considerations

Benzodiazepine Intoxication

Benzodiazepine intoxication may occur with accidental or intentional overdose or in a recreational use setting. Clinically, the manifestations of benzodiazepine intoxication are similar to those of alcohol intoxication (or intoxication involving other sedatives) in that slowed mentation, slurred or dysarthric speech, and ataxia are common. However, some patients will demonstrate a paradoxical response, displaying hyperactive motor behavior and aggressiveness. Any patient manifesting benzodiazepine intoxication requires close observation and monitoring with repeated mental status exams, neurological evaluations, pulse oximetry with range-limit alarms, and blood pressure measurements. Certain clinical history questions need to be addressed, including the time and amount of ingestion, the type of benzodiazepine, and whether other substances were also ingested. Medical history from significant others can be helpful in determining the presence of co-occurring medical and/or psychiatric conditions. Occult trauma, metabolic derangement, infection, and neurological conditions should be ruled out. Chronicity of use should be ascertained to determine the risk that the patient will progress to a withdrawal syndrome (e.g., seizures, delirium). Urine drug screens, metabolic panels, and complete blood counts are essential. Obtaining serum benzodiazepine levels is expensive and usually impractical because of the lengthy delay in acquiring test results. In patients who have not improved after an appropriate length of time, brain imaging should be considered.

Warning Signs of Problematic Use

Identification of patients with problematic benzodiazepine use requires assessment for warning signs, such as requesting early refills or rapid dosage increases, requesting replacement of allegedly lost or stolen prescriptions, and using multiple prescribers to obtain benzodiazepines (Soyka 2017). High-risk patients may claim, for example, that all prior trials of standard noncontrolled medications did not relieve their symptoms or that only one benzodiazepine had helped in the past. "Doctor shopping" is more difficult now with computer-assisted prescription drug monitoring programs for controlled substances, which are utilized by many states. However, some determined individuals acquire multiple identification cards with additional addresses and aliases to circumvent these monitoring programs. Others are adept at changing or forging written prescriptions. DSM-5 criteria for SHA use disorder are provided in Table 20–1.

Benzodiazepine Withdrawal Syndrome

GABA receptors are widely distributed in the CNS. For this reason, GABA system dysfunction can manifest in numerous ways, including clinical signs of withdrawal (Hollister et al. 1961; Soyka 2017). The onset of withdrawal symptoms is related to the total daily dosage and the elimination rate of the benzodiazepine. Physiological dependence can occur within 2–16 weeks of treatment initiation (Rickels et al. 1993). Some patients will experience withdrawal symptoms within 1 or 2 days, whereas others will not experience withdrawal symptoms for a week or longer.

For clinical purposes, withdrawal phenomena can be arbitrarily grouped into three domains: 1) peripheral nervous system symptoms with both sensory and motor abnormalities; 2) CNS symptoms; and 3) autonomic nervous system (ANS) symptoms. These manifestations wax and wane over time and are worsened by stress, fatigue, and other nonspecific factors. Peripheral nervous system symptom manifestations may include pain, paresthesias, dysesthesias, muscle fasciculations, myoclonus, and other involuntary movements. CNS symptom manifestations may include generalized tonic-clonic seizures, delirium (especially in elderly persons), hallucinations, anxiety, insomnia, irritability, hyperactive behaviors, depersonalization, derealization, hyperacusis, photophobia, dysgeusia, and parasomnias. ANS symptom manifestations may include hyperventilation, nausea, vomiting, diaphoresis, tachycardia, and hypertension.

As emphasized previously (see earlier section "Adverse Effects"), the prospective and double-blind controlled clinical trials conducted for FDA approval of benzodiazepines in the treatment of anxiety disorders were short-term studies, and the FDA approval was for short-term use only (i.e., 6–12 weeks). Any patient who takes a benzodiazepine for more than a few weeks is at risk for hazardous use, physical dependence, and possibly SHA use disorder (Janhsen et al. 2015). Although these risks must be considered, Rickels et al. (1990) noted that many individuals have no withdrawal symptoms with abrupt benzodiazepine cessation, just as a significant number of heavy alcohol users experience no withdrawal phenomena on cessation.

Discontinuation Strategies

Many patients end up being chronically maintained on high dosages of benzodi-azepines for years, with the original indication for benzodiazepine use frequently resolved or forgotten. Various societal trends—for example, the rising cost of generic benzodiazepines and the increased control of formulary medications and dosage/strength options by insurance companies—are converging to make it more likely that such patients will voluntarily or involuntarily seek medical treatment for withdrawal from a benzodiazepine and/or that they will dangerously undertake withdrawal on their own. Concerns about benzodiazepine-related falls, motor vehicle accidents, cognitive impairment, and dementia are also growing among public health officials, clinicians, and patients.

Reducing or discontinuing benzodiazepines after long-term use is often challenging, however. This may be due to ongoing clinical indications for continuation as well as the emergence of withdrawal symptoms. Patients often confuse withdrawal symptoms with a return of their previous psychopathology, particularly anxiety and/or insomnia. Some patients develop a "morbid preoccupation" with the details of their symptoms and treatment, further complicating management (Soyka 2017). Consequently, patients often continue to take benzodiazepines for years.

Guidance on discontinuation strategies is widely available and includes not only evidence-based recommendations from scientific studies but also non-evidence-based material from numerous websites, blogs, and published and unpublished treatises accessible to the general public. These non-evidence-based recommendations are often closely read by patients who are taking benzodiazepines or experiencing withdrawal symptoms. There are also a number of self-help books on managing benzodiazepine withdrawal, some written by individuals who have gone through withdrawal, some of whom were health care professionals. Given the plethora of non-evidence-based guidance available, the well-informed clinician is advised to probe patients' knowledge on the topic of benzodiazepine withdrawal prior to developing a treatment plan. Some patients' information may be keenly accurate; however, other patients may be woefully and dangerously misinformed.

Large prospective double-blind trials for the treatment of benzodiazepine or Z-drug withdrawal have not been conducted. However, benzodiazepine taper duration and use of adjunctive agents have been investigated, and two large meta-analyses have been conducted (Baandrup et al. 2018; Parr et al. 2009). In the earlier meta-analysis by Parr et al. (2009), the combination of a benzodiazepine taper over 1 week to 3 months in conjunction with psychosocial treatments showed benefit, although these tapers were highly individualized and not systematic (Parr et al. 2009). Patients receiving concurrent psychosocial treatments consisting of relaxation training, cognitive-behavioral techniques, patient self-monitoring of symptoms, and development of coping skills for recurrent anxiety had significantly better outcomes than did patients treated with benzodiazepine taper alone. In the 2018 Cochrane review, Baandrup et al. (2018) concluded that it was very difficult to make firm treatment recommendations because many of the early studies failed to standardize the reporting of adverse effects, and the study populations of the clinical trials were generally too small and inadequately powered to yield clear conclusions. Baandrup and colleagues likewise refrained from making recommendations on whether patients should be switched from a short-acting to a long-acting benzodiazepine.

Despite the lack of firm recommendations from these Cochrane meta-analyses, several distinguished clinicians and scientists have published recommendations based on their extensive experience. Professor Dr. C. Heather Ashton, a highly respected pharmacologist, physician, and professor at Newcastle University, operated a benzodiazepine discontinuation clinic for over a decade. Her patients endorsed her slow schedules of taper, which often spanned many months and sometimes lasted a year or longer, and she published benzodiazepine dosage conversion tables that are still widely cited (Ashton 2005). Dr. Ashton also favored use of long-half-life over short-half-life benzodiazepines during discontinuation tapers. Gaining patient approval for the tapering regimen and tailoring this schedule to each individual is highly recommended. Professor Dr. Michael Soyka is a clinician and researcher on benzodiazepines and has been professor of psychiatry at Ludwig Maximilian University in Munich, Germany, for over three decades. In his 2017 review, Dr. Soyka provided recommendations similar to those of Dr. Ashton and advised that most patients should be switched to a long-acting benzodiazepine for a taper of about 6 weeks (Soyka 2017).

The Cochrane review of Baandrup et al. (2018) also found little evidence to support the use of adjunctive therapies (e.g., anticonvulsants) during benzodiazepine withdrawal tapering, although the investigators acknowledged that in the previous Cochrane review on this topic (Parr et al. 2009), carbamazepine was recommended as an adjunctive therapy on the basis of evidence from three small clinical trials. This review also noted that the addition of flumazenil was found to increase the risk of seizures, and in one trial, flumazenil was found to precipitate sudden, severe panic attacks (Baandrup et al. 2018; Parr et al. 2009). Similarly, in her 2005 review paper, Dr. Ashton neither encouraged nor discouraged the use of adjunctive therapies, except to say that Z-drugs should not be added because of their side effects, tolerance risk, and risk of misuse (Ashton 2005). In contrast, Dr. Soyka reported moderate-quality evidence for using carbamazepine as adjunctive therapy and also advocated use of psychological adjunctive therapies (Soyka 2017).

Psychiatric Comorbidities

In a paradoxical sense, the treatment of individuals who use SHA drugs and who have other co-occurring substance use or mental disorders is simplified. These patients need to be referred to an intensive outpatient program or to a longer-term residential program. For patients in either environment, any comorbid psychiatric or medical disorders should be evaluated, diagnosed, and treated; intensive psychosocial treatment should be delivered; and, importantly, daily assessments including mental status exams, brief neurological exams, and repeated vital signs should be performed. With the exception of patients receiving medically supervised detoxification treatment, prescribing of benzodiazepines to patients with active substance use disorder(s) (notably, alcohol, opioid, or stimulant use disorders) is unwise. Patients with co-occurring borderline or antisocial personality disorder are also at high risk for early problems with benzodiazepines (Soyka 2017). Serious interactions with alcohol, opioids, and/or other sedative-hypnotics may occur at any point during short-

TABLE 20–3.   Selected benzodiazepine (BZD) drug interactions

Substrate BZDs	Inhibitors	Inducers
CYP2C9/19		
Diazepam	Fluconazole	Carbamazepine
Temazepam	Fluoxetine	Fosphenytoin
Phenobarbital	Isoniazid	Phenytoin
	Modafinil	Rifampin
	Omeprazole	
	Pantoprazole	
CYP3A4		
Alprazolam	Erythromycin	Carbamazepine
Chlordiazepoxide	Fluconazole	Fosphenytoin
Clorazepate	Fluvoxamine	Oxcarbazepine
Diazepam	Isoniazid	Phenobarbital
Estazolam	Ketoconazole	Phenytoin
Flurazepam	Nefazodone	Primidone
Quazepam	Protease inhibitors	Rifampin
Temazepam	(e.g., ritonavir)	
Triazolam		

Note.   CYP= cytochrome P450.

term or long-term benzodiazepine use. If opioid use disorder is present, some patients will require stabilization on an opioid substitution therapy. Antidepressants or mood stabilizers may be necessary to maintain mood stability, and these can often be introduced prior to tapering the benzodiazepine. However, attention to medication interactions is advised (Table 20–3) because of the increased risk of seizures during benzodiazepine withdrawal when patients are concomitantly taking medications that lower the seizure threshold. Ancillary objective monitoring can include urine drug screening, measurement of biomarkers for heavy alcohol use (e.g., percentage carbohydrate deficient transferrin [%CDT]), and administration of standardized diagnostic and quantification scales for anxiety and/or insomnia symptoms may aid in identifying patients who should not use benzodiazepines.

Conclusion

In conclusion, it is important to distinguish between individuals who use benzodiazepines therapeutically and individuals who use them recreationally or in combination with other substances (i.e., polysubstance use). Prescribers should not confuse physical dependence with addictive behaviors. Prescribing of benzodiazepines should be done with particular caution in certain demographic groups, including elderly patients (who are at increased risk of multiple adverse effects, such as cognitive impairment, delirium, falls, and fractures) and individuals with prior substance use disorders. With respect to benzodiazepine prescription, tapering, and withdrawal, the following caveats are advised:

- Prescription of benzodiazepines for periods longer than 6–12 weeks has not been systematically studied in terms of long-term efficacy.
- Patients should to be educated on the potential short- and long-term risks of benzodiazepine use to make an informed decision about treatment.
- Alternative psychological and pharmacological therapies for anxiety and insomnia should be considered before prescribing benzodiazepines. The presence of comorbid psychiatric disorders will influence the withdrawal regimen and will require continued treatment after benzodiazepine discontinuation.
- Once a patient has been taking benzodiazepines for months to years, the benefit/risk ratio and the decision to taper should be weighed carefully by the clinician and the patient. Withdrawal after long-term (i.e., months to years) use of high-dosage benzodiazepines should be undertaken slowly.
- Although benzodiazepines have a critical role in the management of alcohol withdrawal syndrome, careful management is required when prescribing benzodiazepines for dually diagnosed patients, and an alternative treatment plan must be in place for underlying psychiatric disorders.
- Management of benzodiazepine withdrawal requires (at a minimum) patient education, tapering of the benzodiazepine, and psychological treatments. Stopping a benzodiazepine and substituting another class of medication to treat physical dependence is not recommended.

References

Ainsworth S: Mother's little helper still rocking. Nurse Prescribing 11(5):255–256, 2013. Available at: https://www.magonlinelibrary.com/doi/abs/10.12968/npre.2013.11.5.255. Accessed December 26, 2019.

American Geriatrics Society: American Geriatrics Society updated Beers Criteria for potentially inappropriate medication use in older adults. The American Geriatrics Society 2012 Beers Criteria Update Expert Panel. J Am Geriatr Soc 60(4):616–631, 2012 22376048

American Psychiatric Association: Diagnostic and Statistical Manual of Mental Disorders, 4th Edition. Washington, DC, American Psychiatric Association, 1994

American Psychiatric Association: Diagnostic and Statistical Manual of Mental Disorders, 5th Edition. Arlington, VA, American Psychiatric Association, 2013

Ashton H: Benzodiazepine withdrawal: an unfinished story. Br Med J (Clin Res Ed) 288(6424):1135–1140, 1984 6143582

Ashton H: The diagnosis and management of benzodiazepine dependence. Curr Opin Psychiatry 18(3):249–255, 2005 16639148

Baandrup L, Ebdrup BH, Rasmussen JØ, et al: Pharmacological interventions for benzodiazepine discontinuation in chronic benzodiazepine users. Cochrane Database Syst Rev (3):CD011481, 2018 29543325

Bachhuber MA, Hennessy S, Cunningham CO, et al: Increasing benzodiazepine prescriptions and overdose mortality in the United States, 1996–2013. Am J Public Health 106(4):686–688, 2016 26890165

Brandt J, Leong C: Benzodiazepines and Z-drugs: an updated review of major adverse outcomes reported on in epidemiologic research. Drugs R D 17(4):493–507, 2017 28865038

Brower KJ, McCammon RJ, Wojnar M, et al: Prescription sleeping pills, insomnia, and suicidality in the National Comorbidity Survey Replication. J Clin Psychiatry 72(4):515–521, 2011 20868634

Carico R, Zhao X, Thorpe CT, et al: Receipt of overlapping opioid and benzodiazepine prescriptions among veterans dually enrolled in Medicare Part D and the Department of Veterans Affairs: a cross-sectional study. Ann Intern Med 169(9):593–601, 2018 30304353

Center for Behavioral Health Statistics and Quality: 2017 National Survey on Drug Use and Health: Detailed Tables. Rockville, MD, Substance Abuse and Mental Health Services Administration, September 7, 2018. Available at: https://www.samhsa.gov/data/sites/default/files/cbhsq-reports/NSDUHDetailedTabs2017/NSDUHDetailedTabs2017.pdf. Accessed August 7, 2020.

Chouinard G: Issues in the clinical use of benzodiazepines: potency, withdrawal, and rebound. J Clin Psychiatry 65 (suppl 5):7–12, 2004 15078112

Dodds TJ: Prescribed benzodiazepines and suicide risk: a review of the literature. Prim Care Companion CNS Disord 19(2), 2017 28257172

Gellad WF, Zhao X, Thorpe CT, et al: Overlapping buprenorphine, opioid, and benzodiazepine prescriptions among veterans dually enrolled in Department of Veterans Affairs and Medicare Part D. Subst Abus 38(1):22–25, 2017 27925868

He Q, Chen X, Wu T, et al: Risk of dementia in long-term benzodiazepine users: evidence from a meta-analysis of observational studies. J Clin Neurol 15(1):9–19, 2019 30375757

Hesdorffer DC, Berg AT, Kanner AM: An update on antiepileptic drugs and suicide: are there definitive answers yet? Epilepsy Curr 10(6):137–145, 2010 21157540

Hollister LE, Motzenbecker FP, Degan RO: Withdrawal reactions from chlordiazepoxide ("Librium"). Psychopharmacology (Berl) 2(1):63–68, 1961 13715373

International Council for Harmonization: Introductory Guide: MedDRA Version 19.0 (MSSO-DI-6003-19.0.0). March 2016. Available at: https://admin.new.meddra.org/sites/default/files/guidance/file/intguide_19_0_english.pdf. Accessed November 25, 2019.

Janhsen K, Roser P, Hoffmann K: The problems of long-term treatment with benzodiazepines and related substances. Dtsch Arztebl Int 112(1–2):1–7, 2015 25613443

Jembrek MJ, Vlainić J: GABA receptors: pharmacological potential and pitfalls. Curr Pharmaceutical Design 21(34):4943–4959, 2015 26365137

Jones CM, McAninch JK: Emergency department visits and overdose deaths from combined use of opioids and benzodiazepines. Am J Prev Med 49(4):493–501, 2015 26143953

Ladapo JA, Larochelle MR, Chen A, et al: Physician prescribing of opioids to patients at increased risk of overdose from benzodiazepine use in the United States. JAMA Psychiatry 75(6):623–630, 2018 29710086

Lexi-Drugs®: Benzodiazepine comparison table [Internet]. Hudson, OH, Wolters Kluwer Health, 2018. Available at: https://msp.scdhhs.gov/tipsc/sites/default/files/tipSC%20Mar%202018%20benzoequivtable%2042018.pdf. Accessed May 12, 2020.

López-Muñoz F, Ucha-Udabe R, Alamo C: The history of barbiturates a century after their clinical introduction. Neuropsychiatr Dis Treat 1(4):329–343, 2005 18568113

Maust DT, Lin LA, Blow FC: Benzodiazepine use and misuse among adults in the United States. Psychiatr Serv 70(2):97–106, 2019 30554562

Mihic SJ, Mayfield J, Harris RA: Hypnotics and sedatives, in Goodman & Gilman's: The Pharmacological Basis of Therapeutics, 13th Edition. Edited by Brunton LL, Hilal-Dandan R, Knollmann BC. New York, McGraw-Hill Education, 2018, pp 339–354

Park TW, Saitz R, Ganoczy D, et al: Benzodiazepine prescribing patterns and deaths from drug overdose among US veterans receiving opioid analgesics: case-cohort study. BMJ 350:h2698, 2015 26063215

Parr JM, Kavanagh DJ, Cahill L, et al: Effectiveness of current treatment approaches for benzodiazepine discontinuation: a meta-analysis. Addiction 104(1):13–24, 2009 18983627

Paulozzi LJ, Strickler GK, Kreiner PW, et al; Centers for Disease Control and Prevention: Controlled substance prescribing patterns—prescription behavior surveillance system, eight states, 2013. MMWR Surveill Summ 64(9):1–14, 2015 26469747

Posner K, Brown GK, Stanley B, et al: The Columbia–Suicide Severity Rating Scale: initial validity and internal consistency findings from three multisite studies with adolescents and adults. Am J Psychiatry 168(12):1266–1277, 2011 22193671

Rickels K, Schweizer E, Case WG, Greenblatt DJ: Long-term therapeutic use of benzodiazepines, I: effects of abrupt discontinuation. Arch Gen Psychiatry 47(10):899–907, 1990 2222129

Rickels K, Schweizer E, Weiss S, et al: Maintenance drug treatment for panic disorder, II: short- and long-term outcome after drug taper. Arch Gen Psychiatry 50(1):61–68, 1993 8422223

Soyka M: Treatment of benzodiazepine dependence. N Engl J Med 376(12):1147–1157, 2017 28328330

Stephens DN, King SL, Lambert JJ, et al: GABAA receptor subtype involvement in addictive behaviour. Genes Brain Behav 16(1):149–184, 2017 27539865

Stone KL, Ensrud KE, Ancoli-Israel S: Sleep, insomnia and falls in elderly patients. Sleep Med 9 (suppl 1):S18–S22, 2008 18929314

Substance Abuse and Mental Health Services Administration: Key substance use and mental health indicators in the United States: results from the 2017 National Survey on Drug Use and Health (HHS Publ. No. SMA 18-5068, NSDUH Series H-53). Rockville, MD, Center for Behavioral Health Statistics and Quality, SAMHSA, 2018. Available at: https://www.samhsa.gov/data/sites/default/files/cbhsq-reports/NSDUHFFR2017/NSDUHFFR2017.pdf. Accessed June 25, 2020.

Wick JY: The history of benzodiazepines. Consult Pharm 28(9):538–548, 2013 24007886

Xanax (alprazolam) package insert. New York, Pharmacia & Upjohn, 2016

CHAPTER 21

Neurobiology and Treatment of Anabolic-Androgenic Steroid-Related Disorders

Harrison G. Pope Jr., M.D.

Gen Kanayama, M.D., Ph.D.

The anabolic-androgenic steroids (AASs) are a family of hormones that includes the natural male hormone testosterone and hundreds of synthetic relatives of testosterone (Pope et al. 2014b). All AASs possess both anabolic (muscle-building) and androgenic (masculinizing) properties; it is equally correct to refer to these hormones simply as "androgens" (Kanayama et al. 2018a). Testosterone was first isolated in the 1930s, and numerous synthetic AASs were developed over the next decade. By the 1950s, athletes had discovered that AASs would allow them to achieve muscle gains far beyond those attainable by natural means, and AAS use spread rapidly throughout the elite athletic world (Kanayama and Pope 2018). However, it was not until the 1980s that AAS use began to emerge from elite athletics and into the general population. Now, between 3 and 4 million American men, and millions more worldwide, have used these drugs illicitly at some time (Pope et al. 2014a).

There are three common myths about the epidemiology of AAS use (Kanayama and Pope 2012). The first is that AAS use is primarily a problem of doping by athletes. In reality, most AAS users have never used these drugs for any competitive athletic purpose at all, but instead have simply wanted to become leaner and more muscular (Ip et al. 2011; Kanayama and Pope 2012; Parkinson and Evans 2006). A second myth is that girls and women often use AASs. In fact, about 98% of AAS users are male—a finding that is not surprising, given that women rarely aspire to be extremely muscular and are also vulnerable to the masculinizing effects of AASs such as beard growth, deepening of the voice, and masculinization of secondary sexual characteristics (Kanayama et al. 2007; Pope et al. 2014a). The third myth is that AAS use is common among adolescents. However, an analysis of pooled data from nine studies of AAS users, comprising more than 3,000 individuals, found that fewer than 1% of all AAS users began using these drugs prior to age 15 years, and only about 13% before age 18, with age 23 years being the approximate median age at onset of use (Pope et al. 2014a). Thus, contrary to widespread popular belief, AASs represent primarily adult drugs rather than teenage drugs.

In summary, the typical AAS user will be a man between the ages of 20 and 50 years who is using AASs primarily for personal appearance rather than for athletic competition. Because he is an independent adult, and no longer under the observation of parents, teachers, or coaches, his drug use will typically go unnoticed by those around him. Moreover, he will be very unlikely to seek treatment for substance use, and will probably not even disclose his AAS use to clinicians he might encounter. This level of secrecy is illustrated by one study finding that 56% of illicit AAS users had never disclosed their AAS use to any physician they had seen (Pope et al. 2004).

Several factors help to explain why AAS users rarely seek clinical attention. First, many users perceive their AAS use as a positive activity, in combination with intensive exercise and optimal diet as part of the "bodybuilding lifestyle." Commercial and societal forces are partly responsible for this misperception of AASs: muscular male bodies are portrayed as an ideal in advertising, magazines, television, and movies. Even children's action toys, such as G.I. Joe, changed from ordinary-looking men in the 1960s and 1970s to muscle-bound specimens by the 1990s (Pope et al. 1999). Given this societal climate, it is not surprising that AAS users rarely perceive their drug use as representing a psychiatric disorder requiring treatment.

Second, AAS users often have little respect for health professionals. AAS users often regard most clinicians as "geeks" or "pencil-necks" who have no understanding of the bodybuilding world. For example, in the study of Pope et al. (2004), 40% of AAS users reported that they trusted information about AASs from their drug dealers at least as much as information from any physician they had seen. There is some basis for this distrust: for decades, many medical professionals asserted that AASs were ineffective for gaining muscle mass. This claim, based on two decades of flawed studies, caused doctors to lose their credibility among AAS users (Kanayama and Pope 2018). Today, although most clinicians recognize that AASs are effective for gaining muscle mass, they remain largely uninformed about the extent and nature of the AAS-using subculture. Several relatively recent papers have stressed that clinicians should attempt to become more familiar with AASs and AAS-associated syndromes (Goldman et al. 2019; Pope et al. 2017).

Finally, it must be recognized that AASs differ from conventional drugs of abuse in that they do not deliver an immediate "reward" of intoxication when ingested. Instead, AAS users are typically seeking a long-term reward in the form of a more muscular body, athletic success, or admiration from peers or potential sexual partners. Thus, conventional programs or methods for treating substance use, designed to treat individuals who use intoxicating drugs, may be inappropriate unless modified specifically for AAS users (Brower 2009).

Given the considerations discussed above, it is understandable that AAS users rarely request treatment to help them stop using these drugs. Nevertheless, a number of specific situations can bring AAS users to the attention of clinicians. These include 1) AAS dependence syndromes, 2) hypomanic and manic syndromes associated with AAS exposure, 3) syndromes of depression and anxiety associated with AAS withdrawal, 4) body image disorders associated with AAS use, 5) co-occurring substance use disorders, 6) medical conditions associated with long-term AAS use, and 7) forensic situations, such as cases of AAS-induced violence or criminality. In the sections that follow, we begin with a general discussion of the initial identification and assessment of AAS users, and then discuss the seven clinical issues enumerated above.

Identification and Assessment

Identification

AAS use is one of the few types of substance use for which a diagnosis is often suggested simply by looking at the patient. As we have described elsewhere (Kouri et al. 1995), there is a fairly sharp upper limit of muscularity that can be achieved by a lean individual without the help of drugs. We have published a formula to calculate muscularity, expressed as the "fat-free mass index" (FFMI), which clinicians can apply if they know the patient's height, weight, and approximate percentage of body fat (Kouri et al. 1995). Men who have low body fat and who have an FFMI of greater than approximately 26 kg/m^2 are almost certainly using AASs or other performance-enhancing drugs even if they deny such use (Pope and Kanayama 2005). Clinicians who suspect AAS use in any patient should follow several guidelines to take a specific history.

Patient History

The clinician may lead into the topic of AAS use by asking about athletic or fitness-related activities. As discussed above, men ages 20–50 years who lift weights regularly show the highest risk of AAS use (Brower 2009). The clinician can also ask the individual about any use of over-the-counter and mail-order dietary supplements such as vitamins, minerals, amino acids, and creatine. The use of such legal performance- or image-enhancing substances is commonly associated with use of illicit substances such as AASs (Hildebrandt et al. 2011). Another question is whether the patient has ever tried AASs or thought about using them. Patients thinking about AAS use are good candidates for prevention. If the patient is thinking about but is not yet using AASs, the clinician should ask why the patient is interested in using these agents and what has prevented the patient from using them to date. In asking these questions, it is particularly critical that the clinician be nonjudgmental while still discouraging use.

For patients who admit having tried AASs, both the perceived benefits and any adverse consequences are important to determine. The clinician should question the patient about the dates of first use and most recent use, the names and doses of AASs used, the sources of the drugs, and the routes of administration. Patients who inject AASs should be asked about needle sharing, although fortunately this practice now appears to be rare among AAS users (Ip et al. 2011). Most users obtain their drugs by purchasing them either from local illicit dealers or over the Internet. Unlike many other drugs of abuse, such as heroin and cocaine, AASs are legally available without a prescription in many countries outside of the United States. Thus, potential AAS users can easily find Internet sites offering to sell AASs from overseas (Brennan et al. 2013; Cordaro et al. 2011). Drugs purchased through these sites and then shipped by mail into the United States often reach users without being intercepted. Patients and clinicians should remember that drugs obtained from the illicit domestic market and from overseas sources are frequently counterfeit, adulterated, or falsely labeled, and sometimes nonsterile. Thus, the user does not necessarily know what drugs and how much he is taking. The picture is further complicated by what might be called the "gray market" of questionable "dietary supplements," which contain surreptitious illicit AASs or other potentially ergogenic substances (e.g., clenbuterol or selective androgen receptor modulators) that are often inconsistent with the label on the product (Geyer et al. 2008; Parr et al. 2008; Rahnema et al. 2015; Van Wagoner et al. 2017). These supplements are widely available over the Internet and also in stores catering to bodybuilders, who may ingest these substances with little consideration of their potential adverse effects.

Inquiry into patterns of use is also important. Users of illicit AASs typically combine ("stack") multiple types of AASs, including both oral and parenteral forms, to achieve doses that are 10–100 times the amounts ordinarily prescribed for therapeutic indications (Ip et al. 2011; Pope et al. 2014b). Such doses might result in total AAS serum concentrations that are more than 50 times greater than the natural male physiological concentrations of testosterone (Kaufman et al. 2019). AASs are usually taken in "cycles" (courses) of 4–16 weeks or more; individuals often take small doses at the beginning, build to large doses and combinations in the middle, and taper doses at the end of the cycle—a pattern referred to as a "pyramid." The clinician gains useful information by exploring the role of cycling with the individual AAS user: Does the patient cycle off AASs to avoid testing positive on drug screening? Does the patient cycle off AASs to give his body a rest, allowing his endogenous hormonal system a chance to regain normal functioning? Does the patient experience depression or other withdrawal symptoms during "off periods"? Dependent users may eliminate cycling altogether in favor of prolonged, continuous use to avoid withdrawal symptoms (see subsection "AAS Dependence" later in this chapter).

Finally, the clinician should obtain a history of other drug use. Users often combine other drugs with AASs to augment the performance- and image-enhancing effects, as detailed below in the section "Co-occurring Substance Use Disorders" (Hildebrandt et al. 2011; Ip et al. 2011; Pope et al. 2014b). Also, in contradiction to the image of the healthy bodybuilding lifestyle, many AAS users have a history of classical substance use disorders involving cannabis, opiates, cocaine, and other drugs (Dodge and Hoagland 2011; Gårevik and Rane 2010; Kaufman et al. 2019; Skarberg et al. 2009).

Physical Examination

The physical examination is essential to detect the somatic consequences of using AASs. Generalized muscle hypertrophy with a disproportionately large upper torso (neck, shoulders, arms, and chest) is often readily apparent. The skin is examined for acne (on the face, shoulders, and back) and needle marks in large muscles (especially the gluteals, but sometimes the thighs and deltoids). Gynecomastia, caused by metabolic conversion of testosterone and other AASs to estrogen, may be detectable by palpation or even by simple observation in some men. By contrast, the testicles become atrophic as they shut down testosterone production when exogenous AASs are administered in high doses. Male-pattern baldness, hirsutism, hypertension, hepatomegaly, right-upper-quadrant tenderness, jaundice, and prostatic hypertrophy are also possible but are not reliably associated with AAS use. In women, hirsutism, deepening of the voice, and clitoral hypertrophy may be detected.

Mental Status Examination

The clinician should assess the patient's appearance for excessive muscularity as described above, which sometimes can be disguised by oversized clothes, especially when patients with muscle dysmorphia become preoccupied that they do not look big enough and hence wish to hide their bodies (Rohman 2009; Sreshta et al. 2017). The patient's cooperation may vary, depending on his defensiveness about or denial of AAS use. Speech and sensorium are generally normal. However, if the patient is experiencing hypomanic or manic symptoms from current AAS use, he may display irritability, agitation, and possibly grandiose beliefs. Patients experiencing depression from AAS withdrawal may exhibit depressed mood, dysphoria, anxiety, psychomotor retardation, and possible suicidal ideation.

Laboratory Examination

Laboratory abnormalities reported in AAS users are summarized in Table 21–1. Standard urine screens for drugs of abuse do not include AASs, so urine testing for AASs must be performed at a reference laboratory. Such testing can detect only recent AAS use; orally active AASs disappear from the urine within weeks, and most intramuscular preparations, within a few months. However, given the association between AAS use and other illicit drug use, standard urine screens for illicit drugs should also be ordered.

Important blood chemistries include skeletal muscle enzymes, although these can be elevated after intensive weight training even in individuals who do not use AASs. AAS users may occasionally display pronounced elevations of creatine kinase from rhabdomyolysis. Results from standard liver function tests, such as transaminases and lactic dehydrogenase, are nonspecific, because these enzymes are also present in muscle and may be elevated from weight training alone (Dickerman et al. 1999; Pettersson et al. 2008). AAS users may be erroneously thought to have liver disease when in fact their elevated transaminases are entirely muscular in origin. Elevation of chemistries specific to the liver, such as bilirubin and γ-glutamyltransferase, may suggest true hepatic abnormalities.

High-density lipoprotein (HDL) cholesterol is typically decreased during AAS use, particularly when individuals use orally active, 17α-alkylated AASs, such as methandienone (Dianabol), oxymetholone (Anadrol), or stanozolol (Winstrol). The ratio of total cholesterol to HDL, typically considered normal when less than 5.0, may be grossly elevated, with some men in our experience achieving ratios of greater than 20 as a result of extreme decreases in HDL levels. Such high ratios are likely associated with increased atherogenic risk, and may well contribute to the increased prevalence of atherosclerotic disease in older AAS users (Baggish et al. 2017; Santora et al. 2006).

TABLE 21–1.   Laboratory abnormalities in anabolic-androgenic steroid users

Blood work	Abnormalities
Muscle enzymes	↑ ALT, AST, LDH, and CK
Liver function tests	↑ ALT, AST, LDH, GGT, and total bilirubin (caution: ↑ ALT, AST, and LDH are often muscular in origin and do not indicate liver disease)
Cholesterol levels	↓ HDL-C, ↑ LDL-C, ↑ or no change in total cholesterol and triglycerides
Hormonal levels	↑ Testosterone and estradiol (with use of testosterone esters), ↓ testosterone (without use of testosterone esters or during withdrawal), or ↓ LH and FSH
Complete blood count	↑ RBC count, hemoglobin, and hematocrit
Urine testing	
Anabolic-androgenic steroids	Positive
Other drugs of abuse	May be positive
Cardiac testing	
Electrocardiogram	Left ventricular hypertrophy (seen in intensive weight trainers also)
Echocardiogram	↓ Ventricular ejection fraction, impaired diastolic function
Semen analysis	↓ Sperm count and motility, abnormal morphology

Note.   ↑=increased; ↓=decreased; ALT=alanine aminotransferase; AST=aspartate aminotransferase; CK=creatine kinase; FSH=follicle stimulating hormone; GGT=γ-glutamyltransferase; HDL-C=high-density lipoprotein cholesterol; LDH=lactate dehydrogenase; LDL-C=low-density lipoprotein cholesterol; LH=luteinizing hormone; RBC=red blood cell.

AASs also stimulate production of red blood cells, although the magnitude of this effect varies substantially across individuals. In our recent experience, we have seen several men who had hematocrits of 55%–60% while using AASs—placing them at increased risk for thrombotic or hemorrhagic complications.

Blood testosterone concentrations may be grossly elevated in patients who are self-administering exogenous testosterone, with serum concentrations typically several times the upper limit of normal (Pope et al. 2014b). Conversely, testosterone concentrations may be grossly depressed in patients who are administering other types of AASs and hence inhibiting their own endogenous testosterone production. Testosterone levels may also remain depressed for months, and in rare cases even indefinitely, following AAS withdrawal (Christou et al. 2017; Coward et al. 2013; de Souza and Hallak 2011; Kanayama et al. 2015; Rasmussen et al. 2016).

Issues That May Bring AAS Users to Clinical Attention

AAS Dependence

Studies have frequently documented that AASs can create a dependence syndrome, characterized by long-term use of these drugs, often for many years and in spite of adverse effects (Kanayama et al. 2009). AAS dependence may be part of a larger pattern of dependence on appearance- and performance-enhancing drugs, involving other agents in addition to AASs, such as human growth hormone, insulin, and thermogenic agents such as clenbuterol, amphetamines, and thyroid hormones (Hildebrandt et al. 2011). An analysis of pooled data from 10 studies (collectively assessing 1,247 AAS users) found that the mean (95% confidence interval) prevalence of AAS dependence (as defined by criteria adapted from DSM-III [American Psychiatric Association 1980] or DSM-IV [American Psychiatric Association 1994]) was 32.5% (25.4%, 39.7%) (Pope et al. 2014a). Note that with the appearance of DSM-5 (American Psychiatric Association 2013), the term *dependence* is no longer used, and individuals formerly diagnosed as having "AAS dependence" would now generally be diagnosed as having "AAS use disorder, severe." However, we use the term *dependence* in the following text because most of the relevant studies were performed prior to the appearance of DSM-5 and used the term *dependence* to describe this syndrome.

AAS dependence may arise via three different pathways, any or all of which may lead to the syndrome in a given individual (Figure 21–1) (Kanayama et al. 2010). First, there appears to be a "body image" pathway, in which the individual becomes preoccupied with the fear that he will lose muscle size if he stops taking AASs and hence becomes reluctant to discontinue these drugs even for a short interval. Treatment for such symptoms, especially the extreme case of muscle dysmorphia, can likely be performed with cognitive-behavioral therapies or selective serotonin reuptake inhibitors (SSRIs)—treatment modalities that have been found effective for treating other forms of body dysmorphic disorder (Phillips et al. 2008), although not yet specifically tested in muscle dysmorphia, to our knowledge. We discuss muscle dysmorphia in more detail below (see "Body Image Disorders Associated With AAS Use").

In the second potential pathway, use of exogenous AASs leads to suppression of the hypothalamic-pituitary-gonadal (HPG) axis (Christou et al. 2017; Tan and Scally 2009). Thus, when a man discontinues an AAS course, especially if that course has been prolonged, he will likely experience hypogonadism, which in some cases may persist for months or even years after cessation of AASs. Hypogonadism may be associated with loss of sex drive, fatigue, and, occasionally, serious depression; these symptoms may prompt individuals to quickly resume AAS use to make the dysphoric feelings go away. This HPG axis suppression pathway to AAS dependence was first postulated three decades ago (Kashkin and Kleber 1989) and has been increasingly acknowledged in recent years. Indeed, it now appears that protracted severe hypogonadism may be much more common in long-term AAS users than was previously suspected, and that indeed some users may develop irreversible hypogonadism, possibly attributable to the direct toxic effects of long-term AAS exposure on the testes or on other components of the HPG axis (Coward et al. 2013; de Souza and Hallak 2011; Kanayama et al. 2015; Rasmussen et al. 2016). Therefore, in individuals showing AAS withdrawal–associated hypogonadism and expressing a genuine desire not to resume AAS use, it is advisable to institute aggressive endocrinological treatment with agents that stimulate the HPG axis in order to "jump-start" natural endogenous testosterone production and thus reduce the individual's desire to resume illicit exogenous AAS use (Tan and Scally 2009). Such treatment may include clomiphene to stimulate pituitary secretion of luteinizing hormone and follicle-stimulating hormone, together with human chorionic gonadotropin (HCG) to stimulate testicular

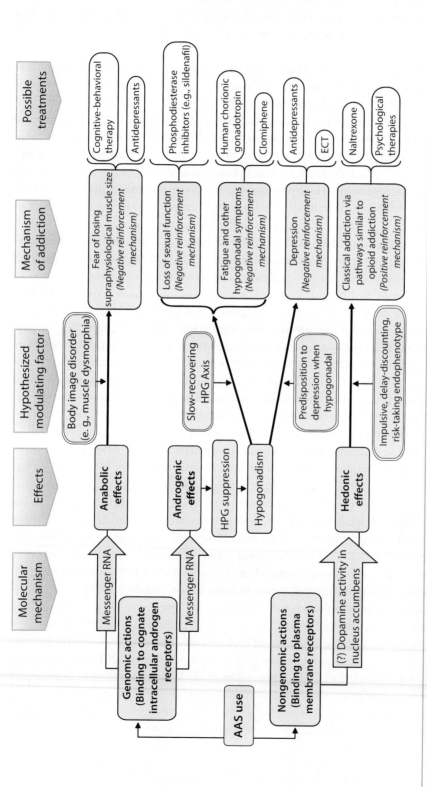

FIGURE 21–1. Three potential pathways that may lead to anabolic-androgenic steroid (AAS) dependence, together with possible therapeutic strategies to address each pathway.

?=hypothesized; ECT=electroconvulsive therapy; HPG=hypothalamic-pituitary-gonadal; RNA=ribonucleic acid.
Source. Reprinted from Kanayama G, Brower KJ, Wood RI, et al.: "Treatment of Anabolic-Androgenic Steroid Dependence: Emerging Evidence and Its Implications." *Drug and Alcohol Dependence* 109:6–13, 2010. Copyright © 2010 Elsevier. Used with permission.

production of testosterone and spermatozoa. Initially, the patient may also require temporary exogenous testosterone administration, typically using one of several commercially available testosterone gels, to maintain adequate testosterone levels while waiting for clomiphene and/or HCG to stimulate resumption of endogenous function. In a typical treatment course of this nature, one would first taper off testosterone, then subsequently discontinue HCG, and then finally taper clomiphene, all while regularly monitoring testosterone levels (Tan and Scally 2009). Individuals still unable to maintain adequate testosterone levels on their own, even after many months of neuroendocrine treatment, may conceivably represent cases of irreversible hypogonadism attributable to a direct toxic effect of AASs, and hence may require testosterone replacement indefinitely. Most psychiatric clinicians will likely wish to seek endocrinological consultation for these interventions.

In the third hypothesized pathway, AASs may induce dependence via a hedonic mechanism, presumably mediated by receptor sites on cell membranes rather than by classical anabolic or androgenic effects that are genomically mediated (i.e., mediated by androgen-receptor complexes that form in the cytoplasm of cells and are then translocated to the cell nucleus, where they augment gene transcription, leading to the production of new proteins). Persuasive evidence for such a hedonic pathway arises from animal studies, which have shown that rats and mice display conditioned place preference for AASs and that male hamsters will self-administer AASs to the point of death (Wood 2008). Interestingly, AAS self-administration in hamsters can be blocked by administration of the opioid antagonist naltrexone (Wood 2008). A number of other clinical and preclinical studies have pointed to interactions between AASs and endogenous as well as exogenous opioids, thus suggesting that the hedonic pathway to AAS dependence may involve opioidergic mechanisms (Nyberg and Hallberg 2012; Wood 2008). One implication of this research is that human AAS dependence might respond, at least in part, to treatments empirically validated for opioid dependence, such as motivational therapies, contingency management, behavioral couples therapy, or behavioral family counseling. Some of these treatments have been successfully used in conjunction with naltrexone in the management of opioid dependence, raising the possibility that the addition of naltrexone might be effective in AAS dependence as well. However, these modalities have not yet been systematically tested in treatment of AAS dependence. For a detailed discussion of each of these three possible pathways to AAS dependence, together with details of potential treatment strategies, we refer the reader to the full article from which Figure 21–1 is taken (Kanayama et al. 2010).

AAS-Induced Hypomania and Mania

Over the last 30 years, a substantial literature has demonstrated that in some individuals, AAS use can produce hypomanic or manic syndromes, sometimes accompanied by aggressive or violent behavior—and, in rare cases, by psychotic symptoms (Hall et al. 2005; Pope and Katz 2003). These effects are rare in individuals taking the equivalent of 300 mg or less of testosterone per week, but they appear to become progressively more common with higher doses, especially those above 1,000 mg/week (Pope and Katz 2003). These syndromes were initially noted in field studies of illicit AAS users, and some investigators questioned whether the effects were in fact due to the

AASs themselves, as opposed to expectational factors, personality variables, or sub-cultural influences. However, several studies have since demonstrated that such syndromes can develop even in non-AAS-using volunteers taking supraphysiological doses of AASs under placebo-controlled double-blind laboratory conditions (Pope and Katz 2003). Therefore, the mood-altering effects of AASs almost certainly have a biological basis, even though these effects can undoubtedly be modified by contextual factors. Hypomanic and manic syndromes appear to be idiosyncratic, with a majority of AAS users displaying few such symptoms, even with high doses of AASs, but with occasional individuals showing severe symptoms, sometimes accompanied by criminal violence (see later subsection "Forensic Situations").

Little has been written about the treatment of AAS-induced hypomania and mania beyond anecdotal reports. Thus, the best treatment recommendations would seem to include removal of the offending agent and temporary treatment, if necessary, with antipsychotics (e.g., risperidone, olanzapine) or mood-stabilizing agents (e.g., lithium, valproate). In general, it appears that manic or hypomanic episodes will remit quickly when AASs are stopped, and clinicians should then be alert for the onset of depressive symptoms associated with abrupt AAS withdrawal. If a patient reports a history of mood disorder prior to AAS use or continues to exhibit manic or psychotic symptoms for more than a few weeks after AASs are stopped, it would seem important to consider the possibility of an underlying major mood disorder independent of AAS use.

AAS Withdrawal–Associated Depression

As mentioned earlier in the subsection "AAS Dependence," hypogonadism related to AAS withdrawal has been increasingly recognized as an important problem in long-term AAS users. During AAS withdrawal, most men do not display marked depressive symptoms, even when their testosterone levels are grossly below the normal range. However, a small number of men develop pronounced depressive symptoms (Schmidt et al. 2004), sometimes accompanied by suicidal ideation and even completed suicide (Pope et al. 2014b). In mild cases of depression, symptoms may remit spontaneously as endogenous testosterone production gradually recovers. However, more severe or prolonged cases of depression may require endocrine interventions to restore HPG axis function, as described earlier (see "AAS Dependence"), together with antidepressant treatment. Depression accompanying AAS withdrawal, which may sometimes linger for months without treatment (Kanayama et al. 2015), appears to respond well to SSRIs such as fluoxetine (Malone and Dimeff 1992). Serotonergic antidepressants may be particularly useful because they may also benefit muscle dysmorphia and other forms of body dysmorphic disorder that may accompany AAS use (Phillips et al. 2008).

Body Image Disorders Associated With AAS Use

Recent years have seen increasing recognition of a form of body dysmorphic disorder called *muscle dysmorphia*, or reverse anorexia nervosa, in which the individual perceives himself to be small and frail, even though he is actually large and muscular (Rohman 2009; Sreshta et al. 2017). Men with muscle dysmorphia often engage in compulsive weight lifting and bodybuilding, even to the exclusion of other activities that they enjoy. They also frequently avoid situations in which their body will be seen by others, such as going to the beach or changing in a locker room, for fear that they look too small. Not surprisingly, such individuals may use AASs to "treat" their self-perceived "deficiency"; paradoxically, however, many describe worsening symptoms of muscle dysmorphia following initiation of AAS use. As mentioned earlier (see "AAS Dependence"), muscle dysmorphia may contribute to AAS dependence, because individuals may become extremely anxious that they are losing muscle size or gaining fat after stopping AAS use, and therefore quickly resume use.

For individuals presenting with muscle dysmorphia or other obsessive concerns about body image or physique, the clinician should always consider and investigate the possibility of AAS use (Murray et al. 2016). Successful treatment of the underlying body image disorder may be helpful in deterring future AAS use; however, individuals with muscle dysmorphia may be reluctant to admit that they have a condition requiring treatment, as is often the case with other forms of body dysmorphic disorder. We are not aware of systematic studies of treatment of muscle dysmorphia per se, but it seems reasonable to follow general principles of treatment of other forms of body dysmorphic disorder, relying on cognitive-behavioral therapy and pharmacological interventions such as SSRIs—modalities of demonstrated efficacy in body dysmorphic disorder generically (Phillips et al. 2008).

Co-Occurring Substance Use Disorders

AAS users frequently use other types of performance- and image-enhancing drugs, including other hormones (e.g., human growth hormone, thyroid hormones, insulin, HCG), agents for fat loss (e.g., clenbuterol, amphetamines, 2,4-dinitrophenol), other drugs with anabolic properties (e.g., selective androgen receptor modulators), and drugs to counteract the side effects of AASs (e.g., aromatase inhibitors and estrogen receptor blockers to counteract gynecomastia caused by esterification of testosterone and other AASs) (Hildebrandt et al. 2011; Pope et al. 2014b). AAS users can obtain abundant information about how to use these various substances both in "underground" guides (Llewellyn 2017) and on the Internet. AAS users also may have substance use disorders involving conventional drugs of abuse, such as cannabis, amphetamines, cocaine, and opioids (Dodge and Hoagland 2011; Sagoe et al. 2015; Skarberg et al. 2009). In particular, the association of AAS use with opioid use may in part reflect similarities between these classes of drugs in their reward mechanisms, as discussed earlier (see "AAS Dependence") (Nyberg and Hallberg 2012; Wood 2008). Consistent with these findings, a recent analysis using directed acyclic graphs—a form of causal modeling similar to the more familiar path diagrams (Hernán and Robins 2019)—found that AAS use contributed significantly to the first-time development of opioid use disorders, but not to the development of other classical substance use disorders (Kanayama et al. 2018b). In our experience, concomitant opioid use disorder is particularly common in North America. We have evaluated many AAS users who were first introduced to oral opioids or intravenous opioid agonist-antagonists such as nalbuphine and who then progressed to intravenous use of classical opioids such as morphine and heroin. We are aware of several cases in which such individuals later died from inadvertent overdoses of intravenous opioids. In Europe, a specific link between AAS use and opioid use appears less prominent, with AAS use more commonly associated with use of other drugs such as cocaine, cannabis, and amphetamines (Gårevik and Rane 2010; Skarberg et al. 2009).

It follows from these observations that clinicians should assess the history of classical substance use disorders in all individuals presenting with AAS use and, conversely, should consider the possibility of AAS use in individuals presenting with classical substance use disorders. In either case, non-AAS substance use disorders in current or former AAS users may require treatment. The reader is referred to relevant corresponding chapters in this volume regarding principles for such treatment. For an in-depth discussion of treatment principles for specific drugs of abuse, the reader is referred to other chapters in this textbook.

Medical Conditions Associated With Long-Term AAS Use

Long-term use of AASs may be associated with a variety of adverse medical complications, the full extent of which is only gradually becoming appreciated. One reason for the still-limited knowledge of these effects, as mentioned earlier, is that AAS use did not become widespread in the general population until the 1980s. Therefore, the oldest of these general-population AAS users—men who first tried AASs at, say, age 20 in the late 1980s—are only now reaching their 50s and entering the age of risk for medical complications of long-term use. We proposed the following analogy in an earlier publication (Kanayama et al. 2008): Imagine that widespread cigarette smoking did not exist until the 1980s and that the great majority of the world's cigarette smokers were still below age 55 today. In that scenario, we would have only a limited recognition of the potential long-term risks of cigarette smoking and, therefore, might substantially underestimate the true amount of morbidity and mortality that would ultimately occur.

An analogous situation may exist with regard to AASs. Recent years have seen growing evidence that AASs produce adverse cardiovascular effects (e.g., cardiomyopathy, atherosclerotic vascular disease, myocardial infarction, cerebrovascular accidents) (Angell et al. 2014; Baggish et al. 2017; Barbosa Neto et al. 2018; Cecchi et al. 2017; Montisci et al. 2012); protracted neuroendocrine disruption (as discussed earlier in "AAS Dependence"); and possible neurotoxicity, as evidenced by studies in AAS users that involved cognitive testing (Kanayama et al. 2013) and neuroimaging (Bjørnebekk et al. 2017; Kaufman et al. 2015; Westlye et al. 2016). Adverse effects on other organ systems, such as the liver and kidney, have also been described and may be associated with cumulative lifetime AAS exposure (Herlitz et al. 2010; Kantarci et al. 2018; Pope et al. 2014b; Solimini et al. 2017).

It follows that aging AAS users may increasingly come to clinical attention as a result of various medical or neurological effects. Thus, substance abuse professionals may receive referrals of such patients from medical clinicians, many of whom may themselves be unfamiliar with illicit AAS use. Such patients may need to discontinue AASs immediately as a result of medical dangers. Many of these patients may never have previously disclosed their AAS use to any clinician, and may be very uncomfortable with the idea of entering treatment and discontinuing AASs. Prompt, knowledgeable, and sympathetic interventions that address all three of the potential AAS dependence pathways described earlier (see Figure 21–1) may be required to achieve a good outcome.

Forensic Situations

AAS users may occasionally come to clinical attention through the courts as a result of violent or criminal behavior. A number of papers have described individuals, often with no prior history of psychiatric disorder, violence, or criminal behavior, who became uncharacteristically violent, and sometimes committed murder, while intoxicated with AASs (Hall et al. 2005; Perry et al. 2003; Pope et al. 2014b). In such cases, AASs are not necessarily the proximal trigger to violence; the direction of causality may sometimes be reversed, in that some individuals may deliberately ingest AASs in preparation for committing a crime, presumably feeling that this will make them stronger and more aggressive (Lundholm et al. 2010).

In some cases of criminal violence, the role of AAS use may be missed because the possibility is never considered. However, AAS use should be suspected when any unusually muscular man is apprehended for violent behavior, especially if it appears that this violence is not characteristic of his usual personality. Such individuals may display manic or hypomanic symptoms, occasionally accompanied by psychotic symptoms, such as paranoid or grandiose delusions (see earlier subsection "AAS-Induced Hypomania and Mania").The clinician's index of suspicion should be raised particularly if such a man rapidly develops vegetative symptoms of depression after being incarcerated, but then improves a few weeks or months later. This pattern may indicate AAS withdrawal, precipitated by the abrupt discontinuation of AASs following incarceration, with a gradual remission of depressive symptoms as suppressed HPG axis function gradually recovers. Of course, this pattern of biological depression must be distinguished from the situational depression associated with incarceration itself.

In cases in which AAS use is acknowledged by the defendant and appears to have been a clear precipitant of criminal behavior, forensic clinicians may be asked to offer an opinion as to whether the defendant exhibited "involuntary intoxication" or "diminished capacity" from AAS use. The legal aspects of this defense are beyond the scope of this chapter. However, it seems clear that if an individual is released and placed on probation after committing a crime that was believed to be associated with AAS use, it may be wise to require random, unannounced, observed urine tests for AASs to ensure that he does not resume these drugs.

Conclusion

Of the various substance use disorders described in this volume, AAS use disorders may be the least familiar to the average clinician. However, the frequency of AAS use disorders, together with the various medical and psychiatric syndromes associated with AAS use, is now beginning to be better recognized. Greater awareness of this problem on the part of clinicians may lead to the detection of many more cases and a better understanding of how best to treat them.

Key take-away points from this chapter can be summarized as follows:

- Anabolic-androgenic steroid (AAS) use must be approached differently from other forms of substance abuse, because AASs do not produce an immediate reward or "high" in the manner of conventional drugs of abuse.

- AAS use has been linked to body dysmorphic disorder.
- AAS users rarely see their drug use as pathological, rarely seek treatment, and may have contempt for physicians.
- AAS users often have a history of substance use disorders involving classical drugs, especially opioids.
- Some individuals experience hypomanic or manic symptoms during AAS exposure and depressive symptoms during AAS withdrawal.
- AASs may produce a well-documented dependence syndrome, for which an animal model exists. This dependence syndrome may arise through several pathways, including a body image pathway, a neuroendocrine pathway, and a hedonic pathway, each of which may dictate specific treatment interventions.

References

American Psychiatric Association: Diagnostic and Statistical Manual of Mental Disorders, 3rd Edition. Washington, DC, American Psychiatric Association, 1980

American Psychiatric Association: Diagnostic and Statistical Manual of Mental Disorders, 4th Edition. Washington, DC, American Psychiatric Association, 1994

American Psychiatric Association: Diagnostic and Statistical Manual of Mental Disorders, 5th Edition. Arlington, VA, American Psychiatric Association, 2013

Angell PJ, Ismail TF, Jabbour A, et al: Ventricular structure, function, and focal fibrosis in anabolic steroid users: a CMR study. Eur J Appl Physiol 114(5):921–928, 2014 24463601

Baggish AL, Weiner RB, Kanayama G, et al: Cardiovascular toxicity of illicit anabolic-androgenic steroid use. Circulation 135(21):1991–2002, 2017 28533317

Barbosa Neto O, da Mota GR, De Sordi CC, et al: Long-term anabolic steroids in male bodybuilders induce cardiovascular structural and autonomic abnormalities. Clin Auton Res 28(2):231–244, 2018 29019018

Bjørnebekk A, Walhovd KB, Jørstad ML, et al: Structural brain imaging of long-term anabolic-androgenic steroid users and nonusing weightlifters. Biol Psychiatry 82(4):294–302, 2017 27616036

Brennan BP, Kanayama G, Pope HG Jr: Performance-enhancing drugs on the web: a growing public-health issue. Am J Addict 22(2):158–161, 2013 23414502

Brower KJ: Anabolic steroid abuse and dependence in clinical practice. Phys Sportsmed 37(4):131–140, 2009 20048550

Cecchi R, Muciaccia B, Ciallella C, et al: Ventricular androgenic-anabolic steroid-related remodeling: an immunohistochemical study. Int J Legal Med 131(6):1589–1595, 2017 28432434

Christou MA, Christou PA, Markozannes G, et al: Effects of anabolic androgenic steroids on the reproductive system of athletes and recreational users: a systematic review and meta-analysis. Sports Med 47(9):1869–1883, 2017 28258581

Cordaro FG, Lombardo S, Cosentino M: Selling androgenic anabolic steroids by the pound: identification and analysis of popular websites on the Internet. Scand J Med Sci Sports 21(6):e247–e259, 2011 21210860

Coward RM, Rajanahally S, Kovac JR, et al: Anabolic steroid induced hypogonadism in young men. J Urol 190(6):2200–2205, 2013 23764075

de Souza GL, Hallak J: Anabolic steroids and male infertility: a comprehensive review. BJU Int 108(11):1860–1865, 2011 21682835

Dickerman RD, Pertusi RM, Zachariah NY, et al: Anabolic steroid-induced hepatotoxicity: is it overstated? Clin J Sport Med 9(1):34–39, 1999 10336050

Dodge T, Hoagland MF: The use of anabolic androgenic steroids and polypharmacy: a review of the literature. Drug Alcohol Depend 114(2–3):100–109, 2011 21232881

Gårevik N, Rane A: Dual use of anabolic-androgenic steroids and narcotics in Sweden. Drug Alcohol Depend 109(1–3):144–146, 2010 20064696

Geyer H, Parr MK, Koehler K, et al: Nutritional supplements cross-contaminated and faked with doping substances. J Mass Spectrom 43(7):892–902, 2008 18563865

Goldman AL, Pope HG, Bhasin S: The health threat posed by the hidden epidemic of anabolic steroid use and body image disorders among young men. J Clin Endocrinol Metab 104(4):1069–1074, 2019 30239802

Hall RC, Hall RC, Chapman MJ: Psychiatric complications of anabolic steroid abuse. Psychosomatics 46(4):285–290, 2005 16000671

Herlitz LC, Markowitz GS, Farris AB, et al: Development of focal segmental glomerulosclerosis after anabolic steroid abuse. J Am Soc Nephrol 21(1):163–172, 2010 19917783

Hernán MA, Robins JM: Causal Inference: What If. November 10, 2019. Available at: https://cdn1.sph.harvard.edu/wp-content/uploads/sites/1268/2019/11/ci_hernanrobins_10nov19.pdf. Accessed November 26, 2019.

Hildebrandt T, Lai JK, Langenbucher JW, et al: The diagnostic dilemma of pathological appearance and performance enhancing drug use. Drug Alcohol Depend 114(1):1–11, 2011 21115306

Ip EJ, Barnett MJ, Tenerowicz MJ, Perry PJ: The Anabolic 500 survey: characteristics of male users versus nonusers of anabolic-androgenic steroids for strength training. Pharmacotherapy 31(8):757–766, 2011 21923602

Kanayama G, Pope HG: Misconceptions about anabolic-androgenic steroid abuse. Psychiatr Ann 42(10):371–375, 2012. Available at: https://www.healio.com/psychiatry/journals/psycann/2012-10-42-10/%7B676601f2-9859-4275-9c14-4178d962986f%7D/misconceptions-about-anabolic-androgenic-steroid-abuse. Accessed January 15, 2020.

Kanayama G, Pope HG Jr: History and epidemiology of anabolic androgens in athletes and non-athletes. Mol Cell Endocrinol 464:4–13, 2018 28245998

Kanayama G, Boynes M, Hudson JI, et al: Anabolic steroid abuse among teenage girls: an illusory problem? Drug Alcohol Depend 88(2–3):156–162, 2007 17127018

Kanayama G, Hudson JI, Pope HG Jr: Long-term psychiatric and medical consequences of anabolic-androgenic steroid abuse: a looming public health concern? Drug Alcohol Depend 98(1–2):1–12, 2008 18599224

Kanayama G, Brower KJ, Wood RI, et al: Anabolic-androgenic steroid dependence: an emerging disorder. Addiction 104(12):1966–1978, 2009 19922565

Kanayama G, Brower KJ, Wood RI, et al: Treatment of anabolic-androgenic steroid dependence: emerging evidence and its implications. Drug Alcohol Depend 109(1–3):6–13, 2010 20188494

Kanayama G, Kean J, Hudson JI, et al: Cognitive deficits in long-term anabolic-androgenic steroid users. Drug Alcohol Depend 130(1–3):208–214, 2013 23253252

Kanayama G, Hudson JI, DeLuca J, et al: Prolonged hypogonadism in males following withdrawal from anabolic-androgenic steroids: an under-recognized problem. Addiction 110(5):823–831, 2015 25598171

Kanayama G, Kaufman MJ, Pope HG Jr: Public health impact of androgens. Curr Opin Endocrinol Diabetes Obes 25(3):218–223, 2018a 29369918

Kanayama G, Pope HG, Hudson JI: Associations of anabolic-androgenic steroid use with other behavioral disorders: an analysis using directed acyclic graphs. Psychol Med 48(15):2601–2608, 2018b 29490719

Kantarci UH, Punduk Z, Senarslan O, et al: Evaluation of anabolic steroid induced renal damage with sonography in bodybuilders. J Sports Med Phys Fitness 58(11):1681–1687, 2018 29148625

Kashkin KB, Kleber HD: Hooked on hormones? An anabolic steroid addiction hypothesis. JAMA 262(22):3166–3170, 1989 2681859

Kaufman MJ, Janes AC, Hudson JI, et al: Brain and cognition abnormalities in long-term anabolic-androgenic steroid users. Drug Alcohol Depend 152:47–56, 2015 25986964

Kaufman MJ, Kanayama G, Hudson JI, Pope HG Jr: Supraphysiologic-dose anabolic-androgenic steroid use: a risk factor for dementia? Neurosci Biobehav Rev 100:180–207, 2019 30817935

Kouri EM, Pope HG Jr, Katz DL, et al: Fat-free mass index in users and nonusers of anabolic-androgenic steroids. Clin J Sport Med 5(4):223–228, 1995 7496846

Llewellyn W: Anabolics, 11th Edition. Jupiter, FL, Molecular Nutrition, 2017

Lundholm L, Käll K, Wallin S, et al: Use of anabolic androgenic steroids in substance abusers arrested for crime. Drug Alcohol Depend 111(3):222–226, 2010 20627426

Malone DA Jr, Dimeff RJ: The use of fluoxetine in depression associated with anabolic steroid withdrawal: a case series. J Clin Psychiatry 53(4):130–132, 1992 1564048

Montisci M, El Mazloum R, Cecchetto G, et al: Anabolic androgenic steroids abuse and cardiac death in athletes: morphological and toxicological findings in four fatal cases. Forensic Sci Int 217(1–3):e13–e18, 2012 22047750

Murray SB, Griffiths S, Mond JM, et al: Anabolic steroid use and body image psychopathology in men: delineating between appearance- versus performance-driven motivations. Drug Alcohol Depend 165:198–202, 2016 27364377

Nyberg F, Hallberg M: Interactions between opioids and anabolic androgenic steroids: implications for the development of addictive behavior. Int Rev Neurobiol 102:189–206, 2012 22748831

Parkinson AB, Evans NA: Anabolic androgenic steroids: a survey of 500 users. Med Sci Sports Exerc 38(4):644–651, 2006 16679978

Parr MK, Koehler K, Geyer H, et al: Clenbuterol marketed as dietary supplement. Biomed Chromatogr 22(3):298–300, 2008 17939172

Perry PJ, Kutscher EC, Lund BC, et al: Measures of aggression and mood changes in male weightlifters with and without androgenic anabolic steroid use. J Forensic Sci 48(3):646–651, 2003 12762541

Pettersson J, Hindorf U, Persson P, et al: Muscular exercise can cause highly pathological liver function tests in healthy men. Br J Clin Pharmacol 65(2):253–259, 2008 17764474

Phillips KA, Didie ER, Feusner J, et al: Body dysmorphic disorder: treating an underrecognized disorder. Am J Psychiatry 165(9):1111–1118, 2008 18765493

Pope HG, Kanayama G: Can you tell if your patient is using anabolic steroids? Current Psychiatry in Primary Care 1:28–34, 2005

Pope HG, Katz DL: Psychiatric effects of exogenous anabolic-androgenic steroids, in Psychoneuroendocrinology: The Scientific Basis of Clinical Practice. Edited by Wolkowitz OM, Rothschild AJ. Washington, DC, American Psychiatric Press, 2003, pp 331–358

Pope HG Jr, Olivardia R, Gruber A, et al: Evolving ideals of male body image as seen through action toys. Int J Eat Disord 26(1):65–72, 1999 10349585

Pope HG, Kanayama G, Ionescu-Pioggia M, et al: Anabolic steroid users' attitudes towards physicians. Addiction 99(9):1189–1194, 2004 15317640

Pope HG Jr, Kanayama G, Athey A, et al: The lifetime prevalence of anabolic-androgenic steroid use and dependence in Americans: current best estimates. Am J Addict 23(4):371–377, 2014a 24112239

Pope HG Jr, Wood RI, Rogol A, et al: Adverse health consequences of performance-enhancing drugs: an Endocrine Society scientific statement. Endocr Rev 35(3):341–375, 2014b 24423981

Pope HG Jr, Khalsa JH, Bhasin S: Body image disorders and abuse of anabolic-androgenic steroids among men. JAMA 317(1):23–24, 2017 27930760

Rahnema CD, Crosnoe LE, Kim ED: Designer steroids—over-the-counter supplements and their androgenic component: review of an increasing problem. Andrology 3(2):150–155, 2015 25684733

Rasmussen JJ, Selmer C, Østergren PB, et al: Former abusers of anabolic androgenic steroids exhibit decreased testosterone levels and hypogonadal symptoms years after cessation: a case-control study. PLoS One 11(8):e0161208, 2016 27532478

Rohman L: The relationship between anabolic androgenic steroids and muscle dysmorphia: a review. Eat Disord 17(3):187–199, 2009 19391018

Sagoe D, McVeigh J, Bjørnebekk A, et al: Polypharmacy among anabolic-androgenic steroid users: a descriptive metasynthesis. Subst Abuse Treat Prev Policy 10:12, 2015 25888931

Santora LJ, Marin J, Vangrow J, et al: Coronary calcification in body builders using anabolic steroids. Prev Cardiol 9(4):198–201, 2006 17085981

Schmidt PJ, Berlin KL, Danaceau MA, et al: The effects of pharmacologically induced hypogonadism on mood in healthy men. Arch Gen Psychiatry 61(10):997–1004, 2004 15466673

Skarberg K, Nyberg F, Engstrom I: Multisubstance use as a feature of addiction to anabolic-androgenic steroids. Eur Addict Res 15(2):99–106, 2009 19182484

Solimini R, Rotolo MC, Mastrobattista L, et al: Hepatotoxicity associated with illicit use of anabolic androgenic steroids in doping. Eur Rev Med Pharmacol Sci 21 (1 suppl):7–16, 2017 28379599

Sreshta N, Pope H, Hudson J, et al: Muscle dysmorphia, in Body Dysmorphic Disorder: Advances in Research and Clinical Practice. Edited by Phillips KA. New York, Oxford University Press, 2017, pp 81–94

Tan RS, Scally MC: Anabolic steroid-induced hypogonadism—towards a unified hypothesis of anabolic steroid action. Med Hypotheses 72(6):723–728, 2009 19231088

Van Wagoner RM, Eichner A, Bhasin S, et al: Chemical composition and labeling of substances marketed as selective androgen receptor modulators and sold via the Internet. JAMA 318(20):2004–2010, 2017 29183075

Westlye LT, Kaufmann T, Alnæs D, et al: Brain connectivity aberrations in anabolic-androgenic steroid users. Neuroimage Clin 13:62–69, 2016 27942448

Wood RI: Anabolic-androgenic steroid dependence? Insights from animals and humans. Front Neuroendocrinol 29(4):490–506, 2008 18275992

Recommended Readings

Brower KJ: Anabolic steroid abuse and dependence in clinical practice. Phys Sportsmed 37(4):131–140, 2009 20048550

Hildebrandt T, Lai JK, Langenbucher JW, et al: The diagnostic dilemma of pathological appearance and performance enhancing drug use. Drug Alcohol Depend 114(1):1–11, 2011 21115306

Kanayama G, Brower KJ, Wood RI, et al: Treatment of anabolic-androgenic steroid dependence: emerging evidence and its implications. Drug Alcohol Depend 109(1–3):6–13, 2010 20188494

Pope HG Jr, Wood RI, Rogol A, et al: Adverse health consequences of performance-enhancing drugs: an Endocrine Society scientific statement. Endocr Rev 35(3):341–375, 2014 24423981

PART IV

Nonpharmacotherapeutic
Treatment Modalities

CHAPTER 22

Psychodynamic Psychotherapy

Edward J. Khantzian, M.D.

With a few exceptions, based primarily on drive theory, the early literature stressed the use of addictive drugs as a regressive pleasurable adaptation and the symbolic meaning of the drugs (Dodes and Khantzian 2016; Khantzian and Treece 1977; Rosenfeld 1965; Yorke 1970). Modern psychodynamic formulations, drawing on a structural model, object relations theory, self psychology, and attachment theory, place emphasis on substance use disorders as a progressive attempt to cope with internal painful emotional processes and threatening external realities. These more recent formulations, elaborated on in this chapter, dating back to the 1960s and 1970s, stressed how disturbances in regulation of affect, sense of self, interpersonal relations, and self-care causes susceptible individuals to succumb to substance use disorders. Such an understanding provides a basis to understand and alleviate these predisposing factors. Employing this perspective in individual and group psychodynamic therapy can be beneficial in helping individuals with substance use disorders to understand and modify these dynamics and overcome their addictive attachments and behaviors (Khantzian 2015).

A Psychodynamic Focus on Addictive Vulnerability

Starting in the 1960s and continuing over the past 50 years, developments in psychoanalytic theory and practice have contributed to their employment in the psychodynamic application, understanding, and treatment of substance use disorders. These

---

Sections on psychodynamics and treatment in this chapter are based in part on two reports (Khantzian 2012, 2015).

contemporary theories have been valuable in deciphering the nature of addictive vulnerability, and this work in turn has provided guidance for treatment approaches that
can remediate the vulnerabilities that predispose to and result from substance use disorders. The recent theories are in contrast to early formulations, which proposed that
psychoanalytic approaches were not suitable for substance use disorders. The developments across time have suggested that substance dependence represents a disorder
of self-regulation involving difficulties in regulating affects, sense of self and self-
esteem, relationships, and behavior. From this perspective, addiction can be considered a special adaptation by which, in the short term, individuals prone to substance
use disorders attempt to alleviate or compensate for their dysregulation disturbances,
a solution that ultimately fails. More often than not, psychodynamic treatment, as explored in this chapter, is not provided as a stand-alone treatment. Combining psychodynamic treatment with group treatments and medication-assisted treatments has
been essential to establishing control over addictive behavior (see later section "Treatment Implications").

Unfortunately, with the exception of the last half of the twentieth century there
have been few psychodynamic explorations or contributions to the study of substance
use disorders. It is safe to say, however, that psychodynamic influences are evident in
contemporary therapies such as cognitive-behavioral therapy, dialectical behavior
therapy, and motivational interviewing. This evidence is especially notable in the humanistic and empathic attitudes exemplified in the evidence-based work of William
Miller and Stephen Rollnick, drawing on the work of Carl Rogers (see Khantzian
2012). Although there are few if any empirical studies validating psychodynamic perspectives on substance use disorders, there are many clinical studies and reports
(practice-based evidence) from all over the world citing and supporting psychodynamic theory and practice; this is particularly apparent on websites such as Research-
Gate, Academia.edu, and Google Scholar.

Affect Regulation

Dysregulation of affects is central in substance use disorders. Recent psychodynamic
views of substance dependence have stressed that individuals with substance use disorders suffer in the extreme with their emotions. At one extreme, affects are elusive, cut
off, and confusing, and at the other, they are intense, threatening, and uncontrollable.
In regard to the first extreme, a range of terms have evolved to characterize the elusive
and discomforting nature of affects; these include *disaffection, alexithymia, anhedonia,*
and *nonfeeling states.* These emotional deficits cause individuals to experience states of
emptiness and thus the inability to use their emotions to guide their reactions and behaviors. Krystal (1988) described a normal developmental line for emotions wherein
affects are at first undifferentiated, somatized, and not verbalized, and subsequently
become differentiated, desomatized, and verbalized. He referred to deficits in the stimulus barrier that made processing of emotions problematic. Krystal's formulations
provided a basis for understanding how emotional deprivation or trauma, whether occurring early or later in life, could produce distortions or deficits in affect experience,
causing individuals to resort to substance use to compensate for these deficits.

At the other extreme, emotions are intense and intolerable. Deficits in affect defense
and drive defense cause individuals with substance use disorders to resort to use of

substances such as opioids and alcohol to help contain these powerful and threatening emotions. Khantzian (1977) stressed how the anti-aggression action of opiates helps to contain such threatening affects, and along similar lines, Wurmser (1974) referred to defects in affect defense, especially violent affect.

Depending on what feelings or affects cause their difficulty, individuals who begin using substances discover what drug suits them best through experimentation. For example, for individuals who are anhedonic or feel empty, the activating, enlivening, and stimulating properties of cocaine or amphetamines are experienced as welcome, whereas for individuals who are unsettled or overwhelmed by intense or threatening feelings, opioids or obliterating doses of alcohol act as correctives (Khantzian 1997). Wieder and Kaplan (1969) coined the term *drug of choice* in describing how adolescents used opiates as prosthetics to manage their anxiety. Milkman and Frosch (1973) studied the role of individuals' ego profiles on their preferential use of opiates versus stimulants. Similarly, Wurmser (1974) and Khantzian (1977) emphasized the use of opiates and high doses of alcohol to control violent and aggressive affects. Patients with substance use disorders experience extreme fluctuations in affect regulation, and therapists can help these patients to access their feelings by using approaches that are more interactive, such as labeling feeling states, drawing out patients' experiences of their feelings, and so on. By asking patients, "What did this drug do for you when you first used it?" therapists can help patients to identify the troubling and/or painful affects that determine their drug of choice (Khantzian 2012).

Patients with substance use disorders make it amply clear that short-term substances of abuse produce relief from confusing and threatening feelings, but it readily becomes apparent that addictive drugs perpetuate and heighten their suffering and distress. Although patients seem to passively endure these consequences as a trade-off for the relief addictive drugs provide, formulations by Gedo (1986), Lichtenberg (1983), and Khantzian and Wilson (1993) suggest that this repetitive aspect of addictive behavior represents attempts to work out early childhood pain and suffering for which there are no words, memories, or mental representation. Thus, the operative changes from relieving suffering to controlling it (Khantzian 1997).

Self-Esteem Regulation

Kohut's (1971, 1977) development of self psychology was groundbreaking in that it provided an understanding of the troubled sense of self and damaged self-esteem that result from faulty parenting and empathic failure in early phases of childhood development. Kohut emphasized how such empathic failures resulted in a disrupted sense of inner harmony, poor self-cohesion, and unending feelings of dis-ease. Although Kohut did not systematically study and treat substance use disorders, he appreciated how individuals with these disorders suffer in this respect and how they adopt defensive postures of counterdependency, bravado, and invincibility to mask feelings of emptiness and inadequacy. Subsequent investigators have pursued how such disturbance plays out with substance use disorders, emphasizing feelings of powerlessness and unimportance as well as compensatory reactions of narcissistic rage and grandiosity (Director 2005; Dodes 1996, 2002). Dodes (1996) linked these dynamics to the idea of substance dependency as a compulsive disorder, thereby making individuals with substance use disorders amenable to conventional psychoanalytic treatment. Defenses of bravado and disdain may shield against and compensate for feelings of shame, low self-worth, and helplessness (Khantzian 2012). These contributions were especially germane in appreciating how reliance on addictive substances serves as a corrective for these individuals' interminable states of fragmentation, lost sense of self, and inability to care about or to love themselves.

This perspective of a fragmented sense of self and feelings of powerlessness provides an understanding of how stimulants, for example, can correct feelings of weakness, or how opiates can contain, soothe, and comfort individuals unable to perform these functions for themselves. Such an appreciation also helps when considering how a person with a substance use disorder might use stimulants to augment or enhance defensive postures of omnipotence and bravado. These dynamics suggest the need for clinicians to see through the defensive posturing as they engage with patients who struggle with substance use disorders and who endure the fragile sense of self that they defend against, and to be prepared to employ individual and group psychotherapies to understand and work on the patients' defenses and underlying vulnerabilities.

Interpersonal Regulation

The troubled and troubling sense of self and self-esteem play out powerfully in the interpersonal relationships of individuals with substance use disorders. In contrast to early psychoanalytic formulations that focused on pathological dependency, contemporary psychodynamic views have focused on problems of isolation and counterdependence (Khantzian 1995). Early life experiences with traumatic abuse and neglect have an impact on self structures and play out later in life in an inability to allow or express wishes for connection, affection, and comfort from others, which these individuals so desperately need but cannot accept or dare. As a result, relational cutoff and loneliness become a tragic way of life, leading some individuals to substitute addictive solutions in place of human ones. Explorations of these early attachment issues help patients and clinicians to understand how such adaptations cause addiction-prone individuals to develop a substance use disorder to deal with the distress and the pain-perpetuating defenses of spurious self-sufficiency, disavowal of need, and counterdependence (Flores 2004; Khantzian 2012; Walant 2002; Weegmann and Cohen 2002).

Bowlby (1973) emphasized that attachment issues persist throughout life, from infancy into adulthood. More recent attachment theorists have placed attachment issues as central in the development of substance use disorders. Walant (2002) elegantly described "normative neglect and abuse," wherein infant and child care is guided more by cultural norms and doctrine than by empathic attunement to the child's needs. For individuals experiencing this normative neglect and abuse, insecure, anxious attachments result, and in particular attachment to addictive drugs. Flores (2004) focused on how secure attachments in early phases of development create a sense of safety, comfort, and well-being, and how, in their absence, attachment to alcohol and drugs becomes likely. In the United Kingdom, Reading (2002) described how attachment theory is fundamental for explaining the interpersonal difficulties of individuals with substance use disorders and their drugs of choice. These investigators have explored and clarified how and why it is that individuals with substance use disorders substitute attachment to addictive substances in place of human attachments. They have also developed empathic individual and group therapeutic tactics and interactive strategies for ameliorating and resolving these patients' pathological connections to addictive drugs and behaviors.

Self-Care Regulation

Early psychoanalytic theorists attributed human self-destructiveness, including dependency on substances, to impaired survival instincts and self-destructive drives (Menninger 1938). Later theorists suggested that this behavior may be more the result of a developmental failure in protective ego and self functions than of impaired survival instincts (Khantzian and Mack 1983). The development of the ego capacity for self-care is crucial for ensuring safety, control of impulses, and a sense of well-being (Khantzian and Mack 1983). Deficits in this function may cause addiction-prone individuals to succumb to the dangers of behaviors leading to substance use disorders and the hazards of experimentation with and continuous use of addictive substances.

In comparison with people without substance use problems, individuals with substance use disorders think and feel differently about potential risks and harms (Khantzian 2012), especially those associated with addictive behavior. For example, these individuals may be or are indifferent to their first experience of inserting a needle into their own veins; they may experience little thought or emotion during injections. Tactfully, the therapist can share with patients his or her own recoil from the idea of self-injection. The clinician initially might consider that these failures and lapses were the function of regression secondary to addictive processes. However, after working long term with patients who misuse drugs, the clinician more often will better appreciate that such patients are constantly remiss or neglectful in attending to daily requirements for medical or dental hygiene, attending to necessary details of license renewals, paying insurance premiums, and performing other important self-care tasks. These underdeveloped self-care capacities remain apparent in long-term treatment even with abstinent patients who are in remission. These deficits in self-care functions malignantly interact with painful affects and suffering associated with troubled self states and interpersonal relationships to make addictive behavior more likely (Khantzian 1997, 2012).

Treatment Implications

The most important treatment advice for psychodynamic therapists and psychoanalysts is that they are misguided and put themselves and their patients at risk if they think that establishing control of or abstinence from unbridled use of alcohol or drugs can wait on working out the dynamics of these disorders. The symptoms of substance use disorders can be life-threatening, and in such cases, an initial focus on establishing control can be critical and essential. Important interventions to help patients achieve control of or abstain from substance use before commencing exploration of underlying dynamics include 12-step programs, moderation management, relapse prevention strategies, group therapy, and rehabilitation confinement. In fact, ongoing patient involvement in 12-step programs and psychodynamically oriented group therapy can work in a complementary and beneficial way with individual psychodynamic psychotherapy to support long-term control of or abstinence from substance use (Khantzian 2014). Additionally, medication-assisted treatments such as methadone, buprenorphine, and naltrexone can be invaluable in reducing or stopping uncontrolled use and regulating the daunting problems of craving and the instability associated with the ravages of chronic drug use (Khantzian 2018). These agents provide biological and emotional stabilization that allow for psychotherapeutic treatment.

Therapeutic modes of impassivity and strictly interpretive approaches can be counterproductive when used with individuals who have substance use disorders. The therapist's empathic attunement to the patient's deficits and complexities in affect experience, self–other difficulties, and self-care failures is central to the therapeutic work. Notwithstanding necessary modifications in technique and practice, the human psychodynamic vulnerabilities involved in individuals with substance use disorders are preeminently amenable to the benefits of therapeutic modes of empathy and understanding, and patients profit from the corrective and transforming experience that psychoanalytic and psychodynamic treatments provide.

Contemporary psychoanalytic theories on dysfunction and deficits in affect regulation, sense of self, interpersonal relations, and self-care regulation have enabled a better understanding of psychopathology beyond early formulations grounded in drive theory, more strictly interpretive approaches, and the exploration of unconscious processes. These advances provide a less speculative and more experience-near observational context that guides practitioners in what needs attending to and therapeutic remediation. These advances are especially germane for a psychodynamic understanding and treatment of substance use disorders.

Therapists need to make appropriate modifications in psychodynamic approaches to better appreciate patients' difficulties in experience, awareness, and expression of feelings that affect them. Clinicians should be prepared to actively assist patients in evoking, labeling, and putting into words what these patients are often unable to express. When patients say that they do not feel anything, the clinician should not necessarily consider this to be denial. Instead, an important aspect of psychotherapy in this context is to help patients via instruction, drawing out and identifying what they cannot do on their own. The contributions of Allen et al. (2008) on "mentalizing"— wherein psychotherapeutic effort is dedicated to helping patients to focus on feelings, thoughts, and behaviors—are preeminently applicable to and beneficial in psychotherapy for patients with substance use disorders. Also, 12-step groups and group therapies naturally, or by design, foster expression and focus on emotions as participants share their experiences of succumbing to and recovering from substance use disorders (Khantzian 2015; Khantzian et al. 1992). When a patient's affects are uncontained, threatening to self and others—feelings and states that can be central to a reliance on addictive substances—therapists should not underestimate the benefit of a strong psychotherapeutic alliance in helping to contain these threatening affects. Therapeutic exploration by the patient and the therapist of the origins, legitimacy, and acceptance of these emotions in psychotherapeutic work can ameliorate the devastating subjective and interpersonal distress that these intense affects generate. Judicious use of modulating medications, such as affect modulators, targeting the unhinging effects of intense violent feelings, which can enable containment and control in order to work on the origins of such intense affect, is recommended (Khantzian 2012).

When therapists are working with patients who have substance use disorders, the use of therapeutic elements of kindness, support, and empathy is extremely important in engaging and helping the patients with their underdeveloped sense of self and low self-esteem. Adopting such an approach can enable both therapist and patient to better appreciate how the patient's damaged sense of self causes subjective confusion, trouble, and elusive connections with self and others. Employment of such a mode of support helps patients to identify and resolve the feelings of powerlessness and defensive rage and the reactions of omnipotence that they so often express and that often play out in treatment. Therapeutic support and kindness are of paramount importance to help the patient and the clinician to identify and better resolve problems with off-putting personality characteristics. Contemporary theories about pathological self formulations can facilitate appreciation and understanding of reactive defenses secondary to feelings of helplessness, as well as feelings of unimportance and inadequacy (Director 2005; Dodes 1996; Khantzian 2012). For patients who seem disengaged and devoid of emotions, the therapist may draw on his or her own energy and liveliness to help activate and enliven patients. In addition, group therapy experiences often can be invaluable in instilling and validating a better sense of self and self-expression (Khantzian 2015).

The sense of a troubled self and low self-esteem significantly contribute to the tendency of individuals with substance use disorders to isolate themselves from and experience difficulties in interpersonal relationships and human attachments. Feelings of unworthiness and unimportance cause individuals so affected to feel disinclined to connect to others. Innovative therapeutic interactions of engagement, activity, and responsiveness, as suggested by Flores (2004), Walant (2002), and Khantzian (2012), are essential in helping patients with their ambivalence about and fear of relationships. Such tactful attention to patients' difficulties around connecting to others can help foster better capacities for human attachments and interdependence. Therapist passivity and detached interpretations when dealing with patients' ambivalence about their attachment issues can leave patients feeling devastatingly alone and not understood. The connections stimulated by individual and group therapy are extremely helpful in understanding and correcting the attachment problems and sense of alienation that addiction-prone patients endure (Khantzian 2015).

Therapeutic attention to the self-care deficits of persons with substance use disorders is essential for successful recovery. Therapists can and should feel comfortable in using and sharing their subjective reactions of alarm and concern with patients when, in the course of psychotherapy, the patients indicate a lack of worry or thoughtfulness about various risky situations and behaviors that unfold in their daily life activities. By focusing on such risky and unthinking behaviors, the therapist working in either individual or group therapy can help patients to develop a growing awareness of how their self-care deficits are involved in their risky and careless tendencies that can lead up to using and relapsing to addictive substances. Ongoing psychotherapy provides opportunities for patients to gain insight and helps them to appreciate the developmental origins of their self-care deficits. Finally, therapists "need to help patients use self-respect, feelings of apprehension/worry, relationships with others, and thoughtfulness as a guide for safe behavior and self-preservation" (Khantzian 2012, p. 278).

Conclusion

In contrast to early psychoanalytic formulations that stressed regressive pleasurable drives and self-destructive motives to explain dependence on alcohol and drugs, more contemporary formulations, drawing on modern theories, consider deficits in affect development, self-esteem, interpersonal relations, and self-care as explanations for substance use disorders. Early theory suggested that substance use disorders were not amenable to psychoanalytic approaches, but recent clinical experiences employing modern understanding and treatment methods show encouraging results in getting at the roots of and effectively treating addictive behavior.

It is of paramount importance that therapists, before addressing the psychodynamics of patients' self-regulation difficulties that are at the roots of substance use disorder, direct their initial clinical efforts toward helping patients to establish control over their excessive and uncontrolled use of drugs and alcohol. Otherwise, patient safety or survival remains at risk. This initial focus is especially important because simply commencing psychotherapy without a focus on the loss of control can create the illusion for patients that they are safe and out of danger.

Early psychoanalytic modes of impassivity, therapeutic detachment, and strictly interpretative techniques are not conducive to building a positive therapeutic relationship with patients who have substance use disorders. In fact, such modes of treatment can be counterproductive and damaging. The therapist's patience, support, kindness, and attunement to the distress that drives addictive behavior provide the foundation for effective psychodynamic psychotherapy. In contrast to early models of impassive psychoanalytic technique, modern psychodynamic psychotherapy employs more interactive, supportive, and interpersonal responsiveness. A premium is placed on assuring comfort and effective connection with patients, thus promoting active empathic attunement to patients' difficulties in managing their affects, self-esteem, interpersonal relations, and self-care issues.

In conclusion, modern psychodynamic theory and practice provide important insights into the suffering and dysfunctions associated with substance use disorders and offer hope and a humanistic foundation for treating and ameliorating the causes and consequences of addictive suffering.

References

Allen JG, Fonagy P, Bateman AW: Mentalizing in Clinical Practice. Washington, DC, American Psychiatric Publishing, 2008

Bowlby J: Attachment and Loss: Volume 2. Separation: Anxiety and Anger. New York, Basic Books, 1973

Director L: Encounters with omnipotence in the psychoanalysis of substance users. Psychoanal Dialogues 15(4):567–586, 2005. Available at: https://www.tandfonline.com/doi/abs/10.1080/10481881509348851. Accessed January 15, 2020.

Dodes LM: Compulsion and addiction. J Am Psychoanal Assoc 44(3):815–835, 1996 8892189

Dodes LM: The Heart of Addiction: A New Approach to Understanding and Managing Alcoholism and Other Addictive Behaviors. New York, Harper Collins, 2002

Dodes LM, Khantzian EJ: Individual psychodynamic psychotherapy, in Clinical Textbook of Addictive Disorders, 4th Edition. Edited by Mack AH, Brady KT, Miller SI, et al. New York, Guilford, 2016, pp 548–562

Flores PJ: Addiction as an Attachment Disorder. New York, Jason Aronson, 2004

Gedo J: Conceptual Issues in Psychoanalysis: Essays in History and Method. Hillsdale, NJ, Analytic Press, 1986

Khantzian EJ: The ego, the self and opiate addiction: theoretical and treatment considerations. NIDA Res Monogr (12):101–117, 1977 97531

Khantzian EJ: Self-regulation vulnerabilities in substance abusers: treatment implications, in The Psychology and Treatment of Addictive Behavior. Edited by Dowling S. New York, International University Press, 1995, pp 17–41

Khantzian EJ: The self-medication hypothesis of substance use disorders: a reconsideration and recent applications. Harv Rev Psychiatry 4(5):231–244, 1997 9385000

Khantzian EJ: Reflections on treating addictive disorders: a psychodynamic perspective. Am J Addict 21(3):274–279, discussion 279, 2012 22494231

Khantzian EJ: A psychodynamic perspective on the efficacy of 12-step programs. Alcoholism Treatment Quarterly 32(2–3):225–236, 2014. Available at: https://www.tandfonline.com/doi/abs/10.1080/07347324.2014.907027. Accessed January15, 2020.

Khantzian EJ: Psychodynamic psychotherapy for the treatment of substance use disorders, in Textbook of Addiction Treatment: International Perspectives. Edited by el-Guebaly N, Kara G, Galanter M, et al. New York, Springer, 2015, pp 811–819

Khantzian EJ: Treating Addiction: Beyond the Pain. New York, Rowman & Littlefield, 2018

Khantzian EJ, Mack JE: Self-preservation and the care of the self. Ego instincts reconsidered. Psychoanal Study Child 38:209–232, 1983 6647652

Khantzian EJ, Treece C: Psychodynamics of drug dependence: an overview, in Psychodynamics of Drug Dependence (NIDA Research Monograph 12). Edited by Blaine JD, Julius DA. Rockville, MD, National Institute on Drug Abuse, 1977, pp 11–25

Khantzian EJ, Wilson A: Substance dependence, repetition and the nature of addictive suffering, in Hierarchical Concepts in Psychoanalysis: Theory, Research, and Clinical Practice. Edited by Wilson A, Gedo JE. New York, Guilford, 1993, pp 263–283

Khantzian EJ, Halliday KS, Golden S, et al: Modified group therapy for substance abusers: a psychodynamic approach to relapse prevention. American Journal on Addictions 1(1):67–76, 1992. Available at: https://onlinelibrary.wiley.com/doi/abs/10.1111/j.1521-0391.1992.tb00008.x. Accessed January 15, 2020.

Kohut H: The Analysis of the Self. New York, International Universities Press, 1971

Kohut H: The Restoration of the Self. New York, International Universities Pres, 1977

Krystal H: Integration and Self-Healing: Affect, Trauma, Alexithymia. Hillsdale, NJ, Analytic Press, 1988

Lichtenberg JD: Psychoanalysis and Infant Research. Hillsdale, NJ, Analytic Press, 1983

Menninger K: Man Against Himself. New York, Free Press, 1938

Milkman H, Frosch WA: On the preferential abuse of heroin and amphetamine. J Nerv Ment Dis 156(4):242–248, 1973 4708884

Reading B: The application of Bowlby's attachment theory to the psychotherapy of addictions, in Psychodynamics of Addiction. Edited by Weegmann M, Cohen R. New York, Wiley, 2002, pp 13–30

Rosenfeld HA: The psychopathology of drug addiction and alcoholism: a critical review of the psychoanalytic literature, in Psychotic States: A Psycho-Analytical Approach. London, Hogarth Press, 1965, pp 217–242

Walant KB: Creating the Capacity for Attachment: Treating Addictions and the Alienated Self. New York, Jason Aronson, 2002

Weegmann M, Cohen R (eds): Psychodynamics of Addiction. New York, Wiley, 2002

Wieder H, Kaplan EH: Drug use in adolescents. Psychodynamic meaning and pharmacogenic effect. Psychoanal Study Child 24:399–431, 1969 5353372

Wurmser L: Psychoanalytic considerations of the etiology of compulsive drug use. J Am Psychoanal Assoc 22(4):820–843, 1974 4420835

Yorke C: A critical review of some psychoanalytic literature on drug addiction. Br J Med Psychol 43(2):141–159, 1970 4910965

CHAPTER 23

Cognitive-Behavioral Therapy

Kathleen M. Carroll, Ph.D.
Brian D. Kiluk, Ph.D.

Cognitive-behavioral treatments are among the most well-defined and rigorously studied behavioral interventions for substance use disorders. Although this chapter will focus primarily on cognitive-behavioral therapy (CBT) approaches, it should be noted that CBT shares several features with the other empirically supported behavioral approaches described in this volume. First, cognitive, behavioral, and motivational therapies are applicable to a broad range of substance use disorders. That is, well-controlled trials have supported their efficacy across alcohol-, stimulant-, marijuana-, and opioid-dependent populations (the latter in conjunction with medications). Second, these approaches were developed from well-founded theoretical traditions with established theories and principles of human behavior. Third, these approaches are highly flexible and can be implemented in a wide range of clinical modalities and settings. Moreover, they are compatible with a variety of pharmacotherapies and, in many cases, foster compliance and enhance the effects of pharmacotherapies including methadone, naltrexone, and disulfiram. Finally, these approaches are relatively brief/short-term and highly focused approaches that emphasize rapid, targeted change in substance use and related problems. Thus, CBT is highly compatible with a rapidly changing health care environment that is increasingly influenced by professional accountability (Humphreys and McLellan 2011).

Support for the work described in this chapter was provided by National Institute on Drug Abuse grants P50 DA09241, U10 DA15831, R01 DA 15969, and R01 DA 030369 and National Institute on Alcohol Abuse and Alcoholism grants R01 AA024122 and R21 AA 021405.

Theoretical Basis

Cognitive-behavioral treatments have their roots in classical behavioral theory and the pioneering work of Pavlov, Watson, Skinner, and Bandura (Craighead et al. 1995). First, Pavlov's work on classical conditioning demonstrated that a previously neutral stimulus could elicit a conditioned response after being paired repeatedly with an unconditioned stimulus. Furthermore, repeated exposure to the conditioned stimulus without the unconditioned stimulus would eventually lead to extinction of the conditioned response. Classical conditioning theory is the basis of several behavioral approaches to substance use treatment, particularly cue exposure approaches.

Second, Skinner's work on operant conditioning demonstrated that behaviors that are positively reinforced are likely to be exhibited more frequently. The field of behavioral pharmacology, which has convincingly demonstrated the reinforcing properties of abused substances in both humans and animals, is grounded in operant conditioning theory and principles. Behavior therapies assume that substance use and related behaviors are learned through their association with the positively reinforcing properties of the substances themselves as well as their secondary association with other environmental stimuli. CBT attempts to disrupt this learned association between drug-related cues or stimuli and drug craving or use by understanding and changing these behavior patterns.

Cognitive-behavioral therapies conceptualize substance use disorders as complex, multidetermined problems, with a number of influences playing a role in the development or perpetuation of the disorder (Marlatt and Donovan 2005). These influences may include family history and genetic factors; the presence of comorbid psychopathology; personality traits such as sensation seeking or impulsivity; and a host of environmental factors, including substance/drug availability and lack of countervailing influences and rewards. Although cognitive-behavioral therapies primarily emphasize the reinforcing properties of substances as central to the acquisition and maintenance of substance abuse and dependence, these etiological influences are seen as heightening risk or vulnerability to the development of substance use problems. For example, some individuals may find substances unusually highly rewarding secondary to genetic vulnerability, comorbid depression, high sensation seeking, and modeling of family and friends who use substances or environments devoid of alternative reinforcers.

Cognitive-behavioral treatments also reflect the pioneering work of Ellis and Beck that emphasized the importance of the person's thoughts and feelings as determinants of behavior (Meichenbaum 1995). CBT evolved in part from dissatisfaction with the extreme positions of radical behaviorism (e.g., emphasis on overt behaviors) and classical psychoanalysis (emphasis on unconscious conflicts or representations). CBT emphasizes how the individual perceives and interprets life events as important determinants of behavior (Meichenbaum 1995), as thoughts, feelings, and expectancies mediate an individual's response to the environment. CBT also seeks to help patients become aware of maladaptive cognitions and "teach them how to notice, catch, monitor, and interrupt the cognitive-affective-behavioral chains and to produce more adaptive coping responses" (Meichenbaum 1995, p. 147).

Empirical Support

Multiple meta-analyses and reviews have concluded that CBT is an effective treatment across a range of substance use disorders (Carroll and Onken 2005; Dutra et al. 2008; Irvin et al. 1999; Magill and Ray 2009). The most recent and comprehensive meta-analysis, which included 53 controlled trials published through 2006 of CBT for adults diagnosed with an alcohol or an illicit drug use disorder, found that CBT produced a small but statistically significant treatment effect (Hedges' $g=0.15$) over control conditions across studies (Magill and Ray 2009). Statistical transformations to a "success percentage" indicated that 58% of patients receiving CBT fared better than patients receiving the comparison condition (Magill and Ray 2009). Although the size of the overall treatment effect across studies was modest, there were some indications of differences according to primary drug of abuse. Specifically, the largest treatment effects were found in studies of marijuana use (moderate effect size, $g=0.51$), whereas smaller effect sizes were found across studies of alcohol, cocaine, stimulants, opiates, or polydrug use (ranging from $g=0.08$ to $g=0.13$). At the time of the meta-analysis, there were far fewer studies evaluating CBT for marijuana use compared with the number evaluating CBT for alcohol or other drug use, and many of these studies combined CBT with other psychosocial treatments to enhance effects (Magill and Ray 2009).

The evidence supporting CBT has been generated from single-site studies, as well as from some of the landmark multisite studies of addiction treatment, such as Project MATCH (Matching Alcoholism Treatments to Client Heterogeneity; Project MATCH Research Group 1997) and Project COMBINE (Combined Pharmacotherapies and Behavioral Interventions for Alcohol Dependence; Anton et al. 2006), the National Institute on Drug Abuse (NIDA) Cooperative Cocaine Treatment Study (Crits-Christoph et al. 1999), and the Marijuana Treatment Project (Babor and Marijuana Treatment Project Research Group 2004). One of the distinguishing features of CBT has been its relative durability of effects, with significant treatment effects persisting through a follow-up period, and in some cases with individuals showing greater improvement after treatment ends (i.e., a "sleeper effect") (e.g., Carroll et al. 1994, 2000; Rawson et al. 2002). CBT has also been shown to be effective in combination with pharmacotherapies for substance use (e.g., Carroll et al. 2004; Schmitz et al. 2001) and has been a widely used platform for pharmacotherapy trials—in other words, constituting the "base" treatment provided to all participants in an effort to enhance treatment retention and medication adherence, and to address other ancillary problems (Carroll 1997; Carroll et al. 2004).

CBT has been combined with other empirically supported treatments for alcohol and drug use disorders, such as motivational interviewing (MI) and contingency management (CM), as a strategy to bolster early treatment engagement and adherence. Several studies have investigated the combination of CBT and MI for various drugs of abuse, including amphetamines (Baker et al. 2005), cocaine (McKee et al. 2007; Rohsenow et al. 2004), methamphetamine (Bux and Irwin 2006), and marijuana (Babor and Marijuana Treatment Project Research Group 2004; Dennis et al. 2004). Although the findings have been mixed with respect to CBT's additive effects on drug use outcomes, there is some evidence to suggest that adding motivational enhancement therapy (MET) to the early stages of CBT can be effective in increasing motivation and improving retention in treatment. Also, given that CM has strong immediate effects on substance use that tend to weaken after the contingencies are terminated (Prendergast et al. 2006), while CBT tends to have more modest effects initially but is comparatively durable, there have been several investigations evaluating various combinations of CBT and CM. Results have largely indicated that CM is associated with better outcomes during the treatment period, but the combination of CM plus CBT may produce greater rates of abstinence during the follow-up period (e.g., Budney et al. 2006; Epstein et al. 2003; Kadden et al. 2007; Petitjean et al. 2014; Rawson et al. 2006).

In contrast to the ample evidence supporting CBT's efficacy, far less is known regarding the mechanisms by which it exerts its effects (Kazdin 2007). Because one of the primary elements of CBT is cognitive and behavioral skills training, most early studies of possible mechanisms of CBT focused on the improvement of these skills as a mediator of treatment effects. However, a seminal review by Morgenstern and Longabaugh (2000) concluded that there was little support for improvement in coping skills as a unique mechanism in CBT for alcohol use disorder. In the years since, promising evidence has emerged in support of acquisition of and improvement in cognitive and behavioral control skills, as well as self-efficacy, as mediators (and potential mechanisms) of CBT's effect on treatment outcomes. For example, improvement in the *quality* of individuals' coping skills following computerized CBT was found to mediate treatment effects on abstinence from drugs, satisfying all criteria in the causal chain (Kiluk et al. 2010). Also, increased self-efficacy has been found to mediate the relationship between drink refusal training (a specific ingredient of CBT) and drinking outcomes (Witkiewitz et al. 2012). However, consistent support for CBT's putative mechanisms of action remains elusive, as it does for many interventions (Emmelkamp et al. 2014).

In addition to skills training, another key component of CBT is emphasis on extrasession practice assignments (hereafter referred to as homework) as a means of facilitating the generalization and maintenance of adaptive behavioral and cognitive skills. The general body of research on homework has indicated a robust relationship between homework completion and positive treatment outcomes (Kazantzis et al. 2010). Although the amount of evidence supporting a homework–outcome relationship in CBT for substance use disorders is relatively sparse across various drugs of abuse, multiple reports have indicated that greater homework completion was associated with reduced drug use (Carroll et al. 2005; Decker et al. 2016; Gonzalez et al. 2006). Moreover, there is evidence to suggest that homework completion is not simply a proxy for motivation or treatment attendance (Decker et al. 2016). While more work in this area is needed, particularly in regard to predictors of homework completion, completion of homework in CBT clearly plays in important role in successful treatment outcomes.

Traditional CBT, including relapse prevention, has been the prevailing empirically based treatment approach for alcohol and drug use disorders for the past 30 years. However, variants of CBT (i.e., "third wave" behavioral therapies) have emerged more recently that focus on the context and function of internal events (e.g., thoughts, feelings, physical sensations) instead of focusing on the content as it relates to substance use. Thus, rather than conveying skills and strategies for changing the verbal content of thoughts, these newer variants of CBT manipulate the context in which such thoughts occur to change the function of these unwanted experiences (Stotts and Northrup 2015). For instance, "contextual CBTs" such as Mindfulness Based Relapse Prevention (MBRP; Bowen et al. 2009), Dialectical Behavior Therapy (DBT; Linehan 1993), and Acceptance and Commitment Therapy (ACT; Hayes et al. 2006) place an emphasis on mindfulness and acceptance strategies to reduce the impact of unpleasant internal triggers on an individual's behavior. Although evidence supporting the efficacy of these approaches for treating alcohol and drug use is still emerging (for reviews, see Dimeff and Linehan 2008; Lee et al. 2015; Li et al. 2017), they do appear to be promising enhancements to traditional CBT (McHugh et al. 2010).

CBT Techniques and Strategies

Specific techniques vary widely depending on the type of cognitive-behavioral treatment used, and there are a variety of manuals, protocols, and training programs available that describe the techniques associated with each approach (Carroll 1998; Monti et al. 1989). Very simply put, however, most CBT approaches attempt to help patients to recognize the situations in which they are most likely to use drugs or alcohol, to avoid those situations when appropriate, and to cope more effectively with a range of problems and problematic behaviors associated with substance use by implementing a range of cognitive and behavioral coping strategies.

Defining Features of CBT

Two key defining features of most cognitive-behavioral approaches to substance use disorders are 1) emphasis on functional analysis of drug use (i.e., attempting to understand drug use with respect to its antecedents and consequences), and 2) emphasis on teaching and implementation of cognitive and behavioral control skills. Cognitive-behavioral approaches include a range of skills for fostering or maintaining abstinence. These typically include strategies for the following:

1. Understanding the patterns that maintain drug use and developing strategies for changing these patterns. This often involves self-monitoring of thoughts and behaviors that take place before, during, and after high-risk situations or episodes of drug use.
2. Fostering the resolution to stop substance use through exploring positive and negative consequences of continued use (also known as the decisional balance technique).
3. Understanding craving and craving cues and developing skills for coping with craving when it occurs. These include a variety of affect regulation strategies (distraction, talking through a craving, "urge surfing," and so on).
4. Recognizing and challenging the cognitions that accompany and maintain patterns of substance use.

5. Increasing self-awareness of the consequences of even small decisions (e.g., which route to take home from work) and identifying "seemingly irrelevant" decisions that can culminate in high-risk situations.
6. Developing problem-solving skills and practicing application of those skills to substance-related and more general problems.
7. Planning for emergencies and unexpected problems and situations that can lead to high-risk situations.
8. Developing skills for assertively refusing offers of drugs as well as for reducing exposure to drugs and drug-related cues.

These basic skills are useful in their application to helping patients control and stop substance use, but it is essential that therapists also point out how these same skills can be applied to a range of other problems. Examples of acquired skills that can be generalized include the following (as illustrated in Table 23–1):

- A functional analysis can be used to understand the determinants of a wide range of behavior patterns.
- Skills used to cope with craving can easily be applied to other aspects of affect control.
- Principles used in the sessions on seemingly irrelevant decisions can easily be adapted to shed light on a wide range of behavioral chains.
- Substance use refusal skills can easily be transferred to more effective and assertive responding in a number of situations.

When therapists are teaching coping skills, it is essential that they emphasize and demonstrate that these skills not only can be immediately applied to control substance use, but also can be extended into general strategies that can be applied to a wide range of situations and problems the patient may encounter in the future.

Broad-spectrum cognitive-behavioral approaches, such as those described by Monti et al. (1989), expand to include interventions targeted toward other problems in the individual's life that are seen as functionally related to substance use. These interventions may include general problem-solving skills, assertiveness training, strategies for coping with negative affects, awareness of anger and anger management, coping with criticism, increasing pleasant activities, enhancing social support networks, and job-seeking skills, among others. In comparison with many other behavioral approaches, CBT is typically highly structured—that is, CBT sessions are generally brief and organized closely around well-specified treatment goals. Each session usually has an articulated agenda, and the clinical discussion remains focused around issues directly related to substance use. Progress toward treatment goals is monitored closely and frequently, with frequent monitoring of substance use through urine toxicology screens, and the therapist takes an active stance throughout treatment. Sessions generally take place within a weekly scheduled therapy "hour." In broad-spectrum cognitive-behavioral approaches, sessions are often organized roughly into thirds (the 20/20/20 rule), with the first third of the session devoted to assessment of the patient's substance use and general functioning in the past week and reporting of current concerns and problems, the second third being more didactic and focusing on skills training and practice; and the final third allowing time for the

TABLE 23–1. Common CBT topics and areas for generalizability	
CBT topic for substance use disorders	Construct taught
Functional analysis	Pattern recognition, "recognize, avoid, cope," temporizing behavior
Coping with craving	Affect and distress tolerance
Refusal skills	Assertiveness, persistence under stress, effective interpersonal behavior, impulse control
Recognizing and coping with thoughts	Cognitive flexibility, cognitive modification
"Seemingly irrelevant" decisions	Decision making, delay discounting
Problem solving	Problem solving, planful behavior
HIV/HCV risk reduction	Generalizability of CBT skills to other areas of behavior

Note. CBT=cognitive-behavioral therapy; HCV=hepatitis C virus.

therapist and the patient to plan for the week ahead and to discuss how the new skills will be implemented (Carroll 1998). The therapeutic relationship is seen as principally collaborative; thus, the role of the therapist is that of consultant, educator, and guide who leads the patient through a functional analysis of his or her substance use, assists in identifying and prioritizing target behaviors, and provides advice and counsel in selecting and implementing strategies to foster the desired behavioral changes. Although CBT is structured and didactic, it is a highly individualized and flexible treatment. That is, rather than viewing CBT treatment as cookbook "psychoeducation," the therapist carefully matches the content, timing, and nature of the presentation of the material to the individual patient. The therapist attempts to provide skills training at the moments the patient is most in need of them. That is, the therapist does not belabor topics such as breaking ties with drug suppliers with a patient who is highly motivated and has been abstinent for several weeks. Similarly, the therapist does not race through material in an attempt to "cover" all of it in a few weeks; for some patients, it may take several weeks to master a basic skill.

Training and Competence in CBT

The growing evidence base for CBT and the increased emphasis on incorporating empirically supported therapies into clinical practice have led to a greater focus on training and dissemination. Although standard methods used to train clinicians to use CBT in clinical efficacy trials have generally been associated with high levels of treatment fidelity and comparatively small levels of variation in treatment delivery, these methods—intensive didactic workshop training plus structured feedback on supervised training cases—have not been commonly used to train clinicians to implement empirically evaluated treatments (Olmstead et al. 2012; Weissman et al. 2006).

To address this issue, a series of studies evaluated the efficacy of clinical training methods by randomly assigning community-based (primarily master's level) clinicians to different training conditions. In a trial evaluating training methods for CBT

(Sholomskas et al. 2005), 78 clinicians were assigned to one of three training conditions: 1) review of the NIDA CBT manual only (Carroll 1998); 2) access to a web-based training site (which included additional frequently asked questions, role-plays, and practice exercises) plus the manual; or 3) a 3-day didactic seminar plus up to three sessions of supervision from a CBT expert trainer based on actual session tapes submitted by the participants plus the manual. Outcomes focused on clinician behavior and included 1) between-group comparisons of the clinicians' ability to demonstrate key CBT techniques based on structured role-plays administered before and after training, and 2) scores on a CBT knowledge quiz. The videotaped role-plays were scored by independent raters who were blind to the participants' training condition as well as to the timing of role-play administration (i.e., pre- vs. posttraining). Scoring was based on adherence/competence ratings of specific CBT techniques from the CBT subscale of the well-validated Yale Adherence and Competence Scale (YACS) (Carroll et al. 2000). Although all groups demonstrated improved adherence and competence scores over time, the only training condition that reached levels of skill consistent with those required of clinicians participating in our CBT efficacy trials was the Manual plus Training plus Supervision condition, with intermediate ratings for the Manual plus Web (Sholomskas et al. 2005). In addition, as shown in Figure 23–1, in comparison with clinicians assigned to the Manual-only condition, a significantly greater percentage of the clinicians assigned to the Manual plus Training plus Supervision condition reached criterion levels for adequate fidelity (54% vs. 15%) (Sholomskas et al. 2005). These findings illustrate that *merely making manuals available to clinicians has little enduring effect on their ability to implement new treatments.* This conclusion has important implications for current efforts to disseminate new treatments: face-to-face training followed by direct supervision and credentialing may be essential for effective implementation of empirically validated therapies.

Looking Ahead: Disseminating CBT Via Technology

A major barrier to effective dissemination of CBT is the lack of a system for training, supervision, and feedback. Although ongoing monitoring and demonstration of clinician skill in delivering treatment and maintaining fidelity to manual guidelines is a methodological requirement for clinical trials evaluating behavioral therapies (Chambless and Hollon 1998; Luborsky and DeRubeis 1984; Rounsaville et al. 2001), systematic monitoring of and feedback on clinicians' implementations of evidence-based therapies is rare in clinical practice (Henggeler et al. 2002; Hoffman and McCarty 2013; Knudsen et al. 2008; Martino et al. 2016; Roche et al. 2007; Sholomskas et al. 2005). Multiple trials evaluating different methods of training clinicians to use evidence-based therapies have demonstrated that monitoring and supervision are significantly more effective than workshop-based training alone for a range of therapies (Beidnas and Kendall 2010; Henggeler et al. 2013; Miller et al. 2004; Schoenwald et al. 2009), including CBT (Rakovshik et al. 2013, 2016; Sholomskas et al. 2005). The lack of supervision and monitoring of clinician implementation of evidence-based treatments in clinical practice suggests that CBT and other evidence-based interventions as typically delivered in clinical practice may bear little resemblance to the more

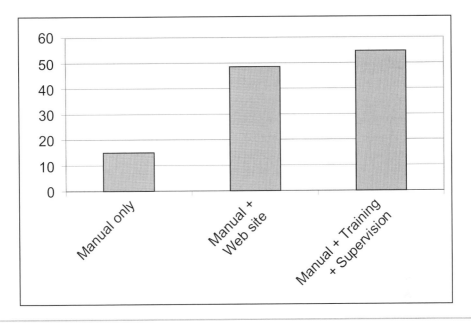

FIGURE 23–1.   Percentage of clinicians trained to certification criterion level.

Note.   See text for description.

Source.   Adapted from Sholomskas DE, Syracuse-Siewert G, Rounsaville BJ, et al.: "We Don't Train in Vain: A Dissemination Trial of Three Strategies of Training Clinicians in Cognitive-Behavioral Therapy." *Journal of Consulting and Clinical Psychology* 73(1):106–115, 2005. Copyright © 2005, American Psychological Association. Used with permission.

closely monitored versions of those treatments implemented in randomized clinical trials demonstrating their efficacy (Martino et al. 2016).

Rapid advancements in the sophistication, speed, and reach of technology have opened up multiple new possibilities for disseminating evidence-based therapies (Bickel et al. 2011; Copeland 2011; Emmelkamp et al. 2014; Gustafson et al. 2011; Kazdin and Blase 2011; Marks et al. 2007; Marsch and Gustafson 2013; Marsch et al. 2014), including cognitive-behavioral therapies. Platforms for delivering addiction interventions via technology are diverse and multiplying rapidly. These include electronic screening and brief interventions (eSBIs) (Carey et al. 2009; Copeland and Martin 2004; Fachini et al. 2012; Gryczynski et al. 2015; Ondersma et al. 2007); web-based multimodule programs and smartphone apps, with and without clinician involvement (Bickel et al. 2008; Gustafson et al. 2014; Suffoletto et al. 2015); treatment delivered "live" via Skype, telephone, or instant messaging (McKay et al. 2004, 2005, 2010, 2011); monitoring via interactive voice response (IVR) and Ecological Momentary Assessment (EMA) and Ecological Momentary Treatment (EMT) platforms (Moore et al. 2013; Morgenstern et al. 2014); and others (Muench 2014). Overall, results from meta-analyses of such interventions are promising (Boumparis et al. 2017; Carey et al. 2009; Riper et al. 2014; Rooke et al. 2010; Tait et al. 2013), but the methodological quality of studies within this young field is variable and often weak (Kiluk et al. 2011).

Our group has developed a computer-assisted version of CBT, called CBT4CBT (computer-based training in cognitive-behavioral therapy). The content of CBT4CBT is based closely on the NIDA CBT manual (Carroll 1998) but is delivered in seven sessions, or modules, and makes extensive use of the multimedia capabilities of computers to convey CBT principles and to illustrate implementation of new cognitive and behavioral strategies (Carroll et al. 2008). Key CBT concepts are taught through short movies, or vignettes, that feature engaging characters in realistic settings confronting a number of challenging situations, as well as a number of interactive games and exercises. Thus, rather than having only the option of listening to their therapists' descriptions (which can sometimes be incomplete or overly abstract), CBT4CBT users are able to view multiple examples of CBT principles being enacted in real-life scenarios (more information is available at CBT4CBT.com).

Seven randomized clinical trials of CBT4CBT have been published in the peer-reviewed literature, all demonstrating its efficacy, durability, and cost-effectiveness relative to a variety of comparison conditions. The earliest trials evaluated CBT4CBT as an add-on to standard outpatient treatment (Carroll et al. 2009) or methadone maintenance (Carroll et al. 2014, 2018). In these studies, CBT4CBT consistently demonstrated significant benefits on reductions in substance use over standard treatment; moreover, these studies demonstrated that CBT4CBT retains key features of clinician-delivered CBT, including the sleeper effect, with durability of effects extending over at least 6 months of follow-up (Carroll et al. 2009, 2014), as well as the ability to convey the targeted skills (Kiluk et al. 2010, 2017). More recent trials with CBT4CBT as a virtual stand-alone treatment (i.e., a 10-minute weekly check-in with a clinician to assess clinical status and use of the program) have demonstrated that CBT4CBT is not only safe, but also significantly more effective than standard outpatient treatment (e.g., weekly group or individual counseling) for individuals with alcohol use disorder (Kiluk et al. 2016) and mixed substance use disorders (Kiluk et al. 2018b).

A culturally adapted version for Spanish-speaking substance users was also recently validated as an add-on to standard care for this important population that often does not have access to evidence-based therapies (Paris et al. 2018). In this study, there was a high proportion of individuals with severe mental illness as well as substance use disorder; the efficacy of CBT4CBT was retained among those with severe mental illness in this sample, underscoring that CBT4CBT may be used in a wide variety of populations. Most recently, a version adapted specifically for individuals enrolled in office-based buprenorphine treatment for opioid use disorder was evaluated, with highly promising results (Shi et al. 2019). A summary of these studies and the evidence supporting CBT4CBT is provided in Table 23–2.

Conclusion

CBT is a behavioral approach that has strong theoretical and empirical support with a variety of substance-abusing populations. In recent years, clinical researchers have urged that CBT approaches be moved more broadly into the clinical community, with the result that a range of practical resources (e.g., books, videotapes, manuals, training resources and programs), as well as web-based versions for ensuring effective implementation in clinical practice, have become available. Moreover, these approaches can be effectively combined and integrated with a variety of other empirically supported behavioral therapies as well as pharmacotherapies. Thus, CBT should be a component of all substance abuse clinicians' repertoire.

TABLE 23–2. Summary of evidence base for **CBT4CBT, 2019**

Version	Safety, efficacy as add-on to standard care	Safety, efficacy as stand-alone	Clinically significant outcome	Demonstration that targeted skills were acquired	Durable effects through 6-month follow-up
Drugs (Carroll et al. 2008, 2009, 2014; Kiluk et al. 2010, 2018b)	X	X	X (DSM symptom count reduction)	X	X
Alcohol (Kiluk et al. 2016, 2018a)	X	X	X (DSM symptom count reduction)	X	X
Spanish (Paris et al. 2018)	X		X (DSM symptom count reduction)	X	X
Buprenorphine (Shi et al. 2019)		X (pilot)	X		

References

Anton RF, O'Malley SS, Ciraulo DA, et al: Combined pharmacotherapies and behavioral interventions for alcohol dependence: the COMBINE Study. JAMA 295(17):2003–2017, 2006 16670409

Babor TF, Marijuana Treatment Project Research Group: Brief treatments for cannabis dependence: findings from a randomized multisite trial. J Consult Clin Psychol 72(3):455–466, 2004 15279529

Baker A, Lee NK, Claire M, et al: Brief cognitive behavioural interventions for regular amphetamine users: a step in the right direction. Addiction 100(3):367–378, 2005 15733250

Beidnas RS, Kendall PC: Training therapists in evidence-based practice: a critical review of studies from a systems-contextual perspective. Clin Psychol (New York) 17(1):1–30, 2010 20877441

Bickel WK, Marsch LA, Marsch LA, et al: Computerized behavior therapy for opioid-dependent outpatients: a randomized controlled trial. Exp Clin Psychopharmacol 16(2):132–143, 2008 18489017

Bickel WK, Christensen DR, Marsch LA: A review of computer-based interventions used in the assessment, treatment, and research of drug addiction. Subst Use Misuse 46(1):4–9, 2011 21190401

Boumparis N, Karyotaki E, Schaub MP, et al: Internet interventions for adult illicit substance users: a meta-analysis. Addiction 112(9):1521–1532, 2017 28295758

Bowen S, Chawla N, Collins SE, et al: Mindfulness-based relapse prevention for substance use disorders: a pilot efficacy trial. Subst Abus 30(4):295–305, 2009 19904665

Budney AJ, Moore BA, Rocha HL, et al: Clinical trial of abstinence-based vouchers and cognitive-behavioral therapy for cannabis dependence. J Consult Clin Psychol 74(2):307–316, 2006 16649875

Bux DA Jr, Irwin TW: Combining motivational interviewing and cognitive-behavioral skills training for the treatment of crystal methamphetamine abuse/dependence. Journal of Gay & Lesbian Psychotherapy 10(3–4):143–152, 2006. Available at: https://www.tandfonline.com/doi/abs/10.1300/J236v10n03_13. Accessed December 21, 2019.

Carey KB, Scott-Sheldon LA, Elliott JC, et al: Computer-delivered interventions to reduce college student drinking: a meta-analysis. Addiction 104(11):1807–1819, 2009 19744139

Carroll KM: Manual-guided psychosocial treatment. A new virtual requirement for pharmacotherapy trials? Arch Gen Psychiatry 54(10):923–928, 1997 9337772

Carroll KM: A Cognitive-Behavioral Approach: Treating Cocaine Addiction. National Institute on Drug Abuse, April 1998. Available at: https://archives.drugabuse.gov/sites/default/files/cbt.pdf. Accessed November 30, 2019.

Carroll KM, Onken LS: Behavioral therapies for drug abuse. Am J Psychiatry 162(8):1452–1460, 2005 16055766

Carroll KM, Rounsaville BJ, Nich C, et al: One-year follow-up of psychotherapy and pharmacotherapy for cocaine dependence. Delayed emergence of psychotherapy effects. Arch Gen Psychiatry 51(12):989–997, 1994 7979888

Carroll KM, Nich C, Sifry RL, et al: A general system for evaluating therapist adherence and competence in psychotherapy research in the addictions. Drug Alcohol Depend 57(3):225–238, 2000 10661673

Carroll KM, Fenton LR, Ball SA, et al: Efficacy of disulfiram and cognitive behavior therapy in cocaine-dependent outpatients: a randomized placebo-controlled trial. Arch Gen Psychiatry 61(3):264–272, 2004 14993114

Carroll KM, Nich C, Ball SA: Practice makes progress? Homework assignments and outcome in treatment of cocaine dependence. J Consult Clin Psychol 73(4):749–755, 2005 16173864

Carroll KM, Ball SA, Martino S, et al: Computer-assisted delivery of cognitive-behavioral therapy for addiction: a randomized trial of CBT4CBT. Am J Psychiatry 165(7):881–888, 2008 18450927

Carroll KM, Ball SA, Martino S, et al: Enduring effects of a computer-assisted training program for cognitive behavioral therapy: a 6-month follow-up of CBT4CBT. Drug Alcohol Depend 100(1–2):178–181, 2009 19041197

Carroll KM, Kiluk BD, Nich C, et al: Computer-assisted delivery of cognitive-behavioral therapy: efficacy and durability of CBT4CBT among cocaine-dependent individuals maintained on methadone. Am J Psychiatry 171(4):436–444, 2014 24577287

Carroll KM, Nich C, DeVito EE, et al: Galantamine and computerized cognitive behavioral therapy for cocaine dependence: a randomized clinical trial. J Clin Psychiatry 79(1):17m11669, 2018 29286595

Chambless DL, Hollon SD: Defining empirically supported therapies. J Consult Clin Psychol 66(1):7–18, 1998 9489259

Copeland J: Application of technology in the prevention and treatment of substance use disorders and related problems: opportunities and challenges. Subst Use Misuse 46(1):112–113, 2011 21190411

Copeland J, Martin G: Web-based interventions for substance use disorders: a qualitative review. J Subst Abuse Treat 26:109–116, 2004 15050088

Craighead WE, Craighead LW, Ilardi SS: Behavioral therapies in historical perspective, in Comprehensive Textbook of Psychotherapy: Theory and Practice. Edited by Bongar BM, Beutler LE. New York, Oxford University Press, 1995, pp 64–83

Crits-Christoph P, Siqueland L, Blaine J, et al: Psychosocial treatments for cocaine dependence: National Institute on Drug Abuse Collaborative Cocaine Treatment Study. Arch Gen Psychiatry 56(6):493–502, 1999 10359461

Decker SE, Kiluk BD, Frankforter T, et al: Just showing up is not enough: homework adherence and outcome in cognitive-behavioral therapy for cocaine dependence. J Consult Clin Psychol 84(10):907–912, 2016 27454780

Dennis M, Godley SH, Diamond G, et al: The Cannabis Youth Treatment (CYT) study: main findings from two randomized trials. J Subst Abuse Treat 27(3):197–213, 2004 15501373

Dimeff LA, Linehan MM: Dialectical behavior therapy for substance abusers. Addict Sci Clin Pract 4(2):39–47, 2008 18497717

Dutra L, Stathopoulou G, Basden SL, et al: A meta-analytic review of psychosocial interventions for substance use disorders. Am J Psychiatry 165(2):179–187, 2008 18198270

Emmelkamp PM, David D, Beckers T, et al: Advancing psychotherapy and evidence-based psychological interventions. Int J Methods Psychiatr Res 23 (suppl 1):58–91, 2014 24375536

Epstein DE, Hawkins WE, Covi L, et al: Cognitive behavioral therapy plus contingency management for cocaine use: findings during treatment and across 12-month follow-up. Psychol Addict Behav 17(1):73–82, 2003 12665084

Fachini A, Aliane PP, Martinez EZ, et al: Efficacy of brief alcohol screening intervention for college students (BASICS): a meta-analysis of randomized controlled trials. Subst Abuse Treat Prev Policy 7:40, 2012 22967716

Gonzalez VM, Schmitz JM, DeLaune KA: The role of homework in cognitive-behavioral therapy for cocaine dependence. J Consult Clin Psychol 74(3):633–637, 2006 16822120

Gryczynski J, Mitchell SG, Gonzales A, et al: A randomized trial of computerized vs. in-person brief intervention for illicit drug use in primary care: outcomes through 12 months. J Subst Abuse Treat 50:3–10, 2015 25282578

Gustafson DH, Shaw BR, Isham A, et al: Explicating an evidence-based, theoretically informed, mobile technology-based system to improve outcomes for people in recovery for alcohol dependence. Subst Use Misuse 46(1):96–111, 2011 21190410

Gustafson DH, McTavish FM, Chih MY, et al: A smartphone application to support recovery from alcoholism: a randomized clinical trial. JAMA Psychiatry 71(5):566–572, 2014 24671165

Hayes SC, Luoma JB, Bond FW, et al: Acceptance and commitment therapy: model, processes and outcomes. Behav Res Ther 44(1):1–25, 2006 16300724

Henggeler SW, Schoenwald SK, Liao JG, et al: Transporting efficacious treatments to field settings: the link between supervisory practices and therapist fidelity in MST programs. J Clin Child Adolesc Psychol 31(2):155–167, 2002 12056100

Henggeler SW, Chapman JE, Rowland MD, et al: Evaluating training methods for transporting contingency management to therapists. J Subst Abuse Treat 45(5):466–474, 2013 23910392

Hoffman KA, McCarty D: Improving the quality of addiction treatment, in Interventions for Addiction: Comprehensive Addictive Behaviors and Disorders, Vol. 3. Edited by Miller PM. San Diego, CA, Academic Press, 2013, pp 579–588

Humphreys K, McLellan AT: A policy-oriented review of strategies for improving the outcomes of services for substance use disorder patients. Addiction 106(12):2058–2066, 2011 21631620

Irvin JE, Bowers CA, Dunn ME, et al: Efficacy of relapse prevention: a meta-analytic review. J Consult Clin Psychol 67(4):563–570, 1999 10450627

Kadden RM, Litt MD, Kabela-Cormier E, et al: Abstinence rates following behavioral treatments for marijuana dependence. Addict Behav 32(6):1220–1236, 2007 16996224

Kazantzis N, Whittington C, Dattilio F: Meta-analysis of homework effects in cognitive and behavioral therapy: a replication and extension. Clinical Psychology: Science and Practice 17(2):144–156, 2010. Available at: https://onlinelibrary.wiley.com/doi/abs/10.1111/j.1468-2850.2010.01204.x. Accessed December 21, 2019.

Kazdin AE: Mediators and mechanisms of change in psychotherapy research. Annu Rev Clin Psychol 3(1):1–27, 2007 17716046

Kazdin AE, Blase SL: Rebooting psychotherapy research and practice to reduce the burden of mental illness. Perspect Psychol Sci 6(1):21–37, 2011 26162113

Kiluk BD, Nich C, Babuscio T, et al: Quality versus quantity: acquisition of coping skills following computerized cognitive-behavioral therapy for substance use disorders. Addiction 105(12):2120–2127, 2010 20854334

Kiluk BD, Sugarman DE, Nich C, et al: A methodological analysis of randomized clinical trials of computer-assisted therapies for psychiatric disorders: toward improved standards for an emerging field. Am J Psychiatry 168(8):790–799, 2011 21536689

Kiluk BD, Devore KA, Buck MB, et al: Randomized trial of computerized cognitive behavioral therapy for alcohol use disorders: efficacy as a virtual stand-alone and treatment add-on compared with standard outpatient treatment. Alcohol Clin Exp Res 40(9):1991–2000, 2016 27488212

Kiluk BD, DeVito EE, Buck MB, et al: Effect of computerized cognitive behavioral therapy on acquisition of coping skills among cocaine-dependent individuals enrolled in methadone maintenance. J Subst Abuse Treat 82:87–92, 2017 29021121

Kiluk BD, Frankforter TL, Cusumano M, et al: Change in DSM-5 alcohol use disorder criteria count and severity level as a treatment outcome indicator: results from a randomized trial. Alcohol Clin Exp Res 42(8):1556–1563, 2018a 29870051

Kiluk BD, Nich C, Buck MB, et al: Randomized clinical trial of computerized and clinician-delivered CBT in comparison with standard outpatient treatment for substance use disorders: primary within-treatment and follow-up outcomes. Am J Psychiatry 175(9):853–863, 2018b 29792052

Knudsen HK, Ducharme LJ, Roman PM: Clinical supervision, emotional exhaustion, and turnover intention: a study of substance abuse treatment counselors in the Clinical Trials Network of the National Institute on Drug Abuse. J Subst Abuse Treat 35(4):387–395, 2008 18424048

Lee EB, An W, Levin ME, et al: An initial meta-analysis of acceptance and commitment therapy for treating substance use disorders. Drug Alcohol Depend 155:1–7, 2015 26298552

Li W, Howard MO, Garland EL, et al: Mindfulness treatment for substance misuse: a systematic review and meta-analysis. J Subst Abuse Treat 75:62–96, 2017 28153483

Linehan MM: Cognitive-Behavioral Treatment of Borderline Personality Disorder. New York, Guilford, 1993

Luborsky L, DeRubeis RJ: The use of psychotherapy treatment manuals: a small revolution in psychotherapy research style. Clinical Psychology Review 4(1):5–14, 1984. Available at: https://www.sciencedirect.com/science/article/pii/0272735884900345?via%3Dihub. Accessed December 21, 2019.

Magill M, Ray LA: Cognitive-behavioral treatment with adult alcohol and illicit drug users: a meta-analysis of randomized controlled trials. J Stud Alcohol Drugs 70:516–527, 2009 19515291

Marks IM, Cavanagh K, Gega L: Hands-On Help: Computer-Aided Psychotherapy (Maudsley Monograph 49). Hove, UK, Psychology Press, 2007

Marlatt GA, Donovan D: Relapse Prevention: Maintenance Strategies in the Treatment of Addictions, 2nd Edition. New York, Guilford, 2005

Marsch LA, Gustafson DH: The role of technology in health care innovation: a commentary. J Dual Diagn 9(1):101–103, 2013 23599690

Marsch LA, Carroll KM, Kiluk BD: Technology-based interventions for the treatment and recovery management of substance use disorders: a JSAT special issue. J Subst Abuse Treat 46(1):1–4, 2014 24041749

Martino S, Paris M Jr, Anez L, et al: The effectiveness and cost of clinical supervision for motivational interviewing: a randomized controlled trial. J Subst Abuse Treat 68:11–23, 2016 27431042

McHugh RK, Hearon BA, Otto MW: Cognitive behavioral therapy for substance use disorders. Psychiatr Clin North Am 33(3):511–525, 2010 20599130

McKay JR, Lynch KG, Shepard DS, et al: The effectiveness of telephone-based continuing care in the clinical management of alcohol and cocaine use disorders: 12-month outcomes. J Consult Clin Psychol 72(6):967–979, 2004 15612844

McKay JR, Lynch KG, Shepard DS, et al: The effectiveness of telephone-based continuing care for alcohol and cocaine dependence: 24-month outcomes. Arch Gen Psychiatry 62(2):199–207, 2005 15699297

McKay JR, Van Horn DH, Oslin DW, et al: A randomized trial of extended telephone-based continuing care for alcohol dependence: within-treatment substance use outcomes. J Consult Clin Psychol 78(6):912–923, 2010 20873894

McKay JR, Van Horn DH, Oslin DW, et al: Extended telephone-based continuing care for alcohol dependence: 24-month outcomes and subgroup analyses. Addiction 106(10):1760–1769, 2011 21545667

McKee SA, Carroll KM, Sinha R, et al: Enhancing brief cognitive-behavioral therapy with motivational enhancement techniques in cocaine users. Drug Alcohol Depend 91(1):97–101, 2007 17573205

Meichenbaum DH: Cognitive-behavioral therapy in historical perspective, in Comprehensive Textbook of Psychotherapy: Theory and Practice. Edited by Bongar BM, Beutler LE. New York, Oxford University Press, 1995, pp 140–158

Miller WR, Yahne CE, Moyers TB, et al: A randomized trial of methods to help clinicians learn motivation interviewing. J Consult Clin Psychol 72(6):1050–1062, 2004 15612851

Monti PM, Rohsenow DJ, Abrams DB, et al: Treating Alcohol Dependence: A Coping Skills Training Guide in the Treatment of Alcoholism. New York, Guilford, 1989

Moore BA, Fazzino T, Barry DT, et al: The recovery line: a pilot trial of automated, telephone-based treatment for continued drug use in methadone maintenance. J Subst Abuse Treat 45(1):63–69, 2013 23375114

Morgenstern J, Longabaugh R: Cognitive-behavioral treatment for alcohol dependence: a review of the evidence for its hypothesized mechanisms of action. Addiction 95(10):1475–1490, 2000 11070524

Morgenstern J, Kuerbis A, Muench F: Ecological momentary assessment and alcohol use disorder treatment. Alcohol Res 36(1):101–109, 2014 26259004

Muench F: The promises and pitfalls of digital technology in its application to alcohol treatment. Alcohol Res 36(1):131–142, 2014 26259008

Olmstead TA, Abraham AJ, Martino S, et al: Counselor training in several evidence-based psychosocial addiction treatments in private US substance abuse treatment centers. Drug Alcohol Depend 120(1–3):149–154, 2012 21831536

Ondersma SJ, Svikis DS, Schuster CR: Computer-based brief intervention: a randomized trial with postpartum women. Am J Prev Med 32(3):231–238, 2007 17236741

Paris M, Silva M, Anez-Nava L, et al: Culturally adapted, web-based cognitive behavioral therapy for Spanish-speaking individuals with substance use disorders: a randomized clinical trial. Am J Public Health 108(11):1535–1542, 2018 30252519

Petitjean SA, Dursteler-MacFarland KM, Krokar MC, et al: A randomized, controlled trial of combined cognitive-behavioral therapy plus prize-based contingency management for cocaine dependence. Drug Alcohol Depend 145:94–100, 2014 25456571

Prendergast M, Podus D, Finney JW, et al: Contingency management for treatment of substance use disorders: a meta-analysis. Addiction 101(11):1546–1560, 2006 17034434

Project MATCH Research Group: Matching alcohol treatments to client heterogeneity: Project MATCH posttreatment drinking outcomes. J Stud Alcohol 58(3):7–29, 1997 8979210

Rakovshik SG, McManus F, Westbrook D, et al: Randomized trial comparing Internet-based training in cognitive behavioural therapy theory, assessment and formulation to delayed-training control. Behav Res Ther 51(6):231–239, 2013 23500894

Rakovshik SG, McManus F, Vazquez-Montes M, et al: Is supervision necessary? Examining the effects of Internet-based CBT training with and without supervision. J Consult Clin Psychol 84(3):191–199, 2016 26795937

Rawson RA, Huber A, McCann M, et al: A comparison of contingency management and cognitive-behavioral approaches during methadone maintenance treatment for cocaine dependence. Arch Gen Psychiatry 59(9):817–824, 2002 12215081

Rawson RA, McCann MJ, Flammino F, et al: A comparison of contingency management and cognitive-behavioral approaches for stimulant-dependent individuals. Addiction 101(2):267–274, 2006 16445555

Riper H, Blankers M, Hadiwijaya H, et al: Effectiveness of guided and unguided low-intensity Internet interventions for adult alcohol misuse: a meta-analysis. PLoS One 9(6):e99912, 2014 24937483

Roche AM, Todd CL, O'Connor J: Clinical supervision in the alcohol and other drugs field: an imperative or an option? Drug Alcohol Rev 26(3):241–249, 2007 17454013

Rohsenow DJ, Monti PM, Martin RA, et al: Motivational enhancement and coping skills training for cocaine abusers: effects on substance use outcomes. Addiction 99(7):862–874, 2004 15200582

Rooke S, Thorsteinsson E, Karpin A, et al: Computer-delivered interventions for alcohol and tobacco use: a meta-analysis. Addiction 105(8):1381–1390, 2010 20528806

Rounsaville BJ, Carroll KM, Onken LS: A stage model of behavioral therapies research: getting started and moving on from stage I. Clinical Psychology: Science and Practice 8:133–142, 2001. Available at: https://onlinelibrary.wiley.com/doi/abs/10.1093/clipsy.8.2.133. Accessed December 21, 2019.

Schmitz JM, Stotts AL, Rhoades HM, et al: Naltrexone and relapse prevention for cocaine-dependent patients. Addict Behav 26(2):167–180, 2001 11316375

Schoenwald SK, Sheidow AJ, Chapman JE: Clinical supervision in treatment transport: effects on adherence and outcomes. J Consult Clin Psychol 77(3):410–421, 2009 19485583

Shi JM, Henry SP, Dwy SL, et al: Randomized pilot trial of Web-based cognitive-behavioral therapy adapted for use in office-based buprenorphine maintenance. Subst Abus 40(2):132–135, 2019 30714880

Sholomskas DE, Syracuse-Siewert G, Rounsaville BJ, et al: We don't train in vain: a dissemination trial of three strategies of training clinicians in cognitive-behavioral therapy. J Consult Clin Psychol 73(1):106–115, 2005 15709837

Stotts AL, Northrup TF: The promise of third-wave behavioral therapies in the treatment of substance use disorders. Curr Opin Psychol 2:75–81, 2015 26693170

Suffoletto B, Kristan J, Chung T, et al: An interactive text message intervention to reduce binge drinking in young adults: a randomized controlled trial with 9-month outcomes. PLoS One 10(11):e0142877, 2015 26580802

Tait RJ, Spijkerman R, Riper H: Internet and computer-based interventions for cannabis use: a meta-analysis. Drug Alcohol Depend 133(2):295–304, 2013 23747236

Weissman MM, Verdeli H, Gameroff MJ, et al: National survey of psychotherapy training in psychiatry, psychology, and social work. Arch Gen Psychiatry 63(8):925–934, 2006 16894069

Witkiewitz K, Donovan DM, Hartzler B: Drink refusal training as part of a combined behavioral intervention: effectiveness and mechanisms of change. J Consult Clin Psychol 80(3):440–449, 2012 22289131

Recommended Readings

Carroll KM, Kiluk BD: Cognitive behavioral interventions for alcohol and drug use disorders: through the stage model and back again. Psychol Addict Behav 31(8):847–861, 2017 28857574

Carroll KM, Rounsaville BJ: A vision of the next generation of behavioral therapies research in the addictions. Addiction 102(6):850–862, 2007 17523974

Kazantzis N, Deane FP, Ronan KR, et al (eds): Using Homework Assignments in Cognitive Behavior Therapy. New York, Routledge Taylor & Francis, 2005

Marlatt GA, Donovan D: Relapse Prevention: Maintenance Strategies in the Treatment of Addictions, 2nd Edition. New York, Guilford, 2005

Miller WR, Carroll KM (eds): Rethinking Substance Abuse: What the Science Shows, and What We Should Do About It. New York, Guilford, 2006

Wright JH, Basco MR, Thase ME: Learning Cognitive-Behavioral Therapy: An Illustrated Guide. Washington, DC, American Psychiatric Publishing, 2005

CHAPTER 24

Contingency Management

Maxine L. Stitzer, Ph.D.

Mary M. Sweeney, Ph.D.

Nancy Petry, Ph.D.[‡]

Introduction: Application of Behavioral Principles in Substance Use Disorder Treatment

An operant behavioral perspective has been very useful in formulating effective strategies to treat individuals with substance use disorders. In this view, drug seeking and drug taking are operant behaviors reinforced by the immediate effects following from drug use, such as euphoria and relief from withdrawal. Therefore, behavioral treatment strategies have focused on emphasizing the positive outcomes following from drug abstinence, such as improved health and relationships, which in the natural environment may be remote and uncertain. Contingency management (CM) interventions make positive consequences for drug abstinence or other desired behaviors more immediate, salient, and predictable. CM developers have turned to monetary-based reinforcers (including goods) because money is a universal reinforcer that can successfully compete with drug reinforcers.

As reviewed in this chapter, CM interventions are efficacious when applied to a variety of clinical populations and highly relevant target behaviors. These target behaviors have included entry and engagement in substance use disorder treatment, abstinence from drugs and alcohol, engagement with needed health care, and adherence to prescribed medication. It is important to utilize effective implementation methods when applying CM to promote positive behavior change. We detail these implementation principles in the chapter, and also outline considerations for patient selection. Finally, we provide a guide to training resources and highlight new digital

---

[‡] Deceased.

delivery tools that may pave the way to more widespread adoption of evidence-based CM treatments.

Attendance at Substance Use Disorder Treatment and Other Clinical Services

Treatment Attendance

CM interventions can be ideal for boosting and sustaining attendance and engagement in substance use disorder (SUD) treatment. For example, Corrigan et al. (2005) compared methods for increasing participation in substance abuse treatment among patients with traumatic brain injury (N=195). Among patients newly enrolled in treatment, the percentage who returned for a second appointment was 84% for those who were told they could receive financial help with transportation or a $20 gift card upon attending, compared with 45% for those who received only appointment reminder phone calls encouraging their attendance. A number of other studies have similarly shown that CM interventions are associated with increased therapy attendance among methadone maintenance patients, adolescent substance users, and patients in community treatment programs (see Petry 2012). Improved attendance, especially early in SUD treatment, may have a positive therapeutic impact, and may also have a positive financial impact on programs that bill on the basis of service delivery. Thus, adoption of CM interventions to improve treatment attendance is both clinically and administratively attractive.

Treatment Linkage

Novel strategies involving CM have been developed to encourage treatment enrollment. For example, Kidorf and colleagues invited individuals with opioid use disorder presenting at a needle exchange program to attend group sessions designed to enhance motivation for treatment entry (Kidorf et al. 2009) or reentry after dropout (Kidorf et al. 2011). One-third were randomly assigned to receive $10–$20 and a bus pass for attending the motivational sessions plus $50 sent directly to any treatment program they joined to defray intake and admission charges. Significantly more participants receiving incentive than nonincentivized control participants entered (52% [n=94] vs. 34% [n=187]) or reentered (64% [n=49] vs. 33% [n=64]) treatment in these studies. Future research should examine how contingent financial incentives may be similarly applied to screening, brief intervention, and referral to treatment programs in general health care settings, including hospitals, primary care practices, and emergency departments, in order to improve suboptimal rates of successful treatment linkage following brief intervention (e.g., Trowbridge et al. 2017).

Other Support Services

Financial incentives can also dramatically improve utilization of a diverse range of potentially beneficial services. In a multisite study conducted within the National Institute on Drug Abuse (NIDA) Clinical Trials Network (CTN) among 801 hospitalized patients with HIV who also used substances (Metsch et al. 2016), participating patients were randomly assigned to receive usual-care referral to community resources (*n*=264) or help from a patient navigator who encouraged and supported their involvement in HIV care and substance abuse treatment, either with (*n*=271) or without (*n*=266) contingent financial incentives targeting a variety of health care and substance use abatement activities. Participants could earn $220 over the 6-month intervention by attending up to 11 sessions with a patient navigator who helped them to reengage in HIV care. Individuals who were offered incentives attended a median of 11 sessions (versus 7 sessions for those without CM) (Metsch et al. 2016). The combination of incentives and patient navigation support was associated with better viral load outcomes compared with usual care at 6-month end of treatment, although not at 12-month follow-up (see "HIV Viral Load" subsection later in chapter). In a study of individuals with comorbid posttraumatic stress disorder (PTSD) and SUD (Schacht et al. 2017), those receiving monetary incentives attended a median of 9 out of 12 sessions (versus 1 session for the control group) and also exhibited larger reductions in PTSD symptom severity over time. Increasing treatment attendance is an important use for CM, because beneficial services can only be delivered to patients who attend treatment sessions.

Drug Abstinence

The use of CM as a treatment strategy for promoting and sustaining drug abstinence has been previously reviewed (Benishek et al. 2014; Lussier et al. 2006; Petry 2012). In this section, we provide an overview of the research supporting this intervention and highlight recent developments in the field.

Treatment of Stimulant Use Disorders

Use of Voucher Reinforcement to Promote Stimulant Abstinence

Stimulant use has been a logical target of CM interventions in the absence of an efficacious medication. Higgins et al. (1994) developed the first CM intervention to promote abstinence from stimulants using drug-negative urine tests as an objective marker of recent drug use. Reinforcers were vouchers (points exchangeable for retail goods) awarded for each stimulant-negative urine sample obtained over a 12-week period of thrice-weekly urine testing. The number of points awarded increased under an escalating schedule for each consecutive negative urine sample and reset to the original low value when a urine result was missing or positive. The total amount available—about $1,000 over a 12-week intervention—was designed to be attractive to patients and to motivate behavior change. The voucher program was combined with an intensive cognitive-behavioral counseling intervention based on the Community Reinforcement Approach (Budney and Higgins 1998).

Clinical trials of this intervention have consistently shown beneficial effects from treatment. For example, in an early study, the percentages of participants completing 24 weeks of treatment were 75% and 40% for those offered intensive counseling with and without the voucher incentive program, respectively (Higgins et al. 1994). Subsequent studies by Higgins and colleagues showed that the contingency linking voucher reinforcement to negative urine results was critical for promoting abstinence, that the intervention had long-term benefits that extended through the 6-month posttreatment follow-up (Higgins et al. 2000), and that outcomes were better when vouchers were combined with an intensive counseling treatment component than when vouchers were given as a stand-alone intervention (Higgins et al. 2003). Voucher reinforcement has also been very effective in promoting cocaine abstinence in patients on methadone maintenance treatment in the United States (e.g., Silverman et al. 2004) and in clinical treatment patients in Spain (García-Fernández et al. 2011). In short, voucher reinforcement combined with psychosocial counseling is well established as an efficacious evidence-based intervention for stimulant use disorder.

Use of Prize-Based Intermittent Reinforcement to Promote Stimulant Abstinence

An alternative efficacious method for delivering CM relies on principles of intermittent reinforcement and was developed with the intent of lowering implementation costs (for reviews, see Benishek et al. 2014 and Petry 2012). The prize-draw intermittent reinforcement approach is also called the "fishbowl method" because, operationally, patients who meet criteria for incentive delivery (e.g., submission of a stimulant-negative urine sample) earn draws from a bowl filled with chips or tickets. As in the voucher program, the amount earned (in this case, the number of draws) escalates over successive instances of the target behavior in order to promote sustained behavior change. In the standard application, about half of the chips in the bowl indicate a prize win and the other half indicate no win ("Good job"). Furthermore, there are three different prize levels: small (worth about $1), large (worth about $20), and jumbo (worth about $100). The number of chips present in the bowl is inversely related to prize value so that there is a much higher chance of winning small than large prizes and only a very small chance of winning the jumbo prize. Cost of the intervention depends on the value of prizes and the probabilities of winning; however, total prize values of $240 or more over an 8-week intervention are needed for efficacy (Petry et al. 2004).

As reviewed by Stitzer et al. (2010), a large multisite trial conducted within the NIDA CTN included two parallel studies among stimulant users either entering outpatient drug-free counseling treatment (N=415) or enrolled in methadone maintenance treatment (N=388). Both studies showed that the intervention was effective when participants could earn up to $400 in prizes over 12 weeks for submitting drug- and alcohol-negative samples (Stitzer et al. 2010). Retention was improved in outpatient drug-free treatment settings (49% of incentive group vs. 35% of control group were retained for 12 weeks), and the intervention significantly increased the number of stimulant-negative urine samples submitted by methadone maintenance patients (54% stimulant-negative results in the incentive group vs. 39% in the control group). This large multisite study was a significant step in establishing the efficacy of the prize-bowl method for treatment of stimulant use.

Treatment of Other Substance Use Disorders

Cannabis

Cannabis is another substance associated with problematic use for which no medications have been approved by the U.S. Food and Drug Administration (FDA), and therefore is a substance for which intervention with CM treatments could be especially useful. Tetrahydrocannabinol (THC) and cannabinoid metabolites can be readily detected via urinalysis, but a challenge is the long half-life of cannabis and its metabolites in the body after use has stopped. This has typically been overcome in CM treatment studies by incorporating a 2-week lead-in period so that the drug can clear the body prior to implementing abstinence contingencies for THC-negative samples (e.g., Budney et al. 2015). The benefits of adding CM for cannabis use to SUD counseling have been demonstrated across several randomized controlled trials in both adolescents (e.g., Stanger et al. 2015) and adults (e.g., Budney et al. 2006). In a study by Budney et al. (2015), 46% of adults with cannabis use disorder (N=59) were abstinent at the end of a 12-week treatment when CM was combined with motivational enhancement and cognitive-behavioral therapy counseling, compared with 12% of those in a comparison group receiving only brief motivational counseling (N=16).

Alcohol

The challenge in treating problematic alcohol use with CM has been detection of recent use, given alcohol's very short half-life. Petry et al. (2000) nevertheless conducted an early study using breath alcohol measures in a group of patients (N=42) entering treatment at a Veterans Health Administration clinic. The study showed that 84% of participants in the CM group (n=19) and 22% of participants in the treatment-as-usual control group (n=23) completed 8 weeks of treatment, and that half as many in the CM group as in the control group reported drinking during the treatment episode. More recent measurement methodologies that make it more feasible to offer CM for alcohol use disorder include Secure Continuous Remote Alcohol Monitoring (SCRAM) bracelets (e.g., Dougherty et al. 2015); longer-lasting alcohol biological markers, particularly ethyl glucuronide (McDonell et al. 2017); and remote breath alcohol monitoring (e.g., Koffarnus et al. 2018). Initial studies using these monitoring techniques have demonstrated that CM interventions have substantial efficacy for individuals with alcohol use disorder (see the later subsection "Delivery Advances Via Digital Therapeutics").

Tobacco

A Cochrane review (Cahill et al. 2015) encompassing 21 trials, including several studies with pregnant women (see the later subsection on pregnant women in "Patient Selection for Contingency Management"), concluded that contingent incentives were effective in improving rates of cigarette smoking cessation and abstinence. One example is a large-scale study by Volpp et al. (2009), in which employees of a large company were randomly assigned to receive information about smoking cessation with or without financial incentives. The incentives included $100 for completing a smoking cessation program, $250 for attaining cessation within 6 months, and $400 for maintaining 6 months of continuous abstinence after the quit. Cessation rates at 9–12 months were 15% for employees offered financial incentives versus 5% for those not offered incentives. Breath carbon monoxide (CO) is by far the most convenient biological measure for detecting recent smoke inhalation, with recent abstinence verified by CO readings of ≤6 parts per million. Like breath alcohol, however, breath CO can be detected for only a few hours after smoke inhalation. Therefore, innovative interventions, including remote breath CO monitoring (e.g., Dallery et al. 2017), have been developed to improve the feasibility of CM implementation with cigarette smokers. Cotinine, the specific metabolite of nicotine, can also be a useful biological marker for long-term cessation. However, this marker cannot be used to validate nonsmoking during nicotine replacement therapy, because the same metabolites occur with both nicotine replacement therapy and combustible tobacco use.

Opioids

Prior research clearly demonstrated that use of illicit heroin during methadone maintenance (Silverman et al. 1996) or methadone detoxification treatment (Robles et al. 2002) can be suppressed by contingent incentive interventions. There may, however, be limits on the ability of contingent incentives to improve outcomes for opioid users enrolled in types of therapy other than methadone. For example, patients in psychosocial counseling treatment programs whose primary abused drug was an opioid (in comparison with patients whose primary drug of abuse was a stimulant, alcohol, or marijuana) were the one subgroup that did not benefit from contingent abstinence incentives targeting the patients' primary problematic substance (Cochran et al. 2015). Furthermore, findings on efficacy of CM with opioid users in buprenorphine treatment have been mixed, with several trials showing positive results but one large trial by Ling et al. (2013) failing to find any effects of CM during buprenorphine treatment (for a review, see Carroll and Weiss 2017). More research is needed to clarify the conditions under which contingent incentives may be useful for suppressing ongoing illicit opioid use observed during various types of background treatment.

Patients' Primary Problematic Substance

A multisite study from the NIDA CTN implemented a clinic-wide intervention that took the novel and clinically appropriate approach of delivering escalating reinforcement under the prize-draw method based on abstinence from the patients' self-identified primary problematic substance, with bonus payments available for abstinence from the entire panel of tested drugs (Campbell et al. 2014). Treatment was delivered via an Internet-based intervention called Therapeutic Education System (TES), which includes both self-administered cognitive-behavioral skills training modules and CM abstinence incentives. As shown in Figure 24–1, the study found significant improvements in during-treatment drug use outcomes for TES versus usual care. The study also observed an important interaction between patient characteristics and treatment outcomes such that significant improvements in treatment outcomes were seen only in patients who were nonabstinent (i.e., actively using drugs) at baseline.

Other Therapeutically Relevant Intervention Targets

Overall, results from the studies discussed in the previous section indicate that CM interventions can be successfully and efficaciously applied to a variety of substance use disorders, with the only requirement being that a convenient objective marker of recent use be available to serve as the target for drug abstinence. In this section, we

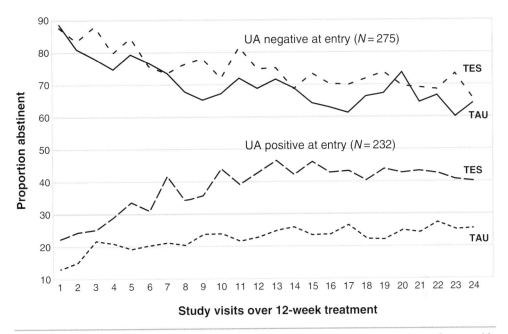

FIGURE 24–1.   Proportion of patients abstinent from 10 drugs and alcohol at twice-weekly study visits during a 12-week trial.

Overall study results showed significant improvement in outcomes with the Therapeutic Education System (TES) relative to treatment as usual (TAU), but there was a significant (post hoc) difference in outcomes as a function of urinalysis (UA) positive versus negative for any drug or alcohol at the time of study randomization.

Source.   Reprinted from Campbell ANC, Nunes EV, et al.: "Internet-Delivered Treatment for Substance Abuse: A Multisite Randomized Controlled Trial." *American Journal of Psychiatry* 171(6):683–690, 2014. Copyright © 2014, American Psychiatric Association. Used with permission.

review CM interventions that have been applied to other important targets for successful substance use disorder treatment.

Medication Adherence

A review (DeFulio and Silverman 2012) and a meta-analysis (Petry et al. 2012b) have summarized the impact of CM interventions on adherence to tuberculosis treatment regimens, hepatitis vaccination, HIV antiretroviral therapy, antipsychotic medications, and naltrexone therapy for the treatment of opioid use disorder. Naltrexone is an especially apt example of a therapy in which CM may be useful in promoting medication adherence, because individuals with opioid use disorder are frequently nonadherent to this highly safe and effective therapy. Jarvis et al. (2017) analyzed a series of three clinical trials evaluating a novel intervention for opioid users in which access to a therapeutic workplace (and hence employment earnings) was contingent on either daily or monthly (i.e., long-acting Vivitrol) naltrexone adherence. The intervention resulted in increased naltrexone adherence and decreased opioid use. Overall, CM appears to be a promising approach to addressing medication adherence. Its utility may be facilitated in the future with the advent of new technologies that allow for remote electronic tracking and video verification of medication ingestion.

HIV Viral Load

The use of financial incentives has also shown promise as an intervention to support better outcomes in persons living with HIV. In a study by El-Sadr et al. (2017), community clinics in two urban communities (37 HIV testing sites and 39 HIV care sites) were randomly assigned to either a financial incentives or a usual-care condition. The investigators found that $70 gift cards provided quarterly, contingent only on suppressed viral loads (i.e., HIV RNA<400 copies/mL), were associated with a small-magnitude but significant improvement in rates of viral suppression and of care continuity among patients already enrolled at the care clinics.

Silverman et al. (2019) conducted a 2-year randomized controlled trial investigating whether a higher-magnitude incentive (up to $10 per day) would be effective in promoting suppression of viral load among people living with HIV. Community HIV patients ($N=102$) with detectable viral loads (i.e., HIV RNA > 400 copies/mL) were randomly assigned to receive either usual care ($n=50$) or financial incentives ($n=52$) contingent upon providing blood samples that showed either reduced or undetectable viral loads. At 3-month assessments over the first year of the study, 72% of blood samples provided by participants in the incentives group showed undetectable viral loads, compared with 39% of blood samples provided by participants in the usual-care group ($n=50$). The higher-magnitude incentive and the rapid delivery of incentives to a prepaid debit card likely contributed to this study's larger effect on viral load relative to prior work.

In the multisite NIDA CTN study by Metsch et al. (2016) involving patients with HIV and substance use (described earlier in chapter; see subsection "Other Support Services"), the treatment group that received support from patient navigators plus incentives contingent upon multiple behaviors (e.g., doctor visits, substance use) had a significantly higher end-of-treatment HIV viral suppression rate (46% [$n=271$]) compared with the group that received treatment as usual (35% [$n=264$]), whereas the suppression rate for the group receiving navigation alone (39% [$n=266$]) was not significantly different from that for usual care (Metsch et al. 2016).

On the basis of these study findings, continued exploration of the use of financial incentives to improve outcomes among persons living with HIV appears warranted.

Implementation Considerations

An effective CM intervention requires contingent reinforcers of sufficient magnitude and immediacy to affect behavior. Several studies (see, e.g., Lussier et al. 2006; Petry et al. 2012a) have demonstrated that a larger magnitude (i.e., the total amount available) of reinforcement is associated with a higher likelihood of behavior change relative to smaller magnitudes. In general, the largest feasible magnitude of reinforcer should be offered. When the value of available reinforcers for reducing drug use drops too low (e.g., below an average of $30 per patient per week over the intervention duration), efficacy may be compromised (Petry 2012; Petry et al. 2004).

It is also important that positive reinforcers be delivered as closely as possible to the time at which the desired behavior is observed, which in the case of drug abstinence is immediately after results of a negative drug test are obtained. One way to achieve such timely delivery is through use of on-site urine testing, because results can be obtained in minutes rather than days. To adequately detect recent drug use, especially in the case of short-acting drugs, testing should be conducted at frequent (e.g., 2–3 times weekly) or unpredictable intervals. Furthermore, although the simplest way to deliver CM is with a fixed-value reinforcer given each time the behavior is observed, it may be ideal to use an escalating schedule in which the reinforcer amount increases as the duration of continuous abstinence increases over time (Budney and Higgins 1998; Higgins et al. 1994). This strategy promotes sustained behavioral change because the value of remaining abstinent increases with consecutive submissions of negative samples, while relapse is prevented because earnings are reset to a lower value if a sample tests positive for the target drug(s).

As a general rule, it is advisable for CM interventions to be kept in place for as long as feasible, because longer-duration interventions (e.g., 6 months or longer) are associated with better outcomes (e.g., Kirby et al. 2013). Abrupt discontinuation at the end of a specified intervention period has been associated with relapse, as would be the case in any chronic relapsing disorder. Thus, gradual withdrawal schedules implementing low-value reinforcers may be advantageous to reduce rates of subsequent relapse (Budney and Higgins 1998; Higgins et al. 1994). Given the strong association between in- and post-treatment abstinence durations (e.g., Higgins et al. 2000), a novel but as yet untested strategy would be to keep incentives in place until the individual has achieved a specified duration of abstinence (e.g., 6 months). Further implementation considerations and strategies for cost-effective interventions can be found in Petry's (2012) guide to CM in substance abuse treatment.

Patient Selection for Contingency Management

A striking finding in the CM literature is that patients with a wide array of demographic and drug use characteristics respond comparably to CM interventions. Similar beneficial effects from CM approaches have been observed for individuals with and without legal problems, with and without concurrent mental health problems, and across income levels typical among treatment-seeking substance users (for a review, see Forster et al. 2019). However, there are some guidelines that identify special populations that are preferred candidates for CM.

Patients With a Poorer Prognosis

In general, patients with a poor prognosis are most likely to benefit from the addition of CM. This principle is nicely illustrated in the study by Campbell et al. (2014). Patients who came to psychosocial counseling treatment while in remission (i.e., testing drug-negative at entry) did not benefit from abstinence incentives with significant short-term (during-treatment) improvement in outcomes, whereas those who tested drug-positive at entry did benefit with improved outcomes. Also, because patients in remission submit a high rate of drug-negative samples, they are costly to the incentive program (Cunningham et al. 2017). If it is possible to prioritize contingent abstinence incentives within a clinical population, preference should be given to currently active users. Alternatively, if it is desirable to offer incentives to all patients, those who are in remission at entry may be offered attendance rather than abstinence incentives. This strategy can improve retention over usual care without degrading drug use outcomes, and can conserve costs by reducing expenditures associated with collecting and screening urine samples (Petry et al. 2012a).

Individuals With Serious Mental Illness

Individuals who use drugs and have serious mental illness also may be especially well served by CM. A study by McDonell et al. (2013) showed the expected improvements in drug use when patients with serious mental illness who had used stimulants within the past 30 days (N=176) were treated with and without an abstinence-contingent prize-bowl procedure (Figure 24–2) in combination with outpatient treatment as usual (consisting of mental health, substance use, housing, and vocational services). In addition to improved drug use outcomes, substantial associated reductions were seen in psychiatric symptoms and hospitalization days (14 vs. 152 total hospital days for contingent vs. noncontingent participants) during the 6 months following randomization. This finding suggests that CM holds considerable promise for producing substantial cost savings for health care delivery services.

Pregnant Women

Pregnant women also represent an important subpopulation for CM intervention, given that the condition is time-limited and that treatment for substance use during pregnancy benefits not only the pregnant woman but also the health of her child. For example, in a study examining the efficacy of a voucher-based CM smoking-cessation intervention among 166 pregnant women, Higgins et al. (2010) found significantly higher smoking-cessation rates at the end of pregnancy (34% vs. 7%) among the women assigned to the contingent condition (n=85), in which financial incentive payments totaling about $400 over 9 months were given contingent on smoking abstinence, in comparison with women assigned to the noncontingent condition (n=81), in which payments were given independent of smoking behavior. These significant group differences in smoking cessation were maintained at 12 and 24 weeks postpartum. Furthermore, infants of women treated with CM had significantly higher birth weights—an important and potentially cost-saving secondary health benefit of smoking cessation during pregnancy.

Delivery Advances Via Digital Therapeutics

Advances in technology have allowed for considerable innovation in the implementation of CM for the treatment of substance use disorders. A program for Internet-based delivery of cognitive-behavioral therapy and CM was described earlier in this chapter (see subsection "Patients' Primary Problematic Substance" in "Treatment of Other Substance Use Disorders" section), along with data from a multisite clinical trial supporting the program's efficacy (Campbell et al. 2014). This evidence-based intervention, originally named Therapeutic Education System (as it is called earlier in this chapter), was reconfigured for delivery as a smartphone application. Under the name reSET™ (www.resetforrecovery.com), this application is the first digital therapeutic to receive FDA clearance for use in the treatment of substance use disorders related to stimulants, cannabis, cocaine, or alcohol. A companion app, reSET-O, is tailored for opioid use disorder patients concurrently receiving buprenorphine.

Another important new technology-based implementation strategy is remote digital monitoring of drug use to facilitate more frequent substance use testing. For ex-

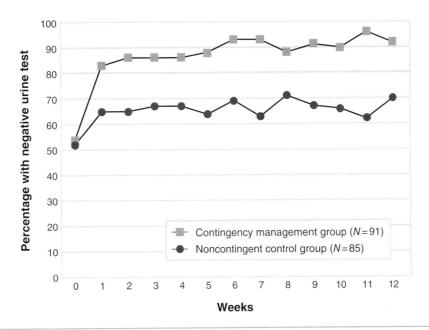

FIGURE 24–2. Percentage of stimulant users with serious mental illness (*N*=176) submitting stimulant-negative urines during each week of a 12-week treatment program.

Patients in contingency management could earn up to $400 in prizes on average under a prize-draw procedure with an escalating schedule of draws; those in the noncontingent group earned an equivalent number of draws independent of urine test results under a yoked control procedure.

Source. Reprinted from McDonell MG, Srebnik D, Angelo F, et al.: "Randomized Controlled Trial of Contingency Management for Stimulant Use in Community Mental Health Patients With Serious Mental Illness." *American Journal of Psychiatry* 170(1):94–101, 2013. Copyright © 2013, American Psychiatric Association. Used with permission.

ample, remote breath alcohol testing addresses the difficulty in obtaining multiple breath alcohol tests daily to verify abstinence from this rapidly metabolized substance. In one recent study (Koffarnus et al. 2018), participants (*N*=40) were provided with breathalyzers and smartphones as needed and were prompted by text messages to submit thrice-daily breathalyzer samples validated by photos. Study staff remotely delivered reinforcers via online accounts for prepaid cards, which facilitated frequent and immediate incentive payments. The 20 participants randomly assigned to receive contingent incentives (up to $350 over 3 weeks) had 85% of days abstinent compared with 35% for the 20 participants in the noncontingent comparison group (Koffarnus et al. 2018). Similar strategies have been implemented with alcohol use (monitored via SCRAM bracelets) and cigarette smoking (via remotely monitored breath CO) (for reviews, see Getty et al. 2019 and McPherson et al. 2018). Such technologies have the potential to more effectively monitor substance use and increase the accessibility of CM treatments.

Dissemination and Training

CM is an evidence-based intervention with over 30 years of research supporting its efficacy in a variety of target behavior applications and clinical populations. Nevertheless, treatment providers have been slow to adopt its use. An exception is the Veterans Health Administration (VHA), which in 2011 modeled the adoption of CM throughout its national network of outpatient SUD clinics. Following intensive clinician training, abstinence incentives primarily targeting stimulant use were implemented in 94 programs involving more than 2,000 patients (DePhilippis et al. 2018). The VHA was especially well suited to adopt CM because most hospitals operate a retail canteen for patients such that canteen vouchers could be used as CM incentives.

Three issues are generally cited as barriers to wider adoption of CM interventions: negative attitudes on the part of staff, a lack of clinician and staff training in the principles and practices of the intervention, and a lack of financial resources in the service delivery system to support financial incentives. Clinician and staff attitudes should continue to improve as implementation becomes more convenient and as CM adoption becomes more widespread. The recent FDA clearance of the prescription digital therapeutic device reSET™ may presage entry of CM into more widespread use in SUD treatment programs. While there may be a variety of ways to raise money for CM implementation, monetary barriers could be significantly lowered if insurance companies agreed to pay for this evidence-based practice as part of a digital therapeutic intervention.

A significant number of resources are available for training. The NIDA CTN has produced two "Blending Products" that contain CM training resources for clinicians (www.bettertxoutcomes.org). Budney and Higgins (1998) published a manual that comprehensively outlines implementation of their Community Reinforcement Approach plus vouchers therapy. Henggeler et al. (2011) provide a manual outlining CM interventions specifically for adolescents. Petry and colleagues have a published manual (Petry 2012; http://contingencymanagement.uchc.edu) that reviews the supporting research and details how to design and implement prize-draw CM interventions in practice settings.

Conclusion

CM is an effective evidence-based intervention based on the principles of reinforcement. It has been shown to be an adaptable treatment approach that promotes positive change across a range of important health behaviors. The material reviewed in this chapter supports the following conclusions:

- Contingency management involving delivery of positive reinforcement is a highly effective intervention that can be used to promote therapeutically desirable behaviors, including treatment attendance and drug abstinence.
- Abstinence incentives have been effectively used in treating stimulant, cannabis, alcohol, and tobacco users and have been found effective in drug users with a wide variety of demographic, psychosocial, and substance use characteristics.
- Both voucher and prize-draw intervention methods are effective, but implementation details are important and interventions must adhere to basic principles of contingent reinforcement to effectively promote behavior change. Specifically, incentives must be of sufficient magnitude and delivered reliably and as close as possible to the behavior targeted for reinforcement.

- Substance use disorder counselors and other health care providers can be trained to implement these highly effective techniques; both training and implementation support resources are available for use in community programs.
- New digital therapeutics may further enhance the feasibility and convenience of incorporating this evidence-based practice into routine clinical care.

References

Benishek LA, Dugosh KL, Kirby KC, et al: Prize-based contingency management for the treatment of substance abusers: a meta-analysis. Addiction 109(9):1426–1436, 2014 24750232

Budney AJ, Higgins ST: A Community Reinforcement Plus Vouchers Approach: Treating Cocaine Addiction. Rockville, MD, National Institute on Drug Abuse, 1998

Budney AJ, Moore BA, Rocha HL, et al: Clinical trial of abstinence-based vouchers and cognitive-behavioral therapy for cannabis dependence. J Consult Clin Psychol 74(2):307–316, 2006 16649875

Budney AJ, Stanger C, Tilford JM, et al: Computer-assisted behavioral therapy and contingency management for cannabis use disorder. Psychol Addict Behav 29(3):501–511, 2015 25938629

Cahill K, Hartmann-Boyce J, Perera R: Incentives for smoking cessation. Cochrane Database Syst Rev (5):CD004307, 2015 25983287

Campbell AN, Nunes EV, Matthews AG, et al: Internet-delivered treatment for substance abuse: a multisite randomized controlled trial. Am J Psychiatry 171(6):683–690, 2014 24700332

Carroll KM, Weiss RD: The role of behavioral interventions in buprenorphine maintenance treatment: a review. Am J Psychiatry 174(8):738–747, 2017 27978771

Cochran G, Stitzer M, Campbell AN, et al: Web-based treatment for substance use disorders: differential effects by primary substance. Addict Behav 45:191–194, 2015 25697725

Corrigan JD, Bogner J, Lamb-Hart G, et al: Increasing substance abuse treatment compliance for persons with traumatic brain injury. Psychol Addict Behav 19(2):131–139, 2005 16011383

Cunningham C, Stitzer M, Campbell AN, et al: Contingency management abstinence incentives: cost and implications for treatment tailoring. J Subst Abuse Treat 72:134–139, 2017 26482136

Dallery J, Raiff BR, Kim SJ, et al: Nationwide access to an Internet-based contingency management intervention to promote smoking cessation: a randomized controlled trial. Addiction 112(5):875–883, 2017 27923264

DeFulio A, Silverman K: The use of incentives to reinforce medication adherence. Prev Med 55 (suppl):S86–S94, 2012 22580095

DePhilippis D, Petry NM, Bonn-Miller MO, et al: The national implementation of contingency management (CM) in the Department of Veterans Affairs: attendance at CM sessions and substance use outcomes. Drug Alcohol Depend 185:367–373, 2018 29524874

Dougherty DM, Lake SL, Hill-Kapturczak N, et al: Using contingency management procedures to reduce at-risk drinking in heavy drinkers. Alcohol Clin Exp Res 39(4):743–751, 2015 25833033

El-Sadr WM, Donnell D, Beauchamp G, et al: Financial incentives for linkage to care and viral suppression among HIV-positive patients: a randomized clinical trial (HPTN 065). JAMA Intern Med 177(8):1083–1092, 2017 28628702

Forster SE, DePhilippis D, Forman SD: "I's" on the prize: a systematic review of individual differences in contingency management treatment response. J Subst Abuse Treat 100:64–83, 2019 30898330

García-Fernández G, Secades-Villa R, García-Rodríguez O, et al: Long-term benefits of adding incentives to the community reinforcement approach for cocaine dependence. Eur Addict Res 17(3):139–145, 2011 21447950

Getty CA, Morande A, Lynskey M, et al: Mobile telephone-delivered contingency management interventions promoting behaviour change in individuals with substance use disorders: a meta-analysis. Addiction 114(11):1915–1925, 2019 31265747

Henggeler SW, Cunningham PB, Rowland MD, et al: Contingency Management for Adolescent Substance Abuse: A Practitioner's Guide. New York, Guilford, 2011

Higgins ST, Budney AJ, Bickel WK, et al: Incentives improve outcome in outpatient behavioral treatment of cocaine dependence. Arch Gen Psychiatry 51(7):568–576, 1994 8031230

Higgins ST, Badger GJ, Budney AJ: Initial abstinence and success in achieving longer term cocaine abstinence. Exp Clin Psychopharmacol 8(3):377–386, 2000 10975629

Higgins ST, Sigmon SC, Wong CJ, et al: Community reinforcement therapy for cocaine-dependent outpatients. Arch Gen Psychiatry 60(10):1043–1052, 2003 14557150

Higgins ST, Bernstein IM, Washio Y, et al: Effects of smoking cessation with voucher-based contingency management on birth outcomes. Addiction 105(11):2023–2030, 2010 20840188

Jarvis BP, Holtyn AF, DeFulio A, et al: Effects of incentives for naltrexone adherence on opiate abstinence in heroin-dependent adults. Addiction 112(5):830–837, 2017 27936293

Kidorf M, King VL, Neufeld K, et al: Improving substance abuse treatment enrollment in community syringe exchangers. Addiction 104(5):786–795, 2009 19413790

Kidorf M, King VL, Peirce J, et al: A treatment reengagement intervention for syringe exchangers. J Subst Abuse Treat 41(4):415–421, 2011 21831559

Kirby KC, Carpenedo CM, Dugosh KL, et al: Randomized clinical trial examining duration of voucher-based reinforcement therapy for cocaine abstinence. Drug Alcohol Depend 132(3):639–645, 2013 23680075

Koffarnus MN, Bickel WK, Kablinger AS: Remote alcohol monitoring to facilitate incentive-based treatment for alcohol use disorder: a randomized trial. Alcohol Clin Exp Res 42(12):2423–2431, 2018 30335205

Ling W, Hillhouse M, Ang A, et al: Comparison of behavioral treatment conditions in buprenorphine maintenance. Addiction 108(10):1788–1798, 2013 23734858

Lussier JP, Heil SH, Mongeon JA, et al: A meta-analysis of voucher-based reinforcement therapy for substance use disorders. Addiction 101(2):192–203, 2006 16445548

McDonell MG, Srebnik D, Angelo F, et al: Randomized controlled trial of contingency management for stimulant use in community mental health patients with serious mental illness. Am J Psychiatry 170(1):94–101, 2013 23138961

McDonell MG, Leickly E, McPherson S, et al: A randomized controlled trial of ethyl glucuronide-based contingency management for outpatients with co-occurring alcohol use disorders and serious mental illness. Am J Psychiatry 174(4):370–377, 2017 28135843

McPherson SM, Burduli E, Smith CL, et al: A review of contingency management for the treatment of substance-use disorders: adaptation for underserved populations, use of experimental technologies, and personalized optimization strategies. Subst Abuse Rehabil 9:43–57, 2018 30147392

Metsch LR, Feaster DJ, Gooden L, et al: Effect of patient navigation with or without financial incentives on viral suppression among hospitalized patients with HIV infection and substance use: a randomized clinical trial. JAMA 316(2):156–170, 2016 27404184

Petry NM: Contingency Management for Substance Abuse Treatment: A Guide to Implementing This Evidence-Based Practice. New York, Taylor & Francis, 2012

Petry NM, Martin B, Cooney JL, et al: Give them prizes, and they will come: contingency management for treatment of alcohol dependence. J Consult Clin Psychol 68(2):250–257, 2000 10780125

Petry NM, Tedford J, Austin M, et al: Prize reinforcement contingency management for treating cocaine users: how low can we go, and with whom? Addiction 99(3):349–360, 2004 1498254

Petry NM, Barry D, Alessi SM, et al: A randomized trial adapting contingency management targets based on initial abstinence status of cocaine-dependent patients. J Consult Clin Psychol 80(2):276–285, 2012a 22229758

Petry NM, Rash CJ, Byrne S, et al: Financial reinforcers for improving medication adherence: findings from a meta-analysis. Am J Med 125(9):888–896, 2012b 22800876

Robles E, Stitzer ML, Strain EC, et al: Voucher-based reinforcement of opiate abstinence during methadone detoxification. Drug Alcohol Depend 65(2):179–189, 2002 11772479

Schacht RL, Brooner RK, King VL, et al: Incentivizing attendance to prolonged exposure for PTSD with opioid use disorder patients: a randomized controlled trial. J Consult Clin Psychol 85(7):689–701, 2017 28414485

Silverman K, Wong CJ, Higgins ST, et al: Increasing opiate abstinence through voucher-based reinforcement therapy. Drug Alcohol Depend 41(2):157–165, 1996 8809505

Silverman K, Robles E, Mudric T, et al: A randomized trial of long-term reinforcement of cocaine abstinence in methadone-maintained patients who inject drugs. J Consult Clin Psychol 72(5):839–854, 2004 15482042

Silverman K, Holtyn AF, Rodewald AM, et al: Incentives for viral suppression in people living with HIV: a randomized clinical trial. AIDS and Behavior 23:2337–2346, 2019. Available at: https://link.springer.com/article/10.1007/s10461-019-02592-8. Accessed July 10, 2020.

Stanger C, Ryan SR, Scherer EA, et al: Clinic- and home-based contingency management plus parent training for adolescent cannabis use disorders. J Am Acad Child Adolesc Psychiatry 54(6):445.e2–453.e2, 2015 26004659

Stitzer ML, Petry NM, Peirce J: Motivational incentives research in the National Drug Abuse Treatment Clinical Trials Network. J Subst Abuse Treat 38 (suppl 1):S61–S69, 2010 20307797

Trowbridge P, Weinstein ZM, Kerensky T, et al: Addiction consultation services—linking hospitalized patients to outpatient addiction treatment. J Subst Abuse Treat 79:1–5, 2017 28673521

Volpp KG, Troxel AB, Pauly MV, et al: A randomized, controlled trial of financial incentives for smoking cessation. N Engl J Med 360(7):699–709, 2009 19213683

CHAPTER 25

Motivational Enhancement

Matisyahu Shulman, M.D.

Katherine Pruzan, Psy.D.

Kenneth M. Carpenter, Ph.D.

In the United States in 2018, approximately 7.8% of adults and 3.8% of adolescents (Substance Abuse and Mental Health Services Administration 2018) met criteria for a current substance use disorder (SUD). SUDs significantly affect the physical and psychological health of the individuals struggling with these problems and of their loved ones. Although evidence-based strategies exist for individuals seeking to change their substance misuse (National Institute on Drug Abuse 2012), only 10%–15% of individuals with a current SUD will come into contact with a treatment professional (Hasin and Grant 2015). Reasons given for not seeking treatment include limited health care coverage, cost concerns, fear that doing so may impact employment, and stigma (Substance Abuse and Mental Health Services Administration 2018). Importantly, approximately 40% of individuals with a current SUD report not being ready to stop using (Substance Abuse and Mental Health Services Administration 2018).

Motivation is a key construct in behavioral medicine and is a particularly salient issue in the treatment of SUDs (e.g., Higgins and Silverman 1999). Prochaska and DiClemente's (1983) transtheoretical Stages of Change model is a useful heuristic for understanding the different cognitive-motivational-behavioral states that individuals demonstrate as they move through the change process. Briefly, the model proposes five stages of change:

1. Individuals may not believe there is a problem with their behavior and may not see a need to change (*precontemplation stage*).

2. As awareness of a problem increases, individuals may begin to weigh the pros and cons of engaging in a specific behavior, a state often described as "ambivalence" (*contemplation stage*).

3. When a state of ambivalence is resolved in the direction of making a change, individuals may then begin to develop a change plan (*preparation stage*).

4. Individuals then embark on successive efforts to change the behavior (*action stage*).

5. The *maintenance stage* characterizes the ongoing efforts to keep momentum and reduce the likelihood of reengaging in previous behavioral patterns (e.g., relapse).

Importantly, this model conceptualizes change as a nonlinear process, characterized by a dynamic back and forth of motivational states as individuals move toward long-term shifts in their behavior. This view differs from change being characterized as a unidirectional shift from being "unmotivated" to being "motivated" and suggests that helping strategies should be sensitive to an individual's position in the change process.

The role that personal motivation plays in the process of recovery has been viewed differently over time, and these evolving perspectives have in turn influenced the strategies used in treatment settings and the advice offered to family members. In his history of addiction treatment and recovery in America, White (2014) proposed that the baseline view was that recovery was not possible unless an individual was ready to change and that the motivation to change was derived from the pain of the person's behavior, thus necessitating the need to "hit bottom." The second perspective focused on the actions of loved ones, who could protect an individual from the painful consequences of his or her substance use and delay the need to change; therefore, teaching loved ones to refrain from rescuing (i.e., "enabling") the individual was seen as an important way to accelerate the pace of change. The third perspective incorporated the view that raising an individual from the "bottom" could be facilitated by a caring confrontation, although pain and threat remained the active ingredients for increasing motivation. More recently, motivational barriers to recovery have been viewed as coming not from the absence of pain but rather from the absence of hope, and empowering relationships developed during the treatment process are seen as important factors for enhancing motivation. These perspectives provide the historical context in which strategies to influence an individual's motivation, particularly during the earlier stages of recovery (i.e., precontemplation, contemplation, and preparation), have been developed and implemented. These perspectives also continue to be found in the current practices of professionals and paraprofessionals, as well as in the advice and strategies offered to family members. As discussed in this chapter, evidence supports the use of some of these strategies but highlights the iatrogenic effects of others.

Seeking help for SUDs is associated with a perceived need for treatment, which is also associated with the presence of psychiatric, medical, and substance comorbidities (Hasin and Grant 2015). These findings suggest that negative emotional and physical sequelae of substance use can influence personal motivation to seek help. Furthermore, teaching family members communication strategies and the strategic use of contingency management (i.e., positive reinforcement, allowing for the negative consequences of substance use, and limit setting) can increase the probability that an individual will engage in treatment (Manuel et al. 2012; Miller et al. 1999a) and improve treatment outcomes (Ariss and Fairbairn 2020; Brigham et al. 2014). Importantly, these findings highlight the potential utility of continued engagement and interaction (i.e., relationships) between concerned individuals as a motivation-enhancing strategy, in contrast to a fully detached, disconnected, punitive stance. The use of certain clinician-guided, -planned, and -scripted family interventions (e.g., Johnson Institute's model for intervention [Johnson 1986]) has also demonstrated some efficacy in increasing treatment enrollment. However, findings of studies examining these types of interventions indicate that a significant proportion of family members do not go through with the intervention meeting, thereby reducing its overall clinical impact (Liepman et al. 1989; Miller et al. 1999a).

A significant body of evidence indicates that the use of confrontation in individual, group, and family-focused interventions does not improve outcomes compared with other treatment strategies and may negatively affect treatment response and engagement (White and Miller 2007). In contrast, certain counseling styles, such as those striving to convey accurate empathy and to minimize confrontational interactions, have been associated with significantly better treatment response (Miller et al. 1993; Moyers and Miller 2013). This evidence highlights the significant role that helper–client interactions play in influencing an individual's personal motivation to engage in the change process. In this chapter, we focus on motivational interviewing (MI) (Miller and Rollnick 2013), a counseling style that aims to establish a collaborative and empathetic approach to helping individuals resolve their ambivalence about change as they move through the change process. MI is aligned with the view that motivation to change can emerge from empowering relationships that instill hope (White 2014). In this chapter, we outline the ingredients of an MI counseling style, important parameters in learning and maintaining proficiency in MI, and recent attempts to extend the utility of MI beyond the clinician's office.

Motivational Interviewing: The Clinical Approach

MI has been defined as "a collaborative conversation style for strengthening a person's own motivation and commitment to change" (Miller and Rollnick 2013, p. 12). Clinicians focus on increasing client *"change talk"*—verbal utterances focused on the client's *desire, ability, reasons,* or *need* to make changes, with the goal of increasing *commitment* statements toward the end of a clinical interaction (remembered by the acronym *DARN-C*; Amrhein 2004). For providers, MI can be conceptualized as a conversation about change that incorporates four key processes (i.e. engaging, focusing, evoking, and planning). While guiding these processes, clinicians adopt a therapeutic stance (i.e., the spirit of MI) to help clients feel comfortable and empowered to explore their ambivalence about making changes. Additionally, a specific set of core therapist skills is used to guide these processes throughout collaborative discussions that aim to bring forth an understanding of the client's perspective and to elicit and strengthen the client's talk about change (Miller and Rollnick 2013).

Relational Components of Motivational Interviewing

MI Spirit is the name given to the stance taken by clinicians to convey an open attitude that will encourage clients to explore reasons for change. It encompasses the relational components of MI and includes four dimensions: partnership, acceptance, compassion, and evocation.

Partnership

The clinician takes a stance of active collaboration with the client that is in the service of the client's own goals. This stance includes conveying that clinician and client are equals with different arenas of expertise that they are collaborating around. This collaboration has been described as a dance with two partners working together and in sync, rather than a wrestling match in which the clinician tries to force the client into change (Miller and Rollnick 2013).

Acceptance

Acceptance in MI is based in Rogerian therapy concepts (Rogers 1961) and differs from the notion of approval. The clinician's stance should convey a belief in the client's absolute worth, including future potential. It also includes support for the client's autonomy: the client's power in making his or her own choices and the client's independence of thought. This stance is in opposition to a therapeutic stance in which the clinician confronts the client and spells out why the client "must" change. Clinicians strive for accurate empathy in interactions with each client, or try to understand each client's own unique reasons for change rather than imposing what they feel should be the client's primary motivators for change. Finally, the clinician's acceptance of the client is demonstrated by the clinician's affirmation of the client's actual strengths and positive efforts (Miller and Rollnick 2013).

Compassion

The clinician displays ongoing compassion for the client, the client's welfare, and the priority of the client's needs as a driving force and motivator of therapeutic change (Miller and Rollnick 2013).

Evocation

Throughout MI guided discussions, the clinician works to pull from the client his or her own motivations and reasons for moving forward. This includes exploring the client's ambivalence about change and highlighting the client's reasons for making changes. It is important that clinicians avoid pushing their own reasons why clients should change, because doing so is likely to undermine the MI process (Miller and Rollnick 2013).

Core Skills of Motivational Interviewing: OARS

In the context of MI Spirit (i.e., a nonjudgmental and accepting stance), clinicians utilize a set of core skills, which are captured by the acronym OARS: open-ended questions, affirmations, reflections, and summary statements (Miller and Rollnick 2013). These components make up the "technical skills" of MI work.

Open-Ended Questions

Within an MI framework, the goal is to rely most heavily on open-ended questions. Open-ended questions cannot be answered with a simple "yes" or "no" and are designed to elicit from the client additional information, context, and room for further exploration of ambivalence (Miller and Rollnick 2013). For example, the closed-ended question "Have you been taking your medications?" can be rephrased as the open-ended question "What has your experience been with medications since we last met?"

Affirmations

With the information gleaned through open-ended questions and reflections, the clinician highlights the client's strengths, efforts, abilities, and what has been going well. This approach is meant to linguistically reinforce desires or efforts to change that are consistent with the client's goals. For example, the therapist might say, "You've worked hard to take several days off from drinking in the last month and felt really proud when you accomplished that" (Miller and Rollnick 2013).

Reflections

Reflections in MI are strategic efforts by the clinician to guess at the client's meaning in a way that further focuses the conversation toward change. Clinicians choose which components of a client's utterances they want to reflect, and these choices provide topics for further evocation and focusing of the session (Miller and Rollnick 2013). Reflections can be either simple (e.g., the clinician provides a paraphrase of the client's words) or complex (e.g., the clinician guesses at the client's additional meanings). As an example, if the client says, "I went out with my friends and had a blast. I don't remember the entire night, though, and one of my friends hasn't spoken to me since—I'm not sure why." A simple reflection from the therapist could be "You don't remember the entire evening." This sticks fairly closely to what the client said, and directs the conversation toward what the client might want to change about substance use. A complex reflection from the same material could be "Substance use contributed to conflict with your friend." In this case, the clinician guesses the meaning and adds it to the reflection, in the hope of moving the conversation forward toward exploring ambivalence and reasons for change. Complex reflections are particularly associated with increased change talk by the client (Magill et al. 2018).

Summary Statements

Summary statements by the clinician allow further focusing of the session (Miller and Rollnick 2013). The clinician can choose client utterances that will highlight the prospect of change and that are most likely to move the conversation toward the client's committing to change. As an example, the clinician might say, "We've discussed a number of items in the past 20 minutes. You at times black out when you drink, and that can lead to your saying or doing things that bother others. You also don't like waking up feeling groggy after drinking." The clinician in this instance may have chosen to omit information about what the client enjoyed about drinking in the past week.

The Four Processes of Motivational Interviewing

The frequency and proportion of MI-consistent skills used by the clinician in sessions are associated with greater change talk by the client (Magill et al. 2018). MI-adherent behaviors have also been shown to increase the strength of change statements during the course of a counseling session (Amrhein et al. 2003). This evidence implies that properly delivered MI provides space for clients to explore their own ambivalence about their current situation and to increase their resolve to make changes.

From an MI perspective, a helpful conversation about change encompasses four processes during which the clinician continuously sets the tone by using the MI Spirit and employing the OARS skills. The clinician's use of the technical skills to facilitate each of the processes can be placed alongside the Stages of Change model (Prochaska and DiClemente 1983; see chapter introduction) to provide a broad heuristic for conceptualizing the arch of MI-informed conversation(s) for both clinician and client.

Engaging: Building a Working Relationship

Engaging underpins any possibility of helping a client move toward change, because a collaborative, autonomy-reinforcing relationship helps clients build awareness of potential areas of change and open up about ways they may be contemplating changes. Clients in precontemplation and contemplation stages can be particularly helped by a clinician's engaging stance, which encourages openness, discussion of the issues surrounding their behaviors, and reasons for seeking a talk with the counselor. This allows individuals to move toward greater readiness to change by discussing the issues surrounding their behavior and their reasons for seeking treatment (Prochaska and DiClemente 1983).

Focusing: Identifying a Specific Set of Changes to Address

Focusing encompasses the clinician's process of strategically narrowing the conversation and helping the client to target an area for potential movement. This process may align with the contemplation stage of change, because clients may require focused thought and discussion before being more actively ready to change. Focusing may also align with earlier or later stages of change. Clients in the precontemplation stage can benefit from conversations eliciting discussion of ways that particular behaviors are or are not serving their needs or values. Clients in the preparation or action stage can benefit from focused discussions on ways they might move toward the changes they have committed themselves to making.

Evoking: Inviting Clients to State Their Own Reasons for Change

During the evoking process, the clinician strategically "invites in" a client's change talk and differentially responds to it. The evoking process links with client change talk around a specific behavior such that the clinician can elicit additional reasons for change and invite the client to commit to a plan. This process thus tends to align with the preparation stage of change—the stage in which most of the clinician's directional effort occurs.

Planning: Developing an Action Plan

In the planning process, the clinician offers guidance, with the client's permission, on how a plan might be put in place for making changes (Miller and Rollnick 2013). The giving of advice by the clinician is always subject to the client's permission, honoring the client's autonomy and choice. The clinician's request for permission before providing advice ensures that the action stage of change aligns with the client's own values; it also encourages future discussion of what did or did not work in action implementation, thereby providing a helpful feedback loop leading to continued movement toward healthier behaviors and a continued positive working relationship with the clinician.

Motivational Enhancement Therapy

Motivational enhancement therapy (MET) is a specific, short-term manualized application of MI relational and technical components. MET was originally developed for the National Institute on Alcohol Abuse and Alcoholism–funded Project MATCH (Matching Alcoholism Treatment to Client Heterogeneity), a 5-year multisite study of alcohol treatments that investigated whether the relative efficacy of different treatments was linked to the characteristics of clients (Miller et al. 1999b). A detailed overview of MET as used in Project MATCH—including client handouts, assessments, and tips for applying MET to other settings—has been provided by Miller et al. (1999b) and is available online free of charge.

The therapy begins with a comprehensive 7- to 8-hour assessment. Following this session, clients receive four individual treatment sessions with a clinician, spread over a period of 12 weeks. Of the four sessions, the first two occur over 2 consecutive weeks and ideally include a significant other as part of the process. These early sessions are meant to provide personalized feedback from the initial assessment, strengthen the client's own commitment to change, elicit feedback and support from the significant other, and make a change plan. The remaining two sessions occur at the midpoint and end point of the treatment period (roughly 6 and 12 weeks after assessment). These sessions help monitor and encourage progress (Miller et al. 1999b). In addition to the MI Spirit and the core skills already discussed (see earlier subsections "Relational Components of Motivational Interviewing" and "Core Skills of Motivational Interviewing"), MET explicitly tethers sessions to personalized feedback based on the comprehensive assessment and provides a menu of choices for how the client might move forward with change. MET can be of benefit to clinicians with limited time or opportunity to elicit change discussions, because it was developed specifically to be a brief intervention with a spread of time in between sessions (Miller et al. 1999b). Brief interventions have been found to have a particularly beneficial impact on alcohol, tobacco, and marijuana use, and when targeting the use of other substances, brief interventions are significantly more effective than a waitlist or no-treatment condition (DiClemente et al. 2017).

Research on Motivational Interviewing

Efficacy

Since the inception of MI, numerous trials have studied MI for its effect on different behaviors. Most reviews have concluded that MI is more effective than no treatment but comparable in efficacy to other psychosocial interventions. For example, in a large meta-analysis, Smedslund et al. (2011) reviewed evidence from 59 trials comparing the efficacy of MI against no treatment, active comparators, or treatment as usual in reducing alcohol and illicit drug use. Their findings were consistent with those from previous reviews (Burke et al. 2003; Lundahl et al. 2010; Rubak et al. 2005) that found MI to be significantly better than no intervention in terms of decreasing substance use immediately following the intervention and at short- and medium-term follow-ups. However, the review of Smedslund et al. (2011) failed to find any long-term effect of MI on substance abuse outcomes (e.g., levels of substance use, treatment retention) among study participants receiving MI in comparison with those receiving treatment as usual and active comparators.

Special Populations

An evaluation of MI for the prevention of alcohol misuse in adolescents (Foxcroft et al. 2016) found that MI was significantly more likely than no intervention to decrease the number of problems related to drinking and the quantity and frequency of alcohol consumption in the short term, although there was no effect on binge drinking. The review failed to find a significant difference in drinking outcomes after 4-month follow-up because MI did not significantly differ from alternative prevention interventions. The effectiveness of MI has been found to be significantly greater in minority populations, including Native Americans and non-white Hispanics, than in the general population (Hettema et al. 2005; Villanueva et al. 2007).

Cost-Effectiveness

Although MI has demonstrated effect sizes similar to those seen with other behavioral interventions, some have argued that MI is preferable to many other behavioral interventions because it requires relatively fewer sessions to demonstrate its effects. For example, in Project MATCH (see subsection "Motivational Enhancement Therapy" above), four MET sessions performed similarly to comparison interventions involving 12 weekly sessions. Also, meta-analyses of trials involving brief interventions (some as brief as 70–90 minutes) that were based on MI principles concluded that these interventions were effective in producing significant improvements in substance use outcomes (i.e., treatment entry, days in treatment, alcohol use) (Dunn et al. 2001; Vasilaki et al. 2006).

Proposed Mechanisms of Action

Two general mechanisms of action have been proposed to explain why the MI approach yields beneficial results (Miller and Rose 2009). The first, termed the *technical model*, postulates that clinician skills that increase a client's talk about change can facilitate shifts in behavior. Self-perception theory has been employed to understand this effect. This theory, grounded in the behavioral model of psychology and propounded by Daryl Bem (1967), models motivation to change as an outgrowth of behaviors that reinforce change. Applied to MI, this theory assumes that clients' speech about the need to change mentally creates and reinforces the desire to change in the individual. As the clinician allows the client to explore his or her ambivalence about a behavior (e.g., alcohol use), the verbalization of the need to decrease the negative behaviors will reinforce the individual's resolve to indeed stop. Theoretical evidence for this hypothesis was found in a trial linking MI-adherent behaviors on the part of the clinician with client change talk and further linking this change talk to decreased drinking days (Magill et al. 2018; Moyers et al. 2009).

The second mechanism of action proposed for MI, termed the *relational model,* postulates that it is not technical behaviors occurring in the interview but rather a general confluence of factors that allows for motivational change. This approach is based in Rogerian thinking (Rogers 1961) that change will occur if the correct conditions are created by the clinician in treatment. One such condition is a supportive, nonthreatening atmosphere in which the client can explore his or her own ambivalence about change. A number of studies have borne out that it is the client-centered, empathetic approach of the clinician, rather than specific clinician behaviors, that most influences drinking outcomes (Magill et al. 2018). A recent secondary analysis showed that both relational and technical elements of MI appear to influence outcomes (Villarosa-Hurlocker et al. 2019).

Motivational Interviewing in Community Practice

The use of MI, since its development, has expanded immensely in the treatment community. Today, many state agencies require the use of MI in SUD and general psychiatric treatment settings, and it is one of the most commonly reported interventions employed by private treatment facilities. For example, in a survey of clinical directors at privately funded substance abuse treatment centers in the United States ($N=345$), 73% of the clinics reporting the use of MI also reported the expectation that all counselors at their programs be proficient in its use (Olmstead et al. 2012).

Training in Motivational Interviewing

Training approaches to MI vary considerably. Studies examining approaches to training include formats ranging from brief 20-minute videos to multiday training programs that include post-workshop training sessions (Madson et al. 2009; Söderlund et al. 2011). A meta-analysis of these studies has found benefit for most training approaches in the immediate term, with improved performance following the training; however, although these are effective for a short period of time, skills deteriorate quickly without booster sessions or ongoing supervision (Walters et al. 2005). Critically, studies have shown that follow-up training sessions that include coaching and/ or feedback can help maintain gains in MI skills after a workshop, although these gains can disappear after several months without such maintenance interventions (Miller et al. 2004). Furthermore, clinician characteristics, such as educational level and verbal proficiency, may guide the optimum approach to post-workshop supervision and coaching efforts (Carpenter et al. 2012). Several issues remain unresolved in terms of training and dissemination, including the more significant cost of providing ongoing training. A trial of three approaches—self-directed learning, "train the trainer," and expert training—found that utilizing an expert trainer to train staff, although more expensive, was also most effective (Olmstead et al. 2011). The significant cost and logistical difficulties of providing expert training remain important barriers to dissemination of high-quality MI in the community. Thus, alternative approaches to ongoing training, such as remote supervision (Smith et al. 2012) and automated ratings and training (Imel et al. 2019), offer promising frameworks for addressing these challenges.

Assessing Motivational Interviewing Fidelity: Rating Scales

The need for a rating system for MI fidelity arises from its nonspecific nature. Unlike with manualized treatments, it is difficult to exactly quantify what is and what is not proper MI practice. Although ratings are important in terms of providing verification of methods in research, they can also play an important role in clinical training and practice in ensuring clinicians' abilities. This is particularly important in light of the disconnect between individuals' actual abilities and their perceptions of their own skill levels. Studies have found little correlation between a clinician's estimation of his or her MI ability and independent ratings of his or her MI skill during counseling sessions (Wain et al. 2015).

Several scales have been developed to measure clinician fidelity to core MI skills and session quality. The first of these, the Motivational Interviewing Skill Code (MISC), was developed in 2001 and requires three "listen-throughs" of a recorded session by an evaluator (Miller et al. 2003). The evaluator rates the clinician using a global score based on 12 session characteristics, 27 behavior counts, and session length. Other coding schemes, such as the Motivational Interviewing Process Code (MIPC; Barsky and Coleman 2001), which provided a framework for systematic observation and evaluation of clinical interviews across 13 MI-consistent dimensions, were developed soon afterward. Due to the complexities of the MISC, a briefer and more efficient rating system was developed using factor analysis to identify the MISC's most relevant components, yielding the Motivational Interviewing Treatment Integrity (MITI) scale. The MITI requires one listen-through of each session and requires the rater to provide ratings of global impression of several elements, along with behavior counts based on the clinician's use of the technical skills (Moyers et al. 2005).

Several additional attempts have been made to develop briefer and more user-friendly measures of clinicians' MI skills through use of standardized prompts. These measures, such as the Video Assessment of Simulated Encounters—Revised (VASE-R; Rosengren et al. 2008), the Computer Assessment of Simulated Patient Interviews (CASPI; Baer et al. 2012), and the Helpful Responses Questionnaire (HRQ; Miller et al. 1991), have been shown to be useful in ascertaining clinician abilities; however, repeated measurement is problematic, a human rater is still required, and the assessments do not capture clinician skill during an actual treatment session. Thus, a rating scale that would allow for the assessment of a clinician's actual in-session skill but would not require a trained rater would greatly assist in implementation of MI in community settings. Attempts also have been made to use natural language processing methods and machine learning to automate the behavioral coding aspects of existing MI rating scales (Atkins et al. 2014; Lord et al. 2015). This approach trains an artificial intelligence program to recognize session quality and replicate the MITI rating system without requiring human input.

Extending Motivational Interviewing Outside the Clinical Office

A small minority of individuals with SUDs will seek help, and even fewer will come into contact with a treatment professional trained in evidence-based treatments (Dimoff et al. 2017; Hasin and Grant 2015). Therefore, the majority of the interactions an individual with an SUD will have will be with nonprofessionals, peers, and family members. There has been growing interest in, as well as data supporting the acceptability and utility of, using community health workers (Dewing et al. 2013) or peer counselors (Shilling et al. 2013) to increase the reach of effective behavioral health programs. MI has been a critical feature of peer-based programs addressing engagement in HIV care among adolescents (Wolfe et al. 2013), adherence to antiviral treatment protocols among HIV-positive patients attending South African (West Cape) clinics (Dewing et al. 2013), heavy drinking among college students (Larimer et al. 2001; Mastroleo et al. 2010), and other mental health issues among older adults (Conner et al. 2015) and military veteran populations (Tsai et al. 2017). Although some studies have provided evidence to suggest that peer counselors can learn MI skills (e.g., reducing use of closed-ended questions) and implement interventions that significantly impact drinking and treatment adherence (Mastroleo et al. 2010), other studies (Dewing et al. 2013; Tsai et al. 2017) have indicated that certain aspects of MI (e.g., decreasing unsolicited advice, facilitating change talk) may be difficult to learn by nonprofessionals. Thus, peer counselors may play an important role in extending the reach of traditionally clinic-based interventions such as MI, although continued work is needed to define the right training structure to help peer counselors to employ the effective communication strategies (e.g., OARS) at a proficient level.

Family systems have also been identified as an important mechanism for addressing motivation in the context of SUDs among children and adults (National Institute on Drug Abuse 2019). Unilateral treatment programs have been developed to help family members implement strategies in their home environment independent of an affected loved one's stage of change and treatment involvement. Such programs have been effective both in enhancing the affected loved one's motivation to seek help and in improving the family members' own well-being. Studies suggest that families can also learn to apply evidence-based treatment strategies as an active adjunct to formal treatment services. For example, Smeerdijk et al. (2014) demonstrated that parents can learn MI skills (e.g., use of affirmations, evocation, empathetic listening) as part of a family support program. Furthermore, when these skills were implemented in the context of parent–child interactions at home, they exerted a significant effect on reducing cannabis use among children who were also receiving treatment for a psychotic disorder (Smeerdijk et al. 2012). In addition, the MI counseling approach has been adapted for use in self-guided programs that aim to help individuals resolve their ambivalence toward change outside of clinical settings (Zuckoff and Gorscak 2015). Together, these findings are encouraging because they highlight the potential utility of MI when placed in the context of self-help efforts and the helping repertoire of peers and family members, which are the types of situations and relationships that will define the majority of interpersonal interactions that individuals will have throughout the process of change. Although further research is needed to elucidate the best methods for training peers and family in MI, these initial studies suggest that the use of strategies for enhancing motivation need not be limited to clinical settings, but rather can be disseminated among clients' wider social networks, thereby increasing the likelihood that interpersonal interactions can be of help as they navigate the dynamic shifts in their personal motivation throughout the process of change.

Conclusion

The conceptualization of motivation and its relationship to the change process has varied over time. However, motivation has remained a critical issue, both for individuals struggling with substance use disorders and for their family members and treatment providers. Studies have highlighted the significant role that interpersonal interactions play in influencing an individual's motivation to change. Motivational interviewing (MI), a collaborative and empathetic counseling style aimed at helping individuals resolve their ambivalence about change, has demonstrated efficacy in reducing substance use in both clinical and nonclinical settings. Learning MI requires the acquisition of a core set of conversational skills for implementation in the context of a collaborative and person-centered therapeutic stance, as well as an awareness of and proficiency in four counseling processes aimed at moving the person toward increased openness to change. Furthermore, ongoing practice and feedback are critical components of training for clinicians and others who desire to build and maintain competency in this approach to helping others.

References

Amrhein PC: How does Motivational Interviewing work? What client talk reveals. Journal of Cognitive Psychotherapy 18(4):323–336, 2004. Available at: https://connect.springer-pub.com/content/sgrjcp/18/4/323. Accessed January 15, 2020.

Amrhein PC, Miller WR, Yahne CE, et al: Client commitment language during motivational interviewing predicts drug use outcomes. J Consult Clin Psychol 71(5):862–878, 2003 14516235

Ariss T, Fairbairn CE: The effect of significant other involvement in treatment for substance use disorders: a meta-analysis. J Consult Clin Psychol 88(6):526–540, 2020 32162930

Atkins DC, Steyvers M, Imel ZE, et al: Scaling up the evaluation of psychotherapy: evaluating motivational interviewing fidelity via statistical text classification. Implement Sci 9:49, 2014 24758152

Baer JS, Carpenter KM, Beadnell B, et al: Computer Assessment of Simulated Patient Interviews (CASPI): psychometric properties of a web-based system for the assessment of motivational interviewing skills. J Stud Alcohol Drugs 73(1):154–164, 2012 22152673

Barsky A, Coleman H: Evaluating skill acquisition in motivational interviewing: the development of an instrument to measure practice skills. J Drug Educ 31(1):69–82, 2001 11338966

Bem D: Self-perception: an alternative interpretation of cognitive dissonance phenomena. Psychological Review 74(3):183–200, 1967. Available at: https://psycnet.apa.org/doiLanding?doi=10.1037%2Fh0024835. Accessed January 16, 2020.

Brigham GS, Slesnick N, Winhusen TM, et al: A randomized pilot clinical trial to evaluate the efficacy of Community Reinforcement and Family Training for Treatment Retention (CRAFT-T) for improving outcomes for patients completing opioid detoxification. Drug Alcohol Depend 138:240–243, 2014 24656054

Burke BL, Arkowitz H, Menchola M: The efficacy of motivational interviewing: a meta-analysis of controlled clinical trials. J Consult Clin Psychol 71(5):843–861, 2003 14516234

Carpenter KM, Cheng WY, Smith JL, et al: "Old dogs" and new skills: how clinician characteristics relate to motivational interviewing skills before, during, and after training. J Consult Clin Psychol 80(4):560–573, 2012 22563640

Conner KO, McKinnon SA, Ward CJ, et al: Peer education as a strategy for reducing internalized stigma among depressed older adults. Psychiatr Rehabil J 38(2):186–193, 2015 25915057

Dewing S, Mathews C, Cloete A, et al: From research to practice: lay adherence counsellors' fidelity to an evidence-based intervention for promoting adherence to antiretroviral treatment in the Western Cape, South Africa. AIDS Behav 17(9):2935–2945, 2013 23666183

DiClemente CC, Corno CM, Graydon MM, et al: Motivational interviewing, enhancement, and brief interventions over the last decade: a review of reviews of efficacy and effectiveness. Psychol Addict Behav 31(8):862–887, 2017 29199843

Dimoff JD, Sayette MA, Norcross JC: Addiction training in clinical psychology: are we keeping up with the rising epidemic? Am Psychol 72(7):689–695, 2017 29016172

Dunn C, Deroo L, Rivara FP: The use of brief interventions adapted from motivational interviewing across behavioral domains: a systematic review. Addiction 96(12):1725–1742, 2001 11784466

Foxcroft DR, Coombes L, Wood S, et al: Motivational interviewing for the prevention of alcohol misuse in young adults. Cochrane Database Syst Rev (7):CD007025, 2016 27426026

Hasin DS, Grant BF: The National Epidemiologic Survey on Alcohol and Related Conditions (NESARC) Waves 1 and 2: review and summary of findings. Soc Psychiatry Psychiatr Epidemiol 50(11):1609–1640, 2015 26210739

Hettema J, Steele J, Miller WR: Motivational interviewing. Annu Rev Clin Psychol 1:91–111, 2005 17716083

Higgins ST, Silverman K: Motivating Behavior Change Among Illicit-Drug Abusers: Research on Contingency Management Interventions. Washington, DC, American Psychological Association, 1999

Imel ZE, Pace BT, Soma CS, et al: Design feasibility of an automated, machine-learning based feedback system for motivational interviewing. Psychotherapy (Chic) 56(2):318–328, 2019 30958018

Johnson VE: Intervention: How to Help Someone Who Doesn't Want Help. Minneapolis, MN, Hazelden Foundation, 1986

Larimer ME, Turner AP, Anderson BK, et al: Evaluating a brief alcohol intervention with fraternities. J Stud Alcohol 62(3):370–380, 2001 11414347

Liepman MR, Nirenberg TD, Begin AM: Evaluation of a program designed to help family and significant others to motivate resistant alcoholics into recovery. Am J Drug Alcohol Abuse 15(2):209–221, 1989 2729227

Lord SP, Sheng E, Imel ZE, et al: More than reflections: empathy in motivational interviewing includes language style synchrony between therapist and client. Behav Ther 46(3):296–303, 2015 25892166

Lundahl BW, Kunz C, Brownell C, et al: A meta-analysis of motivational interviewing: twenty-five years of empirical studies. Research on Social Work Practice 20(2):137–160, 2010. Available at: https://journals.sagepub.com/doi/10.1177/1049731509347850. Accessed January 16, 2020.

Madson MB, Loignon AC, Lane C: Training in motivational interviewing: a systematic review. J Subst Abuse Treat 36(1):101–109, 2009 18657936

Magill M, Apodaca TR, Borsari B, et al: A meta-analysis of motivational interviewing process: technical, relational, and conditional process models of change. J Consult Clin Psychol 86(2):140–157, 2018 29265832

Manuel JK, Austin JL, Miller WR, et al: Community Reinforcement and Family Training: a pilot comparison of group and self-directed delivery. J Subst Abuse Treat 43(1):129–136, 2012 22154038

Mastroleo NR, Turrisi R, Carney JV, et al: Examination of posttraining supervision of peer counselors in a motivational enhancement intervention to reduce drinking in a sample of heavy-drinking college students. J Subst Abuse Treat 39(3):289–297, 2010 20673621

Miller WR, Rollnick S (eds): Motivational Interviewing: Helping People Change, 3rd Edition. New York, Guilford, 2013

Miller WR, Rose GS: Toward a theory of motivational interviewing. Am Psychol 64(6):527–537, 2009 19739882

Miller WR, Hedrick KE, Orlofsky DR: The Helpful Responses Questionnaire: a procedure for measuring therapeutic empathy. J Clin Psychol 47(3):444–448, 1991 2066417

Miller WR, Benefield RG, Tonigan JS: Enhancing motivation for change in problem drinking: a controlled comparison of two therapist styles. J Consult Clin Psychol 61(3):455–461, 1993 8326047

Miller WR, Meyers RJ, Tonigan JS: Engaging the unmotivated in treatment for alcohol problems: a comparison of three strategies for intervention through family members. J Consult Clin Psychol 67(5):688–697, 1999a 10535235

Miller WR, Zweben A, DiClemente CC, et al: Motivational Enhancement Therapy Manual: A Clinical Research Guide for Therapists Treating Individuals With Alcohol Abuse and Dependence, Vol 2. National Institute on Alcohol Abuse and Alcoholism, 1999b. Available at: https://motivationalinterviewing.org/sites/default/files/MATCH.pdf. Accessed December 3, 2019.

Miller WR, Moyers TB, Ernst D, Amrhein P: Manual for the motivational interviewing skill code (MISC). Unpublished manuscript. Albuquerque, NM, Center on Alcoholism, Substance Abuse and Addictions, University of New Mexico, 2003

Miller WR, Yahne CE, Moyers TB, et al: A randomized trial of methods to help clinicians learn motivational interviewing. J Consult Clin Psychol 72(6):1050–1062, 2004 15612851

Moyers TB, Miller WR: Is low therapist empathy toxic? Psychol Addict Behav 27(3):878–884, 2013 23025709

Moyers TB, Martin T, Manuel JK, et al: Assessing competence in the use of motivational interviewing. J Subst Abuse Treat 28(1):19–26, 2005 15723728

Moyers TB, Martin T, Houck JM, et al: From in-session behaviors to drinking outcomes: a causal chain for motivational interviewing. J Consult Clin Psychol 77(6):1113–1124, 2009 19968387

National Institute on Drug Abuse: Principles of Drug Addiction Treatment: A Research-based Guide, 3rd Edition (NIH Publ No 12-4180). Revised December 2012. Available at: https://www.drugabuse.gov/publications/principles-drug-addiction-treatment-research-based-guide-third-edition/preface. Accessed July 13, 2020.

National Institute on Drug Abuse: Treatment Approaches for Drug Addiction DrugFacts. January 2019. Available at: https://www.drugabuse.gov/publications/drugfacts/treatment-approaches-drug-addiction. Accessed July 1, 2020.

Olmstead T, Carroll KM, Canning-Ball M, et al: Cost and cost-effectiveness of three strategies for training clinicians in motivational interviewing. Drug Alcohol Depend 116(1–3):195–202, 2011 21277713

Olmstead TA, Abraham AJ, Martino S, et al: Counselor training in several evidence-based psychosocial addiction treatments in private U.S. substance abuse treatment centers. Drug Alcohol Depend 120(1–3):149–154, 2012 21831536

Prochaska JO, DiClemente CC: Stages and processes of self-change of smoking: toward an integrative model of change. J Consult Clin Psychol 51(3):390–395, 1983 6863699

Rogers C: On Becoming a Person: A Therapist's View of Psychotherapy. Boston, Houghton Mifflin, 1961

Rosengren DB, Hartzler B, Baer JS, et al: The Video Assessment of Simulated Encounters–Revised (VASE-R): reliability and validity of a revised measure of motivational interviewing skills. Drug Alcohol Depend 97(1–2):130–138, 2008 18499356

Rubak S, Sandbaek A, Lauritzen T, et al: Motivational interviewing: a systematic review and meta-analysis. Br J Gen Pract 55(513):305–312, 2005 15826439

Shilling V, Morris C, Thompson-Coon J, et al: Peer support for parents of children with chronic disabling conditions: a systematic review of quantitative and qualitative studies. Dev Med Child Neurol 55(7):602–609, 2013 23421818

Smedslund G, Berg RC, Hammerstrøm KT, et al: Motivational interviewing for substance abuse. Cochrane Database Syst Rev (5):CD008063, 2011 21563163

Smeerdijk M, Keet R, Dekker N, et al: Motivational interviewing and interaction skills training for parents to change cannabis use in young adults with recent-onset schizophrenia: a randomized controlled trial. Psychol Med 42(8):1627–1636, 2012 22152121

Smeerdijk M, Keet R, de Haan L, et al: Feasibility of teaching motivational interviewing to parents of young adults with recent-onset schizophrenia and co-occurring cannabis use. J Subst Abuse Treat 46(3):340–345, 2014 24157087

Smith JL, Carpenter KM, Amrhein PC, et al: Training substance abuse clinicians in motivational interviewing using live supervision via teleconferencing. J Consult Clin Psychol 80(3):450–464, 2012 22506795

Söderlund LL, Madson MB, Rubak S, et al: A systematic review of motivational interviewing training for general health care practitioners. Patient Educ Couns 84(1):16–26, 2011 20667432

Substance Abuse and Mental Health Services Administration: Key Substance Use and Mental Health Indicators in the United States: Results From the 2017 National Survey on Drug Use and Health (HHS Publ. No. SMA 18-5068, NSDUH Series H-53). Rockville, MD, Center for Behavioral Health Statistics and Quality, SAMHSA, 2018. Available at: https://www.samhsa.gov/data/sites/default/files/cbhsq-reports/NSDUHFFR2017/NSDUHFFR2017.pdf. Accessed June 25, 2020.

Tsai J, Klee A, Shea N, et al: Training peer specialists with mental illness in motivational interviewing: a pilot study. Psychiatr Rehabil J 40(4):354–360, 2017 27786521

Vasilaki EI, Hosier SG, Cox WM: The efficacy of motivational interviewing as a brief intervention for excessive drinking: a meta-analytic review. Alcohol Alcohol 41(3):328–335, 2006 16547122

Villanueva M, Tonigan JS, Miller WR: Response of Native American clients to three treatment methods for alcohol dependence. J Ethn Subst Abuse 6(2):41–48, 2007 18192203

Villarosa-Hurlocker MC, O'Sickey AJ, Houck JM, et al: Examining the influence of active ingredients of motivational interviewing on client change talk. J Subst Abuse Treat 96:39–45, 2019 30466547

Wain RM, Kutner BA, Smith JL, et al: Self-report after randomly assigned supervision does not predict ability to practice motivational interviewing. J Subst Abuse Treat 57:96–101, 2015 25963775

Walters ST, Matson SA, Baer JS, et al: Effectiveness of workshop training for psychosocial addiction treatments: a systematic review. J Subst Abuse Treat 29(4):283–293, 2005 16311181

White WL: Slaying the Dragon: The History of Addiction Treatment and Recovery in America, 2nd Edition. Bloomington, IL, Chestnut Health Systems, 2014

White WL, Miller WR: The use of confrontation in addiction treatment: history, science, and time for change. Counselor (Deerfield Beach) 8(4):12–30, 2007. Available at: http://www.williamwhitepapers.com/pr/2007ConfrontationinAddictionTreatment.pdf. Accessed January 16, 2020.

Wolfe H, Haller DL, Benoit E, et al: Developing PeerLink to engage out-of-care HIV+ substance users: training peers to deliver a peer-led motivational intervention with fidelity. AIDS Care 25(7):888–894, 2013 23230862

Zuckoff A, Gorscak B: Finding Your Way to Change: How the Power of Motivational Interviewing Can Reveal What You Want and Help You Get There. New York, Guilford, 2015

CHAPTER 26

Alcoholics Anonymous and Twelve-Step Facilitation

Richard K. Ries, M.D.

The goal of this chapter is to help clinicians better engage and support patients with co-occurring or primary alcohol or drug problems through use of 12-step programs to enhance treatment outcomes and recovery. "Twelve-step programs" refers to Alcoholics Anonymous (AA) and its spin-offs—Narcotics Anonymous (NA), Cocaine Anonymous (CA), and others that are based on the 12 steps to recovery elucidated in the original Alcoholics Anonymous meetings and "Big Book," developed in the 1930s in the eastern United States. Currently, there are more than 100,000 different AA meetings a week in the United States, and lesser numbers of NA, CA, and other "Anonymous" meetings. Meetings can be found in almost all countries of the world, are led by their own members, do not involve cross-talk, and generally follow the 12 steps and 12 traditions of AA (www.aa.org/pages/en_US/index). Meetings can occur throughout the day, but most are in the evenings and last 60–90 minutes. McCrady and Tonnigan (2014) have provided a detailed discussion of Anonymous programs and the research base supporting these programs, and an updated Cochrane review has demonstrated the efficacy of 12-step programs (Kelly et al. 2020).

Twelve-step facilitation (TSF) is an evidence-based intervention program with a large research base; a therapy manual (Nowinski et al. 1992, 1999); a web-based training site (Sholomskas and Carroll 2006); and an adaptation, with a manual, for group work with stimulant users (Daley et al. 2011). TSF is a valuable therapeutic program that is easily accessible to practicing psychiatrists and other mental health professionals, and both research and practice reveal that active referral makes a difference (Donovan and Floyd 2008; Manning et al. 2012).

TSF has been demonstrated to be very helpful to many individuals. Fifteen percent of the general population may be diagnosed with a substance use disorder (SUD) (13% with alcohol abuse, with or without other drug abuse) at some time in their lives (Kessler et al. 2005), and somewhere between 20% and 50% of typical psychiatric inpatients or outpatients will have a current, episodic, or past history of an SUD (Center for Substance Abuse Treatment 2005). For example, approximately 50% of patients with bipolar disorder will experience alcohol or drug problems, and research has shown that those with active substance use are more likely to be nonadherent to medication and to experience a wide variety of other problems, including suicide attempts and more frequent decompensations (Comtois et al. 2004). Research has shown that these problems improve with sobriety and that 12-step involvement enhances medication adherence (Weiss et al. 2005). Furthermore, Worley et al. (2012) reported that compared with a cognitive-behavioral approach, TSF improved depression independently of substance-related outcomes for depressed patients with SUDs. When treating a patient with a comorbid mental disorder who has relapsed to or developed an SUD, the clinician is faced with several options: try to manage the patient on his or her own, refer the patient for outside substance use treatment while continuing to treat him or her, or refer the patient to another service or an addiction specialist for management of both disorders. In our experience, many clinicians would rather continue working with most of their patients; however, many assess their weekly, biweekly, or monthly visits as just not potent enough to deal with an active addiction as well as a comorbid mental disorder.

For patients who have developed a severe SUD, have lost control, and are at serious risk for adverse consequences, referral to a specialized inpatient or outpatient program may be the best choice. However, many patients may have a less severe SUD or may not want addiction treatment to show up on their insurance or health records. Furthermore, participating in concurrent, outside professional treatment may present other problems, including problems with cost, location, transportation, time, and potentially conflicting treatment messages. Even if outside referral is made but the patient returns when stable, there is a good chance that 12-step programs will be part of the patient's ongoing treatment plan. In any case, almost all residential treatment programs in the United States have a strong 12-step orientation and are geared toward the patient's continuation with 12-step attendance after discharge.

Adding Twelve-Step Facilitation to Ongoing Psychiatric Treatment

A typical treatment plan would include integration of the patient's usual psychiatric therapy and medications with the principles, content, and support offered in 12-step meetings such as AA and NA. TSF is a method for helping the patient both get to and productively use 12-step meetings, as well as a way for the clinician to learn and use key concepts about 12-step meetings as part of overall therapy. This integrated treatment plan, which is not indicated or possible for all individuals, has some significant advantages in terms of its impact on addictions: no or low cost, ready availability in most communities, anonymity to insurance and others, long-term support that will not go away with a change or end in insurance benefits, and, importantly, an ongoing relationship with the treating clinician. Patients with comorbid alcohol use disorder and psychiatric disorders may have become socially isolated and will benefit from 12-step meetings' social support, particularly support that does not endorse substance use. For example, research in individuals with alcohol use disorder has shown that compared with support from a patient's own family, nondrinking support from other 12-step meeting participants is associated with over three times greater abstinence (Kaskutas et al. 2002). Addiction treatment programs that are 12-step based have been shown to yield reduced costs in continuing care (Humphreys and Moos 2007). Further evidence of the benefit of 12-step-oriented approaches in treatment programs was provided by Morgenstern (2004), who found that promotion of a 12-step orientation was associated with a greater decrease in substance use at 6 months posttreatment than was the use of cognitive-behavioral therapy; this finding was also supported by the recent Cochrane meta-analysis of Kelly et al. (2020).

Furthermore, 12-step programs endorse taking personal responsibility for one's own recovery behavior, relinquishing denial of illness (denial of illness also occurs for many psychiatric disorders), and helping others to recover (thus developing both empathy and self-esteem). These elements of 12-step recovery are applicable to treatment of and recovery from psychiatric disorders, in addition to addiction recovery (Minkoff 1989). Nevertheless, patients and physicians may resist this approach because of some common misperceptions, including beliefs that 12-step programs oppose use of medication and require certain religious beliefs.

Starting Out

The first step in helping patients go to 12-step meetings is for clinicians to work on a simple program to enhance their own familiarity with meetings as well as 12-step content. There are three easy ways to do this:

1. *Read AA material.* Introductory material is available at the AA website (www.aa.org) or in print. After reading through this material, the clinician will be in a much stronger position for referring patients to AA and the website because the clinician will be able to talk about his or her actual experience with this material and with this site. Basic orientation requires 15–30 minutes. Other material is on the website, including *Alcoholics Anonymous*, the "Big Book" of AA, now in its fourth edition (Alcoholics Anonymous World Services 2001). Printed materials can be obtained by calling a local AA phone number. This same approach applies to NA materials (www.na.org).
2. *Read the TSF manual.* The *Twelve Step Facilitation Therapy Manual* (Nowinski et al. 1999) can be obtained online (https://pubs.niaaa.nih.gov/publications/project-match/match01.pdf) or in print from the National Institute on Alcohol Abuse and Alcoholism.
3. *Go to a meeting as a professional guest.* There is no better way to learn about AA (or other 12-step programs) than by going to an actual meeting as a professional guest. A clinician merely needs to call the AA phone number in virtually any telephone directory throughout the United States (and many other countries) and

identify him- or herself as a doctor or other health care provider who would like a guide to take him or her to a local AA meeting as a professional guest. Most AA communities have standing committees of members whose job it is to do this, and often some of them are recovering health care professionals themselves. Many communities now also have online virtual meetings, and these can be found by calling the AA, NA or other Intergroup numbers (which are easily located via an online search) or by accessing local websites.

Core Elements of the Twelve-Step Facilitation Manual

Much of the material that follows is adapted from the *Twelve Step Facilitation Therapy Manual* (Nowinski et al. 1999; see also Carroll 2018). What is offered here might be considered a primer for the manual, with editorial comments and additions for psychiatrists regarding treating patients with co-occurring addiction and other psychiatric disorders. In addition, we have included some references to other "self-help" groups as well as to issues related to opioids in the last section of this chapter. In Project MATCH (Matching Alcoholism Treatments to Client Heterogeneity), TSF was designed to be implemented in 12 sequential sessions over about 3 months. However, for the practicing psychiatric clinician, it is more likely that real-world TSF will occur off and on over the course of patients' treatment, which for some may be weeks or months and for others may be years.

Acceptance

The first step of AA—admitting that one is powerless over alcohol and that one's life has become unmanageable—may seem daunting to some patients and even to some clinicians.

Providing a corollary to this first step for patients with other psychiatric disorders can be useful. For example, in the case of bipolar disorder, this admission might read as follows: "I came to believe I was powerless over untreated bipolar disorder and my life had become unmanageable." Dual Recovery Anonymous (DRA) (1993–2009), or "Double Trouble," is a 12-step program for persons with comorbid addiction and other psychiatric disorders. The first of DRA's 12 steps reads as follows: "We admitted we were powerless over our dual illness of chemical dependency and emotional or psychiatric illness—that our lives had become unmanageable."

Most psychiatrists are familiar with the patient with a mental disorder (e.g., depression, mania, schizophrenia) who understands that he or she has a disorder, accepts it, and does everything in his or her power to stay well, but over time comes to believe that he or she no longer has the disorder and then decreases or stops taking medications and receiving therapy and decompensates to the disorder. The same process can hold for individuals with addictions. Clinical experience shows that relapsing back into denial of illness happens for both psychiatric and addiction disorders and is not something that is dealt with once for all time. Quite often, denial can creep back intermittently and lead to serious problems. By continually concentrating on acceptance of illness, 12-step members re-inoculate themselves against denial. For example, each time members of AA, DRA, or another 12-step program speak in meetings, they introduce themselves by saying "Hi, my name is Rick, and I am a recovering alcoholic." In dual-disorder AA or DRA meetings, the speaker might say, "Hi, my name is Rick, and I am a recovering bipolar alcoholic." The power in this phrase is its direct challenge to denial; 12-step meetings strongly emphasize that denial can re-emerge if it is not actively and regularly challenged. AA further endorses the strong message that although an individual may not be responsible for his or her genetics or illness, the person is very much responsible for engaging in recovery behaviors, and this extends to psychiatric treatment and recovery as well.

Cognitions

Both addictions and other psychiatric conditions may affect cognition or cause patients to display denial in different ways. For example, grandiosity in mania leads the patient to believe that he or she "knows better" and can handle anything, whereas nihilism in depression leads the patient to believe that he or she is not worth treatment and that nothing matters anyway. Alcohol or drugs may magnify either of these cognitive distortions as well as disinhibiting actions around the cognitions, such as suicide or violence toward others.

Emotions

A version of the AA view of emotions and how to deal with them is described in Topic 8, HALT (**H**ungry, **A**ngry, **L**onely, **T**ired), of the TSF manual (Nowinski et al. 1999, pp. 79–86) but is too lengthy to fully review here. It may be surprising to the reader to find that many elements of Marlatt and Gordon's (1985) relapse prevention and Linehan's (1993) dialectical behavioral therapy have a good deal of overlap with AA content and principles in terms of analyzing how certain emotions lead to certain behaviors and how to handle them.

HALT is an AA mnemonic and slogan that not only captures common emotional relapse states but also suggests action, as in "HALT before you do something you do not really want to do." This model is quite compatible with the cognitive-behavioral approach that many therapists apply in treating addictive or other psychiatric disorders. When reviewing psychiatric symptoms or substance use or craving since a patient's previous visit, the psychiatrist might integrate the HALT mnemonic by asking, "Have there been any episodes of feeling hungry, angry, lonely, or tired since your last visit, and did these affect either your drug craving or your psychiatric condition, and if so, how did you handle them?" By using the AA verbiage, the psychiatrist is indicating to the patient that he or she supports AA and that the psychiatrist's therapy is meant to be integrated with what the patient is getting through AA.

In the treatment of patients with co-occurring disorders, the term *self-medication* may emerge as a patient's self-reported behavioral strategy for dealing with his or her emotions or illness, or it may even be invoked by some clinicians. Unfortunately, this term has the potential to confuse both the psychiatrist and the patient. Virtually all research conducted on the matter shows that abuse or dependent use of substances makes major psychiatric disorders worse, resulting in increased symptoms, decompensation, emergency room visits, and homelessness—none of which would be desired as "medication" outcomes (Center for Substance Abuse Treatment 2005). Furthermore, patients who invoke the term *self-medication* have an increased likelihood of suicidal ideation and suicide attempts (Bolton et al. 2006). In fact, research has shown that when an individual with bipolar disorder who is in a manic state claims to be self-medicating, he or she is most likely aiming to become even more euphoric, and that patients who use the term *self-medication* have worse prognoses for recovery (Weiss 2004). Such terminology allows concrete-thinking patients to say to themselves, "Well, the psychiatrist said I self-medicated, so I guess I will take his medications [lithium, antipsychotics, etc.] on Monday through Friday and my medications [crack and alcohol] on the weekend. After all, it's all medication."

Social Issues

Identifying persons who are supportive of recovery and avoiding those who are not are important elements of TSF. Such awareness is especially important in choosing certain AA meetings that may be more supportive of co-occurring issues and in selecting a sponsor. If an individual has comorbidities, the sponsor either should also have co-occurring disorders or should be supportive and understanding of these issues. In larger communities, most local meeting schedules list dual-disorder meetings.

Spirituality

Spirituality has been defined as "that which gives people meaning and purpose in life" (Puchalski et al. 2004, p. 689). The element of spirituality is what distinguishes AA from orientations that approach addiction recovery solely on the basis of physical and behavioral consequences of disease, as well as from formal religious practices (Galanter 2007). The book *Alcoholics Anonymous* repeatedly mentions a "program of recovery" and associates recovery with terms such as *spiritual experience* and *spiritual awakening* (Alcoholics Anonymous World Services 1976). A spiritual orientation is inherent in four of the steps, which include the word *God*. However, both of the key AA texts (Alcoholics Anonymous World Services 1976, 1984) dedicate great effort to differentiating traditional concepts of God from the AA spiritual concept of a higher power.

Both *spirituality* and *God* can have many different meanings, and either word can attract or repel individuals, depending on their associations. A patient who balks at a specific interpretation of these terms might be open to working under another interpretation. During discussions with a patient about his or her previous experiences with 12-step programs (or simply about what he or she might have heard about them), the issue of God or the spiritual element in these programs usually comes up fairly quickly. (Special care needs to be taken in working with psychotic patients who experience religious delusions.) The clinician should try to explore the person's associations to key words by using open-ended questions:

- What do you know or think about the term *spirituality*? How do you think it is used in AA [or another 12-step program the individual may have attended or heard about]?
- How about the term *higher power*? Has this concept ever been helpful to you? If not, let's see if we can figure out how it might be helpful. What is the difference to you between the terms *higher power* and *God*?

- Your addiction to alcohol/drugs, by definition, has been stronger than your own willpower. Do you recognize your dependence as a power greater than yourself? If so, then what are some examples of this?
- Recovery from this substance dependence has clearly been "greater than yourself," since you have not been able to attain it on your own, even after numerous tries. What does this mean to you?
- The wisdom and experience from those in 12-step meetings with successful long-term recovery are clearly greater than your own. Are you willing to use this help? Is this a power greater than yourself?

When speaking with an individual who seems resistant to discussing God, the clinician may find it helpful to explain that use of the term *God* is not a requirement for membership in AA or other 12-step programs and that some individuals prefer to use the terms *my higher power* or *the power of my AA group*. In fact, most larger communities have agnostic and atheist AA groups. In the context of the 12-step process, spirituality can be thought of as the willingness to change. It can also be defined as connectedness with other people and with what is meaningful in a person's life.

"Wreckage of the Past"

Analyzing and understanding the "wreckage of the past"—a typical AA phrase—should be navigated as part of taking a good history for both addiction and other psychiatric issues. The purpose is to help challenge the patient's denial. Although AA steps make it clear that the cocaine-abusing patient who sold his or her parents' television should acknowledge substance use problems and make restitution, a trickier situation is the manic patient who by choice cuts down on medications to "get an edge" and then spends the entire limit of the family's credit cards on unnecessary, impulsive items. Is the latter scenario an illness issue, a moral issue, or both? The AA approach says that although an individual may not be responsible for having the illness, he or she is very responsible for managing its recovery. Facing up to the wreckage of the past, whether from addictions, other psychiatric disorders, or both, is a basic part of recovery. Although restitution of money or other concrete objects can be made, self-forgiveness for hurting others, such as in the examples above, is more difficult. The individual and the therapist must work together on this task.

Role of the Therapist

The primary role of the TSF therapist is as a facilitator of the patient's acceptance of his or her SUD and of the patient's commitment to the fellowship of a 12-step program as the preferred path of recovery. However, when the facilitator is also a psychiatric practitioner (and often a prescriber as well), explaining the nature of co-occurring psychiatric illnesses, medications, and other therapies is also important (this becomes TSF-COD [Co-Occurring Disorders]).

The psychiatric practitioner can productively use the patient's attendance and participation at 12-step meetings and the patient's understanding of the meeting discussions as therapeutic material for both addiction and other psychiatric disorders. With such discussion, the psychiatrist is both demonstrating support for the patient's attending meetings and helping the patient to integrate the material. The clinician should keep in mind that first-time attendees or patients with social anxiety may be reluctant to speak or meet with other members. Basic meeting-involvement coaching might include asking questions such as the following: What meetings did you attend since the last session? Did you arrive early, on time, or late for meetings? Where exactly were the meetings? Where did you sit? Did you stay for the whole meeting? Were you able to pay attention the whole time?

Discussion of the patient's answers to these questions may uncover resistance and nonattendance as well as psychiatric problems that might be interfering with attendance, such as paranoia or social phobia. Dealing with the causes of nonattendance and resistance then becomes part of the therapeutic work, which can include use of medications, motivational interviewing, cognitive-behavioral techniques, or other specific cognitive approaches. Initiation of a discussion about AA involvement using such approaches is briefly illustrated below:

- *Motivational interviewing:* So, you thought about going to a meeting last night but didn't quite get there…. What do you think you might have gained if you had gone? What would have been the downside of going?
- *Cognitive-behavioral therapies and AA facilitation:* So, you thought about going to a meeting last night but didn't quite get there…. Let's examine what you said to yourself to convince yourself not to go, and then work out a strategy to get you there next time.
- *Twelve-step disease model facilitation:* So, you thought about going to a meeting last night but didn't quite get there…. What was responsible for your not getting there—was it you, or was it your disease? That kind of experience is the illness at work; it's the disease that tells you that you don't have a disease. Who is someone you could have called?
- *More detailed attendance questions:* Did you offer to help with setup or cleanup at the meeting? Did you talk to anyone before or after the meeting? What were some key issues you heard discussed at the meeting? How did these issues apply to you? Did you say something in the meeting? What was it like to talk or want to talk, but be unable or afraid to talk? Let's rehearse right here what you could say.
- *An example of a specific co-occurring disorders intervention (panic disorder and social phobia):* So, you thought about going to a meeting last night but were afraid you would panic if you were called on, so you didn't go. Let's work out a strategy (see Tonigan et al. 2010):
  - Prescribe a medication for social phobia (e.g., selective serotonin reuptake inhibitor, gabapentin). Note that an alcoholic patient should not receive benzodiazepines for anxiety management (see Alcoholics Anonymous World Services 1984; Wolitzky-Taylor et al. 2011).
  - Help the patient rehearse something very simple to say in meetings (in the patient's own words), with visualization, such as "Hi, I'm Rick, and I'm glad to be here." Have the patient carry a written card or write this phrase on his or her hand. Rehearse this again and again in session and have the patient practice at home.

– Let the patient know that there is no requirement for individuals to say anything during meetings; even if called on, he or she can just pass. For highly anxious performance-challenged patients, a 10- to 20-mg dose of propranolol before meetings may help, until the patient is more comfortable.

Naturally, a number of other types of issues can arise with respect to initiating AA treatment. Table 26–1 presents some common problems and offers solutions that may guide a clinician in his or her facilitation of AA participation. Table 26–2 provides specific questions and topics whose discussion can further help to facilitate a patient's involvement in treatment.

Sponsors

Sponsors are more senior AA members who help newer members to understand and "work" the 12-step program. Sponsors are a key part of 12-step recovery; experienced members sometimes volunteer to be sponsors to new members, or new members may ask a more senior member to be their "temporary" sponsor. Some clinicians choose to meet the patient's sponsor so that the sponsor and clinician can be sure that they are on the same side and are providing consistent information to the individual seeking treatment. Such a meeting would occur only with the patient's approval and only during a session with the patient present. Other clinicians prefer not to meet the patient's sponsor, but it is still important to encourage a constructive relationship between patient and sponsor. A patient may not feel comfortable with the original choice of sponsor and may discuss this in therapy. If such a discussion takes place, the therapist can explore the patient's concerns; this discussion may help the patient to relate more comfortably to his or her sponsor or to decide to find a new sponsor.

Some patients are resistant to the idea of getting a sponsor, and this can be a problem. For those with more serious psychiatric disorders, it is best, but not absolutely necessary, that their sponsors also have co-occurring disorders. If the sponsor has personal experience with co-occurring disorders, then problems relating to psychiatric diagnosis, symptoms, and treatments, especially medications, are usually avoided, and psychiatric treatments will be reinforced rather than resisted by the sponsor. Patients are more likely to meet sponsors who are similar to them by going to DRA, dual-diagnosis AA meetings, or other variants of 12-step meetings that focus on persons with co-occurring disorders. Many AA schedules in larger communities even list dual diagnosis as a qualifier for certain meetings.

Other Self-Help Groups and Issues Related to Opioids

Although the Anonymous programs are ubiquitous in most communities and are the most widely available of the self-help groups, there are a growing number of alternatives. One fairly widespread group is SMART Recovery (www.smartrecovery.org), which is more cognitive-behaviorally based, and certain patients prefer the language

TABLE 26–1. Engaging individuals with Alcoholics Anonymous (AA) resistance

Problem	Solution
The patient has had previous bad experiences with treatment for alcohol dependence, and AA is guilty by association.	Explore these issues and interpret the resistance of guilt by association.
The patient has had a previous bad experience with AA directly (e.g., he or she might have met someone at a meeting and then drunk with him or her; the patient might have gone to a meeting and felt that he or she did not fit in with the other attendees).	Explore what happened and the patient's role in this. Talk about matching meetings to the patient.
The patient has had a previous bad experience due to symptoms of co-occurring psychiatric problems (e.g., social phobia, paranoia).	Explore this, and explain that you will help the patient develop a strategy to deal with these symptoms. Explain to the patient that an AA meeting is about the safest place there is to exhibit symptoms publicly because it is a supportive and nonconfrontational environment.
The patient has had very little previous experience with AA, but stopped attending meetings, used alcohol or drugs, and concluded that meetings "don't work."	Explain that the patient's previous attendance and involvement could not be considered an adequate "dose." Illustrate this point with one of the following analogies, selecting the analogy that the patient is most likely to hear or understand, given his or her clinical history: • *Antibiotic model:* Would it be safe to conclude that an antibiotic was ineffective after taking only one-third of the dose for only one-third of the time prescribed? • *Diabetes model:* Would it be safe to conclude that a diabetes treatment was ineffective after taking the medicine only half the time and eating chocolate cake between doses? • *Bipolar model:* Would it be safe to conclude that a bipolar medication was ineffective after taking only one-third of the prescribed dose or skipping doses altogether for weeks at a time?

TABLE 26–2. **Core topics and questions to elicit discussion about patients' previous treatment experiences**

Sobriety

"Tell me about the times you have been abstinent from both drugs and alcohol."

"What seemed to work and what did not work for 1) addictions, 2) psychiatric problems, and 3) both problems?"

Treatment

"Tell me about times you have stopped or cut down on use in the past."

"Tell me about your previous treatments? What seemed to work and what didn't?"

Twelve-step meetings

"What have been your experiences with Alcoholics Anonymous (AA)?"

"Have you ever gone to meetings? If so, when?"

"How involved and committed were you? Did you ever try '90 in 90' (90 meetings in 90 days)?"

"Did you go to the same meeting regularly (e.g., weekly for several months)? Tell me about these meetings and the people you met there."

"Did you get a sponsor? If so, how, and what was he or she like? Did he or she help, and if so, how? If not, why not—what got in the way? Did this sponsor know that you had a dual disorder or that you were also taking medications?"

"Did you ever 'work the steps'? If so, which steps?"

"How fully 'plugged-in' did you ever get with AA? Did the people in your group know you? Did you know them? Did you ever do any 'service'? If so, tell me about your service."

If the patient answers mostly "yes" to the above 12-step questions, analyze what happened to the patient's 12-step relationship.

If the patient answers mostly "no" to the above 12-step questions, make your position clear on why you are a strong advocate of AA by stating, "Most people with more than a few months of sobriety are regularly using AA" and "The more involved with AA you are, the more likely it is that you will have a positive outcome and that your psychiatric disorder will improve."

and structure of these groups to those of 12-step groups. Less widely available groups include Women for Sobriety (https://womenforsobriety.org), which is aimed at women and their issues (women's AA meetings are more commonly available), and Medication Assisted Recovery Services (MARS; http://marsproject.org), which is based on peer support for persons taking medication-assisted treatment for addictions. Also, the addiction treatment organization Hazelden has developed the COR-12 training program as well as an app that integrates 12-step principles with opioid medication–assisted treatment (www.hazelden.org/web/public/opioid-recovery-app.page).

We suggest that when clinicians recommend 12-step or other self-help programs to persons taking medication-assisted treatment, they should take much the same approach as the one we have outlined for co-occurring psychiatric disorders and medications. Specifically, clinicians should coach patients on *not* talking about their treatment medications, but rather focusing on their addiction problems and issues. Although psychiatric medications may have become more commonly accepted and even supported in many meetings, opioid treatment medications are less well known and may be misunderstood and even discouraged. It is important that clinicians ask their patients who attend meetings about issues discussed that they found especially meaningful. Asking questions about meetings helps the clinician to integrate the treatments and shows patients that clinicians value what happens in meetings.

Conclusion

Twelve-step facilitation is an evidence-based intervention program with proven benefit for persons with substance use disorders, which this chapter has shown can be integrated into treatment for co-occurring psychiatric and substance use disorders. The following key points summarize the information presented in this chapter:

- Co-occurring substance use disorders and other psychiatric disorders are common, and mental health practitioners can enhance outcomes for both disorders by applying the principles of twelve-step facilitation (TSF).
- TSF is not Alcoholics Anonymous (AA) and is not endorsed by AA. Rather, it is an evidence-based therapy conducted by the clinician to help a patient begin to attend and benefit from 12-step meetings, including AA.
- TSF for co-occurring disorders is a practical enhancement of TSF that includes typical psychiatric issues and treatment but has not been separately tested.
- Twelve-step approaches and meetings are widely available, inexpensive, and provide long-term, recovery-based help for patients with substance use disorders.
- Twelve-step approaches to relinquishment of denial and acceptance of the chronic and often relapsing illness of substance use disorder are also appropriate for and benefit patients with most other psychiatric disorders.
- The official policy of AA is supportive of participants seeing psychiatrists and taking psychiatric medications for other mental disorders; however, a good deal of variability exists among individual 12-step communities, with some offering dual-disorder meetings and others being neutral or even hostile toward the idea of psychiatric treatment of comorbid substance use and other mental disorders.
- Development of dual-disorder TSF skills is an effective way for mental health practitioners to stay productively involved with their dual-disorder patients, offers a good model of integrated care, and allows delivery of low-cost but high-frequency psychosocial support to the patient.

References

Alcoholics Anonymous World Services: Alcoholics Anonymous. New York, Alcoholics Anonymous World Services, 1976

Alcoholics Anonymous World Services: Alcoholics Anonymous, 4th edition. New York, Alcoholics Anonymous World Services, 2001

Alcoholics Anonymous World Services: Twelve Steps and Twelve Traditions. New York, Alcoholics Anonymous World Services, 1984

Bolton J, Cox B, Clara I, et al: Use of alcohol and drugs to self-medicate anxiety disorders in a nationally representative sample. J Nerv Ment Dis 194(11):818–825, 2006 17102705

Carroll KM: Twelve step facilitation approaches, in The ASAM Principles of Addiction Medicine, 6th Edition. Edited by Miller SC, Fiellin DA, Rosenthal RN, Saitz R. Baltimore, MD, Lippincott Williams & Wilkins, 2018, pp 1027–1031

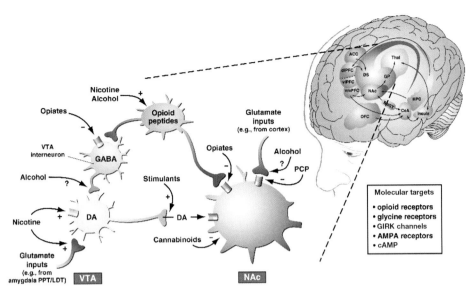

PLATE 1. Neurocircuitry associated with the addiction cycle, part 1: the *binge/intoxication* stage.

Reinforcing effects of drugs may engage associative mechanisms and reward neurotransmitters in the nucleus accumbens (NAc) shell and core and then engage stimulus-response habits that depend on the dorsal striatum (DS). Two major neurotransmitters that mediate the rewarding effects of drugs of abuse are dopamine (DA) and opioid peptides. Drugs of abuse, despite diverse initial actions, produce some common effects on the ventral tegmental area (VTA) and the NAc *(inset)*. Stimulant drugs act at DA terminals to either interfere with DA reuptake (cocaine) or increase DA release (methamphetamine). Opioids activate the NAc by inhibiting γ-aminobutyric acid (GABA) interneurons in the VTA, which disinhibit VTA DA neurons. Opioids also act directly on opioid receptors on NAc neurons and converge within some NAc neurons. The actions of other drugs remain more conjectural. Nicotine appears to activate VTA DA neurons directly by stimulating nicotinic acetylcholine receptors on these neurons and indirectly by stimulating nicotinic acetylcholine receptors on glutamatergic nerve terminals that innervate DA cells. Alcohol, by promoting $GABA_A$ receptor function, may inhibit GABAergic terminals in the VTA and hence disinhibit VTA DA neurons. Alcohol may similarly inhibit glutamatergic terminals that innervate NAc neurons. Many additional mechanisms (not shown) are proposed for alcohol. Cannabinoid mechanisms are complex and involve the activation of cannabinoid CB_1 receptors (which, like dopamine D_2 and opioid receptors, are G_i protein–linked) on glutamatergic and GABAergic nerve terminals in the NAc and on NAc neurons themselves. Phencyclidine (PCP) may act by inhibiting postsynaptic N-methyl-D-aspartate (NMDA) glutamate receptors in the NAc. Finally, some evidence indicates that nicotine and alcohol may activate endogenous opioid pathways and that nicotine, alcohol, and other drugs of abuse (such as opioids) may activate endogenous cannabinoid pathways (not shown).

ACC=anterior cingulate cortex; AMPA=α-amino-3-hydroxy-5-methyl-4-isoxazolepropionic acid; BNST= bed nucleus of the stria terminalis; cAMP=cyclic adenosine monophosphate; CeA=central nucleus of the amygdala; dlPFC=dorsolateral prefrontal cortex; GP=globus pallidus; GIRK=G protein–coupled inwardly rectifying K⁺ (potassium); HPC=hippocampus; OFC=orbitofrontal cortex; PPT/LDT=peduncular pontine tegmentum/lateral dorsal tegmentum; Thal=thalamus; vlPFC=ventrolateral prefrontal cortex; vmPFC= ventromedial prefrontal cortex.

The "Molecular targets" box lists key molecular targets that may convey genetic and epigenetic plasticity to the neurocircuits described in this figure.

Source. Modified with permission from Nestler EJ: "Is There a Common Molecular Pathway for Addiction?" *Nature Neuroscience* 8(11):1445–1449, 2005.

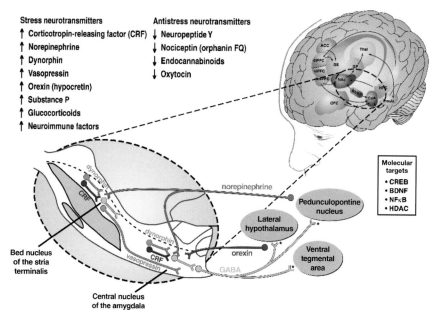

Stress neurotransmitters
↑ Corticotropin-releasing factor (CRF)
↑ Norepinephrine
↑ Dynorphin
↑ Vasopressin
↑ Orexin (hypocretin)
↑ Substance P
↑ Glucocorticoids
↑ Neuroimmune factors

Antistress neurotransmitters
↓ Neuropeptide Y
↓ Nociceptin (orphanin FQ)
↓ Endocannabinoids
↓ Oxytocin

Molecular targets
• CREB
• BDNF
• NFκB
• HDAC

PLATE 2. Neurocircuitry associated with the addiction cycle, part 2: the *withdrawal/negative affect* stage.

The negative emotional state of withdrawal may engage activation of the extended amygdala. The extended amygdala is composed of several basal forebrain structures, including the bed nucleus of the stria terminalis (BNST), the central nucleus of the amygdala (CeA), and possibly a transition area in the medial portion (shell) of the nucleus accumbens (NAc) *(inset)*. Major neurotransmitters in the extended amygdala that are hypothesized to play a role in negative reinforcement are corticotropin-releasing factor (CRF), norepinephrine, and dynorphin. The extended amygdala has major projections to the hypothalamus and the brain stem. The negative emotional state of withdrawal engages activation of the extended amygdala. Neurotransmitter systems engaged in the neurocircuitry of the extended amygdala *(listed at top left)* that convey negative emotional states are indicated by *upward arrows,* and neurotransmitter systems that may buffer negative emotional states *(listed at top center)* are indicated by *downward arrows.* The magnified section *(blue oval enclosed in dashes)* shows the extended amygdala in detail. *Green/blue pathways* *(see asterisks)* indicate glutamatergic projections.

ACC=anterior cingulate cortex; BDNF=brain-derived neurotrophic factor; CREB=cyclic adenosine monophosphate response element–binding protein; dlPFC=dorsolateral prefrontal cortex; DS=dorsal striatum; GABA=γ-aminobutyric acid; GP=globus pallidus; HDAC=histone deacetylase; HPC=hippocampus; NFκB=nuclear factor κB; OFC=orbitofrontal cortex; Thal=thalamus; vlPFC=ventrolateral prefrontal cortex; vmPFC=ventromedial prefrontal cortex.

The "Molecular targets" box lists key molecular targets that may convey genetic and epigenetic plasticity to the neurocircuits described in this figure.

Source.   Adapted from George and Koob 2013 (brain); Koob 2008 (diagram).

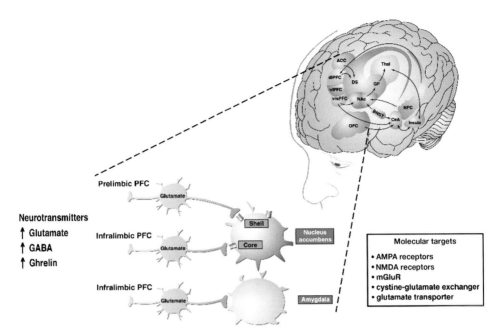

PLATE 3. Neurocircuitry associated with the addiction cycle, part 3: the *preoccupation/anticipation* stage.

The preoccupation/anticipation stage involves processing of conditioned reinforcement in the basolateral amygdala and processing of contextual information in the hippocampus (HPC). Executive control depends on the prefrontal cortex (PFC) and includes the representation of contingencies, the representation of outcomes, the presentation of values, and subjective states (i.e., craving and, presumably, feelings) associated with drugs. These subjective states, termed *drug craving* in humans, involve activation of the orbitofrontal cortex (OFC), anterior cingulate cortex (ACC), and temporal lobe, including the amygdala, in functional imaging studies. A major neurotransmitter involved in the preoccupation/anticipation stage is glutamate, which is localized in pathways from the frontal regions and the basolateral amygdala that project to the ventral striatum *(inset)*. An increase in the activity of prelimbic and infralimbic cortices in the PFC is hypothesized to initiate and inhibit the reinstatement of drug-seeking behavior. Prelimbic glutamate projections to the nucleus accumbens (NAc) shell are hypothesized to contribute to incentive salience and habit formation. Infralimbic glutamate projections to the NAc core are hypothesized to contribute to the inhibition of drug seeking. Infralimbic glutamate projections to the amygdala are hypothesized to contribute to the inhibition of brain stress systems. A combination of high prelimbic and low infralimbic glutamate activity may drive drug seeking by driving craving and disinhibiting restraints on impulsivity and compulsivity (for a review, see Kalivas 2009).

AMPA=α-amino-3-hydroxy-5-methyl-4-isoxazolepropionic acid; BNST=bed nucleus of the stria terminalis; CeA=central nucleus of the amygdala; dlPFC=dorsolateral prefrontal cortex; DS=dorsal striatum; GABA=γ-aminobutyric acid; GP=globus pallidus; mGLu=metabotropic glutamate; NMDA=N-methyl-D-aspartate; Thal=thalamus; vlPFC=ventrolateral prefrontal cortex; vmPFC=ventromedial prefrontal cortex.

The "Molecular targets" box lists key molecular targets that may convey genetic and epigenetic plasticity to the neurocircuits described in this figure.

Source. Adapted from George and Koob 2013.

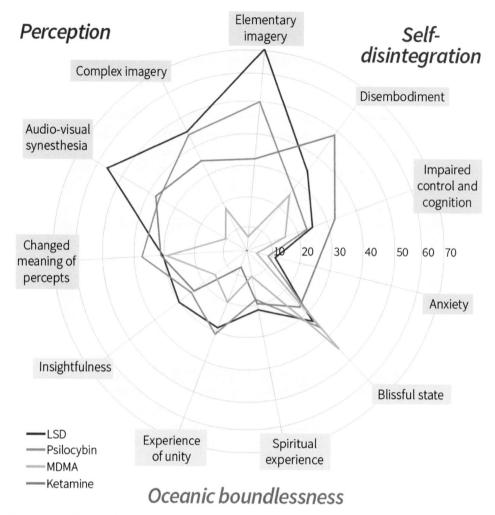

Perception

Complex imagery

Audio-visual synesthesia

Changed meaning of percepts

Insightfulness

LSD
Psilocybin
MDMA
Ketamine

Experience of unity

Elementary imagery

Self-disintegration

Disembodiment

Impaired control and cognition

10   20   30   40   50   60   70

Anxiety

Blissful state

Spiritual experience

Oceanic boundlessness

PLATE 4. Psychoactive effects of common hallucinogens according to the Five Dimensions of Altered States of Consciousness (5D-ASC) scale.

Data mapped in the figure were compiled from separate trials, each administering a single psychoactive substance. The 5D-ASC dimensions of psychoactive effects studied—oceanic boundlessness, ego disintegration, and perception—each contain elements of the perceptual, experiential, and mystical-type/transpersonal effects discussed in chapter text. LSD=lysergic acid diethylamide; MDMA=3,4-methylenedioxymethamphetamine.

Source.   Reprinted from "The Psychedelic Experience According to the 5D-ASC Scale" (chart) in Marlene Rupp, "The Psychedelic Experience," *Sapiensoup Blog*, June 27, 2017. Available at: https://sapiensoup.com/psychedelic-experience. Accessed June 19, 2020. Used with permission.

Center for Substance Abuse Treatment: Substance Abuse Treatment for Persons With Co-Occurring Disorders. A Treatment Improvement Protocol TIP 42 (DHHS Publ No SMA-05-3992). Rockville, MD, Substance Abuse and Mental Health Services Administration, 2005

Comtois KA, Russo JE, Roy-Byrne P, et al: Clinicians' assessments of bipolar disorder and substance abuse as predictors of suicidal behavior in acutely hospitalized psychiatric inpatients. Biol Psychiatry 56(10):757–763, 2004 15556120

Daley DC, Stuart Baker MA, Donovan DM, et al: A combined group and individual 12-step facilitative intervention targeting stimulant abuse in the NIDA Clinical Trials Network: STAGE-12. J Groups Addict Recover 6(3):228–244, 2011 22859917

Donovan DM, Floyd AS: Facilitating involvement in twelve-step programs. Recent Dev Alcohol 18:303–320, 2008 19115776

Dual Recovery Anonymous: The Twelve Steps of Dual Recovery Anonymous, 1993–2009. Available at: http://www.draonline.org/ dra_steps.html. Accessed December 3, 2019.

Galanter M: Spirituality and recovery in 12-step programs: an empirical model. J Subst Abuse Treat 33(3):265–272, 2007 17889297

Humphreys K, Moos RH: Encouraging post-treatment self-help group involvement to reduce demand for continuing care services: two-year clinical and utilization outcomes. Alcohol Clin Exp Res 31(1):64–68, 2007 17207103

Kaskutas LA, Bond J, Humphreys K: Social networks as mediators of the effect of Alcoholics Anonymous. Addiction 97(7):891–900, 2002 12133128

Kelly JF, Humphreys K, Ferri M: Alcoholics Anonymous and other 12-step programs for alcohol use disorder. Cochrane Database Syst Rev (3):CD012880, 2020 32159228

Kessler RC, Chiu WT, Demler O, et al: Prevalence, severity, and comorbidity of 12-month DSM-IV disorders in the National Comorbidity Survey Replication. Arch Gen Psychiatry 62(6):617–627, 2005 15939839

Linehan MM: Cognitive Behavioral Treatment of Borderline Personality Disorder. New York, Guilford, 1993

Manning V, Best D, Faulkner N, et al: Does active referral by a doctor or 12-step peer improve 12-step meeting attendance? Results from a pilot randomised control trial. Drug Alcohol Depend 126(1–2):131–137, 2012 22677458

Marlatt GA, Gordon JR (eds): Relapse Prevention: Maintenance Strategies in the Treatment of Addictive Behaviors. New York, Guilford, 1985

McCrady BS, Tonnigan S: Recent research into twelve-step programs, in The ASAM Principles of Addiction Medicine, 5th Edition. Edited by Ries RK, Fiellin DA, Miller SC, et al. Alphen aan den Rijn, The Netherlands, Wolters Kluwer, 2014, pp 1043–1064

Minkoff K: An integrated treatment model for dual diagnosis of psychosis and addiction. Hosp Community Psychiatry 40(10):1031–1036, 1989 2807203

Morgenstern J: Pathogenesis and Treatment of Alcoholism. PsycCRITIQUES. Washington, DC, American Psychological Association, 2004

Nowinski J, Baker S, Carroll K: Twelve Step Facilitation Therapy Manual: A Clinical Research Guide for Therapists Treating Individuals With Alcohol Abuse and Dependence. NIAAA Project MATCH Monograph Series, Vol 1; DHHS Publ. No. (ADM) 92-1893. Rockville, MD, National Institute on Alcohol Abuse and Alcoholism, 1992

Nowinski J, Baker S, Carroll K: Twelve Step Facilitation Therapy Manual: A Clinical Research Guide for Therapists Treating Individuals With Alcohol Abuse and Dependence. Project MATCH Monograph Series, Vol 1; NIH Publ. No. 94-3722. Reprinted 1999. Available at: https://pubs.niaaa.nih.gov/publications/projectmatch/match01.pdf. Accessed June 30, 2020.

Puchalski CM, Dorff RE, Hendi IY: Spirituality, religion, and healing in palliative care. Clin Geriatr Med 20(4):689–714, vi–vii, 2004 15541620

Sholomskas DE, Carroll KM: One small step for manuals: computer-assisted training in twelve-step facilitation. J Stud Alcohol 67(6):939–945, 2006 17061013

Tonigan JS, Book SW, Pagano M, et al: 12-step therapy and women with and without social phobia: a study of the effectiveness of 12-step therapy to facilitate AA engagement. Alcohol Treat Q 28(2):151–162, 2010 21423569

Weiss RD: Treating patients with bipolar disorder and substance dependence: lessons learned. J Subst Abuse Treat 27(4):307–312, 2004 15610832

Weiss RD, Ostacher MJ, Otto MW, et al: Does recovery from substance use disorder matter in patients with bipolar disorder? J Clin Psychiatry 66(6):730–735, quiz 808–809, 2005 15960566

Wolitzky-Taylor K, Operskalski JT, Ries R, et al: Understanding and treating comorbid anxiety disorders in substance users: review and future directions. J Addict Med 5(4):233–247, 2011 22042216

Worley MJ, Tate SR, Brown SA: Mediational relations between 12-step attendance, depression and substance use in patients with comorbid substance dependence and major depression. Addiction 107(11):1974–1983, 2012 22578037

Recommended Readings

Nowinski J, Baker S, Carroll K: Twelve Step Facilitation Therapy Manual: A Clinical Research Guide for Therapists Treating Individuals With Alcohol Abuse and Dependence. Project MATCH Monograph Series, Vol 1; NIH Publ. No. 94-3722. Reprinted 1999. Available at: https://pubs.niaaa.nih.gov/publications/projectmatch/match01.pdf. Accessed June 30, 2020.

Puchalski CM, Dorff RE, Hendi IY: Spirituality, religion, and healing in palliative care. Clin Geriatr Med 20(4):689–714, vi–vii, 2004 15541620

Sholomskas DE, Carroll KM: One small step for manuals: computer-assisted training in twelve-step facilitation. J Stud Alcohol 67(6):939–945, 2006 17061013

Tonigan JS, Book SW, Pagano M, et al: 12-Step therapy and women with and without social phobia: a study of the effectiveness of 12-Step therapy to facilitate AA engagement. Alcohol Treat Q 28(2):151–162, 2010 21423569

Weiss RD: Treating patients with bipolar disorder and substance dependence: lessons learned. J Subst Abuse Treat 27(4):307–312, 2004 15610832

Weiss RD, Ostacher MJ, Otto MW, et al: Does recovery from substance use disorder matter in patients with bipolar disorder? J Clin Psychiatry 66(6):730–735, 2005 15960566

CHAPTER 27

Family Therapy

Peter Steinglass, M.D.

In a paper published in the *Quarterly Journal of Studies on Alcohol* in 1953, Thelma Whalen claimed to have identified four specific patterns of behavior in wives of alcoholic men that she hypothesized might be causative in the onset and/or perpetuation of their husbands' abusive drinking. The concept Whalen advanced was that the deep-seated intrapsychic conflicts these women were experiencing were being resolved via their marriage to alcoholic men. Pejorative names were given to these wifely patterns, such as "Suffering Susan," a name meant to describe a woman who was satisfying a need for self-punishment, or "Punitive Polly," a name coined to connote a woman who would seek out a man she could dominate to satisfy her own intrapsychic needs.

Whalen's (1953) paper reflected a pervasive view held among many clinicians at the time that wives and families of patients with serious psychiatric disorders often had a negative influence in that they either caused or tended to exacerbate the patient's symptomatology. In the case of alcohol-related disorders, the implication was that increased relapse rates in particular could be attributed to ways in which spouses and families were undermining recovery. Furthermore, Whalen suggested that in many instances spousal psychopathology might be an etiological factor in the onset and perpetuation of chronic alcohol misuse. Whalen's clinical vignettes purportedly provided examples of this linkage.

Similar hypotheses were also prevalent as explanations for chronic opioid addiction. A frequently mentioned hypothesis was that women married to drug-addicted men were attracted to these men out of desire to partner with men they considered weak (Taylor et al. 1966). Once again, the suggestion was that personality disorders in these women led them to select marriages in which they felt they could dominate their opioid-addicted spouses, and perpetuating their husbands' chronic opioid use served one of their central psychopathological needs.

In these hypotheses regarding substance use disorders (SUDs)—both alcohol use disorder (AUD) and opioid use disorder (OUD)—the implication was that psycho-pathology in these women was somehow responsible for the emergence and main-tenance of their spouses' addictive behaviors. By extension, therapeutic strategies for patients based on these hypotheses called for the separation of users from spouses and families. Marital and/or family therapy was thought to be not only unhelpful but also potentially counterproductive.

Subsequently, over the next several decades, others working in the addiction field began noting the profound negative impact that excessive alcohol and drug use had on families (Hurcom et al. 2000). Perhaps the greatest attention was given to the in-creased incidence of domestic violence associated with these disorders (Chase et al. 2003; Chermack et al. 2008), but the linkage between SUDs and substantially higher rates of sexual abuse (especially of children), legal difficulties and incarceration, fi-nancial crises, divorce, work disruptions, and the like all pointed to the profound neg-ative impact of these conditions on family life (Copello et al. 2005).

Although no one was arguing that SUDs were the only factors leading to such pow-erful family events as physical abuse or family breakups, assumptions that there might be a direct link between alcohol and/or drug abuse and increased marital and family problems were unavoidable because of the markedly increased rates of these events in families in which SUDs were also present. Additionally, SUDs have been found to cre-ate in families a myriad of emotional responses, including grief, despair, helplessness, hopelessness, and uncertainty about the future. More recently, the growing opioid epi-demic in the United States over the past decade has amplified public awareness of the profoundly negative effects of excessive drug use on families, particularly on children and their caregivers, secondary to opioid and heroin overdoses.

While many clinicians seemed to be arguing that families were negative influences in the lives of patients with SUDs, the data on the impact of SUDs on family life sug-gested something quite different—namely, that families have a powerful stake not only in successful SUD treatment but also in treatment approaches that address the needs of all family members, not only those of the substance users. Put another way, clinicians should think of families as natural allies in their efforts to design and im-plement family-focused interventions for SUD treatment, rather than subverters of the therapeutic process.

This change in how families living with SUDs were viewed—from considering them as dysfunctional potential contributors to the onset and/or perpetuation of sub-stance abuse to thinking of them as distressed individuals struggling to cope with the sequelae of an SUD—has paralleled similar shifts in thinking among family thera-pists about how to approach treatment for families dealing with major psychiatric or chronic medical conditions (Heru 2006; Patterson and Garwick 1994). What makes these newer models significantly different from earlier ideas is that they move away from describing the difficulties apparent in these families as problems residing solely in individual family members. Instead, these models use as their starting point the ex-amination of patterns of interaction directly related to a family's efforts to cope with a chronic psychiatric or medical disorder. This view, in turn, has ushered in a different perspective on the potential value of family therapy for any chronic psychiatric or medical condition, including a substance use disorder.

Overview of Family Therapy SUD Treatment Models

Virtually all of the wide array of family-focused treatment approaches for SUDs rely heavily on one or more of three conceptual models: family systems, family behavioral, and/or social network therapies. Although these models have many differences in theoretical orientation and clinical techniques, they all share the conviction that treatment should include the patient *and* the family together. In some instances, this has meant working with the entire family. In other instances, it has meant targeting an important subsystem of the family, such as a marital couple or a parent-child dyad. However, regardless of who is in the room, the emphasis is on changing maladaptive interaction patterns of behavior that might inadvertently be maintaining alcohol and/or drug use behavior. In other words, the therapist's interest is not so much on etiology (i.e., what started the substance use behavior) as on family behaviors that either reinforce or attenuate substance use on the part of the patient with an SUD.

Also, many of the techniques used by family therapists to treat SUDs have been based on findings from empirical research. For example, the initial efforts on the part of both cognitive-behavioral and family systems researchers focused on the design and implementation of observational studies in which behavior could be measured and analyzed. The data emerging from these studies in turn were used by clinicians as the basis for many of the more important family-focused treatment models for addiction disorders. As one example, Steinglass and colleagues used their findings from home observation studies of alcoholic families (Steinglass 1981) to incorporate three aspects of family behavior—in-home daily routines, family rituals such as holiday celebrations or vacations, and family problem-solving styles—as foci for the assessment component of their family systems treatment model (Steinglass 2009; Steinglass et al. 1987).

Another example of influential new data involved findings about differences in interactional behavior during periods of intoxication versus sobriety, especially findings suggesting that behaviors appearing only during periods of active substance use had adaptive as well as negative consequences for the families being studied (Jacob and Leonard 1988; Steinglass 1979). These findings then led to the development of interviewing techniques aimed at helping families to better appreciate the complexity of their patterns of behavior in relation to substance use (McCrady 2012).

Family Systems Approaches

Family systems models, while utilizing many behavioral techniques as part of their clinical approach, pay particular attention to patterns of behavior used by families to control the challenges associated with chronic substance misuse. Comparable attention is paid to the choices families make over time that result in substance use becoming an issue around which much of family life is now organized. Three additional components are viewed as critical to the family systems approach: 1) a therapeutic stance that emphasizes therapist neutrality, the use of nonpathologizing language with patients and families, and family–therapist collaboration (rather than a hierarchical approach in which the therapist takes the position of "expert" and unilaterally defines the treatment goals for the family); 2) a belief that central to the success of treatment is the ability to ascertain both individual- and family-level beliefs about the role of alcohol use in family life; and 3) a conviction that therapy, to be effective, must include a credible action plan for addressing the drinking behavior itself that is embraced by the entire family.

Examples of treatment approaches that have relied heavily on family systems concepts include those of Treadway (1989), those of Steinglass et al. (1987), and the Systemic-Motivational Therapy model proposed by Steinglass (2009), an approach that integrates family systems ideas with those of motivational interviewing (Miller and Rollnick 2013) and harm reduction (Marlatt et al. 2011). Both the Treadway model and those proposed by Steinglass and colleagues focus primarily on adult AUD.

Two other models, Functional Family Therapy (FFT) (Alexander et al. 2013) and Multidimensional Family Therapy (MDFT) (Liddle et al. 2001, 2018), have emerged as promising approaches for treating adolescent drug problems. Although eclectic in their designs, both models draw substantially on family systems concepts, are evidence based and manual driven, and have been successfully used in treating complex clinical situations (e.g., dual diagnosis, antisocial behavior) affecting adolescents within a family context. Furthermore, both approaches have been successfully used with families representing a wide range of ethnic and cultural groups, as well as in diverse treatment settings.

The overlap between the FFT and MDFT models is considerable in that both approaches can be thought of as short-term, highly structured, strengths-based family intervention models that focus on risk and protective factors at both the individual and the family level. Of the two models, MDFT deserves particular attention, not only because its impact on reducing adolescent alcohol and cannabis drug use has been shown to be long-standing (Liddle 2016) but also because it has been identified as one of the more promising approaches to the treatment of adolescent OUD when used in conjunction with medications for OUD (Waldron and Turner 2008).

In the MDFT approach, therapy is conceptualized as occurring in four different treatment domains: the adolescent alone, the parent alone, the family together, and the adolescent's community. Therefore, an MDFT therapist might at one point be having individual sessions with the adolescent patient, but at other points be seeing the adolescent in conjoint sessions with his or her family, teachers, employers, and so forth. In each of these "domains," the focus is on 1) establishing a nonjudgmental treatment environment; 2) promoting change in emotions, thoughts, and behaviors (of both adolescents and other family members); and 3) using techniques to enhance motivation for change.

Family Behavioral Approaches

Family behavioral models extend classical conditioning and cognitive-behavioral principles to an examination of the relationship between interpersonal behavior and substance use. Concepts of reciprocity, coercion, and reinforcement are applied to an analysis of the contingencies that help explain how patterns of interaction behavior may influence the acute and chronic phases of SUDs. Examples of family behavioral approaches include the cognitive-behavioral model outlined by McCrady and colleagues (Epstein and McCrady 1998, 2009; McCrady 2012) and the Behavioral Marital Therapy model described by O'Farrell and Fals-Stewart (2006). Both of these approaches have been manualized and have been subjected to multiple randomized clinical trials (RCTs), with uniformly positive results (McCrady et al. 2016; O'Farrell and Clements 2012). Sometimes these approaches have been tested as stand-alone treatments, but they have also been tested as components of more complex treatment protocols, a strategy that more closely reflects how marital and family therapy are currently incorporated into residential and outpatient SUD treatment programs.

Social Network Therapy Approaches

Approaches based on concepts of social network therapy, which is not strictly thought of as family therapy, should also be mentioned. These models, best represented by the Network Therapy model proposed by Galanter (1999), take advantage of the potential power not only of families but also of larger social support systems in motivating patients to seek treatment and to maintain changes in substance use behavior. (A more detailed description of social network approaches can be found in Chapter 28, "Network Therapy.")

Summary of Family Therapy Models

Although family systems, family behavioral, and social network therapy approaches represent different ways of working with SUD problems from a family-based perspective, it is unusual to find any of these treatment approaches practiced in "pure" form in clinical settings. Instead, most clinicians use both family systems and family behavioral concepts when working with families of patients with SUDs, and also at times rely on information gathered from patients' larger social and extended family networks. In fact, the models themselves have considerable overlap in the techniques employed. Furthermore, because family therapy is often only one of many treatment components included in most residential and intensive outpatient programs (alongside individual and group therapy components, 12-step groups, and the like), the family therapy component is often designed to be integrated with these other components, rather than being implemented in "pure" form.

SUD Marital and Family Therapy Outcome Research

Multiple reports over the past 25 years together build a compelling case for greater inclusion of family-focused approaches in SUD treatment. By now, well over 100 RCTs and a number of meta-analyses have been published examining outcome differences between marital and family therapy (MFT) approaches and a wide variety of comparison treatments, including individual counseling/therapy, group therapy, psychoeducation, and treatment-as-usual conditions (Copello et al. 2005; O'Farrell and Clements 2012; Shadish and Baldwin 2003; Templeton et al. 2010). In virtually all studies, MFT has proven to be superior to—or, at the very least, equal in effectiveness to—the comparison treatments in regard to the outcome of reduced substance use. Furthermore, as noted later in this section, MFT has the added advantage of improving the functioning of *all* family members, not only that of the patient with an SUD.

The target population for the family component of these RCTs has most frequently been the marital dyad, but parent–child dyads and whole families have also been studied. In most instances, families studied have had one member diagnosed with an SUD (either alcohol or an opioid drug), but some studies have included polydrug users and families with more than one member with an SUD diagnosis. Although the vast majority of RCTs have focused on families dealing with an AUD, studies of family therapy models for treating OUD have increased in recent years (Liddle 2016; Waldron and Turner 2008). However, despite the increased use of medication-assisted treatment of OUD in clinical practice, RCTs to date have not included guidelines regarding how such medication regimens are being incorporated into family therapy study protocols. Presumably, this issue of combined treatment will receive greater attention going forward as evidence showing the effectiveness of family therapy approaches such as MDFT gains wider recognition.

Findings from the numerous outcome studies can be grouped into four main categories:

1. When the challenge is how to effectively engage treatment-resistant patients, the involvement of family members (especially parents and/or spouses) early in the assessment phase significantly improves participation rates of alcohol- or drug-abusing family members in subsequent treatment. Programs specifically designed to work with spouses and/or parents around engagement issues have produced dramatic results, in some cases achieving success rates as high as 80% in subsequent agreement of patients to participate in treatment.

   To date, the most comprehensive overview of these outcome data remains a review paper in which Stanton (2004) examined results from 19 outcome studies of 10 different approaches for working with family members to facilitate patient engagement in substance abuse treatment. Overall, findings from these studies demonstrated impressive results (engagement rates greater than 65%) for family approaches compared with waitlist control conditions (engagement rates averaging 6%). Similarly impressive evidence of effectiveness in relation to engagement of adolescents with substance misuse has been reported when approaches have been modified to work with the parents of these adolescents (Liddle 2004).

2. The active inclusion of family members during the assessment/diagnostic phase of treatment substantially increases the accuracy of the clinical picture. In particular, being able to access clinical information from family members as well as the patient provides a far more reliable picture of SUD-related variables such as quantity and frequency of use, safety issues, typical behavior when intoxicated, and the impact of the SUD on family, work, social relationships, and physical health. Studies have shown that because patients with SUDs frequently minimize their substance use and deny its negative sequelae, being able to access information from other family members provides clinicians with a more complete picture of the magnitude of substance use and its impact on patient and family life (McCrady et al. 2013). These data, in turn, are invaluable in making decisions about treatment options, such as whether a residential treatment program is necessary.

3. Many RCTs as well as less rigorous clinical reports of a wide variety of family therapy approaches for SUD treatment have consistently indicated significant improvement in functioning not only for patients but also for other family members participating in therapy sessions (O'Farrell and Fals-Stewart 2006). Although outcome measures in these various studies have understandably focused primarily on posttreatment quantity and frequency measures of substance use, family ther-

apy outcome studies have been distinguished by the multidimensional nature of functional outcomes in the study designs. These studies typically have included measures of individual adjustment of nonpatient family members (including children) as well as measures of overall couple and/or family psychosocial functioning. A particularly impressive set of findings has indicated that participation in marital and/or family therapy is associated with dramatic reductions in incidence rates of posttreatment domestic violence; these findings held regardless of whether the initiator of the violence was a male or a female patient with an SUD (O'Farrell et al. 2004; Schumm et al. 2009).

Most of the findings regarding benefits of therapy for nonpatient family members have come from effectiveness and efficacy studies of the Behavioral Marital Therapy (BMT) (O'Farrell and Clements 2012) and Motivational Enhancement Therapy (MET) models (Miller et al. 1992) as applied to AUD. Furthermore, these studies have almost exclusively focused on treatment of marital dyads. However, studies of both FFT (Alexander et al. 2013) and MDFT (Liddle et al. 2001) have generated impressive evidence supporting their utility as treatments for OUD, and these models have been applied to treatment of parent–child as well as marital dyads.

To date, far fewer studies have included treatment approaches stemming from family systems models where the target for treatment (and conceptualization of outcome measures) is the family as a unit. Perhaps the most ambitious effort thus far was a study in which a manualized family systems–based treatment was compared with a modified version of cognitive-behavioral therapy and a treatment-as-usual condition (Rohrbaugh et al. 1995). Results were considered difficult to interpret, however, in part because the majority of subjects were families in which the patient with an SUD had been mandated to treatment secondary to arrests for driving under the influence.

This focus on evaluating treatment outcomes not only for the patient but also for the participating family members is one of the features of MFT approaches that clearly differentiate them from individual or group therapy approaches. Also, this focus parallels an argument made by MFT researchers studying the effectiveness of MFT for a wide range of psychiatric and medical conditions: active involvement of family members in therapy significantly improves functioning not only for identified patients but also for many other nonpatient individuals in the family (Baucom et al. 2012; Dixon et al. 2001; Orford et al. 2013). For this reason, it often has been argued that family therapy is significantly more cost-effective than treatments targeting individual patients alone (O'Farrell et al. 1996), an argument that certainly is supported by the SUD treatment outcome data noted above.

4. A number of studies have focused on treatment adherence as an important "active ingredient" contributing to the overall effectiveness of family-based treatment approaches. One of the more compelling examples of this emphasis is the use of an "Antabuse contract" (O'Farrell et al. 1995), which was developed as a key component of the BMT model described by O'Farrell and Fals-Stewart (2006). In this approach, the patient with an SUD and a spouse or partner design a protocol together that specifies how they will monitor disulfiram (Antabuse) adherence. As it turns out, having the spouse or partner actively involved in this process very significantly increases patient adherence, which in turn presumably has a positive effect on subsequent abstinence.

Components of Family Therapy SUD Treatment

Although family therapy SUD treatment models differ somewhat in their approach, the most salient aspect in all of these models is their emphasis on actively involving spouses and/or other family members at each phase of the treatment process: engagement, assessment, detoxification, postdetoxification stabilization, and rehabilitation. Because some of the more striking contrasts between family and individual therapy approaches can be seen during the engagement, assessment, and detoxification phases of treatment, these phases deserve further explication.

Engagement

As underscored in the previous section, "SUD Marital and Family Therapy Outcome Research," a particularly compelling example of the usefulness of family-based approaches to SUD treatment is demonstrated by the dramatic improvement in engagement of patients with treatment-resistant SUD when these models are used. Although a wide variety of approaches have been proposed, two models in particular deserve special attention because their success rates have been so notable.

1. Community Reinforcement and Family Training (CRAFT): The central focus of CRAFT is working with spouses or concerned significant others in the family to teach methods of positive reinforcement of non-substance-use behavior and ways to restructure everyday life to emphasize abstinence as a central component of family behavior (Meyers et al. 1998; Smith and Meyers 2004). An extension of an earlier approach called Community Reinforcement Training (CRT) (Sisson and Azrin 1989), which focused on training family members how to avoid confrontation around substance use behavior, CRAFT also incorporates techniques similar to those used by other successful treatment engagement programs such as motivational interviewing. A detailed manual on how to implement CRAFT in outpatient settings is available (Smith and Meyers 2004) and has been used widely for staff training in the method.

   In one example of the power of the CRAFT approach, an RCT was carried out in which CRAFT was compared with Al-Anon facilitation (Timko et al. 2012) and the Johnson Institute family intervention approach (Johnson 1986). CRAFT (n=45) achieved a 64% success rate in subsequent engagement of the patients in the study, whereas the engagement rates of the Al-Anon (n=45) and the Johnson Intervention (n=40) legs of the study were 13% and 30%, respectively (Miller et al. 1999).

   Although CRAFT was originally designed for use in situations in which the patient with an SUD is an adult (most typically a spouse or parent), more recently clinicians have been applying CRAFT to work with parents of substance-abusing adolescents. Given the difficulties often experienced in engaging adolescent substance users in treatment, the positive reports of clinicians using CRAFT in this situation have been particularly encouraging (Kirby et al. 2015).

2. A Relational Intervention Sequence for Engagement (ARISE): ARISE is a graduated stepwise approach (three stages of increasing intensity depending on when engagement successfully occurs) in which family members and other important

members of the patient's social network are mobilized with the specific goal of supporting the patient's engagement in SUD treatment (Landau et al. 2000). Central to the effectiveness of ARISE is its emphasis on minimizing the use of confrontational techniques and maximizing the use of collaborative, open communication to address denial. In this regard, ARISE has major overlaps with techniques recommended by Galanter (1999) as key components of his Network Therapy approach.

Like CRAFT, ARISE has a detailed instructional manual (Garrett and Landau 1999), and formal training is available. Although controlled outcome studies of the ARISE program have not yet been conducted, Landau and colleagues have reported findings from a clinical trial of ARISE involving 110 patients with alcohol and drug use disorders; in this trial, 83% of patients subsequently engaged in extended treatment (Landau 2011; Landau et al. 2004). Landau and colleagues have also emphasized that ARISE should be thought of as a highly cost-effective program for dealing with patients with SUDs who decline to receive treatment, in that the average amount of telephone and session time required by the clinicians implementing ARISE in their study was 1.5 hours, an obviously low figure to achieve such high engagement rates.

Considering the impressive results for programs such as CRAFT and ARISE in engaging treatment-resistant patients, it is disappointing that these programs have not been more widely implemented in clinical settings. Instead, two other programs for spouses, children, and/or parents struggling with a treatment-resistant family member—Al-Anon/Alateen and the Johnson Intervention—continue to dominate the addictions field.

Although Al-Anon and Alateen programs have been reported to be helpful in improving functioning of participating members, they have not yet been shown to improve patient engagement in treatment (Timko et al. 2012). Their central message to family members regarding maintenance of a "loving detachment" from the patient's substance misuse behavior makes these programs quite different from most marriage and family therapy models, as well as programs such as CRAFT or ARISE. Also, it has been argued that participation in Al-Anon groups may have the unintended consequences of increasing marginalization within the family and pathologizing non-substance-using participants through the use of terms such as "enabling" and "codependency" (Young and Timko 2015).

The Johnson Intervention (Johnson 1986), a method that has been widely touted by its developers as efficacious for dealing with treatment resistance in the addiction field, relies on duplicity in getting the patient with an SUD to the intervention session and on confrontational exchanges once the patient has been brought to the intervention session. This method is clearly very different from the collaborative, positive-reinforcement exchanges between patient and family members advocated by approaches such as CRAFT and ARISE. The Johnson Intervention has been almost exclusively applied in situations in which the goal is to engineer the immediate enrollment of a highly resistant patient with an SUD in an intensive residential treatment program. This goal is quite different from the goals of approaches such as CRAFT or ARISE. The actual success rates of the Johnson Intervention, like those of most clinical techniques, vary widely depending on the training and skill of the interventionist;

however, when subjected to more systematic review (O'Farrell and Clements 2012), this approach has a disappointing track record as an engagement strategy (e.g., treatment engagement rates of 25%–30%).

Furthermore, when compared with other routes of engagement in/referral to treatment, the Johnson Intervention has substantially higher rates of relapse when patients transition from residential to outpatient treatment (Loneck et al. 1996). When these relatively low success rates are combined with the frequent reports of negative impacts on family relationships attendant on the coercive strategies central to the Johnson Intervention, it is not surprising that this method remains highly controversial.

Assessment

Although assessment strategies may vary somewhat across family therapy models, family therapists contend that because assessment is invariably carried out with both patient and family members present, this approach significantly improves the quality and accuracy of the reported data. For example, information about the quantity and frequency of substance use, triggers for use, behavior changes with substance use, and evidence of withdrawal symptoms or blackouts can be better understood when questions are asked to multiple family members rather than to the patient alone.

Family-based assessment strategies also emphasize aspects of behavior particularly salient to the interface between substance use and family life. As one example, in the treatment approaches advocated by Steinglass and colleagues, explicit questions are asked about the impact of the patient's substance use on the family's daily life (routines) and important family rituals (e.g., holiday celebrations, vacations), as well as its role in family problem-solving strategies (Steinglass 2009; Steinglass et al. 1987). In each of these areas, the goal is to better understand how family behavior has become altered or organized around the on/off cycling of sober/intoxicated interactional behavior, how substance use is talked about within the family (if at all), and how family members' beliefs about the benefits as well as the costs of substance use contribute to SUD chronicity.

As another example, detailed descriptions obtained from marital dyads about sequential interactional behavior during periods of active substance use are critical to interventions used by behavioral marital therapists that are designed to interrupt negative stimulus-response patterns and reinforce positive responses to situations in which substance use is being suppressed (O'Farrell and Fals-Stewart 2006). Information obtained from only one spouse would most likely be highly skewed and thus misleading, and subsequent attempts to alter marital interactions in a more productive direction could then be seriously undermined.

Detoxification

One of the more unique aspects of family-based substance abuse treatment models is the approach to the detoxification phase of treatment. Regardless of whether their treatment goal is abstinence or harm reduction, most family-based models assume that the goal can be best achieved if negotiated with other family members present.

The most commonly used approach involves patients and family members in discussions directed at designing a contract to facilitate eliminating or reducing substance use. In some cases, the contract is a limited one, such as the previously mentioned spousal contract for Antabuse use adherence (O'Farrell et al. 1995) (see section "SUD Marital and Family Therapy Outcome Research"), but in other cases, a more ambitious family-based contract is aimed not only at addressing the patient's substance misuse but also at "detoxifying" the psychosocial environment of the entire family.

An example of the latter approach would be the "family detoxification" model described by Steinglass et al. (1987), in which the family together designs a contract directed at living substance free for a predetermined period of time. Framed by the therapist as an "experiment" to enhance the family's understanding of how its life has become organized around substance use, the contract is also intended as a vehicle for challenging family members' beliefs about their helplessness to facilitate behavioral change. A more recent version of this "family-level detoxification" approach proposed by Steinglass (2009) has incorporated concepts from both motivational interviewing and harm reduction approaches to foster a better appreciation of the role of ambivalence about behavior change vis-à-vis substance use and to make significant reductions in substance use (rather than total abstinence) a credible outcome goal for the family detoxification contracting process.

Assessment is significantly improved when it is carried out with the whole family present, and the same rationale applies to involvement of the family in detoxification contracting. Independent of whether substance misuse started because of the behavior of one individual within the family, by the time it has reached a chronic phase, it has become a central organizer of so many aspects of family life that enlisting the entire family in the detoxification (or harm reduction) process is an obvious route to follow.

Conclusion

With the accumulated research data and clinical experience in family therapy approaches to SUD treatment, a compelling case can be made for the incorporation of family-based interventions as core components of treatment of SUDs. For example, even as far back as 2002, Miller and Wilbourne (2002) reviewed what they at the time considered to be the most impressive evidence-based approaches to SUD treatment and pointed out that in the vast majority of cases (9 of the 11 examples cited), involvement of families and/or social networks were identified as key ingredients contributing to treatment success. Subsequent reviews of the treatment outcome literature have only strengthened support for the effectiveness of family-focused therapy models (Liddle 2016; McCrady et al. 2016; O'Farrell and Clements 2012).

Although it is encouraging that appreciation of the potential value of including family therapy as a core component of SUD treatment programs is now coming from multiple directions, it is also the case that systemic or behavioral family therapy approaches continue to be underutilized in most residential and intensive outpatient programs. Instead, the more typical situation is one in which parallel rather than integrated programs are designed for patients and family members, with little to no opportunities for patient and nonpatient family members to participate together in therapy sessions.

Additionally, SUD clinicians' attitudes toward families too often remain negative and pathologizing. For example, the continuing widespread use of the terms *enabler* and *codependency* may send families the message that they are part of the problem rather than a valuable resource for the patient. Another example is the tendency in most residential programs to urge families to avoid contact with the patient with an SUD until the third or fourth week of the program, perhaps inadvertently giving the family the message that until the patient is fully stabilized, interactions with other family members would be potentially toxic rather than supportive.

A number of factors have contributed to this marginalization of family-focused treatment approaches to substance use disorders. At the top of the list are health care systems built around the diagnosis and treatment of individuals, and health insurance policies that often exclude reimbursement for couples and family therapy. Equally important, however, is the minimal training that addiction professionals receive in family systems assessment and treatment, as well as the parallel paucity of attention paid to substance use issues in most marital and family therapy graduate training programs.

As a consequence of this systemwide marginalization, most addiction therapists are only peripherally aware of the advances made in family therapy approaches to SUD treatment, and most family therapists still think of addiction treatment as being limited to individual therapy, pharmacotherapy, and self-help groups. Given this situation, there would appear to be ample room for an exploration of integrative approaches that bring together some of the newer ideas in family therapy on the one hand and SUD treatment on the other.

References

Alexander JF, Waldron HB, Robbins MS, et al: Functional Family Therapy for Adolescent Behavior Problems. Washington, DC, American Psychological Association, 2013

Baucom DH, Porter LS, Kirby JS, et al: Couple-based interventions for medical problems. Behav Ther 43(1):61–76, 2012 22304879

Chase KA, O'Farrell TJ, Murphy CM, et al: Factors associated with partner violence among female alcoholic patients and their male partners. J Stud Alcohol 64(1):137–149, 2003 12608494

Chermack ST, Murray RL, Walton MA, et al: Partner aggression among men and women in substance use disorder treatment: correlates of psychological and physical aggression and injury. Drug Alcohol Depend 98(1–2):35–44, 2008 18554825

Copello AG, Velleman RD, Templeton LJ: Family interventions in the treatment of alcohol and drug problems. Drug Alcohol Rev 24(4):369–385, 2005 16234133

Dixon L, McFarlane WR, Lefley H, et al: Evidence-based practices for services to families of people with psychiatric disabilities. Psychiatr Serv 52(7):903–910, 2001 11433107

Epstein EE, McCrady BS: Behavioral couples treatment of alcohol and drug use disorders: current status and innovations. Clin Psychol Rev 18(6):689–711, 1998 9779329

Epstein EE, McCrady BS: A Cognitive-Behavioral Treatment Program for Overcoming Alcohol Use Problems: Therapist Guide. New York, Oxford University Press, 2009

Galanter M: Network Therapy for Alcohol and Drug Abuse. New York, Guilford, 1999

Garrett J, Landau J: A Relational Intervention Sequence for Engagement ARISE: Manual for Certified ARISE Interventionists. Albany, NY, Linking Human Systems, 1999

Heru AM: Family psychiatry: from research to practice. Am J Psychiatry 163(6):962–968, 2006 16741194

Hurcom C, Copello A, Orford J: The family and alcohol: effects of excessive drinking and conceptualizations of spouses over recent decades. Subst Use Misuse 35(4):473–502, 2000 10741538

Jacob T, Leonard KE: Alcoholic-spouse interaction as a function of alcoholism subtype and alcohol consumption interaction. J Abnorm Psychol 97(2):231–237, 1988 3385076

Johnson VE: How To Help Someone Who Doesn't Want Help. Center City, MN, Hazelden Publishing, 1986

Kirby KC, Versek B, Kerwin ME, et al: Developing Community Reinforcement and Family Training (CRAFT) for parents of treatment-resistant adolescents. J Child Adolesc Subst Abuse 24(3):155–165, 2015 25883523

Landau J: The ARISE intervention and continuum of care: engaging substance abusers and their families in treatment and long-term recovery. Familiendynamik 36(2):132–141, 2011. Available at: https://arise-network.com/wp-content/uploads/2017/08/ARISEInterventionandContinuumofCare2010.pdf. Accessed January 11, 2020.

Landau J, Garrett J, Shea RR, et al: Strength in numbers: the ARISE method for mobilizing family and network to engage substance abusers in treatment. A Relational Intervention Sequence for Engagement. Am J Drug Alcohol Abuse 26(3):379–398, 2000 10976664

Landau J, Stanton MD, Brinkman-Sull D, et al: Outcomes with the ARISE approach to engaging reluctant drug- and alcohol-dependent individuals in treatment. Am J Drug Alcohol Abuse 30(4):711–748, 2004 15624546

Liddle HA: Family-based therapies for adolescent alcohol and drug use: research contributions and future research needs. Addiction 99 (suppl 2):76–92, 2004 15488107

Liddle HA: Multidimensional Family Therapy: evidence base for transdiagnostic treatment outcomes, change mechanisms, and implementation in community settings. Fam Process 55(3):558–576, 2016 27565445

Liddle HA, Dakof GA, Parker K, et al: Multidimensional family therapy for adolescent drug abuse: results of a randomized clinical trial. Am J Drug Alcohol Abuse 27(4):651–688, 2001 11727882

Liddle HA, Dakof GA, Rowe CL, et al: Multidimensional Family Therapy as a community-based alternative to residential treatment for adolescents with substance use and co-occurring mental health disorders. J Subst Abuse Treat 90:47–56, 2018 29866383

Loneck B, Garrett JA, Banks SM: The Johnson Intervention and relapse during outpatient treatment. Am J Drug Alcohol Abuse 22(3):363–375, 1996 8841685

Marlatt GA, Larimer ME, Witkiewitz K: Harm Reduction: Pragmatic Strategies for Managing High Risk Behaviors, 2nd Edition. New York, Guilford, 2011

McCrady BS: Treating alcohol problems with couple therapy. J Clin Psychol 68(5):514–525, 2012 22504611

McCrady BS, Owens M, Brovko JM: Couples and family treatment methods, in Addictions: A Comprehensive Guidebook. Edited by McCrady BS, Epstein EE. New York, Oxford University Press, 2013, pp 454–481

McCrady BS, Wilson AD, Muñoz RE, et al: Alcohol-focused behavioral couple therapy. Fam Process 55(3):443–459, 2016 27369809

Meyers RJ, Miller WR, Hill DE, et al: Community Reinforcement and Family Training (CRAFT): engaging unmotivated drug users in treatment. J Subst Abuse 10(3):291–308, 1998 10689661

Miller WR, Rollnick S: Motivational Interviewing: Helping People Change, 3rd Edition. New York, Guilford, 2013

Miller WR, Wilbourne PL: Mesa Grande: a methodological analysis of clinical trials of treatments for alcohol use disorders. Addiction 97(3):265–277, 2002 11964100

Miller WR, Zweben A, DiClemente CC, Rychtanik RG: Motivational Enhancement Therapy Manual: A Clinical Guide for Therapists Treating Individuals With Alcohol Abuse and Dependence. Project MATCH Monograph Series Vol 2 (DHS Publ. No. [ADM] 92-1894). Rockville, MD, National Institute on Alcohol Abuse and Alcoholism, 1992. Available at: https://motivationalinterviewing.org/sites/default/files/MATCH.pdf. Accessed July 29, 2020.

Miller WR, Meyers RJ, Tonigan JS: Engaging the unmotivated in treatment for alcohol problems: a comparison of three strategies for intervention through family members. J Consult Clin Psychol 67(5):688–697, 1999 10535235

O'Farrell TJ, Clements K: Review of outcome research on marital and family therapy in treatment for alcoholism. J Marital Fam Ther 38(1):122–144, 2012 22283384

O'Farrell T, Fals-Stewart W: Behavioral Couples Therapy for Alcoholism and Drug Abuse. New York, Guilford Press, 2006

O'Farrell TJ, Allen JP, Litten RZ: Disulfiram (Antabuse) contracts in treatment of alcoholism. NIDA Res Monogr 150:65–91, 1995 8742773

O'Farrell TJ, Choquette KA, Cutter HSG, et al: Cost-benefit and cost-effectiveness analyses of behavioral marital therapy as an addition to outpatient alcoholism treatment. J Subst Abuse 8(2):145–166, 1996 8880657

O'Farrell TJ, Murphy CM, Stephan SH, et al: Partner violence before and after couples-based alcoholism treatment for male alcoholic patients: the role of treatment involvement and abstinence. J Consult Clin Psychol 72(2):202–217, 2004 15065955

Orford J, Velleman R, Natera G, et al: Addiction in the family is a major but neglected contributor to the global burden of adult ill-health. Soc Sci Med 78:70–77, 2013 23268776

Patterson JM, Garwick AW: The impact of chronic illness on families: a family systems perspective. Annals of Behavioral Medicine 16(2):131–142, 1994. Available at: https://psycnet.apa.org/record/1995-06087-001. Accessed January 11, 2020.

Rohrbaugh MJ, Shoham V, Spungen C, et al: Family systems therapy in practice: a systemic couples therapy for problem drinking, in Comprehensive Textbook of Psychotherapy: Theory and Practice. Edited by Bongar B, Beutler LE. New York, Oxford University Press, 1995, pp 228–253

Schumm JA, O'Farrell TJ, Murphy CM, et al: Partner violence before and after couples-based alcoholism treatment for female alcoholic patients. J Consult Clin Psychol 77(6):1136–1146, 2009 19968389

Shadish WR, Baldwin SA: Meta-analysis of MFT interventions. J Marital Fam Ther 29(4):547–570, 2003 14593694

Sisson RW, Azrin NH: The community reinforcement approach, in Handbook of Alcoholism Treatment Approaches: Effective Alternatives. Edited by Hester RK, Miller WR. Elmsford, NY, Pergamon Press, 1989, pp 242–258

Smith JE, Meyers RJ: Motivating Substance Abusers to Enter Treatment: Working With Family Members. New York, Guilford, 2004

Stanton MD: Getting reluctant substance abusers to engage in treatment/self-help: a review of outcomes and clinical options. J Marital Fam Ther 30(2):165–182, 2004 15114946

Steinglass P: An experimental treatment program for alcoholic couples. J Stud Alcohol 40(3):159–182, 1979 449341

Steinglass P: The alcoholic family at home. Patterns of interaction in dry, wet, and transitional stages of alcoholism. Arch Gen Psychiatry 38(5):578–584, 1981 7235860

Steinglass P: Systemic-motivational therapy for substance abuse disorders: an integrative model. Journal of Family Therapy 31(2):155–174, 2009. Available at: https://onlinelibrary.wiley.com/doi/abs/10.1111/j.1467-6427.2009.00460.x. Accessed January 11, 2020.

Steinglass P, Bennett LA, Wolin SJ, et al: The Alcoholic Family. New York, Basic Books, 1987

Taylor SD, Wilbur M, Osnos R: The wives of drug addicts. Am J Psychiatry 123(5):585–591, 1966 5921668

Templeton L, Velleman R, Russell C: Psychological interventions with families of alcohol misusers: a systematic review. Addiction Research & Theory 18(6):616–648, 2010. Available at: https://www.tandfonline.com/doi/abs/10.3109/16066350903499839?src=recsys&journalCode=iart20. Accessed January 11, 2020.

Timko C, Young LB, Moos RH: Al-Anon family groups: Origins, conceptual basis, outcomes, and research opportunities. Journal of Groups in Addiction & Recovery 7(2–4):279–296, 2012. Available at: https://www.tandfonline.com/doi/abs/10.1080/1556035X.2012.705713. Accessed February 10, 2020.

Treadway D: Before It's Too Late: Working With Substance Abuse in the Family. New York, Norton, 1989

Waldron HB, Turner CW: Evidence-based psychosocial treatments for adolescent substance abuse. J Clin Child Adolesc Psychol 37(1):238–261, 2008 18444060

Whalen T: Wives of alcoholics: four types observed in a family service agency. Q J Stud Alcohol 14(4):632–641, 1953 13121236

Young LB, Timko C: Benefits and costs of alcoholic relationships and recovery through Al-Anon. Subst Use Misuse 50(1):62–71, 2015 25268181

CHAPTER 28

Network Therapy

Marc Galanter, M.D.

Psychotherapy for people dependent on alcohol and other drugs presents unique problems for the office-based practitioner. Among these are the ever-present vulnerability to relapse to substance use and the high dropout rates. To address these problems, therapists can consider how engaging the input of people close to an addicted person can help in achieving a stable abstinence and dealing with the vulnerability to dropout from treatment. As I discuss in this chapter, the input of people close to the patient can help to reveal triggers to drug use that may not be apparent to the patient. For willing patients, or ones who have family and friends who can cooperate, the Network Therapy approach can be most valuable.

The Network Therapy Approach

The Network Therapy approach can be useful in addressing a broad range of patients with the following clinical hallmarks of addictive illness: First, when they initiate consumption of their addictive agent, be it alcohol, cocaine, opiates, or depressant drugs, they frequently cannot limit that consumption to a reasonable and predictable level; this phenomenon has been termed *loss of control* by clinicians who treat persons dependent on substances (Jellinek 1963). Second, they may have consistently demonstrated relapse to the agent of abuse; that is, they have attempted to stop using the substance for varying periods of time but have returned to it, despite a specific intent to avoid it.

This treatment approach is not necessary for those people with substance use disorders who can learn to set limits on their use of alcohol or drugs; their disorder may be treated as a behavioral symptom in a more traditional psychotherapeutic fashion. The approach also is not directed toward those patients for whom the addictive pattern is most unmanageable, such as addicted people with unusual destabilizing circumstances such as homelessness, severe character pathology, or psychosis. These patients may need special supportive care such as inpatient detoxification or long-term residential treatment.

Network Therapy Technique

Three key elements are integrated in the Network Therapy technique. The first is a cognitive-behavioral approach to relapse prevention, which has been considered valuable in addiction treatment (Beck et al. 1993; Marlatt and Gordon 1985). Emphasis in this approach is placed on triggers to relapse and behavioral techniques for avoiding them, in preference to exploring underlying psychodynamic issues.

Second, support from the patient's natural social network is engaged in treatment. Peer support in Alcoholics Anonymous (AA) has long been shown to be an effective vehicle for promoting abstinence, and the idea of the therapist's intervening with family and friends in starting treatment was employed in one of the early ambulatory techniques specific to addiction (Johnson 1986). The involvement of spouses (McCrady et al. 1991) has since been shown to be effective in enhancing the outcome of professional therapy.

Third, the orchestration of resources to provide community reinforcement suggests a more robust treatment intervention by providing support for drug-free rehabilitation (Azrin et al. 1982). Khantzian (1988) pointed to the "primary care therapist" as one who functions in a direct coordinating and monitoring role in order to combine psychotherapeutic and mutual support elements. This role of overall management of circumstances outside as well as inside the office session is employed to maximize the effectiveness of the intervention.

Cognitive-Behavioral Therapy

Cognitive-behavioral therapy (CBT) has been shown to be effective for a wide variety of substance use disorders, including dependence on alcohol (Morgenstern and Longabaugh 2000), marijuana (Stephens et al. 2002), and cocaine (Carroll 1998). CBT is premised on the original findings by Wikler (1973) on conditioning models of drug seeking in subjects addicted to heroin.

The CBT approach is goal oriented and focuses on current circumstances in the patient's life. In Network Therapy, salient past experiences can also be referenced in both individual and conjoint sessions. CBT sessions are typically structured so that, for example, patients begin each Network Therapy session with a recounting of recent events directly relevant to their addiction and recovery.

The process of guided recall is particularly important because it allows the therapist, in both individual and conjoint sessions, to guide the patient to recognize a sequence of conditioned stimuli (triggers) that play a role in drug seeking. Such triggers may not initially be apparent to the patient or network members but, through encouragement and prompting, can emerge over the course of an exploration of the circumstances that have led to substance use, either in the past or in a recent "slip."

Social Support

Social support has been studied in a variety of data sets in relation to recovery from substance use disorders. For example, in the federal Project MATCH (Matching Alcoholism Treatment to Client Heterogeneity), researchers compared three modalities:

12-step facilitation, motivational enhancement, and cognitive-behavioral approaches. In a secondary analysis of findings from this multisite study, it was found that certain aspects of social support were most predictive of abstinence outcomes (Zywiak et al. 2002). Non-substance-using supportive participants are important to a long-term clinical outcome. In fact, a large number of network members, when their participation is effectively maintained over time, can counter a variety of circumstances that may undermine a patient's abstinence. Additionally, they can provide varied aspects of support relative to the patient's experience in recovery.

Community Reinforcement

Family involvement in substance abuse treatment has long been shown to be effective in improving outcomes, and numerous approaches make use of social network involvement in treatment, including Behavioral Couples Therapy (Fals-Stewart et al. 2000), Marital Therapy (O'Farrell 1986), and the Community Reinforcement Approach (Azrin et al. 1982; Meyers et al. 2003). More specifically, the Community Reinforcement and Family Training (CRAFT) program (Smith and Meyers 2004) includes many aspects of treatment that are also employed in Network Therapy. The CRAFT approach was developed to encourage individuals with problem drinking to enter therapy and reduce their alcohol consumption, in part by eliciting the support of concerned others, as well as to enhance satisfaction with life among members of a patient's social network who were concerned about the patient's drinking. Like Network Therapy, the CRAFT program includes a functional analysis to understand the patient's substance use with respect to its antecedents and consequences. Also like Network Therapy, the CRAFT program serves to minimize reciprocal blaming and defensiveness among the patient's concerned significant others, and to promote the patient's sobriety-oriented activities.

The Initial Encounter: Starting the Network

When starting Network Therapy with a patient, the therapist should ask the patient to bring his or her spouse or a close friend to the first session. Patients with substance use disorder often dislike certain things they hear when they first come for treatment and may deny or rationalize, even if they have voluntarily sought help. Because of patients' denial of their problem, a significant other is essential both for history taking and for implementing a viable treatment plan. A close relative or spouse can often cut through a patient's denial in a way that an unfamiliar therapist cannot, and can therefore be invaluable in setting a standard of realism in dealing with the addiction.

Some patients make it clear that they wish to come to the initial session alone. This desire is often associated with their wish to preserve the option of continued substance abuse and their fear that an alliance with others will be established to prevent this. Although a delay may be tolerated for a session or two, the therapist should communicate unambiguously at the outset the following points: 1) optimal treatment can be undertaken only on the basis of a therapeutic alliance built around the addiction issue and enlisting the support of significant others, and 2) the patient is expected to bring in a network of close friends and/or relatives within a session or two at the most.

The therapist should be available for consultation on the phone and should encourage the patient to call if problems arise. This accessibility makes the therapist's commitment clear and sets the tone for a "team effort." Therapist availability begins to undercut one reason for relapse: the patient's sense of being on his or her own if unable to manage a situation. The astute therapist, however, will avoid spending excessive time with patients on the telephone or in emergency sessions. Therefore, the patient needs to develop a support network that can handle the majority of problems involved in day-to-day assistance and should expect the therapist to respond only to occasional questions involving interpreting the terms of the understanding among the therapist, the patient, and support network members. If the therapist questions the ability of the patient and network to manage the period between the initial sessions, the first few scheduled sessions may be arranged at intervals of only 1–3 days. Also, frequent appointments should be scheduled at the outset if a pharmacological detoxification with benzodiazepines is indicated, so that the patient need never manage more than a few days' medication at a time.

It is essential that the network be forged into a working group capable of providing the necessary support for the patient between the initial sessions. Network size can range from one to several persons close to the patient. Contacts between network members at this early stage typically include telephone calls (at the therapist's or patient's initiative), dinner arrangements, and social encounters and should be preplanned to a fair extent during the joint session. These encounters are most often undertaken at the time when alcohol or drug use is likely to occur. In planning meetings, the therapist should clarify to network members that relatively little unusual effort will be required for the long term, and that after the patient is stabilized, members' participation will amount to little more than attendance at infrequent meetings with the patient and therapist. This explanation is reassuring to those network members who are unable to make a major time commitment to the patient as well as to those patients who do not want to be placed in a dependent position.

Defining the Network's Membership

Establishing a network is a task undertaken with the active collaboration of the patient and the therapist. The two, aided by those parties who join the network initially, must search for the right balance of members; however, the therapist must carefully promote the choice of appropriate network members, just as the platoon leader selects the individuals who will go into combat. The network will be crucial in determining the balance of the therapy. The process of determining network membership is not without problems, and the therapist must think in a strategic fashion of the interactions that might take place among network members. The following case vignette illustrates this task.

A 25-year-old graduate student had been abusing cocaine since high school, in part by drawing funds from his affluent family, who lived in a remote city. At two points in the process of establishing his support network, the reactions of his live-in girlfriend, who worked with the therapist from the outset, were particularly important. Both she and the patient moved on to evaluating the patient's elderly friend, whom the patient initially preferred to exclude, despite the fact that his girlfriend thought him appropriate. It later turned out that the friend was perceived as a potentially disapproving representative of the parental generation. The therapist encouraged the patient to accept the friend as a network member nonetheless, so as to round out the range of relationships within the group, and spelled out the rationale for this friend's inclusion. The friend did turn out to be caring and supportive, particularly after he was helped to understand the nature of the addictive process.

Defining the Network's Task

In Network Therapy, the therapist's relationship to the network is like that of a task-oriented team leader, rather than that of a family therapist oriented toward insight. The network is established to implement a straightforward task—that of aiding the therapist in sustaining the patient's abstinence. The network must be directed with the same clarity of purpose that a task force is directed in any effective organization. Competing and alternative goals must be suppressed, or at least prevented from interfering with the primary task.

Unlike family members involved in traditional family therapy, network members are not led to expect symptom relief or self-realization for themselves. The therapist's clarification of this prevents the development of competing goals for the network's meetings. It also assures the members protection from having their own motives scrutinized and thereby supports their continuing involvement without the threat of an assault on their psychological defenses. Because network members have—kindly—volunteered to participate, their motives must not be impugned. Their constructive behavior should be commended. It is useful to acknowledge and express appreciation for the contribution they are making to the therapy. There is always a counterproductive tendency on their part to minimize the value of their contribution. The network must, therefore, be structured as an effective working group with high morale. This is not always easy, as demonstrated in the following case vignette.

> A single woman served as an executive in a large family-held business—except when her alcohol problem led to protracted binges. Her father, brother, and sister were prepared to banish her from the business but decided that they would first seek consultation. Because they had initiated the contact with the clinician, the father, brother, and sister were included in the initial network and indeed were very helpful in stabilizing the patient. Unfortunately, however, the father was a domineering figure who intruded in all aspects of the business, evoking angry outbursts from his children. The children's typical reactions of petulance provoked rancorous tirades from the father in return. The situation came to a head when both of the patient's siblings angrily petitioned the therapist to exclude the father from the network. However, the therapist decided to support the father's membership in the group, pointing out the constructive role he had played in getting the therapy started. The hubbub did, in fact, quiet down with time. The children became less provocative themselves as the group responded to the therapist's pleas for civil behavior.

Use of Alcoholics Anonymous

Use of mutual help modalities is desirable whenever appropriate. For the person with alcohol use disorder, participation in AA is strongly encouraged. Groups such as Narcotics Anonymous, Pills Anonymous, and Cocaine Anonymous are modeled after AA and play a similarly useful role for individuals with drug use disorders. Some patients are more easily convinced to attend AA meetings; others may be more reluctant to do so. The therapist should mobilize the support network as appropriate to continue pressuring the patient to attend AA for a reasonable trial.

Use of Pharmacotherapy in the Network Format

For the individual with alcohol use disorder, disulfiram may be of marginal help in maintaining abstinence when used in a traditional counseling context (Fuller et al. 1986), but it becomes much more valuable when carefully integrated into work with the patient and network, particularly when the drug is taken under observation (Table 28–1). A similar circumstance applies to the use of oral or depot naltrexone for stabilizing abstinence in an opioid-dependent person.

An important consideration is how the support network can be used to deal with recurrences of alcohol use, when in fact the patient's prior association with these same persons did not prevent the patient from drinking. The following case example illustrates how this may be done when social resources are limited. In this vignette, a specific protocol was arranged with the network members to monitor a patient's adherence to a disulfiram regimen.

> A 33-year-old public relations executive had moved from a remote city 3 years before coming to treatment. She had no long-standing close relationships in the current city, a circumstance not uncommon for a single person with alcohol use disorder in a setting removed from her origins. The woman presented with a 10-year history of heavy drinking that had increased in severity since her arrival, no doubt associated with her social isolation. Six months before the beginning of treatment, she had attended AA meetings for 2 weeks and remained abstinent during that time; however, she had then relapsed, and became discouraged about the possibility of maintaining abstinence. At the outset of treatment, it was necessary for the therapist to reassure the patient that her prior relapse was in large part a function of not having established sufficient outside supports (including more sound relationships within AA) and of having seen herself as a failure after only one slip. Together, the therapist and the patient came up with the idea of bringing into the network an old friend of the patient whom she saw occasionally and whom she felt she could trust. A schedule was then established wherein the patient would attend therapy sessions twice a week and would see her friend once each weekend. On each of these thrice-weekly occasions, she would take disulfiram under observation.

Meeting Arrangements

For at least the first month of therapy, it is important that the clinician see the patient with the network group on a weekly basis. Unstable circumstances demand more frequent contacts with the network. After the supportive network is established, sessions can be tapered off to biweekly and then to monthly intervals.

To sustain the continuing commitment of the group, particularly between therapist and network members, network sessions should be held every 3 months or so for the duration of the individual therapy. Once the patient has stabilized, the meetings tend to address day-to-day issues less often. Individuals meetings may begin with the patient's recounting of the drug situation. Reflections on the patient's progress and goals, or sometimes on relations among the network members, may then be dis-

TABLE 28–1.	**Format for medication observation by network members**

1. Have the patient take the medication every morning in front of a network member.
2. Have the patient take the pills so that the other person can observe the patient swallowing it.
3. Have the observer write down the time of day the pills were taken on a list prepared by the therapist.
4. Have the observer bring the list to the therapist's office at each network session.
5. Have the observer leave a message on the therapist's answering machine on any day in which the patient did not take the pills in a way that allowed ingestion to be clearly observed. This issue will then be dealt with by the therapist and the patient, eliminating the need for network members to serve as reinforcers.

cussed. In any case, two things are essential: that network members contact the therapist if they are concerned about the patient's possible use of substances, and that the therapist contact the network members if the therapist becomes concerned about a potential relapse.

Adapting Individual Therapy to Network Treatment

The fact that network sessions are scheduled on a weekly basis at the outset of treatment is likely to limit the number of individual contacts. Indeed, if network sessions are held once a week, the patient may not be seen individually for a period of time. The patient may perceive this as a deprivation unless the individual therapy is presented as an opportunity for further growth predicated on achieving stable abstinence, which is assured through work with the network.

When the individual therapy does begin, the traditional objectives of therapy must be arranged so as to accommodate the goals of the substance abuse treatment. For insight-oriented therapy, clarification of unconscious motivations is a primary objective; for supportive therapy, the bolstering of established constructive defenses is primary. In the therapeutic context that is described here, however, the following objectives are given precedence.

Of first importance is the need to address exposure to substances of abuse or exposure to cues that might precipitate substance use. This can be done in conjunction with the network. Both patient and therapist should also be sensitive to this matter in individual sessions and should explore these situations as they arise. Second, a stable social context in an appropriate social environment—one conducive to abstinence with minimal disruption of life circumstances—should be supported. For a considerable period of time, the patient will be highly vulnerable to exacerbations of the addictive illness and in some respects must be viewed with the considerable caution with which one treats the recently compensated person with psychosis.

After these priorities have been attended to, psychological conflicts that the patient must resolve, relative to his or her own growth, are considered. As the therapy continues, these conflicts come to assume a more prominent role. In the earlier phases of therapy, such conflicts often directly reflect issues associated with the patient's previous substance use.

A Longer Course of Treatment

The following case vignette illustrates how a network was engaged in treating a patient in long-term care for his addiction problem.

> A 22-year-old man had been using heroin intranasally on and off for 3 years, but for the past 6 months had additionally been "sniffing" large doses at least twice daily. At the initial encounter, the therapist asked the patient for permission to engage collateral support for the patient due to concern about the patient's reliability. The therapist asked if they could both speak on the phone with a friend or a close family member of the patient's who could be a resource for him until the next session. The patient agreed to their calling a cousin with whom he had a close relationship and who had repeatedly expressed concern over his drug use. The three agreed that the cousin would meet the patient for dinner right before the next scheduled session and would then come with the patient to that session.
>
> This patient was a good candidate for Network Therapy; his continuous dependence on heroin had lasted less than a year, a period insufficient to meet candidacy requirements for maintenance on buprenorphine or methadone. It would be desirable to avoid long-term dependence on an opioid if possible, and in fact the patient did not wish to pursue that option anyway. His network consisted of three people: his cousin, a close friend, and an uncle 20 years his senior, whom he viewed as a mentor and friend.
>
> A second component of the treatment was to provide protection from relapse by having the patient take oral naltrexone twice weekly (on Monday and Wednesday), and three on a third occasion (Friday). He would take the medication in front of his cousin, who lived only one block away from him. This naltrexone regimen was continued over the course of the ensuing 10 months, and after that, on the patient's own recognizance. He did indeed maintain abstinence over 1 year of subsequent ongoing psychotherapy for general adaptive issues, and was found to be abstinent and in continuing therapy for 3 years after that.

Principles of Network Therapy

Table 28–2 presents a set of guidelines for applying Network Therapy. These principles can be adapted to the needs of a given patient and to the relative availability of potential network members.

Research on Network Therapy

An initial chart review was conducted on a series of 60 patients dependent on substances, with follow-up appointments scheduled through the period of treatment and up to 1 year thereafter (Galanter 1993). In another study, a Network Therapy training sequence was developed for psychiatric residents and then evaluated (Galanter et al. 1997a, 2002). The residents, inexperienced in drug treatment, achieved results similar to those reported for experienced professionals employing other modalities (Carroll et al. 1994; Higgins et al. 1993).

Glazer et al. (2003) reviewed videotaped Network Therapy sessions for 21 patients addicted to cocaine and rated the quality of the patient–therapist alliance using the

TABLE 28–2.	**Principles of Network Therapy**

1. Start a network as soon as possible with at least two people selected by the therapist and the patient together.

2. Manage the network with care, explaining the addictive process and maintaining nonjudgmental support for the patient.

3. Keep the network's agenda focused on addiction recovery issues, with the patient reporting relevant alcohol- or drug-use-related events, and with the entire group focusing on potential triggers.

4. Augment network sessions with individual patient sessions during which more general issues can also be addressed with the patient.

5. Include medication for substance use disorders in the overall plan, and clarify to network members how medications work.

6. Employ 12-step groups and other group modalities as appropriate to augment network and individual sessions.

Penn Helping Alliance Rating Scale (Alexander and Luborsky 1986) and the Working Alliance Inventory (Horvath and Greenberg 1989). Anther study conducted in a community-based addictions treatment clinic (Keller and Galanter 1999) used essentially the same Network Therapy training sequence developed by Galanter et al. (1997a) for psychiatry residents. Psychiatrists and other professionals could be offered training by a distance-learning method using the Internet, a medium that offers the advantage of not being fixed in either time or location (Galanter et al. 1997b). In an additional study, Galanter et al. (2004) evaluated the impact of Network Therapy relative to a control condition (medical management) among patients who were inducted onto buprenorphine for 16 weeks and then tapered to zero dose.

In a program referred to as behavioral naltrexone therapy, Rothenberg et al. (2002) adapted Network Therapy and combined it with relapse prevention and a voucher reinforcement system for use in the treatment of patients dependent on opioids who were enrolled in a 6-month course of treatment with naltrexone. Copello et al. (2002) combined elements of Network Therapy with social aspects of the Community Reinforcement Approach and relapse prevention in a program referred to as Social Behaviour and Network Therapy (SBNT) for the treatment of persons with "alcohol problems" (Dale et al. 2011). Additional studies involving this study sample were conducted to assess cost-effectiveness (UKATT Research Team 2005), clients' perceptions of change in alcohol drinking behaviors, and drinking goal preference (Adamson et al. 2010). Copello et al. (2006) adapted SBNT for persons presenting with drug problems.

Conclusion

In summary, family and peer support can be added to an ongoing treatment to better engage the patient with an SUD. This can yield better retention and improved cooperation in achieving a goal of abstinence.

References

Adamson SJ, Heather N, Morton V, et al: Initial preference for drinking goal in the treatment of alcohol problems, II: Treatment outcomes. Alcohol Alcohol 45(2):136–142, 2010 20130150

Alexander LB, Luborsky L: The Penn Helping Alliance Scales, in The Psychotherapeutic Process: A Research Handbook (Guilford Clinical Psychology And Psychotherapy Series). Edited by Greenberg LS, Pinsof WM. New York, Guilford, 1986, pp 325–366

Azrin NH, Sisson RW, Meyers R, et al: Alcoholism treatment by disulfiram and community reinforcement therapy. J Behav Ther Exp Psychiatry 13(2):105–112, 1982 7130406

Beck AT, Wright FD, Newman CF, et al: Cognitive Therapy of Substance Abuse. New York, Guilford, 1993

Carroll KM: A Cognitive-Behavioral Approach: Treating Cocaine Addiction. Rockville, MD, National Institute on Drug Abuse, 1998

Carroll KM, Rounsaville BJ, Gordon LT, et al: Psychotherapy and pharmacotherapy for ambulatory cocaine abusers. Arch Gen Psychiatry 51(3):177–187, 1994 8122955

Copello A, Orfor J, Hodgson R, et al: Social Behaviour and Network Therapy basic principles and early experiences. Addict Behav 27(3):345–366, 2002 12118625

Copello A, Williamson E, Orford J, et al: Implementing and evaluating Social Behaviour and Network Therapy in drug treatment practice in the UK: a feasibility study. Addict Behav 31(5):802–810, 2006 16024177

Dale V, Coulton S, Godfrey C, et al: Exploring treatment attendance and its relationship to outcome in a randomized controlled trial of treatment for alcohol problems: secondary analysis of the UK Alcohol Treatment Trial (UKATT). Alcohol 46(5):592–599, 2011 21733833

Fals-Stewart W, O'Farrell TJ, Feehan M, et al: Behavioral couples therapy versus individual-based treatment for male substance-abusing patients. An evaluation of significant individual change and comparison of improvement rates. J Subst Abuse Treat 18(3):249–254, 2000 10742638

Fuller RK, Branchey L, Brightwell DR, et al: Disulfiram treatment of alcoholism. A Veterans Administration cooperative study. JAMA 256(11):1449–1455, 1986 3528541

Galanter M: Network Therapy for substance abuse: a clinical trial. Psychotherapy: Theory, Research, Practice, Training 30(2):251–258, 1993. Available at: https://psycnet.apa.org/record/1994-34913-001. Accessed January 11, 2020.

Galanter M, Keller DS, Dermatis H: Network therapy for addiction: assessment of the clinical outcome of training. Am J Drug Alcohol Abuse 23:355–367, 1997a 9261485

Galanter M, Keller DS, Dermatis H: Using the Internet for clinical training: a course on Network Therapy for substance abuse. Psychiatr Serv 48(8):999–1000, 1008, 1997b 9255829

Galanter M, Dermatis H, Keller D, et al: Network Therapy for cocaine abuse: use of family and peer supports. Am J Addict 11(2):161–166, 2002 12028746

Galanter M, Dermatis H, Glickman L, et al: Network Therapy: decreased secondary opioid use during buprenorphine maintenance. J Subst Abuse Treat 26(4):313–318, 2004 15182896

Glazer SS, Galanter M, Megwinoff O, et al: The role of therapeutic alliance in Network Therapy: a family and peer support-based treatment for cocaine abuse. Subst Abus 24(2):93–100, 2003 12766376

Higgins ST, Budney AJ, Bickel WK, et al: Achieving cocaine abstinence with a behavioral approach. Am J Psychiatry 150(5):763–769, 1993 8480823

Horvath AO, Greenberg LS: Development and validation of the Working Alliance Inventory. Journal of Counseling Psychology 36(2):223–233, 1989. Available at: https://psycnet.apa.org/doiLanding?doi=10.1037%2F0022-0167.36.2.223. Accessed September 21, 2020.

Jellinek EM: The Disease Concept of Alcoholism. New Haven, CT, Hillhouse, 1963

Johnson VE: Intervention: How to Help Someone Who Doesn't Want Help. Minneapolis, MN, Hazelden Foundation, 1986

Keller DS, Galanter M: Technology transfer of Network Therapy to community-based addictions counselors. J Subst Abuse Treat 16(2):183–189, 1999 10023618

Khantzian EJ: The primary care therapist and patient needs in substance abuse treatment. Am J Drug Alcohol Abuse 14(2):159–167, 1988 3177338

Marlatt GA, Gordon JR (eds): Relapse Prevention: Maintenance Strategies in the Treatment of Addictive Behaviors. New York, Guilford, 1985

McCrady BS, Stout R, Noel N, et al: Effectiveness of three types of spouse-involved behavioral alcoholism treatment. Br J Addict 86(11):1415–1424, 1991 1777736

Meyers RJ, Smith JE, Lash DN: The community reinforcement approach. Recent Dev Alcohol 16:183–195, 2003 12638638

Morgenstern J, Longabaugh R: Cognitive-behavioral treatment for alcohol dependence: a review of evidence for its hypothesized mechanisms of action. Addiction 95(10):1475–1490, 2000 11070524

O'Farrell TJ: Marital therapy in the treatment of alcoholism, in Clinical Handbook of Marital Therapy. Edited by Jacobson NS, Gurman AS. New York, Guilford, 1986, pp 513–535

Rothenberg JL, Sullivan MA, Church SH, et al: Behavioral naltrexone therapy: an integrated treatment for opiate dependence. J Subst Abuse Treat 23(4):351–360, 2002 12495797

Smith JE, Meyers RJ: Motivating Substance Abusers to Enter Treatment: Working With Family Members. New York, Guilford, 2004

Stephens RS, Babor TF, Kadden R, et al: The Marijuana Treatment Project: rationale, design and participant characteristics. Addiction 97 (suppl 1):109–124, 2002 12460133

UKATT Research Team: Effectiveness of treatment for alcohol problems: findings of the randomised UK Alcohol Treatment Trial (UKATT). BMJ 331(7516):541–543, 2005 16150764

Wikler A: Dynamics of drug dependence. Implications of a conditioning theory for research and treatment. Arch Gen Psychiatry 28(5):611–616, 1973 4700675

Zywiak WH, Longabaugh R, Wirtz PW: Decomposing the relationships between pretreatment social network characteristics and alcohol treatment outcome. J Stud Alcohol 63(1):114–121, 2002 11925053

CHAPTER 29

Digitally Delivered Therapies

Sarah E. Lord, Ph.D.

Katherine M. Seavey, B.A.

Alan J. Budney, Ph.D.

Lisa A. Marsch, Ph.D.

The significant science-to-practice translational gap is a long-standing issue in health care, and the translation of demonstrated evidence-based treatment for substance use disorders (SUDs) to broad delivery is no exception. Current initiatives in the United States emphasize greater focus on successful dissemination and implementation strategies for delivering empirically supported treatments to close the gap (Onken et al. 2014). Digital technology offers a promising platform for broad dissemination of evidence-based approaches to treatment of SUDs and related conditions.

Digital therapeutic approaches can address many of the traditional barriers to delivery of evidence-based treatment, including limited access and reach as well as challenges to maintaining fidelity and engagement. The relative ubiquity of digital technologies expands the potential for reaching broad audiences with evidence-based care. Accessibility of mobile technology continues to grow rapidly: over 5 billion people globally own mobile devices, of which over 50% are smartphones (Taylor and Silver 2019). A majority (95%) of adults in the United States own a mobile phone of some kind, and 77% have smartphones (Anderson 2019). Smartphone accessibility is greater in advanced economies relative to emerging economies, and ownership is higher among younger and more educated groups relative to older and less educated groups (Anderson 2019). Internet use is nearly universal in most advanced economies and is growing rapidly in emerging economies. Access to, and thus usage of, the Internet is somewhat lower in rural regions in the United States relative to urban areas, primarily due to less developed wireless and broadband infrastructure in rural regions (Perrin 2019). Despite continued access disparities, largely along socioeconomic lines, there is good evidence that disenfranchised populations, such as those with SUDs, can access digital technologies and would use them for treatment and recovery support (Bonar et al. 2018; Lord et al. 2016; Milward et al. 2015).

The accessibility of Internet, social media, mobile applications, and text messaging technologies offers the possibility of expanding the reach of evidence-based treatment to broad population bases. Digital therapeutic approaches, accessible through computers, tablets, or mobile phones, transcend the time and geographic boundaries of traditional clinical practice settings, so that treatment and support are available 24/7, when and where people need it. The wide use of digital devices also opens opportunities for empowering individuals to be more actively involved in their own care.

The automated, self-directed nature of digital therapeutic approaches also helps to ensure that core treatment components are delivered with fidelity. Data capture and usage tracking capabilities of digital technologies allow stakeholders to assess what components of a program are used and for how long, and can be used to evaluate intervention fidelity and to measure therapeutic "dose" in evaluations of treatment impact. Different media (e.g., text, audio, video, animation) can also be incorporated into digital therapeutics to appeal to a broad range of learning styles and to promote engagement (Milward et al. 2018). In this chapter, we describe the existing evidence supporting the efficacy of digital therapeutic approaches to SUDs and related conditions across the treatment continuum and highlight directions for innovative research in this area.

Evidence-Based Digital Treatment Approaches for Substance Use Conditions

There is strong and growing evidence for digital therapeutic approaches targeting SUDs and related conditions across the care continuum (Marsch et al. 2014b; Sugarman et al. 2017). These digital behavioral health approaches have demonstrated efficacy in identifying symptoms (Butler et al. 2001; Lord et al. 2011; McNeely et al. 2016), evoking positive behavioral change (Campbell et al. 2014; Carroll et al. 2008, 2009, 2014; Marsch et al. 2014a), and facilitating recovery support (Gonzales et al. 2014; Gustafson et al. 2014). The empirical literature includes studies of digital therapeutic approaches evaluated in a variety of ways, including as stand-alone treatment approaches, as adjuncts to clinician-delivered treatment, or as replacements for certain aspects of care, across a range of patient or client populations and in diverse settings. There is consistent evidence demonstrating that when digital interventions are developed well, and are in concert with the needs of target end-users, they can produce outcomes comparable to, and in some cases better than, the effects of interventions delivered by trained clinicians (Marsch et al. 2014b). In the following sections we describe the state of the science with regard to empirically tested digital approaches for SUD treatment across the care continuum.

Screening and Assessment

The majority of research on digital approaches to screening and assessment has focused on translation of existing validated instruments to digital forms, primarily web-based programs and mobile applications. For example, the Addiction Severity Index–Multimedia Version (ASI-MV; Butler et al. 2001) is a translation of the widely used Addiction Severity Index (McLellan et al. 1992) to an interactive, multimedia web-based format that includes video-guided delivery of assessment content to promote client self-report and engagement. The ASI-MV program demonstrated strong psychometric properties when compared with nondigital assessment approaches (Butler et al. 2001), and it has been widely used in SUD treatment settings. The Comprehensive Health Assessment for Teens (CHAT; Lord et al. 2011) is a web-based, self-report comprehensive substance use assessment for adolescents that has demonstrated good to excellent psychometric properties when compared with other validated self-report instruments in studies with clinical and nonclinical adolescent populations.

The Screener and Opioid Assessment for Patients with Pain—Revised (SOAPP-R) is a brief computerized self-report tool to facilitate assessment and planning for patients with chronic pain who are being considered for long-term opioid treatment (Butler et al. 2009a; Weiner et al. 2015). The tool has been studied extensively in pain populations, with established psychometric properties and good predictive accuracy for identifying which patients will engage in aberrant medication-related behavior (Finkelman et al. 2017, 2019). A companion digital tool, the brief version of the Current Opioid Misuse Measure (COMM-9; McCaffrey et al. 2019), can be used to help clinicians identify whether a patient currently on long-term opioid therapy may be engaging in aberrant opioid-related behavior.

The **T**obacco, **A**lcohol, **P**rescription Medication, and Other **S**ubstance Use Tool (TAPS; McNeely et al. 2016) is a two-part web-based substance use screening and brief assessment tool adapted from validated instruments and specifically developed for use in primary care settings. The TAPS tool can be administered by a clinician interviewer or completed by patients on a computer or tablet at a clinic or through a patient portal. In psychometric studies with adult patients in primary care, TAPS demonstrated high sensitivity for detecting problematic tobacco and marijuana use; moderate sensitivity for detecting tobacco, marijuana, and alcohol SUDs; and good validity when compared with similar nondigital instruments (McNeely et al. 2016; Schwartz et al. 2017).

The examples described above are just a few of the many empirically supported and psychometrically sound digital screening tools available for use in a range of practice settings (e.g., primary care, specialty care, community care) as a frontline strategy to identify SUDs and related risks among diverse patient populations. Digital screening and assessment approaches allow for standardization of assessment processes for identification of treatment needs. There is also solid evidence indicating that individuals are more likely to be honest about sensitive risk behaviors when reporting on a digital device relative to in-person interviews (Butler et al. 2009b). Use of digital screening and assessment tools in primary care or emergency department waiting rooms has resulted in increased rates of both screening and identification of patients with substance use problems (Harris et al. 2016; Spirito et al. 2016). Screening results can be automatically imported into electronic health records, and clinical protocols built into electronic health records can prompt delivery of an appropriate intervention (Tai and McLellan 2012).

Brief Interventions

Much of the early work with digital therapeutic approaches targeted problematic alcohol use in college students and focused on translation of screening and brief intervention harm-reduction models to online platforms. These programs include features to support identification of personal risk behaviors and consequences and provision of normative feedback, relevant education, and motivational enhancement and cognitive-behavioral strategies to promote self-management skills. Numerous studies of brief digital interventions have demonstrated their short-term positive effects on alcohol and other substance use and related consequences. We describe several examples below.

Drinker's Checkup is single-session digital intervention based on principles of normative feedback that has demonstrated efficacy for reducing alcohol use and associated risks, particularly among heavy drinkers (Hester et al. 2012). The electronic Alcohol eCHECKUP TO GO, formerly known as e-CHUG, utilizes risk assessment and personalized normative feedback to highlight drinking patterns and build motivation to change (Walters et al. 2007). Controlled studies demonstrated that college students who received Alcohol eCHECKUP TO GO significantly reduced their alcohol consumption and experienced fewer alcohol-related consequences compared with those who received assessment only, and the impact was strongest for high-risk drinkers (Doumas et al. 2011; Walters et al. 2007). In studies with high school ninth graders, students assigned to receive the Alcohol eCHECKUP TO GO intervention showed greater reductions in positive alcohol expectancies and frequency of drinking in comparison with those who received standard substance use education (Doumas et al. 2014a), but effects were not maintained at 6 months (Doumas et al. 2014b). A study with high school seniors showed significant reductions in weekly and peak drinking quantities and in frequency of drinking to intoxication in the Alcohol eCHECKUP TO GO group relative to the assessment-only control group, but only for students who reported recent heavy drinking (Doumas et al. 2017). Use of motivational text message boosters can enhance outcomes (Tahaney and Palfai 2017).

A number of evidence-based brief digital interventions target marijuana and other substances. For example, Marijuana eCHECKUP TO GO (formerly known as e-TOKE) produced greater reductions in college students' perceptions of the extent of peer cannabis use and in reported marijuana-related consequences relative to assessment-only conditions; there were no group differences in rates of cannabis initiation or use (Palfai et al. 2014). A brief digital motivational intervention with adolescent cannabis users in primary care yielded short-term reductions in cannabis-related consequences and other drug use compared with enhanced usual care (Walton et al. 2013). In another study with adolescents in primary care, this brief digital intervention produced lower rates of cannabis use initiation and lower frequency of use at 3 and 6 months compared with usual care (Walton et al. 2014).

The Motivational Enhancement System (MES; Ondersma et al. 2005) addresses substance use is perinatal and postpartum women. This single-session intervention utilizes principles of motivational interviewing to engage women in active change of their substance use behaviors. An animated narrator provides normative feedback about participants' substance use, guides evaluation of pros and cons of use, and assists in goal setting (Ondersma et al. 2005). Studies have demonstrated modest short-term impacts on motivation to change and reductions in use of alcohol, tobacco, and illicit substances by perinatal women (Ondersma et al. 2005, 2012, 2016).

In sum, brief digital interventions have demonstrated positive short-term impacts on substance-related perceptions and substance use behaviors. The most consistent results have been found for alcohol use, and positive impacts are generally most pronounced among high-risk drinkers. A salient mechanism of action of many brief interventions is alteration of perceptions of social norms regarding use. Although there is a need for studies to demonstrate the reproducibility of these positive findings for brief digital interventions across populations, the brevity, ease of use, and self-directed nature of these interventions position them as important first-line approaches for problematic substance use and as tools to build motivation to seek more intensive treatment.

Digital Treatment Interventions

A number of self-guided digital treatment interventions for SUDs, each derived from existing empirically supported clinician-delivered treatment approaches, have been evaluated in randomized clinical trials. Reduce Your Use is a self-guided web-based treatment for cannabis use and related problems based on cognitive-behavioral therapy (CBT) and motivational interviewing. In a randomized trial of the program with adults motivated to reduce their cannabis use, individuals in the treatment group showed significantly greater reductions in cannabis use compared with those in a web-based cannabis education control condition (Rooke et al. 2013). Can Reduce is an eight-module CBT-based intervention that has been evaluated as a stand-alone treatment and in combination with online chat counseling. This self-guided program produced significant short-term reductions in cannabis use, particularly when augmented by chat counseling sessions (Schaub et al. 2015).

Computer-Based Training for Cognitive Behavioral Therapy (CBT4CBT) is a self-guided web-based CBT intervention for SUDs that has been extensively evaluated in controlled trials and has consistently demonstrated positive effects on substance use behaviors (Carroll et al. 2008). Over six sessions, CBT4CBT assists users in identifying patterns of substance use and developing coping skills. Video and other multimedia content are used to promote engagement and learning. CBT4CBT has been evaluated as an adjunct to clinician-delivered treatment and as a stand-alone treatment.

In a study conducted in a community treatment setting, participants who received CBT4CBT in addition to counselor-delivered treatment as usual (TAU) demonstrated greater reductions in substance use during treatment compared with those who received counselor treatment alone; reductions in substance use were maintained at 6 months postintervention (Carroll et al. 2009). Similar results were found in a replication study conducted with cocaine-dependent clients receiving methadone maintenance therapy (Carroll et al. 2014). A randomized controlled trial compared CBT4CBT plus TAU, CBT4CBT as a stand-alone treatment with weekly clinician monitoring, and TAU only in treatment-seeking clients with alcohol use disorder (Kiluk et al. 2016). Participants who received CBT4CBT plus TAU achieved greater reductions in overall drinking and heavy drinking over time, and were more likely to complete treatment, in comparison with those who received TAU only. CBT4CBT has been adapted to include a module with information about buprenorphine therapy (CBT4CBT-Buprenorphine). Participants who received CBT4CBT-Buprenorphine as an adjunct to standard buprenorphine therapy submitted significantly more drug-negative urine tests relative to those who received buprenorphine therapy only (Shi et al. 2019).

The Therapeutic Education System (TES) (Bickel et al. 2008) is a self-guided intervention, available on web and mobile platforms, that is based on the Community Reinforcement Approach (CRA) and CBT for treating SUDs. TES includes more than 65 modules targeting coping skills related to SUDs and psychosocial functioning as well as HIV prevention. Modules include video and other multimedia features and interactive exercises to reinforce skill acquisition and learning. Knowledge consolidation is facilitated through fluency learning techniques.

TES has been evaluated in numerous randomized controlled trials and has demonstrated positive treatment outcomes for opioid, cannabis, and methamphetamine use disorders, as well as reductions in HIV risk behaviors, with results comparable to those produced by clinician-delivered evidence-based treatment. The intervention has most often been evaluated as an adjunct to or a replacement for a component of clinician-delivered treatment. In an initial trial, TES as an adjunct to standard drug counseling produced superior opioid and cocaine abstinence outcomes compared with standard counseling only, and it performed just as well as a completely therapist-delivered CRA/CBT treatment condition (Bickel et al. 2008).

In a study of clients receiving treatment at a methadone maintenance program, participants who received TES with reduced clinician time were abstinent for more weeks and provided more drug-free urine samples than did participants who received clinician-delivered treatment only (Marsch et al. 2014a). Treatment retention and time to dropout were similar between groups. The positive impact on outcomes was most pronounced among participants with extensive treatment histories (Kim et al. 2016). Another multisite study compared prison inmates with SUDs who received therapist-delivered behavior therapy with inmates who received TES as a stand-alone treatment. Although no differences were found for drug relapse, reductions in HIV risk behavior, or criminality, participants rated TES more favorably than the therapist-delivered treatment (Chaple et al. 2014).

In a large multisite National Institute on Drug Abuse (NIDA) Clinical Trials Network study conducted in outpatient treatment settings, participants who received TES with reduced clinician time demonstrated significantly greater rates of abstinence from substances at posttreatment and lower treatment dropout rates relative to participants who received the intensive counseling intervention only (Campbell et al. 2014). Treatment effects on abstinence were strongest among participants who were not abstinent at baseline (Campbell et al. 2014). This study formed the foundation of the process leading to market authorization approval of a mobile version of TES (called reSET® [Pear Therapeutics, Boston, MA]) by the U.S. Food and Drug Administration (FDA). The reSET® mobile app is indicated for use as a prescription-only adjunctive treatment for clients with SUDs. A second prescription digital therapeutic tool based on TES and targeted specifically for persons with opioid use disorder (called reSET-O® [Pear Therapeutics]) was subsequently cleared for marketing by the FDA.

In sum, there is strong and growing support for intensive digital treatment approaches for SUDs. The most rigorously evaluated digital approaches demonstrate outcomes on par with clinician-delivered treatments. Existing evidence suggests that positive outcomes are strongest when the digital treatment is provided in conjunction with clinician-delivered care to augment or replace a component of clinician-delivered counseling. One mechanism of action for digital treatment approaches appears to be through improvement of coping self-efficacy. Although there is some support for the utility of stand-alone digital treatment interventions, more research is needed to identify what contexts and conditions are associated with optimal effectiveness across diverse populations and settings.

Recovery Support

There is also growing evidence for the utility of digital relapse prevention and recovery support interventions following intensive treatment. The Addiction Comprehensive Health Enhancement Support System (A-CHESS) is a smartphone application created to help clients develop and maintain motivation for abstinence, and it connects clients with resources to cope with cravings, withdrawal symptoms, and high-risk situations to avoid relapse (Gustafson et al. 2014). In a randomized controlled trial among clients with alcohol use disorder discharged from residential treatment, participants who received A-CHESS had higher odds of reported abstinence from alcohol over the 8-month intervention period and fewer reported risky drinking days at 4-month follow-up relative to participants who received TAU (Gustafson et al. 2014). The impact of A-CHESS on reduction in risky drinking days was mediated by involvement in outpatient addiction treatment (Glass et al. 2017).

Educating and Supporting Inquisitive Youth in Recovery (ESQYIR; Gonzales et al. 2014) is a program that harnesses the ubiquity of mobile phones and text messaging as a popular mode of communication among young people to support addiction recovery. This 12-week mobile text messaging aftercare intervention targets youth (ages 12–24) transitioning out of community-based substance use treatment programs. Participants receive daily texts related to self-monitoring of risks and wellness recovery support tips, as well as education and social support resource information. In a randomized controlled pilot study, youths who participated in the mobile intervention were significantly less likely to relapse to their primary drug than were those in the aftercare-as-usual group, both during the intervention period and at 90-day follow-up. Compared with youths in the standard aftercare group, those who received the ESQYIR intervention also reported significantly lower substance use problem severity and were more likely to participate in extracurricular recovery behaviors (Gonzales et al. 2014). These positive results were sustained at both 6- and 9-month postintervention follow-up (Gonzales et al. 2016). This aftercare intervention highlights how the widely accessible, universal, and familiar features of digital devices can be harnessed to effectively support recovery.

Summary: Digital Therapeutics Across the Care Continuum for Substance Use Disorders

Research demonstrates the promise of digital therapeutic approaches across the care continuum for SUDs. These digital approaches have the potential to reach broad audiences with highly individualized care that can be tailored to an individual's needs, preferences, culture, learning style, stage of recovery, and clinical trajectory over time. Individuals can control the pace of their treatment, and clinicians can augment their treatment practices with digital therapeutic tools to allow them to work at their highest level of training, to work with more clients, and to focus more intensively on high-need clients. There are exciting opportunities for research to identify strategies for bundling evidence-supported digital therapeutic tools to efficiently address substance use treatment needs across the care continuum.

Advancing the Field: Future Directions

Emerging Technologies and Novel Methods

The digital therapeutic approaches described to this point largely represent translation of evidence-based clinician-delivered treatment approaches to digital platforms. Technological innovations and novel analytic approaches and study designs are advancing the potential for treatment delivery to new and exciting dimensions. For example, mobile and wearable sensing technologies and complex machine learning strategies create opportunities for passive identification of substance use behaviors and associated risks, overcoming the limitations of self-report (e.g., bias, burden). Recent work demonstrates how deep neural networking machine learning and social media content can be harnessed to accurately predict alcohol use risk (Hassanpour et al. 2019). Other studies have demonstrated how mobile phone and wearable sensing technologies can be used to predict stress (Mishra et al. 2020) and to model depression dynamics (Wang et al. 2018). These innovative data collection and processing capabilities introduce the possibility of intervening with a person at the moment of greatest risk—or "just in time"—as detailed by Nahum-Shani et al. (2018). The capability to intervene precisely when an individual is most in need is a hallmark of personalized medicine and a defining goal for future research focused on digital therapeutic approaches for SUDs and related conditions. Passive sensing and ecological momentary assessment technologies also allow for ongoing assessment of physiological, psychological, and behavioral mediator, moderator, and outcome indicators, which can advance insight into important mechanisms of action of digital therapeutics.

A challenge with digital therapeutic tools developed in the research space is that technological advances outpace the science. By the time a digital intervention has been rigorously evaluated, the technology may be outdated and not compatible with newer technologies being used by individuals or health care systems. There are also a myriad of mobile apps addressing SUDs and related conditions developed in the commercial space and readily available in app stores; many of these apps have commercial-grade design appeal and technology but no empirical support for producing positive change. Research can be advanced in this area through the use of novel study designs, including Sequential Multiple Assignment Randomized Trial (SMART; Collins et al. 2007) and micro-randomized trial (MRT; Klasnja et al. 2015) designs, to accelerate the pace of evaluation studies and develop adaptive interventions to optimally meet individual needs.

Promoting Uptake of Digital Therapeutics

Despite the growing empirical support for digital therapeutic approaches for SUDs, adoption of these approaches, like that of many treatment innovations, has been slow. Current implementation science frameworks can help to identify barriers to and facilitators of successful adoption and sustainable implementation of digital therapeutic approaches (Damschroder et al. 2009). These barriers and facilitators include features of the digital interventions themselves, characteristics of individuals using the digital technologies, and characteristics of organizations and of the broader external implementation context.

Digital therapeutic tools that are perceived by end users as being easy to use, appealing, relevant, and adaptable and as offering clear advantages over other treatment alternatives are more likely to be adopted and used (Lord et al. 2016). Awareness of and attitudes toward digital therapeutic approaches also influence uptake. For example, perceived social norms can play a powerful role in what people do. Clinicians' perceptions of other clinicians using TES influenced their own intentions to use the program in the future (Buti et al. 2013). Strategies to promote end-user buy-in, such as involving stakeholders in the intervention development process and conducting small-scale rollout pilots prior to full adoption, can help to promote adoption (Lord et al. 2016). Initiatives are currently under way to improve public awareness of existing digital therapeutic tools. For example, the Center for Technology and Behavioral Health (CTBH), a NIDA-designated Center of Excellence, maintains a continually updated compendium of summaries of empirical studies of digital therapeutic tools for SUDs and related conditions (www.c4tbh.org) (Lord et al. 2019).

Client access to appropriate technology should also be a consideration in any initiative aimed at use of a digital therapeutic approach (Lord et al. 2016). Whereas most people in the United States own a smartphone, access disparities still exist. Local technology infrastructure, including wireless and broadband capacity, can impact the relative compatibility of a given digital therapeutic in a given location. For example, many rural regions of the United States have limited or no broadband and wireless capabilities (Perrin 2019), which can pose challenges to broad use of digital therapeutic approaches in these regions. Perceived costs of digital therapeutic tools and lack of reimbursement models for use of digital therapeutic approaches for SUDs are also barriers to adoption (Ramsey et al. 2016). Billing systems and reimbursement structures for digital therapeutics are still in early development, but progress has been made in regard to reimbursement codes for SUD screening and FDA approval of digital therapeutic devices that allows for prescription, and coverage, of these tools.

Implementation science frameworks can inform the next generation of research to further the understanding of how to optimize adoption and sustain implementation of digital therapeutics across broad population bases and in diverse systems of care. Use of innovative study designs, such as hybrid effectiveness–implementation designs (Curran et al. 2012), can help elucidate key strategies to promote implementation while maintaining intervention effectiveness. Research initiatives that include identification and evaluation of relevant facilitators of and barriers to implementation across the stages of digital therapeutic development research, from the outset, can advance the field of digital therapeutics for SUDs by helping to speed translation of research findings into practice. Collaboration among researchers, clients, clinicians, health care administrators, policy makers, and developers can help ensure that future digital therapeutic approaches are supported by high-quality evidence while also meeting the needs of multilevel end users, increasing the likelihood of successful scale-up of digital therapeutics for SUDs to broader systems of care.

Conclusion

Digital therapeutics have great potential to reach broad populations of persons with SUDs and related conditions with science-based treatment. These tools can overcome many of the barriers to clinician-delivered care by providing improved treatment fidelity and replicability across populations and care settings, as well as accessibility to care where and when people need it the most. There are many opportunities for the next generation of science in digital therapeutics to advance the application of these tools more broadly, including studies to elucidate treatment heterogeneity (e.g., What works for whom, how, and when?) and to build cumulative knowledge about implementation of digital therapeutics with diverse populations and in different health care settings (e.g., What works for whom, and where?).

References

Anderson M: Mobile Technology and Home Broadband 2019. Washington, DC, Pew Research Center, June 13, 2019. Available at: https://www.pewresearch.org/internet/2019/06/13/mobile-technology-and-home-broadband-2019/. Accessed October 22, 2020.
Bickel WK, Marsch LA, Buchhalter AR, et al: Computerized behavior therapy for opioid-dependent outpatients: a randomized controlled trial. Exp Clin Psychopharmacol 16(2):132–143, 2008 18489017
Bonar EE, Koocher GP, Benoit MF, et al: Perceived risks and benefits in a text message study of substance abuse and sexual behavior. Ethics Behav 28(3):218–234, 2018 29632430
Buti AL, Eakins D, Fussell H, et al: Clinician attitudes, social norms and intentions to use a computer-assisted intervention. J Subst Abuse Treat 44(4):433–437, 2013 23021495
Butler SF, Budman SH, Goldman RJ, et al: Initial validation of a computer-administered Addiction Severity Index: the ASI-MV. Psychol Addict Behav 15(1):4–12, 2001 11255937
Butler SF, Budman SH, Fernandez KC, et al: Cross-validation of a screener to predict opioid misuse in chronic pain patients (SOAPP-R). J Addict Med 3(2):66–73, 2009a 20161199
Butler SF, Villapiano A, Malinow A: The effect of computer-mediated administration on self-disclosure of problems on the Addiction Severity Index. J Addict Med 3(4):194–203, 2009b 20161486
Campbell AN, Nunes EV, Matthews AG, et al: Internet-delivered treatment for substance abuse: a multisite randomized controlled trial. Am J Psychiatry 171(6):683–690, 2014 24700332

Carroll KM, Ball SA, Martino S, et al: Computer-assisted delivery of cognitive-behavioral therapy for addiction: a randomized trial of CBT4CBT. Am J Psychiatry 165(7):881–888, 2008 18450927

Carroll KM, Ball SA, Martino S, et al: Enduring effects of a computer-assisted training program for cognitive behavioral therapy: a 6-month follow-up of CBT4CBT. Drug Alcohol Depend 100(1–2):178–181, 2009 19041197

Carroll KM, Kiluk BD, Nich C, et al: Computer-assisted delivery of cognitive-behavioral therapy: efficacy and durability of CBT4CBT among cocaine-dependent individuals maintained on methadone. Am J Psychiatry 171(4):436–444, 2014 24577287

Chaple M, Sacks S, McKendrick K, et al: Feasibility of a computerized intervention for offenders with substance use disorders: a research note. J Exp Criminol 10:105–127, 2014 24634641

Collins LM, Murphy SA, Strecher V: The Multiphase Optimization Strategy (MOST) and the Sequential Multiple Assignment Randomized Trial (SMART): new methods for more potent eHealth interventions. Am J Prev Med 32 (5 suppl):S112–S118, 2007 17466815

Curran GM, Bauer M, Mittman B, et al: Effectiveness-implementation hybrid designs: combining elements of clinical effectiveness and implementation research to enhance public health impact. Med Care 50(3):217–226, 2012 22310560

Damschroder LJ, Aron DC, Keith RE, et al: Fostering implementation of health services research findings into practice: a consolidated framework for advancing implementation science. Implement Sci 4:50, 2009 19664226

Doumas DM, Kane CM, Navarro TB, et al: Decreasing heavy drinking in first-year students: evaluation of a web-based personalized feedback program administered during orientation. Journal of College Counseling 14(1):5–20, 2011. Available at: https://onlinelibrary.wiley.com/doi/10.1002/j.2161-1882.2011.tb00060.x. Accessed January 11, 2020.

Doumas DM, Esp S, Turrisi R, et al: A test of the efficacy of a brief, web-based personalized feedback intervention to reduce drinking among 9th grade students. Addict Behav 39(1):231–238, 2014a 24148137

Doumas DM, Hausheer R, Esp S, et al: Reducing alcohol use among 9th grade students: 6 month outcomes of a brief, web-based intervention. J Subst Abuse Treat 47(1):102–105, 2014b 24666810

Doumas DM, Esp S, Flay S, Bond L: A randomized controlled trial testing the efficacy of a brief online alcohol intervention for high school seniors. J Stud Alcohol Drugs 78(5):706–715, 2017 28930058

Finkelman MD, Jamison RN, Kulich RJ, et al: Cross-validation of short forms of the Screener and Opioid Assessment for Patients with Pain–Revised (SOAPP-R). Drug Alcohol Depend 178:94–100, 2017 28645065

Finkelman MD, Jamison RN, Magnuson B, et al: Computer-based testing and the 12-item Screener and Opioid Assessment for Patients With Pain–Revised: a combined approach to improving efficiency. Journal of Applied Biobehavioral Research 24(1):e12145, 2019. Available at: https://onlinelibrary.wiley.com/doi/full/10.1111/jabr.12145. Accessed January 11, 2020.

Glass JE, McKay JR, Gustafson DH, et al: Treatment seeking as a mechanism of change in a randomized controlled trial of a mobile health intervention to support recovery from alcohol use disorders. J Subst Abuse Treat 77:57–66, 2017 28476273

Gonzales R, Ang A, Murphy DA, et al: Substance use recovery outcomes among a cohort of youth participating in a mobile-based texting aftercare pilot program. J Subst Abuse Treat 47(1):20–26, 2014 24629885

Gonzales R, Hernandez M, Murphy DA, Ang A: Youth recovery outcomes at 6 and 9 months following participation in a mobile texting recovery support aftercare pilot study. Am J Addict 25(1):62–68, 2016 26689171

Gustafson DH, McTavish FM, Chih MY, et al: A smartphone application to support recovery from alcoholism: a randomized clinical trial. JAMA Psychiatry 71(5):566–572, 2014 24671165

Harris SK, Knight JR Jr, Van Hook S, et al: Adolescent substance use screening in primary care: validity of computer self-administered versus clinician-administered screening. Subst Abus 37(1):197–203, 2016 25774878

Hassanpour S, Tomita N, DeLise T, et al: Identifying substance use risk based on deep neural networks and Instagram social media data. Neuropsychopharmacology 44(3):487–494, 2019 30356094

Hester RK, Delaney HD, Campbell W: The college drinker's check-up: outcomes of two randomized clinical trials of a computer-delivered intervention. Psychol Addict Behav 26(1):1–12, 2012 21823769

Kiluk BD, Devore KA, Buck MB, et al: Randomized trial of computerized cognitive behavioral therapy for alcohol use disorders: efficacy as a virtual stand-alone and treatment add-on compared with standard outpatient treatment. Alcohol Clin Exp Res 40(9):1991–2000, 2016 27488212

Kim SJ, Marsch LA, Acosta MC, et al: Can persons with a history of multiple addiction treatment episodes benefit from technology delivered behavior therapy? A moderating role of treatment history at baseline. Addict Behav 54:18–23, 2016 26657820

Klasnja P, Hekler EB, Shiffman S, et al: Microrandomized trials: an experimental design for developing just-in-time adaptive interventions. Health Psychol 34S:1220–1228, 2015 26651463

Lord SE, Trudeau KJ, Black RA, et al: CHAT: development and validation of a computer-delivered, self-report, substance use assessment for adolescents. Subst Use Misuse 46(6):781–794, 2011 21174498

Lord S, Moore SK, Ramsey A, et al: Implementation of a substance use recovery support mobile phone app in community settings: qualitative study of clinician and staff perspectives of facilitators and barriers. JMIR Ment Health 3(2):e24, 2016 27352884

Lord SE, Seavey KM, Oren SD, et al: Digital presence of a research center as a research dissemination platform: reach and resources. JMIR Ment Health 6(4):e11686, 2019 30950800

Marsch LA, Guarino H, Acosta M, et al: Web-based behavioral treatment for substance use disorders as a partial replacement of standard methadone maintenance treatment. J Subst Abuse Treat 46(1):43–51, 2014a 24060350

Marsch LA, Lord SE, Dallery J (eds): Behavioral Healthcare and Technology: Using Science-Based Innovations to Transform Practice. New York, Oxford University Press, 2014b

McCaffrey SA, Black RA, Villapiano AJ, et al: Development of a brief version of the Current Opioid Misuse Measure (COMM): the COMM-9. Pain Med 20(1):113–118, 2019 29237039

McLellan AT, Kushner H, Metzger D, et al: The Fifth Edition of the Addiction Severity Index. J Subst Abuse Treat 9(3):199–213, 1992 1334156

McNeely J, Wu LT, Subramaniam G, et al: Performance of the Tobacco, Alcohol, Prescription medication, and other Substance use (TAPS) tool for substance use screening in primary care patients. Ann Intern Med 165(10):690–699, 2016 27595276

Milward J, Day E, Wadsworth E, et al: Mobile phone ownership, usage and readiness to use by patients in drug treatment. Drug Alcohol Depend 146:111–115, 2015 25468818

Milward J, Drummond C, Fincham-Campbell S, et al: What makes online substance-use interventions engaging? A systematic review and narrative synthesis. Digit Health 4:2055207617743354, 2018 29942622

Mishra V, Pope G, Lord S, et al: Continuous detection of physiological stress with commodity hardware. ACM Transactions on Computing for Healthcare 1(2):30, 2020. Available at: https://dl.acm.org/doi/10.1145/3361562. Accessed August 4, 2020.

Nahum-Shani I, Smith SN, Spring BJ, et al: Just-in-time adaptive interventions (JITAIs) in mobile health: key components and design principles for ongoing health behavior support. Ann Behav Med 52(6):446–462, 2018 27663578

Ondersma SJ, Chase SK, Svikis DS, et al: Computer-based brief motivational intervention for perinatal drug use. J Subst Abuse Treat 28(4):305–312, 2005 15925264

Ondersma SJ, Svikis DS, Lam PK, et al: A randomized trial of computer-delivered brief intervention and low-intensity contingency management for smoking during pregnancy. Nicotine Tob Res 14(3):351–360, 2012 22157229

Ondersma SJ, Svikis DS, Thacker LR, et al: A randomised trial of a computer-delivered screening and brief intervention for postpartum alcohol use. Drug Alcohol Rev 35(6):710–718, 2016 27004474

Onken LS, Carroll KM, Shoham V, et al: Reenvisioning clinical science: unifying the discipline to improve the public health. Clin Psychol Sci 2(1):22–34, 2014 25821658

Palfai TP, Saitz R, Winter M, et al: Web-based screening and brief intervention for student marijuana use in a university health center: pilot study to examine the implementation of eCHECKUP TO GO in different contexts. Addict Behav 39(9):1346–1352, 2014 24845164

Perrin A: Digital Gap Between Rural and Nonrural America Persists. Washington, DC, Pew Research Center, May 31, 2019. Available at: https://www.pewresearch.org/fact-tank/2019/05/31/digital-gap-between-rural-and-nonrural-america-persists/. Accessed October 22, 2020.

Ramsey A, Lord S, Torrey J, et al: Paving the way to successful implementation: identifying key barriers to use of technology-based therapeutic tools for behavioral health care. J Behav Health Serv Res 43(1):54–70, 2016 25192755

Rooke S, Copeland J, Norberg M, et al: Effectiveness of a self-guided Web-based cannabis treatment program: randomized controlled trial. J Med Internet Res 15(2):e26, 2013 23470329

Schaub MP, Wenger A, Berg O, et al: A Web-based self-help intervention with and without chat counseling to reduce cannabis use in problematic cannabis users: three-arm randomized controlled trial. J Med Internet Res 17(10):e232, 2015 26462848

Schwartz RP, McNeely J, Wu LT, et al: Identifying substance misuse in primary care: TAPS Tool compared to the WHO ASSIST. J Subst Abuse Treat 76:69–76, 2017 28159441

Shi JM, Henry SP, Dwy SL, et al: Randomized pilot trial of Web-based cognitive-behavioral therapy adapted for use in office-based buprenorphine maintenance. Subst Abus 40(2):132–135, 2019 30714880

Spirito A, Bromberg JR, Casper TC, et al: Reliability and validity of a two-question alcohol screen in the pediatric emergency department. Pediatrics 138(6):e20160691, 2016 27940674

Sugarman DE, Campbell ANC, Iles BR, et al: Technology-based interventions for substance use and comorbid disorders: an examination of the emerging literature. Harv Rev Psychiatry 25(3):123–134, 2017 28475504

Tahaney KD, Palfai TP: Text messaging as an adjunct to a web-based intervention for college student alcohol use: a preliminary study. Addict Behav 73:63–66, 2017 28478315

Tai B, McLellan AT: Integrating information on substance use disorders into electronic health record systems. J Subst Abuse Treat 43(1):12–19, 2012 22154827

Taylor K, Silver L: Smartphone Ownership Is Growing Rapidly Around the World, But Not Always Equally. 2019. Available at: http://www.pewglobal.org/2019/02/05/smartphone-ownership-is-growing-rapidly-around-the-world-but-not-always-equally. Accessed December 4, 2019.

Walters ST, Vader AM, Harris TR: A controlled trial of web-based feedback for heavy drinking college students. Prev Sci 8(1):83–88, 2007 17136461

Walton MA, Bohnert K, Resko S, et al: Computer and therapist based brief interventions among cannabis-using adolescents presenting to primary care: one year outcomes. Drug Alcohol Depend 132(3):646–653, 2013 23711998

Walton MA, Resko S, Barry KL, et al: A randomized controlled trial testing the efficacy of a brief cannabis universal prevention program among adolescents in primary care. Addiction 109(5):786–797, 2014 24372937

Wang R, Wang W, daSilva A, et al: Tracking depression dynamics in college students using mobile phone and wearable sensing. Proceedings of the ACM Interactive, Mobile, Wearable and Ubiquitous Technologies 2(1):1–26, 2018. Available at: https://dl.acm.org/doi/10.1145/3191775. Accessed January 11, 2020.

Weiner SG, Horton LC, Green TC, et al: Feasibility of tablet computer screening for opioid abuse in the emergency department. West J Emerg Med 16(1):18–23, 2015 25671003

CHAPTER 30

Mindfulness, Exercise, and Other Alternative Therapies

Sarah Bowen, Ph.D.

Adam D. Wilson, M.S.

Cameron S. Laue, B.A.

Approaches to the treatment of substance use disorders (SUDs) continue to develop and shift, as does the research supporting these approaches. Although what are often referred to as "alternative" approaches—such as meditation, exercise, yoga, music therapy, and acupuncture—have likely long been integrated into treatment programs, the evidence base underlying these approaches is relatively recent. Research has been growing on the use of mindfulness meditation, exercise, and other "mind and body" practices such as yoga, acupuncture, and tai chi as complements to extant treatment models or as alternatives to standard SUD treatment. In this chapter we offer a brief overview of these alternative approaches.

Mindfulness

Contemplative practices have long been a part of addiction treatment programs, most notably in 12-step approaches, in which both prayer and meditation are included as part of the steps. Early investigations of specific forms of meditation, such as Transcendental Meditation, in addiction treatment can be found as far back as the 1970s (e.g., Marlatt and Marques 1977). A more recent meta-analysis assessing several forms of meditation on a range of psychological variables suggests that these practices have effects across a range of outcomes, particularly negative affective states (Sedlmeier et al. 2012). The fact that meditation as an adjunctive approach to treating addiction continues to be studied reflects its considerable promise for SUD treatment. However, there are gaps in the evidence base, and findings from studies have been mixed (Grant et al. 2017). The multiple and diverse forms of meditation being studied, as well as the range of treatment populations and settings, may account for some of these inconsistencies (Gryczynski et al. 2018). In recent years, the most thoroughly studied approach in relation to substance use has been mindfulness meditation.

Mindfulness practices have their roots in many ancient traditions, most notably Buddhism (Hart 1987). This traditional Eastern-based approach has garnered growing visibility and support via systematic programs of research. Mindfulness meditation instruction is intended to develop a present-focused and nonjudgmental awareness. This awareness fosters insight into the nature of reality, including the relationships among thoughts, emotions, and behaviors and the causes and conditions of suffering, which are thought to be rooted in craving and aversion (Hart 1987). Thus, these practices might benefit individuals experiencing the craving and compulsive behavior that characterize addiction.

Although these practices date back thousands of years, only relatively recently have they acquired a prominent role in traditional Western psychology and medicine. In the context of contemporary psychology, mindfulness has been described as a kind, gentle, and curious awareness of experience (Grossman 2010). Although the practices are typically secularized to suit a contemporary medical context, there have been a few studies of these practices in their original form. For example, an ancient practice of an intensive 10-day Vipassana meditation course, taught in its traditional Buddhist form, was assessed in a trial with incarcerated adults and showed evidence of significant reductions in substance use and improvements in psychosocial outcomes when compared with the treatment-as-usual (TAU) condition (Bowen et al. 2006). The majority of trials, however, examine the effects of secularized, manualized mindfulness training. Systematic reviews of secularized mindfulness practices incorporated into various forms of mental health treatment show promising outcomes across several populations and disorders (Chiesa and Serretti 2017). The past decade has witnessed numerous studies specific to addiction treatment, including multiple randomized controlled trials (RCTs) supporting mindfulness practices as a beneficial addition to or a primary base for treatment of SUDs, with several newly developed programs integrating cognitive-behavioral approaches with mindfulness practice for people with problematic alcohol and substance use patterns.

For example, one study found a lower likelihood of relapse and significantly fewer days of substance use or heavy drinking at 1-year follow-up among study participants assigned to a mindfulness-based relapse prevention program compared with those assigned to either a 12-step-based standard aftercare program or a cognitive-behavioral relapse prevention program (Bowen et al. 2014). A similar study in a residential addiction treatment program for women referred by the criminal justice system found significantly fewer drug use days and fewer legal and medical problems among women randomly assigned to mindfulness-based relapse prevention compared with those assigned to standard relapse prevention (Witkiewitz et al. 2014). One study, specifically focused on cigarette smoking, found that in comparison with participants receiving TAU, participants who received mindfulness training were more likely to maintain smoking abstinence during the 4 months following treatment, and maintained a greater overall reduction in use (Brewer et al. 2011).

A related group of studies assessed a Mindfulness-Oriented Recovery Enhancement (MORE) program for patients with chronic pain who were at risk of developing, or were in treatment for, opioid use disorder. In samples of long-term prescription opioid users, reductions in chronic pain symptoms and in levels of opioid misuse risk were significantly greater among participants in the MORE program than among participants in an active control condition (Garland et al. 2014b).

Other studies have attempted to shed light on how mindfulness practice affects primary addiction outcomes. Mechanistic studies of the MORE program point to increased autonomic and electrocortical responses to natural reward cues that were also associated with the effects of MORE on decreasing pain severity (Garland et al. 2013, 2014a). Other studies have suggested that mindfulness practice may help individuals develop coping skills by promoting awareness and acceptance of craving, thereby diminishing the urge to immediately alleviate the associated discomfort. Thus, mindfulness training may exert its effects by attenuating the link between craving and substance use (Brewer et al. 2013).

Although research in this area has seen significant growth over the past decade, much work remains to be done to adapt these programs for use in diverse populations and to gain a better understanding of the neuropsychological, physiological, and behavioral mechanisms that underlie the changes seen in the trials.

Exercise

The potential role of exercise in the treatment of addictions is another emerging field of study. The degree to which physical exercise may have direct and indirect effects on wellness, behavior modification, and self-direction is a relatively understudied area in SUD treatment research. There is, however, a small body of literature, dating back to the early 1970s, that reports both positive and negative findings in regard to the benefits of adding physical exercise as an adjuvant to acute treatment episodes. Reviews of these efforts (Giesen et al. 2015; Zschucke et al. 2012) provide tentative and preliminary support for the efficacy of exercise as an adjunct to traditional treatment. A meta-analysis (Wang et al. 2014) involving 22 RCTs published between 1990 and 2013 examined the effects of physical exercise on SUD treatment outcomes for nicotine, alcohol, heroin, cocaine, or polysubstance use. Findings indicated that exercise produced significant increases in abstinence rates, reductions in anxiety and depression, and amelioration of withdrawal symptoms. In contrast, a multisite trial (Trivedi et al. 2017) examining exercise as an adjunctive intervention specifically for individuals diagnosed with stimulant use disorder found no significant differences between the intervention and control groups in percentages of stimulant-abstinent days over the last 8 weeks of the 12-week study.

The alcohol use disorder (AUD) treatment literature includes approximately 20 RCTs and nonrandomized controlled trials investigating the impact of physical exercise on AUD- or health-related outcomes. However, as Hallgren et al. (2017) have pointed out, the overwhelming majority of these studies either were conducted at an inpatient SUD treatment facility or measured the acute biological effects of a single session of exercise, making it difficult to determine conclusively whether exercise had a measurable effect on alcohol consumption, recovery, or relapse. The studies also differed with respect to type, duration, and intensity of exercise, as well as measured outcomes of interest, but the results were generally suggestive of a positive benefit.

In an early trial that examined both exercise and meditation in a sample of college student "high-volume drinkers" who averaged 45 drinks or more per month (Murphy et al. 1986), participants were randomly assigned to one of three conditions: 1) 70 minutes of group running three times per week for 8 weeks, 2) 20 minutes of meditation two times per day for 8 weeks, or 3) a pre- and post-assessment-only condition with self-tracking of alcohol consumption behavior. Participants assigned to the exercise condition showed, in addition to the expected significant improvements in fitness, a significant decrease in alcohol consumption at posttreatment compared with the assessment-only control group. There were no significant differences in posttreatment alcohol consumption between participants in the exercise condition and those in the meditation condition, or between participants in the meditation condition and those in the control condition.

An earlier small randomized trial (Gary and Guthrie 1972) tested an adjunctive jogging intervention versus a TAU control condition at an inpatient treatment facility for AUD. Although the inpatient nature of the sample precluded assessment of alcohol consumption, the investigators found that the jogging intervention produced significant benefits for both self-image and body image in addition to the expected significant improvement in physical fitness among the intervention sample. Similar early trials (Luedke 1978; McKelvy et al. 1980) investigating physical health and fitness improvements resulting from exercise among individuals hospitalized for AUD might best be viewed as feasibility studies, with outcomes suggesting that individuals with AUD can safely exercise and will likely see physical fitness gains, but without measured outcomes related to alcohol consumption or alcohol-related consequences, cravings, or affect.

In another early study, 58 inpatients enrolled in an AUD treatment center participated in a daily fitness program involving 6 weeks of five-times-per-week exercise (Sinyor et al. 1982). At the follow-up evaluation 3 months after discharge from the center, there were significant differences in abstinence rates between participants in the intervention group (69.3% abstinent) and those in the control group (36.9% abstinent).

Palmer et al. (1988) were one of the first groups to apply recommendations from the American College of Sports Medicine with regard to a graded aerobic exercise program (60 minutes per day, three times per week, for 4 weeks, at 60%–80% of participants' age-predicted maximal heart rate) as a treatment intervention for inpatient adults with AUD. Although the study design precluded assessment of postintervention alcohol consumption, results from this time-staggered controlled trial of exercise for inpatients with AUD ($N=53$) showed significant decreases ($P<0.01$) in state anxiety and trait anxiety, as well as significant decreases in depression, in the exercise group as compared with the TAU control group.

More recent trials have similarly found promising effects for exercise. For example, Ussher et al. (2004) conducted a within-subject counterbalanced crossover comparison trial of the effect of brief aerobic exercise on alcohol urges and mood among adults who had recently completed alcohol detoxification in a hospital-based clinic. Participants ($N=20$) were randomly assigned to 10 minutes of either moderate-intensity (experimental) or very-light-intensity (control) exercise on a stationary bicycle on day 1 of the trial, and were then switched to the other condition on day 2; measurements of alcohol urges and mood were taken immediately before, during (at 5 minutes), and at three time points after exercise. Relative to baseline measurements, there was a significant decline in alcohol urges for the experimental condition versus the control condition during exercise. However, no significant differences were found between the conditions at assessment time points after the exercise session had ended.

The majority of these trials were conducted in inpatient settings or with non-treatment-seeking college students; therefore, most of the evidence in support of adjunctive exercise in AUD treatment is limited to positive findings around reductions in craving, reductions in depression and anxiety-related symptomatology, improvements in self-concept and internal locus of control, and improvements in various measures of physical health. To date, only one RCT of aerobic exercise in an AUD sample has been conducted in an outpatient setting (Brown et al. 2014). In this study, physically sedentary patients with AUD were randomly assigned to a 12-week moderate-intensity group aerobic exercise intervention or a "brief advice to exercise" control intervention. Results indicated significantly lower frequency and intensity of alcohol use both during and at the end of treatment among participants assigned to the exercise condition compared with those assigned to the control condition, and a significant inverse relationship was seen between minutes of exercise and heavy-drinking days at the 6-month postbaseline follow-up.

Currently, however, there is no consensus in the field as to what constitutes an optimal "dose" of exercise. Two meta-analyses (Barton and Pretty 2010; Carayol et al. 2013) suggested that 90–120 minutes of aerobic activity per week was ideal, whereas another study (Ratey and Hagerman 2008) was more prescriptive in its recommendations, advocating that episodes of exercise optimally should contain a series of five maximal-effort 30- to 40-second sprints, with each sprint followed by 5 minutes of gentle low-intensity aerobic movement before the next maximal effort.

Also unresolved are questions around what mechanisms of action might be driving the link between physical exercise and improvements in psychopathology generally and in SUD specifically. One of the most promising proposed mechanisms of action for these efficacy outcomes is the potential stimulating effect of exercise on brain-derived neurotrophic factor (BDNF), a protein critically implicated in neurogenesis and in the sustenance of new neurons and neural connections (Szuhany et al. 2015). Stimulation of BDNF may promote changes in the neural pathways associated with addictive behavior, altered responses to cue-related craving, and learned acquisition of coping and other behavioral skills (Olsen et al. 2015). Although the conceptual basis for this mechanism has been tested and demonstrated in animal models, no extant studies in the literature have directly tested associations among physical exercise, BDNF, and SUD recovery in humans.

Along with upregulation of BDNF, a number of other potential mechanisms of action, including the previously mentioned reductions in anxiety, depression, and other psychopathology, have been proposed as mediating factors in the positive effects of physical activity on SUD outcomes. Proposed mechanisms have included increases in coping repertoire, reductions in acute craving, attenuated stress reactivity, improvements in affective instability, and neurochemical changes related to endogenous opioid, glutamate, and dopamine transmission (Zschucke et al. 2012).

Other Alternative Approaches

Yoga, acupuncture, and tai chi and qigong fall within the category of mind and body practices as defined by the National Center for Complementary and Integrative Health. Each of these complementary and alternative medicine (CAM) treatments, although less thoroughly examined than exercise or mindfulness-based treatment approaches for treating SUDs, has garnered excitement as a promising therapy for use in the treatment of SUDs and in relapse prevention (Behere et al. 2009). However, methodological issues remain problematic in research on these approaches, as is the case with several other "alternative" approaches; in their review, Posadzki et al. (2016) noted "the need for more quality primary randomized clinical trials...to determine the therapeutic usefulness of CAM" (p. 79).

Yoga

Yoga has been described as "a part of Ayurvedic medicine that can consist of one or more of the following: specific postures, breathing exercises, body cleansing, mindfulness meditation, and lifestyle modifications" (Posadzki and Ernst 2011, p. 632). One of the most widely practiced complementary health approaches in recent years (Clarke et al. 2015), yoga has become increasingly integrated into traditional health care settings, with particular utility as an adjunctive therapy in the management of disorders with more chronic-type profiles such as SUDs. Assessment of psychological correlates of mood is one avenue by which yoga treatment may inform treatment outcomes; indeed, many yoga intervention studies in substance-using populations collect such measures as a primary outcome. An RCT studying the effect of a 4-week yoga intervention in addition to TAU among 66 men enrolled in addiction treatment in India found significant reductions in depression and improvements in sleep quality, with a simultaneous increase in self-esteem, in the treatment group. In contrast, men in the waitlist control group also demonstrated significant decreases in depression and improvements in sleep quality but showed no significant increases on self-esteem measures (Devi and Singh 2016).

Yoga has also been employed as an adjunctive therapy in populations with a primary psychiatric disorder associated with increased substance use risk behaviors but without a formal clinical diagnosis. In a pilot RCT investigating whether participation in a yoga intervention would decrease the risk of engagement in substance abuse behaviors for women with posttraumatic stress disorder (PTSD), participants who had completed both alcohol and drug screening assessments were randomly assigned to either a 12-session yoga intervention or an assessment-only control condition. Results indicated a trend-level (not statistically significant) decrease in alcohol and drug use risk among participants assigned to the yoga intervention relative to those assigned to the assessment-only condition (Reddy et al. 2014). Reported substance use has also been used as a primary outcome measure in studies investigating yoga as an adjunctive treatment for alcohol dependence. In a research study examining the effects of a 10-week adjunctive yoga intervention among individuals in outpatient treatment for alcohol dependence in Sweden (Hallgren et al. 2014), participants were randomly assigned to receive either TAU (consisting of standard psychological and pharmacological treatments for alcohol dependence) or TAU with the addition of the yoga intervention (consisting of a weekly group yoga session, with participants encouraged to practice outside of the class once a day). Greater reductions in alcohol consumption were evident at 6-month follow-up for the TAU-plus-yoga group relative to the TAU-only group, although the results were not statistically significant (Hallgren et al. 2014).

Quality of life (QOL) is often used as an outcome measure in SUD studies examining the effectiveness of yoga, with yoga associated with well-being promotion. Both QOL measures and drug urine screening results were used as primary outcome measures in a study on the effects of Sudarshan Kriya yoga (SKY), "a simple rhythmic breathing technique [that] benefits a wide range of clinical conditions including substance use" (Dhawan et al. 2015, p. 144), in a sample of individuals with opioid dependence. Participants were randomly assigned to either TAU only or TAU plus 12 hours (over 3 days) of the SKY program. The study goal was to assess whether SKY in addition to TAU would help maintain abstinence and improve QOL, with follow-up time points at 3 and 6 months, providing a more longitudinal understanding of sustained abstinence. A total of 55 individuals completed the TAU-plus-SKY course, while a control group of 29 completed TAU only. SKY significantly increased QOL measures relative to the control group, with no relapse based on urine screening at the 6-month follow-up time point (Dhawan et al. 2015).

Acupuncture

The early research on acupuncture as a treatment for drug withdrawal and abstinence was promising but lacked rigor and power. More recently, two large well-designed RCTs demonstrated no differences in abstinence or treatment retention among acupuncture, sham acupuncture, or relaxation for participants with alcohol dependence (Bullock et al. 2002) or cocaine dependence (Margolin et al. 2002). Subsequent research has been similarly inconclusive, with variability in treatment types as well as in results. Specific auricular acupuncture points, specified by the National Acupuncture Detoxification Association (NADA) protocol (Brumbaugh 1993), are now commonly used in Western treatment. A 2016 RCT examined the effects of an auricular acupuncture intervention in 260 individuals with substance abuse and psychiatric comorbidity (Ahlberg et al. 2016). Of the 280 participants, 80 were randomly assigned to the NADA protocol, 80 to a local protocol adapted from the NADA protocol, and 120 to a relaxation control protocol. Although every group improved significantly on measures of sleep problems and anxiety symptoms over the course of treatment, there were no group differences by treatment, and the effect sizes were small. A 2017 study employed the NADA protocol as an adjunct to traditional treatment for 100 participants at a substance abuse service center (Carter et al. 2017). Of the 100 participants, 50 were randomly assigned to TAU with the addition of the NADA protocol, and the other 50 were randomly assigned to the TAU-only group. Participants assigned to the TAU-plus-NADA protocol group had to receive at least two treatments to be included in the statistical analysis, with the group averaging 10 treatment sessions. In comparison with individuals participating in the TAU-only condition, those participating in the TAU-plus-NADA group showed significantly higher QOL scores and significantly decreased alcohol use at 3-month and 6-month follow-ups (Carter et al. 2017).

Tai Chi and Qigong

Tai chi and qigong are mind and body movement approaches that share many characteristics and are based on wellness practices from ancient China, with a number of putative health benefits (Jahnke et al. 2010). A new exercise category—meditative movement—has been created to accommodate these practices (Larkey et al. 2009). Although RCTs have examined the health benefits of tai chi and qigong in domains such as physical function, psychological symptoms, and QOL, there is minimal literature on their effectiveness in substance use treatment. Only one RCT has been published to date. Li et al. (2002) conducted a study examining qigong therapy as an adjunct to inpatient detoxification of heroin users. Participants were randomly assigned to one of the following: 1) the qigong treatment group (practicing 2.5 hours daily for 10 days), 2) a medication group receiving lofexidine hydrochloride in a step-down withdrawal protocol over the course of the 10 days, or 3) a nontreatment group receiving neither. From the first day of the study, the qigong group demonstrated significantly lower symptom scores than the other two groups. In addition, the qigong group had negative urine screens by day 5 of the intervention, whereas the medication treatment group did not demonstrate negative urine screens until day 9. Overall, the study results suggested that qigong therapy aided in accelerating the detoxification process and alleviating withdrawal symptoms for the qigong treatment group relative to the medication group and the control group (Li et al. 2002).

Summary of Other Alternative Approaches

The yoga, acupuncture, tai chi, and qigong RCTs described above show to varying degrees the potential of specific mind and body approaches as adjunctive therapies in substance use. However, the evidence base for each approach is undermined by several key methodological limitations: variability in standardization of treatment approach, variability in outcome measurement, poor study design (i.e., lack of blinding, inadequate informed consent), and lack of control groups.

These approaches have not been well studied in comparison with other integrative techniques such as mindfulness or exercise, but all of these CAM approaches are in beginning stages. There are study results suggesting promise, and the recent growth in the literature suggests that the field of substance use treatment is increasingly looking to such approaches to complement or offer as alternatives to the more traditional 12-step or cognitive-behavioral therapy–based treatments for SUDs.

Conclusion

Although the body of research on mindfulness and alternative therapies for SUDs is still relatively young, the traditions and practices from which these interventions are drawn have been around for centuries, and some even for millennia. Integration of these approaches into contemporary evidence-based treatment models can potentially capitalize on both ancient and modern wisdom and science. As empirical evidence supporting alternative interventions grows, perhaps these therapies will shift from "alternative" to standard components of practice in the field, thereby enhancing and advancing SUD treatment.

References

Ahlberg R, Skårberg K, Brus O, et al: Auricular acupuncture for substance use: a randomized controlled trial of effects on anxiety, sleep, drug use and use of addiction treatment services. Subst Abuse Treat Prev Policy 11(1):24, 2016 27451854

Barton J, Pretty J: What is the best dose of nature and green exercise for improving mental health? A multi-study analysis. Environ Sci Technol 44(10):3947–3955, 2010 20337470

Behere RV, Muralidharan K, Benegal V: Complementary and alternative medicine in the treatment of substance use disorders—a review of the evidence. Drug Alcohol Rev 28(3):292–300, 2009 21462415

Bowen S, Witkiewitz K, Dillworth TM, et al: Mindfulness meditation and substance use in an incarcerated population. Psychol Addict Behav 20(3):343–347, 2006 16938074

Bowen S, Witkiewitz K, Clifasefi SL, et al: Relative efficacy of mindfulness-based relapse prevention, standard relapse prevention, and treatment as usual for substance use disorders: a randomized clinical trial. JAMA Psychiatry 71(5):547–556, 2014 24647726

Brewer JA, Mallik S, Babuscio TA, et al: Mindfulness training for smoking cessation: results from a randomized controlled trial. Drug Alcohol Depend 119(1–2):72–80, 2011 21723049

Brewer JA, Elwafi HM, Davis JH: Craving to quit: psychological models and neurobiological mechanisms of mindfulness training as treatment for addictions. Psychol Addict Behav 27(2):366–379, 2013 22642859

Brown RA, Abrantes AM, Minami H, et al: A preliminary, randomized trial of aerobic exercise for alcohol dependence. J Subst Abuse Treat 47(1):1–9, 2014 24666811

Brumbaugh AG: Acupuncture: new perspectives in chemical dependency treatment. J Subst Abuse Treat 10(1):35–43, 1993 8450571

Bullock ML, Kiresuk TJ, Sherman RE, et al: A large randomized placebo controlled study of auricular acupuncture for alcohol dependence. J Subst Abuse Treat 22(2):71–77, 2002 11932132

Carayol M, Bernard P, Boiché J, et al: Psychological effect of exercise in women with breast cancer receiving adjuvant therapy: what is the optimal dose needed? Ann Oncol 24(2):291–300, 2013 23041586

Carter K, Olshan-Perlmutter M, Marx J, et al: NADA ear acupuncture: an adjunctive therapy to improve and maintain positive outcomes in substance abuse treatment. Behav Sci (Basel) 7(2):37, 2017 28621706

Chiesa A, Serretti A: Mindfulness based cognitive therapy for psychiatric disorders: a systematic review and meta-analysis, in Mindfulness: Clinical Applications of Mindfulness and Acceptance: Specific Interventions for Psychiatric, Behavioural, and Physical Health Conditions, Vol III. Edited by Gaudiano BA. New York, Routledge/Taylor & Francis Group, 2017, pp 157–187

Clarke TC, Black LI, Stussman BJ, et al: Trends in the use of complementary health approaches among adults: United States, 2002–2012. Natl Health Stat Rep (79):1–16, 2015 25671660

Devi NJ, Singh TB: A randomized control trial of the effect of yoga on quality of sleep, self-esteem and depression in substance abuser. International Journal of Multidisciplinary Approach and Studies 3(4):11–17, 2016. Available at: http://ijmas.com/upcomingissue/02.04.2016.pdf. Accessed January 11, 2020.

Dhawan A, Chopra A, Jain R, et al: Effectiveness of yogic breathing intervention on quality of life of opioid dependent users. Int J Yoga 8(2):144–147, 2015 26170596

Garland EL, Froeliger B, Zeidan F, et al: The downward spiral of chronic pain, prescription opioid misuse, and addiction: cognitive, affective, and neuropsychopharmacologic pathways. Neurosci Biobehav Rev 37(10 Pt 2):2597–2607, 2013 23988582

Garland EL, Froeliger B, Howard MO: Effects of mindfulness-oriented recovery enhancement on reward responsiveness and opioid cue-reactivity. Psychopharmacology (Berl) 231(16):3229–3238, 2014a 24595503

Garland EL, Manusov EG, Froeliger B, et al: Mindfulness-oriented recovery enhancement for chronic pain and prescription opioid misuse: results from an early stage randomized controlled trial. J Consult Clin Psychol 82(3):448–459, 2014b 24491075

Gary V, Guthrie D: The effect of jogging on physical fitness and self-concept in hospitalized alcoholics. Q J Stud Alcohol 33(4):1073–1078, 1972 4648626

Giesen ES, Deimel H, Bloch W: Clinical exercise interventions in alcohol use disorders: a systematic review. J Subst Abuse Treat 52:1–9, 2015 25641736

Grant S, Colaiaco B, Motala A, et al: Mindfulness-based relapse prevention for substance use disorders: a systematic review and meta-analysis. J Addict Med 11(5):386–396, 2017 28727663

Grossman P: Mindfulness for psychologists: paying kind attention to the perceptible. Mindfulness 1(2):87–97, 2010. Available at: https://link.springer.com/article/10.1007/s12671-010-0012-7. Accessed January 11, 2020.

Gryczynski J, Schwartz RP, Fishman MJ, et al: Integration of Transcendental Meditation® (TM) into alcohol use disorder (AUD) treatment. J Subst Abuse Treat 87:23–30, 2018 29471923

Hallgren M, Romberg K, Bakshi A-S, Andréasson S: Yoga as an adjunct treatment for alcohol dependence: a pilot study. Complement Ther Med 22(3):441–445, 2014 24906582

Hallgren M, Vancampfort D, Giesen ES, et al: Exercise as treatment for alcohol use disorders: systematic review and meta-analysis. Br J Sports Med 51(14):1058–1064, 2017 28087569

Hart W: The Art of Living: Vipassana Meditation as Taught by S.N. Goenka. New York, HarperCollins, 1987

Jahnke R, Larkey L, Rogers C, et al: A comprehensive review of health benefits of qigong and tai chi. Am J Health Promot 24(6):e1–e25, 2010 20594090

Larkey L, Jahnke R, Etnier J, et al: Meditative movement as a category of exercise: implications for research. J Phys Act Health 6(2):230–238, 2009 19420401

Li M, Chen K, Mo Z: Use of qigong therapy in the detoxification of heroin addicts. Altern Ther Health Med 8(1):50–54, 56–59, 2002 11795622

Luedke K-H: Sporttherapie bei Alkoholkranken. Das Deutsche Gesundheitswesen 33(27):1264–1266, 1978

Margolin A, Kleber HD, Avants SK, et al: Acupuncture for the treatment of cocaine addiction: a randomized controlled trial. JAMA 287(1):55–63, 2002 11754709

Marlatt GA, Marques JK: Meditation, self-control, and alcohol use, in Behavioral Self Management: Strategies, Techniques, and Outcomes. Edited by Stuart RB. New York, Brunner/Mazel, 1977, pp 117–153

McKelvy PL, Stein CA, Bertini AB: Heart-rate response to a conditioning program for young, alcoholic men. Phys Ther 60(2):184–187, 1980 7355149

Murphy TJ, Pagano RR, Marlatt GA: Lifestyle modification with heavy alcohol drinkers: effects of aerobic exercise and meditation. Addict Behav 11(2):175–186, 1986 3526824

Olsen VV, Lugo RG, Sütterlin S: The somatic marker theory in the context of addiction: contributions to understanding development and maintenance. Psychol Res Behav Manag 8:187–200, 2015 26185474

Palmer J, Vacc N, Epstein J: Adult inpatient alcoholics: physical exercise as a treatment intervention. J Stud Alcohol 49(5):418–421, 1988 3216644

Posadzki P, Ernst E: Yoga for asthma? A systematic review of randomized clinical trials. J Asthma 48(6):632–639, 2011 21627405

Posadzki P, Khalil MMK, AlBedah A, et al: Complementary and alternative medicine for addiction: an overview of systematic reviews. Focus on Alternative and Complementary Therapies 21(2):69–81, 2016. Available at: https://onlinelibrary.wiley.com/doi/abs/10.1111/fct.12255. Accessed January 11, 2020.

Ratey JJ, Hagerman E: Spark: The Revolutionary New Science of Exercise and the Brain. New York, Little, Brown, 2008

Reddy S, Dick AM, Gerber MR, et al: The effect of a yoga intervention on alcohol and drug abuse risk in veteran and civilian women with posttraumatic stress disorder. J Altern Complement Med 20(10):750–756, 2014 25211372

Sedlmeier P, Eberth J, Schwarz M, et al: The psychological effects of meditation: a meta-analysis. Psychol Bull 138(6):1139–1171, 2012 22582738

Sinyor D, Brown T, Rostant L, et al: The role of a physical fitness program in the treatment of alcoholism. J Stud Alcohol 43(3):380–386, 1982 7121004

Szuhany KL, Bugatti M, Otto MW: A meta-analytic review of the effects of exercise on brain-derived neurotrophic factor. J Psychiatr Res 60:56–64, 2015 25455510

Trivedi MH, Greer TL, Rethorst CD, et al: Randomized controlled trial comparing exercise to health education for stimulant use disorder: results from the CTN-0037 STimulant Reduction Intervention Using Dosed Exercise (STRIDE) study. J Clin Psychiatry 78(8):1075–1082, 2017 28199070

Ussher M, Sampuran AK, Doshi R, et al: Acute effect of a brief bout of exercise on alcohol urges. Addiction 99(12):1542–1547, 2004 15585045

Wang D, Wang Y, Wang Y, et al: Impact of physical exercise on substance use disorders: a meta-analysis. PLoS One 9(10):e110728, 2014 25330437

Witkiewitz K, Warner K, Sully B, et al: Randomized trial comparing mindfulness-based relapse prevention with relapse prevention for women offenders at a residential addiction treatment center. Subst Use Misuse 49(5):536–546, 2014 24611849

Zschucke E, Heinz A, Ströhle A: Exercise and physical activity in the therapy of substance use disorders. ScientificWorldJournal 2012:901741, 2012 22629222

PART V

Public Health Issues

CHAPTER 31

The U.S. Opioid Crisis

Wilson M. Compton, M.D., M.P.E.
Christopher M. Jones, Pharm.D., Dr.P.H.

The U.S. opioid crisis is an extraordinary public health concern that emerged approximately two decades ago and has accelerated over the past decade (Jalal et al. 2018). It is a significant driver of the unprecedented downturn in life expectancy among Americans (Dowell et al. 2017). In 2018 alone, nearly 47,000 people died from an overdose involving opioids in the United States (Hedegaard et al. 2020). In addition, the economic impacts of the opioid crisis are estimated at more than $500 billion per year in the United States (Council of Economic Advisers 2017).

Although it involves compounds that are closely similar in terms of their pharmacological properties, the opioid overdose epidemic in the United States is really two sets of intertwined issues: misuse of and addiction to prescription opioid analgesics, which predominated in the first decade of the crisis, and, more recently, use of and addiction to illicit opioids (Figure 31–1). Within the rubric of illicit opioid use, a further distinction can be drawn between the resurgent use of heroin and the problem of both deliberate and unintentional administration of even more potent synthetic opioid drugs (i.e., illicitly made fentanyl and its analogs). A rapid rise in deaths involving these synthetic opioids, beginning in 2013, marked a "third wave" of the opioid crisis (Jones et al. 2018).

We begin this chapter by briefly describing the pharmacological properties of opioids and their actions in the central nervous system. We then go on to review the epidemiology and history of the intertwined components of the opioid crisis and the public health measures necessary to curb it.

Disclaimer: The findings and conclusions in this chapter are those of the authors and do not necessarily reflect the views of the National Institute on Drug Abuse of the National Institutes of Health, the Centers for Disease Control and Prevention, or the U.S. Department of Health and Human Services.

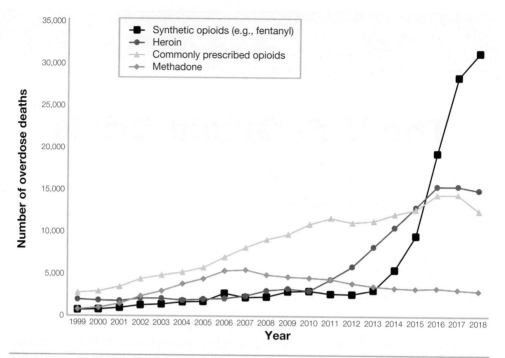

FIGURE 31–1. Opioid-related overdose deaths, by drug category: United States, 1999–2018.

Source.   Data from Hedegaard et al. 2020.

Opioid Neurobiology

Prescription opioids and illicit opioids like heroin and illicitly made fentanyl are pharmacologically quite similar. They interact with endogenous opioid systems that regulate several functions via three types of G protein–coupled receptors: mu (μ), delta (δ), and kappa (κ). Principally, they are potent agonists at the μ-opioid receptor (Valentino and Volkow 2018). μ-Opioid receptors are particularly concentrated in areas of the brain involved in processing pain and reward. The close coupling of these two effects underlies the inherent risks of misuse associated with use of opioids for analgesia. Whereas the neurobiology of the euphoria produced by drugs and other pleasurable activity is still poorly understood, the reinforcement component has been well studied: Activation of the μ-opioid receptor in reward circuits leads to a surge in the release of dopamine, which reinforces the learned (conditioned) association between the euphoria and the act of seeking and taking the drug. Decoupling of the pain-relieving functions from the rewarding functions of the μ-opioid receptor is currently a target of research to develop so-called biased agonists that trigger an analgesic response at the μ receptor without a reward response (Valentino and Volkow 2018).

μ-Opioid receptors are also concentrated in brain stem areas that control respiration, and this involvement accounts for the life-threatening danger of overdose, as μ-opioid receptor agonists suppress respiration (Valentino and Volkow 2018). In addition, μ-opioid receptors are found in brain circuits that handle emotion regulation, and this connection may contribute to their rewarding effects and to the motivation for misuse of opioids in order to help regulate mood.

The misuse liability of a particular opioid compound is a function of several factors, including the compound's binding affinity for the μ-opioid receptor, its ease of crossing the blood–brain barrier (lipophilicity), and other pharmacokinetic and physicochemical characteristics that determine how easily the opioid can be administered through nonoral routes such as injection and insufflation (Comer et al. 2008). Consequently, despite the molecular similarities between prescription and illicit opioids and their shared ability to produce analgesia and reward, their euphorigenic properties may differ, as may their patterns of symptoms produced by withdrawal.

Scope and Epidemiology

Classic epidemiological models focus on three key domains that can help to explain the spread and impact of diseases or conditions: host, agent, and environment domains (Centers for Disease Control and Prevention 2012). Within the host domain are individual susceptibility factors, including genetic background and specific behaviors that may put an individual at risk. The agent constitutes the external causal factor (i.e., the disease-causing substance, toxin, or infectious agent) and how it operates. The environmental domain encompasses factors external to the agent and host that can influence the host's susceptibility, including factors in both the physical and the social realms. An important component of all aspects of opioid epidemiology is market forces—that is, the economic incentives that motivate sellers of opioids and influence substance use patterns through their behaviors. To address this essential component within the typical host-agent-environment model for understanding opioid epidemiology, a fourth domain, the "vector," was added to the model. As has been described in tobacco epidemiology (Giovino 2002), this vector highlights the active role of product purveyors. For opioids, this means considering the behaviors of pharmaceutical companies and of physicians and other prescribers in the case of prescription opioids and illicit opioid sellers in the case of heroin and illicitly produced synthetic opioids. These vectors contribute to and influence both the extent and the spread of the opioid crisis and must be considered when planning responses. As illustrated in Figure 31–2, this host-agent-vector-environment (HAVE) model has been incorporated into the discussion in this chapter and is an essential heuristic for understanding the opioid crisis in the United States.

In 2018, 10.3 million Americans (age 12 years or older) reported having misused opioids (defined as misuse of prescription opioids and/or use of heroin) in the past year; more than 2.0 million met criteria for a past-year opioid use disorder (OUD) (Substance Abuse and Mental Health Services Administration 2019). More males than females misused opioids; 4.0% of males (5.35 million) reported past-year misuse of opioids in 2018, compared with 3.0% of females (4.9 million). Opioid misuse and OUD have always been uncommon among adolescents, and that remains the case: in 2018, 0.4% of those ages 12–17 years had an OUD. Young adults (ages 18–25 years), however, show the highest rates of opioid misuse and OUD, with 0.9% having an OUD in 2018, compared with 0.7% of adults age 26 years or older (Substance Abuse and Mental Health Services Administration 2019).

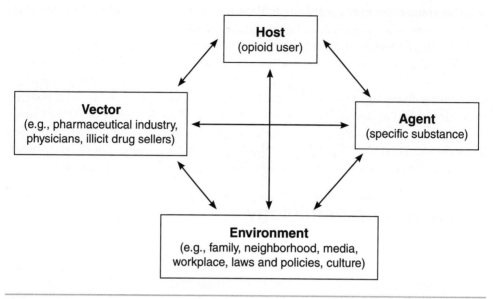

FIGURE 31–2.   Host-agent-vector-environment model.

Certain socioeconomic factors, such as poverty, are correlated with opioid misuse. Approximately 5.5% of individuals living at less than 100% of the federal poverty level (2.19 million) misused opioids in 2018, compared with 4.2% (2.28 million) of people between 100% and 199% of the federal poverty level and 3.2% (5.75 million) of those at 200% or more of the federal poverty level (Substance Abuse and Mental Health Services Administration 2019). Ethnic groups vary significantly, with opioid misuse being most prevalent (5.8%) among non-Hispanic American Indians/Alaska Natives and non-Hispanic whites (4.0%), less prevalent among non-Hispanic African Americans (3.7%) and Hispanics/Latinos (3.6%), and least prevalent (1.4%) among non-Hispanic Asians (Substance Abuse and Mental Health Services Administration 2019). There is also tremendous geographic variability in the rates of drug overdose (Figure 31–3) and of opioid misuse and OUD (Substance Abuse and Mental Health Services Administration 2019) due to a range of demographic factors having to do with health care infrastructure, opioid prescribing, treatment availability, availability of naloxone, penetration by drug traffickers, and so forth. For example, in 2018, while there were 6.9 drug overdose fatalities per 100,000 persons in South Dakota, there were 51.5 per 100,000 in West Virginia (Hedegaard et al. 2020).

Mental illnesses, especially mood disorders, often co-occur with OUD. Of the 9.3 million American adults who misused opioid medications in 2018, 45.7% (4.2 million) had a mental illness in the past year, and 17.1% (1.6 million) had a serious mental illness in the past year (Substance Abuse and Mental Health Services Administration 2019). The rates of co-occurring mental illness were even higher for individuals with a past-year OUD, with 65.7% having any mental illness in the past year and 28.6% having serious mental illness in the past year (Substance Abuse and Mental Health Services Administration 2019). In 2017, 4.0% of opioid overdose deaths were categorized as intentional overdoses (i.e., suicides); however, this likely is an underestimate, given the difficulties in assessing overdose death intent. According to data from the

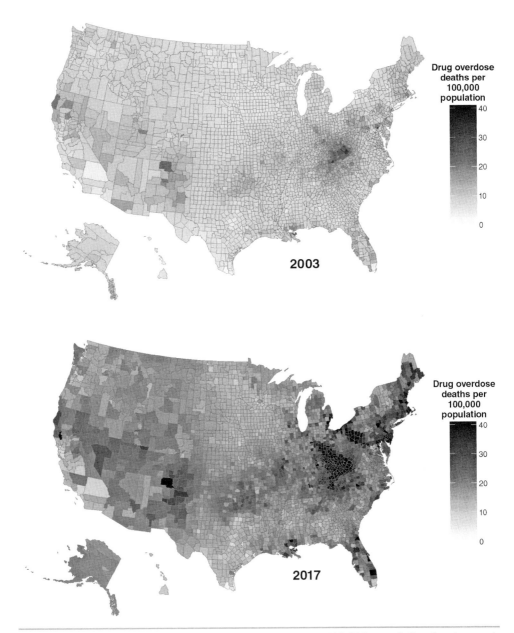

FIGURE 31–3. Estimated age-adjusted death rates per 100,000 population for drug poisoning (overdose), by U.S. county: 2003 and 2017.

Source. Reprinted from Rossen LM, Bastian B, Warner M, et al.: "Drug Poisoning Mortality: United States, 1999–2017," Centers for Disease Control and Prevention, National Center for Health Statistics, 2019. Images designed by Bastian B, Rossen L, Keralis JM, Chong Y. Available at: https://www.cdc.gov/nchs/data-visualization/drug-poisoning-mortality/. Accessed July 11, 2020.

Nationwide Emergency Department Sample for the years 2006–2011, just over half of emergency department visits for opioid poisonings by adults (53.50%) involved unintentional poisonings, leaving nearly half (46.5%) either intentional or undetermined (Tadros et al. 2015). In 2018, 17.3% of adults who had misused opioids (1.6 million people) reported having serious thoughts of suicide, 6.6% (0.6 million) made a suicide plan, and 3.2% (0.3 million) attempted suicide (Substance Abuse and Mental Health Services Administration 2019).

OUD is also highly comorbid with pain. Chronic pain and the emotional distress associated with it may dysregulate the brain's reward and stress circuitry, raising the risk for opioid misuse and OUD (Garland et al. 2013). One study estimated that 10% of patients treated for chronic pain misuse prescription opioids (Garland et al. 2013). In primary care settings, the prevalence of DSM-IV (American Psychiatric Association 1994)–defined opioid dependence (i.e., "addiction") was estimated to range from 3% to 17% (Vowles et al. 2015). Suicidal ideation is also common among patients with chronic pain (Cheatle 2011); overdose is the most commonly reported means of planned suicide among patients with chronic pain who report having suicidal ideation. Estimates from death certificate data indicate that at least 9% of suicide decedents were suffering from chronic pain at the time of their death (Petrosky et al. 2018).

Untreated OUD in pregnant women can also lead to serious complications for the baby, including fetal death and infants born physically dependent on opioids (neonatal abstinence syndrome [NAS])—a serious condition potentially requiring an extended stay in a neonatal intensive care unit. Incidence of NAS among hospital deliveries increased fourfold between 1999 and 2013 (from 1.5 to 6.0 per 1,000 births; Ko et al. 2016). The neonates of mothers treated for OUD during their pregnancy with methadone or buprenorphine also require care for NAS, although NAS in these neonates is less severe (Fajemirokun-Odudeyi et al. 2006).

In recent years, increased attention has been focused on the intersection of the opioid crisis, injection drug use, and the transmission of infectious diseases (e.g., HIV, viral hepatitis) and bacterial infections (e.g., endocarditis). The 2014–2015 HIV outbreak in Scott County, Indiana, in which more than 180 cases of HIV were identified within a short period of time, was the most severe recent outbreak of HIV detected in the United States (Peters et al. 2016). In addition, hepatitis C virus infections have been increasing in the United States over the past decade, with particularly large increases in the states most heavily impacted by the opioid crisis (Zibbell et al. 2018). Most recently, Centers for Disease Control and Prevention (CDC) researchers have identified a connection between increasing rates of invasive methicillin-resistant staphylococcus aureus infections and injection drug use, including opioid injection (Jackson et al. 2018).

Prescription Opioid Misuse

Prescription drug misuse is very different from other drug use issues because it is intricately intertwined with the health care system and with a parallel health issue affecting many Americans: pain. It was through pain and shifting philosophies of pain treatment that today's opioid crisis first took hold.

Physicians and other health care providers had discovered from historical experience the dangerous addictiveness of opioid drugs and for decades were reluctant to use these drugs to treat most pain conditions. Beginning in the 1980s, however, there were calls from some physicians and patient advocacy groups that not enough was being done to treat pain, both in cancer and palliative care patients and more generally. A now-notorious one-paragraph letter in the *New England Journal of Medicine* in 1980 stated that among a large sample of hospitalized patients who had been given opioids, only four developed an addiction to these drugs (Porter and Jick 1980). Despite the fact that this report focused on inpatient administration of opioids, it was later cited widely to support less hesitation in the use of opioids in *outpatient* settings, outside of end-of-life care (Leung et al. 2017). In the early 1990s, advocacy groups, including the American Pain Society, encouraged physicians to treat pain as a "fifth vital sign," and the Joint Commission began to require hospitals to assess all patients' pain. Pain rating scales became ubiquitous in doctor's offices and emergency rooms. Meanwhile, pharmaceutical companies were developing a new generation of extended-release opioid analgesics that contained more opioid per pill but were purported to be less addicting. In 1996, Purdue Pharma's OxyContin (oxycodone) was approved and went on the market.

These shifting attitudes and policies related to the assessment of pain occurred in the context of a medical education system that did not adequately train health care providers in pain care and addiction. According to a 2011 study, many medical schools at that time offered less than 5 hours of training in pain management, with some offering no training (Mezei et al. 2011). One survey of 246 graduate medical trainees (i.e., residents and fellows) found that only 17% felt confident in their ability to assess and manage chronic noncancer pain (Yanni et al. 2010). Additionally, most physicians lacked training in recognizing the signs of medication misuse in their patients and in screening for misuse and addiction. Opioids increasingly began to be prescribed for chronic noncancer pain, despite a lack of evidence supporting their efficacy or safety for patients with these conditions (Reuben et al. 2015). It also became common for patients to go home from emergency rooms, hospitals, and dental offices with prescriptions for enough opioids to last several weeks to a month to treat their acute pain, yet often only needing to take a few pills before their pain could be managed with over-the-counter medications (Bartels et al. 2016). As a result of these shifts in practice, sales of prescription opioids increased fourfold between 1999 and 2010 (Reuben et al. 2015). Unused pills were then readily available for diversion and misuse. Whereas about a third of people who misuse prescription opioids get them from their own prescription, more than half report obtaining them from family members or friends who have opioid prescriptions (Substance Abuse and Mental Health Services Administration 2019).

In addition to increases in the absolute numbers of opioid prescriptions written during the 1990s and 2000s, how opioids were prescribed began to change, with opioids increasingly prescribed at higher doses, for longer durations, and in combination with benzodiazepines—all of which are now well recognized as risk factors for overdose (Gwira Baumblatt et al. 2014; Hwang et al. 2016). Apart from the likelihood of dependence and the risk of addiction when opioids are given long-term, there is also the real possibility that prolonged opioid administration will perpetuate the condition it is intended to treat by increasing pain sensitization (i.e., opioid-induced hyperalgesia) (Roeckel et al. 2016). Chronic administration of opioids may even shift the source of pain from the injured periphery to the central nervous system (Young Casey et al. 2008).

It was originally thought that individuals at risk of prescription opioid misuse and addiction were overwhelmingly confined to those using diverted prescription opioids, and it was even believed that pain had a protective effect against becoming addicted to these medications. But while it remains true that only a minority of patients with pain who are prescribed opioids become addicted, it is nevertheless the case that some do. Overdose risk is also not unique to patients who misuse diverted opioids; patients receiving opioids for pain can also overdose. Multiple studies have shown that the risk of a fatal overdose rises with increased daily dose of an opioid, and many of these deaths may involve the concurrent use of benzodiazepines, which appear to exacerbate respiratory depression (Jones and McAninch 2015).

Methadone prescribed for pain has proven particularly dangerous from an overdose standpoint. It became a popular pain treatment option in the early 2000s because of its long half-life and the fact that it was less expensive than OxyContin and other extended-release opioids. However, methadone's long duration in the body, slow onset of action, and complicated pharmacokinetics made it particularly difficult to manage medically and particularly prone to lead to accidental overdose; it caused a high number of overdose deaths as a result (Jones et al. 2016). At its peak for involvement in overdose deaths in the mid- to late 2000s, methadone was involved in approximately 30% of overdose deaths (Hedegaard et al. 2020), although that percentage has declined in recent years as prescribing of methadone for pain has decreased (Jones et al. 2016); in 2018, only 6.5% of opioid deaths involved methadone (Hedegaard et al. 2020). These data remind us that the particular pharmacology of the specific opioid matters.

The 1990s and 2000s also saw the development of "rogue" pain clinics (sometimes called "pill mills") where opioids were prescribed and dispensed in large quantities and with minimal clinical indications (Rigg et al. 2010). The practice of obtaining prescriptions from multiple physicians (i.e., "doctor shopping") also had become a significant contributor to the opioid crisis and was shown to be disproportionately associated with overdose deaths (Peirce et al. 2012). Florida, a state with a well-documented prescription opioid problem, largely due to its high proliferation of pill mills, responded to this threat by enacting a series of major policy changes that resulted in a 27% decline in overdose deaths between 2010 and 2012 (Johnson et al. 2014).

Illicit Opioids

Heroin

The growing population of individuals who were misusing or had become addicted to prescription opioids created a new market in the United States for heroin (Compton et al. 2016). Heroin's effects are similar to those of prescription opioids when the latter are taken via alternative routes of administration such as injection, and heroin can be much less expensive. According to Muhuri et al. (2013), an estimated 4% of people who recently initiated misuse of prescription opioids initiated heroin use within the next 5 years.

Based on data from patients admitted to treatment programs in the 2000s, three-quarters of individuals presenting for treatment of OUD had initiated misuse with prescription opioids, even if they later switched to heroin (Cicero et al. 2014). This was in stark contrast to previous generations of people addicted to opioids, who had principally initiated use with heroin; furthermore, the demographics of opioid misuse and addiction also had shifted, now comprising a greater proportion of whites, females, and residents of suburban and rural areas than in previous decades, especially among new initiates (90% of whom were white). In recent years, among patients admitted to treatment programs for OUD, those with onset of opioid use since 2010 (coinciding with the influx of historically high-purity and low-cost heroin) are increasingly likely to report that heroin was their first opioid of misuse (Cicero et al. 2017).

The increased difficulty of obtaining diverted prescription opioids among people addicted to them has certainly contributed to expanded heroin use, but market forces related to illicit drug trafficking have also played an enormous role. As described by journalist Sam Quinones in *Dreamland,* Mexican drug cartels were ready to satisfy the demands of the emerging market for illicit opioids by using new, "pizza delivery"–like ways of marketing heroin to potential suburban buyers who otherwise might have been wary of engaging with the illicit drug trade (Quinones 2015). Increased drug trafficking in areas with historically high demand for prescription opioids has also been noted (U.S. Department of Justice 2018). The heroin being sold recently, made from poppies grown in Mexico, is also of higher purity than had been available previously (U.S. Department of Justice 2018). The relatively lower price of heroin (and now fentanyl, as described below) compared with prescription opioids may also have contributed to the transition from prescription opioids to heroin and other illicit opioids.

Fentanyl and Other Synthetic Opioids

From 2010 to 2018, deaths involving fentanyl and other synthetic opioids increased more than tenfold, from 3,007 (14.3% of opioid-related deaths) to 31,335 (67.0%) (Hedegaard et al. 2020; Jones et al. 2018). Synthetic opioids are now twice as likely as prescription opioids or heroin to be involved in overdose deaths (Hedegaard et al. 2020).

Fentanyl and its analogs are synthesized in a laboratory and thus are relatively inexpensive to produce and result in a higher profit margin than heroin (U.S. Department of Justice 2018). Fentanyl and its analogs are often manufactured in China and then smuggled into the United States either via international mail and express consignment systems or via delivery to traditional drug trafficking organizations across the southern and northern borders (U.S. Department of Justice 2018). The high potency of these compounds makes them particularly attractive to dealers and smugglers, because a high street value is seen in very small quantities. But this potency also explains their lethality. Dealers often adulterate heroin with synthetic opioids and also adulterate other illicit drugs (e.g., cocaine, methamphetamine, counterfeit prescription analgesics, benzodiazepines), extending risk beyond people who use opioids.

While it remains uncertain how many synthetic opioid–related deaths involve opioid users who actively and knowingly use fentanyl or an analog, a study in New Hampshire that interviewed people (*N*=76) who used opioids about their practices and attitudes toward heroin versus fentanyl found that 25% of these individuals specifically sought fentanyl or heroin laced with fentanyl over other opioids (Meier et al. 2017). Many other users reported preferring heroin or a specific prescription opioid but found that in their region, alternatives without fentanyl were hard to obtain. A study of people living in West Virginia in 2018 who inject drugs found that among persons who had ever used fentanyl (*N*=311), 43.4% reported preferring fentanyl-containing drugs (Mazhnaya et al. 2020). Factors associated with preferring fentanyl included being younger (adjusted Prevalence Ratio [PrR] for each additional year of age: 0.98; 95% confidence interval [CI]: 0.97–1.00), being female (PrR: 1.45; 95% CI:

1.14–1.83), having increased drug use in the past 6 months (PrR: 1.28; 95% CI: 1.01–1.63), and having injected fentanyl in the past 6 months (PrR: 1.89; 95% CI: 1.29–2.75).

Public Health Responses

Public health efforts to reduce the number of deaths from opioid overdoses require approaching the problem from a range of angles, including prevention, treatment, and harm reduction. Such efforts also require addressing how pain is managed and treated, given that pain is so tightly intertwined with opioid misuse and OUD. The public health response should be comprehensive, so as to address both the upstream drivers and downstream consequences of opioid misuse and to prevent a shift to abuse of other substances. This response should also be balanced, to ensure that efforts to constrain the prescribing of opioids are implemented in tandem with 1) appropriate tapering protocols (for assisting patients in discontinuing opioid use) and 2) expanded access to non-opioid pain treatments. A complete discussion of the numerous public health interventions undertaken to address the opioid crisis is beyond the scope of this chapter; thus, in the remainder of this section, we will limit our focus to five critical strategies: 1) health care provider education, training, and guidance; 2) prescription drug monitoring programs; 3) primary prevention of substance use, including opioid misuse; 4) improving access to and use of naloxone; and 5) expanding the use of medication-assisted treatment for OUD (and syringe service programs as part of an overall effort to minimize negative health outcomes).

Provider Education

Physicians and other health care providers receive little training in pain care or in substance use and addiction in most medical and health professional schools, and lack of provider preparedness in these areas has been partly blamed for the emergence of the opioid crisis (Mezei et al. 2011; Yanni et al. 2010). Thus, a core component of the public health response to the opioid crisis is providing additional education, training, and guidance to strengthen health care provider competencies in pain care and addiction management. In 2016, the CDC released its Guideline for Prescribing Opioids for Chronic Pain, which is particularly relevant for patients being considered for chronic pain treatment in primary care settings (Dowell et al. 2016). This guideline (Table 31–1) is intended to inform clinical practice but does not constitute a set of regulations, nor are its recommendations intended to supplant clinical experience and training. To assist with implementation of the guideline and integration of its recommendations and quality improvement measures into clinical practice, the CDC has developed provider and patient education and training resources as well as a Quality Improvement and Coordinated Care Resource website (Centers for Disease Control and Prevention 2018).

Prescription Drug Monitoring Programs

Another intervention and clinical tool to reduce inappropriate or excessive prescribing, reduce diversion, and facilitate identification of individuals at risk for overdose

TABLE 31–1.   **Summary of CDC Guideline for Prescribing Opioids for Chronic Pain**

When prescribing opioid pain relievers for acute pain:
- Providers should prescribe the lowest effective dosage possible.
- Providers should prescribe no greater quantity than needed for the expected duration of pain severe enough to require opioid pain relievers (3 or fewer days will usually be sufficient).

When prescribing opioid pain relievers for chronic pain:
- Non-opioid therapies are preferred for chronic pain.
- If opioids are prescribed, they should be used in combination with non-opioid therapy such as cognitive-behavioral therapy, exercise therapy, and/or non-opioid pharmacological therapy such as nonsteroidal anti-inflammatory drugs (NSAIDs) and acetaminophen; avoid concurrent prescribing of other opioids and benzodiazepines if possible.
- Prior to beginning prescription opioid therapy, establish treatment goals and discuss risks and realistic benefits.
- Reassess risks and benefits throughout treatment; continue prescription opioids only if pain and functioning meaningfully improve.
- Use prescription drug monitoring programs (PDMPs) to determine whether patients are using other opioids.

Prescription opioid selection, dosage, and follow-up:
- Prescribe immediate-release opioids instead of long-acting/extended-release opioids.
- Start low and go slow—Prescribe opioids with the lowest possible effective dosage; reassess individual benefits and risks when considering increasing dosage to ≥50 morphine milligram equivalents (MME)/day; avoid increasing dosage to ≥90 MME/day unless justified.
- Evaluate benefits and harms within 1–4 weeks of starting opioid therapy for chronic pain or after dosage escalation, and discuss considerations for discontinuation of opioid therapy.

Assessing risk and addressing harms of opioid use:
- Prior to beginning opioid therapy and periodically during therapy, evaluate risk factors for opioid-related harms. Risk factors include sleep-disordered breathing, pregnancy, kidney disease, age ≥65 years, mental health conditions, substance use disorder, or prior nonfatal overdose.
- Incorporate strategies to mitigate risk; offer naloxone when patient is at increased risk of opioid overdose.
- Ask patients about their drug and alcohol use via a validated screening tool such as the single-question screener, the Drug Abuse Screening Test (DAST), or the Alcohol Use Disorders Identification Test (AUDIT).
- Use urine drug screening to test for concurrent illicit drug use.
- Offer evidence-based treatment for opioid use disorder.

Source.   Adapted from Dowell et al. 2016.

is the implementation of prescription drug monitoring programs (PDMPs). PDMPs are state-based databases that collect information on all dispensed controlled prescription drugs. They now exist in some fashion in all 50 states plus the District of Columbia, and their use has been associated with reduced opioid prescribing (Lin et al. 2018). However, evidence for the effectiveness of PDMPs in reducing overdoses has been somewhat mixed and seems to depend on how fully they are implemented and used by clinicians (Fink et al. 2018).

Prevention Programs

In addition to a focus on changing clinical practice behaviors, efforts to reduce demand among individuals who are misusing opioids as well as to prevent initiation in the first place are essential. Evidence-supported prevention interventions that target known risk factors for substance use and boost protective factors can have an effect as early as infancy. Prevention programs that help parents with parenting skills, for instance, have shown significant effects on ameliorating the toxic effects of social disadvantage on brain development and behavior (Brody et al. 2017). Several programs delivered in community or school settings in childhood, during middle school, and in high school have shown effectiveness in reducing substance use and other related problem behaviors, including middle-school interventions that have specifically demonstrated an impact on reducing prescription opioid misuse (Compton et al. 2019). In general, these programs use a positive youth development and resilience approach that focuses on developmental competencies, and the positive impacts that these early adolescent programs provide demonstrated a long-term protective effect against prescription opioid misuse into young adulthood (Compton et al. 2019).

Naloxone Distribution Programs

Wider access to the overdose-reversal drug naloxone is another pillar of the public health response to curb the opioid overdose epidemic. The opioid antagonist naloxone, when administered promptly, can dislodge opioid agonists from μ-opioid receptors and restore breathing in someone who has overdosed. In Massachusetts communities where overdose education and naloxone distribution programs were implemented, opioid overdose death rates were reduced 27%–46% (Walley et al. 2013). A probabilistic analysis found layperson naloxone distribution programs to be effective in preventing overdose deaths, to increase quality-adjusted life years, and to be highly cost-effective (Coffin and Sullivan 2013). Use of harm-reduction practices such as co-prescribing of naloxone as a routine part of opioid treatment (especially for patients receiving higher dosages or longer-term opioid prescriptions, receiving concomitant benzodiazepines, or having other risk factors for overdose) as well as pharmacist-initiated dispensing of naloxone under laws such as standing orders have also been increasing in recent years. Studies have found these measures to be beneficial in reducing opioid-related adverse events and overdose deaths (Abouk et al. 2019; Coffin et al. 2016). Critics of harm-reduction approaches have claimed that wider naloxone availability may lead to increased opioid misuse, but the Massachusetts research, consistent with prior research, did not find such an effect (Walley et al. 2013). Finally, with the increasing numbers of overdoses from potent synthetic opioids, emergency personnel are finding that multiple naloxone administrations are sometimes necessary to counteract overdoses of these drugs or to prevent a subsequent overdose once the initial naloxone administration wears off (Faul et al. 2017). Thus, expansion of naloxone access, including ensuring that multiple doses are available to first responders and lay personnel, is increasingly important in the response to the opioid crisis.

Removal of Barriers to Medications for Opioid Use Disorder Treatment

Expanding access to effective treatment for OUD is a crucial part of ending the crisis. Principally this means increasing the use of effective medications (buprenorphine, methadone, and naltrexone) for treating OUD. These medications have been shown in study after study to significantly reduce the risk of overdose, relapse, and other adverse health and social outcomes of opioid addiction; however, these treatments are markedly underutilized and even when implemented are not used for long enough by enough patients (Williams et al. 2019). When they are prescribed, agonists are often given for too short a duration to be effective—often less than 90 days. In addition, multiple barriers to prescribing buprenorphine for OUD treatment exist, such as lack of insurance coverage and reimbursement, lack of access to additional prescribers (both specialists and general practice clinicians) or behavioral health providers, lack of provider self-efficacy in managing patients with OUD, and regulatory concerns (Jones and McCance-Katz 2019).

Brief Intervention and Referral to Treatment

In addition to expanding access to medications in primary care settings, making increased use of medications in emergency departments and criminal justice settings can have a lifesaving impact among those at highest risk. Initiation of buprenorphine treatment among patients seeking care in the emergency department with linkage to a buprenorphine provider in the community has been shown to be effective in reducing subsequent opioid use and increasing treatment engagement (D'Onofrio et al. 2017). Given the significant increase in risk of overdose following the first few weeks after release from incarceration due to lost opioid tolerance (Binswanger et al. 2007), increased utilization of medications in justice settings stands to substantially reduce overdose deaths. Research has shown that expansion of medications in this setting reduces subsequent opioid use, increases treatment engagement after release from prison, and reduces the risk of overdose (Green et al. 2018; Kinlock et al. 2007).

Syringe Services Programs

Given the rising rates of opioid injection and related infectious disease transmission, expanding access to syringe services programs (SSPs) is an evidence-based strategy to reduce the spread of infectious diseases and to improve other health outcomes among people who inject drugs. SSPs have been shown to reduce injection-related risk behaviors and to decrease HIV, hepatitis C virus (HCV), and hepatitis B virus (HBV) transmission (MacArthur et al. 2014). SSPs directly lower the risk of injection-related harms by decreasing needle sharing and reuse, reducing the prevalence of blood-borne infectious agents in needles available for reuse, and, in some SSPs, directly providing treatment for HIV and HCV as well as medication-assisted treatment for OUD (Des Jarlais et al. 2015). Indirectly, SSPs lower the risk of injection-related harms by linking individuals to substance use treatment; offering harm-reduction education services, including testing, counseling, and linkage to treatment for infectious diseases; and providing condoms and education on safe sexual practices (Des Jarlais et al. 2015).

Conclusion

The opioid crisis that has unfolded and evolved in the United States over the first two decades of the twenty-first century has been remarkably lethal. The roots of the opioid crisis are complex and inextricably entangled with the health care system, especially in its treatment of another serious health problem: pain. Although failures of the health care system—such as lack of training in pain management and lack of caution in using a class of medications that was known to be addictive—precipitated the rise in opioid misuse and addiction over the past two decades, a wider range of social and economic forces has helped to perpetuate the crisis and has altered its character. The opioid crisis can now be said to include multiple drug crises involving compounds that are closely related chemically but require different and coordinated responses.

References

Abouk R, Pacula RL, Powell D: Association between state laws facilitating pharmacy distribution of naloxone and risk of fatal overdose. JAMA Intern Med 179(6):805–811, 2019 31058922

American Psychiatric Association: Diagnostic and Statistical Manual of Mental Disorders, 4th Edition. Washington, DC, American Psychiatric Association, 1994

Bartels K, Mayes LM, Dingmann C, et al: Opioid use and storage patterns by patients after hospital discharge following surgery. PLoS One 11(1):e0147972, 2016 26824844

Binswanger IA, Stern MF, Deyo RA, et al: Release from prison—a high risk of death for former inmates. N Engl J Med 356(2):157–165, 2007 17215533

Brody GH, Gray JC, Yu T, et al: Protective prevention effects on the association of poverty with brain development. JAMA Pediatr 171(1):46–52, 2017 27893880

Centers for Disease Control and Prevention: Principles of Epidemiology in Public Health Practice, Third Edition. Atlanta, GA, 2012. Available at: https://www.cdc.gov/csels/dsepd/ss1978/SS1978.pdf. Accessed June 29, 2020.

Centers for Disease Control and Prevention: Implementing the CDC Guideline for Prescribing Opioids for Chronic Pain. 2018. Available at: https://www.cdc.gov/drugoverdose/pdf/prescribing/CDC-DUIP-QualityImprovementAndCareCoordination-508.pdf. Accessed December 5, 2019.

Cheatle MD: Depression, chronic pain, and suicide by overdose: on the edge. Pain Med 12 (suppl 2):S43–S48, 2011 21668756

Cicero TJ, Ellis MS, Surratt HL, et al: The changing face of heroin use in the United States: a retrospective analysis of the past 50 years. JAMA Psychiatry 71(7):821–826, 2014 24871348

Cicero TJ, Ellis MS, Kasper ZA: Increased use of heroin as an initiating opioid of abuse. Addict Behav 74:63–66, 2017 28582659

Coffin PO, Sullivan SD: Cost-effectiveness of distributing naloxone to heroin users for lay overdose reversal. Ann Intern Med 158(1):1–9, 2013 23277895

Coffin PO, Behar E, Rowe C, et al: Nonrandomized intervention study of naloxone coprescription for primary care patients receiving long-term opioid therapy for pain. Ann Intern Med 165(4):245–252, 2016 27366987

Comer SD, Sullivan MA, Whittington RA, et al: Abuse liability of prescription opioids compared to heroin in morphine-maintained heroin abusers. Neuropsychopharmacology 33(5):1179–1191, 2008 17581533

Compton WM, Jones CM, Baldwin GT: Relationship between nonmedical prescription opioid use and heroin use. N Engl J Med 374(2):154–163, 2016 26760086

Compton WM, Jones CM, Baldwin GT, et al: Targeting youth to prevent later substance use disorder: an underutilized response to the US opioid crisis. Am J Public Health 109(S3):S185–S189, 2019 31242006

Council of Economic Advisers: The Underestimated Cost of the Opioid Crisis. November 2017. Available at: https://www.whitehouse.gov/sites/whitehouse.gov/files/images/The%20Underestimated%20Cost%20of%20the%20Opioid%20Crisis.pdf. Accessed December 5, 2019.

Des Jarlais DC, Nugent A, Solberg A, et al: Syringe service programs for persons who inject drugs in urban, suburban, and rural areas—United States, 2013. MMWR Morb Mortal Wkly Rep 64(48):1337–1341, 2015 26655918

D'Onofrio G, Chawarski MC, O'Connor PG, et al: Emergency department-initiated buprenorphine for opioid dependence with continuation in primary care: outcomes during and after intervention. J Gen Intern Med 32(6):660–666, 2017 28194688

Dowell D, Haegerich TM, Chou R: CDC guideline for prescribing opioids for chronic pain—United States, 2016. MMWR Recomm Rep 65(1):1–49, 2016 26987082

Dowell D, Arias E, Kochanek K, et al: Contribution of opioid-involved poisoning to the change in life expectancy in the United States, 2000–2015. JAMA 318(11):1065–1067, 2017 28975295

Fajemirokun-Odudeyi O, Sinha C, Tutty S, et al: Pregnancy outcome in women who use opiates. Eur J Obstet Gynecol Reprod Biol 126(2):170–175, 2006 16202501

Faul M, Lurie P, Kinsman JM, et al: Multiple naloxone administrations among emergency medical service providers is increasing. Prehosp Emerg Care 21(4):411–419, 2017 28481656

Fink DS, Schleimer JP, Sarvet A, et al: Association between prescription drug monitoring programs and nonfatal and fatal drug overdoses: a systematic review. Ann Intern Med 168(11):783–790, 2018 29801093

Garland EL, Froeliger B, Zeidan F, et al: The downward spiral of chronic pain, prescription opioid misuse and addiction: cognitive, affective and neuropsychopharmacologic pathways. Neurosci Biobehav Rev 37(10 Pt 2):2597–2607, 2013 23988582

Giovino GA: Epidemiology of tobacco use in the United States. Oncogene 21(48):7326–7340, 2002 12379876

Green TC, Clarke J, Brinkley-Rubinstein L, et al: Postincarceration fatal overdoses after implementing medications for addiction treatment in a statewide correctional system. JAMA Psychiatry 75(4):405–407, 2018 29450443

Gwira Baumblatt JA, Wiedeman C, Dunn JR, et al: High-risk use by patients prescribed opioids for pain and its role in overdose deaths. JAMA Intern Med 174(5):796–801, 2014 24589873

Hedegaard H, Miniño AM, Warner M: Drug Overdose Deaths in the United States, 1999–2018. NCHS Data Brief, No. 356. Hyattsville, MD, National Center for Health Statistics, January 2020. Available at: https://www.cdc.gov/nchs/data/databriefs/db356-h.pdf. Accessed July 11, 2020.

Hwang CS, Kang EM, Kornegay CJ, et al: Trends in the concomitant prescribing of opioids and benzodiazepines, 2002–2014. Am J Prev Med 51(2):151–160, 2016 27079639

Jackson KA, Bohm MK, Brooks JT, et al: Invasive methicillin-resistant staphylococcus aureus infections among persons who inject drugs—six sites, 2005–2016. MMWR Morb Mortal Wkly Rep 67(22):625–628, 2018 29879096

Jalal H, Buchanich JM, Roberts MS, et al: Changing dynamics of the drug overdose epidemic in the United States from 1979 through 2016. Science 361(6408):eaau1184, 2018 30237320

Johnson H, Paulozzi L, Porucznik C, et al: Decline in drug overdose deaths after state policy changes—Florida, 2010–2012. MMWR Morb Mortal Wkly Rep 63(26):569–574, 2014 24990490

Jones CM, McAninch JK: Emergency department visits and overdose deaths from combined use of opioids and benzodiazepines. Am J Prev Med 49(4):493–501, 2015 26143953

Jones CM, McCance-Katz EF: Characteristics and prescribing practices of clinicians recently waivered to prescribe buprenorphine for the treatment of opioid use disorder. Addiction 114(3):471–482, 2019 30194876

Jones CM, Baldwin GT, Manocchio T, et al: Trends in methadone distribution for pain treatment, methadone diversion, and overdose deaths—United States, 2002–2014. MMWR Morb Mortal Wkly Rep 65(26):667–671, 2016 27387857

Jones CM, Einstein EB, Compton WM: Changes in synthetic opioid involvement in drug overdose deaths in the United States, 2010–2016. JAMA 319(17):1819–1821, 2018 29715347

Kinlock TW, Gordon MS, Schwartz RP, et al: A randomized clinical trial of methadone maintenance for prisoners: results at 1-month post-release. Drug Alcohol Depend 91(2–3):220–227, 2007 17628351

Ko JY, Patrick SW, Tong VT, et al: Incidence of neonatal abstinence syndrome—28 states, 1999–2013. MMWR Morb Mortal Wkly Rep 65(31):799–802, 2016 27513154

Leung PTM, Macdonald EM, Stanbrook MB, et al: A 1980 letter on the risk of opioid addiction. N Engl J Med 376(22):2194–2195, 2017 28564561

Lin HC, Wang Z, Boyd C, et al: Associations between statewide prescription drug monitoring program (PDMP) requirement and physician patterns of prescribing opioid analgesics for patients with non-cancer chronic pain. Addict Behav 76:348–354, 2018 28898808

MacArthur GJ, van Velzen E, Palmateer N, et al: Interventions to prevent HIV and hepatitis C in people who inject drugs: a review of reviews to assess evidence of effectiveness. Int J Drug Policy 25(1):34–52, 2014 23973009

Mazhnaya A, O'Rourke A, White RH, et al: Fentanyl preference among people who inject drugs in West Virginia. Subst Use Misuse 55(11):1774–1780, 2020 32441202

Meier A, Moore SK, Saunders EC, et al: Understanding Opioid Overdoses in New Hampshire. NDEWS Hotspot Report, June 2017. Available at: https://umd.app.box.com/v/NDEWS-HotSpot-Report-June-2017. Accessed December 5, 2019.

Mezei L, Murinson BB; Johns Hopkins Pain Curriculum Development Team: Pain education in North American medical schools. J Pain 12(12):1199–1208, 2011 21945594

Muhuri PK, Gfroerer JC, Davies MC: Associations of Nonmedical Pain Reliever use and Initiation of Heroin Use in the United States. Substance Abuse and Mental Health Services Administration, CBHSQ Data Review, August 2013. Available at: https://www.samhsa.gov/data/sites/default/files/DR006/DR006/nonmedical-pain-reliever-use-2013.htm. Accessed December 5, 2019.

Peirce GL, Smith MJ, Abate MA, et al: Doctor and pharmacy shopping for controlled substances. Med Care 50(6):494–500, 2012 22410408

Peters PJ, Pontones P, Hoover KW, et al: HIV infection linked to injection use of oxymorphone in Indiana, 2014–2015. N Engl J Med 375(3):229–239, 2016 27468059

Petrosky E, Harpaz R, Fowler KA, et al: Chronic pain among suicide decedents, 2003–2014: findings from the National Violent Death Reporting System. Ann Intern Med 169(7):448–455, 2018 30208405

Porter J, Jick H: Addiction rare in patients treated with narcotics. N Engl J Med 302(2):123, 1980 7350425

Quinones S: Dreamland: The True Tale of America's Opiate Epidemic. New York, Bloomsbury Press, 2015

Reuben DB, Alvanzo AA, Ashikaga T, et al: National Institutes of Health Pathways to Prevention Workshop: the role of opioids in the treatment of chronic pain. Ann Intern Med 162(4):295–300, 2015 25581341

Rigg KK, March SJ, Inciardi JA: Prescription drug abuse and diversion: role of the pain clinic. J Drug Issues 40(3):681–702, 2010 21278927

Roeckel LA, Le Coz GM, Gavériaux-Ruff C, Simonin F: Opioid-induced hyperalgesia: cellular and molecular mechanisms. Neuroscience 338:160–182, 2016 27346146

Substance Abuse and Mental Health Services Administration: Results From the 2018 National Survey on Drug Use and Health: Detailed Tables. Center for Behavioral Health Statistics and Quality, August 20, 2019. Available at: https://www.samhsa.gov/data/report/2018-nsduh-detailed-tables. Accessed July 7, 2020.

Tadros A, Layman SM, Davis SM, et al: Emergency visits for prescription opioid poisonings. J Emerg Med 49(6):871–877, 2015 26409674

U.S. Department of Justice: National Drug Threat Assessment. Drug Enforcement Administration, October 2018. Available at: https://www.dea.gov/sites/default/files/2018-11/DIR-032-18%202018%20NDTA%20final%20low%20resolution.pdf. Accessed December 5, 2019.

Valentino RJ, Volkow ND: Untangling the complexity of opioid receptor function. Neuropsychopharmacology 43(13):2514–2520, 2018 30250308

Vowles KE, McEntee ML, Julnes PS, et al: Rates of opioid misuse, abuse, and addiction in chronic pain: a systematic review and data synthesis. Pain 156(4):569–576, 2015 25785523

Walley AY, Xuan Z, Hackman HH, et al: Opioid overdose rates and implementation of overdose education and nasal naloxone distribution in Massachusetts: interrupted time series analysis. BMJ 346:f174, 2013 23372174

Williams AR, Nunes EV, Bisaga A, et al: Development of a cascade of care for responding to the opioid epidemic. Am J Drug Alcohol Abuse 45(1):1–10, 2019 30675818

Yanni LM, McKinney-Ketchum JL, Harrington SB, et al: Preparation, confidence, and attitudes about chronic noncancer pain in graduate medical education. J Grad Med Educ 2(2):260–268, 2010 21975631

Young Casey C, Greenberg MA, Nicassio PM, et al: Transition from acute to chronic pain and disability: a model including cognitive, affective, and trauma factors. Pain 134(1–2):69–79, 2008 17504729

Zibbell JE, Asher AK, Patel RC, et al: Increases in acute hepatitis C virus infection related to a growing opioid epidemic and associated injection drug use, United States, 2004 to 2014. Am J Public Health 108(2):175–181, 2018 29267061

U.S. Department of Justice, National Drug Control Strategy, 2016; Substance Abuse and Mental Health Services Administration.

CHAPTER 32

Cannabis Policy and Use

Arthur Robin Williams, M.D., M.B.E.

Legal access to cannabis in the United States, whether for medical or recreational purposes, has changed dramatically since the late 1990s, driven mostly by reforms at the state level. As of 2018, it became more common for states to have medical cannabis programs than to not have them. Additionally, almost a dozen states now allow legal recreational access for adults. Our nation has not had such widespread legal access to cannabis for almost 100 years. Many important questions remain unanswered, such as how this expanded access to what has become a multitude of cannabis-based products will change rates of 1) adolescent and adult use, 2) adverse events due to cannabis use (e.g., motor vehicle accidents, unintentional poisonings [Cooper and Williams 2018]), and 3) development of cannabis use disorder and related treatment admissions. In this chapter we provide a brief history of cannabis laws in the United States and the ever-evolving medical and recreational markets.

Theoretical Impact of Policy on Cannabis Use

In general, as drugs become cheaper and more available, rates of use increase. Every intoxicant, including cannabis, theoretically has its own demand curve related to the population's perception of harm related to its use, costs of use, and legal risks of obtaining and possessing the drug (Caulkins et al. 2012a). Like that for other market goods, the price elasticity of demand for a given drug affects its consumption (Nordstrom and Kleber 2011). *Price elasticity of demand* refers to the percentage change in quantity demanded for a given good divided by the percentage change in price. Consumption of nonessential goods (e.g., gourmet chocolate) tends to be more price-elastic, whereas consumption of staples (e.g., toilet paper) tends to be price-inelastic. Young adults and adolescents tend to exhibit greater price elasticity than older adults.

Price elasticity and overall demand for a drug may also depend on whether a given drug functions as a complement to or a substitute for similar products. For instance, convincing arguments can be made that cannabis and alcohol function both as complements to and as substitutes for one another (Anderson and Rees 2011, 2014). Some pro-legalization advocates suggest that increased consumption of cannabis will lead to decreases in the demand for alcohol, because cannabis is a substitute good. Indeed, some analyses suggest that alcohol-related traffic fatalities dropped (by around 10%) following the implementation of medical cannabis programs in some states (Anderson and Rees 2011, 2014), although drivers involved in fatal crashes were more likely to test positive for cannabis after implementation of medical cannabis laws in comparison with before passage of such laws (Salomonsen-Sautel et al. 2014). However, epidemiological studies have found that states with medical cannabis programs may show increases in alcohol consumption, because heavy-drinking and binge-drinking behaviors can be complementary to cannabis use and thus positively associated (Anderson and Rees 2014; Choi 2014).

Cannabis Policy: A Brief Modern History

Until the 1914 Harrison Narcotics Act, drug control laws that restricted access to intoxicants were left up to the states (Musto 1999). Cannabis prohibition did not arise on a national scale until the passage of the Marihuana Tax Act of 1937, which required users to register to pay tax on purchases and superseded all state-level laws (Table 31–1). Although the federal government had regulated the clear labeling of cannabis-based tinctures and pharmaceuticals under the Pure Food and Drugs Act of 1906 (the legislation that created the U.S. Food and Drug Administration), it did not attempt to restrict access to cannabis until the Marihuana Tax Act. The resulting regulations for physician prescription of cannabis "were so complicated that [physicians were] not likely to [prescribe] it" (Musto 1999), and sales of cannabis between individuals were otherwise banned by the new legislation. As a result, law enforcement officials began to criminally prosecute Americans nationwide for selling and possessing cannabis. These efforts are now widely condemned as intentionally targeting Mexican immigrants, as indicated by the title of the act.

A new cultural era for cannabis arose in the 1960s, in part led by the psychedelic guru Timothy Leary. In 1969, the U.S. Supreme Court invalidated the Marihuana Tax Act on the grounds that the requirement of registration was a form of self-incrimination (and thus was unconstitutional according to the Fifth Amendment). In response, President Richard Nixon and Congress passed the Controlled Substances Act in 1970, creating the scheduling system for what are now known as controlled substances under the U.S. Department of Justice. As a result, cannabis was classified as a "Schedule I" substance, meaning that it has no accepted medical uses and great addictive liability. Publicly released documents from the Nixon administration have since confirmed long-held suspicions that the criminalization of cannabis was in part politically motivated to suppress the votes of African Americans and liberals, who were perceived to have higher rates of cannabis use at the time.

TABLE 32–1. Timeline of cannabis-related laws and major pertinent historical events

Milestone	Year	Significance
Pure Food and Drugs Act	1906	Created a role for federal regulation (i.e., superseding many states' own laws) of product labeling of commonly used substances to prevent the manufacture, sale, or transportation of adulterated, misbranded, or unsafe food and drugs. Prior to the law, consumers often bought pharmaceuticals over the counter with unknown amounts of narcotics and adulterants. Precursor to the establishment of the U.S. Food and Drug Administration.
Harrison Narcotic Act	1914	Required physicians prescribing narcotics (opium and/or cocaine derivatives) to register annually with the federal government. Although it did not apply to cannabis, the Harrison Act became the model for drug regulation (i.e., prohibition) at the federal level.
Marihuana Tax Act	1937	The federal government's first attempt to effectively prohibit the possession or use of cannabis. The act imposed strict registration and reporting requirements and exorbitant taxes on recreational cannabis as opposed to medically authorized use.
Federally licensed cannabis cultivation	1968	The University of Mississippi was contracted under the U.S. Drug Enforcement Administration as the sole source of cannabis for government use such as National Institutes of Health–funded research.
Controlled Substances Act	1970	Passed as part of the Comprehensive Drug Abuse Prevention and Control Act, the CSA created the scheduling system for addictive substances and led to the classification of cannabis under the DEA and FDA as a "Schedule I" substance, meaning that it has no therapeutic value and high addictive liability.
Beginning of the "War on Drugs"	1971	President Nixon declared, "America's public enemy number one in the U.S. is drug abuse. In order to fight and defeat this enemy, it is necessary to wage a new, all-out offensive," initiating what is colloquially referred to as the "War on Drugs" with a growing emphasis on law enforcement approaches and interdiction.
First Medical Cannabis Program	1996	California voters passed Proposition 215 to protect the legal rights of patients and their caregivers to possess cannabis (for medical purposes) with a physician's recommendation.
Gonzales v. Raich (U.S. Supreme Court)	2005	In a 6–3 opinion delivered by Justice Stevens, the U.S. Supreme Court held that the commerce clause gave Congress authority to prohibit the local cultivation and use of cannabis, despite state laws to the contrary.

TABLE 32–1. **Timeline of cannabis-related laws and major pertinent historical events** *(continued)*

Milestone	Year	Significance
The Ogden memo	2009	U.S. Deputy Attorney General Ogden released a memo stating that the U.S. Department of Justice would not target "individuals whose actions are in clear and unambiguous compliance with existing state laws providing for the medical use of cannabis," leading state legislatures (rather than popular vote via referenda) to pass medical cannabis program legislation, expand state-licensed production, and open dispensaries for medical cannabis.
First U.S. state legalization of recreational cannabis	2012	In November 2012, voters in Washington and Colorado passed amendments to allow recreational production, sales, and possession of cannabis by adults over the age of 21 years. Alaska, Oregon, and Washington, D.C., joined them in 2014.
Canada legalizes marijuana for adult recreational use	2018	In October 2018, recreational cannabis became legal in Canada, making it the second country in the world to legalize cannabis (following Uruguay). Canadian adults may possess up to 30 grams (~1 ounce) of dried cannabis and up to 4 home-grown marijuana plants. Edibles and other cannabis-infused products remain illegal.

CSA=Controlled Substances Act; DEA=U.S. Drug Enforcement Association; FDA=U.S. Food and Drug Administration.
Source. Adapted from Courtwright 2002; Williams 2016.

Medical Cannabis Programs

Given the explosive growth of what is fast becoming a billion-dollar industry with many for-profit stakeholders, it is easy to forget that efforts to legalize "medical marijuana" were initially promoted as compassionate care for severely and terminally ill patients whose illnesses had not responded to conventional treatments and who were at risk of legal jeopardy if found in possession of cannabis (which remained illegal under all state and federal laws until 1996, when California first passed its medical cannabis law). Typically, these efforts were simply meant to protect the rights of patients using cannabis to treat symptoms such as nausea, cachexia, or spasticity (Hill 2015b). As of March 2020, 33 states (and the District of Columbia) have authorized legal protections for the possession of cannabis for medicinal purposes, with many states going much further, in some cases creating state agencies to license the production, manufacturing, and dispensing of medical cannabis and derivative products.

States vary greatly in the requirements and provisions allowable under their medical cannabis laws (Pacula and Sevigny 2014). Although physicians have rarely been involved in crafting medical cannabis laws or regulations for resultant medical cannabis programs, they are tasked in all participating states with "recommending" the use of cannabis to eligible individuals, who then commonly must seek registration in a medical cannabis program (Sevigny et al. 2014). More than two million Americans are estimated to be participating in medical cannabis programs among the 27 operational programs as of May 2018 (Procon.org 2018), and these numbers are thought to have increased as programs continue to expand into new states.

Official rates of enrollment for all medical cannabis programs were notably low before 2009 (Anderson and Rees 2014), given the great uncertainty around the prospect of federal prosecution of medical cannabis programs and enrolled patients (Bachhuber et al. 2014). Following the release of the "Ogden memo" by the U.S. Department of Justice in 2009, which provided uniform guidance to focus federal prosecutions and helped relieve states' concerns over possible investigations by clarifying federal intentions to refrain from interfering with lawfully run medical cannabis programs (Ogden 2009; Sznitman and Zolotov 2015), states operationalized dispensaries in greater numbers, facilitating consequent expansion of patient enrollment (Bachhuber et al. 2014; Pacula et al. 2015).

In many states, individuals receive recommendations for cannabis from physicians whom they have seen for a single visit, from whom they receive no diagnosis, and with whom they do not follow up for ongoing care, yet little research has assessed how medical cannabis program policies vary across states with respect to basic tenets of medical practice and pharmaceutical regulation (Sevigny et al. 2014; Wilkinson and D'Souza 2014).

Considerable variation exists in the medical orientation of medical cannabis programs, and this has a large impact on the number of participants, with more loosely regulated programs typically enrolling many more customers (Williams et al. 2016). Although just over half of medical cannabis programs require a bona fide doctor–patient relationship, other common elements of clinical practice, such as those involving controlled substances, are much less common, including 30-day refill limits on cannabis and linkage to state prescription drug monitoring programs. Additionally, very few states require any sort of physician certification through a state-based licensing or training program specific to medical cannabis (Williams et al. 2016). Finally, only a handful of states limit cannabis use to nonsmoked forms (e.g., cannabis-based edibles or tinctures), although such limitations may be more common among recently passed programs in more conservative states (e.g., Iowa, Louisiana, West Virginia). Many alternatives to smoking whole-plant cannabis now exist—notably, vaporization with small portable devices that use pods of cannabis-containing oils—obviating the need for smoked cannabis (Hill 2015b; Kalant 2008), which nonetheless remains allowable in most states with medical cannabis programs.

In sum, more than half of medical cannabis programs depart from a basic medical model; these states allow either home cultivation of cannabis or other forms of procurement outside of state-licensed manufacturing sites and do not include practices consistent with the basic standards of clinical care. Such differences in program regulation may be related to the process by which medical cannabis programs were established in each state; early programs were mostly passed before the year 2009 by voter initiatives in Western states with low population density and depart from a medical model. Voter initiatives in many states (e.g., propositions in California) are typically difficult to scale back or regulate once passed (Caulkins et al. 2012b). More recent programs enacted by Midwestern and Northeastern state legislatures since 2009 are more highly regulated and more adherent to a medical model (Williams et al. 2016). These more recent programs typically require several years between initial passage and full implementation of a state-licensed manufacturing and dispensary system (in contrast to earlier programs, which simply permitted home cultivation or authorized legal protection for possession) (Pacula et al. 2014).

The effects of dispensaries on rates of cannabis use, heavy use, and use of high-potency strains, as well as on associated changes in prices, have received some attention in the medical and policy literature (Anderson and Rees 2014; Cerdá et al. 2012; Pacula et al. 2015). Findings from epidemiological studies have been mixed in associating passage of medical cannabis laws with postimplementation changes in prevalence of use among adolescents and adults (Cerdá et al. 2012; Williams et al. 2017). One study found that the presence of operating dispensaries was associated with increased rates of heavy use of cannabis (Pacula et al. 2015). A subsequent report, however, found no relationship between the opening of dispensaries and rates of cannabis use (Anderson and Rees 2014). All of these studies were conducted against the backdrop of increasing rates of adult cannabis use nationwide, making it more difficult to parse out the impact of heterogeneous state laws.

Medical cannabis programs that establish dispensaries are mixed in their allowance of other means of cannabis procurement. For instance, many of the early medical cannabis programs implemented in states with higher rates of recreational cannabis use allowed home cultivation in addition to dispensaries (Sevigny et al. 2014). Such arrangements may confound the impact of dispensaries on access to cannabis. While the presence of dispensaries may increase access (especially access to high-potency cannabis products) and/or reduce costs (and may concomitantly increase use or heavy use of cannabis), lower rates of program enrollment may result from state-licensed dispensaries when they are the exclusive route of access to medical cannabis. It may be that the mere presence of dispensaries has less influence on rates of use than eligibility requirements restricting who legitimately qualifies as a medical cannabis patient. If so, restrictions on access have direct implications for the role of physicians as gatekeepers (Appel 2008; Gambino 2013; Wilkinson and D'Souza 2014).

Indications for Medical Cannabis

Until the past few years, states tended to include a common set of qualifying indications for participation in a medical cannabis program, including diagnoses such as cancer, HIV/AIDS, epilepsy, and amyotrophic lateral sclerosis accompanied by complications such as severe pain, nausea, and cachexia (Institute of Medicine et al. 1999). Recently, there has been a dramatic increase in the number of indications qualifying for medical cannabis, with many states frequently amending and expanding their lists of qualifying conditions (Williams 2016). Despite 20 years of medical cannabis programs, there remains limited high-quality evidence supporting the use of cannabis for many of the purposes for which participants seek program enrollment (Hill 2015b; National Academies of Sciences, Engineering, and Medicine 2017). However, there has been a growing literature demonstrating effectiveness of cannabis-based products for the treatment of various pain syndromes (National Academies of Sciences, Engineering, and Medicine 2017), and virtually all states now list pain syndromes in one form or another as an allowable indication (Williams 2016). For instance, two systematic reviews found that high-quality evidence for the benefits of cannabinoids was limited to severe pain syndromes, neuropathic pain, and spasticity such as that due to multiple sclerosis (Hill 2015b; Whiting et al. 2015). Of note, many "medical marijuana" clinical studies are actually trials investigating U.S. Food and Drug Administration–approved medications (e.g., dronabinol, nabilone) rather than smoked whole-plant cannabis.

To date, there is no evidence suggesting a psychiatric indication for medical cannabis use. Rather, several studies of moderate to high quality suggest that regular, and especially heavy, use of cannabis can cause and worsen affective, anxiety, and psychotic symptoms (Crippa et al. 2009; Degenhardt et al. 2003; Moore et al. 2007; Volkow et al. 2014). Nonetheless, posttraumatic stress disorder (PTSD) has now been adopted by several states as an indication for qualification in a medical cannabis program (Bonn-Miller et al. 2014). Unfortunately, there is emerging concern that cannabis use can worsen PTSD (similar to the effect on depression and anxiety) and that cannabis use disorder is much harder to treat in patients with PTSD (Boden et al. 2013). Additionally, patients with a comorbid mental illness such as a mood, anxiety, or substance use disorder are generally considered poor candidates for medical cannabis given its side-effect profile (Hill 2015a; Whiting et al. 2015).

There is currently a disconnect between evidence-based indications for medical cannabis and the qualifications for which patients seek enrollment in medical cannabis programs (Williams 2016). In fact, hundreds of thousands of medical cannabis program participants in states with looser regulations are thought to have been enrolled through medical cannabis specialty clinics staffed with their own physicians, who certify patients as being eligible for a medical cannabis permit based largely on patient self-report (Crombie 2012). Initial studies of these program participants showed that the typical medical cannabis patient was a young male with a nonspecific chronic or severe pain indication, without a formal diagnosis or prior trials of conventional treatments, and with a history of recreational cannabis use, rather than an older adult with a terminal illness under intensive medical care (Bachhuber et al. 2014; Boden et al. 2013; Bonn-Miller et al. 2014; Reinarman et al. 2011). These trends are likely different in more tightly regulated and medicalized states; for instance, the average age of medical cannabis participants in New York State's highly regulated program is above 50.

It is often difficult to differentiate between cannabis users based on medical versus recreational use (Walsh et al. 2013). In other words, historically the great majority of medical cannabis users have histories of recreational use, and the recreational users in the studies endorse motivations for recreational cannabis use—such as help with pain, anxiety, and sleep—that are comparable to those endorsed by medical cannabis program participants (Kim et al. 2018). A study in a Michigan dispensary ($N=348$) found that 87% of patients were enrolled for "pain relief" and that many of the patients concomitantly used opioids for pain (Ilgen et al. 2013). About half of those patients also reported wanting to cut down on their use of prescription pain pills, suggesting that medical cannabis programs may be a venue for identifying patients with difficulty controlling opioid use. In fact, amid worsening opioid-related overdose rates, New York State has now authorized reduction in opioid use as a qualifying condition for medical cannabis access.

Physician Liability

Despite the growing presence of medical cannabis programs across the country and the tremendous increase in participant enrollment since 2009, there remain uncertainties about the legal liability, however remote, of physicians who recommend or certify patients for participation (Lazar and Murphy 2014). After California first legalized medical cannabis in 1996, the federal government threatened to take away the medical licenses of physicians who recommended the use of cannabis and raided some medical cannabis clinics. A subsequent U.S. Court of Appeals ruling in the case of *Conant v. Walters* (2002) restrained the federal government from revoking a physician's U.S. Drug Enforcement Administration (DEA) license to prescribe controlled substances or conducting an investigation of a physician if the basis for the government's action was solely the physician's recommendation of the use of medical cannabis. The U.S. Supreme Court denied an appeal; therefore, physicians maintained the right to discuss cannabis with their patients, in keeping with long-standing freedom-of-speech protections for physicians.

The legal implications of certifying patients (or certifying caregivers, as is required of physicians in some states) for medical cannabis also remain unclear, given the differences between the views of states and those of the federal government. Cannabis is classified as a Schedule I substance, meaning that federal agencies (largely the DEA) have concluded that it has no currently accepted medical use and possesses a high potential for abuse. The prescription, supply, and sale of cannabis remain illegal under federal law, according to the Controlled Substances Act of 1970. Furthermore, it is not known to what extent, if any, a physician who certifies a patient for medical cannabis may be held liable for negative outcomes (e.g., motor vehicle crashes, psychiatric adverse effects) (D'Souza and Ranganathan 2015). It is not known whether malpractice insurance would cover liability attributable to physicians certifying or recommending medical cannabis for their patients, and little case law exists on the matter.

Physicians working in the Veterans Affairs Healthcare System (VA) operate under different rules, given that the VA is federally managed. As a result, VA physicians are banned from recommending medical cannabis to patients who ask about it, even in states with legal medical cannabis programs. Even though VA physicians cannot certify their patients for medical cannabis, veterans have the option of going outside of VA services and finding private physicians to help them gain access. In 2010, the U.S. Department of Veterans Affairs announced that veterans who participated in medical cannabis programs would no longer be disqualified from enrolling in substance abuse treatment and pain control programs through the VA.

Given the more than 1 million participants in medical cannabis programs, the lack of data on these programs is a strong argument for better and more consistent state reporting on programs as well as for longitudinal research. Many medical and professional societies have called for high-quality research into the potential therapeutic applications of cannabis. There is also a need for further population-level research to assess the impact of medical cannabis programs once enacted.

Recreational Cannabis

United States

As of June 2019, the recreational use of cannabis and cannabis-derived products by adults older than 21 years has been legalized in 14 states and territories. In addition, dozens of states have reduced or eliminated criminal penalties for the possession of cannabis (i.e., for personal consumption), so that possession is treated more like a traffic ticket (in general, no threat of felony convictions or incarceration). The enforcement of these reformed laws varies, however. For instance, even though New York State "decriminalized" cannabis possession decades ago, it was common practice until the 2010s for law enforcement officials to arrest individuals for cannabis possession during stop-and-frisk procedures.

As with medical cannabis laws, states and jurisdictions differ in their legislation allowing for recreational access and will likely experience different population-level effects of their reforms based on how they regulate cannabis production, sales, and advertising. There are several models of legalization that do not a priori involve corporate commercialization (Reuter 2014). Primarily, there are two options available, which have not yet garnered much attention but have the potential to provide routes of legalization that may limit widespread increases in cannabis use by avoiding mass commercialization and marketing: 1) state monopoly systems and 2) "grow your own" policies that prohibit commercial sales but permit "gifting" of small amounts of cannabis (Reuter 2014).

Allowing for the sale of cannabis in commercial stores (versus state-operated stores) would likely lead to much higher rates of use, and possibly higher rates of heavy use as well. An example from alcohol control policy reform in Washington State gives insight. Costco was a major funder of a 2011 initiative to dismantle Washington State's requirement that liquor be sold only through state-licensed stores. As a result, liquor sales increased despite higher privatized prices when the number of stores selling liquor in the state mushroomed from 330 to 1,500 (Room 2014).

It is difficult to predict what these states will experience regarding changes in price for recreational cannabis. The expectation of full legalization is that it would significantly drop prices for cannabis due to decreased risk, increased automation, and economies of scale. The typical price elasticity of demand (percentage change in consumption divided by percentage change in price) for cannabis has a wide range, depending on the population studied, although among youth, it is roughly the same as the corresponding estimated ranges for cigarette price elasticity, suggesting that youth will be highly price-sensitive (Caulkins et al. 2012b). If this is the case, and cannabis does become cheaper after full legalization, it is likely that youth will consume greater quantities unless taxes or other state interventions artificially increase the costs of use.

Consumption of cannabis, like consumption of other drugs of abuse, is heavily concentrated among a minority of the heaviest users. As a result, it is the response of these users to changes in price that is most influential in determining how a price change will affect the overall quantity of cannabis consumed. For tobacco and alcohol, the elasticity of the total quantity consumed among heavy users is thought to be double that of the general population, meaning that they are more sensitive to small changes in price (Caulkins et al. 2012b). Based on the evidence available for cannabis, Pacula and Sevigny (2014) estimated that the total price elasticity of demand around the current price of cannabis might be between −0.4 and −1.2.

Owing to the complexities of the intermingled finances of the emerging legal commercial market and persistent black market activity, it is unlikely that there is one pricing scheme or tax rate that simultaneously maximizes tax revenues and minimizes consumption, given the inevitable rise in illicit activity that accompanies higher prices (as is seen currently with cigarette sales and illegal trafficking across state lines). A public health approach would ideally consider tax rates that also reflect tetrahydrocannabinol potency or even the full cannabinoid profile of the product, so that products with greater individual- and population-level risks are disproportionately taxed, thereby incentivizing safer consumption practices.

International Perspectives

International examples can provide insight into some of the decisions that U.S. states are facing when reforming cannabis laws and how different policies can affect the public.

For instance, the Netherlands has chosen not to enforce laws pertaining to cannabis, leading to a de facto legalization of adult possession and use (Nordstrom and Kleber 2011; Pardo 2014). Technically, under Dutch law, the wholesale cultivation, processing, and "backdoor" sale of cannabis to retail outlets remain illegal, and this law is intermittently enforced, keeping prices elevated (Pardo 2014; Transform Drug Policy Foundation 2009). Under this system, commercial advertising began to expand, and cannabis use among Dutch youth increased by 200% between 1984 and 1992 (whereas use decreased by 66% during this time in the United States) (Nordstrom and Kleber 2011). As a result, in 1996 the Dutch Parliament attempted to close some of the "coffee shops," ban advertising, and reduce the amount of cannabis customers could buy in order to decelerate rising rates of use.

The Dutch experience suggests that once mass marketing is allowed, it will affect rates of use; therefore, once a substance has been legalized, commercial interests will greatly influence any attempts to rein in activity, especially in the United States, which has a track record of protecting corporations' rights to free speech and broad leeway for advertising (Caulkins et al. 2012a; Nordstrom and Kleber 2011). Currently, coffee shops in the Netherlands are banned from advertising in mass media. This restriction was intended to limit use among youth; however, such a ban would not necessarily hold up to judicial scrutiny in the United States. Additional reforms have been attempted in the Dutch system in recent years, such as requiring proof of residence, but these policies have been inconsistently enforced (Hill 2015a).

Recreational cannabis became legal in Canada on October 17, 2018, making Canada the second country in the world to legalize it (in addition to Uruguay). Under Canadian law, adults age 19 years or older (18 years in some provinces) can now possess, carry, and share (with other adults) up to 30 grams (just over one ounce) of dried cannabis, enough to fill dozens of joints. They are also permitted a maximum of four homegrown marijuana plants per household, although this varies by province. Initially, edibles and other cannabis-infused products remained illegal for the first year, but these were approved for sale beginning in December 2019. This closely watched legal revolution in our nearest neighboring country will offer opportunities to assess the impact of recreational cannabis laws in settings outside the United States but with similar culture, perhaps as a precursor to federal reform at home.

Conclusion

Although physicians do not have the legal authority to prescribe medical cannabis anywhere in the United States (because marijuana remains a Schedule I controlled substance), more than half of states now permit physicians to "recommend" cannabis for medical purposes to patients who have a qualifying condition. However, states are inconsistent in their medical cannabis program regulations, and qualifying indications bear little relationship to the current evidence base. To date, there are no psychiatric disorders with high-quality evidence for benefits from long-term use of cannabis. Meanwhile, there is a growing literature indicating that heavy or prolonged cannabis use can worsen symptoms of psychotic, anxiety, mood, trauma-related, and substance use disorders (Volkow et al. 2014). Furthermore, the liability to physicians who recommend cannabis use to patients is unknown and may change as state and federal policies evolve under different political climates.

Although a growing number of states have legalized adult use of recreational cannabis, no state currently allows individuals to transport cannabis across state lines. States that now allow both medical cannabis and recreational sales are struggling with models of production, sales, and taxation that minimize risks to the public while also constraining black market activity. As state policies continue to evolve, and new users of all ages continue to initiate cannabis use, especially heavy daily use, states will serve as natural experiments for clinicians, researchers, and policymakers to better understand pathways leading to cannabis use disorder and other related adverse outcomes of heavy cannabis use.

References

Anderson MD, Rees DI: Medical Marijuana Laws, Traffic Fatalities, and Alcohol Consumption. Discussion Paper Series, Forschungsinstitut zur Zukunft der Arbeit, No. 6112, November 2011. Available at: http://ftp.iza.org/dp6112.pdf. Accessed December 5, 2019.

Anderson DM, Rees DI: The role of dispensaries: the devil is in the details. J Policy Anal Manage 33(1):235–240, 2014 24358532

Appel J: "Physicians are not bootleggers": the short, peculiar life of the medicinal alcohol movement. Bull Hist Med 82(2):355–386, 2008 18622072

Bachhuber MA, Saloner B, Cunningham CO, et al: Medical cannabis laws and opioid analgesic overdose mortality in the United States, 1999–2010. JAMA Intern Med 174(10):1668–1673, 2014 25154332

Boden MT, Babson KA, Vujanovic AA, et al: Posttraumatic stress disorder and cannabis use characteristics among military veterans with cannabis dependence. Am J Addict 22(3):277–284, 2013 23617872

Bonn-Miller MO, Boden MT, Bucossi MM, et al: Self-reported cannabis use characteristics, patterns and helpfulness among medical cannabis users. Am J Drug Alcohol Abuse 40(1):23–30, 2014 24205805

Caulkins JP, Hawken A, Kilmer B, et al: Cannabis Legalization: What Everyone Needs to Know. New York, Oxford University Press, 2012a

Caulkins JP, Kilmer B, MacCoun RJ, et al: Design considerations for legalizing cannabis: lessons inspired by analysis of California's Proposition 19. Addiction 107(5):865–871, 2012b 21985069

Cerdá M, Wall M, Keyes KM, et al: Medical marijuana laws in 50 states: investigating the relationship between state legalization of medical marijuana and marijuana use, abuse and dependence. Drug Alcohol Depend 120(1–3):22–27, 2012 22099393

Choi A: The impact of medical marijuana laws on cannabis use and other risky health behaviors. Doctoral Dissertation, Cornell University, Department of Policy Analysis and Management, New York, December 1, 2014

Conant v. Walters, 309 F.3d 629 (9th Cir. 2002)

Cooper ZD, Williams AR: Cannabis and cannabinoid intoxication and toxicity, in Cannabis Use Disorder. Edited by Montoya I, Weiss S. New York, Springer, 2018, pp 103–112

Courtwright D: Forces of Habit: Drugs and the Making of the Modern World. Cambridge, MA, Harvard University Press, 2002

Crippa JA, Zuardi AW, Martín-Santos R, et al: Cannabis and anxiety: a critical review of the evidence. Hum Psychopharmacol 24(7):515–523, 2009 19693792

Crombie N: Medical marijuana: a few high-volume doctors approve most patients. The Oregonian/Oregon Live, December 29, 2012. Available at: https://www.oregonlive.com/health/2012/12/medical_marijuana_a_few_high-v.html. Accessed September 3, 2020.

Degenhardt L, Hall W, Lynskey M: Exploring the association between cannabis use and depression. Addiction 98(11):1493–1504, 2003 14616175

D'Souza DC, Ranganathan M: Medical marijuana: is the cart before the horse? JAMA 313(24):2431–2432, 2015 26103026

Gambino M: During prohibition your doctor could write you a prescription for booze. Smithsonian.com, October 7, 2013. Available at: http://www.smithsonianmag.com/history/during-prohibition-your-doctor-could-write-you-prescription-booze-180947940/?no-ist. Accessed December 5, 2019.

Hill KP: Cannabis: The Unbiased Truth About the World's Most Popular Weed. Center City, MN, Hazelden, 2015a

Hill KP: Medical marijuana for treatment of chronic pain and other medical and psychiatric problems: a clinical review. JAMA 313(24):2474–2483, 2015b 26103031

Ilgen MA, Bohnert K, Kleinberg F, et al: Characteristics of adults seeking medical marijuana certification. Drug Alcohol Depend 132(3):654–659, 2013 23683791

Institute of Medicine; Joy JE, Watson SJ Jr, et al (eds): Cannabis and Medicine: Assessing the Science. Washington, DC, National Academy Press, 1999

Kalant H: Smoked marijuana as medicine: not much future. Clin Pharmacol Ther 83(4):517–519, 2008 18349871

Kim J, Coors ME, Young SE, et al: Cannabis use disorder and male sex predict medical cannabis card status in a sample of high risk adolescents. Drug Alcohol Depend 183:25–33, 2018 29223914

Lazar K, Murphy S: DEA targets doctors linked to medical marijuana. The Boston Globe, June 6, 2014

Moore TH, Zammit S, Lingford-Hughes A, et al: Cannabis use and risk of psychotic or affective mental health outcomes: a systematic review. Lancet 370(9584):319–328, 2007 17662880

Musto DF: The American Disease: Origins of Narcotic Control. New York, Oxford University Press, 1999

National Academies of Sciences, Engineering, and Medicine: The Health Effects of Cannabis and Cannabinoids: The Current State of Evidence and Recommendations for Research. Washington, DC, National Academies Press, 2017

Nordstrom BR, Kleber HD: Clinical and societal implications of drug legalization, in Lowinson and Ruiz's Substance Abuse: A Comprehensive Textbook. Edited by Ruiz P, Strain E. Philadelphia, PA, Lippincott Williams & Wilkins, 2011, pp 1032–1043

Ogden DW: Memorandum for Selected United States Attorneys: Investigations and Prosecutions in States Authorizing the Medical Use of Cannabis. U.S. Department of Justice, Office of the Deputy Attorney General. October 19, 2009. Available at: https://www.justice.gov/archives/opa/blog/memorandum-selected-united-state-attorneys-investigations-and-prosecutions-states. Accessed December 5, 2019.

Pacula RL, Sevigny EL: Marijuana liberalization policies: why we can't learn much from policy still in motion. J Policy Anal Manage 33(1):212–221, 2014 24358530

Pacula RL, Hunt P, Boustead A: Words can be deceiving: a review of variation among legally effective medical marijuana laws in the United States. J Drug Policy Anal 7(1):1–19, 2014 25657828

Pacula RL, Powell D, Heaton P, et al: Assessing the effects of medical marijuana laws on marijuana use: the devil is in the details. J Policy Anal Manage 34(1):7–31, 2015 25558490

Pardo B: Cannabis policy reforms in the Americas: a comparative analysis of Colorado, Washington, and Uruguay. Int J Drug Policy 25(4):727–735, 2014 24970383

Procon.org: Number of Legal Medical Marijuana Patients. May 17, 2018. Available at: https://medicalmarijuana.procon.org/view.resource.php?resourceID=005889. Accessed December 5, 2019.

Reinarman C, Nunberg H, Lanthier F, et al: Who are medical marijuana patients? Population characteristics from nine California assessment clinics. J Psychoactive Drugs 43(2):128–135, 2011 21858958

Reuter P: The difficulty of restricting promotion of legalized marijuana in the United States. Addiction 109(3):353–354, 2014 24524313

Room R: Legalizing a market for cannabis for pleasure: Colorado, Washington, Uruguay and beyond. Addiction 109(3):345–351, 2014 24180513

Salomonsen-Sautel S, Min SJ, Sakai JT, et al: Trends in motor vehicle crashes before and after marijuana commercialization in Colorado. Drug Alcohol Depend 140:137–144, 2014 24831752

Sevigny EL, Pacula RL, Heaton P: The effects of medical marijuana laws on potency. Int J Drug Policy 25(2):308–319, 2014 24502887

Sznitman SR, Zolotov Y: Cannabis for therapeutic purposes and public health and safety: a systematic and critical review. Int J Drug Policy 26(1):20–29, 2015 25304050

Transform Drug Policy Foundation: After the War on Drugs: Blueprint for Regulation. 2009. Available at: https://transformdrugs.org/wp-content/uploads/2018/10/Blueprint.pdf. Accessed December 9, 2019.

Volkow ND, Baler RD, Compton WM, et al: Adverse health effects of marijuana use. N Engl J Med 370(23):2219–2227, 2014 24897085

Walsh Z, Callaway R, Belle-Isle L, et al: Cannabis for therapeutic purposes: patient characteristics, access, and reasons for use. Int J Drug Policy 24(6):511–516, 2013 24095000

Whiting PF, Wolff RF, Deshpande S, et al: Cannabinoids for medical use: a systematic review and meta-analysis. JAMA 313(24):2456–2473, 2015 26103030

Wilkinson ST, D'Souza DC: Problems with the medicalization of marijuana. JAMA 311(23):2377–2378, 2014 24845238

Williams AR: Medical and recreational marijuana policy: from prohibition to the rise of regulation, in Marijuana and Mental Health. Edited by Compton MT. Arlington, VA, American Psychiatric Publishing, 2016, pp 39–70

Williams AR, Olfson M, Kim JD, et al: Older, less regulated medical marijuana programs have much greater enrollment rates. Health Aff (Millwood) 35(3):480–488, 2016 26953303

Williams AR, Santaella-Tenorio J, Mauro CM, et al: Loose regulation of medical marijuana programs associated with higher rates of adult marijuana use but not cannabis use disorder. Addiction 112(11):1985–1991, 2017 28600874

CHAPTER 33

HIV/AIDS and Hepatitis C Virus

Andrea Norcini Pala, Ph.D.

Robert H. Remien, Ph.D.

Globally, approximately 37 million people are living with HIV. Since the introduction of effective antiretroviral drugs, rates of new infections have declined, and HIV has became a manageable chronic illness for many. However, this improved survival and quality of life requires sustained adherence to complex medication regimens to achieve HIV viral load suppression, limit HIV-induced immune impairment, and prevent infection—in particular, coinfection with the hepatitis C virus (HCV), which carries the potential for more serious medical consequences than are seen with HIV or HCV infection alone. Depression and problematic use of substances (especially alcohol) are the conditions most commonly associated with acquisition and progression of HIV and/or HCV infection. Although often overlooked, these mental health problems can increase the risk of HIV or HCV treatment failure as well as the risk of immunosuppression, cardiovascular disease, liver disease, and premature death.

In this chapter, we review the epidemiology and the physical and mental health consequences of coinfection with HIV and HCV, as well as the negative effects of co-occurring substance use and intersecting forms of societal stigma on clinical outcomes among people living with HIV–HCV coinfection.

Epidemiology of HIV–HCV Coinfection

The tremendous advances in HIV treatment during the past three decades radically changed the natural course of the illness for most people living with HIV (Slaymaker et al. 2014). The first cases of HIV infection in the early 1980s rapidly progressed to acquired immunodeficiency syndrome (AIDS), characterized by severe immunological impairment and resulting in elevated vulnerability to life-threatening comorbidities (e.g., viral infections, cancers) (Deeks 2011). With the advent of combination anti-retroviral therapy (cART) in 1996, AIDS-defining comorbidities became rarer. Concurrently, the life quality and life expectancy of people living with HIV markedly improved (Slaymaker et al. 2014). As survival rates improved, rates of early onset of aging-related complications (e.g., cardiovascular disease, cancer) and premature mortality increased exponentially among people living with HIV, especially among those with HCV coinfection (Deeks 2011).

Worldwide, there are approximately 37 million people living with HIV, 2 million of whom live with HCV coinfection (Platt et al. 2016). Eastern Europe and Central Asia bear the highest burden of HIV–HCV coinfection, with more than 600,000 diagnoses (Platt et al. 2016), followed by sub-Saharan Africa, which accounts for more than 70% of the global HIV epidemic. In the United States, rates of new HIV infections have decreased in recent years among white men who have sex with men (MSM), heterosexual men and women, and people who inject drugs, while they have remained stable or have increased for black and Latino MSM (Centers for Disease Control and Prevention 2017). Since 2012, HCV infections have continued to increase, with a current prevalence of 25% among the 1.2 million people living with HIV in the United States (Centers for Disease Control and Prevention 2017). In addition to the alarmingly high rates of HIV–HCV coinfection, there remains a substantial number of people with undiagnosed or untreated HIV or HCV monoinfection or HIV–HCV coinfection (Torian et al. 2018).

The overlapping transmission modes of HIV and HCV contribute to the high prevalence of coinfection. Both viruses are blood-borne, transmitted through direct contact with infected blood (e.g., needle sharing) (Sulkowski 2008). People who inject drugs have a disproportionately high prevalence of HIV–HCV coinfection due to sharing of drug injection equipment (e.g., contaminated needles). While sexual transmission of HCV is rare among HIV-negative individuals, the risk increases in the context of HIV infection. U.S. rates of sexually transmitted HCV among people living with HIV have increased in the past few years, especially in black HIV-positive MSM (Yaphe et al. 2012). HIV increases vulnerability to HCV acquisition, likely due to HIV effects on the immune system (Sulkowski 2008). Thus, sustained adherence to cART is critical to achieve HIV viral load suppression, limit HIV-induced immune impairment, and, consequently, reduce HCV acquisition and negative clinical consequences of HIV–HCV coinfection.

Sustained viral suppression is a key goal of both HIV and HCV treatment, not only to prevent medical complications for the individual but also to prevent HIV transmission to sexual partners (Eisinger and Fauci 2018; Wyles et al. 2018). Current guidelines recommend early cART initiation, given the net benefits in terms of reduced morbidity and mortality for people living with HIV and the reduced likelihood of transmission to others (Eisinger and Fauci 2018). While HIV infection remains incurable, HCV can be eradicated through direct-acting antiviral (DAA) therapy (McGinley et al. 2017). Rates of DAA therapy–induced virological response—that is, sustained virological response (SVR), the marker of HCV eradication, consisting of undetectable HCV load for more than 12 weeks—are above 90% (McGinley et al. 2017). Before 2011 (i.e., before the availability of DAA therapy), HCV therapy consisted of interferon (IFN)–α injection alone or in combination with ribavirin, an antiviral medication (McGinley et al. 2017). IFN-based therapy, however, had SVR rates of only 50% (Pearlman and

Traub 2011) and severe side effects such as depressive symptoms interfering with adherence to HCV and/or HIV therapy (Fialho et al. 2017; Vancassel et al. 2018). DAA therapy represents an improvement over IFN-α therapy, with fewer or no side effects, higher rates of success, and more rapid SVR achievement (McGinley et al. 2017). However, in some countries in Eastern Europe and Central Asia, the availability of DAA therapy is limited, mainly as a result of the elevated cost, approximately $84,000 for a 12-week course of treatment (Maistat et al. 2017). It is critical to increase access to DAA therapy and cART, given their strong potential to reduce the burden of HIV–HCV coinfection (Operskalski and Kovacs 2011).

Physical Health Consequences of HIV–HCV Coinfection

Compared with the general population, people living with HIV or HCV have disproportionately higher rates of other medical complications (e.g., diabetes), which are even higher in the context of HIV–HCV coinfection (Operskalski and Kovacs 2011). The complex HIV and HCV interaction dramatically increases vulnerability to noncommunicable diseases including metabolic disorders (e.g., diabetes), bone disorders (e.g., osteoporosis), kidney disease, cardiovascular disease, neurological disorders, and cancer, including hepatocellular carcinoma (Operskalski and Kovacs 2011). HCV, in turn, may promote progression of HIV infection (e.g., a smaller CD4+ increase following cART initiation) (Inshaw et al. 2015). HIV and HCV cause significant immunological impairment that greatly contributes to the development of potentially fatal medical complications.

HIV, directly, and HCV, indirectly, weaken the immune system. HIV causes depletion and functional impairment of CD4+ cells, immune cells contributing to antiviral response (Sant and McMichael 2012). The effect of HIV on CD4+ cells increases the risk of other viral infections, including HCV. Furthermore, the risk of developing chronic HCV infection is higher for people living with HIV than for HIV-negative individuals (Hernandez and Sherman 2011). Coinfection with HCV, in turn, amplifies HIV-induced immune activation, accelerating the aging process and the development of aging-related noncommunicable diseases (e.g., cardiovascular disease, cancer).

HIV-induced immune activation consists of persistent immunological response despite HIV viral suppression (Deeks 2011). Following viral infection, T helper (Th) cells (e.g., CD4+) release cytokines (i.e., small proteins) to coordinate the body's immunological response (Modrow et al. 2013). Th1 cells release pro-inflammatory cytokines (e.g., INF-γ, tumor necrosis factor [TNF]–α) to activate other immune cells. Th2 cells, in contrast, release anti-inflammatory cytokines (e.g., interleukin [IL]–10 and IL-4) to inhibit the release of pro-inflammatory cytokines (Modrow et al. 2013). Th1 and Th2, respectively, upregulate and downregulate inflammation through a self-regulatory mechanism that, however, HIV infection alters, leading to elevated levels of anti-inflammatory and some pro-inflammatory cytokines (i.e., IL-6, IL-1, and TNF-α). IFN-γ, which plays a critical role in the spontaneous clearance of HCV (Ahlenstiel et al. 2010), decreases during chronic HIV infection. Due to HIV-induced Th1/Th2 imbalance, people living with HIV develop a greater vulnerability to HCV acquisition and chronic infection (Shmagel et al. 2016).

HIV–HCV coinfection exacerbates HIV-induced chronic inflammation (Swaminathan et al. 2014), increasing the risk for immunosuppression and potentially fatal medical complications. Immunosuppression consists of progressive numeric loss and functional impairment of CD4+ cells, which have been associated with neurological infections and diseases, several types of cancer, and cancer-specific mortality (Shmagel et al. 2016). Chronic inflammation activates the kynurenine pathway, leading to tryptophan depletion, which exacerbates immunosuppression (Boasso et al. 2007). The indoleamine 2,3-dioxygenase (IDO) enzyme, in particular, transforms tryptophan into its immunosuppressive and neurotoxic metabolite kynurenine (Boasso et al. 2007; Lawson et al. 2011). Chronic inflammation and elevated kynurenine levels contribute to the slower CD4+ cell recovery after cART initiation among people living with HIV and HCV compared with people living with HIV alone (Inshaw et al. 2015).

Optimal adherence to cART is critical to achieve viral suppression, yet a sizable proportion of people living with HIV worldwide (more than 30% in one meta-analysis [Bezabhe et al. 2016]) do not achieve that level of adherence. With the early medication regimens, 95% adherence to cART was considered necessary to suppress HIV viral replication (Viswanathan et al. 2015). More recent studies have shown that with the newer and more "forgiving" regimens, viral suppression is achievable with cART adherence as low as 80% (Viswanathan et al. 2015). However, even with these newer regimens, people living with HIV who are not 100% adherent to cART have been found to have higher pro-inflammatory cytokine levels despite viral suppression (Castillo-Mancilla et al. 2016). To improve clinical outcomes among people living with HIV–HCV coinfection, and, more generally, among people living with HIV, it is essential to assess not only the levels of, but also the potential barriers to, cART adherence in routine health care settings, with subsequent implementation of interventions to improve adherence when needed.

Factors interfering with cART and DAA therapy adherence include regimen complexity, side effects, toxicity, and mental illness and other psychosocial factors (e.g., stigma) (Shuper et al. 2016; Turan et al. 2017). Regimen complexity depends on the number of pills that need to be taken, the dosing schedule, and potential food restriction to ensure treatment efficacy (Bezabhe et al. 2016; Shuper et al. 2016). Side effects and toxicity due to drug interactions can negatively affect adherence to HIV and HCV treatment (Bezabhe et al. 2016). Although adherence levels might be expected to be lower among people living with HIV–HCV coinfection compared with those living with HIV or HCV monoinfection, some studies have found that adherence levels among people living with HIV–HCV coinfection are similar to levels among people living with HIV or HCV monoinfection (Townsend et al. 2016). Depression and problematic alcohol and substance use, on the other hand, remain major barriers to HIV and HCV medication adherence (Fialho et al. 2017; Ironson et al. 2015).

Mental Health in the Context of HIV–HCV Coinfection

Mental health impairment due to psychiatric distress (e.g., subclinical depressive symptoms) or psychiatric disorders (e.g., major depressive disorder) is significantly more prevalent among people who are living with HIV and HCV, not only in comparison with the general population but also in comparison with people who are living with HIV or HCV monoinfection (Fialho et al. 2017; O'Cleirigh et al. 2015). Depression and problematic use of substances (especially alcohol) are the conditions most commonly associated with acquisition and progression of HIV and/or HCV infection (O'Cleirigh et al. 2015; Sood et al. 2014). Although often overlooked, depression and problematic substance use are potentially dangerous conditions that can increase the risk of HIV or HCV treatment failure (i.e., persistence of a detectable viral load) as well as the risk of immunosuppression, cardiovascular disease, liver disease, and premature death (Deeks 2011; Ironson et al. 2015; Pence et al. 2018).

Chronic inflammation caused by HIV–HCV coinfection may contribute both to the high rates of depression and to the effects of depression and problematic substance use on clinical outcomes. Chronic inflammation alters the synthesis of neurotransmitters (i.e., serotonin and dopamine) involved in the pathogenesis of depression and the reinforcement of problematic substance use (Dantzer et al. 2011; Vancassel et al. 2018). Because tryptophan is the precursor of serotonin, inflammation-induced tryptophan depletion lowers serotonin levels (Lawson et al. 2011). There is evidence that higher levels of IL-6 and kynurenine among people living with HIV and IFN-α treatment among people living with HCV are both associated with severe depressive symptoms (Martinez et al. 2014; Norcini Pala et al. 2016; Vancassel et al. 2018). Although DAA therapy has replaced IFN-α treatment, study findings confirm the role of pro-inflammatory cytokines and the kynurenine pathway in the development of depression in individuals with HIV or HCV monoinfection.

In addition to affecting serotonin, chronic inflammation interferes with dopamine synthesis and the activity of dopaminergic neurons, which are involved in the pathogenesis of anhedonia, fatigue, and neurocognitive impairment (e.g., working memory deficit) (Vancassel et al. 2018). Pro-inflammatory cytokines prevent the phenylalanine hydroxylase (PAH) enzyme from metabolizing the amino acid phenylalanine into dopamine (Vancassel et al. 2018). In addition, lower dopamine levels can lead to use of alcohol and other substances (e.g., methamphetamine) that are capable of inducing dopamine surges (Deserno et al. 2015). Prolonged use of these substances, however, further impairs dopaminergic neuron activity and mental health status (Deserno et al. 2015).

Problematic substance use as well as depression can further affect serotonin and dopamine synthesis by exacerbating HIV- or HCV-induced chronic inflammation directly and indirectly, through behavioral and stress-related mechanisms. For example, people living with HIV–HCV coinfection who engage in problematic use of alcohol (Fuster et al. 2014) or morphine (El-Hage et al. 2011) have been shown to have higher levels of pro-inflammatory cytokines. Among people living with HIV who use heroin, the response to pathogens is significantly impaired, and this impairment can increase the risk of, for example, HCV coinfection (Meijerink et al. 2015). Depression and problematic substance use can increase levels of chronic inflammation through behavioral pathways, including poor adherence to health care and medication regimens such as cART and DAA therapy (Remien et al. 2007; Turan et al. 2017). Poor medication adherence, in turn, is associated with having a detectable HIV or HCV viral load as well as having elevated inflammatory levels despite viral HIV suppression (Castillo-Mancilla et al. 2016).

Depression, problematic substance use, medication nonadherence, and HIV and HCV coinfection or monoinfection share similar psychosocial risk factors, including discrimination and other forms of stigma (e.g., internalized stigma) (Bogart et al. 2013; Turan et al. 2017; Wray et al. 2016). People living with HIV–HCV coinfection often carry the burden of multiple stigmas associated with characteristics such as sexual orientation, gender, race or ethnicity, income level, or HIV and/or HCV status. Intersecting stigmas detrimentally affect everyday life, social relationships, and mental and physical health (Turan et al. 2017). Among people living with HIV, discrimination (e.g., racial, sexual) has been associated with depressive symptoms, problematic substance use, and high-risk sexual behaviors as well as with poorer HIV-related outcomes (i.e., detectable viral load, lower CD4+ cell count) (Bogart et al. 2013; Wray et al. 2016). The effects of discrimination on clinical outcomes are likely mediated by depression and problematic substance use, cART nonadherence, and stress-related biological mechanisms (Turan et al. 2017). However, these biological mechanisms remain poorly understood.

According to the minority stress theory, the experience of discrimination causes chronic stress that can ultimately affect hypothalamic-pituitary-adrenal (HPA) axis activity, leading to dysregulation of cortisol, the anti-inflammatory "stress hormone" (Brody et al. 2015; Hatzenbuehler and McLaughlin 2014). Biological (e.g., pro-inflammatory cytokines), environmental (e.g., noise), and psychosocial (e.g., discrimination) stressors can activate the HPA axis (Zunszain et al. 2011). Prolonged exposure to stressors alters HPA axis activity, leading to dysregulated release and impaired anti-inflammatory activity of cortisol (Zunszain et al. 2011). Furthermore, cortisol activates the tryptophan 2,3-dioxygenase (TDO) enzyme, which, similarly to IDO, depletes tryptophan (Zunszain et al. 2011). The resulting chronic inflammation and cortisol dysregulation cause massive tryptophan depletion, kynurenine synthesis, and neurotransmitter (i.e., serotonin, dopamine) deficit.

Conclusion

HIV–HCV coinfection remains a major global public health challenge (Deeks 2011; Platt et al. 2016). Eastern Europe, Central Asia, and sub-Saharan Africa bear the highest burden of HIV–HCV coinfection, yet the availability of DAA therapy is still limited (Kharsany and Karim 2016; Platt et al. 2016). Although people who inject drugs remain the population at highest risk of HIV–HCV coinfection globally, there has been a significant increase in rates of sexually transmitted HIV–HCV coinfection among black and Latino MSM in the United States (Centers for Disease Control and Prevention 2015; Platt et al. 2016). Unlike HIV-negative individuals, people living with HIV are likely to acquire HCV through high-risk sexual behaviors (Yaphe et al. 2012). The increased susceptibility to HCV may stem from HIV-induced immune impairment (Hernandez and Sherman 2011; Sant and McMichael 2012). Therefore, to prevent medical complications as well as HIV and/or HCV transmission to sexual partners, it is critical that people living with HIV achieve and sustain HIV and HCV viral suppression through strict adherence to cART and DAA therapy (Eisinger and Fauci 2018; Wyles et al. 2018).

Treatments for HIV and HCV have led to tremendous improvements in life quality and life expectancy for people living with HIV–HCV coinfection, although immunosuppression and accelerated aging processes contribute to the development of potentially fatal medical complications, including kidney disease, cardiovascular disease, neurological disorders, and cancer (Operskalski and Kovacs 2011). Elevated inflammation levels despite HIV and/or HCV viral suppression cause depletion and functional impairment of CD4+ cells (Sant and McMichael 2012). Nonadherence to cART and DAA therapy exacerbates HIV-induced inflammation levels (Modrow et al. 2013; Shmagel et al. 2016). In this context, IDO and TDO activation triggered by pro-inflammatory cytokines increases kynurenine levels, which negatively affect CD4+ cells as well as the brain (Boasso et al. 2007; Jenabian et al. 2016; Lawson et al. 2011).

The neurotoxicity of kynurenine and its metabolites, coupled with serotonin and dopamine deficits, dramatically increases the risk of developing depression and reinforces problematic substance use (Lawson et al. 2011; Vancassel et al. 2018). The effects of pro-inflammatory cytokines on IDO, TDO, and PAH greatly contribute to the high rates of depression among people living with HIV–HCV coinfection or with HIV/HCV monoinfection compared with the general population (Fialho et al. 2017; Ironson et al. 2015; O'Cleirigh et al. 2015). Concurrently, depression and problematic substance use, as well as stress caused by psychosocial factors (e.g., intersecting stigmas), further exacerbate HIV- or HCV-induced chronic inflammation both directly and indirectly—for example, through nonadherence to cART and DAA therapy (Remien et al. 2007; Turan et al. 2017). Problematic alcohol and substance use directly amplifies HIV- or HCV-induced cytokine dysregulation (El-Hage et al. 2011; Fuster et al. 2014). Chronic stress not only promotes depression and problematic substance use but also reduces access and adherence to health care and medication treatment and affects inflammation levels through stress-related biological mechanisms (e.g., HPA axis dysregulation) (Brody et al. 2015; Hatzenbuehler and McLaughlin 2014; Turan et al. 2017).

Despite the advances made in treatments for HIV and HCV, there remains a need for additional work to address the gaps in integration of evidence-based mental health and substance use treatment services into all HIV and HCV prevention and care settings. The evidence discussed in this chapter clearly suggests that it is critical to integrate mental health and substance use screening and treatment into clinical as well as community-based services. Partnerships among researchers, clinicians, policymakers, and community advocates and stakeholders can facilitate such integration. Integration of mental health and substance use screening and care into these settings will lead to better outcomes for HIV/HCV prevention and care efforts, improving the lives of vulnerable populations and protecting the public health.

References

Ahlenstiel G, Titerence RH, Koh C, et al: Natural killer cells are polarized toward cytotoxicity in chronic hepatitis C in an interferon-alfa-dependent manner. Gastroenterology 138(1):325–35.e1, 2, 2010 19747917

Bezabhe WM, Chalmers L, Bereznicki LR, et al: Adherence to antiretroviral therapy and virologic failure: a meta-analysis. Medicine (Baltimore) 95(15):e3361, 2016 27082595

Boasso A, Herbeuval JP, Hardy AW, et al: HIV inhibits CD4+ T-cell proliferation by inducing indoleamine 2,3-dioxygenase in plasmacytoid dendritic cells. Blood 109(8):3351–3359, 2007 17158233

Bogart LM, Landrine H, Galvan FH, et al: Perceived discrimination and physical health among HIV-positive Black and Latino men who have sex with men. AIDS Behav 17(4):1431–1441, 2013 23297084

Brody GH, Yu T, Miller GE, et al: Discrimination, racial identity, and cytokine levels among African-American adolescents. J Adolesc Health 56(5):496–501, 2015 25907649

Castillo-Mancilla JR, Brown TT, Erlandson KM, et al: Suboptimal adherence to combination antiretroviral therapy is associated with higher levels of inflammation despite HIV suppression. Clin Infect Dis 63(12):1661–1667, 2016 27660234

Centers for Disease Control and Prevention: Surveillance for Viral Hepatitis—United States, 2014. Viral Hepatitis Statistics and Surveillance, 2015. Available at: http://www.cdc.gov/hepatitis/statistics/2014surveillance/index.htm. Accessed December 10, 2019.

Centers for Disease Control and Prevention: HIV Among African American Gay and Bisexual Men. 2017. Available at: https://www.cdc.gov/hiv/group/msm/bmsm.html. Accessed December 10, 2019.

Dantzer R, O'Connor JC, Lawson MA, et al: Inflammation-associated depression: from serotonin to kynurenine. Psychoneuroendocrinology 36(3):426–436, 2011 21041030

Deeks SG: HIV infection, inflammation, immunosenescence, and aging. Annu Rev Med 62(1):141–155, 2011 21090961

Deserno L, Beck A, Huys QJM, et al: Chronic alcohol intake abolishes the relationship between dopamine synthesis capacity and learning signals in the ventral striatum. Eur J Neurosci 41(4):477–486, 2015 25546072

Eisinger RW, Fauci AS: Ending the HIV/AIDS pandemic. Emerg Infect Dis 24(3):413–416, 2018 29460740

El-Hage N, Dever SM, Fitting S, et al: HIV-1 coinfection and morphine coexposure severely dysregulate hepatitis C virus-induced hepatic proinflammatory cytokine release and free radical production: increased pathogenesis coincides with uncoordinated host defenses. J Virol 85(22):11601–11614, 2011 21900165

Fialho R, Pereira M, Rusted J, et al: Depression in HIV and HCV co-infected patients: a systematic review and meta-analysis. Psychol Health Med 22(9):1089–1104, 2017 28100073

Fuster D, Cheng DM, Quinn EK, et al: Inflammatory cytokines and mortality in a cohort of HIV-infected adults with alcohol problems. AIDS 28(7):1059–1064, 2014 24401638

Hatzenbuehler ML, McLaughlin KA: Structural stigma and hypothalamic-pituitary-adrenocortical axis reactivity in lesbian, gay, and bisexual young adults. Ann Behav Med 47(1):39–47, 2014 24154988

Hernandez MD, Sherman KE: HIV/hepatitis C coinfection natural history and disease progression. Curr Opin HIV AIDS 6(6):478–482, 2011 22001892

Inshaw J, Leen C, Fisher M, et al: The impact of HCV infection duration on HIV disease progression and response to cART amongst HIV seroconverters in the UK. PLoS One 10(7):e0132772, 2015 26225723

Ironson G, O'Cleirigh C, Kumar M, et al: Psychosocial and neurohormonal predictors of HIV disease progression (CD4 cells and viral load): a 4 year prospective study. AIDS Behav 19(8):1388–1397, 2015 25234251

Jenabian M-A, Mehraj V, Costiniuk CT, et al: Influence of hepatitis C virus sustained virological response on immunosuppressive tryptophan catabolism in ART-treated HIV/HCV coinfected patients. J Acquir Immune Defic Syndr 71(3):254–262, 2016 26436613

Kharsany ABM, Karim QA: HIV infection and AIDS in sub-Saharan Africa: current status, challenges and opportunities. Open AIDS J 10:34–48, 2016 27347270

Lawson MA, Kelley KW, Dantzer R: Intracerebroventricular administration of HIV-1 Tat induces brain cytokine and indoleamine 2,3-dioxygenase expression: a possible mechanism for AIDS comorbid depression. Brain Behav Immun 25(8):1569–1575, 2011 21620953

Maistat L, Kravchenko N, Reddy A: Hepatitis C in Eastern Europe and Central Asia: a survey of epidemiology, treatment access and civil society activity in eleven countries. Hepatol Med Policy 2(1):9, 2017 30288322

Martinez P, Tsai AC, Muzoora C, et al: Reversal of the kynurenine pathway of tryptophan catabolism may improve depression in ART-treated HIV-infected Ugandans. J Acquir Immune Defic Syndr 65(4):456–462, 2014 24220289

McGinley J, Schofield J, Garthwaite M, et al: Hepatitis C therapy delivered within and by a community addiction service: real life data shows SVR rates >90%. J Hepatol 66 (1 suppl):S512, 2017. Available at: https://www.journal-of-hepatology.eu/article/S0168-8278(17)31426-5/fulltext. Accessed December 22, 2019.

Meijerink H, Indrati A, Utami F, et al: Heroin use is associated with suppressed pro-inflammatory cytokine response after LPS exposure in HIV-infected individuals. PLoS One 10(4):e0122822, 2015 25830312

Modrow S, Falke D, Truyen U, et al: Molecular Virology. New York, Springer, 2013

Norcini Pala A, Steca P, Bagrodia R, et al: Subtypes of depressive symptoms and inflammatory biomarkers: an exploratory study on a sample of HIV-positive patients. Brain Behav Immun 56:105–113, 2016 26883521

O'Cleirigh C, Magidson JF, Skeer MR, et al: Prevalence of psychiatric and substance abuse symptomatology among HIV-infected gay and bisexual men in HIV primary care. Psychosomatics 56(5):470–478, 2015 25656425

Operskalski EA, Kovacs A: HIV/HCV co-infection: pathogenesis, clinical complications, treatment, and new therapeutic technologies. Curr HIV/AIDS Rep 8(1):12–22, 2011 21221855

Pearlman BL, Traub N: Sustained virologic response to antiviral therapy for chronic hepatitis C virus infection: a cure and so much more. Clin Infect Dis 52(7):889–900, 2011 21427396

Pence BW, Mills JC, Bengtson AM, et al: Association of increased chronicity of depression with HIV appointment attendance, treatment failure, and mortality among HIV-infected adults in the United States. JAMA Psychiatry 75(4):379–385, 2018 29466531

Platt L, Easterbrook P, Gower E, et al: Prevalence and burden of HCV co-infection in people living with HIV: a global systematic review and meta-analysis. Lancet Infect Dis 16(7):797–808, 2016 26922272

Remien RH, Exner TM, Morin SF, et al: Medication adherence and sexual risk behavior among HIV-infected adults: implications for transmission of resistant virus. AIDS Behav 11(5):663–675, 2007 17243012

Sant AJ, McMichael A: Revealing the role of CD4(+) T cells in viral immunity. J Exp Med 209(8):1391–1395, 2012 22851641

Shmagel KV, Saidakova EV, Shmagel NG, et al: Systemic inflammation and liver damage in HIV/hepatitis C virus coinfection. HIV Med 17(8):581–589, 2016 27187749

Shuper PA, Joharchi N, Irving H, et al: Differential predictors of ART adherence among HIV-monoinfected versus HIV/HCV-coinfected individuals. AIDS Care 28(8):954–962, 2016 26971360

Slaymaker E, Todd J, Marston M, et al: How have ART treatment programmes changed the patterns of excess mortality in people living with HIV? Estimates from four countries in East and Southern Africa. Glob Health Action 7(1):22789, 2014 24762982

Sood S, Wong D, Holmes A, et al: Depression in a real world population of hepatitis C patients. Journal of Gastroenterology, Pancreatology, and Liver Disorders 1(2):1–3, 2014. Available at: https://symbiosisonlinepublishing.com/gastroenterology-pancreatology-liverdisorders/gastroenterology-pancreatology-liverdisorders09.php. Accessed December 22, 2019.

Sulkowski MS: Viral hepatitis and HIV coinfection. J Hepatol 48(2):353–367, 2008 18155314

Swaminathan G, Pascual D, Rival G, et al: Hepatitis C virus core protein enhances HIV-1 replication in human macrophages through TLR2, JNK, and MEK1/2-dependent upregulation of TNF-alpha and IL-6. FEBS Lett 588(18):3501–3510, 2014 25131930

Torian LV, Felsen UR, Xia Q, et al: Undiagnosed HIV and HCV infection in a New York City emergency department, 2015. Am J Public Health 108(5):652–658, 2018 29565667

Townsend K, Petersen T, Gordon LA, et al: Effect of HIV co-infection on adherence to a 12-week regimen of hepatitis C virus therapy with ledipasvir and sofosbuvir. AIDS 30(2):261–266, 2016 26691547

Turan B, Hatcher AM, Weiser SD, et al: Framing mechanisms linking HIV-related stigma, adherence to treatment, and health outcomes. Am J Public Health 107(6):863–869, 2017 28426316

Vancassel S, Capuron L, Castanon N: Brain kynurenine and BH4 pathways: relevance to the pathophysiology and treatment of inflammation-driven depressive symptoms. Front Neurosci 12:499, 2018 30140200

Viswanathan S, Detels R, Mehta SH, et al: Level of adherence and HIV RNA suppression in the current era of highly active antiretroviral therapy (HAART). AIDS Behav 19(4):601–611, 2015 25342151

Wray TB, Pantalone DW, Kahler CW, et al: The role of discrimination in alcohol-related problems in samples of heavy drinking HIV-negative and positive men who have sex with men (MSM). Drug Alcohol Depend 166:226–234, 2016 27481457

Wyles DL, Kang M, Matining RM, et al: Similar low rates of HCV recurrence in HCV/HIV- and HCV-infected participants who achieved SVR after DAA treatment: interim results from the ACTG A5320 Viral Hepatitis C Infection Long-Term Cohort Study (V-HICS). Open Forum Infect Dis 5(6):ofy103, 2018 29977962

Yaphe S, Bozinoff N, Kyle R, et al: Incidence of acute hepatitis C virus infection among men who have sex with men with and without HIV infection: a systematic review. Sex Transm Infect 88(7):558–564, 2012 22859499

Zunszain PA, Anacker C, Cattaneo A, et al: Glucocorticoids, cytokines and brain abnormalities in depression. Prog Neuropsychopharmacol Biol Psychiatry 35(3):722–729, 2011 20406665

CHAPTER 34

Nicotine and Public Health

K. Michael Cummings, Ph.D., M.P.H.

Ron Borland, Ph.D., FASSA

David Braak, M.D. candidate

Tobacco use is the most prevalent cause of premature morbidity and mortality in the world. Factory-made cigarettes are by far the predominant form of tobacco consumed and the most lethal, responsible for the premature deaths of over half of long-term users. This chapter reviews shifting trends in the tobacco marketplace, the role of nicotine in cigarette addiction, the successes and limitations of traditional public health interventions to reduce smoking, and the potential opportunity to minimize the harms of smoking with the emergence of potentially lower-risk, noncombustible alternative nicotine-delivery products. Since 2000, the evolving marketplace of lower-risk nicotine products in combination with the advent of regulatory authority over tobacco products has provided new opportunities to dramatically transform the cigarette business in ways that were never imagined when the war on tobacco was raging decades ago. However, this opportunity requires embracing risk-proportionate regulation and taxation policies and providing consumers with accurate public messaging on products' relative risks. A regulatory framework based on sound science that encourages and rewards new or existing manufacturers for investing in consumer-acceptable lower-risk products to replace cigarettes offers the potential to complement existing smoking-control measures and interventions.

Tobacco Products, Nicotine, and Health Risks

The nicotine product market is global and rapidly evolving. However, efforts to control the marketplace of nicotine products are typically conducted at the local level so as to be tailored to address the unique set of products and issues that relate to a particular country. In this chapter we briefly discuss the evolving marketplace of nicotine products and then focus on historical and recent efforts to control the harms caused by tobacco products in the United States since the mid-1960s.

Tobacco use is the leading preventable cause of death worldwide (World Health Organization 2017). The tobacco products covered in this chapter fall into two broad groups: those that are smoked (i.e., combusted) and those that are not smoked (i.e., noncombusted or smokeless). The combusted category includes factory-made cigarettes and other products in which the tobacco is burned, such as roll-your-own cigarettes, cigars and cigarillos, pipes, bidis (small, hand-rolled cigarettes made of tobacco and wrapped in a tendu or temburni leaf), and kreteks (cigarettes made with a blend of tobacco and cloves). The noncombusted category of nicotine products includes various forms of oral tobacco (e.g., chewing tobacco, moist and dry snuff) and, more recently, heated tobacco products (e.g., IQOS and Eclipse are in a class of products that heat processed tobacco leaf to create an aerosol, which users inhale into their lungs). Also included in the noncombusted category are tobacco-derived nicotine vaping products, as well as the longer-established smoking cessation products known as nicotine replacement therapies (NRTs).

In 2017, global sales of nicotine-containing products were estimated at $785 billion (Foundation for a Smoke-Free World 2019). Factory-made cigarettes dominated the market, accounting for 89.1% of retail nicotine sales worldwide, followed by other smoked tobacco products (6.7%), oral tobacco (1.6%), nicotine vaping products (1.5%), heated tobacco products (0.8%), and medicinal nicotine products (0.3%) (Foundation for a Smoke-Free World 2019). The United States is the largest vaping market in the world. In 2017, nicotine vaping products accounted for approximately 4% of the nicotine product market in the United States (Foundation for a Smoke-Free World 2019).

In 2017, six companies controlled about 80% of the cigarette market worldwide (Foundation for a Smoke-Free World 2019) (Figure 34–1). The remainder of the market consisted of smaller private and state and semi-state-affiliated companies that typically control the smaller regional markets.

While trends in cigarette sales vary by region of the world, with some regions trending upward and others declining, overall sales have been dropping at an annual rate of about 2% since 2000 (Foundation for a Smoke-Free World 2019). In some countries, this is because cigarettes are being displaced by other categories of nicotine products (Foundation for a Smoke-Free World 2019; Lund et al. 2011; Ramström et al. 2016). For example, in Sweden, snus, a type of smokeless tobacco engineered to minimize toxicants, has displaced cigarettes as the main tobacco product consumed (Ramström et al. 2016). A similar trend is evident in Norway (Lund et al. 2011). Technological innovation, particularly in the nicotine vaping category, is also disrupting cigarette sales in various regions around the world (Sweanor and Yach 2013). In the United States and the United Kingdom, use of nicotine vaping products has increased rapidly over the past decade to the point that vaping products have displaced NRT as the most popular smoking cessation aid used by adult smokers (Beard et al. 2016; Caraballo et al. 2017). The overall impact of vaping products on cigarette sales is hard to determine; however, in the United States, quit ratios, which had been unchanged for decades, have started to inch up, in parallel with the growing availability of nicotine vaping products (Gitchell et al. 2017). (*Quit ratio* refers to the ratio of former smokers to ever smokers, with *ever smokers* defined as those who report having smoked at least 100 cigarettes during their lifetime.) A similar and perhaps even more dramatic

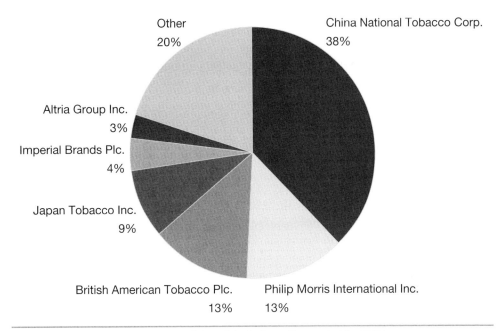

FIGURE 34–1. Company share of the global cigarette market in 2017.

Company volume share of cigarette stick equivalents based on Euromonitor Passport for World by Retail Volume and Value; and Foundation estimates. British American Tobacco pro forma acquisition of Reynolds American. Japan Tobacco pro forma acquisitions of Mighty Corp and Donskoy Tabak.

Source. Reprinted from Chart 1 (Global nicotine ecosystem company volume share in 2017; p. 11) in "Global Trends in Nicotine" by the Foundation for a Smoke-Free World, based on Foundation estimates and data from Euromonitor International, 2018. Available at: https://www.smokefreeworld.org/wp-content/uploads/2019/08/fsfw-report-trends-in-nicotine-1005201811.pdf. Accessed May 11, 2020. Used with permission of the Foundation for a Smoke-Free World and Euromonitor International.

shift in cigarette sales may also be occurring in Japan and other countries following the introduction and wide-scale marketing of heated tobacco products (Gerzog and Kanada 2018; Tabuchi et al. 2016).

Although both combusted and noncombusted tobacco products pose health risks to users, the two categories confer vastly different levels of risk (Abrams et al. 2018; Institute of Medicine 2001; National Center for Chronic Disease Prevention and Health Promotion Office on Smoking and Health 2014). Combusted tobacco products are by far the most dangerous category of tobacco product, with cigarettes being responsible for an estimated 6 million deaths annually worldwide, and for about 520,000 deaths annually in the United States (National Center for Chronic Disease Prevention and Health Promotion Office on Smoking and Health 2014; World Health Organization 2017). The health risks of noncombusted nicotine delivery products are clearly lower than the risks from smoked tobacco (Abrams et al. 2018; Institute of Medicine 2001; McNeill et al. 2018; National Academies of Sciences, Engineering, and Medicine 2018; National Center for Chronic Disease Prevention and Health Promotion Office on Smoking and Health 2014; Rodu and Cole 2004). Sweden has the lowest level of mortality from smoking-related diseases of all countries in the European Union, despite having similar overall rates of tobacco use. Among the Swedish population, especially among men, the primary mode of tobacco use is consumption of snus (a nonfermented type of moist powdered tobacco that is placed under the upper lip) (Ramström et al. 2016; Rodu and Cole 2004). This finding underscores the fact that the type of nicotine tobacco product used will make a difference in terms of disease risks. Although it is too early to know the long-term health risks and/or benefits of nicotine vaping and heated tobacco products, studies show that when used correctly, these products produce lower levels of biomarkers of exposure to toxicants typically found in cigarette smoke; therefore, given the known dose-response effects of smoking-related harms, a large reduction in harm would be expected (McNeill et al. 2018; National Academies of Sciences, Engineering, and Medicine 2018).

The smoke from factory-made cigarettes is especially dangerous, because it is engineered to be mildly acidic, allowing the smoke to be readily inhaled deep into the airways, with less discomfort than the alkaline smoke from burned tobacco in large cigars (U.S. Department of Health and Human Services 2010). With every puff, the burning tobacco produces a complex mixture of more than 9,000 chemicals, including toxins known to cause cancer and inflammation leading to other serious diseases (Rodgman and Perfetti 2016). The negative consequences of smoking are well established; it increases the risks for various types of cancers, especially cancer of the lung, and is a major contributing cause of heart disease, stroke, and chronic obstructive pulmonary disease (National Center for Chronic Disease Prevention and Health Promotion Office on Smoking and Health 2014).

Most of the harm from smoking and other tobacco products is the result of long-term use over years and decades due to nicotine dependence (Abrams et al. 2018; Institute of Medicine 2001; McNeill et al. 2018; National Academies of Sciences, Engineering, and Medicine 2018; National Center for Chronic Disease Prevention and Health Promotion Office on Smoking and Health 2014; Rodu and Cole 2004; U.S. Department of Health and Human Services 2010). Nicotine itself is not especially harmful, but it is the drug in tobacco that causes the neuroadaptive changes in the brain that lead to dependence, which in turn makes it difficult for individuals to stop using tobacco products (Henningfield and Keenan 1993; Orleans and Slade 1993; U.S. Department of Health and Human Services 1988). The mode of nicotine delivery in a tobacco product is strongly associated with the product's abuse liability (Abrams et al. 2018; Henningfield and Keenan 1993; Institute of Medicine 2001; McNeill et al. 2018; National Academies of Sciences, Engineering, and Medicine 2018; National Center for Chronic Disease Prevention and Health Promotion Office on Smoking and Health 2014; Orleans and Slade 1993; Rodu and Cole 2004; U.S. Department of Health and Human Services 1988). Aerosolized nicotine delivered into the large surface area of the lungs permits rapid uptake of nicotine into the bloodstream, allowing it to reach the brain within 10 seconds (Henningfield and Keenan 1993; Orleans and Slade 1993; U.S. Department of Health and Human Services 1988). Smoke and nicotine that are held in the mouth and not inhaled into the airways have lower abuse liability, because the surface area for nicotine absorption is smaller in the mouth than in the lungs. Nicotine absorbed through a patch placed on the skin has an even lower potential for creating nicotine abuse. The more alkaline smoke (i.e., pH above 8.0) of tobacco typically found in large cigars means that the smoke is unpleasant to inhale, preventing lung delivery of the nicotine, thereby lowering the abuse liability of these cigars relative to factory-made cigarettes (Burns 1998; Teague 1973).

The capability to deliver nicotine into the airways, along with other smoke toxicants, is what makes cigarettes so highly addictive and dangerous (Abrams et al.

2018; Institute of Medicine 2001; McNeill et al. 2018; National Academies of Sciences, Engineering, and Medicine 2018; National Center for Chronic Disease Prevention and Health Promotion Office on Smoking and Health 2014; Rodu and Cole 2004; U.S. Department of Health and Human Services 2010). In the average smoker, the nicotine in the blood acts upon the central nervous system, producing an instantaneous sensation that can be described as both stimulating and relaxing (Henningfield and Keenan 1993; Orleans and Slade 1993; Senkus 1976; U.S. Department of Health and Human Services 1988). However, the effects of nicotine are relatively short-lived, with nicotine blood levels dropping soon after the smoker has finished a cigarette (Henningfield and Keenan 1993; Orleans and Slade 1993; U.S. Department of Health and Human Services 1988). Within 15–30 minutes after finishing a cigarette, a smoker who has developed a tolerance for nicotine will often experience mild symptoms of nicotine withdrawal (e.g., nervousness, anxiety, fatigue) and a craving for another cigarette (Henningfield and Keenan 1993; Orleans and Slade 1993; U.S. Department of Health and Human Services 1988).

Determinants of Tobacco Use

There is little doubt today that the nicotine in tobacco is the primary reason why most smokers continue to expose themselves to known toxins in smoke on a daily basis (Abrams et al. 2018; Henningfield and Keenan 1993; National Center for Chronic Disease Prevention and Health Promotion Office on Smoking and Health 2014; Orleans and Slade 1993; Senkus 1976; U.S. Department of Health and Human Services 1988, 2010). Most smokers begin smoking during their teenage years and struggle to quit as adults (National Center for Chronic Disease Prevention and Health Promotion Office on Smoking and Health 2014). Response to nicotine is also likely genetically influenced, with some individuals being predisposed to become dependent if exposed to nicotine and others being apparently immune to the addictive effects of nicotine (Liu et al. 2019; National Cancer Institute 2009; Senkus 1976). Some nicotine users clearly benefit from the self-medicating effects of nicotine, such as alleviation of stress, anxiety, depression, and symptoms of other mental disorders (e.g., schizophrenia), which likely explains the higher rates of smoking in individuals with these conditions (Niaura 2016).

Researchers have found that the strength of an individual's nicotine dependence is a key predictor of how likely that individual is to relapse after discontinuing use of a tobacco product (Borland et al. 2010; Strong et al. 2015). A simple way to screen for nicotine dependence is to ask the patient whether he or she uses a nicotine-containing product every day or on some days (Strong et al. 2015). Virtually all persistent daily smokers are nicotine dependent to some degree; however, level of dependence is best assessed by asking smokers 1) how many cigarettes they smoke daily and 2) at what time they smoke their first cigarette each day, as both of these questions assess individual variation in the pharmacokinetics of nicotine (Borland et al. 2010; Strong et al. 2015).

In 2017, the prevalence of smoking was estimated to be 13.9% among U.S. adults ages 18 years and older (National Center for Health Statistics 2018). By contrast, in 1965, 42% of U.S. adults were current smokers (Cummings and Proctor 2014). However, in 1965, concurrent use of different types of nicotine-containing tobacco products was less common than it is today. A U.S. national survey conducted in 2013 and 2014 found that approximately 28% of adults were current users of at least one type of tobacco product, and that among tobacco product users, about 38% reported using multiple products concurrently (Kasza et al. 2017).

The social environment plays an important moderating role in determining how innate biological factors involved in nicotine dependence actually get expressed at the population level (Cummings and Proctor 2014; Cummings et al. 2009). In other words, having a genetic predisposition conferring susceptibility to nicotine dependence does not automatically guarantee that an individual will become a smoker or be unable to stop smoking. The environment in which one lives can be an important influence as to whether tobacco use is taken up and continued. The importance of the social environment in influencing trends in tobacco use behaviors is illustrated in a study that monitored the smoking habits of 12,067 individuals over a 30-year period as part of the Framingham Heart Study (Christakis and Fowler 2008). In this study, trends in smoking behavior were strongly linked to an individual's social ties. Smokers whose social networks included an increasing share of nonsmokers or former smokers were much more likely to stop smoking over time, whereas smokers whose social ties were mainly to other smokers continued to smoke. Socioeconomic status, gender, and religious beliefs also are strongly linked to tobacco use in some parts of the world (Cummings et al. 2009). For example, the state of Utah, which has a large concentration of Mormons, has the lowest rates of smoking in the United States (Cummings et al. 2009). Finally, how smoking is portrayed in the mass media can have an influence on how smoking is perceived and used (National Cancer Institute 2008).

Public Health Interventions to Reduce Cigarette Smoking

The solution to the cigarette smoking problem lies in changing the smoking behaviors of individuals, changing the social contexts that affect incentives for smoking, and changing the behavior of the cigarette industry to prevent it from acting in ways that counter the goals of public health in terms of both the types of products developed and sold and the ways that such products are promoted (Cummings et al. 2009).

Public health interventions that have the greatest chance of reducing smoking in the population are those that reach the most smokers (International Agency for Research on Cancer 2008). Highly efficacious interventions that reach only a tiny fraction of the target population will not have a sizable impact on rates of smoking in the population at large. This is one of the reasons that past research has shown that the most potent demand-reducing influences on smoking have been interventions that impact virtually all smokers repeatedly, such as higher taxes on tobacco products, comprehensive bans on advertising, mandated pack warnings, mass media campaigns, and smoke-free policies (Institute of Medicine 2007; International Agency for Research on Cancer 2008; National Cancer Institute 2008; U.S. Department of Health and Human Services 1989). Similarly, despite ample evidence supporting the efficacy of different smoking cessation treatments, there is not much evidence to support the idea that any of these therapies have dramatically influenced rates of smoking in the population at large, because too few smokers use them when they try to quit (Jamal et al. 2016).

Public health interventions to reduce smoking can be grouped into three broad categories, according to their primary objectives (Figure 34–2): 1) interventions intended to directly influence smokers and potential smokers by increasing public awareness of the health risks of smoking via mass media campaigns and product warnings, and by providing direct support (in the form of stop-smoking services and aids) to promote behavioral change; 2) interventions affecting when and where people can use tobacco products (i.e., smoke-free laws); and 3) interventions targeting the tobacco product marketplace, including efforts aimed at controlling pricing, placement (i.e., where and how tobacco can be accessed), promotion (i.e., advertisement and marketing constraints), and product types (i.e., rules about what kinds of products can be sold).

The challenge is to apply rigorous science to ensure that the most appropriate and effective mix of strategies for controlling tobacco use are adopted and effectively implemented. In the following section, we summarize evidence regarding the effectiveness of public health intervention approaches as applied to cigarette smoking.

Interventions Intended to Directly Influence Smokers

Consumer Education

Consumer education about the health risks of smoking has been an important focus of public health efforts to reduce smoking (Institute of Medicine 2007; International Agency for Research on Cancer 2008; National Cancer Institute 2008; U.S. Department of Health and Human Services 1989). Public health efforts to discourage cigarette use accelerated in the mid-1960s, coinciding with the release of the 1964 report of the Surgeon General's Advisory Committee (Cummings and Proctor 2014). In 1966, the first cautionary label appeared on cigarette packs, stating that cigarette smoking "may be hazardous to your health" (U.S. Department of Health and Human Services 1989). The warnings were updated in 1970 and again in 1985, although the effectiveness of these warnings has been the subject of much scientific debate (U.S. Department of Health and Human Services 1989). Warnings on packs provide repeated reminders about the harms of smoking. Research indicates that warning labels on cigarette packs can be a salient means of communicating with smokers, although their effectiveness depends on their size and comprehensiveness (Fong et al. 2009).

Research indicates that anti-tobacco mass media campaigns, when adequately funded, can be effective in reducing cigarette consumption (National Cancer Institute 2008). The first large-scale national counter-advertising campaign to educate the U.S. public about the health risks of tobacco use occurred between 1967 and 1970, when the Federal Communications Commission mandated that licensees who broadcast cigarette commercials provide free media time for anti-smoking public service announcements under the fairness doctrine (National Cancer Institute 2008; U.S. Department of Health and Human Services 1989). Subsequently, studies in several states and other countries confirmed that adequately resourced mass media campaigns aimed at educating the public about the risks of smoking could lead to reductions in cigarette consumption (National Cancer Institute 2008). Educational interventions in

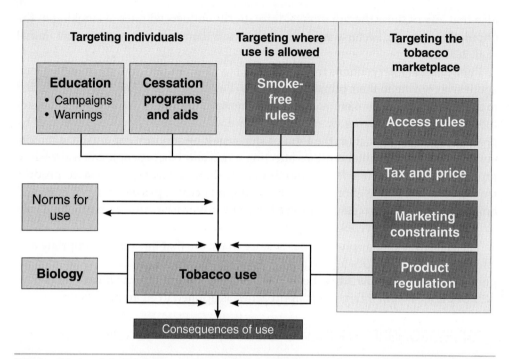

FIGURE 34–2.   Primary influences on tobacco use, as targeted by public health interventions.

The figure shows the main modes of action for tobacco control. Most strategies target tobacco use, but product regulation, by altering the harm profile of the product, can also impact on the level of harm generated by any given level of use.

schools also improve knowledge about the risks of smoking, although these interventions have limited effectiveness in discouraging smoking uptake (Pierce et al. 2010).

Consumer education efforts have changed public perceptions regarding smoking and health in the United States. A 1966 poll found that only 40% of Americans recognized smoking as a major cause of lung cancer. In 2001, this same question ("Would you say that cigarette smoking is definitely, probably, probably not, or definitely not a major source of lung cancer, or that you don't have an opinion either way?") was asked in a Gallup Poll, and this time, 71% of Americans said that smoking was a major cause of lung cancer (Cummings and Proctor 2014). Today, most smokers concede that smoking poses serious risks to health; however, recognition of the relative health risks of different tobacco products remains incomplete and confused (Kozlowski and Abrams 2016). Additionally, there are still many misconceptions; for example, many smokers believe that noncombustible tobacco products, such as smokeless tobacco and nicotine vaping products, pose the same health risks as cigarette smoking, contrary to scientific evidence (Fong et al. 2019).

Cessation Assistance

Although less-dependent smokers can often quit unassisted, more-dependent smokers typically require help to achieve abstinence from smoking. Comprehensive reviews of the efficacy of different smoking cessation treatments indicate that provision of both pharmacotherapy and counseling support for all quit attempts helps to optimize rates of cessation (Abrams and Niaura 2003; Aubin et al. 2014; Clinical Practice Guideline Treating Tobacco Use and Dependence 2008 Update Panel, Liaisons, and Staff 2008). The most effective pharmacotherapies are varenicline and a combination of NRT products, typically patches accompanied by an oral product for dealing with situational temptations (Aubin et al. 2014). Cognitive-behavioral treatments delivered individually or in groups of smokers (either by phone or using a range of automated and semiautomated personalized advice programs) can also be effective for helping smokers quit (Abrams and Niaura 2003). Combining the use of optimal pharmacotherapy with cognitive-behavioral treatment has been shown to yield the best outcomes (Clinical Practice Guideline Treating Tobacco Use and Dependence 2008 Update Panel, Liaisons, and Staff 2008). However, even with optimized treatments, quitting success is boosted only 1.5- to 3-fold over what is already a low baseline for sustained quitting success (Abrams and Niaura 2003; Aubin et al. 2014; Clinical Practice Guideline Treating Tobacco Use and Dependence 2008 Update Panel, Liaisons, and Staff 2008). Thus, whereas some progress has been made in prompting smokers to use evidence-based nicotine dependence treatments in their quit attempts, there is still a lot of room for improvement. In 1986, the vast majority (>90%) of quit attempts were made without any form of outside assistance (i.e., cold turkey); today, that percentage has been reduced to about 60% (Fiore et al. 1990; Jamal et al. 2016). However, there are wide disparities in who gets access to evidence-based stop-smoking treatments based on income and insurance status (Caraballo et al. 2017; Jamal et al. 2016).

Interventions Affecting When and Where People Can Use Tobacco Products

Until the early 1980s, smoking was permitted nearly everywhere (Cummings and Proctor 2014). Today, smokers are largely prevented (and in many states, completely prevented) from smoking in enclosed public spaces and workplaces, and increasingly also in shared public outdoor settings.

These laws have been successful in protecting nonsmokers, as they are generally highly complied with and now accepted by smokers (International Agency for Research on Cancer 2008). They have also helped to redefine the social context for smoking, making it less acceptable and less convenient, thus contributing to the general denormalization of smoking (Cummings and Proctor 2014; Cummings et al. 2009; International Agency for Research on Cancer 2008). Smoke-free policies can increase motivation to quit, may help to discourage uptake of smoking, and may help those who have quit to stay smoke-free (International Agency for Research on Cancer 2008).

Interventions Targeting the Tobacco Product Marketplace

Efforts to intervene in the tobacco market directly can be organized around the four P's of marketing: price, promotion, place, and product (International Agency for Research on Cancer 2008).

Price

Price controls include a range of policies affecting the structure of the tobacco product market by impacting the costs of producing and marketing tobacco products. Interventions that alter incentives to smoke can have a powerful impact on smoking rates. It is well recognized in economic theory, as well as in everyday life, that incentives can influence behavior. Thus, policies that make cigarettes more costly to purchase should discourage smoking. The main way those outside the tobacco industry can influence price is via taxes on tobacco products. Considerable economic research over the past three decades has demonstrated that increasing cigarette prices is associated with lower rates of cigarette consumption (International Agency for Research on Cancer 2008). Cigarette tax increases have been shown to promote quit attempts, prevent nonsmokers (especially youth) from becoming smokers, keep former smokers from relapsing back to smoking, and reduce the amount consumed by continuing smokers (International Agency for Research on Cancer 2008). Taxes are not the only way to influence the price of tobacco products. Anything that affects the costs of manufacturing and marketing cigarettes will contribute to cigarette prices. For example, policies that affect marketing of tobacco products, such as rules dictating minimum package size, banning product sampling, or restricting use of coupons and price promotion, can affect the price the consumer pays for cigarettes. Additionally, product regulation and litigation are business expenses that add to the cost of cigarettes and typically get passed along to smokers in the price they pay for a pack of cigarettes. Differential tax and regulatory policies for different types of tobacco products are one way to influence demand for different types of products (i.e., higher taxes on combustible tobacco versus noncombustible tobacco products) (Chaloupka et al. 2015).

Promotional Controls

Promotional controls on the marketing of cigarettes in the United States date back to 1971, when broadcast (i.e., radio and television) advertising of cigarettes was prohibited (U.S. Department of Health and Human Services 1989). The 1998 Master Settlement Agreement further limited the placement of advertising on billboards and in youth-oriented magazines (National Cancer Institute 2008). The Family Smoking Prevention and Tobacco Control Act (referred to as the Tobacco Control Act), signed into law on June 22, 2009, gave the U.S. Food and Drug Administration (FDA) the authority to control the marketing of tobacco products by prohibiting distribution of free product samples, sales to minors (i.e., <18 years of age), and product claims (U.S. Food and Drug Administration 2009). Research has shown that cigarette packaging serves as a vital channel for product communications (International Agency for Research on Cancer 2008). The Tobacco Control Act gave the FDA the authority to regulate tobacco product warnings and to set rules related to the placement and appearance of warnings to ensure that consumers are not misled (U.S. Food and Drug Administration 2009). In 2010, the FDA banned the use of terms such as "low tar," "light," "ultralight," and "mild" on cigarette packages and in advertising because of evidence suggesting that many smokers perceived these terms to mean that the cigarettes were less dangerous compared with other cigarettes, when in fact there was no strong scientific evidence to support such an interpretation (Yong et al. 2011). In 2017, the FDA negotiated an agreement with R.J. Reynolds (now owned by British American Tobacco [BAT]) to eliminate the use of descriptors such as "natural" and "100% additive-free" on packaging and in advertising for Natural American Spirit (NAS) cigarettes, because research found that many consumers were misled into believing that the NAS cigarettes were less dangerous to smoke compared with other brands of cigarettes (Neuhauser and Simoneau 2017). Although the effects of these restrictions are difficult to quantify, research shows that comprehensive restrictions on cigarette promotions do exert downward pressure on consumption (International Agency for Research on Cancer 2008). Industry documents reveal a strategic interest in placing marketing advertisements in locations where young people congregate (Cummings et al. 2002).

Place Controls

Place controls are policies that reduce the availability of tobacco products by limiting the number and/or types of retail outlets where products can be sold and by restricting whom they can be sold to—for example, banning sales to young people and requiring that buyers show proof of age (International Agency for Research on Cancer 2008; U.S. Department of Health and Human Services 1989). Bans on cigarette vending machines (except in adult-only venues) also target youth access (National Cancer Institute 2008; U.S. Food and Drug Administration 2009). In some countries (e.g., France), tobacco products can be sold only through licensed tobacconists (International Agency for Research on Cancer 2008). In the United States, some pharmacy chains have adopted policies of not selling tobacco, but there are few additional constraints on the types of locations where tobacco products can be sold, making tobacco one of the most accessible products for consumers. The 2009 Tobacco Control Act prohibited the distribution of free product samples, but otherwise the distribution of tobacco products remained largely under state and local jurisdictional control (U.S. Food and Drug Administration 2009).

Product Controls

Product controls include rules about what types of products can be sold (e.g., some jurisdictions have banned the sale of flavored tobacco products), disclosure of information about products, requirements for testing products, and mandated performance standards for products (International Agency for Research on Cancer 2008; U.S. Food and Drug Administration 2009). This is an area where there is likely to be more activity in the future, as is discussed later in this chapter (see section "What Does the Future Hold?").

The Status of Tobacco Control in the United States

Current estimates suggest that there were about 63 million former smokers in the United States in 2017, which was nearly twice the number of current cigarette smokers in the U.S. adult population (i.e., 36.5 million, of whom 83% were daily smokers [Kasza et al. 2017]). Population trends in adult smoking cessation rates can be tracked by comparing annual quit ratios (i.e., the proportion of former smokers among ever smokers) from the U.S. National Health Interview Survey (NHIS). As shown in Figure 34–3, NHIS quit ratios increased steadily between 1965 and the late 1980s, and then leveled off and remained relatively flat until around 2010, at which time they started to increase again.

The period from 1990 to 2010 encompassed a time when interventions to promote smoking cessation were ramped up in the United States (International Tobacco Control Project 2014). For example, several new smoking cessation treatments were in-

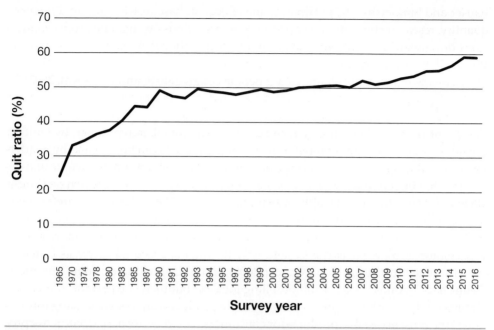

FIGURE 34–3. Trends in quit ratios: National Health Interview Survey (NHIS), 1965–2016.

Line graph showing quit ratios (i.e., percentage of ever smokers[a] who quit smoking) among NHIS respondents ages 18 years or older for each survey year during the period 1965–2016. In the United States beginning in 1965, quit ratio trends increased steadily up until 1990; then plateaued, with virtually no change between 1990 and 2010; and then began to increase again in 2010, corresponding to the time period when e-cigarettes started to become popular.

[a]Ever smokers=individuals who reported having smoked at least 100 cigarettes during their lifetime.

Source.   National Health Interview Survey, National Center for Health Statistics, public use data, 1965–2016; provided by the National Center for Chronic Disease Prevention and Health Promotion, Office on Smoking and Health, October 19, 2018.

troduced during this period, such as nicotine patches (1991), prescription inhalers (1996), nasal spray (1994), sublingual tablets (1999), lozenges (2002), and the non-nicotine prescription medications bupropion SR (i.e., Zyban, 1998) and varenicline (i.e., Chantix, 2006) (Clinical Practice Guideline Treating Tobacco Use and Dependence 2008 Update Panel, Liaisons, and Staff 2008). In 1996, the FDA approved the switch of nicotine gum and the nicotine patch from prescription to over-the-counter status in an effort to increase smokers' access to smoking cessation aids (Clinical Practice Guideline Treating Tobacco Use and Dependence 2008 Update Panel, Liaisons, and Staff 2008). Smoking cessation treatment guidelines were also issued around this time (1998 and 2008) and were widely disseminated, and a national network of state-run telephone-based quit lines was established and widely promoted (Clinical Practice Guideline Treating Tobacco Use and Dependence 2008 Update Panel, Liaisons, and Staff 2008). In addition, the period from 1990 to 2010 also encompassed a time during which cigarette prices increased dramatically, smoke-free polices became widely adopted, and anti-smoking mass media campaigns were implemented (Institute of Medicine 2007; International Tobacco Control Project 2014; National Cancer Institute 2008). However, despite these interventions, quit ratios remained largely unchanged from 1990 to 2010, suggesting that these sets of interventions had little impact on helping smokers to quit.

The relatively dismal population trends in quit ratios, coupled with evidence from cohort studies tracking rates of smoking cessation, reinforces the importance of nicotine dependence as a barrier to sustained quitting, especially for daily smokers (Henningfield and Keenan 1993; Orleans and Slade 1993; U.S. Department of Health and Human Services 1988, 2010). By the end of the 1980s, it is likely that most of those for whom quitting was easy would have quit, leaving a more dependent group. On any given quit attempt, fewer than 10% of attempters succeed in remaining smoke-free for more than 6 months; these rates are even lower when restricted to persistent daily smokers who exhibit high levels of nicotine dependence (Jamal et al. 2016; U.S. Department of Health and Human Services 1988). The apparent increase in quit rates during this decade may be due to greater mass education and to the emergence of alternative nicotine products that appeal to consumers.

Public health interventions aimed at curbing cigarette consumption in the United States have been fairly successful in preventing youth from taking up smoking, protecting nonsmokers from exposure to secondhand smoke, and motivating smokers to quit, but they have been less successful in facilitating the ability of daily smokers to actually sustain quitting (National Center for Chronic Disease Prevention and Health Promotion Office on Smoking and Health 2014). Despite impressive reductions in smoking prevalence rates over the last half-century, there still remains a large number of adult daily smokers (i.e., over 30 million) whose preventable deaths from smoking are unlikely to be averted unless public health interventions to control smoking are modified in ways that help smokers to refrain from smoking (Jeon et al. 2018; National Center for Chronic Disease Prevention and Health Promotion Office on Smoking and Health 2014).

Current treatments for nicotine dependence have limited efficacy, and while there are some novel treatment approaches under investigation, it is impossible to predict when and if such treatments will be available (Gómez-Coronado et al. 2018). Most smokers are motivated to quit and are looking for options to help them stop smoking (Sweanor and Yach 2013). Population surveys show that more than 90% of smokers regret their decision to start smoking; in addition, 70% say that they would like to stop, and more than half of adult smokers make at least one quit attempt (lasting 1 day or longer) each year (Fong et al. 2004; Jamal et al. 2016). It should also be noted that estimates of quitting activity by smokers are likely to be grossly underestimated in surveys, since the vast majority of quit attempts are of short duration (i.e., ≤1 day), and short-duration quit attempts are often not recalled by smokers when asked about quitting efforts over the previous year (Borland et al. 2012).

What Does the Future Hold?

The two big changes that are likely to shape tobacco use most in the coming years are the emergence of new nicotine-delivering products and the new FDA comprehensive plan for regulating tobacco and nicotine. Signed into law on June 22, 2009, the Family Smoking Prevention and Tobacco Control Act gave the FDA the authority to regulate the design, production, marketing, and advertising of tobacco products (U.S. Food and Drug Administration 2009). The Tobacco Control Act originally applied only to cigarettes, roll-your-own cigarettes, and smokeless tobacco, but in August 2016 it was extended to include other tobacco products (i.e., cigars, other smoked tobacco, nicotine vaping products). The Tobacco Control Act requires manufacturers to register and disclose ingredients used in the manufacturing of tobacco products and requires manufacturers to notify and seek approval from the FDA for any changes in product design (U.S. Food and Drug Administration 2009). The Tobacco Control Act also requires the FDA to establish product performance standards intended to protect the public's health (U.S. Food and Drug Administration 2009).

In 2017, the FDA commissioner announced a new national comprehensive nicotine management strategy (Gottlieb and Zeller 2017) that included two main parts: 1) reducing the abuse liability of combustible tobacco products by establishing a very-low-threshold nicotine standard and 2) increasing the availability of potentially less harmful nicotine-delivery products (i.e., both tobacco and medicinal nicotine products).

The low average success rates for quitting smoking are the result of how cigarettes are engineered in ways to make them hard to stop using (U.S. Department of Health and Human Services 2010). As one cigarette company acknowledged, "We cannot ever be comfortable selling a product which most of our customers would stop using if they could.... If the exit gate from our market should suddenly open, we could be out of business almost overnight" (Teague 1982, p. 2). This same document also noted that "most of those who have smoked for any significant time would like to stop smoking" (Teague 1982, p. 1). The feasibility of reducing and controlling the nicotine levels in cigarettes has existed for decades, as demonstrated in the business records from different cigarette manufacturers shown in Table 34–1.

Scientific studies comparing test cigarettes with different amounts of nicotine in the tobacco rod have found that smokers who were switched to cigarettes with lower nicotine levels (e.g., 0.3, 0.4, and 0.5 mg nicotine per gram of tobacco filler) reported smoking fewer cigarettes, getting less satisfaction from the cigarettes smoked, and having overall lower desire for cigarettes in comparison with smokers who were given cigarettes with nicotine levels greater than 0.5 mg nicotine per gram of filler (U.S. Food and Drug Administration 2018).

In the past, cigarette companies were able to secretly manipulate other elements of cigarette design so as to ensure that smokers would get sufficient amounts of nicotine from the cigarettes despite low machine-measured nicotine levels (National Cancer Institute 2001). However, the Tobacco Control Act explicitly restricted the ability of manufacturers to manipulate other elements of product design that could potentially negate the impact of a low-nicotine standard (U.S. Food and Drug Administration 2009).

Thus, establishing a very-low-nicotine product standard should make it easier for smokers who wish to stop smoking to do so, and will make it less likely that nonsmokers who experiment with smoking will go on to become daily smokers. One recent study estimated that in the first year of a low-nicotine-policy standard, 20% of adult smokers in the United States would stop smoking as a result of the policy (Apelberg et al. 2018).

Rapidly evolving technologies in the development of lower-risk nicotine delivery products have the potential to transform the combustion tobacco sector (Abrams et al. 2018; Foundation for a Smoke-Free World 2019; Gerzog and Kanada 2018; Sweanor and Yach 2013; Tabuchi et al. 2016). The demand for noncombustible nicotine delivery products in the United States is evident from the rapid growth of the noncombustible

TABLE 34–1. **The role of nicotine in cigarette design: evidence from corporate documents**

Date	Source	Quote[a]
December 9, 1935	American Tobacco Company (1935)	It is quite possible to "de-nicotinize" a cigarette by chemical and thermal methods. (www.industrydocumentslibrary.ucsf.edu/tobacco/docs/sxwv0024)
November 2, 1959	R.J. Reynolds (Rodgman 1959)	The physiological requirements of the smoker with respect to nicotine can be met by the application of the optimum amount of nicotine to the extracted tobacco. (www.industrydocumentslibrary.ucsf.edu/tobacco/docs/fxkp0034)
July 17, 1963	Brown & Williamson (Yeaman 1963)	Moreover, nicotine is addictive. We are, then, in the business of selling nicotine, an addictive drug effective in the release of stress mechanisms. (www.industrydocumentslibrary.ucsf.edu/tobacco/docs/rhxp0042)
September 18, 1963	Brown & Williamson (Brown & Williamson Tobacco Corp. and Griffith 1963)	It may be well to remind you, however, that we have a research program in progress to obtain, by genetic means, any level of nicotine desired. (www.industrydocumentslibrary.ucsf.edu/tobacco/docs/jglw0200)
February 1, 1965	Phillip Morris (Tamol 1965)	Determine minimum nicotine required to keep human smoker "hooked." (www.industrydocumentslibrary.ucsf.edu/tobacco/docs/qynn0226)
May 24, 1971	R.J. Reynolds (Laurene 1971)	Habituating level of nicotine (how low can we go?) (www.industrydocumentslibrary.ucsf.edu/tobacco/docs/tjvk0191)
April 14, 1972	R.J. Reynolds (Teague 1972)	Research activities need to more precisely define the minimum amount of nicotine required for "satisfaction" in terms of dose levels, dose frequency, dosage form and the like. (www.industrydocumentslibrary.ucsf.edu/tobacco/docs/stdb0184)
July 22, 1977	Lorillard (Schultz 1977)	The level of nicotine in the smoke required to produce the desired results is an unknown factor, however, we have estimated it to be in the neighborhood of 0.4–0.5 mg per cigarette. (www.industrydocumentslibrary.ucsf.edu/tobacco/docs/gxbv0035)

TABLE 34–1. **The role of nicotine in cigarette design: evidence from corporate documents** *(continued)*

Date	Source	Quote[a]
June 30, 1978	Phillip Morris (Gullotta et al. 1978)	For quite some time we have been interested in finding out how smokers would react to cigarettes with normal levels of tar and very low levels of nicotine.... The tobacco used to make these cigarettes was treated for 25 min. with steam and ammonia to reduce the total alkaloids from 1.56% to 0.07%. (www.industrydocumentslibrary.ucsf.edu/tobacco/docs/srdv0184)
February 13, 1980	Lorillard (Smith 1980)	Determine the minimum level of nicotine that will allow continued smoking. (www.industrydocumentslibrary.ucsf.edu/tobacco/docs/kpmv0035)
January 18, 1982	Phillip Morris (Gullotta and Schultz 1982)	[A] threshold [for nicotine effects] exists somewhere between 0.1 and 0.3 mg of nicotine. (www.industrydocumentslibrary.ucsf.edu/tobacco/docs/tnbx0108)

[a]Links to source documents come from the University of California San Francisco Library's Truth Tobacco Industry Documents collection.

tobacco market segment, especially nicotine vaping products, since 2010 (Foundation for a Smoke-Free World 2019). Quit ratios, which had been flat for nearly two decades between 1990 and 2010, began to increase after 2010, coinciding with the growing popularity of electronic cigarettes (see Figure 34–3). One study estimated that if all adult smokers in the United States who were unable to quit combustible cigarettes were to switch to electronic cigarettes, more than 6.6 million deaths could be averted, and 87 million years of life lost would then be avoided (Levy et al. 2017).

The growing popularity of nicotine vaping products among adult smokers and the emerging evidence of their effectiveness for smoking cessation have spurred investor interest, increased product innovation, and, most importantly, generated competition among companies vying for a share of the nicotine market (Foundation for a Smoke-Free World 2019; Hajek et al. 2019). The three major cigarette companies in the United States (i.e., Philip Morris USA, BAT, and Imperial Brands PLC), which for decades have monopolized the nicotine product marketplace, are for the first time being challenged for market share (Foundation for a Smoke-Free World 2019). Cigarette manufacturers have responded to this threat by introducing their own nicotine vaping products. However, in comparison with the cigarette business, the nicotine vaping product sector is more diverse and is largely independent of cigarette manufacturers (Foundation for a Smoke-Free World 2019). Nonetheless, efforts to transform the cigarette business will remain unrealized without public health interventions to encourage smokers to switch away from combustible tobacco products (Gottlieb and Zeller 2017).

A regulatory approach based on a "continuum of risk" philosophy that supports product innovations by incentivizing the development and marketing of lower-risk nicotine-containing products holds promise for reducing the harm caused by smoking and use of other combustible tobacco products (Abrams et al. 2018; Gottlieb and Zeller 2017). Nicotine, although not benign, is not directly responsible for the cancers caused by tobacco and the lung and heart disease that kill almost half a million Americans each year (Abrams et al. 2018; Niaura 2016; Sweanor and Yach 2013). In summary, embracing risk-proportionate tobacco product regulation and taxation policies and providing consumers with accurate public messaging on products' relative risks offers the potential for public health to dramatically transform the cigarette business in ways that could save millions of lives in the coming decades.

References

Abrams DB, Niaura R: The Tobacco Dependence Treatment Handbook: A Guide to Best Practices. New York, Guilford, 2003

Abrams DB, Glasser AM, Villanti AC, et al: Managing nicotine without smoke to save lives now: evidence for harm minimization. Prev Med 117:88–97, 2018 29944902

American Tobacco Company: Improving the Taste and Character of Cigarette Tobacco With a View to Removing Irritants and Producing a Light Smoke. A Chapter in Laboratory Research. December 9, 1935. Available at: https://www.industrydocuments.ucsf.edu/docs/#id=sxwv0024. Accessed December 20, 2019.

Apelberg BJ, Feirman SP, Salazar E, et al: Potential public health effects of reducing nicotine levels in cigarettes in the United States. N Engl J Med 378(18):1725–1733, 2018 29543114

Aubin HJ, Luquiens A, Berlin I: Pharmacotherapy for smoking cessation: pharmacological principles and clinical practice. Br J Clin Pharmacol 77(2):324–336, 2014 23488726

Beard E, West R, Michie S, Brown J: Association between electronic cigarette use and changes in quit attempts, success of quit attempts, use of smoking cessation pharmacotherapy, and use of stop smoking services in England: time series analysis of population trends. BMJ 354:i4645, 2016 27624188

Borland R, Yong H-H, O'Connor RJ, et al: The reliability and predictive validity of the Heaviness of Smoking Index and its two components: findings from the International Tobacco Control Four Country study. Nicotine Tob Res 12 (suppl):S45–S50, 2010 20889480

Borland R, Partos TR, Yong HH, et al: How much unsuccessful quitting activity is going on among adult smokers? Data from the International Tobacco Control Four Country cohort survey. Addiction 107(3):673–682, 2012 21992709

Brown & Williamson Tobacco Corporation; Griffith RB: Letter From RB Griffith to John Kirwan Regarding Neil Gilliam's Presentation at Chelwood. September 18, 1963. Available at: https://www.industrydocuments.ucsf.edu/docs/#id=jglw0200. Accessed December 20, 2019.

Burns DM: Cigar Smoking: Overview and Current State of the Science. Smoking and Tobacco Control Monograph No. 9. U.S. Department of Health and Human Services, National Institutes of Health, National Cancer Institute, 1998. Available at: https://cancercontrol.cancer.gov/brp/tcrb/monographs/9/m9_1.pdf. Accessed December 20, 2019.

Caraballo RS, Shafer PR, Patel D, et al: Quit methods used by US adult cigarette smokers, 2014–2016. Prev Chronic Dis 14:E32, 2017 28409740

Chaloupka FJ, Sweanor D, Warner KE: Differential taxes for differential risks—toward reduced harm from nicotine-yielding products. N Engl J Med 373(7):594–597, 2015 26267620

Christakis NA, Fowler JH: The collective dynamics of smoking in a large social network. N Engl J Med 358(21):2249–2258, 2008 18499567

Clinical Practice Guideline Treating Tobacco Use and Dependence 2008 Update Panel, Liaisons, and Staff: A clinical practice guideline for treating tobacco use and dependence: 2008 update. A U.S. Public Health Service report. Am J Prev Med 35(2):158–176, 2008 18617085

Cummings KM, Proctor RN: The changing public image of smoking in the United States: 1964–2014. Cancer Epidemiol Biomarkers Prev 23(1):32–36, 2014 24420984

Cummings KM, Morley CP, Horan JK, et al: Marketing to America's youth: evidence from corporate documents. Tob Control 11 (suppl 1):I5–I17, 2002 11893810

Cummings KM, Fong GT, Borland R: Environmental influences on tobacco use: evidence from societal and community influences on tobacco use and dependence. Annu Rev Clin Psychol 5:433–458, 2009 19327036

Fiore MC, Novotny TE, Pierce JP, et al: Methods used to quit smoking in the United States. Do cessation programs help? JAMA 263(20):2760–2765, 1990 2271019

Fong GT, Hammond D, Laux FL, et al: The near-universal experience of regret among smokers in four countries: findings from the International Tobacco Control Policy Evaluation Survey. Nicotine Tob Res 6 (suppl 3):S341–S351, 2004 15799597

Fong GT, Hammond D, Hitchman SC: The impact of pictures on the effectiveness of tobacco warnings. Bull World Health Organ 87(8):640–643, 2009 19705020

Fong GT, Elton-Marshall T, Driezen P, et al: U.S. adult perceptions of the harmfulness of tobacco products: descriptive findings from the 2013–14 baseline wave 1 of the path study. Addict Behav 91:180–187, 2019 30502927

Foundation for a Smoke-Free World: Global Trends in Nicotine. 2019. Available at: https://www.smokefreeworld.org/advancing-industry-transformation/global-trends-nicotine. Accessed November 11, 2019.

Gerzog B, Kanada P: Takeaways from Philip Morris International Inc's 2018 Investor Day. Wells Fargo Equity Research, October 1, 2018

Gitchell JG, Shiffman S, Sembower MA: Trends in serious quit attempts in the United States, 2009–14. Addiction 112(5):897–900, 2017 27933678

Gómez-Coronado N, Walker AJ, Berk M, et al: Current and emerging pharmacotherapies for cessation of tobacco smoking. Pharmacotherapy 38(2):235–258, 2018 29250815

Gottlieb S, Zeller M: A nicotine-focused framework for public health. N Engl J Med 377(12):1111–1114, 2017 28813211

Gullotta FP, Schultz CJ: Repetitive Smoking and the Pattern Reversal Evoked Potential. January 18, 1982. Available at: https://www.industrydocuments.ucsf.edu/docs/#id=tnbx0108. Accessed December 20, 2019.

Gullotta FP, Levy CJ, Dunn WL: Behavioral Research Laboratory 1978 Annual Review—Part 1 and Philip Morris U.S.A. July 30, 1978. Available at: https://www.industrydocuments.ucsf.edu/docs/#id=srdv0184. Accessed December 20, 2019.

Hajek P, Phillips-Waller A, Przulj D, et al: A randomized trial of e-cigarettes versus nicotine-replacement therapy. N Engl J Med 380(7):629–637, 2019 30699054

Henningfield JE, Keenan RM: Nicotine delivery kinetics and abuse liability. J Consult Clin Psychol 61(5):743–750, 1993 8245272

Institute of Medicine: Clearing the Smoke: Assessing the Science Base for Tobacco Harm Reduction. Washington, DC, National Academies Press, 2001

Institute of Medicine: Ending the Tobacco Problem: A Blueprint for the Nation. Washington, DC, National Academies Press, 2007

International Agency for Research on Cancer: Methods for Evaluating Tobacco Control Policies. Lyon, France, International Agency for Research on Cancer, 2008

International Tobacco Control Project: ITC United States National Report Waves 1 to 8 (2002–2011). University of Waterloo, Waterloo, Ontario, Canada and Medical University of South Carolina, Charleston, South Carolina, United States, February 2014. Available at: https://www.itcproject.org/resources/view/1538. Accessed December 20, 2019.

Jamal A, King BA, Neff LJ, et al: Current cigarette smoking among adults—United States, 2005–2015. MMWR Morb Mortal Wkly Rep 65(44):1205–1211, 2016 27832052

Jeon J, Holford TR, Levy DT, et al: Smoking and lung cancer mortality in the United States from 2015 to 2065: a comparative modeling approach. Ann Intern Med 169(10):684–693, 2018 30304504

Kasza KA, Ambrose BK, Conway KP, et al: Tobacco-product use by adults and youths in the United States in 2013 and 2014. N Engl J Med 376(4):342–353, 2017 28121512

Kozlowski LT, Abrams DB: Obsolete tobacco control themes can be hazardous to public health: the need for updating views on absolute product risks and harm reduction. BMC Public Health 16:432, 2016 27221096

Laurene AH: Possible IBT Projects. May 24, 1971. Available at: https://www.industrydocuments.ucsf.edu/docs/#id=tjvk0191. Accessed December 20, 2019.

Levy DT, Borland R, Villanti AC, et al: The application of a decision-theoretic model to estimate the public health impact of vaporized nicotine product initiation in the United States. Nicotine Tob Res 19(2):149–159, 2017 27613952

Liu M, Jiang Y, Wedow R, et al; 23andMe Research Team; HUNT All-In Psychiatry, et al: Association studies of up to 1.2 million individuals yield new insights into the genetic etiology of tobacco and alcohol use. Nat Genet 51(2):237–244, 2019 30643251

Lund KE, Scheffels J, McNeill A: The association between use of snus and quit rates for smoking: results from seven Norwegian cross-sectional studies. Addiction 106(1):162–167, 2011 20883459

McNeill A, Brose LS, Calder R, et al: Evidence Review of E-Cigarettes and Heated Tobacco Products 2018. A Report Commissioned by Public Health England. Public Health England, 6. 2018. Available at: https://assets.publishing.service.gov.uk/government/uploads/system/uploads/attachment_data/file/684963/Evidence_review_of_e-cigarettes_and_heated_tobacco_products_2018.pdf. Accessed December 20, 2019.

National Academies of Sciences, Engineering, and Medicine: Public Health Consequences of E-Cigarettes. Washington, DC, National Academies Press, 2018

National Cancer Institute: Risks Associated With Smoking Cigarettes With Low Tar Machine-Measured Yields of Tar and Nicotine. Smoking and Tobacco Control Monograph 13. U.S. Department of Health and Human Services, National Institutes of Health, National Cancer Institute, 2001. Available at: https://cancercontrol.cancer.gov/brp/tcrb/monographs/13/m13_complete.pdf. Accessed December 20, 2019.

National Cancer Institute: The Role of the Media in Promoting and Reducing Tobacco Use. Tobacco Control Monograph No. 19. U.S. Department of Health and Human Services, National Institutes of Health, National Cancer Institute, 2008. Available at: https://cancercontrol.cancer.gov/brp/tcrb/monographs/19/m19_complete.pdf. Accessed December 20, 2019.

National Cancer Institute: Phenotypes and Endophenotypes: Foundations for Genetic Studies of Nicotine Use and Dependence. Smoking and Tobacco Control Monograph 20. U.S. Department of Health and Human Services, National Institutes of Health, National Cancer Institute, 2009. Available at: https://cancercontrol.cancer.gov/brp/tcrb/monographs/20/m20_entire_acc.pdf. Accessed December 20, 2019.

National Center for Chronic Disease Prevention and Health Promotion Office on Smoking and Health: The Health Consequences of Smoking—50 Years of Progress: A Report of the Surgeon General. Atlanta, GA, Centers for Disease Control and Prevention, 2014

National Center for Health Statistics: National Health Interview Survey, 1997–September 2017, Sample Adult Core Component. Atlanta, GA, U.S. Department of Health and Human Services, Centers for Disease Control and Prevention, National Center for Health Statistics, 2018

Neuhauser MA, Simoneau A: Memorandum of Understanding. U.S. Food and Drug Administration Center for Tobacco Products and RAI Services Company/Santa Fe Natural Tobacco Company, Inc., January 19, 2017

Niaura R: Re-Thinking Nicotine and Its Effects. Schroeder Institute, Truth Initiative, 2016. Available at: http://vapit.it/wp-content/uploads/2016/12/ReThinking-Nicotine.pdf. Accessed December 20, 2019.

Orleans CT, Slade J: Nicotine Addiction: Principles and Management. New York, Oxford University Press, 1993

Pierce JP, Distefan JM, Hill D: Adolescent smoking, in Tobacco: Science, Policy and Public Health, 2nd Edition. Edited by Boyle P, Gray N, Henningfield J, et al. New York, Oxford University Press, 2010, pp 313–324

Ramström L, Borland R, Wikmans T: Patterns of smoking and snus use in Sweden: implications for public health. Int J Environ Res Public Health 13(11):E1110, 2016 27834883

Rodgman A: The Optimum Composition of Tobacco and Its Smoke. November 2, 1959. Available at: https://www.industrydocuments.ucsf.edu/docs/#id=jglw0200. Accessed December 20, 2019.

Rodgman A, Perfetti TA: The Chemical Components of Tobacco and Tobacco Smoke. New York, CRC Press, 2016

Rodu B, Cole P: The burden of mortality from smoking: comparing Sweden with other countries in the European Union. Eur J Epidemiol 19(2):129–131, 2004 15074568

Schultz FJ: 2 Mg Product. July 22, 1977. Available at: https://www.industrydocuments.ucsf.edu/docs/#id=gxbv0035. Accessed December 20, 2019.

Senkus M: Smoking Satisfaction. R.J. Reynolds, 1976. Available at: https://www.industrydocumentslibrary.ucsf.edu/tobacco/docs/lxfv0093. Accessed December 20, 2019.

Smith RE: U.S Exhibit 34,328, Memo, Re: Goal of the RT Information Task Force, Richard E. Smith, Lorillard Inc. February 13, 1980. Available at: https://www.industrydocuments.ucsf.edu/docs/#id=kpmv0035. Accessed December 20, 2019.

Strong DR, Messer K, Hartman SJ, et al: Measurement of multiple nicotine dependence domains among cigarette, non-cigarette and poly tobacco users: insights from item response theory. Drug Alcohol Depend 152:185–193, 2015 26005043

Sweanor D, Yach D: Looking for the next breakthrough in tobacco control and health. S Afr Med J 103(11):810–811, 2013 24148163

Tabuchi T, Kiyohara K, Hoshino T, et al: Awareness and use of electronic cigarettes and heat-not-burn tobacco products in Japan. Addiction 111(4):706–713, 2016 26566956

Tamol RA: Phillip Morris Records. February 1, 1965. Available at: https://www.industrydocuments.ucsf.edu/docs/#id=qynn0226. Accessed December 20, 2019.

Teague CE: Research Planning Memorandum on the Future of the Tobacco Business and the Crucial Role of Nicotine Therein. April 14, 1972. Available at: https://www.industrydocuments.ucsf.edu/docs/#id=stdb0184. Accessed December 20, 2019.

Teague CE: Implication and Activities Arising From Correlation of Smoke pH With Nicotine Impact, Other Smoke Qualities, and Cigarette Sales. R.J. Reynolds, 1973. Available at: https://www.industrydocumentslibrary.ucsf.edu/tobacco/docs/xphv0094. Accessed December 20, 2019.

Teague CE: Nordine Study. R.J. Reynolds, 1982. Available at: https://www.industrydocumentslibrary.ucsf.edu/tobacco/docs/jtjc0094. Accessed December 20, 2019.

U.S. Department of Health and Human Services: The Health Consequences of Smoking: Nicotine Addiction. A Report of the Surgeon General. Atlanta, GA, U.S. Department of Health and Human Services, Centers for Disease Control and Prevention, Office on Smoking and Health, 1988

U.S. Department of Health and Human Services: Reducing the Health Consequences of Smoking: 25 Years of Progress. A Report of the Surgeon General. Atlanta, GA, U.S. Department of Health and Human Services, Centers for Disease Control and Prevention, Office on Smoking and Health, 1989

U.S. Department of Health and Human Services: How Tobacco Smoke Causes Disease: The Biology and Behavioral Basis for Smoking-Attributable Disease: A Report of the Surgeon General. Atlanta, GA, U.S. Department of Health and Human Services, Centers for Disease Control and Prevention, National Center for Chronic Disease Prevention and Health Promotion, Office on Smoking and Health, 2010. Available at: https://www.ncbi.nlm.nih.gov/books/NBK53017/. Accessed October 19, 2020.

U.S. Food and Drug Administration: Family Smoking Prevention and Tobacco Control Act. June 22, 2009. Available at: https://www.fda.gov/TobaccoProducts/Labeling/RulesRegulationsGuidance/ucm262084.htm. Accessed December 20, 2019.

U.S. Food and Drug Administration: Tobacco product standard for nicotine level of combusted cigarettes. Fed Regist 83(52):11818–11843, 2018. Available at: https://www.federalregister.gov/documents/2018/03/16/2018-05345/tobacco-product-standard-for-nicotine-level-of-combusted-cigarettes. Accessed December 22, 2019.

World Health Organization: WHO Report on the Global Tobacco Epidemic 2011. 2017. Available at: http://www.who.int/tobacco/global_report/2011/en/. Accessed December 20, 2019.

Yeaman A: The Optimum Composition of Tobacco and Its Smoke. July 17, 1963. Available at: https://www.industrydocuments.ucsf.edu/docs/#id=rhxp0042. Accessed December 20, 2019.

Yong HH, Borland R, Cummings KM, et al: Impact of the removal of misleading terms on cigarette pack on smokers' beliefs about "light/mild" cigarettes: cross-country comparisons. Addiction 106(12):2204–2213, 2011 21658140

CHAPTER 35

Prevention of Substance Use Disorders

Katrina E. Champion, Ph.D.

Nicola C. Newton, Ph.D.

Maree Teesson, Ph.D.

Substance use continues to pose substantial public health problems worldwide, despite significant advances in prevention science over the past 20 years. In the United States, an estimated 19.7 million people age 12 years or older had a substance use disorder in 2017. Of these, 14.5 million people had an alcohol use disorder and 7.5 million people had an illicit drug use disorder, with the most common illicit drug use disorder being for marijuana (4.1 million people) (Substance Abuse and Mental Health Services Administration 2018). Concerted prevention efforts are needed to minimize the devastating effects of substance use disorders on individuals, families, and communities and to reduce the substantial associated burden of disease and social and economic costs. Indeed, a considerable proportion of global disease, disability, and mortality can be attributed to the use of alcohol and other drugs. Globally, in 2016, 99.2 million disability-adjusted life years (DALYs)—or 4.2% of all DALYs—were attributable to alcohol use, and 31.8 million DALYs—or 1.3% of all DALYs—were attributable to illicit drug use (Degenhardt et al. 2018). The burden of disease attributed to alcohol and other drugs is great among young people ages 15–24 years (Mokdad et al. 2016), which corresponds with the typical period of onset of substance-related problems. Although effective prevention provides an opportunity to avert the substantial burden associated with substance use disorders and related harms, further research is needed to strengthen the evidence base and to improve the implementation, scalability, and sustainability of substance use prevention efforts.

In this chapter we attempt to summarize the current state of the evidence in relation to substance use prevention, including when and where prevention efforts should be deployed. The evidence base for substance use prevention delivered outside of school settings is not as strong as that for preventive measures delivered within schools, largely due to a lack of high-quality evaluations and gold-standard randomized controlled trials (RCTs) examining prevention programs in nonschool settings. The focus of this chapter is therefore on school-based prevention, although other important approaches, such as community, family, and mass media interventions, are also discussed. The potential of new approaches, such as web-based and mobile health interventions, is also highlighted.

A Developmental Approach to Prevention

Adolescence is an important transitional period characterized by major change, identity formation, and shifting social, emotional, and educational challenges. It is a time when young people typically acquire greater autonomy over their lifestyle choices, while exposure to risk behaviors, such as substance use, increases. In addition to greater exposure, an increased risk for substance use in adolescence can be partly attributed to diminished self-control (Casey 2015) and a peak in sensation seeking (Steinberg 2005). Adolescence represents a peak period of substance use initiation, and interventions targeting this period, prior to the establishment of harmful patterns of use and the development of substance use disorders, can have a unique impact. For these reasons, the focus of most existing substance use prevention efforts to date has been on adolescents.

For prevention efforts targeting substance use and related harms to be optimally effective, they must be delivered at developmentally appropriate times and should be guided by knowledge about the developmental progression of substance use (Botvin and Griffin 2007). This approach enables prevention efforts to be matched to the developmental needs and competencies of the target population. Optimal developmental timing can be conceptualized as encompassing two key phases (McBride 2003):

- *Inoculation phase (before initiation of substance use):* Interventions delivered immediately before the onset of substance use (McBride 2003) can be effective in halting or delaying the progression from experimental use to more harmful use (Botvin and Griffin 2007). Absorbing knowledge and increasing skills during this phase has the potential to modify young people's behavioral patterns and responses in later drug-related situations (McBride 2003).
- *Early relevance phase (as exposure increases):* Interventions delivered during initial exposure to substance use can enable individuals to apply the skills and knowledge taught within prevention programs in meaningful and practical ways in their own lives (McBride 2003).

Although these phases provide a guide for intervention timing, it is important to note that there is substantial global variation in the extent to which different substances are used and in the average age at which onset of use occurs. For this reason, timing of preventive interventions should take into account local prevalence data for specific drugs (McBride 2003).

Levels of Prevention

A widely used classification system for substance use preventive interventions now exists as part of a continuum of care spanning prevention, treatment, and maintenance. Adopted by the U.S. Institute of Medicine (Mrazek and Haggerty 1994), this system separates prevention efforts into three types according to level of risk—namely, *universal, selective,* and *indicated* efforts. In the context of substance use prevention, *universal* interventions are those that target an entire population (e.g., a whole classroom, school, or community), without prior screening for risk factors. Universal school-based prevention programs aim to halt or delay the onset of substance use and related harms by targeting an entire class or grade, regardless of students' individual levels of risk (Foxcroft and Tsertsvadze 2011b). *Selective* prevention programs target their interventions to specific subsets of the population that have been identified as being at an increased risk of developing a substance use disorder (Griffin and Botvin 2010). This might include, for example, young people who exhibit personality traits shown to increase the risk of substance use problems (Conrod 2016) or adolescents living in communities with high rates of crime or poverty. Finally, *indicated* prevention programs, also commonly referred to as "early intervention," target individuals who are already showing early signs or symptoms of substance use problems but who do not yet meet criteria for a substance use disorder diagnosis.

In weighing the relative benefits of the different levels of substance use prevention, universal prevention programs are advantageous in that they have the potential to be widely implemented and carry a low risk of stigmatizing individuals. They typically produce small to modest effects (Faggiano et al. 2014; Foxcroft and Tsertsvadze 2011b); however, small effect sizes at the population level have been associated with significant economic savings (Caulkins et al. 2004). Selective prevention programs generally yield larger effects in comparison with universal interventions; however, they require prior identification of at-risk individuals, which may lead to stigmatization (Offord 2000). Finally, indicated prevention programs can be costly to deliver in terms of time and money, but they provide preventive interventions to those individuals who need them most.

Evidence-Based Approaches to Substance Use Prevention

Multiple risk factors for substance use have been identified, including genetic, individual, family, school, and community factors (Griffin and Botvin 2010). For this reason, preventive interventions must be diverse in the risk factors that they aim to address and in the settings in which they are delivered. Traditionally, interventions are delivered to families, individuals, and groups in homes, schools, and communities, as well as through mass media and public policy initiatives (Bühler and Thrul 2015; Griffin and Botvin 2010).

School-Based Interventions

Probably the most widely used approach to substance use prevention is universal school-based drug education. Schools are an appropriate setting in which to deliver universal substance use preventive interventions because they possess both the infrastructure to deliver alcohol and other drug education and the appropriate social and learning environment to attenuate risks. Outside of the family environment, the school is the primary setting within which the development of children and young people can be directed and shaped.

Universal Interventions

Universal school-based substance use education programs are usually delivered in the classroom and are aligned with the health curriculum. Systematic reviews have demonstrated that universal school-based prevention programs can be effective in reducing substance use among adolescents; however, effects are typically modest (Das et al. 2016; Foxcroft and Tsertsvadze 2011b; Mewton et al. 2018; Strøm et al. 2014). In terms of universal alcohol use prevention programs, a Cochrane review (Foxcroft and Tsertsvadze 2011b) found that six out of eleven alcohol-specific school-based interventions produced positive effects for alcohol use outcomes when compared with a standard curriculum. Small yet positive effects have also been demonstrated for universal school-based prevention programs for illicit substances (Das et al. 2016; Faggiano et al. 2014).

According to the literature, the most effective universal school-based substance use prevention programs adopt what is known as a comprehensive social influence approach. This approach uses three key social influence principles—1) information provision, 2) normative education about the prevalence of substance use among peers, and 3) resistance skills training (Faggiano et al. 2014)—in conjunction with strategies to build social competence or life skills (Sussman et al. 2004). Social competence strengthening strategies aim to equip students with generic life skills such as assertiveness, decision making, problem solving, and coping tactics. Table 35–1 summarizes characteristics of effective prevention programs that use a comprehensive social influence approach, as reported in the recently updated International Drug Prevention Standards (United Nations Office on Drugs and Crime 2018).

Two large studies that used social influence and social competence principles are the *Unplugged* program in Europe (Vigna-Taglianti et al. 2014) and Botvin's *Life Skills Training* (LST) program in the United States (Botvin and Griffin 2014). *Unplugged* was a 12-lesson program delivered to 12- to 14-year-olds by trained teachers. The program was evaluated as part of a Europe-wide RCT (EU-Dap) and was found to be effective in reducing tobacco use, cannabis use, and episodes of drunkenness among adolescents (Vigna-Taglianti et al. 2014). The LST program was a universal prevention program that aimed to teach students generic social skills, personal self-management skills, and AOD (alcohol and other drug) resistance skills. The intervention consisted of 15 lessons delivered by a trained classroom teacher or health professional. LST has been evaluated in multiple RCTs, including among both urban minority and rural populations. Findings from these trials have shown LST to be effective in reducing smoking, binge drinking, and cannabis use and have also demonstrated positive effects on normative beliefs about substance use and refusal skills (Botvin and Griffin 2014).

TABLE 35–1.   **Characteristics of effective and ineffective substance use prevention programs utilizing a social influence approach**

Characteristics associated with efficacy or effectiveness	Characteristics associated with a lack of efficacy or adverse effects
• Use of interactive delivery methods	• Use of noninteractive delivery methods, such as lecturing
• Delivery by trained facilitators (including trained peers)	• Emphasis on information-giving, particularly fear arousal
• Delivery through a series of structured sessions (typically 10–15) once a week, often with provision of booster sessions over multiple years	• Delivery primarily through unstructured dialogue sessions
• Focus on dispelling misconceptions that substance use is "normal" and that "most people" engage in such use	• Focus primarily on building of self-esteem and emotional education
• Aim to influence perceptions of risk associated with substance use, with emphasis on immediate consequences	• Aim to influence ethical/moral decision making or values
• Provide opportunities to learn and practice personal and social skills (e.g., coping, decision making, resistance strategies)	• Use of testimonials from ex–drug users

Source.   United Nations Office on Drugs and Crime 2018.

Although school-based programs have been shown to be effective and universal interventions can reach larger numbers of students, there are often significant barriers to the implementation and sustainability of these programs. Limited resources in terms of time, money, and teacher training mean that many schools are unable to implement evidence-based prevention programs (Bumbarger and Perkins 2008), especially those in geographically isolated or low-socioeconomic-status areas. Although not a problem specific to school settings, resource limitations can also impede ongoing and sustainable implementation of substance use prevention programs, which can be costly and unachievable for many schools (Hawkins et al. 2015).

Finally, much of the research on school-based prevention programs comes from high-income countries in North America, Europe, and Australia, with little evidence from low- and middle-income countries.

Selective Interventions

One example of a *selective* school-based preventive intervention is *Preventure* (Conrod 2016), a personality-targeted intervention designed for high-risk youth who exhibit one of four personality traits that have been found to be associated with substance use and psychopathology: 1) hopelessness (low mood; feelings of worthlessness; negative beliefs about oneself, the world, and the future); 2) anxiety sensitivity (fear of anxiety-related physical sensations); 3) impulsivity (rapid decision making and action, poor response inhibition); and 4) sensation seeking (elevated need for stimulation and intolerance of boredom). *Preventure* consists of two 90-minute group sessions delivered by trained facilitators in a school setting. Based on principles derived from cognitive-behavioral therapy and motivational interviewing, the intervention aims to teach young people personality-specific coping skills to prevent the use of alcohol and drugs. The effectiveness of *Preventure* in preventing adolescent drinking has been demonstrated in a number of RCTs worldwide (Conrod 2016). Most recently, an Australian evaluation of *Preventure* found it to be effective in reducing drinking, binge drinking (5+ standard drinks), and alcohol-related harms among high-risk students, with effects lasting up to 3 years following the intervention (Newton et al. 2016). This trial also demonstrated that *Preventure* was as effective as a universal alcohol-focused intervention in reducing population-level drinking and binge-drinking rates (despite the fact that *Preventure* was a selective program delivered to approximately 45% of the population) and that *Preventure* was superior to the universal intervention in reducing alcohol-related harm, likely due to its focus on factors that lead high-risk youth to misuse alcohol (Newton et al. 2016; Teesson et al. 2017). In addition, a trial in the United Kingdom found *Preventure* to be effective in improving mental health outcomes in high-risk youth, with significant reductions in depressive, anxiety, and conduct disorder symptoms reported up to 2 years following the interventions (Conrod 2016).

Community-Based Interventions

Community-based prevention approaches typically include multicomponent interventions delivered to whole communities, community mobilization strategies, or "community coalitions" to promote positive youth development (Bühler and Thrul 2015; Gates et al. 2006). Such approaches can be tailored to target specific risks in specific communities and to address an array of different types of risk factors, and preventive messages can be reinforced through multiple delivery methods. However, community-based interventions are often very resource intensive and are difficult to implement with high fidelity. In addition, although there is some research to support the efficacy of community-based approaches in preventing substance use (Bühler and Thrul 2015; Hawkins et al. 2014b), the evidence is mixed, and high-quality trials evaluating community approaches are lacking (Gates et al. 2006; Mewton et al. 2018).

Communities That Care (CTC) is perhaps the best-known community-based approach to adolescent substance use prevention. CTC aims to address and prevent multiple youth problem behaviors, including substance use, risky sexual behavior, violence, and school dropout, through whole-community change. Rather than assigning communities specific interventions to implement with youth, CTC trains local community members to choose which evidence-based activities to implement, based on the unique needs of people in the community (Hawkins et al. 2014a). Findings from trials of CTC in the United States indicate that communities that received the CTC intervention showed reductions in risk factors for substance use as well as delayed initiation of delinquent behavior from 2 to 5 years after implementation (Hawkins et al. 2008). Eight years after beginning the program, youth in the communities that were randomly assigned to CTC were more likely to have abstained from alcohol and drug use compared with youth in the control communities (Hawkins et al. 2014a). Effects were also demonstrated in terms of reducing violence and delinquency. However, long-term evaluations of CTC found that although the initiative may have been effective in preventing the onset of alcohol and drug use, it was not effective in reducing the frequency of use after youth had initiated substance use. In fact, there was an iatrogenic effect among a very small number of adolescents in relation to ecstasy use, with those in the CTC communities reporting higher prevalence of past-month ecstasy use compared with those in the control communities. It is not clear whether this finding was related to the intervention or to other variables in the community. More evidence is needed to fully support community-based interventions for substance use prevention.

Family-Based Interventions

Parents are significant sources of information for young people and can play an important role in delaying the onset of substance use in adolescents (Ryan et al. 2010). Parent- or family-based preventive interventions provide an opportunity to target risk factors associated with peer, social, and family influences. This includes programs focused on provision of skills to parents (e.g., communication, rule setting, monitoring), strategies for improving family dynamics, and combined student–parent interventions (Yap et al. 2017). Evidence suggests that parent-based interventions (i.e., those focused solely on parents) can be effective in preventing substance use by improving parent–child communication, rule setting, and monitoring (Kuntsche and Kuntsche 2016). In addition, a recent review (Mewton et al. 2018) concluded that there was good evidence to suggest that family-based universal prevention programs were effective in delaying and reducing alcohol use, as well as emerging evidence that these programs were effective in reducing illicit drug use. Combined student- and parent-based prevention programs have also been shown to produce beneficial effects in terms of adolescent substance use outcomes (Foxcroft and Tsertsvadze 2011a; Hickman et al. 2014; Newton et al. 2017); however, effects are often small (Das et al. 2016).

One example of an effective combined student and parent prevention program with particularly good effect sizes is the Prevention of Alcohol Use in Students (PAS) program developed by researchers in the Netherlands (Koning et al. 2009). Based on the theory of planned behavior and social cognitive theory, this program includes both student- and parent-based intervention components. In the program, parents of high school students are invited to attend a face-to-face informational meeting at the beginning of the school year, where they receive information about alcohol use among adolescents and the important role of parental attitudes and behavior. Parents are then encouraged as a group to agree upon a set of strict rules regarding alcohol use. Two weeks after the parents' meeting, they are provided with an information leaflet and a copy of the agreed-upon rules. Six months after the parent component is delivered, students (ages 12–13 years) complete a four-lesson online intervention focused on increasing alcohol refusal skills, followed by a booster lesson 1 year later. Evaluations of the PAS program found that in comparison with students in the control condition, students who received the PAS intervention reported a delay in the onset of alcohol use, weekly alcohol use, and heavy weekly alcohol use, as well as less alcohol consumption and heavy weekend alcohol consumption up to 50 months postbaseline (Koning et al. 2011).

Although not the case for the PAS program, a key barrier for parent- or family-based prevention efforts is that these efforts require active parent involvement, and parental participation is often low. Attempts to increase parental participation by addressing barriers, such as lack of time, costs, child care, and transport issues, are critical for the success of combined student and parent interventions. It is also often the case that the adolescents who are most at risk of substance use or related problems may not have strong family role models or parents likely to participate in an intervention.

Mass Media Interventions

Mass media interventions involve the use of advertisements and media campaigns to shape patterns of substance use, influence intentions to use, and modify awareness, knowledge, and attitudes (Allara et al. 2015). Advantages of these approaches include their wide reach, broad dissemination capacity, and well-documented ability to engage the interest of young people. However, mass media interventions can be costly, and evidence regarding their effectiveness in improving substance use outcomes is not promising (Mewton et al. 2018), with some reviews finding no evidence of beneficial effects and others suggesting that these interventions may even *increase* substance use (Allara et al. 2015).

eHealth Interventions

Web-based interventions have several advantages over traditional prevention programs, including increased youth engagement, fidelity, and scalability. These advantages, in conjunction with increased accessibility to the Internet and technology, have led to the emergence of web-based prevention programs spanning a range of public issues, including substance use. Systematic reviews of online and computer-based universal substance use prevention programs (Champion et al. 2013, 2016b) have found that online interventions can be effective in reducing alcohol and other drug use among adolescents; however, further research in this space is needed (Das et al. 2016; Mewton et al. 2018). The majority of programs in these reviews were delivered in the school setting. Indeed, online school-based prevention programs have the potential to overcome many of the implementation barriers commonly encountered by teachers, because trained professionals are not required for their delivery, and teachers typically need little or no training to implement the programs. The portability of the Internet also suggests that online programs could be easily delivered to youth in other settings, such as the home or community. For example, one web-based program to prevent cannabis use was delivered in a primary care setting, which has the potential to reach high-risk youth who are likely to be missed by interventions delivered in schools (Walton et al. 2014).

One effective web-based substance use prevention program is *Climate Schools*. The *Climate Schools* programs are universal school-based interventions based on a comprehensive social influence approach (see Table 35–1). The programs use cartoon storylines and web-based delivery to engage and maintain student interest and to overcome implementation barriers. Four separate modules—covering education about alcohol, cannabis, psychostimulants, and new psychoactive substances—have been developed and evaluated. To date, seven RCTs of the *Climate Schools* courses have been conducted across Australia (Newton et al. 2009, 2010; see also Champion et al. 2016a; Teesson et al. 2017, 2020; Vogl et al. 2009, 2014), and a pilot trial has been conducted in the United Kingdom (Newton et al. 2014). These trials have found that in comparison with control students who received their usual health and drug education at school, students who received the *Climate Schools* courses showed significant improvements in alcohol- and drug-related knowledge and reductions in alcohol use, binge-drinking frequency, cannabis use, and alcohol-related harms up to 3 years following the interventions.

In addition to web-based interventions, interventions delivered via other digital media also offer great potential for preventing substance use and related harms. For example, there is some evidence to support the use of computerized serious educational games (i.e., video games developed primarily for educational purposes) as a prevention strategy (Rodriguez et al. 2014). Mobile health (mHealth) interventions, such as smartphone applications and text messaging, are commonly used to target a wide range of health behaviors in adults and represent a rapidly growing area among youth (Dute et al. 2016). mHealth interventions are a particularly promising intervention tool for young people, given that smartphone use is extensive among adolescents (Pew Research Center 2019), which may lead to increased engagement and uptake. Mobile technology appears to be a largely untapped medium for adolescent substance use prevention. Few rigorous studies have been conducted; therefore, strong conclusions about the efficacy of mHealth preventive interventions for youth substance use cannot yet be made. However, the limited evidence base that does exist suggests that mHealth substance use interventions are well accepted by adolescents and have the potential to produce promising results (Badawy and Kuhns 2017; Kazemi et al. 2017). As technology continues to advance, new intervention opportunities for preventing substance use and related harms are also likely to emerge.

Conclusion

Substance use is a significant public health problem worldwide. Fortunately, much of the burden of disease associated with alcohol and other drug use can be averted through targeted use of evidence-based prevention strategies. Regardless of the delivery setting, prevention strategies focused on drug use among young people must be implemented early, during developmentally appropriate periods. Effective school-, family-, community-, and Internet-based substance use interventions do exist; however, further rigorous research—including trials in low- and middle-income countries and more studies evaluating online and mHealth interventions—is needed to strengthen the evidence base. Finally, substance use prevention is just one piece of the puzzle; such interventions must be implemented as part of a holistic approach to positive youth development that considers multiple facets of young people's environments and lifestyles.

References

Allara E, Ferri M, Bo A, et al: Are mass-media campaigns effective in preventing drug use? A Cochrane systematic review and meta-analysis. BMJ Open 5(9):e007449, 2015 26338836
Badawy SM, Kuhns LM: Texting and mobile phone app interventions for improving adherence to preventive behavior in adolescents: a systematic review. JMIR Mhealth Uhealth 5(4):e50, 2017 28428157

Bava S, Tapert SF: Adolescent brain development and the risk for alcohol and other drug problems. Neuropsychol Rev 20(4):398–413, 2010 20953990

Botvin GJ, Griffin KW: School-based programmes to prevent alcohol, tobacco and other drug use. Int Rev Psychiatry 19(6):607–615, 2007 18092239

Botvin GJ, Griffin KW: Life skills training: preventing substance misuse by enhancing individual and social competence. New Dir Youth Dev 2014(141):57–65, 2014 24753278

Bühler A, Thrul J: Prevention of Addictive Behaviours. Luxembourg, European Monitoring Centre for Drugs and Drug Addiction, 2015

Bumbarger B, Perkins D: After randomised trials: issues related to dissemination of evidence-based interventions. Journal of Children's Services 3(2):55–64, 2008. Available at: https://www.emerald.com/insight/content/doi/10.1108/17466660200800012/full/html. Accessed December 22, 2019.

Casey BJ: Beyond simple models of self-control to circuit-based accounts of adolescent behavior. Annu Rev Psychol 66(1):295–319, 2015 25089362

Caulkins JP, Pacula RL, Paddock S, et al: What we can—and cannot—expect from school-based drug prevention. Drug Alcohol Rev 23(1):79–87, 2004 14965889

Champion KE, Newton NC, Barrett EL, et al: A systematic review of school-based alcohol and other drug prevention programs facilitated by computers or the Internet. Drug Alcohol Rev 32(2):115–123, 2013 23039085

Champion KE, Newton NC, Stapinski LA, et al: Effectiveness of a universal Internet-based prevention program for ecstasy and new psychoactive substances: a cluster randomized controlled trial. Addiction 111(8):1396–1405, 2016a 26880476

Champion KE, Newton NC, Teesson M: Prevention of alcohol and other drug use and related harm in the digital age: what does the evidence tell us? Curr Opin Psychiatry 29(4):242–249, 2016b 27153124

Conrod PJ: Personality-targeted interventions for substance use and misuse. Curr Addict Rep 3(4):426–436, 2016 27909645

Das JK, Salam RA, Arshad A, et al: Interventions for adolescent substance abuse: an overview of systematic reviews. J Adolesc Health 59(4S):S61–S75, 2016 27664597

Degenhardt L, Charlson F, Ferrari A, et al: The global burden of disease attributable to alcohol and drug use in 195 countries and territories, 1990-2016: a systematic analysis for the Global Burden of Disease Study 2016. Lancet Psychiatry 5(12):987–1012, 2018 30392731

Dute DJ, Bemelmans WJE, Breda J: Using mobile apps to promote a healthy lifestyle among adolescents and students: a review of the theoretical basis and lessons learned. JMIR Mhealth Uhealth 4(2):e39, 2016 27150850

Faggiano F, Minozzi S, Versino E, et al: Universal school-based prevention for illicit drug use. Cochrane Database Syst Rev (12):CD003020, 2014 25435250

Foxcroft DR, Tsertsvadze A: Universal family-based prevention programs for alcohol misuse in young people. Cochrane Database Syst Rev (9):CD009308, 2011a 21901733

Foxcroft DR, Tsertsvadze A: Universal school-based prevention programs for alcohol misuse in young people. Cochrane Database Syst Rev (5):CD009113, 2011b 21563171

Gates S, McCambridge J, Smith LA, et al: Interventions for prevention of drug use by young people delivered in non-school settings. Cochrane Database Syst Rev (1):CD005030, 2006 16437511

Griffin KW, Botvin GJ: Evidence-based interventions for preventing substance use disorders in adolescents. Child Adolesc Psychiatr Clin N Am 19(3):505–526, 2010 20682218

Hawkins J, Jenson J, Catalano R, et al: Unleashing the Power of Prevention. Washington, DC, Institute of Medicine of the National Academies, 2015

Hawkins JD, Brown EC, Oesterle S, et al: Early effects of Communities That Care on targeted risks and initiation of delinquent behavior and substance use. J Adolesc Health 43(1):15–22, 2008 18565433

Hawkins JD, Catalano RF, Kuklinski MR: Communities That Care, in Encyclopedia of Criminology and Criminal Justice. Edited by Bruinsma G, Weisburd D. New York, Springer, 2014a, pp 393–408

Hawkins JD, Oesterle S, Brown EC, et al: Youth problem behaviors 8 years after implementing the Communities That Care prevention system: a community-randomized trial. JAMA Pediatr 168(2):122–129, 2014b 24322060

Hickman M, Caldwell DM, Busse H, et al: Individual-, Family-, and School-Level Interventions for Preventing Multiple Risk Behaviours Relating to Alcohol, Tobacco and Drug Use in Individuals Aged 8 to 25 Years. 2014. Available at: https://www.politopedia.cl/wp-content/uploads/2016/06/Individual-family-and-school-level-interventions-for-preventing-multiple-risk-behaviours-relating-to-alcohol-tobacco-and-drug-use-in-individuals-aged-8-to-25-years.The-Cochrane-library.Noviembre-2014-1.pdf. Accessed December 20, 2019.

Kazemi DM, Borsari B, Levine MJ, et al: A systematic review of the mHealth interventions to prevent alcohol and substance abuse. J Health Commun 22(5):413–432, 2017 28394729

Koning IM, Vollebergh WA, Smit F, et al: Preventing heavy alcohol use in adolescents (PAS): cluster randomized trial of a parent and student intervention offered separately and simultaneously. Addiction 104(10):1669–1678, 2009 21265908

Koning IM, van den Eijnden RJ, Verdurmen JE, et al: Long-term effects of a parent and student intervention on alcohol use in adolescents: a cluster randomized controlled trial. Am J Prev Med 40(5):541–547, 2011 21496753

Kuntsche S, Kuntsche E: Parent-based interventions for preventing or reducing adolescent substance use—a systematic literature review. Clin Psychol Rev 45:89–101, 2016 27111301

McBride N: A systematic review of school drug education. Health Educ Res 18(6):729–742, 2003 14654505

Mewton L, Visontay R, Chapman C, et al: Universal prevention of alcohol and drug use: an overview of reviews in an Australian context. Drug Alcohol Rev 37 (suppl 1):S435–S469, 2018 29582489

Mokdad AH, Forouzanfar MH, Daoud F, et al: Global burden of diseases, injuries, and risk factors for young people's health during 1990–2013: a systematic analysis for the Global Burden of Disease Study 2013. Lancet 387(10036):2383–2401, 2016 27174305

Mrazek P, Haggerty R: Reducing Risks for Mental Disorders: Frontiers for Preventive Intervention Research. Washington, DC, National Academy Press, 1994

Newton NC, Vogl LE, Teesson M, et al: CLIMATE Schools: alcohol module: cross-validation of a school-based prevention programme for alcohol misuse. Aust N Z J Psychiatry 43(3):201–207, 2009 19221908

Newton NC, Teesson M, Vogl LE, et al: Internet-based prevention for alcohol and cannabis use: final results of the Climate Schools course. Addiction 105(4):749–759, 2010 20148791

Newton NC, Conrod PJ, Rodriguez DM, Teesson M: A pilot study of an online universal school-based intervention to prevent alcohol and cannabis use in the UK. BMJ Open 4(5):e004750, 2014 24840248

Newton NC, Conrod PJ, Slade T, et al: The long-term effectiveness of a selective, personality-targeted prevention program in reducing alcohol use and related harms: a cluster randomized controlled trial. J Child Psychol Psychiatry 57(9):1056–1065, 2016 27090500

Newton NC, Champion KE, Slade T, et al: A systematic review of combined student- and parent-based programs to prevent alcohol and other drug use among adolescents. Drug Alcohol Rev 36(3):337–351, 2017 28334456

Offord DR: Selection of levels of prevention. Addict Behav 25(6):833–842, 2000 11125774

Pew Research Center: Mobile Fact Sheet. June 12, 2019. Available at: https://www.pewresearch.org/internet/fact-sheet/mobile/. Accessed December 20, 2019.

Rodriguez DM, Teesson M, Newton NC: A systematic review of computerised serious educational games about alcohol and other drugs for adolescents. Drug Alcohol Rev 33(2):129–135, 2014 24329810

Ryan SM, Jorm AF, Lubman DI: Parenting factors associated with reduced adolescent alcohol use: a systematic review of longitudinal studies. Aust N Z J Psychiatry 44(9):774–783, 2010 20815663

Steinberg L: Cognitive and affective development in adolescence. Trends Cogn Sci 9(2):69–74, 2005 15668099

Strøm HK, Adolfsen F, Fossum S, et al: Effectiveness of school-based preventive interventions on adolescent alcohol use: a meta-analysis of randomized controlled trials. Subst Abuse Treat Prev Policy 9(1):48, 2014 25495012

Substance Abuse and Mental Health Services Administration: Key Substance Use and Mental Health Indicators in the United States: Results From the 2017 National Survey on Drug Use and Health (HHS Publ. No. SMA 18-5068, NSDUH Series H-53). Rockville, MD, Center for Behavioral Health Statistics and Quality, SAMHSA, 2018. Available at: https://www.samhsa .gov/data/sites/default/files/cbhsq-reports/NSDUHFFR2017/NSDUHFFR2017.pdf. Accessed June 25, 2020.

Sussman S, Earleywine M, Wills T, et al: The motivation, skills, and decision-making model of "drug abuse" prevention. Subst Use Misuse 39(10–12):1971–2016, 2004 15587955

Teesson M, Newton NC, Slade T, et al: Combined universal and selective prevention for adolescent alcohol use: a cluster randomized controlled trial. Psychol Med 47(10):1761–1770, 2017 28222825

Teesson M, Newton NC, Slade T, et al: Combined prevention for substance use, depression, and anxiety in adolescence: a cluster-randomised controlled trial of a digital online intervention. The Lancet Digital Health 2(2):e74–e84, 2020. Available at: https://www.thelancet.com/ journals/landig/article/PIIS2589-7500(19)30213-4/fulltext. Accessed July 8, 2020.

United Nations Office on Drugs and Crime: International Standards on Drug Use Prevention, 2nd Edition. Vienna, Austria, United Nations, 2018

Vigna-Taglianti FD, Galanti MR, Burkhart G, et al: "Unplugged," a European school-based program for substance use prevention among adolescents: overview of results from the EU-Dap trial. New Dir Youth Dev 2014(141):67–82, 2014 24753279

Vogl L, Teesson M, Andrews G, et al: A computerized harm minimization prevention program for alcohol misuse and related harms: randomized controlled trial. Addiction 104(4):564–575, 2009 19335655

Vogl LE, Newton NC, Champion KE, Teesson M: A universal harm-minimisation approach to preventing psychostimulant and cannabis use in adolescents: a cluster randomised controlled trial. Subst Abuse Treat Prev Policy 9:24, 2014 24943829

Walton MA, Resko S, Barry KL, et al: A randomized controlled trial testing the efficacy of a brief cannabis universal prevention program among adolescents in primary care. Addiction 109(5):786–797, 2014 24372937

Yap MBH, Cheong TWK, Zaravinos-Tsakos F, et al: Modifiable parenting factors associated with adolescent alcohol misuse: a systematic review and meta-analysis of longitudinal studies. Addiction 112(7):1142–1162, 2017 28178373

PART VI

Special Populations

CHAPTER 36

Substance-Related Disorders in Women

Grace Hennessy, M.D.

Constance Guille, M.D.

Shelly F. Greenfield, M.D., M.P.H.

Sex and gender differences play a significant role in the epidemiology, risk and protective factors, onset, and development of substance use disorders (SUDs), as well as in access to and outcomes of SUD treatment. According to the National Institutes of Health, *sex* refers to "biological differences between females and males, including chromosomes, sex organs, and endogenous hormonal profiles," whereas *gender* refers to "socially constructed and enacted roles and behaviors which occur in a historical and cultural context and vary across societies and over time" (National Institutes of Health 2019, paragraph 2). Although SUDs remain more prevalent in men than in women, the gender gap has been narrowing overall at an increasing rate, and especially for more recent birth cohorts in the United States; this holds true across most substances, including alcohol, marijuana, opioids, stimulants, and smoked tobacco as well as other nicotine delivery systems. There are also gender disparities in seeking and obtaining treatment and in treatment retention. Although the main outcomes in some SUD medication and behavioral treatment studies demonstrate equivalence in men and women, in other studies, the efficacy of treatments for use disorders involving specific substances, such as tobacco, vary by sex and gender. In addition, certain clinical characteristics that are associated with treatment outcomes often vary by gender and may, therefore, have a disproportionate effect on women's SUD treatment outcomes. The effects of factors such as co-occurring psychiatric disorders, history of trauma, education, and financial independence, among other factors that differentially affect men and women, can be more significant for women's SUD treatment outcomes and require consideration in gender-specific treatment for women. Hormonal and neuroendocrine effects, including variations in craving, use, and treatment outcomes across the menstrual cycle, are understudied. In addition, women of reproductive age have specific risks to reproductive health and pregnancy if they are using substances or have a SUD. Pregnancy and the perinatal period require specific attention to treatment of both maternal and child outcomes. In this chapter, we review the epidemiology, biological factors, co-occurring psychiatric disorders, and treatment of SUDs in women, including during pregnancy and the perinatal period.

Epidemiology

According to the 2017 National Survey on Drug Use and Health (Substance Abuse and Mental Health Services Administration 2018b), 62% of females ages 12 years and older reported drinking alcohol in the past year, compared with 67% of males. Marijuana had the second-highest percentage of past-year use (25% for females vs. 34% for males), followed by cigarettes (20% vs. 26%), cocaine (1% vs. 1.3%), and opioids (0.1% vs. 0.2%). Although males continue to have higher past-year substance use percentages than females, the gender gap has narrowed over time, especially in the youngest age cohorts.

Data from the National Epidemiologic Survey on Alcohol and Related Conditions (NESARC) revealed an overall increase in alcohol use, high-risk drinking (defined as exceeding the daily drinking guidelines at least weekly in the past 12 months), and alcohol use disorder (AUD) in the United States between the survey periods of 2001–2002 and 2012–2013 (Grant et al. 2017). When these data are broken down by gender, a worrisome trend among women relative to men emerges. Women's 12-month alcohol use increased 16%, high-risk drinking increased 58%, and AUD increased 84%. In comparison, the percentage increases for men were 7%, 15%, and 35%, respectively, between the survey periods. One prior study that used data from the NESARC and the National Longitudinal Alcohol Epidemiologic Survey found lower rates of abstaining from alcohol and higher rates of AUD among women born after, compared with women born before, World War II (Grucza et al. 2008), and current data suggest a continuing trend of rising rates of alcohol use among women during the first decade of the twenty-first century. More recent reports document a steep rise in alcohol-related liver disease in young adult women as well as deaths secondary to alcohol-related liver cirrhosis in this cohort that is likely related to the overall increase in women's alcohol consumption (Doycheva et al. 2017; Yoon and Chen 2018).

Another worrisome trend is the increased prevalence of binge drinking by high school girls and adult women. Table 36–1 summarizes the prevalence, frequency, and intensity of binge drinking by women ages 18 years and older during a 1-month period in 2011 (Centers for Disease Control and Prevention 2013). As shown in the table, binge drinking is highly prevalent among young adult women of reproductive age (ages 18–34 years). Among high school girls in grades 9–12 (data not shown in table), the prevalence of current alcohol use was 37.9% and the prevalence of binge drinking was 19.8% (Centers for Disease Control and Prevention 2013).

Similar gender trends have been reported for other substances. For example, of the 42 million Americans who smoked cigarettes in 2012, approximately 48% (20 million) were women and girls age 12 years or older (U.S. Department of Health and Human Services 2014). Although men continue to smoke in greater numbers than women, women are now as likely as men to die from diseases caused by smoking, and the rel-

TABLE 36–1. **Past-month prevalence, frequency, and intensity of binge drinking among women ages 18 years and older: United States, 2011**

Age group	Prevalence	Frequency[1]	Intensity[2]
All age groups surveyed	12.5%	3.2	5.7
18–24 years	24.2%	3.6	6.4
25–34 years	19.9%	3.0	6.0
35–44 years	14.5%	3.0	5.5
44–64 years	9.5%	3.3	5.1
≥65 years	2.5%	3.4	4.2

[1]Average number of binge-drinking episodes per month.
[2]Average largest number of drinks consumed by binge drinkers on any occasion in the past month.
Source. Adapted from Centers for Disease Control and Prevention 2013.

ative risk of developing coronary artery disease and chronic obstructive pulmonary disease is greater for currently smoking females than for currently smoking males.

A study examining data from the National Survey on Drug Use and Health for the years 2011–2015 found similar increases in the prevalence of cocaine use for females and males (John and Wu 2017), with a 20% increase in cocaine use among all individuals ages 12 years and older over that period; however, the prevalence of past-year cocaine use increased by 32% in women, compared with an increase of only 17% in men. The same survey also found that prevalence estimates of weekly cocaine use increased 60% for women and 47% for men during this same time period. In spite of this increased overall use, the prevalence of cocaine use disorder decreased 16% among women but increased 13% among men.

Significant gender differences have also emerged regarding heroin and prescription opioids (Table 36–2). Between 1991 and 2017, women's use of heroin increased to rates that are similar to those of men. Women are more likely than men to be prescribed opioids in their lifetime, women are decreasing their nonmedical opioid use at a slower rate than men, and women have had a greater increase in prescription opioid deaths relative to men over time (Centers for Disease Control and Prevention 2017; Cicero et al. 2014; Hirschtritt et al. 2017; Marsh et al. 2018). The slower rate of decline in nonmedical opioid use among women may be associated with gender-specific factors such as the greater likelihood for women to report chronic pain and the greater likelihood for women with chronic pain to be prescribed opioids in general. Men are more likely than women to die of prescription opioid overdose; however, the percentage of prescription opioid deaths between 1999 and 2016 increased more than 596% among women, compared with an increase of 312% among men (Centers for Disease Control and Prevention 2017). Women between the ages of 25 and 54 years are more likely than any other age group of women to go to an emergency department for opioid misuse or opioid use disorder (OUD), yet women between the ages of 45 and 54 years have the highest risk of any age group of dying from a prescription opioid overdose (Centers for Disease Control and Prevention 2017).

In addition to population studies across all ages, studies of adolescents reveal more marked narrowing and in some instances complete closing of the gender gap in substance use. According to the 2017 Monitoring the Future study, the most notable

TABLE 36–2.	Gender differences in use of heroin and misuse of prescription opioids

Heroin

Rates of heroin use among women have increased steadily since the 1960s and were equal to rates among men by 2010 (Cicero et al. 2014).

Prescription opioids

The decline in nonmedical opioid use has been slower among women than among men (Marsh et al. 2018).

Women are more likely than men to be prescribed opioids (54% vs. 46%) during their lifetime (Hirschtritt et al. 2017).

Men are more likely than women to die of prescription opioid use (Centers for Disease Control and Prevention 2017).

Prescription opioid deaths between 1999 and 2016 increased more for women (596%) than for men (312%) (Centers for Disease Control and Prevention 2017).

changes in the gender gap among tenth graders since 1991 were in past-month prevalence of alcohol use, binge drinking, cigarette smoking, and marijuana use (Table 36–3) (Johnston et al. 2018a, 2018b). By 2017, the prevalence of binge drinking among tenth-grade females exceeded that among their male counterparts, whereas the rate of cigarette smoking remained equivalent.

Although cigarette use among all adolescents is declining, nicotine vaping (usually via an electronic cigarette) is on the rise, with 16% of all tenth graders and 19% of all twelfth graders reporting nicotine vaping in the past 30 days in 2017, the first year in which data on nicotine vaping were collected (Johnston et al. 2018a, 2018b). Female and male tenth graders had a similar 30-day prevalence (approximately 8.1% for each gender), but nicotine vaping prevalence among twelfth graders showed a clear gender difference, with fewer females than males reporting 30-day use (8.1% vs. 14.3%) (Johnston et al. 2018b). One of the more consistent trends in tobacco use since 1991 is that compared with their male counterparts, females in grades 10 and 12 report much lower usage rates for smokeless tobacco (snuff and chew) and dissolvable tobacco as well as for large and small cigars (Johnston et al. 2018b).

Between 1991 and 2017, there was an overall downward trend in drug use other than marijuana for all tenth graders (from 12.2% in 1991 to 9.4% in 2017) and twelfth graders (from 16.2% to 13.3%) (Johnston et al. 2018b). In general, males in grades 10 and 12 report higher rates of other drug use compared with females, although females in these grades are more likely than males to report misuse of prescription drugs such as amphetamines, sedatives, and tranquilizers. One notable exception is the consistently greater annual misuse of prescription opioids by males than by females in grade 12 (Johnston et al. 2018b).

There is concern that the historical gender gap in substance use and SUDs, which has been characterized by a higher prevalence in men, is also decreasing globally (McHugh et al. 2018). Internationally, SUD epidemiological survey results vary and are influenced by culture, by policies that affect women's ability to access substances, and by the acceptability of substance use by women. The World Health Organization's World Mental Health Surveys, for example, found that the decrease of traditional gender roles (often defined by factors such as women's representation in the

TABLE 36–3. **Changes in past-month prevalence of alcohol use, binge drinking, cigarette smoking, and marijuana use among tenth graders: 1991 and 2017**

	Alcohol use		Binge drinking		Cigarette smoking		Marijuana use	
	1991	2017	1991	2017	1991	2017	1991	2017
Male	45.5%	17.1%	24.1%	9.0%	20.8%	5.0%	10.1%	15.3%
Female	40.2%	19.2%	18.1%	10.5%	20.7%	4.9%	7.3%	15.8%
Gender difference[a]	5.3%	–2.1%	6.0%	–1.5%	0.1%	0.1%	2.8%	–0.5%

[a]Negative percentage indicates that prevalence rates in females exceed those in males.
Source. Adapted from Johnston et al. 2018a, 2018b.

workforce, access to contraception, etc.) is associated with smaller male/female differences in SUDs (Seedat et al. 2009). Although variations exist across cultures, men are generally more likely than women to have access to substances, and this appears to explain most of the gender variance in substance use prevalence. When studies control for men's greater access to substances, however, the likelihood of gender differences in substance use is diminished (McHugh et al. 2018).

Course of Illness

Although women have traditionally initiated substance use at later ages than men (Greenfield et al. 2010; Keyes et al. 2010), this difference appears to be declining. One reason why this is particularly troubling is that a number of research studies have shown that women transition more rapidly from initiation of substance use to substance-related problems, and from substance-related problems to first treatment episode (Hernandez-Avila et al. 2004). This phenomenon of a more rapid progression in women from use to disorder—a compressed course of SUD—has been called the "telescoping effect" and has been demonstrated for alcohol, cocaine, marijuana, and prescription opioid use (but not for heroin) (McHugh et al. 2018). A telescoping effect for alcohol was not found in one large population-based analysis (Keyes et al. 2010). However, the telescoping effect may be less evident in population-based studies (which include women with a wide range of substance use severity) than in studies of treatment samples (which can include subsets of women who are particularly vulnerable to developing severe illness) (McHugh et al. 2018).

Biological Factors

Sex differences in the physiological effects of alcohol are well documented. Compared with men, women have lower concentrations of gastric alcohol dehydrogenase, the primary enzyme for alcohol metabolism, and a lower total percentage of body water (McHugh et al. 2018). As a result, women have higher blood alcohol levels and report greater levels of intoxication after consuming alcohol amounts equivalent to those consumed by men (McHugh et al. 2018). This higher blood alcohol level for each ounce of alcohol consumed may be one factor contributing to women's increased risk of adverse medical consequences, such as alcohol-related liver disease for any level of alcohol consumption, alcohol-induced cancers, and cardiomyopathy (Agabio et al. 2016a). Compared with women without an AUD, women with an AUD are more likely to report sexual dysfunction, irregular menses, and early menopause (Nolen-Hoeksema and Hilt 2006).

Gender and sex differences in medical consequences of use have also been documented for other substances. Among people who smoke tobacco, women have a higher risk than men of tobacco-related heart disease, lung disease, and health problems (Agabio et al. 2016a). Women with heroin dependence are at greater risk than men of contracting hepatitis C and HIV (Agabio et al. 2016a), which may be associated with the finding that women are more likely than men to inject with a previously used needle (Greenfield et al. 2010). In addition, rates of attempted suicides and overall mortality rates have been shown to be higher for women than for men with heroin dependence (Agabio et al. 2016a).

There are also gender and sex differences in the symptoms of withdrawal from specific substances. For example, in research studies, women rate nicotine withdrawal symptoms, such as anger, depression, anxiety, and cigarette craving, as being more severe than do men (Pang and Leventhal 2013; Xu et al. 2008). Concerns about weight gain and social isolation after smoking cessation are more likely to be obstacles to smoking cessation for women than for men (Greenfield et al. 2010). In a study of gender differences in cannabis withdrawal symptoms, women had higher-severity scores than did men on measures of withdrawal symptoms such as headaches, hot flashes, nausea, sleep disturbances, and mood swings (Sherman et al. 2017). In regard to substance use relapse, some studies of relapse to alcohol, cocaine, and tobacco use have shown that women are more likely than men to relapse in response to negative affect, may be more sensitive than men to drug-related cues that can trigger relapse, and have a longer period of substance use before the next quit attempt (Hudson and Stamp 2011).

Menstrual cycle phases may contribute to sex differences in the acute and long-term effects of alcohol and other drugs. For example, some studies have found that women in the follicular phase are more likely than those in the luteal phase to report drug liking and pleasant subjective effects, but other studies did not find such fluctuations across the menstrual cycle; therefore, the associations among substance craving, substance use, and menstrual cycle phase remain unclear (McHugh et al. 2018). Because of these mixed findings, the emphasis has shifted from examining the two traditional phases of the menstrual cycle to examining the fluctuating levels of ovarian hormones over the two phases, with a focus on progesterone (Allen et al. 2016). Several studies have shown that administration of oral progesterone to normally menstruating women during the follicular phase reduces craving for and the positive subjective effects of both nicotine and tobacco when compared with placebo (Peltier and Sofuoglu 2018). Additionally, studies of postpartum women treated with progesterone found lower rates of relapse to cocaine (Yonkers et al. 2014) and a greater likelihood of abstinence, a slower rate of relapse, and lower craving scores for tobacco (Forray et al. 2017). Although these results are promising, future studies of progesterone in women with SUDs will be needed to confirm these findings and to determine progesterone's effectiveness for these and other substances.

Co-Occurring Psychiatric Disorders

Gender differences in psychiatric disorders and their relationship to the onset of substance use begin to emerge during adolescence. For example, depression increases the risk of substance use in adolescent females, whereas conduct disorder and attention-deficit disorder increase the risk of substance use in adolescent males (Kuhn 2015). In one study, adolescent females were more likely to report drinking alcohol to cope with depressed mood, whereas adolescent males were more likely to report alcohol use as a way to have more fun at parties (Kuntsche and Müller 2012). Adult women with SUDs have also been shown to have a higher prevalence of depression and anxiety disorders when compared with men, and women often report using substances as a way to manage negative affective states (Greenfield et al. 2007). Co-occurring other psychiatric disorders are more frequent in treatment-seeking women with SUDs than their male counterparts, with women more likely than men to have three or more co-occurring diagnoses (Brady et al. 2009).

Trauma exposure, posttraumatic stress disorder (PTSD), and substance use are strongly associated among women. Research has shown a clear relationship between a history of trauma and the development of SUDs in women (Hien et al. 2005), and women with substance use problems are more likely than their male counterparts to report childhood sexual abuse in particular (Kuhn 2015). The development of PTSD as a result of childhood sexual trauma and other traumas is highly correlated with and often precedes the development of SUDs in women (McHugh et al. 2018). Studies have found that more than 50% of women receiving SUD treatment have histories of childhood physical or sexual abuse, and a high percentage have symptoms that meet criteria for PTSD (Brady et al. 2004; Greenfield et al. 2010). Ongoing substance use to manage symptoms of PTSD may, in turn, result in an increased risk of both experiencing sexual victimization and engaging in risky sexual behaviors (McHugh et al. 2018).

Finally, eating disorders, including anorexia nervosa, bulimia nervosa, and binge-eating disorder, are more common in women than in men in the general population and are particularly common among women with SUDs (Cohen et al. 2010). The strongest associations between SUDs and eating disorders involve bulimic behaviors, such as binge eating, purging, and laxative use (Spindler and Milos 2007). Almost one-third of women entering SUD treatment report binge eating, and women who are diagnosed with SUDs, binge-eating disorder, and PTSD have more severe clinical courses and worse treatment outcomes than women with SUDs and PTSD but no eating disorder pathology (Cohen et al. 2010). These findings highlight the importance of assessing eating disorder behaviors and symptoms, and other co-occurring psychiatric disorders, in women seeking treatment for SUDs.

Treatment

In general, women are less likely than men to seek and receive SUD treatment (Greenfield et al. 2007), a finding that is demonstrated in U.S. population–based treatment data. Although overall rates of treatment among individuals with SUDs in the United States are low, the rates are even lower among women. In 2015, for example, only 10.4% of an estimated 7.9 million women with SUDs received treatment, compared with 11.1% of men with SUDs (Center for Behavioral Health Statistics and Quality 2016). Adult women with AUD, in particular, are less likely than men with AUD to utilize SUD treatment, although this gender difference in treatment entry has not been systematically demonstrated for other substance-related disorders such as OUD and cannabis use disorder (McHugh et al. 2018). Few gender disparities have been demonstrated in the main outcomes of multisite randomized clinical trials of medication or behavioral treatments for SUDs; however, main outcome analyses rarely examine other endpoints that vary by gender, such as functional status, or they may exclude individuals with co-occurring other psychiatric disorders, which are more prevalent in women. There may also be some differences in the long-term course of recovery for women compared with men (Greenfield et al. 2007). Two studies of individuals diagnosed with AUD, for example, found that women were more likely than men to be abstinent at 7- and 16-year follow-ups (Satre et al. 2007; Timko et al. 2006) and that self-help involvement had a stronger association with decreases in drinking for women than for men (Timko et al. 2006).

Although gender itself may not predict SUD treatment outcome overall in multisite randomized clinical trials of specific behavioral or medication treatments, several gender-specific factors can affect treatment outcomes (Greenfield et al. 2007). For example, co-occurring disorders such as depression, anxiety, and PTSD, as well as a history of trauma, may disproportionately affect treatment outcomes among women because these disorders are more prevalent among women than among men. SUD treatment that takes into account gender-specific factors for women may be of greater benefit than traditional programs in improving engagement, retention, substance reduction, and other treatment outcomes.

Gender-Specific Treatment

There is converging evidence that SUD treatment that specifically addresses the needs of women is associated with higher rates of treatment completion and improved outcomes for women (Greenfield et al. 2007; Grella 2008). Women in gender-specific SUD treatment also report greater treatment satisfaction, decreased sex-role stereotyping, greater feelings of safety, greater group cohesion, and enhanced comfort and support within the treatment group (Greenfield et al. 2013). The Women's Recovery Group (WRG) was developed in response to these findings and is an empirically supported, manual-based group therapy that specifically addresses the needs of women with SUDs, including co-occurring psychiatric disorders, partners, caregiving roles, effects of substances on women's health, and trauma histories (Greenfield 2016). WRG studies demonstrated clinically meaningful decreases in substance use during and after treatment and have found that the WRG was as effective as a mixed-gender drug counseling group control condition in reducing substance use (Greenfield 2016; Greenfield et al. 2014). Additionally, women in the WRG reported that communication among their same-gender peers felt safer and more supported and that they were able to discuss important topics relevant to their recovery such as sexuality, trauma histories, partners, and caregiving roles, in a way that was not possible in the mixed-gender group (Greenfield et al. 2013). Furthermore, women who experienced the greatest level of support, as measured by group affiliation, had better clinical outcomes at 6 months posttreatment compared with women who experienced lower group affiliation. Finally, the best 6-month outcomes were among those women exposed to the highest group affiliation in the WRG group compared with women in the mixed-gender control group (Valeri et al. 2018).

In one large multisite trial, women receiving Seeking Safety, a manualized cognitive-behavioral group therapy for individuals with co-occurring PTSD and SUDs (Najavits 2002), had significant reductions in PTSD and substance use, but these were not reliably different from those of women in the control group (Hien et al. 2009). However, another analysis of these data demonstrated that women in the Seeking Safety group also had more rapid reductions in PTSD severity, which were further associated with significant reductions in substance use (Morgan-Lopez et al. 2014). These studies highlight the importance of treatments tailored to the specific clinical needs of women with SUDs.

The number of women with substance use and other psychiatric disorders who are in the U.S. correctional system has continued to rise, and there is emerging awareness of the need for gender-responsive programming for this population (Covington and Bloom 2007). A gender-responsive treatment (GRT) program based on curricula developed by Covington was implemented within this population, with 28 modules covering a range of topics of specific relevance to women's recovery, such as trauma. The standard therapeutic community (TC) curriculum focuses on positive values and socialization but does not address gender- or trauma-related issues. In an efficacy trial, incarcerated women (*N*=55) were randomly assigned to receive either GRT or TC. GRT participants had significantly greater reductions in drug use, were more likely to remain in aftercare, and were less likely to be reincarcerated when compared with TC participants (Messina et al. 2010).

Pharmacotherapy

A growing body of literature has reported gender differences in the response to medications approved for the treatment of SUDs. These gender differences are especially striking in regard to pharmacotherapies for smoking cessation. For example, bupropion, an antidepressant and smoking cessation aid, is more effective in women than in men, whereas nicotine replacement therapies (NRTs) are more effective in men (Perkins 2001). More recent studies demonstrated that varenicline, a selective nicotinic receptor partial agonist, was significantly more effective for smoking cessation than nicotine transdermal patch and bupropion for women than for men both in clinical trials (Smith et al. 2016) and in studies of real-world effectiveness (Smith et al. 2017; Walker et al. 2016). One study showed that varenicline was 46% more efficacious in women than in men at end of treatment and 34% more efficacious at 6 months posttreatment (McKee et al. 2016). Despite these findings, in clinical practice women are less likely than men to be prescribed varenicline, a circumstance that may be related to lack of clinician awareness or possibly to concerns about varenicline use during pregnancy (Walker et al. 2016).

Gender differences in treatment response have also been shown for medications used to treat OUD and AUD. When men and women are given the same medication dose of buprenorphine, a μ-opioid receptor partial agonist used to treat OUD, women attain significantly higher plasma levels (Moody et al. 2011). Additionally, compared with men, women treated with naltrexone, a μ-opioid receptor antagonist used to treat both OUD and AUD, are more likely to experience certain medication-induced side effects (e.g., nausea) and to experience greater side-effect sensitivity during the luteal phase than the follicular phase of the menstrual cycle (Roche and King 2015). Gender differences in the safety and efficacy of disulfiram for the treatment of AUD have not been evaluated because insufficient numbers of women entered these clinical trials (Agabio et al. 2016b). Although adequate numbers of women were recruited for studies of acamprosate and nalmefene, two other medications used to treat AUD, no gender differences in the safety and efficacy of these medications have been found (Agabio et al. 2016b).

In several off-label trials of medications for the treatment of cocaine and cannabis use disorders, there have been a few examples of worse outcomes among women treated with medication compared with placebo. For example, women with cocaine dependence who were treated with buspirone had increased cocaine use compared with women in the placebo group (Winhusen et al. 2014), and buspirone treatment for women with cannabis dependence was associated with fewer cannabinoid-negative urines when compared with placebo (McRae-Clark et al. 2015). Similarly, a placebo-controlled trial of vilazodone found that women in the medication group were more likely than placebo-treated women to have cannabinoid-positive urine tests and higher creatinine-adjusted cannabinoid levels (McRae-Clark et al. 2016). It should be noted that these medications had no significant effects on cocaine and cannabis use in the full sample of men and women.

Barriers to Treatment

Despite the availability of effective treatments for women with SUDs, women frequently encounter barriers to accessing and completing treatment (Greenfield 2016). Women often cite feelings of shame and embarrassment and intense stigma as impediments to seeking SUD treatment. Women may also attribute their substance use to family or personal problems or to mood and anxiety symptoms and seek care for these other problems, contributing to the lack of detection and treatment of their substance use problem. Another barrier to treatment for women with SUDs is that their families and partners may not support their actively seeking or engaging in treatment. Data from studies of heterosexual women have shown that a male partner's substance use may also directly interfere with a woman's ability to seek treatment. In addition, women's caregiving roles in families can interfere with their ability to seek and engage in treatment. Other barriers to treatment for women include lack of financial resources for treatment, lack of child or elder care, lack of information about treatment options and their efficacy, and lack of reliable transportation, as well as the need for integrated treatment of co-occurring trauma and psychiatric disorders, and for specialized treatment services during pregnancy and the perinatal period. It is crucial for treatment programs to recognize these barriers and to work with women to overcome them.

Pregnancy and the Perinatal Period

Screening and Assessment for Substance Use During Pregnancy

In the 2017 National Survey on Drug Use and Health, 14.7% of pregnant women reported past-month use of tobacco, 11.5% alcohol, and 8.5% an illicit drug (Substance Abuse and Mental Health Services Administration 2018b). Early identification of SUDs in pregnant women is vital to improving the health and well-being of mothers and their infants and children (ACOG Committee on Health Care for Underserved Women and American Society of Addiction Medicine 2012). Professional health organizations recommend screening for SUDs at the initial prenatal care visit and at several points throughout the prenatal care schedule to facilitate early identification of SUDs and implementation of prenatal and substance abuse treatment.

A number of screening instruments have been validated for the detection of substance use in pregnant women. These include the Substance Use Risk Profile of Pregnancy (SURP-P) (Knight et al. 2003), the Wayne Indirect Drug Use Questionnaire (WIDUS) (Beatty et al. 2014), the CRAFFT Questionnaire (Chang et al. 2011), and the 5Ps Prenatal Substance Abuse Screen for Alcohol and Drugs Questionnaire (Watson et al. 2003). The T-ACE (Sokol et al. 1989) and the TWEAK (Russell et al. 1996) are two screening instruments that can help identify alcohol use during pregnancy.

Following screening and identification of perinatal use or misuse of tobacco, alcohol, prescription medications, or illicit substances, providers play a vital role in counseling women on the importance of avoiding substances, in supporting their efforts to implement behavioral change, and in referring pregnant women with SUDs to specialized treatment. Although Screening, Brief Intervention, and Referral to Treatment (SBIRT) is normally clinician delivered, a recent randomized controlled trial (RCT) demonstrated that computer-based delivery of SBIRT resulted in a significant decrease in days of primary substance use compared with enhanced usual care among pregnant and nonpregnant women receiving care in a reproductive clinic (Martino et al. 2018).

Pregnancy represents an ideal time for women to enter treatment for any SUD. Pregnant women can obtain health insurance through Medicaid programs because prenatal care is considered an essential benefit, and women are often motivated toward treatment in an effort to invest in the health and well-being of their future children (Davis and Yonkers 2012). Comprehensive prenatal and SUD treatment for pregnant women not only reduces maternal morbidity and mortality but also results in fewer deliveries of preterm, small-for-gestational-age, and low-birthweight infants (Pinto et al. 2010). Unfortunately, there is a dearth of comprehensive treatment programs for pregnant women with SUDs (Terplan et al. 2015a). It is important for providers to consider barriers to care, including stigma, guilt, and shame, for pregnant women with SUDs (Jones et al. 2014). Providers can help reduce these sources of stress by projecting a caring and nonjudgmental attitude that can ultimately build trust and rapport as well as facilitate effective communication. Fear of child welfare consequences is also a potent barrier to care for this population, and providers need to be aware of their states' reporting requirements and the legal consequences of perinatal substance use so that women are informed and can work collaboratively with their providers to ensure the best possible outcomes for their infants (Jones et al. 2014).

A thorough patient history is the gold standard for diagnosing SUDs. For each substance of use identified, it is important to determine the extent of the use (e.g., duration and frequency of use, route of administration) and the sources of financial support for the use in order to identify high-risk behaviors (e.g., theft, prostitution, drugs for sex) that need also to be addressed (Jones et al. 2014). Screening for trauma and comorbid mental problems is critical to the assessment and treatment of perinatal SUDs. Urine drug screens have limited utility in the diagnosis of SUDs, have a high rate of false positives (5%), and may not detect semisynthetic opioids (White and Black 2007).

Management of Pregnant Patients With Substance Use Disorders

As we discuss in this section, a wide variety of behavioral interventions have been evaluated for the reduction of perinatal substance use and should be included as part of an overall treatment plan. Table 36–4 summarizes the behavioral therapies and their benefits for reducing perinatal substance use.

Tobacco

The harms of smoking for the mother, the fetus, and the newborn are well established. Smoking during pregnancy has been associated with increased risk for ectopic pregnancy, miscarriage, placental abruption, low birth weight, prematurity, and infant mortality (Forray 2016). Secondhand smoke has also been associated with adverse effects on the newborn, including increased risks for respiratory and ear infections, cognitive impairments, behavioral problems, and sudden infant death syndrome (Forray 2016).

In addition to effective behavioral treatments (see Table 36–4), pharmacotherapies for nicotine cessation for nonpregnant populations include NRT, bupropion, varenicline, and electronic nicotine delivery systems (ENDS). No studies to date have evaluated the efficacy of varenicline or ENDS for pregnant women with nicotine use disorder, and only one small study has evaluated bupropion. In RCTs, NRT has been found to be no more effective than placebo for smoking cessation in pregnant women (Coleman et al. 2015).

Given the lack of efficacy of NRT in reducing perinatal nicotine use, NRT is not routinely recommended for pregnant women with nicotine use disorder. However, women with a history of being able to abstain from tobacco use with NRT may want to consider the use of NRT during pregnancy after carefully weighing the risks of continued nicotine use versus the use of NRT.

Alcohol

Of all prenatal substance exposures, exposure to alcohol has the most well-established adverse fetal and child health effects. It is well known that alcohol use during pregnancy is associated with fetal alcohol syndrome (FAS), characterized by growth retardation, characteristic facial features, and central nervous system problems (Pruett et al. 2013). Considered one of the most common and preventable causes of birth defects, FAS causes 5,000–12,000 new cases of intellectual disability in the United

TABLE 36–4. **Behavioral interventions for the reduction of perinatal substance use**

Targeted substance	Behavioral therapy	Summary of benefit
Tobacco	Contingency management, motivational interviewing, and psychoeducation	Modest benefit with all modalities (Levitt et al. 2007), with contingency management being the most beneficial (Chamberlain et al. 2013; Ierfino et al. 2015)
Alcohol	Motivational enhancement therapy, brief psychodynamic psychotherapy, interpersonal psychotherapy, educational interventions, family-focused therapy, professional group education, self-help, and cognitive-behavioral therapy	Modest benefit with all modalities, but no modality is clearly more effective than another (Stade et al. 2009)
Cannabis	Motivational interviewing, cognitive-behavioral therapy, and contingency management	Evaluated in adult nonpregnant women with some benefit (Forray 2016)
Opioids	Motivational interviewing, cognitive-behavioral therapy, and contingency management	Modest benefit with all modalities, with contingency management being the most beneficial (Terplan et al. 2015b)
Stimulants	Motivational interviewing, cognitive-behavioral therapy, and contingency management	Modest benefit with all modalities, with contingency management being the most beneficial (Terplan et al. 2015b)

States annually (Pruett et al. 2013). The neurobehavioral sequelae of FAS are well characterized in the *Diagnostic and Statistical Manual of Mental Disorders*, 5th Edition (DSM-5), and are described as a neurodevelopmental disorder associated with prenatal alcohol exposure (American Psychiatric Association 2013, p. 86). The neurobehavioral sequelae of FAS manifest during childhood and cause significant distress or impairment in multiple areas of functioning. No amount of alcohol use is considered safe during pregnancy, because evidence for the safety of even low to moderate alcohol use in pregnancy is inconclusive (Henderson et al. 2007).

A wide variety of behavioral interventions have been evaluated for the reduction of alcohol use in pregnancy, including motivational enhancement therapy, brief psychodynamic psychotherapy, interpersonal psychotherapy, educational interventions, family-focused therapy, professional group education, self-help, and cognitive-behavioral therapy (DeVido et al. 2015). The majority of studies have demonstrated some benefit for these interventions, including increased abstinence and/or reduction in alcohol consumption, among pregnant women (Stade et al. 2009).

The U.S. Food and Drug Administration (FDA) has approved three medications—naltrexone, disulfiram, and acamprosate—for the treatment of AUD in nonpregnant populations. To our knowledge, there are no RCTs evaluating the efficacy of pharmacological interventions for the treatment of perinatal AUD. Preclinical data suggest that perinatal use of the opioid receptor blocker naltrexone may lead to long-term alterations in the μ-opioid receptor in the developing fetus (Zagon et al. 1998), but there are not adequate studies examining the reproductive effects and safety of this drug in pregnant women in general or in pregnant women with AUD. The safety of disulfiram during pregnancy has likewise not been established. Furthermore, the maternal, fetal, and obstetric effects of a disulfiram–alcohol reaction are unknown. Similarly, the safety of acamprosate in pregnancy has not been established in preclinical and clinical studies.

Pharmacological treatments for perinatal AUD are not routinely recommended due to the paucity of efficacy and safety data. To our knowledge, no studies to date have systematically examined the effects of perinatal alcohol withdrawal or of benzodiazepine treatment for perinatal alcohol withdrawal. The literature examining the risks of benzodiazepine use during pregnancy shows inconsistent associations with fetal malformations (DeVido et al. 2015). Recent data in this area, however, are more reassuring and demonstrate that prospective cohort studies are less likely than case–control studies to show an association between fetal malformations and benzodiazepine use, likely due to recall bias associated with case–control studies (DeVido et al. 2015). Long-term use of benzodiazepines during pregnancy, particularly at higher dosages, is associated with benzodiazepine withdrawal syndrome in the newborn (DeVido et al. 2015). Clinicians and patients need to weigh the risks of benzodiazepine exposure against the risks of alcohol withdrawal or continued alcohol use during pregnancy.

Cannabis

The prevalence of cannabis use during pregnancy is increasing, particularly among young adult women (Brown et al. 2017). Studies evaluating the obstetric risks and long-term outcomes associated with cannabis use during pregnancy have included four systematic reviews and meta-analyses and four published prospective cohort studies (Mark and Terplan 2017). Although these studies have limitations, collectively the data support an association between perinatal cannabis use and slightly lower birth weights, increased rates of neonatal intensive care unit admissions, and potential adverse effects on executive functioning in the child (Mark and Terplan 2017). Importantly, the reduced birth weight associated with cannabis use is not characterized as "low birth weight," and its clinical significance is unclear. It is also unknown whether the executive function effects associated with cannabis are a direct result of perinatal cannabis exposure or are moderated by environment factors. Future prospective studies are needed to examine cannabis exposure in pregnancy, particularly with respect to timing and amount of exposure and type of cannabis used. Providers are encouraged to screen for cannabis use in pregnant patients, to inform women of the known risks associated with perinatal marijuana use, and to provide evidence-based psychotherapy to support reduction of perinatal cannabis use (Mark and Terplan 2017).

Opioids

Perinatal OUD is associated with substantial maternal, fetal, and newborn risks. It is associated with the risk of unintentional overdose and death, as seen in the general population, but is additionally associated with considerable maternal, obstetric, fetal, and newborn morbidity and mortality, including a 4.6-fold increased risk for maternal death at delivery (Maeda et al. 2014). A well-known consequence of opioid use during pregnancy is the newborn opioid withdrawal syndrome, also known as neonatal abstinence syndrome, with 60% of newborns born to pregnant women with OUD exhibiting withdrawal following delivery (Patrick et al. 2012). The incidence of newborn opioid withdrawal syndrome in the United States increased from 1.2 per 1,000 hospital births in 2000 to 8 per 1,000 hospital births in 2014 (Patrick et al. 2015).

The standard of care for the treatment of perinatal OUD includes pharmacotherapy with either methadone or buprenorphine (Substance Abuse and Mental Health Services Administration 2018a) as part of a comprehensive treatment program that provides prenatal care and psychological interventions for relapse prevention. Pharmacotherapy such as methadone has been the recommended standard of care since the early 1990s (U.S. Department of Health and Human Services 1997), and more recent studies support buprenorphine as another treatment option (Jones et al. 2010). The American College of Obstetricians and Gynecologists recommends the use of methadone or buprenorphine as part of the standard of care for pregnant women with OUD (ACOG Committee on Health Care for Underserved Women and American Society of Addiction Medicine 2012). A Cochrane review of studies comparing the efficacy of methadone versus buprenorphine for the treatment of perinatal OUD did not conclude that one pharmacotherapy is superior to the other (Minozzi et al. 2013). Therefore, selection of methadone or buprenorphine is largely driven by patient preference, feasibility, and prior treatment response. Pregnant women should be prescribed naloxone, and partners and family members should be educated on the administration of this drug in the context of a life-threatening overdose.

Medication-assisted withdrawal, or opioid taper or detoxification, is not recommended during pregnancy. In the largest systematic review to date, which involved 1,126 pregnant women with OUD who underwent opioid detoxification, rates of successful detoxification (9%–100%) and illicit drug use (0%–100%) were widely variable (Terplan et al. 2018). Prior work suggested that rates of relapse following opioid detoxification in pregnancy are likely high. Similarly, the risks of fetal and newborn complications associated with opioid withdrawal during pregnancy are largely unknown due to the significant bias and poor to fair quality of prior studies (Terplan et al. 2018). Despite the recommendation against medication-assisted withdrawal, women may still want to pursue this treatment approach in the hope of mitigating the risk of newborn opioid withdrawal syndrome. So that women can make an informed treatment choice, it is critical that providers present balanced information about the risks of medication-assisted withdrawal for the pregnant woman, including the risks of relapse to opioids and the risks of methadone or buprenorphine stabilization and treatment. Untreated OUD in pregnancy carries with it the risks associated with ongoing use of opioids, including intoxication and withdrawal cycles; the risks of infection through infected needles or unprotected sexual encounters; and the risk of poor adherence to recommended prenatal care. A shared decision-making tool is available to assist patients and providers in this treatment choice (Guille et al. 2019).

Stimulants

The use of stimulants such as cocaine and methamphetamine during pregnancy has been associated with a number of adverse obstetric and birth outcomes. For example, perinatal cocaine use has been associated with premature rupture of membranes, placental abruption, prematurity, and low birth weight (Addis et al. 2001; Gouin et al. 2011). Similarly, perinatal methamphetamine use has been associated with gestational hypertension, preeclampsia, low birth weight, prematurity, and intrauterine fetal demise (Wright et al. 2015). Research findings on the long-term effects of cocaine or methamphetamine use have been inconsistent, with some studies finding no long-term effects of cocaine use during pregnancy (Frank et al. 2001) and others finding an association with later language, motor, or cognitive difficulties (Bandstra et al. 2004; Chaplin et al. 2010). Methamphetamine use during pregnancy has been associated with developmental and behavioral effects in the growing child; however, many of these studies did not control for important postnatal environmental factors that are associated with substance use and may negatively impact child development (Forray 2016).

Postnatal Care of Mother–Infant Dyad

The postnatal period is highly demanding and challenging for every parent. Women with SUDs have additional challenges that can make this time even more stressful, including lack of social support, unstable housing, financial difficulties, psychiatric comorbidities, history of early childhood or past trauma, and/or current interpersonal violence. Also, in many states, Medicaid insurance will terminate during the postpartum period, rendering women without other insurance unable to access ongoing SUD treatment. Stressful life events are one of the greatest risk factors for relapse to substance use among women, and relapse adds to the risk of interruption of the mother–infant dyad. These potential stressors are apparent during pregnancy and should prompt implementation of a supportive, dyadic-centered treatment plan prior to delivery; the clinician should devise a plan for continuing treatment postpartum and for managing prescription pain medications routinely prescribed at the time of delivery. Plans for the immediate postpartum period should address medical comorbidities, such as hepatitis C, that cannot be addressed during pregnancy. It is highly encouraged that women in recovery breast-feed their infants. Breast feeding has significant benefits for both mother and newborn, has been shown to reduce the need for newborn opioid withdrawal treatment (Welle-Strand et al. 2013), and further supports the need for dyadic-centered newborn services.

Conclusion

There are many domains with important sex and gender differences that affect SUDs; examples include epidemiology; biological, metabolic, and physiological responses to substances; health effects; co-occurring other psychiatric disorders; and gender-specific factors that affect access to and outcomes of treatment. Among women with SUDs, important differences in SUD craving, use, and treatment outcome can occur with varying levels of ovarian hormones. For women with SUDs, pregnancy and the perinatal period require special attention to optimize maternal and neonatal outcomes.

References

ACOG Committee on Health Care for Underserved Women, American Society of Addiction Medicine: ACOG Committee Opinion No. 524: Opioid abuse, dependence, and addiction in pregnancy. Obstet Gynecol 119(5):1070–1076, 2012 22525931

Addis A, Moretti ME, Ahmed Syed F, et al: Fetal effects of cocaine: an updated meta-analysis. Reprod Toxicol 15(4):341–369, 2001 11489591

Agabio R, Campesi I, Pisanu C, et al: Sex differences in substance use disorders: focus on side effects. Addict Biol 21(5):1030–1042, 2016a 27001402

Agabio R, Pani PP, Preti A, et al: Efficacy of medications approved for the treatment of alcohol dependence and alcohol withdrawal syndrome in female patients: a descriptive review. Eur Addict Res 22(1):1–16, 2016b 26314552

Allen AM, McRae-Clark AL, Carlson S, et al: Determining menstrual phase in human biobehavioral research: a review with recommendations. Exp Clin Psychopharmacol 24(1):1–11, 2016 26570992

American Psychiatric Association: Diagnostic and Statistical Manual of Mental Disorders, 5th Edition. Arlington, VA, American Psychiatric Association, 2013

Bandstra ES, Vogel AL, Morrow CE, et al: Severity of prenatal cocaine exposure and child language functioning through age seven years: a longitudinal latent growth curve analysis. Subst Use Misuse 39(1):25–59, 2004 15002943

Beatty JR, Chase SK, Ondersma SJ: A randomized study of the effect of anonymity, quasi-anonymity, and Certificates of Confidentiality on postpartum women's disclosure of sensitive information. Drug Alcohol Depend 134:280–284, 2014 24246900

Brady KT, Back SE, Coffey SF: Substance abuse and posttraumatic stress disorder. Current Directions in Psychological Science 13(5):206–209, 2004. Available at: https://journals.sagepub.com/doi/10.1111/j.0963-7214.2004.00309.x. Accessed February 6, 2020.

Brady KT, Back SE, Greenfield SF (eds): Women and Addiction: A Comprehensive Handbook. New York, Guilford, 2009

Brown QL, Sarvet AL, Shmulewitz D, et al: Trends in marijuana use among pregnant and non-pregnant reproductive-aged women, 2002–2014. JAMA 317(2):207–209, 2017 27992619

Center for Behavioral Health Statistics and Quality: Key Substance Use and Mental Health Indicators in the United States: Results From the 2015 National Survey on Drug Use and Health (HHS Publ No SMA-16-4984, NSUH Series H-51). 2016. Available at: https://www.samhsa.gov/data/sites/default/files/NSDUH-FFR1-2015/NSDUH-FFR1-2015/NSDUH-FFR1-2015.htm. Accessed December 27, 2019.

Centers for Disease Control and Prevention: Vital signs: binge drinking among women and high school girls—United States, 2011. MMWR Morb Mortal Wkly Rep 62(1):9–13, 2013 23302817

Centers for Disease Control and Prevention: Prescription Painkiller Overdoses: A Growing Epidemic Especially Among Women. Vital Signs, 2017. Available at: https://www.cdc.gov/vitalsigns/prescriptionpainkilleroverdoses/index.html. Accessed December 27, 2019.

Chamberlain C, O'Mara-Eves A, Oliver S, et al: Psychosocial interventions for supporting women to stop smoking in pregnancy. Cochrane Database Syst Rev (10):CD001055, 2013 24154953

Chang G, Orav EJ, Jones JA, et al: Self-reported alcohol and drug use in pregnant young women: a pilot study of associated factors and identification. J Addict Med 5(3):221–226, 2011 21844837

Chaplin TM, Freiburger MB, Mayes LC, et al: Prenatal cocaine exposure, gender, and adolescent stress response: a prospective longitudinal study. Neurotoxicol Teratol 32(6):595–604, 2010 20826209

Cicero TJ, Ellis MS, Surratt HL, et al: The changing face of heroin use in the United States: a retrospective analysis of the past 50 years. JAMA Psychiatry 71(7):821–826, 2014 24871348

Cohen LR, Greenfield SF, Gordon S, et al: Survey of eating disorder symptoms among women in treatment for substance abuse. Am J Addict 19(3):245–251, 2010 20525031

Coleman T, Chamberlain C, Davey MA, et al: Pharmacological interventions for promoting smoking cessation during pregnancy. Cochrane Database Syst Rev (12):CD010078, 2015 26690977

Covington SS, Bloom BE: Gender responsive treatment and services in correctional settings. Women and Therapy 29(3–4):9–33, 2007. Available at: https://www.tandfonline.com/doi/abs/10.1300/J015v29n03_02. Accessed February 6, 2020.

Davis KJ, Yonkers KA: Making lemonade out of lemons: a case report and literature review of external pressure as an intervention with pregnant and parenting substance-using women. J Clin Psychiatry 73(1):51–56, 2012 22316576

DeVido J, Bogunovic O, Weiss RD: Alcohol use disorders in pregnancy. Harv Rev Psychiatry 23(2):112–121, 2015 25747924

Doycheva I, Watt KD, Rifai G, et al: Increasing burden of chronic liver disease among adolescents and young adults in the USA: a silent epidemic. Dig Dis Sci 62(5):1373–1380, 2017 28194666

Forray A: Substance use during pregnancy. F1000Res 5:F1000 Faculty Rev-887, 2016 27239283

Forray A, Gilstad-Hayden K, Suppies C, et al: Progesterone for smoking relapse prevention following delivery: a pilot, randomized, double-blind study. Psychoneuroendocrinology 86:96–103, 2017 28926762

Frank DA, Augustyn M, Knight WG, et al: Growth, development, and behavior in early childhood following prenatal cocaine exposure: a systematic review. JAMA 285(12):1613–1625, 2001 11268270

Gouin K, Murphy K, Shah PS, et al: Effects of cocaine use during pregnancy on low birthweight and preterm birth: systematic review and metaanalyses. Am J Obstet Gynecol 204(4):340.e1–340.e12, 2011 21257143

Grant BF, Chou SP, Saha TD, et al: Prevalence of 12-month alcohol use, high-risk drinking, and DSM-IV alcohol use disorder in the United States, 2001–2002 to 2012–2013: results from the National Epidemiologic Survey on Alcohol and Related Conditions. JAMA Psychiatry 74(9):911–923, 2017 28793133

Greenfield SF: Treating Women With Substance Use Disorders: The Women's Recovery Group Manual. New York, Guilford, 2016

Greenfield SF, Brooks AJ, Gordon SM, et al: Substance abuse treatment entry, retention, and outcome in women: a review of the literature. Drug Alcohol Depend 86(1):1–21, 2007 16759822

Greenfield SF, Back SE, Lawson K, Brady KT: Substance abuse in women. Psychiatr Clin North Am 33(2):339–355, 2010 20385341

Greenfield SF, Cummings AM, Kuper LE, et al: A qualitative analysis of women's experiences in single-gender versus mixed-gender substance abuse group therapy. Subst Use Misuse 48(9):750–760, 2013 23607675

Greenfield SF, Sugarman DE, Freid CM, et al: Group therapy for women with substance use disorders: results from the Women's Recovery Group Study. Drug Alcohol Depend 142:245–253, 2014 25042759

Grella CE: From generic to gender-responsive treatment: changes in social policies, treatment services, and outcomes of women in substance abuse treatment. J Psychoactive Drugs 40 (suppl 5):327–343, 2008 19256044

Grucza RA, Bucholz KK, Rice JP, Bierut LJ: Secular trends in the lifetime prevalence of alcohol dependence in the United States: a re-evaluation. Alcohol Clin Exp Res 32(5):763–770, 2008 18336633

Guille C, Jones HE, Abuhamad A, et al: Shared decision-making tool for treatment of perinatal opioid use disorder. Psychiatric Research and Clinical Practice 1(1):27–31, 2019. Available at: https://prcp.psychiatryonline.org/doi/10.1176/appi.prcp.20180004. Accessed February 6, 2020.

Henderson J, Gray R, Brocklehurst P: Systematic review of effects of low-moderate prenatal alcohol exposure on pregnancy outcome. BJOG 114(3):243–252, 2007 17233797

Hernandez-Avila CA, Rounsaville BJ, Kranzler HR: Opioid-, cannabis- and alcohol-dependent women show more rapid progression to substance abuse treatment. Drug Alcohol Depend 74(3):265–272, 2004 15194204

Hien D, Cohen L, Campbell A: Is traumatic stress a vulnerability factor for women with substance use disorders? Clin Psychol Rev 25(6):813–823, 2005 15967556

Hien DA, Wells EA, Jiang H, et al: Multisite randomized trial of behavioral interventions for women with co-occurring PTSD and substance use disorders. J Consult Clin Psychol 77(4):607–619, 2009 19634955

Hirschtritt ME, Delucchi KL, Olfson M: Outpatient, combined use of opioid and benzodiazepine medications in the United States, 1993–2014. Prev Med Rep 9:49–54, 2017 29340270

Hudson A, Stamp JA: Ovarian hormones and propensity to drug relapse: a review. Neurosci Biobehav Rev 35(3):427–436, 2011 20488201

Ierfino D, Mantzari E, Hirst J, et al: Financial incentives for smoking cessation in pregnancy: a single-arm intervention study assessing cessation and gaming. Addiction 110(4):680–688, 2015 25727238

John WS, Wu LT: Trends and correlates of cocaine use and cocaine use disorder in the United States from 2011 to 2015. Drug Alcohol Depend 180:376–384, 2017 28961544

Johnston LD, Miech RA, O'Malley PM, et al: Demographic Subgroup Trends Among Adolescents in the Use of Various Licit and Illicit Drugs, 1975–2017 (Monitoring for the Future Occasional Paper No. 90). Ann Arbor, MI, University of Michigan, 2018a

Johnston LD, Miech RA, O'Malley PM, et al: Monitoring for the Future, National Survey Results on Drug Use 1975–2017: 2017 Overview, Key Findings on Adolescent Drug Use. Ann Arbor, MI, University of Michigan, 2018b

Jones HE, Kaltenbach K, Heil SH, et al: Neonatal abstinence syndrome after methadone or buprenorphine exposure. N Engl J Med 363(24):2320–2331, 2010 21142534

Jones HE, Deppen K, Hudak ML, et al: Clinical care for opioid-using pregnant and postpartum women: the role of obstetric providers. Am J Obstet Gynecol 210(4):302–310, 2014 24120973

Keyes KM, Martins SS, Blanco C, et al: Telescoping and gender differences in alcohol dependence: new evidence from two national surveys. Am J Psychiatry 167(8):969–976, 2010 20439391

Knight JR, Sherritt L, Harris SK, et al: Validity of brief alcohol screening tests among adolescents: a comparison of the AUDIT, POSIT, CAGE, and CRAFFT. Alcohol Clin Exp Res 27(1):67–73, 2003 12544008

Kuhn C: Emergence of sex differences in the development of substance use and abuse during adolescence. Pharmacol Ther 153:55–78, 2015 26049025

Kuntsche E, Müller S: Why do young people start drinking? Motives for first-time alcohol consumption and links to risky drinking in early adolescence. Eur Addict Res 18(1):34–39, 2012 22142752

Levitt C, Shaw E, Wong S, et al: Systematic review of the literature on postpartum care: effectiveness of interventions for smoking relapse prevention, cessation, and reduction in postpartum women. Birth 34(4):341–347, 2007 18021150

Maeda A, Bateman BT, Clancy CR, et al: Opioid abuse and dependence during pregnancy: temporal trends and obstetrical outcomes. Anesthesiology 121(6):1158–1165, 2014 25405293

Mark K, Terplan M: Cannabis and pregnancy: maternal child health implications during a period of drug policy liberalization. Prev Med 104:46–49, 2017 28528172

Marsh JC, Park K, Lin YA, et al: Gender differences in trends for heroin use and nonmedical prescription opioid use, 2007–2014. J Subst Abuse Treat 87:79–85, 2018 29433788

Martino S, Ondersma SJ, Forray A, et al: A randomized controlled trial of screening and brief interventions for substance misuse in reproductive health. Am J Obstet Gynecol 218(3):322.e1–322.e12, 2018 29247636

McHugh RK, Votaw VR, Sugarman DE, et al: Sex and gender differences in substance use disorders. Clin Psychol Rev 66:12–23, 2018 29174306

McKee SA, Smith PH, Kaufman M, et al: Sex differences in varenicline efficacy for smoking cessation: a meta-analysis. Nicotine Tob Res 18(5):1002–1011, 2016 26446070

McRae-Clark AL, Baker NL, Gray KM, et al: Buspirone treatment of cannabis dependence: a randomized, placebo-controlled trial. Drug Alcohol Depend 156:29–37, 2015 26386827

McRae-Clark AL, Baker NL, Gray KM, et al: Vilazodone for cannabis dependence: a randomized, controlled pilot trial. Am J Addict 25(1):69–75, 2016 26685701

Messina N, Grella CE, Cartier J, et al: A randomized experimental study of gender-responsive substance abuse treatment for women in prison. J Subst Abuse Treat 38(2):97–107, 2010 20015605

Minozzi S, Amato L, Bellisario C, et al: Maintenance agonist treatments for opiate-dependent pregnant women. Cochrane Database Syst Rev (12):CD006318, 2013 24366859

Moody DE, Fang WB, Morrison J, et al: Gender differences in pharmacokinetics of maintenance dosed buprenorphine. Drug Alcohol Depend 118(2–3):479–483, 2011 21515002

Morgan-Lopez AA, Saavedra LM, Hien DA, et al: Indirect effects of 12-session seeking safety on substance use outcomes: overall and attendance class-specific effects. Am J Addict 23(3):218–225, 2014 24724878

Najavits LM: Seeking Safety: A Treatment Manual for PTSD and Substance Abuse. New York, Guilford, 2002

National Institutes of Health: Sex and Gender. Office of Research on Women's Health, 2019. Available at: https://orwh.od.nih.gov/sex-gender. Accessed December 27, 2019.

Nolen-Hoeksema S, Hilt L: Possible contributors to the gender differences in alcohol use and problems. J Gen Psychol 133(4):357–374, 2006 17128956

Pang RD, Leventhal AM: Sex differences in negative affect and lapse behavior during acute tobacco abstinence: a laboratory study. Exp Clin Psychopharmacol 21(4):269–276, 2013 23834551

Patrick SW, Schumacher RE, Benneyworth BD, et al: Neonatal abstinence syndrome and associated health care expenditures: United States, 2000–2009. JAMA 307(18):1934–1940, 2012 22546608

Patrick SW, Davis MM, Lehman CU, et al: Increasing incidence and geographic distribution of neonatal abstinence syndrome: United States 2009 to 2012. J Perinatol 35(8):667, 2015 26219703

Peltier MR, Sofuoglu M: Role of exogenous progesterone in the treatment of men and women with substance use disorders: a narrative review. CNS Drugs 32(5):421–435, 2018 29761343

Perkins KA: Smoking cessation in women. Special considerations. CNS Drugs 15(5):391–411, 2001 11475944

Pinto SM, Dodd S, Walkinshaw SA, et al: Substance abuse during pregnancy: effect on pregnancy outcomes. Eur J Obstet Gynecol Reprod Biol 150(2):137–141, 2010 20227162

Pruett D, Waterman EH, Caughey AB: Fetal alcohol exposure: consequences, diagnosis, and treatment. Obstet Gynecol Surv 68(1):62–69, 2013 23322082

Roche DJ, King AC: Sex differences in acute hormonal and subjective response to naltrexone: the impact of menstrual cycle phase. Psychoneuroendocrinology 52:59–71, 2015 25459893

Russell M, Martier SS, Sokol RJ, et al: Detecting risk drinking during pregnancy: a comparison of four screening questionnaires. Am J Public Health 86(10):1435–1439, 1996 8876514

Satre DD, Blow FC, Chi FW, et al: Gender differences in seven-year alcohol and drug treatment outcomes among older adults. Am J Addict 16(3):216–221, 2007 17612826

Seedat S, Scott KM, Angermeyer MC, et al: Cross-national associations between gender and mental disorders in the World Health Organization World Mental Health Surveys. Arch Gen Psychiatry 66(7):785–795, 2009 19581570

Sherman BJ, McRae-Clark AL, Baker NL, et al: Gender differences among treatment-seeking adults with cannabis use disorder: clinical profiles of women and men enrolled in the Achieving Cannabis Cessation–Evaluating N-acetylcysteine Treatment (ACCENT) study. Am J Addict 26(2):136–144, 2017 28152236

Smith PH, Bessette AJ, Weinberger AH, et al: Sex/gender differences in smoking cessation: a review. Prev Med 92:135–140, 2016 27471021

Smith PH, Zhang J, Weinberger AH, et al: Gender differences in the real-world effectiveness of smoking cessation medications: findings from the 2010–2011 Tobacco Use Supplement to the Current Population Survey. Drug Alcohol Depend 178:485–491, 2017 28715776

Sokol RJ, Martier SS, Ager JW: The T-ACE questions: practical prenatal detection of risk-drinking. Am J Obstet Gynecol 160(4):863–870, 1989 2712118

Spindler A, Milos G: Links between eating disorder symptom severity and psychiatric comorbidity. Eat Behav 8(3):364–373, 2007 17606234

Stade BC, Bailey C, Dzendoletas D, et al: Psychological and/or educational interventions for reducing alcohol consumption in pregnant women and women planning pregnancy. Cochrane Database Syst Rev (2):CD004228, 2009 19370597

Substance Abuse and Mental Health Services Administration: Clinical Guidance for Treating Pregnant and Parenting Women With Opioid Use Disorder and Their Infants (HHS Publ No SMA-18-5054). 2018a. Available at: https://store.samhsa.gov/system/files/sma18-5054.pdf. Accessed December 27, 2019.

Substance Abuse and Mental Health Services Administration: Key Substance Use and Mental Health Indicators in the United States: Results From the 2017 National Survey on Drug Use and Health (HHS Publ. No. SMA 18-5068, NSDUH Series H-53). Rockville, MD, Center for Behavioral Health Statistics and Quality, SAMHSA, 2018b. Available at: https://www.samhsa.gov/data/sites/default/files/cbhsq-reports/NSDUHFFR2017/NSDUHFFR2017.pdf. Accessed June 25, 2020.

Terplan M, Longinaker N, Appel L: Women-centered drug treatment services and need in the United States, 2002–2009. Am J Public Health 105(11):e50–e54, 2015a 26378825

Terplan M, Ramanadhan S, Locke A, et al: Psychosocial interventions for pregnant women in outpatient illicit drug treatment programs compared to other interventions. Cochrane Database Syst Rev (4):CD006037, 2015b 25835053

Terplan M, Laird HJ, Hand DJ, et al: Opioid detoxification during pregnancy: a systematic review. Obstet Gynecol 131(5):803–814, 2018 29630016

Timko C, Debenedetti A, Moos BS, et al: Predictors of 16-year mortality among individuals initiating help-seeking for an alcoholic use disorder. Alcohol Clin Exp Res 30(10):1711–1720, 2006 17010138

U.S. Department of Health and Human Services: Effective Medical Treatment of Opiate Addiction. National Institutes of Health Consensus Conference Statement, November 17–19, 1997. Available at: https://consensus.nih.gov/1997/1998treatopiateaddiction108html.htm. Accessed December 27, 2019.

U.S. Department of Health and Human Services: The Health Consequences of Smoking—50 Years of Progress: A Report of the Surgeon General. 2014. Available at: https://www.cdc.gov/tobacco/data_statistics/sgr/50th-anniversary/index.htm. Accessed December 27, 2019.

Valeri L, Sugarman DE, Reilly ME, et al: Group therapy for women with substance use disorders: in-session affiliation predicts women's substance use treatment outcomes. J Subst Abuse Treat 94:60–68, 2018 30243419

Walker NJ, van Woerden HC, Kiparoglou V, et al: Gender difference and effect of pharmacotherapy: findings from a smoking cessation service. BMC Public Health 16(1):1038, 2016 27716223

Watson E, Barnes H, Brown E, et al: Alcohol Screening Assessment in Pregnancy: The ASAP Curriculum. Cambridge, MA, Institute for Health and Recovery, 2003

Welle-Strand GK, Skurtveit S, Jansson LM, et al: Breastfeeding reduces the need for withdrawal treatment in opioid-exposed infants. Acta Paediatr 102(11):1060–1066, 2013 23909865

White R, Black ML: Pain Management Testing Reference. Washington, DC, AACC Press, 2007

Winhusen TM, Kropp F, Lindblad R, et al: Multisite, randomized, double-blind, placebo-controlled pilot clinical trial to evaluate the efficacy of buspirone as a relapse-prevention treatment for cocaine dependence. J Clin Psychiatry 75(7):757–764, 2014 24911028

Wright TE, Schuetter R, Tellei J, Sauvage L: Methamphetamines and pregnancy outcomes. J Addict Med 9(2):111–117, 2015 25599434

Xu J, Azizian A, Monterosso J, et al: Gender effects on mood and cigarette craving during early abstinence and resumption of smoking. Nicotine Tob Res 10(11):1653–1661, 2008 18988078

Yonkers KA, Forray A, Nich C, et al: Progesterone reduces cocaine use in postpartum women with a cocaine use disorder: a randomized, double-blind study. Lancet Psychiatry 1(5):360–367, 2014 25328863

Yoon YH, Chen CM: Surveillance Report #111: Liver Cirrhosis Mortality in the United States: National, State, and Regional Trends, 2000–2015. April 2018. Available at: https://pubs.niaaa.nih.gov/publications/surveillance111/Cirr15.pdf. Accessed December 27, 2019.

Zagon IS, Tobias SW, Hytrek SD, et al: Opioid receptor blockade throughout prenatal life confers long-term insensitivity to morphine and alters mu opioid receptors. Pharmacol Biochem Behav 59(1):201–207, 1998 9443556

CHAPTER 37

Substance-Related Disorders in Adolescents

Amanda T. Roten, M.D.

Kevin M. Gray, M.D.

Adolescence is a unique stage of human development. The World Health Organization defines an adolescent as an individual between the ages of 10 and 19 years; however, many suggest that a broader age range would be more appropriate. Sawyer et al. (2018) proposed the age range of 10–24 years, given that brain development continues into the early 20s and that a broader age range may be more reflective of societal structure. Although there are differing views on exact age ranges, adolescence is universally seen as the transitional period between childhood and adulthood that encompasses extensive biological, psychological, and social changes.

The biological changes in adolescence are at least in part driven by changes in the endocrine system and secretion of hormones. The onset of puberty can be seen as a signal of the start of adolescence, although puberty alone does not define adolescence. Changes during this time include physical growth and development of secondary sex characteristics. Unique changes in the brain, including synaptic pruning, myelination, and a decrease in the gray matter volume, also occur during adolescence (Sawyer et al. 2018; Spear 2013). Psychosocial changes include development of higher-level reasoning skills, moral development, an increase in ability to use abstract thinking, an increase in the desire for autonomy, a focus on the development of identity, an increase in empathy, and an increasing importance placed on peer relationships (World Health Organization 2014).

Substance use has the potential to both affect and be affected by the changes noted above during adolescence. Therefore, it is imperative to consider substance use disorders (SUDs) in adolescence within the lens of development and with the expectation that there can be significant differences in substance use and/or disorders in adolescents compared with adults. This chapter highlights some of the unique issues surrounding substance use and SUDs in this population.

Many adolescents use substances to at least some extent, with 47.8% using any illicit drug and 58.5% using alcohol by grade 12 (Miech et al. 2018). Although most adolescents do not meet criteria for an SUD, there are reasons for concern with any level of use during this developmental stage, suggesting that clinical strategies should be employed across the spectrum of use. For individuals seeking treatment for non-substance-related psychiatric disorders, psychoeducation should include reviewing the effects that substance use may have on mood, anxiety, and/or other disorders.

Substance use in adolescents is heterogeneous and highly prevalent, with a potential for both acute and chronic adverse outcomes. There are unique challenges to targeting substance use in adolescence, but there also are unique opportunities to intervene to increase the likelihood of positive outcomes that have the potential to impact the longer-term life trajectory.

Epidemiology

Substance use initiation typically occurs during adolescence (Yuan et al. 2015). According to the Monitoring the Future survey (Johnston et al. 2018), which has followed substance use in adolescents yearly since 1975, illicit drug use peaked in 1981 (lifetime prevalence of 66% in 1981). The prevalence then decreased until around 1992 and then started increasing until the late 1990s, at which time there was a decline again, followed by stabilization. In 2018, alcohol was the most commonly used substance among adolescents, and marijuana the most commonly used illicit substance. Rates of "vaping" (e-cigarette use) have increased rapidly among adolescents since the introduction of these products to the market. The 2018 prevalence rates of past-year and current daily use of selected substances are summarized in Tables 37–1 and 37–2, respectively.

Monitoring the Future questionnaires also inquire about perceived risk of harm associated with substance use, substance availability, and other related domains. In general, perceived risk of harm is inversely correlated with use in adolescents (Miech et al. 2018). In addition, a number of factors influence the risk of initiating substance use and developing SUDs in adolescents. Whitesell et al. (2013) reviewed the available literature and divided risk factors into three categories: familial, social, and individual. Within these three categories are factors such as family history of substance abuse, child maltreatment, association with peers who use substances, and being diagnosed with attention-deficit/hyperactivity disorder and/or depression. These and other risk factors are listed in Table 37–3.

Adolescents can also develop substance use disorders. In a nationally representative sample of more than 10,000 adolescents ages 13–18 years (Merikangas et al. 2010), 11.4% met criteria, based on a diagnostic interview, for an SUD as described in the *Diagnostic and Statistical Manual of Mental Disorders,* Fourth Edition (DSM-IV; American Psychiatric Association 1994). Of this sample, 8.9% met criteria for a nonalcohol SUD and 6.4% met criteria for alcohol use disorder. The median age at onset of SUDs (15 years) is older than the median age at onset of several non-substance-related psychiatric disorders, including anxiety, mood, and disruptive behavior disorders (Merikangas et al. 2010). Initiation of substance use during adolescence can increase the risk

TABLE 37–1. **Prevalence of past-year use of selected substances, 2017**

Substance	8th graders	10th graders	12th graders
Alcohol (any use)	18.7%	37.8%	53.3%
Alcohol (been drunk)	6.5%	20.9%	33.9%
Marijuana	10.5%	27.5%	35.9%
Synthetic marijuana	1.6%	2.9%	3.5%
Vaping (any)	17.6%	32.3%	37.3%
Vaping (nicotine)	10.9%	24.7%	29.7%
Vaping (marijuana)	4.4%	12.4%	13.1%
Vaping (flavoring only)	15.1%	24.7%	25.7%
Amphetamines	3.7%	5.7%	5.5%
Inhalants	4.6%	2.4%	1.6%
Over-the-counter cough/cold medicines	2.8%	3.3%	3.4%
Cocaine	0.8%	1.5%	2.3%
Heroin	0.3%	0.2%	0.4%
Opioids other than heroin	Not assessed	Not assessed	3.4%

Source. Adapted from Miech et al. 2018.

TABLE 37–2. **Prevalence of daily use of selected substances among U.S. adolescents, 2017**

Substance	8th graders	10th graders	12th graders
Marijuana	0.7%	3.4%	5.8%
Alcohol	0.1%	0.5%	1.2%
Cigarettes	0.8%	1.8%	3.6%

Source. Adapted from Miech et al. 2018.

of addiction. For example, about 9% of individuals who use marijuana will become addicted; this number increases to 16.7% for individuals who start using marijuana in adolescence (Volkow et al. 2014). Additionally, the lifetime prevalence of alcohol use disorder is four to six times higher among individuals who began drinking before age 15 years than among those who began drinking at age 21 years or later (Grant and Dawson 1997).

By late adolescence, 78.2% of youth have used alcohol at least once (Swendsen et al. 2012). Because the rate of experimentation is high, it is important to recognize that although only a portion of individuals with lifetime use will develop acute or chronic problems from use, any use in adolescents warrants clinical attention given the severity of and variability in potential adverse outcomes. The consequences of even sporadic substance use can be severe. In 2016, 15% of drivers in fatal motor vehicle accidents with a blood alcohol content of 0.08 g/dL or greater were 16–20 years of age (National Highway Traffic Safety Administration 2017). Substance use also is associ-

TABLE 37–3. **Factors influencing risk of substance use and substance use disorders in adolescents**

Familial	Social	Individual
• Childhood maltreatment • Family history of substance abuse • Marital status of parents • Level of parental education • Parent–child relationships • Socioeconomic status	• Deviant peer relationships • Perceived popularity (especially identification of oneself as being popular) • Bullying • Association with gangs	• Posttraumatic stress disorder • Attention-deficit/hyperactivity disorder • Depression

ated with increased risk for unintentional injuries, homicide, and suicide, which are all leading causes of death among adolescents (Bonnie and O'Connell 2004). Although the prevalence of past-year use of heroin and other opioids among adolescents is relatively low (see Table 37–1 earlier in chapter), opioids are responsible for more fatal overdoses in adolescents than any other substances (Curtin et al. 2017).

The emergence of vaping is also notable. Vaping, the act of inhaling and exhaling the aerosol ("vapor") produced by e-cigarettes or pod devices, has increased since 2011, when its use was almost nonexistent among adolescents. Vaping devices can be used to deliver nicotine, cannabinoids, or other products and are often supplied with flavors and packaging that are appealing to youth. Although the decline in traditional tobacco cigarette smoking among adolescents over the last three decades is a remarkable public health achievement, clinicians must be attentive to the rising popularity of vaping and consider the potential for adverse consequences (Barrington-Trimis and Leventhal 2018; Barrington-Trimis et al. 2018).

In adolescents as in adults, co-occurrence of psychiatric disorders with SUDs is common. Among adolescents with SUDs, about 76% (Kandel et al. 1999) of those ages 14–18 years and 64% of those ages 13–17 years (Wu et al. 2011) also meet criteria for a co-occurring psychiatric disorder. In a group of adolescents ages 13–17 years seen in various settings in a tertiary-care academic center, 25% had an SUD. This can be further broken down into 13.5% with one SUD and 11.7% with more than one (Wu et al. 2011). Wu and colleagues found that mood disorders were the most common comorbidity in their research sample of more than 1,000 children and adolescents diagnosed with SUD. Other common comorbidities were conduct disorders and attention-deficit/hyperactivity disorder (Wu et al. 2011). In this same study, Wu et al. also found that adolescents with a non-substance-related psychiatric disorder in addition to an SUD used more inpatient care resources than did those with a non-substance-related psychiatric disorder alone (43% vs. 21%). These findings converge with those of Roberts et al. (2007), who identified elevated rates of co-occurring psychiatric disorders, most commonly mood and disruptive behavior disorders, among youth with SUDs in an epidemiological survey; comorbidity was associated with worse functional impairment.

Neurobiology

Adolescence is marked by substantial changes in the brain, involving alterations in multiple regions at different rates and times. Generally, the first regions of the brain to mature are the subcortical regions, including the nucleus accumbens; the prefrontal cortex is the last region to fully mature. In addition, the striatum develops in a curvilinear progression, whereas the prefrontal cortex develops linearly (Casey and Jones 2010). Disparities or imbalances in the relative maturity or functioning of different cortical regions are thus heightened during adolescence. The prefrontal cortex is crucial in cognitive control, whereas the subcortical regions are important in reward seeking (Casey and Jones 2010). During a developmental window in which subcortical development outpaces prefrontal development, adolescents often show a tendency to overvalue immediate reward rather than considering longer-term consequences; this phenomenon of subcortical maturity before prefrontal cortex maturity is sometimes referred to as "bottom-up" control versus "top-down" control, and it increases vulnerability to substance use.

Use of substances amid ongoing development of the brain's reward systems is associated with increased risk of lifetime SUDs. In addition, substance use during adolescence has been associated with a variety of lasting adverse neurocognitive outcomes (Casey and Jones 2010; Meier et al. 2012). A number of ongoing multisite longitudinal studies seek to elucidate the predictors and consequences of adolescent substance use, with a particular focus on neurobiology, neurodevelopment, and cognition. These studies include the National Consortium on Alcohol and Neurodevelopment in Adolescence, which is following more than 800 youths across five different sites in the United States over at least 10 years (http://ncanda.org); the IMAGEN study, which has followed 2,000 youths from England, Ireland, Germany, and France for the past 10 years (https://imagen-europe.com); and the Adolescent Brain Cognitive Development study (http://abcdstudy.org), which in 2015 completed initial enrollment of 11,875 youths across 21 U.S. sites who will be followed for at least 10 years. These large-scale studies will allow for a complex understanding of how demographic, social, genetic, and environmental factors play a role in the impact of substance use on brain development.

Although adolescents may be more susceptible than adults to the long-term negative effects of substance use, there is evidence that they are less susceptible to aversive effects during intoxication. This lower susceptibility can place adolescents at increased risk of rapidly increasing use and of developing tolerance and other symptoms of SUDs as well as long-term sequelae of use during adolescence (Sharma and Morrow 2016). For example, studies have shown that adolescent rats are less susceptible than adult rats to the motor, behavioral, and acute withdrawal effects of alcohol (Casey and Jones 2010) and that adolescent rats are less sensitive than adult rats to withdrawal from nicotine and to the aversive effects of nicotine (Yuan et al. 2015). The implication of these findings is that human adolescents may likewise be less likely to experience negative effects from use of a substance and therefore be more likely to continue using that substance. In contrast, adults may be more likely to experience negative effects during intoxication and as a result be less likely to use that substance again.

Prevention

Preventing or delaying substance use onset has the potential to yield substantial public health benefits. Over the last several decades, a number of large-scale programs have sought, with mixed results, to prevent adolescent substance use and its associated consequences. Generally speaking, prevention programs aim to reduce modifiable risk factors and to enhance modifiable protective factors to reduce the likelihood of substance use (Harrop and Catalano 2016). Interventions with some support include parenting-focused (Allen et al. 2016), school-based teacher-led (Lize et al. 2017), and peer-led prevention programs (MacArthur et al. 2016). Examples of school-based programs with some supportive evidence include Positive Action, LifeSkills Training, Project Toward No Drug Abuse, Blues Program (Cognitive-Behavioral Group Depression Prevention), and Brief Alcohol Screening and Intervention for College Students. Examples of evidence-based family programs include Multisystemic Therapy and Functional Family Therapy (Harrop and Catalano 2016).

Screening and Assessment

Given the significant implications of adolescent substance use, it is imperative that adolescents at risk or those who are using are identified as early as possible to allow for appropriate intervention. The American Academy of Pediatrics, the American Psychiatric Association, and the American Academy of Child and Adolescent Psychiatry have all recommended screening for substance use at routine visits (Borus et al. 2016; Levy et al. 2011).

Screening, Brief Intervention, and Referral to Treatment (SBIRT) is a model used among adults in primary care (Levy et al. 2016). Screening involves using a validated tool to identify individuals at risk of developing an SUD. Brief intervention includes reinforcement for making positive choices as well as using motivational interviewing tools to encourage change. This component often involves a discussion about specific changes an individual is considering and the scheduling of a follow-up visit to assess for these changes. Finally, for individuals who are at moderate to high risk of developing an SUD, providers may consider referral for treatment (Levy et al. 2011). Although the U.S. Preventive Services Task Force cites a lack of evidence for the use of SBIRT with adolescents, the American Academy of Pediatrics and the Substance Abuse and Mental Health Services Administration both recommend the routine use of SBIRT in adolescent patients (Chadi et al. 2018; Levy et al. 2016).

Ideally, screening for substance use should be brief and easy for both the clinician and the patient, given the need to screen universally among adolescents. Multiple screening tools have been validated in this age group (for a review, see Borus et al. 2016). The CRAFFT, an extensively studied tool, consists of six simple questions—related to the words *car, relax, alone, forget, friends,* and *trouble*—that can be asked (Knight et al. 2002; Pilowsky and Wu 2013). Other useful screening tools include the Problem Oriented Screening Instrument for Teenagers (POSIT; Knight et al. 2001); the Screening to Brief Intervention (S2BI; Levy et al. 2014); the Brief Screener for Tobacco, Alcohol, and Other Drugs (BSTAD; Kelly et al. 2014); the NIAAA Youth Alcohol

Screen (Linakis et al. 2019); and the Alcohol Use Disorders Identification Test (AUDIT; Liskola et al. 2018). Levy et al. (2014) found that the S2BI, which consists of single questions about the frequency of use of eight categories of substances, was sensitive and specific in identifying SUDs and their severity. It is worth noting that the CAGE screening tool (**c**ut down, **a**nnoyed, **g**uilty, **e**ye opener) validated for screening adults does not have the same supportive evidence for screening adolescents, and the questions may not be developmentally relevant (Knight et al. 2002).

Although screening is an important initial component of assessment, the gold standard for assessment of psychiatric diagnoses is the clinical interview. The clinician should use nonjudgmental wording and discuss the terms and limits of confidentiality. Age at first use, frequency of use, most recent use, context of use, perceived benefits of use, and problems associated with use are important to assess for each substance. An initial individual interview with the adolescent is recommended. Collateral information from parents can be gathered after the initial interview with the adolescent. This information may be extremely helpful and may yield evidence of adverse consequences the adolescent has not acknowledged that may be diagnostically important.

There are some notable distinctions in the clinical presentations of substance use in adolescents versus adults. Whereas adolescents can suffer both acute and chronic consequences from substance use, adults with substance use tend to experience more chronic consequences, including significant economic and relationship challenges (Gonzales-Castaneda and Kaminer 2016). Adolescents and adults can also differ in their likelihood of meeting certain criteria for SUDs. For example, youth are more likely to develop tolerance quickly but are less likely to experience withdrawal symptoms (Kaminer and Winters 2015). These nuances may lead to either under- or over-identification of substance-related impairments in adolescents, with either of these errors having potential negative consequences.

Objective drug testing using laboratory techniques can be useful in the initial assessment as well as in monitoring progress. However, these tests should be used in the context of a full evaluation, including self-report, and the limitations of drug tests should be kept in mind. Such limitations include variable (and often short) windows of detection for many substances. In work with adolescent patients, it is crucial to obtain consent or assent to urine drug testing and to determine with the patient prior to the testing how the results of the drug testing will be communicated. This discussion includes obtaining permission or assent from the adolescent to share the results with parents and making a plan with the patient and parents for that disclosure. During these discussions, it can be helpful for the clinician to identify potential benefits of drug testing, which can include gaining back the trust of parents or other parties, receiving contingent praise and rewards, and indicating engagement in treatment (Bukstein et al. 2005; Hadland and Levy 2016).

Treatment

A variety of individual, group, and family modalities of psychosocial treatment have been developed to target adolescent SUDs. These interventions span a wide range, from brief single-session feedback to complex, extended, multimodal strategies. Most are conducted in outpatient clinical settings, and many are developmentally adapted from previously established adult-targeted treatments.

Although there may be value in targeting earlier stages of substance experimentation, brief stand-alone interventions appear insufficiently effective when adolescents present with SUDs. Limited therapeutic effects on SUDs have been shown for SBIRT (Young et al. 2014), school-based (Carney et al. 2016), and motivational interviewing (Li et al. 2016) interventions. Similarly, studies examining the utility of mobile technology–delivered brief interventions have yielded mixed findings, with one meta-analysis indicating a small positive effect size for text messaging interventions (Mason et al. 2015). When provided as part of SUD treatment, brief intervention strategies should be used as components of a more intensive and extended treatment model.

The efficacy of psychosocial interventions has been the subject of comprehensive reviews (Hogue et al. 2014; Waldron and Turner 2008). Treatments with the most well-established efficacy include ecological family-based treatment (e.g., Multisystemic Therapy, Multidimensional Family Therapy, Functional Family Therapy), group cognitive-behavioral therapy (CBT), and individual CBT. There is also evidence to support the efficacy of behavioral family therapy and motivational enhancement therapy (MET). These modalities can be delivered as stand-alone treatments, but they also are routinely combined to enhance outcomes. Some patients and families might be more amenable and/or responsive to a particular modality or modalities, and a particular patient's clinical presentation may indicate the relative merits of various modalities. Among combined treatments, evidence is strongest for combined MET and CBT and for combined MET, CBT, and behavioral family therapy (Hogue et al. 2014). Overall, these interventions are associated with reduction or cessation of substance use during treatment, but effect sizes are modest, and few adolescents achieve long-term abstinence. Behavioral treatment contingency management can be used as a complement to the aforementioned therapies to enhance abstinence outcomes during treatment (Stanger et al. 2015, 2016).

Addressing co-occurring psychiatric disorders while engaging adolescents in SUD treatment is an essential component of care. Psychosocial treatments are often effectively delivered in group settings, although efforts should be undertaken to minimize the risk for iatrogenic effects of groups, particularly when they include adolescents with co-occurring conduct disorder and/or more serious substance involvement than others in the group (Macgowan and Wagner 2005).

Candidate pharmacotherapies have been tested for their potential utility in complementing psychosocial and behavioral treatments (Hammond and Gray 2016). Buprenorphine-naloxone is now approved by the U.S. Food and Drug Administration (FDA) for treating opioid use disorder in adolescents as young as age 16 years, based on trials demonstrating improved treatment retention and outcomes with this medication. To date, no other pharmacotherapies have demonstrated sufficient evidence to support FDA approval for their use in treating adolescent SUDs, but some have demonstrated positive findings in randomized controlled trials, including sustained-release bupropion or the nicotine patch for tobacco use disorder, N-acetylcysteine for cannabis use disorder, and naltrexone for alcohol use disorder. In general, pharmacotherapies should be considered for adolescents with moderate or severe SUDs that are not adequately responsive to psychosocial treatments.

Conclusion

Adolescence is a developmental stage with elevated risk for substance initiation, progression to SUDs, and lasting consequences from use. The rates of adolescent use of various substances have vacillated over time, with the use of alcohol, marijuana, and tobacco-related products generally being the most prevalent. Prevention of substance use during adolescence is a critical public health priority, and evaluation and management of adolescents who use substances are similarly important. Recent research has demonstrated a number of effective screening and evaluation tools to identify problematic substance use in adolescents, and a number of efficacious treatment modalities have been developed for SUDs. Ongoing research is focused on strategies to enhance the effectiveness and reach of prevention and treatment programs.

References

Allen ML, Garcia-Huidobro D, Porta C, et al: Effective parenting interventions to reduce youth substance use: a systematic review. Pediatrics 138(2):e20154425, 2016 27443357

American Psychiatric Association: Diagnostic and Statistical Manual of Mental Disorders, 4th Edition. Washington, DC, 1994

Barrington-Trimis JL, Leventhal AM: Adolescents' use of "pod mod" e-cigarettes—urgent concerns. N Engl J Med 379(12):1099–1102, 2018 30134127

Barrington-Trimis JL, Kong G, Leventhal AM, et al: E-cigarette use and subsequent smoking frequency among adolescents. Pediatrics 142(6):e20180486, 2018 30397165

Bonnie RJ, O'Connell ME (eds): Reducing Underage Drinking: A Collective Responsibility. National Research Council (U.S.) and Institute of Medicine (U.S.) Committee on Developing a Strategy to Reduce and Prevent Underage Drinking. Washington, DC, National Academies Press, 2004

Borus J, Parhami I, Levy S: Screening, Brief Intervention, and Referral to Treatment. Child Adolesc Psychiatr Clin N Am 25(4):579–601, 2016 27613340

Bukstein OG, Bernet W, Arnold V, et al; Work Group on Quality Issues: Practice parameter for the assessment and treatment of children and adolescents with substance use disorders. J Am Acad Child Adolesc Psychiatry 44(6):609–621, 2005 15908844

Carney T, Myers BJ, Louw J, et al: Brief school-based interventions and behavioural outcomes for substance-using adolescents. Cochrane Database Syst Rev (1):CD008969, 2016 26787125

Casey BJ, Jones RM: Neurobiology of the adolescent brain and behavior: implications for substance use disorders. J Am Acad Child Adolesc Psychiatry 49(12):1189–1201, quiz 1285, 2010 21093769

Chadi N, Bagley SM, Hadland SE: Addressing adolescents' and young adults' substance use disorders. Med Clin North Am 102(4):603–620, 2018 29933818

Curtin SC, Tejada-Vera B, Warner M: Drug Overdose Deaths Among Adolescents Aged 15–19 in the United States: 1999–2015 (NCHS Data Brief, No 282). Hyattsville, MD, National Center for Health Statistics, 2017

Gonzales-Castaneda R, Kaminer Y: Youth Recovery for Substance Use Disorders and Co-Occurring Disorders: Implications of Developmental Perspectives on Practice, Assessment, Definitions, and Measurement. National Academy of Sciences, August 16, 2016. Available at: https://sites.nationalacademies.org/cs/groups/dbassesite/documents/webpage/dbasse_173832.pdf. Accessed January 3, 2020.

Grant BF, Dawson DA: Age at onset of alcohol use and its association with DSM-IV alcohol abuse and dependence: results from the National Longitudinal Alcohol Epidemiologic Survey. J Subst Abuse 9:103–110, 1997 9494942

Hadland SE, Levy S: Objective testing: urine and other drug tests. Child Adolesc Psychiatr Clin N Am 25(3):549–565, 2016 27338974

Hammond CJ, Gray KM: Pharmacotherapy for substance use disorders in youths. J Child Adolesc Subst Abuse 25(4):292–316, 2016 28082828

Harrop E, Catalano RF: Evidence-based prevention for adolescent substance use. Child Adolesc Psychiatr Clin N Am 25(3):387–410, 2016 27338963

Hogue A, Henderson CE, Ozechowski TJ, et al: Evidence base on outpatient behavioral treatments for adolescent substance use: updates and recommendations 2007–2013. J Clin Child Adolesc Psychol 43(5):695–720, 2014 24926870

Johnston LD, Miech RA, O'Malley PM, et al: Monitoring the Future national survey results on drug use, 1975–2017: Overview, key findings on adolescent drug use. Ann Arbor, MI, Institute for Social Research, University of Michigan, 2018. Available at: https://eric.ed.gov/?id=ED589762. Accessed June 29, 2020.

Kaminer Y, Winters KC: DSM-5 criteria for youth substance use disorders: lost in translation? J Am Acad Child Adolesc Psychiatry 54(5):350–351, 2015 25901770

Kandel DB, Johnson JG, Bird HR, et al: Psychiatric comorbidity among adolescents with substance use disorders: findings from the MECA Study. J Am Acad Child Adolesc Psychiatry 38(6):693–699, 1999 10361787

Kelly SM, Gryczynski J, Mitchell SG, et al: Validity of brief screening instrument for adolescent tobacco, alcohol, and drug use. Pediatrics 133(5):819–826, 2014 24753528

Knight JR, Goodman E, Pulerwitz T, et al: Reliability of the Problem Oriented Screening Instrument for Teenagers (POSIT) in adolescent medical practice. J Adolesc Health 29(2):125–130, 2001 11472871

Knight JR, Sherritt L, Shrier LA, et al: Validity of the CRAFFT substance abuse screening test among adolescent clinic patients. Arch Pediatr Adolesc Med 156(6):607–614, 2002 12038895

Levy SJ, Kokotailo PK; Committee on Substance Abuse: Substance use screening, brief intervention, and referral to treatment for pediatricians. Pediatrics 128(5):e1330–e1340, 2011 22042818

Levy S, Weiss R, Sherritt L, et al: An electronic screen for triaging adolescent substance use by risk levels. JAMA Pediatr 168(9):822–828, 2014 25070067

Levy SJ, Williams JF; Committee on Substance Use and Prevention: Committee on Substance Use and Prevention: substance use screening, brief intervention, and referral to treatment. Pediatrics 138(1):e20161211, 2016 27325634

Li L, Zhu S, Tse N, et al: Effectiveness of motivational interviewing to reduce illicit drug use in adolescents: a systematic review and meta-analysis. Addiction 111(5):795–805, 2016 26687544

Linakis JG, Bromberg JR, Casper TC, et al; Pediatric Emergency Care Applied Research Network: Predictive validity of a 2-question alcohol screen at 1-, 2-, and 3-year follow-up. Pediatrics 143(3):e20182001, 2019 30783022

Liskola J, Haravuori H, Lindberg N, et al: AUDIT and AUDIT-C as screening instruments for alcohol problem use in adolescents. Drug Alcohol Depend 188:266–273, 2018 29803033

Lize SE, Iachini AL, Tang W, et al: A meta-analysis of the effectiveness of interactive middle school cannabis prevention programs. Prev Sci 18(1):50–60, 2017 27785662

MacArthur GJ, Sean H, Deborah M C, et al: Peer-led interventions to prevent tobacco, alcohol and/or drug use among young people aged 11–21 years: a systematic review and meta-analysis. Addiction 111(3):391–407, 2016 26518976

Macgowan MJ, Wagner EF: Iatrogenic effects of group treatment on adolescents with conduct and substance use problems: a review of the literature and a presentation of a model. J Evidence-Based Soc Work 2(1–2):79–90, 2005 20396587

Mason M, Ola B, Zaharakis N, et al: Text messaging interventions for adolescent and young adult substance use: a meta-analysis. Prev Sci 16(2):181–188, 2015 24930386

Meier MH, Caspi A, Ambler A, et al: Persistent cannabis users show neuropsychological decline from childhood to midlife. Proc Natl Acad Sci USA 109(40):E2657–E2664, 2012 22927402

Merikangas KR, He JP, Burstein M, et al: Lifetime prevalence of mental disorders in U.S. adolescents: results from the National Comorbidity Survey Replication—Adolescent Supplement (NCS-A). J Am Acad Child Adolesc Psychiatry 49(10):980–989, 2010 20855043

Miech RA, Schulenberg JE, Johnston LD, et al: National Adolescent Drug Trends in 2018. Ann Arbor, MI, Monitoring the Future, 2018

National Highway Traffic Safety Administration: Traffic Safety Facts: 2016 Data. Alcohol-Impaired Driving. National Center for Statistics and Analysis, October 2017. Available at: https://crashstats.nhtsa.dot.gov/Api/Public/ViewPublication/812450. Accessed December 28, 2019.

Pilowsky DJ, Wu L-T: Screening instruments for substance use and brief interventions targeting adolescents in primary care: a literature review. Addict Behav 38(5):2146–2153, 2013 23454877

Roberts RE, Roberts CR, Xing Y: Comorbidity of substance use disorders and other psychiatric disorders among adolescents: evidence from an epidemiologic survey. Drug Alcohol Depend 88 (suppl 1):S4–S13, 2007 17275212

Sawyer SM, Azzopardi PS, Wickremarathne D, et al: The age of adolescence. Lancet Child Adolesc Health 2(3):223–228, 2018 30169257

Sharma A, Morrow JD: Neurobiology of adolescent substance use disorders. Child Adolesc Psychiatr Clin N Am 25(3):367–375, 2016 27338961

Spear LP: Adolescent neurodevelopment. J Adolesc Health 52 (2 suppl 2):S7–S13, 2013 23332574

Stanger C, Ryan SR, Scherer EA, et al: Clinic- and home-based contingency management plus parent training for adolescent cannabis use disorders. J Am Acad Child Adolesc Psychiatry 54(6):445–453.e2, 2015 26004659

Stanger C, Lansing AH, Budney AJ: Advances in research on contingency management for adolescent substance use. Child Adolesc Psychiatr Clin N Am 25(4):645–659, 2016 27613343

Swendsen J, Burstein M, Case B, et al: Use and abuse of alcohol and illicit drugs in U.S. adolescents: results of the National Comorbidity Survey–Adolescent Supplement. Arch Gen Psychiatry 69(4):390–398, 2012 22474107

Volkow ND, Baler RD, Compton WM, et al: Adverse health effects of marijuana use. N Engl J Med 370(23):2219–2227, 2014 24897085

Waldron HB, Turner CW: Evidence-based psychosocial treatments for adolescent substance abuse. J Clin Child Adolesc Psychol 37(1):238–261, 2008 18444060

Whitesell M, Bachand A, Peel J, et al: Familial, social, and individual factors contributing to risk for adolescent substance use. J Addict 2013:579310, 2013 24826363

World Health Organization: Adolescence: A Period Needing Special Attention. 2014. Available at: h3ttp://apps.who.int/adolescent/second-decade/section2. Accessed December 28, 2019.

Wu L-T, Gersing K, Burchett B, et al: Substance use disorders and comorbid Axis I and II psychiatric disorders among young psychiatric patients: findings from a large electronic health records database. J Psychiatr Res 45(11):1453–1462, 2011 21742345

Young MM, Stevens A, Galipeau J, et al: Effectiveness of brief interventions as part of the Screening, Brief Intervention and Referral to Treatment (SBIRT) model for reducing the nonmedical use of psychoactive substances: a systematic review. Syst Rev 3:50, 2014 24887418

Yuan M, Cross SJ, Loughlin SE, et al: Nicotine and the adolescent brain. J Physiol 593(16):3397–3412, 2015 26018031

CHAPTER 38

Substance-Related Disorders in Patients With Chronic Pain

Kelly S. Barth, D.O.

Allison J. Smith, M.D.

The management of chronic pain, which involves various psychological, psychiatric, and medical comorbidities, has long been a challenge. The increase in opioid prescribing by physicians to treat pain over the last three decades and the subsequent increase in opioid misuse and overdose deaths have emphasized the challenges relating to treating comorbid pain and substance use disorders.

In the early 1990s, the "first wave" of the opioid crisis in the United States was kindled by the sharp increase in medical prescription of opioids to manage pain, which paralleled a subsequent marked increase in the nonmedical use of opioids, peaking at 2.7 million new users per year in 2002 (Kolodny et al. 2015). The opioid crisis continued to evolve from prescription opioids to heroin ("second wave," starting approximately in 2010) and fentanyl ("third wave," starting approximately in 2013), and the cumulative death toll from overdoses involving opioids from 1999 to 2018 was almost 450,000, representing a sixfold increase in opioid-related overdose mortality (Centers for Disease Control and Prevention 2018).

The nationwide response to the opioid crisis has included initiatives to distribute naloxone for overdose reversal, to improve access to treatment of opioid use disorder (OUD), and to reduce opioid prescribing. However, the experiences gained from the evolving opioid crisis and various response initiatives have highlighted numerous questions and challenges involving the relationship between pain and addiction. In this chapter, we explore these questions as well as clinical implications and opportunities in the relationship between pain and addiction.

Chronic Pain and Opioids: Shortcomings of the Biomedical Model

Chronic pain, often defined as pain lasting longer than 3 months or past the normal time for tissue healing, is a highly prevalent and disabling condition affecting approximately 18% of adults in the United States (about 40 million people) (Pitcher and Purser 2019). Chronic pain prevalence increases with age, with nearly 40% of U.S. adults ages 55 years and older reporting chronic pain (Johannes et al. 2010). Chronic pain is associated with an annual cost estimated at $560–$635 billion, is accompanied by impaired physical and mental functioning and reduced quality of life, and is the leading cause of disability in the United States (Institute of Medicine Committee on Advancing Pain Research 2011).

Chronic pain is a poorly understood condition with numerous psychiatric, psychological, and medical comorbidities, making the management complicated within a traditional biomedical model. This situation has prompted recommendations from expert guidelines to ideally manage chronic pain from a "biopsychosocial" framework within an interdisciplinary or interprofessional team (Dowell et al. 2016). Ironically, application of the biopsychosocial model to chronic pain management is not new. In the 1950s, Henry Beecher was a pioneer in pain management who first recognized the impact of psychosocial factors on chronic pain while serving in the Army Medical Corps during World War II. He realized, from interviews with soldiers and nonsoldiers, that their highly variable pain experiences were mediated by the meaning they assigned to their injuries (Beecher 1956). In the 1960s and 1970s, the health care community first distinguished acute and chronic pain as separate entities and subsequently developed behavioral and rehabilitative approaches specific to chronic pain. These approaches were considered revolutionary at the time because basic changes in behavior among patients in chronic pain led to a reduction in the use of analgesic medications and improved functioning during treatment (Main et al. 2015). In response to the growing evidence in support of biopsychosocial treatment for chronic pain, the number of interprofessional pain programs in the United States grew over the next two decades to over 1,000 programs in 1999 at their peak (Schatman 2015). However, after the 1990s, due to the rise in the use of opioid analgesics and economic forces favoring interventional pain management (Jeffery et al. 2011), the number of interprofessional pain programs decreased, with only about 90 programs remaining in 2015 (outside military and Veterans Administration centers) (Schatman 2015).

The nation is now reeling from the effects of overreliance on prescription opioids for the management of a complicated biopsychosocial disease. In the face of the opioid crisis, as prescriptions for opioid analgesics are now being curbed across the nation (Dart et al. 2015), there is renewed national interest in interprofessional pain programs. In fact, the Centers for Disease Control and Prevention guidelines for pain in 2016 (Dowell et al. 2016) cited interprofessional pain programs, such as pain rehabilitation programs, as evidence-based alternatives to prescribing opioids for chronic pain. Additionally, concern has grown about the unintended consequences of tapering patients off long-term opioid analgesics (i.e., gradually reducing the dosage and discontinuing the opioid), including patient abandonment, acute withdrawal, uncontrolled pain, and even suicide (Dowell et al. 2019). This concern has fueled an increased need for programs that can provide a higher level of care for patients who are suffering with poorly controlled pain while taking long-term opioids, those who are struggling to taper from long-term opioid analgesics, and those who might benefit from opioid rotation (i.e., switching from one opioid analgesic to another to improve clinical outcomes) (Crouch et al. 2019).

During the opioid crisis, the need to measure and define the risk and prevalence of substance use disorders (SUDs) among those with chronic pain became critical. Estimates of SUDs in chronic pain populations vary greatly, from 3% to 48% (Morasco et al. 2011), and when looking solely at OUD among those with chronic pain, prevalence estimates still vary widely, from less than 1% to 26% (Banta-Green et al. 2009). This variability can be partly attributed to problems with imprecise terminology and definitions. When precise definitions are used, OUD rates among individuals with pain have generally averaged less than 8%, whereas rates of substance abuse and misuse and of substance-related aberrant behaviors have ranged from 15% to 26% (Volkow and McLellan 2016). Prescribers tend to estimate rates of OUD and/or opioid misuse in the 20%–24% range (Barry et al. 2010), and even if relatively low in prevalence, there is general dissatisfaction with the management of chronic pain and the belief that patients with comorbid pain and SUDs consume more of the providers' time and energy than those without this complicated comorbidity. Importantly, due to high variability in the prevalence of SUD comorbidity with chronic pain and the fact that individuals with SUD are generally excluded from pain clinical trials (Morasco et al. 2011), limited evidence exists to guide clinicians in efficient and effective screening and treatment of SUD in individuals with chronic pain or in the management of chronic pain in individuals with SUDs.

When managing patients with comorbid chronic pain and SUDs, clinicians optimally need to manage both conditions to improve outcomes (Chang and Compton 2013), but there are unique challenges with regard to the setting in which patients are seeking treatment. Although it is known that treatment of addiction can be just as effective in individuals with chronic pain as it is in those without pain (Weiss et al. 2011), identification of addiction in individuals who are actively seeking opioid treatment for pain remains a challenge for the medical provider. First, there is an inherent disincentive for patients to confide symptoms of addiction to a prescriber for fear of losing their opioid prescriptions. Second, many symptoms of SUDs (e.g., poor functioning, loss of control, continued use despite consequences, aberrant behaviors) can be attributed to or rationalized as undertreated pain.

For patients with SUDs in an addiction treatment setting who are suffering with chronic pain, it is important to manage chronic pain because untreated and undertreated pain is a significant risk factor for relapse to substance use (Stromer et al. 2013). However, most addiction providers, like providers from most specialties, receive little training in the area of opioid and non-opioid pain management and are appropriately apprehensive about prescribing or recommending opioids to patients with SUDs due to concerns about activating misuse, addiction, or diversion (Morasco et al. 2011). Methadone, a full-agonist opioid that can treat both severe pain and OUD, can be prescribed for the treatment of addiction only within an opioid treatment program (methadone clinic), entry to which may be logistically and financially unattainable for some patients. Whereas buprenorphine/naloxone can provide relief of chronic pain in the setting of OUD (Weiss et al. 2011), for patients who do not receive good pain relief with buprenorphine/naloxone, the next step up to methadone maintenance remains logistically challenging and inaccessible to some patients. All of these challenges place patients with SUDs at risk for undertreatment of pain (Chang and Compton 2013).

Terminology of Chronic Pain and Substance Use Disorders

To appropriately identify and diagnose SUDs in patients with chronic pain, clinicians need to understand the differences among opioid tolerance, physical dependence, and addiction. The repeated administration of any opioid predictably leads to physiological counteradaptations that cause *tolerance* and *physical dependence. Tolerance* is defined as a diminished effect with continued use of the same dose, and the need for increased amounts of a substance to reach the desired effect. The phenomenon of tolerance creates the primary conundrum of prescribing long-term opioids for chronic pain—namely, that increasingly higher dosages are typically needed to maintain the same level of pain relief (Buntin-Mushock et al. 2005). The solution for tolerance could simply be to increase the dose. However, because tolerance develops more rapidly for some drug effects, such as analgesia and euphoria, but more slowly for other effects, such as respiratory depression, dosage escalation differentially increases risk for respiratory depression (Volkow and McLellan 2016). Tolerance generally resolves after discontinuation of the opioid, usually within days to weeks, depending on the type of opioid, the dosage, and the exposure duration.

Physical dependence is the state of adaptation in which one experiences symptoms of physical withdrawal (e.g., muscle aches, insomnia, chills, diarrhea, restlessness, nausea/vomiting) if the opioid dosage is abruptly reduced or the drug is discontinued. Withdrawal symptoms also vary considerably in length and severity, depending on the type of opioid, the dosage taken, and the exposure duration (Volkow and McLellan 2016).

Addiction is different from dependence or tolerance in that it is a primary, chronic neurobiological disease with genetic, psychosocial, and environmental factors characterized by impaired control over a substance, compulsive use, cravings, and continued use despite negative consequences (Chang and Compton 2013). The neurobiological processes underlying addiction are different from those responsible for tolerance and physical dependence, and the clinical consequences differ. Addiction generally develops slowly (e.g., over months), but it is not a predictable result of opioid consumption, because addiction occurs in only a small proportion of individuals who are exposed to opioids (Volkow and McLellan 2016). Once addiction does develop, it often becomes a chronic illness that typically does not remit with opioid discontinuation alone. However, because there is no diagnostic biomarker for OUD, the diagnosis of OUD along the progression from tolerance/dependence to OUD/addiction relies on clinical assessment.

Part of the confusion in terminology stems from the use of the term *opioid dependence* in earlier editions of the *Diagnostic and Statistical Manual of Mental Disorders* (DSM). DSM-5, the current edition of DSM (American Psychiatric Association 2013), combines the DSM-IV categories of substance abuse and substance dependence into a single entity, substance use disorder, with severity rated on a continuum from mild to severe. However, in DSM-5, tolerance and withdrawal are no longer counted as criteria when diagnosing SUD for individuals taking opioids (or other prescribed medications such as benzodiazepines or stimulants) solely under "appropriate medical supervision." Therefore, if someone who is taking prescription opioids presents solely with symptoms of opioid dependence or tolerance, it would generally *not* be appropriate to diagnose OUD or to treat the individuals with a medication for OUD. However, the "opioid dependence" terminology continues to linger in electronic medical records (EMRs) and in ICD-9 and ICD-10 coding, which creates confusion among clinicians and challenges accuracy for research utilizing data extraction from coding or EMR data.

Opioid Use, Pain, and Reward

Genetic vulnerability to addiction accounts for at least 35%–40% of the risk associated with addiction (Volkow and McLellan 2016). In a classic addiction model, opioids can activate the brain's dopamine reward pathway and promote continued use during the early stages of opioid addiction (positive reinforcement) in individuals genetically or epigenetically predisposed to addiction. Repeated exposure to the drug can lead to physical dependence and daily use to avoid symptoms of withdrawal (negative reinforcement). Continued prolonged use can produce long-lasting changes in the brain that likely drive the compulsive drug-seeking behaviors and subsequent adverse consequences that are the hallmarks of addiction (Kalivas et al. 2005). It was once thought that pain was protective against the development of addiction in individuals with pain, but subsequent research has disproved that notion (Volkow and McLellan 2016). In fact, the negative reinforcement of opioids is compounded by the relief of pain (with opioids or non-opioids), a mechanism that interestingly also involves activation of the dopamine reward system (Mayer et al. 2018). In an individual with pain and a high level of anxiety (related or unrelated to the pain), use of an opioid can relieve the pain and anxiety (directly or secondarily), again compounding the negative reinforcement and rewarding the behavior of taking opioids. One can imagine that for individuals with these comorbidities, an opioid can be profoundly rewarding from both positive- and negative-reinforcement standpoints, and that patterns of learning to avoid pain, anxiety, and withdrawal can become deeply ingrained for patients experiencing chronic pain. This multiplying effect of reward and relief learning highlights the importance of a biopsychosocial approach to pain treatment, particularly for individuals with OUD, to address the underlying learned behaviors that strongly reinforce addiction and pain avoidance.

Pain in the Medical Setting: Preventing Misuse and Addiction During Opioid Pain Management

Pain guidelines for many years have recommended non-opioid pharmacological and nonpharmacological therapy as first-line treatments for chronic pain (Barth et al.

2017). As alternatives to opioids, non-opioid analgesics for chronic pain generally yield small to moderate short-term effects on pain and small effects on functioning (Chou et al. 2017). Recently, cannabis and cannabidiol (CBD) have become increasingly popular for the medical management of pain with increasing legalization, and many patients report positive analgesic effects from cannabis and CBD. Medical researchers also have been investigating whether CBD can beneficially augment treatment for OUD (Hurd et al. 2019). According to recent controlled trials and meta-analyses of cannabinoids for pain (which are limited by the overall poor quality of the body of literature on the safety and efficacy of medical cannabinoids), it is postulated that cannabinoids generally provide modest relief of neuropathic and cancer-related pain, with small effect sizes that tend to diminish over time (Stockings et al. 2018; Whiting et al. 2015). Significant side effects can occur, including cognitive impairment (with both acute and chronic cannabis use) and increased risk of anxiety, depression, and psychosis (with regular cannabis use) (Hill 2015). Additionally, reports of spontaneous pain reduction among patients taking cannabinoids are correlated with the magnitude of the drug high, suggesting that some level of intoxication is required for cannabis to have an analgesic effect (van de Donk et al. 2019). In one study investigating the utility of CBD *without* relevant tetrahydrocannabinol content for chronic pain, analgesic effects were not different for CBD and placebo, a finding that prompts speculation that for pain and in SUD, self-reported positive effects may be related to improvement of anxiety, mood, and/or insomnia, or to a placebo effect (Hurd et al. 2019; van de Donk et al. 2019).

In contrast to the avid uptake of cannabinoids in the United States, the uptake of evidence-based nonpharmacological treatments for pain has been slow, due to issues involving access to care and treatment beliefs, among others (Becker et al. 2017). Access to and coverage for these treatments are improving, and patients and clinicians are encouraged to make themselves aware of what nonpharmacological resources are available in their community, because utilizing non-opioid pain treatments is the clearest way to mitigate risks associated with opioid use.

If opioids are deemed necessary and appropriate for the management of a patient's chronic pain, in order to mitigate risk, clinicians should first conduct a comprehensive patient history and risk assessment, which can include use of a validated screening questionnaire such as the Revised Screener and Opioid Assessment for Patients with Pain (SOAPP-R; Butler et al. 2008) or the Opioid Risk Tool (ORT; Webster and Webster 2005). The clinician should also evaluate the impact of pain on the patient's functioning (physical and emotional), enjoyment of life, and mood, and should identify known risk factors for addiction, many of which are also risk factors for the development of chronic pain (Table 38–1).

Once risk factors are identified, an important (but often overlooked) step is to address any treatable risk factors or conditions that are poorly controlled (e.g., depression, posttraumatic stress disorder [PTSD], sleep-disordered breathing, insomnia) prior to initiating opioid treatment. Effective treatment of these conditions can often relieve pain. Also, as discussed in the previous section, when a person with poorly controlled depression or anxiety takes an opioid for chronic pain, it is difficult to determine which symptom the opioid is relieving. It is important to identify and treat OUD if present, as well as to screen for other SUDs or for sedative-hypnotic use.

TABLE 38–1.	Factors associated with the risk of chronic pain and addiction
Factor	**Risk[b]**
Medication-related factors	
Daily dosage >100 morphine milligram equivalents	Addiction[1]
Long-term (>3 months) opioid use	Addiction,[1] chronic pain[2]
Patient-related factors	
Depression	Addiction,[1] chronic pain[2]
Abuse/trauma history[a]	Addiction,[3] chronic pain[3]
Genetic vulnerability	Addiction,[1] chronic pain[2]
Comorbid tobacco use	Addiction,[1] chronic pain[2]
Sleep disturbances	Addiction,[1] chronic pain[2]
Low socioeconomic status	Addiction[1]
Involvement in legal system	Addiction[3]
Female gender	Chronic pain[2]
Adolescent age	Addiction[1]

[a]History of abuse or violence in a domestic or public setting; history of sexual violence; history of childhood neglect or sexual or physical abuse.
[b]References for risk data: [1]Volkow and McLellan 2016; [2]van Hecke et al. 2013; [3]Chang and Compton 2013.

Once comorbid conditions are being managed as well as they can be, opioid prescribing guidelines (reviewed in more detail in Chapter 31, "The U.S. Opioid Crisis") recommend that the clinician initiating opioid treatment should start by prescribing an immediate-release formulation and should limit the dosage to the lowest effective level for the shortest effective duration (for both acute and chronic pain) to mitigate risk. Also, the clinician should regularly reassess the effectiveness of the opioid and should taper the dosage if effectiveness is no longer being achieved. Clinicians should review their own state's prescription drug monitoring program (PDMP) database at each patient visit and prior to prescribing any controlled substance.

Differential Diagnosis of the Poorly Functioning Patient With Pain

Although the risk mitigation strategies discussed in the previous section are advisable, several challenging scenarios that occur in the treatment of patients with chronic pain highlight the clinical conundrum of applying guidelines to individual patient care. In a commonly encountered scenario, a patient reports initially responding well to opioids (possibly prescribed by another provider) but after some time is no longer receiving benefit from the medication and is now experiencing increased pain and poor physical and/or psychosocial functioning; the patient might even be running out of opioids early or experiencing withdrawal symptoms between doses. When this occurs, a provider may discuss with the patient the clinical guideline recommendation that opioids be tapered when a patient is experiencing poor functioning that is suspected to be related to chronic opioid use and the risks of opioids are felt to outweigh the benefits. The patient or family may attribute the poor functioning to worsening pain (and not to tolerance, depression, anxiety, or addiction). Rather than tapering off opioids, the patient or family may actually seek an increase in the opioid dosage to alleviate the patient's suffering in the short term. Additionally, due to fears of worsening pain or fears of experiencing withdrawal, the patient or family might feel understandable apprehension about an opioid taper. One helpful approach has been to provide education to the patient and/or family, informing them that many people do not experience withdrawal or an increase in pain with a slow opioid taper, and in fact, many feel improved on lower dosages of opioids or off opioids altogether. Apprehension about tapering can be successfully addressed with effective communication, education, and a good patient–provider alliance.

It is necessary in this scenario for the clinician to correctly recognize and diagnose the cause(s) of the patient/s functional impairment and aberrant behaviors in order to provide appropriate treatment and optimize outcomes. The differential diagnosis for a poorly functioning patient experiencing chronic pain can include the following: psychiatric comorbidity (e.g., depression, PTSD, early-life trauma), psychological comorbidity (e.g., "chemical coping" or personality disorder), addiction (to opioids or otherwise), tolerance, and other causes (e.g., undertreated pain, disease progression, opioid-induced hyperalgesia). It is important for clinicians to attempt to clarify which of these conditions is present so as to offer the appropriate treatment; however, clinicians also need to acknowledge that this effort may require a trial-and-error process because there are few, if any, biomarkers for these conditions. For example, if psychiatric or psychological comorbidity (e.g., depression, PTSD, personality disorder, "chemical coping") is identified, the condition should be treated with psychotherapy and/or psychotropic medications, and pain should then be reassessed. If addiction (i.e., an SUD) is diagnosed, targeted addiction therapy and appropriate medications should be initiated. If undertreated pain ("pseudo-addiction") is suspected as the etiology of aberrant behaviors or poor functioning, the clinician could try an increase in medication, because undertreated pain can provoke drug-seeking or aberrant behaviors. In this case, adequately treating the pain with an increase in the opioid dosage (if clinically appropriate) or a multimodal mechanism should eliminate the aberrant behaviors and/or improve functioning. However, the issue of tolerance, and plans for how to address and/or prevent it, need to be discussed at these early stages of chronic pain treatment.

Differentiating undertreated pain or disease progression from tolerance is difficult. For the clinician who suspects, from careful history taking, that a patient is developing tolerance and is beginning to experience functional difficulties as a result, there exists no "best practice" approach for addressing the problem. In the past, the answer to tolerance was to increase the dosage or rotate the patient to a different opioid, but with the recent discovery of dose-related associations with overdose risk, increasing the opioid dosage to address tolerance (or disease progression) has become a less valid option. Clinicians and prescribers receive little, if any, education on how to effectively accomplish opioid rotation. Some patients taking opioid analgesics might prefer to continue taking an ineffective dosage rather than tapering off or rotating to another medication. However, the downstream effects of this approach are not known. Some patients might want to taper off their pain medications but fear the pain and withdrawal symptoms they will suffer, and therefore may require more support than can be provided through routine outpatient care. Although there are interprofessional pain programs available in the United States that incorporate opioid tapering (Sletten et al. 2015) and there is some research suggesting that it is possible for individuals to successfully reduce their prescription opioid dosages as outpatients (Darnall et al. 2018), more research is needed—including well-designed trials evaluating opioid rotation and medically supported withdrawal—to devise effective discontinuation plans for individuals who have developed tolerance to opioid pain medications.

Opioid-induced hyperalgesia (OIH) is a clinical concern that frequently arises for the poorly functioning patient taking opioids. From animal and human studies, it is known that continuous long-term exposure to opioids can cause sympathetic stimulation, dysregulation of the hypothalamic-pituitary-adrenal axis, and activation of the proinflammatory immune system, any of which can lead to an increased perception of pain (Chu et al. 2008). Strictly defined, OIH is a paradoxical state of nociceptive sensitization that can occur after exposure to an opioid. This state results in an increase in sensitivity to painful stimuli as the patient receives more opiates. In theory, OIH pain should diminish after closely supervised withdrawal from opioids, although study results have been mixed and it is not clear to what degree opioid dosage tapering improves pain responses and outcomes, if at all. The mechanism of OIH has been better described in animal literature, but the precise molecular mechanism of OIH varies substantially even in basic science studies. The central glutamatergic system is thought to be the most likely mechanism (Lee et al. 2011). In the clinical literature addressing pain and addiction, there is considerable overlap in descriptions of the mechanisms of OIH and opioid tolerance, although most clinical studies are limited by the presence in patients of underlying acute and/or chronic pain and/or addiction, which can also alter pain thresholds and perception (Lee et al. 2011). Additionally, in clinical studies, little is done to control for other comorbidities that can alter pain sensitivity, such as insomnia, early-life trauma, PTSD, or mood disorders. Given that we lack both well-defined evidence for OIH in humans and a clear understanding of how or whether OIH differs from opioid tolerance, it remains important to clinically screen and treat patients with chronic pain for the common psychiatric, psychological, and medical comorbidities (discussed above) that can affect pain perception, tolerance, and sensitivity.

Buprenorphine and Methadone in the Management of Pain and Addiction

Significant evidence demonstrates that buprenorphine and methadone are effective medications for the treatment of OUD (Schuckit 2016). Both are also effective pain medications. Buprenorphine is a partial μ-opioid receptor agonist, a nociceptin (opioid receptor–like 1 receptor) agonist (spinal cord level), and a κ-opioid receptor antagonist that has been shown to have antidepressant effects and antihyperalgesic effects (involving spinal dynorphin and *N*-methyl-D-aspartate activity). Two buprenorphine products—a patch formulation (Butrans) and a buccal film (Belbuca)—have received U.S. Food and Drug Administration (FDA) approval for the treatment of severe pain that requires long-term opioid treatment (in the ambulatory setting). A waiver is not required to prescribe these buprenorphine products for pain, which decreases barriers to the medication's use in pain populations, although insurance coverage barriers remain. Buprenorphine has many benefits, including a high affinity for and slow dissociation from the μ-opioid receptor, which make it an excellent withdrawal medication; a ceiling effect on respiratory depression and euphoria; and a lower propensity to induce tolerance. Transitioning from long-term opioid medication to buprenorphine has shown preliminary promise in clinical chronic pain populations and small research pilot studies (Daitch et al. 2014). However, as a partial μ-opioid receptor agonist, buprenorphine may not achieve the magnitude of analgesia achieved with full agonists, and therefore buprenorphine may leave pain undertreated. Buprenorphine is also long-acting, so for individuals who experience intermittent or "breakthrough" pain (e.g., patients with sickle cell disease), buprenorphine may not provide adequate analgesia and may block the effects of short-acting full agonists. Buprenorphine, as an initial opioid therapy or a rotation agent, deserves more investigation to assess whether it can be an appropriate risk-mitigation strategy when opioids are indicated for patients with pain that is nonresponsive to non-opioid treatment or for individuals who have developed tolerance to long-term opioid treatment. Our clinical experience suggests that the more symptoms of tolerance and/or addiction a patient has, the more likely it is that the patient will have a good overall pain/quality-of-life response to treatment with buprenorphine, although research is ongoing in this area.

Methadone has been approved by the FDA for the treatment of both OUD and severe pain. It is important to note that for treating OUD, methadone can only be prescribed within a certified opioid treatment program (e.g., a methadone clinic). In the treatment of chronic pain (including for patients with comorbid OUD), caution must be used when prescribing methadone, especially during treatment initiation, given its long and variable half-life (8–59 hours) and narrow therapeutic window, especially when combined with central nervous system depressants such as sedatives, hypnotics, other opioids, and alcohol. In addition, methadone can cause QTc prolongation, and it is metabolized by the cytochrome P450 system, which increases risks for medication interactions and adverse effects when taken with certain commonly prescribed medications (e.g., antibiotics). Moreover, methadone, when used for addiction in an opioid treatment program, is not yet reported in PDMPs in most states and does not test positive for opioids on most routine urine toxicology screens; therefore, clinicians must rely on patients to disclose that they are taking methadone to avoid potentially dangerous medication interactions.

Because the duration of its analgesic action is 4–8 hours, methadone prescribed for pain is generally dosed every 8 hours (as opposed to once daily when prescribed for addiction in an opioid treatment program), and steady-state plasma concentrations are not attained for 3–5 days (or longer for some). For those with comorbid pain and OUD, the once-daily initial dosing of methadone in opioid treatment programs can leave patients with undertreated pain, which can increase risk of relapse. There has been interest and advocacy during the evolving opioid crisis and the coronavirus disease 2019 (COVID-19) pandemic to consider allowing prescribers outside of opioid treatment programs to use methadone for the treatment of OUD, which could allow for more flexible dosing, but research is ongoing in this area.

Management of Acute, Perioperative, and Postoperative Pain in Patients Being Treated for Opioid Use Disorder

Patients who are taking medications for OUD are at particular risk for undertreatment of acute pain and perioperative pain, and good communication and coordination of care are necessary to decrease this risk. Before patients taking naltrexone (a full opioid antagonist) undergo elective procedures, it is important for providers to discuss pain management with the patient, surgeon, and anesthesiologist. As with all patients, attempts to use non-opioids should be made whenever possible. When an elective surgery is planned, the procedure should be scheduled at least 72 hours after the last oral naltrexone dose and at least 4 weeks after receipt of a naltrexone injection. For emergency procedures or unexpected severe pain (e.g. after a motor vehicle accident), regional anesthesia, conscious sedation, or general anesthesia can be considered (Alford et al. 2006).

After surgery, patients receiving methadone maintenance therapy should continue taking their verified daily dose, and short-acting opioids should be added for relief of acute postoperative pain (Alford et al. 2006). Patients may require higher dosing of opioids (i.e., dosages that are 1.5 times higher than usual) due to increased pain sensitivity and opioid cross-tolerance and may require pain medications at shorter intervals. It has been shown that opioid analgesics may be used safely for postsurgical pain in patients receiving methadone maintenance therapy without increasing the risk of relapse (Kantor et al. 1980).

There is a lack of consensus regarding acute and perioperative pain management for patients already taking buprenorphine. Treatment with opioids for patients taking buprenorphine is complicated due to buprenorphine's variable half-life (20–72 hours) and its high affinity for the μ-opioid receptor, which results in competition with and potential displacement of full-agonist opioids. Potential treatment options include the following: 1) continue buprenorphine and add short-acting opioids (mounting evidence for this; may not inhibit full-agonist analgesia); 2) discontinue buprenorphine, use normal (or slightly higher) opioid analgesia, and titrate to effect, with a plan to resume buprenorphine after the acute pain no longer requires full-agonist opioid analgesia; 3) divide buprenorphine dosages and administer a dose every 6–8 hours and/or use supplemental buprenorphine to take advantage of its analgesic pain properties; and 4) convert buprenorphine to methadone (which binds less tightly to μ-opioid receptors) at 30–40 mg/day to prevent withdrawal, and add short-acting opioids, with a plan to switch back to buprenorphine prior to discharge (Alford et al. 2006). If the decision is made to discontinue buprenorphine before an elective surgery, it is important to coordinate with the anesthesiology team, because institutional practices vary in regard to when to hold the last dose of buprenorphine preoperatively. Some hospitals have a "5-day rule" (Stern 2015) for major surgeries, in which case buprenorphine would be held for 5 days prior to surgery and the patient would be covered with extended-release and long-acting opioids until surgery (e.g., sustained-release morphine 15 mg bid). However, some institutions and case studies have reported success with holding buprenorphine for shorter periods of time for less-major surgeries (e.g., 1–2 days preoperatively [Stern 2015]) or even continuing buprenorphine for minor or unexpected procedures (Book et al. 2007).

Gender Differences in Chronic Pain and Addiction

From 1999 to 2017, drug overdose deaths among women ages 30–64 years increased by 260% in the United States (VanHouten et al. 2019). The significant gender differences in addiction and chronic pain have important implications for optimal pain and addiction management. Women represent up to 80% of the chronic pain population (Fillingim et al. 2009), and there are physiological, neurological, and hormonal differences in the ways that men and women perceive, experience, respond to, and cope with pain. In comparison with men, women show increased sensitivity to laboratory pain (Fillingim et al. 2009), and women rate their pain as being higher in intensity and unpleasantness (Alqudah et al. 2010). Women are more likely than men to start using opioids in medical settings, and opioids for pain are more commonly recommended to women than to men (Fillingim et al. 2009). Compared with men with SUDs, women with SUDs have higher rates of psychiatric comorbidities (Chen et al. 2011), and women with OUD report greater use of opioids to cope with negative emotions and pain (McHugh et al. 2013). Furthermore, women are more likely than men to develop prescription (vs. heroin) OUD (Center for Behavioral Health Statistics and Quality 2018), and rates of OUD are increasing more rapidly in women than in men. From 1999 to 2015, prescription OUD increased 471% in women versus 218% in men, and from 2002 to 2013, heroin use increased 100% in women versus 50% in men (VanHouten et al. 2019). Additionally, perinatal opioid use and neonatal withdrawal syndrome rates are increasing, with implications for both mother and newborn. However, it is known that women are less likely than men to enter traditional SUD treatment programs (Greenfield et al. 2007; McHugh et al. 2019). Perhaps because the initial pathway to opioid use and development of OUD for women more often involves the medical setting (i.e., in the course of seeking treatment for chronic pain), women with OUD appear to preferentially seek treatment for their problematic use in that setting, whereas men with OUD are more likely to seek treatment in the addiction setting. There are ongoing studies to determine whether gender-based treatment is more effective than combined treatment in both pain and addiction settings.

Conclusion

The identification of SUDs, and in particular OUD, in individuals with pain conditions can be challenging, but being able to do so is important. The contribution of inappropriate prescribing by physicians to the current opioid crisis is partly attributable to lack of training in the recognition of SUDs, the management of opioids, and the treatment of chronic pain. Additionally, lack of access to evidence-based non-opioid treatments for chronic pain, including biopsychosocial treatment programs, has increased providers' reliance on opioids for chronic pain. Treatment of pain in individuals who have a comorbid SUD (active or in remission) is an area that requires more exploration, but it is known that both conditions must be addressed and appropriately treated to achieve maximal functional improvement and pain relief. Correctly identifying and treating OUD in patients with pain can be the most effective initial approach to improving outcomes in the comorbid population. More research is needed to provide guidance in evidence-based approaches to chronic pain conditions, particularly in regard to evaluating outcomes of opioid tapering and improving access to non-opioid and nonpharmacological treatments for chronic pain.

References

Alford DP, Compton P, Samet JH: Acute pain management for patients receiving maintenance methadone or buprenorphine therapy. Ann Intern Med 144(2):127–134, 2006 16418412

Alqudah AF, Hirsh AT, Stutts LA, et al: Sex and race differences in rating others' pain, pain-related negative mood, pain coping, and recommended medical help. J Cyber Ther Rehabil 3(1):63–70, 2010 21499447

American Psychiatric Association: Diagnostic and Statistical Manual of Mental Disorders, 5th Edition. Arlington, VA, American Psychiatric Association, 2013

Banta-Green CJ, Merrill JO, Doyle SR, et al: Opioid use behaviors, mental health and pain—development of a typology of chronic pain patients. Drug Alcohol Depend 104(1–2):34–42, 2009 19473786

Barry DT, Irwin KS, Jones ES, et al: Opioids, chronic pain, and addiction in primary care. J Pain 11(12):1442–1450, 2010 20627817

Barth KS, Guille C, McCauley J, et al: Targeting practitioners: a review of guidelines, training, and policy in pain management. Drug Alcohol Depend 173 (suppl 1):S22–S30, 2017 28363316

Becker SA, Cummins M, Davis A, et al: NMC Horizon Report: 2017 Higher Education Edition. The New Media Consortium, 2017. Available at: https://files.eric.ed.gov/fulltext/ED582134.pdf. Accessed January 8, 2020.

Beecher HK: Relationship of significance of wound to pain experienced. J Am Med Assoc 161(17):1609–1613, 1956 13345630

Book SW, Myrick H, Malcolm R, et al: Buprenorphine for postoperative pain following general surgery in a buprenorphine-maintained patient. Am J Psychiatry 164(6):979, 2007 17541066

Buntin-Mushock C, Phillip L, Moriyama K, et al: Age-dependent opioid escalation in chronic pain patients. Anesth Analg 100(6):1740–1745, 2005 15920207

Butler SF, Fernandez K, Benoit C, et al: Validation of the Revised Screener and Opioid Assessment for Patients with Pain (SOAPP-R). J Pain 9(4):360–372, 2008 18203666

Center for Behavioral Health Statistics and Quality: Results from the 2017 National Survey on Drug Use and Health: Detailed Tables. Rockville, MD, Substance Abuse and Mental Health Services Administration, Center for Behavioral Health Statistics and Quality, September 7, 2018. Available at: https://www.samhsa.gov/data/sites/default/files/cbhsq-reports/NSDUHDetailedTabs2017/NSDUHDetailedTabs2017.pdf. Accessed August 7, 2020.

Centers for Disease Control and Prevention: Understanding the Epidemic. National Center for Injury Prevention and Control, December 19, 2018. Available at: https://www.cdc.gov/drugoverdose/epidemic/index.html. Accessed January 8, 2020.

Chang YP, Compton P: Management of chronic pain with chronic opioid therapy in patients with substance use disorders. Addict Sci Clin Pract 8(1):21, 2013 24341916

Chen KW, Banducci AN, Guller L, et al: An examination of psychiatric comorbidities as a function of gender and substance type within an inpatient substance use treatment program. Drug Alcohol Depend 118(2–3):92–99, 2011 21514751

Chou R, Deyo R, Friedly J, et al: Nonpharmacologic therapies for low back pain: a systematic review for an American College of Physicians Clinical Practice Guideline. Ann Intern Med 166(7):493–505, 2017 28192793

Chu LF, Angst MS, Clark D: Opioid-induced hyperalgesia in humans: molecular mechanisms and clinical considerations. Clin J Pain 24(6):479–496, 2008 18574358

Crouch T, Goble L, Sletten C, Barth KS: Cognitive-behavioral therapy for chronic pain, in Bonica's Management of Pain, 5th Edition. Edited by Fishman S, Ballantyne J, Rathmell JP, et al. Baltimore, MD, Lippincott, Williams & Wilkins, 2019, pp 1405–1413

Daitch D, Daitch J, Novinson D, et al: Conversion from high-dose full-opioid agonists to sublingual buprenorphine reduces pain scores and improves quality of life for chronic pain patients. Pain Med 15(12):2087–2094, 2014 25220043

Darnall BD, Ziadni MS, Stieg RL, et al: Patient-centered prescription opioid tapering in community outpatients with chronic pain. JAMA Intern Med 178(5):707–708, 2018 29459978

Dart RC, Surratt HL, Cicero TJ, et al: Trends in opioid analgesic abuse and mortality in the United States. N Engl J Med 372(3):241–248, 2015 25587948

Dowell D, Haegerich TM, Chou R: CDC guideline for prescribing opioids for chronic pain— United States, 2016. JAMA 315(15):1624–1645, 2016 26977696

Dowell D, Haegerich T, Chou R: No shortcuts to safer opioid prescribing. N Engl J Med 380(24):2285–2287, 2019 31018066

Fillingim RB, King CD, Ribeiro-Dasilva MC, et al: Sex, gender, and pain: a review of recent clinical and experimental findings. J Pain 10(5):447–485, 2009 19411059

Greenfield SF, Brooks AJ, Gordon SM, et al: Substance abuse treatment entry, retention, and outcome in women: a review of the literature. Drug Alcohol Depend 86(1):1–21, 2007 16759822

Hill KP: Medical marijuana for treatment of chronic pain and other medical and psychiatric problems: a clinical review. JAMA 313(24):2474–2483, 2015 26103031

Hurd YL, Spriggs S, Alishayev J, et al: Cannabidiol for the reduction of cue-induced craving and anxiety in drug-abstinent individuals with heroin use disorder: a double-blind randomized placebo-controlled trial. Am J Psychiatry 176(11):911–922, 2019 31109198

Institute of Medicine Committee on Advancing Pain Research: Relieving Pain in America: A Blueprint for Transforming Prevention, Care, Education, and Research. Washington, DC, National Academies Press, 2011

Jeffery MM, Butler M, Stark A, et al: Multidisciplinary Pain Programs for Chronic Non-Cancer Pain. Minnesota Evidence-Based Practice Center. Rockville, MD, Agency for Healthcare Research and Quality, 2011

Johannes CB, Le TK, Zhou X, et al: The prevalence of chronic pain in United States adults: results of an Internet-based survey. J Pain 11(11):1230–1239, 2010 20797916

Kalivas PW, Volkow N, Seamans J: Unmanageable motivation in addiction: a pathology in prefrontal-accumbens glutamate transmission. Neuron 45(5):647–650, 2005 15748840

Kantor TG, Cantor R, Tom E: A study of hospitalized surgical patients on methadone maintenance. Drug Alcohol Depend 6(3):163–173, 1980 6107237

Kolodny A, Courtwright DT, Hwang CS, et al: The prescription opioid and heroin crisis: a public health approach to an epidemic of addiction. Annu Rev Public Health 36:559–574, 2015 25581144

Lee YC, Nassikas NJ, Clauw DJ: The role of the central nervous system in the generation and maintenance of chronic pain in rheumatoid arthritis, osteoarthritis and fibromyalgia. Arthritis Res Ther 13(2):211, 2011 21542893

Main CJ, Keefe FJ, Jensen MP, et al: Fordyce's Behavioral Methods for Chronic Pain and Illness: Republished With Invited Commentaries. Philadelphia, PA, Lippincott Williams & Wilkins, 2015

Mayer D, Kahl E, Uzuneser TC, et al: Role of the mesolimbic dopamine system in relief learning. Neuropsychopharmacology 43(8):1651–1659, 2018 29453443

McHugh RK, Devito EE, Dodd D, et al: Gender differences in a clinical trial for prescription opioid dependence. J Subst Abuse Treat 45(1):38–43, 2013 23313145

McHugh RK, Kneeland ET, Edwards RR, et al: Pain catastrophizing and distress intolerance: prediction of pain and emotional stress reactivity. J Behav Med 2:1–7, 2019 31376099

Morasco BJ, Gritzner S, Lewis L, et al: Systematic review of prevalence, correlates, and treatment outcomes for chronic non-cancer pain in patients with comorbid substance use disorder. Pain 152(3):488–497, 2011 21185119

Pitcher SN, Purser DC: Oral Anaerobic Glutathione Supplement in Liposome Suspension. United States Patent Publ No 10272130. April 30, 2019. Available at: https://patentscope.wipo.int/beta/en/detail.jsf?docId=US241524619&_cid=B26-K55F2X-36741-1. Accessed January 8, 2020.

Schatman ME: The American chronic pain crisis and the media: about time to get it right? J Pain Res 8:885–887, 2015 26719722

Schuckit MA: Treatment of opioid-use disorders. N Engl J Med 375(4):357–368, 2016 27464203

Sletten CD, Kurklinsky S, Chinburapa V, et al: Economic analysis of a comprehensive pain rehabilitation program: a collaboration between Florida Blue and Mayo Clinic Florida. Pain Med 16(5):898–904, 2015 25645237

Stern E: Buprenorphine and the Anesthesia Considerations: A Literature Review. Nurse Anesthesia Capstones, March 2015. Available at: http://accurateclinic.com/wp-content/uploads/2016/08/Buprenorphine-And-The-Anesthesia-Considerations_-A-Literature-Rev-2015.pdf. Accessed January 8, 2020.

Stockings E, Campbell G, Hall WD, et al: Cannabis and cannabinoids for the treatment of people with chronic noncancer pain conditions: a systematic review and meta-analysis of controlled and observational studies. Pain 159(10):1932–1954, 2018 29847469

Stromer W, Michaeli K, Sandner-Kiesling A: Perioperative pain therapy in opioid abuse. Eur J Anaesthesiol 30(2):55–64, 2013 23241915

van de Donk T, Niesters M, Kowal MA, et al: An experimental randomized study on the analgesic effects of pharmaceutical-grade cannabis in chronic pain patients with fibromyalgia. Pain 160(4):860–869, 2019 30585986

van Hecke O, Torrance N, Smith BH: Chronic pain epidemiology—where do lifestyle factors fit in? Br J Pain 7(4):209–217, 2013 26516524

VanHouten JP, Rudd RA, Ballesteros MF, et al: Drug overdose deaths among women aged 30–64 Years—United States, 1999–2017. MMWR Morb Mortal Wkly Rep 68(1):1–5, 2019 30629574

Volkow ND, McLellan AT: Opioid abuse in chronic pain—misconceptions and mitigation strategies. N Engl J Med 374(13):1253–1263, 2016 27028915

Webster LR, Webster RM: Predicting aberrant behaviors in opioid-treated patients: preliminary validation of the Opioid Risk Tool. Pain Med 6(6):432–442, 2005 16336480

Weiss RD, Potter JS, Fiellin DA, et al: Adjunctive counseling during brief and extended buprenorphine-naloxone treatment for prescription opioid dependence: a 2-phase randomized controlled trial. Arch Gen Psychiatry 68(12):1238–1246, 2011 22065255

Whiting PF, Wolff RF, Deshpande S, et al: Cannabinoids for medical use: a systematic review and meta-analysis. JAMA 313(24):2456–2473, 2015 26103030

CHAPTER 39

Substance Use and Related Disorders in Sexual and Gender Minority Populations

Jeremy D. Kidd, M.D., M.P.H.

Maria is a 47-year-old Latina lesbian woman employed as a research assistant at a local university who was referred by her primary care provider for alcohol use disorder. Maria states that she began drinking alcohol shortly before her twenty-first birthday and typically drank 1–3 beers 1–2 times per month with friends. Over the past year, her drinking has increased to 6–10 beers 4–5 days per week. She feels ashamed about her drinking and as a result spends less time with friends and more time alone. Her work performance has deteriorated, and her wife, Susan, has expressed concern that she seems more "down" when she drinks.

Are rates of hazardous alcohol use and alcohol use disorder different among lesbian women? How might Maria's lesbian identity and life experiences relate to her current alcohol use? How might a clinician change the diagnostic assessment and treatment plan in response to these sociocultural factors? These are some of the issues addressed in this chapter. The term *sexual and gender minority* (SGM) refers to *sexual minority* (SM) individuals (e.g., lesbian, gay, bisexual, queer) and *gender minority* (GM) individuals (e.g., transgender, genderqueer) (see next section of this chapter for more details on terminology). SGM people are a diverse group by age, race/ethnicity, religious background, and nationality. Furthermore, SGM identities represent normal variations of

The author wishes to thank Dr. Petros Levounis for providing commentary on a draft of this chapter.

human sexual orientation and gender identity. Since the beginning of the modern SGM rights movement in 1969, advocates have achieved numerous legislative and societal advances (e.g., increased media representation, legal same-gender marriage in the United States and elsewhere globally, expanded insurance coverage of gender-affirming health care for GM individuals). However, SGM people still face numerous challenges. According to a report by the National Academy of Medicine (2011), SGM individuals experience discrimination and harassment across the lifespan and face multiple health disparities. These include disproportionately high rates of tobacco, alcohol, and drug use. By recognizing the unique health needs of SGM individuals, clinicians can intervene on health disparities in this marginalized population.

I begin this chapter with an overview of key concepts related to sexual orientation and gender identity. I then review the epidemiology of substance use among SGM individuals. Next, I introduce Minority Stress Theory as a conceptual model for explicating SGM health disparities, and then discuss clinical considerations that are important when working with SGM patients. Finally, I highlight several concrete recommendations for delivering culturally responsive substance use disorder (SUD) treatment to SGM patients. Several case examples are provided throughout the chapter to illustrate these topics.

Definitions and Key Concepts

SGM populations are defined by two related but distinct aspects of identity: 1) sexual orientation and 2) gender identity. *Sexual orientation* comprises sexual attraction, sexual behavior, and sexual identity. For many people, these concepts align (e.g., a woman who identifies as a lesbian, is attracted to women, and engages in romantic/sexual relationships with women). However, for others, behavior and identity diverge. Terms such as *men who have sex with men* and *women who have sex with women* refer to individuals who engage in sexual activity with people of the same gender as themselves, regardless of their sexual identity. Sexual identity labels include *heterosexual/straight, lesbian, gay, bisexual,* and *queer.* The word *queer,* which was historically used pejoratively to denigrate SGM people, deserves further explanation. Beginning in the 1980s, some SGM scholars and activists began reclaiming *queer* as a positive identity label. Today, queer individuals use this word in various ways—some as an umbrella term for all SGM people and others as a specific but diverse identity that rejects societal privileging of heterosexuality and embraces a nonbinary conceptualization of sex and gender.

Gender identity is one's internal sense of being a man, a woman, another gender (e.g., genderqueer, nonbinary), or no gender. *Gender expression* is how gender identity is displayed externally and in society, a process that varies across cultures. Gender expression includes (but is not limited to) clothing and mannerisms as well as the name and gender pronoun (e.g., *he, she, they*[1]) one uses. Gender identity is distinct from *sex,* a biological construct defined on an anatomic, genetic, or hormonal basis. In the

---

[1] Some people have a gender identity that is outside the female/male binary. Such individuals may use *they* as a singular pronoun or another pronoun entirely (e.g., *hir* or *zie*) to best reflect their gender identity.

United States and many parts of the world, sex is assigned at birth (male or female) based on external genitalia. GM individuals (e.g., transgender people) have a gender identity that differs from the sex that they were assigned at birth. For some GM individuals, this incongruence creates distress, or *gender dysphoria,* for which they may seek psychological, hormonal, or surgical treatments. In contrast, *cisgender* refers to individuals whose gender identity and sex assigned at birth align.

Notably, sexual orientation and gender identity are distinct (though often related) aspects of a person's identity. For example, although GM individuals are minorities in terms of their gender identity, they may or may not be minorities in terms of their sexual orientation. Depending on the romantic/sexual partners to whom they are attracted, some GM individuals identify as heterosexual/straight. Others may identify as gay/lesbian, bisexual, or another sexual orientation.

Epidemiology of Substance Use Among SGM People

> Marcus is a single 29-year-old white gay man who was raised Catholic and is living in a large urban area, where he is employed as a restaurant manager. His chief complaint is "I can't focus at work anymore." The clinical evaluation suggests the possibility of attention-deficit/hyperactivity disorder. However, when the clinician asks him about substance use, Marcus reports using crystal methamphetamine (crystal meth) 3–4 times per week. He began using crystal meth 3 years earlier at weekend parties and during sex because "it felt amazing." This is still the primary context in which he uses, but he is now using more frequently. Marcus has sex exclusively with men and does not wear condoms. He was recently diagnosed with syphilis and received treatment. The clinician asks Marcus if he has considered making any changes in his crystal meth use. He replies, "Yeah, I know it's not good for me. Honestly, though, I can't imagine having sex without it."

This clinical scenario is one example of how substance use may differ among some SGM populations in comparison with other populations. In this example, Marcus began using crystal meth in the context of sex to heighten sexual pleasure. This type of crystal meth use is common among a subset of SM men, particularly in urban areas of the United States. However, it differs from how crystal meth is used in other populations and in more rural regions. These differences are perhaps influenced by particular cultural norms or experiences. Additionally, rates of substance use differ between SGM and non-SGM individuals. Figure 39–1 compares rates of past-year tobacco, alcohol, and drug use among SM and heterosexual individuals, using data from the 2015 National Survey on Drug Use and Health (NSDUH) (Medley et al. 2016). In the following subsections, these differences and some of the unique sociocultural influences on substance use by SGM people will be considered.

Tobacco/Nicotine

In the United States, SM adults report higher rates of past-30-day tobacco/e-cigarette use in comparison with heterosexual adults (32% vs. 21%) (Medley et al. 2016). This is true both when comparing SM men with heterosexual men (27%–37% vs. 17%) and when comparing SM women with heterosexual women (25%–44% vs. 13%–17%)

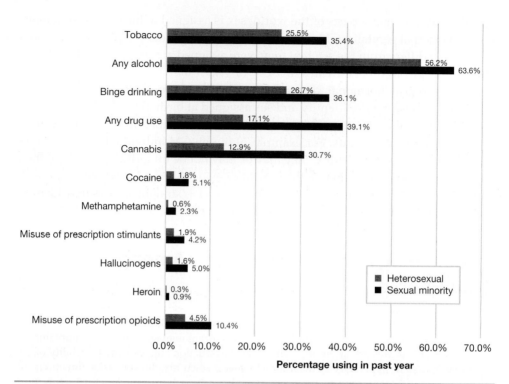

FIGURE 39–1. Past-year substance use among heterosexual and sexual minority adults: U.S. National Survey on Drug Use and Health, 2015.

Note. Sexual minority adults are those who self-identify as being lesbian, gay, or bisexual. Sexual majority adults are those who self-identify as being heterosexual or straight.

Source. Data from Medley G, Lipari RN, Bose J, et al.: Sexual orientation and estimates of adult substance use and mental health: results from the 2015 National Survey of Drug Use and Health. 2016. Available at: https://www.samhsa.gov/data/sites/default/files/NSDUH-SexualOrientation-2015/NSDUH-Sexual-Orientation-2015/NSDUH-SexualOrientation-2015.htm. Accessed October 13, 2018.

(Centers for Disease Control and Prevention 2018b; Johnson et al. 2016). Although bisexual women also have significantly higher rates of smoking in comparison with heterosexual women (36% vs. 13%–17%) (Centers for Disease Control and Prevention 2018b; Johnson et al. 2016), findings are less consistent for bisexual men (Lee et al. 2009). Similar to SM adults, SM youth are nearly twice as likely as heterosexual youth to report current tobacco/e-cigarette use (19% vs. 10%) (Kann et al. 2016). GM individuals report even higher rates of tobacco use (33%–83%) (Kidd et al. 2018a).

The history of tobacco marketing to SGM populations may help explain these disparities (Stevens et al. 2004). In the 1990s, internal documents from R.J. Reynolds Tobacco Company, made public as a result of the Master Settlement Agreement, revealed an internal marketing campaign known as Project SCUM (SubCulture Urban Marketing), later renamed Project Sourdough. These documents describe a multipronged effort to target tobacco marketing toward SGM people and other minority populations in San Francisco's Castro and Tenderloin districts. For many public health researchers, this revelation exemplified the interaction of sociocultural factors and neurobiology that influences SUD disparities between SGM and non-SGM populations.

Alcohol

In general, SM individuals report significantly higher rates of binge drinking (defined as more than 4 drinks for women or 5 drinks for men on a single occasion) than do heterosexual individuals (36% vs. 27%) and slightly higher rates of heavy drinking (defined as 5 or more episodes of binge drinking on 5 or more days in the past month) (8.2% vs. 7.1%) (Medley et al. 2016). When results are stratified by gender, sexual orientation disparities persist. Alcohol use disparities are even more pronounced between SM women and heterosexual women (Hughes et al. 2016). In comparison with cisgender youth, GM youth are at higher risk for past 30-day alcohol use (27% vs. 16%) and binge drinking (19% vs. 8%) (De Pedro et al. 2017). GM adults report higher rates of binge drinking (33%) (Scheim et al. 2016) compared with the general U.S. population (17%) (Centers for Disease Control and Prevention 2018a). Rates of hazardous drinking among GM individuals may differ by sex assigned at birth, although findings are inconsistent. Some studies have reported higher rates among GM women (i.e, who identify as women but were assigned male at birth) (Downing and Przedworski 2018), whereas others have found more hazardous drinking among GM men (i.e., who identify as men but were assigned female at birth) (Kidd et al. 2019; Scheim et al. 2016).

Cannabis

SM individuals, in comparison with heterosexual individuals, report higher rates of past-year cannabis use (31% vs. 13%) and cannabis use disorder (4% vs. 1%) (Medley et al. 2016). These disparities persist when SM women are compared with heterosexual women (33% vs. 10%) and SM men are compared with heterosexual men (27% vs. 16%) (Medley et al. 2016). GM individuals also report high rates of past-3-month cannabis use (24%), with higher rates among GM men (31%) than among GM women (19%) (Gonzalez et al. 2017).

Stimulants and "Club Drugs"

SM individuals, in comparison with heterosexual individuals, report higher rates of past-year cocaine/stimulant use (5% vs. 2%) (Medley et al. 2016). "Club drugs," named for their frequent use at dance clubs and music festivals, include psychostimulants such as methamphetamine (crystal meth) and methylenedioxymethamphetamine (MDMA; commonly called ecstasy), as well as hallucinogens such as γ-hydroxybutyrate (GHB), γ-butyrolactone (GBL), and lysergic acid diethylamide (LSD). Use of club drugs, especially crystal meth, is common among a particular subset of SM men. Although the 2015 NSDUH found that 2.3% of SM adults reported past-year methamphetamine use (vs. 0.6% of heterosexual individuals) (Medley et al. 2016), other studies suggested that SM men may be up to 20 times more likely than heterosexual men to use crystal meth (Reback et al. 2012). Data from GM individuals are limited, but GM women may be more likely than those in the general population to use crystal meth (Scheim et al. 2016). Crystal meth use among SM men and GM women is often associated with unprotected anal intercourse. In fact, the HIV infection risk for SM men who use crystal meth is double that for SM men who do not use crystal meth (Buchacz et al. 2005) and is perhaps 3 times higher among GM women who use crystal meth in comparison with GM women who do not use crystal meth (Santos et al. 2014). Rajasingham et al. (2012) provided a detailed overview of crystal meth use among SM men, including reasons for use and potential behavioral interventions. Self-reported reasons for use of crystal meth among SM men included enhanced sexual pleasure, increased energy, improved self-confidence and self-esteem, improved ability to meet sexual partners, better coping with grief, and feeling more attractive. Few studies have investigated use of club drugs among SM women. In a study of 1,104 women recruited from dance clubs in New York City, Parsons et al. (2006) found that SM women reported significantly higher lifetime use rates of ecstasy, cocaine, methamphetamine, and LSD in comparison with heterosexual women; however, the overall magnitude of use among SM women is still not clear.

Opioids

Despite increased attention from medical professionals and policy makers to the current opioid crisis, data on opioid use among SGM individuals are extremely limited. According to the 2015 NSDUH, 2% of SM individuals reported problematic use of prescription pain medications, compared with 0.7% of heterosexual individuals (Medley et al. 2016). Few studies have examined gender differences in opioid use among SM individuals. One recent study examined the data further and found that bisexual adults were at particularly high risk for past-month opioid use and that bisexual women were at the highest risk (Duncan et al. 2019). No data are available on opioid use among GM individuals. Additionally, it is not clear how the national epidemic of opioid overdose deaths is impacting SGM individuals.

Racial/Ethnic Differences in Substance Use in SGM Populations

Few studies have examined racial/ethnic differences in substance use among SGM individuals (Kidd et al. 2018b), but several trends have emerged, particularly for SM youth. For example, although young SM men generally report higher rates of substance use compared with young heterosexual men, Swann et al. (2017) found that young black SM men reported a more gradual trajectory of increase in alcohol, cannabis, and noncannabis drug use compared with young white SM men. In contrast, compared with young white SM men, young Latino SM men reported a steeper trajectory of increase in alcohol use but a more gradual increase in drug use. Using data from the Youth Risk Behavior Surveillance Survey, Talley et al. (2016) found that Asian SM youth were more likely than Asian heterosexual youth to report lifetime drinking. Racial/ethnic minority SM youth have also reported higher levels of stigma and discrimination (Bruce et al. 2014), which are associated with worse substance use outcomes. These are only a few examples of the ways that having multiple minority identities can impact health disparities, possibly via multiple marginalization.

Minority Stress Theory: A Model for Explicating Risk and Protective Factors for SGM Populations

Minority Stress Theory (Meyer 2003) is an evidence-based conceptual model used to explicate a wide variety of health disparities, including substance use, for SGM populations. In Minority Stress Theory, individuals from stigmatized minority populations experience a unique type of stress (i.e., minority stress) in response to discrimination, internalized stigma, and societal prejudice. Minority stress is additive to the general stress experienced by all individuals. For SGM individuals, minority stress can take many forms (e.g., housing/employment discrimination, family rejection, hate violence victimization, discriminatory laws/policies) and can affect SGM individuals in myriad ways. For example, stigma against SGM people can disrupt central family and peer relationships, leading to decreased social support. In New York City, 13%–36% of homeless youth identify as SGM, and many are homeless due to family rejection (New York City Commission on Lesbian, Gay, Bisexual, Transgender, and Questioning Runaway and Homeless Youth 2010). Family rejection is itself a predictor of hazardous substance use among both SGM adolescents (Kidd et al. 2018b) and SGM adults (Klein and Golub 2016). Conversely, adolescents' attachment to their parents, enrollment in college, feeling of belonging at school, and early SM self-identification are protective against substance use among SM youth and young adults (Kidd et al. 2018b). Social support may also be protective, but this depends on the perceived substance use norms of the support system.

Heterosexism is the societal privileging of heterosexuality and heterosexual relationships over other identities. Heterosexism can cause SGM individuals to view themselves as inferior, a feeling known as *internalized heterosexism*. In turn, internalized heterosexism is associated with higher rates of substance use and of anxiety and depressive symptoms (Meyer 2003). Among SM individuals, higher levels of discrimination are also associated with increased likelihood of having an SUD (Slater et al. 2017). Among GM individuals, discrimination and harassment are associated with higher odds of past-3-month tobacco use (Kidd et al. 2018a), hazardous alcohol use (Gonzalez et al. 2017), and heavy cannabis use (Gonzalez et al. 2017).

Structural factors, such as laws and policies, are increasingly recognized as risk and protective factors for SGM individuals. For example, rates of alcohol and drug use disorders (along with rates of depressive and anxiety disorders) are significantly higher in U.S. states with anti-SGM laws (e.g., constitutional prohibitions on same-gender marriage) (Hatzenbuehler et al. 2010) and in U.S. states that lack pro-SGM protections (e.g., SGM-inclusive nondiscrimination ordinances) (Hatzenbuehler et al. 2009). Similarly, among SGM adolescents and young adults, those with access to SGM-inclusive antibullying policies or supportive high school programs such as Gay-Straight Alliances were found to engage in more frequent resource seeking and discussion of topics related to mental health and substance use, compared with those without access to these affirming policies and programs (Poteat et al. 2017). Interestingly, these programs are associated with improved health outcomes among both SGM *and* heterosexual students (Poteat et al. 2017).

Key Clinical Considerations in SUD Treatment With SGM Patients

Thomas is a 52-year-old black GM man (identifies as a man but was assigned female at birth). He recently completed an inpatient alcohol detoxification program and is seeking residential treatment for alcohol use disorder. Thomas came out as transgender when he was 21 years old and has lived openly as a man since that time. He started gender-affirming hormone treatment with testosterone at age 23. He has struggled since age 18 to limit his alcohol use and has previously attended outpatient treatment programs but, he says, "It never stuck." During the intake process, Thomas meets with a physician, Dr. Bob, who requests permission to perform a physical examination. Trying to preempt any awkwardness, Thomas explains to Dr. Bob that he is transgender. Dr. Bob is visibly uncomfortable and stammers, "Oh…well, we might need to have you stay with the women then." Dr. Bob also explains that while in treatment, Thomas will need to cover up his tattoos and might consider keeping his transgender identity a secret "because other patients might not understand…. It'll just be smoother that way." Thomas finishes the intake process but leaves the program the following day.

The fundamentals of providing psychopharmacological and psychosocial SUD treatments apply to SGM patients just as they do to heterosexual, cisgender patients. However, as illustrated in the case of Thomas, the experiences of SGM individuals in addiction treatment may be different from those of their non-SGM peers. In this section, I discuss key topics for clinicians to consider when evaluating and treating SGM patients that can improve the therapeutic alliance and facilitate a more nuanced understanding of substance use in this patient population.

Coming Out: Revealing One's SGM Identity to Others

Despite societal advances and increased media representation of SGM people, most institutions (e.g., schools, religious institutions, workplaces) still operate on the implicit assumption that people are heterosexual, a bias known as heterosexism. *Coming out* refers to the process of disclosing one's SGM identity to others. In popular culture, coming out is often portrayed as a single, climactic moment in an SGM individual's life. In reality, coming out is an iterative process. With each new interpersonal interaction, SGM individuals make decisions about whether and how to disclose these parts of their identity. Considerations may include the type of relationship (e.g., friend vs. coworker), the anticipated reaction of the other person, and the perceived consequences of rejection. Even if these calculations become less stressful over time, coming out is often still an active process to some extent. Furthermore, the relationship between disclosure and substance use is complicated. Although some studies have found an association between earlier self-disclosure and lower risk for substance use, this association is moderated by the outcome of the disclosure (i.e., affirmation or rejection) (Kidd et al. 2018b). Therefore, coming out is an individualized decision. Psychiatrists and other health professionals can provide validation and a supportive, safe, affirming environment in which to explore these decisions, while still respecting patient autonomy in deciding whether and when to come out.

SGM patients also make decisions about coming out when they seek medical or psychiatric care. In fact, fear of discrimination from health care providers leads many GM people to delay seeking necessary care (Glick et al. 2018). Therefore, it is important that health care professionals create an SGM-affirming environment. Clinicians should routinely ask patients about their sexual orientation and gender identity, rather than making assumptions or waiting for patients to self-disclose. This approach includes asking about and consistently using the patient's preferred name and gender pronouns (e.g., *he, she, they*). If patients appear confused by name and pronoun questions, providers can use their own names and pronouns as examples. Table 39–1 provides sample

TABLE 39–1. Sample interview and clinic form questions for asking patients about their sexual orientation and gender identity

	Interview Questions	Clinic Form Questions
	Prefaced by: I ask all of my patients these questions. It helps me get to know you better and provide you with the best care possible.	
Sexual orientation	People use different words to describe their sexual orientation, such as straight, gay, or bisexual. How would you describe your sexual orientation?	Which of the following best describes your sexual orientation? ❏ Heterosexual/Straight ❏ Homosexual/Gay/Lesbian ❏ Bisexual ❏ Queer ❏ None of these labels describe me. → Please tell us more about your sexual orientation.
Gender identity	People describe their gender in different ways. These include words like *man, woman,* or another label altogether. How would you describe your gender?	**2-Step Method** 1. What was your sex assigned at birth (on your original birth certificate)? ❏ Male ❏ Female ❏ Other[a] 2. Which of the following best describes your current gender identity? (Check all that apply.) ❏ Male ❏ Female ❏ Transmale/transman/FTM ❏ Transfemale/transwoman/MTF ❏ Genderqueer/nonbinary/ gender nonconforming ❏ Different identity → Please state:
Legal and preferred name	You chart lists your name as [Name], but some people have another name that they use. What name would you like me to use?	Legal Name (the name listed on your insurance card): Preferred Name (if different from above):
Gender pronoun	I would like to be respectful. What pronouns do you use? For example, I use [pronoun].	Pronoun (e.g., he, she, they):

Note. FTM=female-to-male; MTF=male-to-female.
[a]Some states allow an X or other nonbinary marker on birth certificates.

questions that can be incorporated into a clinical interview or the demographic forms completed by patients in many health care settings. (For a review of the two-question method of assessing gender identity [which has been recommended by the World Professional Association for Transgender Health for use when asking patients about gender identity], readers are referred to Deutsch et al. 2013.)

Families: Support Versus Rejection

As described earlier, many SGM people still experience negative reactions from their families of origin (e.g., biological or adoptive parents) after coming out. Responses can range from derogatory remarks to increased emotional distance to outright rejection. Family rejection can lead to homelessness (New York City Commission on Lesbian, Gay, Bisexual, Transgender, and Questioning Runaway and Homeless Youth 2010) and increased risk for SUDs and other psychiatric illnesses (Kidd et al. 2018b; Klein and Golub 2016). Asking about family-of-origin relationships can help clinicians understand potential early-life stressors for SGM individuals, stressors that may continue to influence their substance use. Conversely, SGM identity affirmation is protective against substance use (Poteat et al. 2017). Many SGM individuals receive affirmation from people outside of their families of origin. Such "chosen families" may include romantic partners (with or without legal recognition) and close friends. In an open-ended manner, clinicians can ask SGM patients about their support systems. If the treatment being provided typically involves family members, the clinician should consider inviting SGM patients to include members of their chosen family.

Gender-Affirming Health Care: Working With Gender Minority Patients

As described earlier, some GM individuals seek gender-affirming psychological, hormonal (e.g., estrogen, testosterone), and/or surgical (e.g., mastectomy, vaginoplasty, phalloplasty) treatments to reduce gender incongruence and alleviate gender dysphoria. Although SUDs are not an absolute contraindication for these treatments, there are relevant clinical considerations. For example, both tobacco use and estrogen/testosterone treatment are associated with increased cardiovascular risk (Streed et al. 2017), highlighting the importance of smoking cessation counseling (Kidd et al. 2018a). Mental health care providers may also be asked to conduct evaluations prior to gender-affirming surgery. These might include screening for SUDs, providing psychoeducation about associated risks, and facilitating treatment. Assessing the impact of active substance use on surgical risk is best done in consultation with the patient's surgeon. More information on this type of psychiatric evaluation can be obtained from the World Professional Association for Transgender Health (2011).

HIV and Hepatitis C: Where Substance Use Meets Sexual Health

Despite decreasing HIV infection rates in the United States, HIV remains a major public health issue. Incident HIV infection rates remain particularly high among black and Latinx men who have sex with men and among GM women (Centers for Disease

Control and Prevention 2018c, 2018d). Health care providers working with these populations can provide crucial psychoeducation on safer sex practices, including condom use and pre- and postexposure prophylaxis (PrEP and PEP). PrEP and PEP are evidence-based methods for preventing HIV infection that involve taking antiretroviral medications on a regular basis before any potential HIV exposure occurs (PrEP) or taking medications shortly after a potential exposure occurs (PEP). In addition to unprotected sex, injection drug use is a major risk factor for HIV and hepatitis C transmission. Individuals who inject drugs can reduce their infection risk by refraining from sharing or reusing syringes. Policies that facilitate access to clean syringes (e.g., syringe services programs, over-the-counter availability) can help reduce infection risk. Randomized controlled trial data also support the use of PrEP for individuals who share syringes (Choopanya et al. 2013). The Centers for Disease Control and Prevention (2018e) recommends that people who inject drugs be offered vaccination against viral hepatitis A and B as well as testing for HIV and hepatitis C at least annually (see also Chapter 33, "HIV/AIDS and Hepatitis C Virus").

Inpatient and Residential Treatments: Concerns Among SGM Patients

As described in the case vignette presented at the beginning of this section, Thomas is a GM man seeking residential addiction treatment. Although policies and treatment philosophies vary, residential SUD treatment (i.e., detoxification and/or rehabilitation) programs can present unique challenges for SGM individuals such as Thomas. Some treatment programs incorporate religious language and scripture that may be stigmatizing of SGM people. Even when such programs are not overtly hostile to SGM identities, SGM people may find this religious focus uncomfortable, particularly if they have previously encountered stigma from religious communities. Consequently, SGM patients may feel compelled to hide their sexual orientation or gender identity in order to receive treatment. In doing so, they are forced to withhold part of their identity from treatment staff and peers, potentially hindering effective treatment. Additionally, some residential treatment programs restrict the types of items patients can bring with them. Prohibited items can include jewelry, makeup, and certain types of clothing that may be important parts of gender expression for GM individuals. Although it is understandable that programs must have some guidelines (e.g., prohibiting clothing with drug-related images), more restrictive policies can marginalize GM (and many SM) individuals, forcing them to choose between gender affirmation and SUD treatment.

Many SUD treatment programs, whether residential or outpatient programs, provide treatment separately to men and women. In residential programs, dormitory and restroom/shower facilities are often separated by gender. For GM individuals, such policies can create significant anxiety and may increase barriers to treatment. Systems of care and clinical guidelines in this area continue to evolve. Ideally, in a treatment program that separates patients on the basis of gender, GM individuals would be offered housing and treatment in accordance with their gender identity, rather than their sex assigned at birth, unless a patient desires a different arrangement. For example, a GM man (who identifies as a man but was assigned female at birth) would be offered housing and treatment with other men. For individuals with nonbinary gender identities (e.g., genderqueer), principles of patient-centered care can be applied to involve the patient in decision making related to housing and treatment.

Psychiatric Comorbidity: Higher Rates Among SGM Individuals

For SGM individuals, as is generally the case for all patients, it is important to screen for comorbid psychiatric disorders, because failure to identify co-occurring conditions reduces the person's chance of receiving appropriate treatment. When a psychiatric illness co-occurs with SUD, treatment should address both sets of problems. Generally speaking, rates of depressive and anxiety disorders are 2–4 times higher among SM individuals than among heterosexual/straight individuals (Kerridge et al. 2017). Table 39–2 presents rates of DSM-5 psychiatric disorders by sexual orientation among participants in the 2012–2013 National Epidemiologic Survey on Alcohol and Related Conditions–III (Kerridge et al. 2017). It is likely that prevalences are even higher among SGM individuals with SUDs. Because minority stress is a risk factor for the development of both SUDs and other psychiatric disorders (Hatzenbuehler et al. 2009, 2010; Meyer 2003), clinicians should ask SGM patients about their experiences of discrimination, stigma, and maltreatment. Doing so allows clinicians to provide support and validation that can strengthen the therapeutic alliance. This line of questioning also helps clinicians to better understand the particular contexts in which substance use occurs, because minority stressors can trigger cravings and increase relapse risk.

Self-Disclosure by Health Care Providers: Whether, When, and How

For clinicians, disclosing one's own sexual orientation or gender identity to patients is a consideration in treating both SGM and heterosexual, cisgender patients. Some patients may ask directly about a provider's identity. Others may make more indirect inquiries, such as "I hope you and your wife have a nice vacation…" or "I went to this [gay] bar The Eagle last night. Have you been there?" For many providers, such inquiries can provoke anxiety and confusion about how to respond. Levounis and Anson (2012) have discussed this issue in detail and have presented a framework for considering self-disclosure (summarized in Table 39–3). Considerations include the therapist's comfort with their own identity and with being "out" in a professional setting, the phase and frame of the treatment (e.g., monthly medication management vs. weekly psychotherapy), the patient's comfort with their own identity, and the potential consequences of disclosure. Whereas some patients may feel uncomfortable knowing their health care provider's sexual orientation or gender identity, other patients may derive benefit from the therapist's modeling of self-disclosure in a nonstigmatizing, self-affirming manner.

Sexual Function and Dysfunction: More Than Just Safe Sex

In some cases, sexual functioning (e.g., desire, arousal, orgasm) can be negatively impacted by acute substance (e.g., opioid, cocaine) intoxication, long-term sequelae of

TABLE 39–2. **12-Month prevalences of DSM-5 psychiatric disorders by sexual orientation among participants in the 2012–2013 National Epidemiologic Survey on Alcohol and Related Conditions (NESARC-III)**

Disorder	Heterosexual/ Straight, %	Gay/ Lesbian, %	Bisexual, %	Unsure,[a] %
Major depressive disorder	10.0	18.0	24.0	20.5
Persistent depressive disorder (dysthymia)	3.0	6.8	8.9	6.4
Bipolar I disorder	1.5	2.2	5.2	5.5
Panic disorder	2.8	7.9	10.8	12.7
Social phobia	2.7	6.6	11.1	8.6
Generalized anxiety disorder	5.1	9.6	14.0	11.2
Posttraumatic stress disorder	4.4	6.7	17.9	13.8
Borderline personality disorder	10.9	19.8	36.4	32.8
Schizotypal personality disorder	5.9	11.2	25.9	22.2

[a]Unsure participants reported questioning their sexual orientation in some way.
Source. Adapted from Kerridge BT, Pickering RP, Saha TD, et al: "Prevalence, Sociodemographic Correlates and DSM-5 Substance Use Disorders and Other Psychiatric Disorders Among Sexual Minorities in the United States." *Drug and Alcohol Dependence* 170:82–92, 2017.

TABLE 39–3. **Considerations for providers in self-disclosing their sexual orientation or gender identity to patients**

Considerations in favor of direct disclosure	Considerations against direct disclosure
• Treatment just beginning and patient feels comfortable asking about provider's identity.	• Indirect inquiries communicate patient's discomfort with knowing provider's identity.
• Provider identifies as SGM, and patient has identified "coming out" or normalizing SGM thoughts/feelings as a treatment goal.	• Treatment is psychodynamic and the patient's fantasies about the provider's identity produce material that warrants further exploration.
• Patient indirectly expresses continued curiosity about provider's identity.	• Patient is particularly defended against exploring their sexual orientation or gender identity.
• Provider or clinic advertises as SGM-oriented.	• Patient expresses violent views about SGM people or identities and provider is SGM.
• Not disclosing would undermine patient–provider relationship.	
• Patient's misinterpretation of provider's refusal to disclose might reinforce patient's feelings of self-hatred.	• Provider has significant unresolved feelings about their own sexual orientation or gender identity.

SGM=sexual and gender minority.
Source. Adapted from Levounis P, Anson AJ: "Sexual Identity in Patient–Therapist Relationships," in *The LGBT Casebook.* Edited by In Levounis P, Drescher J, Barber M. Washington, DC, American Psychiatric Association Publishing, 2012, pp 73–83. Used with permission.

substance use (e.g., uncontrolled diabetes in the setting of alcohol use disorder), or SUD treatment itself (e.g., methadone maintenance) (Zaazaa et al. 2013). In other cases, substances may be used to overcome sexual dysfunction (e.g., poppers/inhaled nitrites, crystal meth) or to alleviate anticipatory anxiety about sexual activity (e.g., alcohol, benzodiazepines). Inquiring about sexual activity, sexual satisfaction, and sexual dysfunction can help providers better understand patients' substance use. Because sexual dysfunction may serve as a trigger for substance use, clinicians should inquire about medical conditions (e.g., diabetes mellitus, hypertension, chronic pain), psychiatric disorders (e.g., major depressive disorder), and medications (e.g., serotonergic antidepressants and antipsychotics) that may affect sexual functioning. Finally, sexual functioning changes with age (Thompson et al. 2011; Wight et al. 2012); for example, individuals assigned female at birth may experience postmenopausal reductions in vaginal lubrication that make penetrative vaginal sex uncomfortable. Individuals assigned male at birth may experience erectile dysfunction or greater difficulty in achieving orgasm. Health care providers can assist these patients in understanding these age-related changes and in many cases can recommend treatment to help mitigate their impact on sexual satisfaction. For GM individuals, gender-affirming hormone therapy may affect sexual functioning: estrogen can cause erectile dysfunction and reduced libido, whereas testosterone may lead to increased libido and decreased vaginal lubrication (World Professional Association for Transgender Health 2011). Alternatively, gender-affirming medical/surgical care may make sexual activity more enjoyable by reducing gender dysphoria (van de Grift et al. 2017). Although the relationship between sexual functioning and substance use is not unique to SGM individuals, treatment providers can foster an affirming therapeutic relationship with SGM patients by using inclusive language and avoiding heterosexist assumptions.

Smartphone Apps: Sex and Drugs in the Twenty-First Century

Over the past 10 years, smartphone apps such as Grindr, Scuff, Jack'd, Hornet, and Chappy have changed the ways that SGM individuals, particularly SM men, find sexual partners outside of the typical bar and party culture. Using geolocation technology, app users can exchange texts, photos, and videos in real time with nearby app users. Public health officials are exploring ways to use apps for health promotion (e.g., safer sex education). However, recent studies have highlighted how such apps may also facilitate "chemsex"—the practice of combining sexual activity with the use of drugs such as crystal meth (Anzani et al. 2018). As described earlier, crystal meth use among SM men and GM women increases the risk for unprotected sex and HIV infection (Buchacz et al. 2005; Santos et al. 2014). Therefore, clinicians can better understand stimulant use among SGM individuals by expanding sexual history taking to include discussions about how patients meet sexual partners (including via smartphone apps) and how sexual activity might relate to drug use. For example, behavioral therapies for crystal meth addiction often include limiting the use of websites and smartphone apps that facilitate "chemsex."

Trauma: An All-Too-Common Life Experience in SGM Populations

As detailed earlier, trauma can take many forms (e.g., emotional, sexual, physical) and is a consideration when working with SGM patients. Hate crimes are a particular type of crime in which victims are targeted because of their identity. According to the U.S. Federal Bureau of Investigation (2018), crimes motivated by sexual orientation and gender identity bias represented 16.7% and 2.2%, respectively, of all reported hate crimes in 2018. These figures are likely to be underestimates, because reporting is voluntary and varies by state and locality. GM individuals, particularly GM women of color, are especially at risk for hate violence. Even when individuals do not experience violence or discrimination, fear of victimization or harassment is common (Veldhuis et al. 2018) and can impact health outcomes. Therefore, when screening for trauma, clinicians should ask questions about harassment or violence motivated by anti-SGM bias.

Given the prevalence of violence victimization in SGM populations, it is not surprising that rates of posttraumatic stress disorder (PTSD) are also disproportionately higher among SGM individuals than in the general population (Kerridge et al. 2017). PTSD may increase substance use risk. For example, in a study of young GM women in San Francisco, those with PTSD were twice as likely as those without PTSD to report drug use (Rowe et al. 2015). Screening for traumatic experiences and trauma-related disorders among SGM patients with SUDs can improve detection and allow clinicians to provide trauma-informed SUD treatment, taking into account the ways in which such experiences might affect substance use and relapse risk.

Summary of Recommendations for Providing SGM-Affirming SUD Treatment

The following are strategies for providing SGM-affirming SUD treatment, regardless of the treatment setting:

- Ask all patients about their sexual orientation and gender identity (see Table 39–1). Asking routinely reduces the risk of making false assumptions.
- Ask about support systems broadly. Remember that friends and chosen family may be influential supports for SGM people.
- Update intake forms to ask about legal name, preferred name, and gender pronouns (see Table 39–1). Including such questions helps staff members to avoid mistakes and demonstrates to patients that your treatment program is affirming and inclusive.
- Use gender-neutral language (e.g., *partner*) when asking about romantic or sexual partners.
- Use gender-neutral pronouns (e.g., *they*) and avoid gendered salutations (e.g., *Mr.* and *Ms.*) until you know how a patient identifies.
- Identify and address anti-SGM bias and stigma in your workplace.

- Gently correct colleagues if they are disrespectful (e.g., use the incorrect name or pronoun for a patient). Everyone makes mistakes, and correcting these helps create a culture of respect.
- Respect SGM individuals' autonomy in defining their identity and making decisions about disclosure, while providing a safe and affirming environment in which they can explore these questions.

References

Anzani A, Di Sarno M, Prunas A: Using smartphone apps to find sexual partners: a review of the literature. Sexologies 27(3):e61–e65, 2018. Available at: https://www.sciencedi-rect.com/science/article/abs/pii/S1158136018300719. Accessed April 24, 2020.

Bruce D, Stall R, Fata A, et al: Modeling minority stress effects on homelessness and health disparities among young men who have sex with men. J Urban Health 91(3):568–580, 2014 24807702

Buchacz K, McFarland W, Kellogg TA, et al: Amphetamine use is associated with increased HIV incidence among men who have sex with men in San Francisco. AIDS 19(13):1423–1424, 2005 16103774

Centers for Disease Control and Prevention: Alcohol and Public Health: Data and Maps. 2018a. Available at: https://www.cdc.gov/alcohol/data-stats.htm. Accessed January 8, 2020.

Centers for Disease Control and Prevention: Current cigarette smoking among adults—United States, 2016. MMWR Morb Mortal Wkly Rep 67(2):53–59, 2018b 29346338

Centers for Disease Control and Prevention: HIV/AIDS: Basic Statistics. 2018c. Available at: https://www.cdc.gov/hiv/basics/statistics.html. Accessed January 8, 2020.

Centers for Disease Control and Prevention: HIV among transgender people. 2018d. Available at: https://www.cdc.gov/hiv/group/gender/transgender/index.html. Accessed January 8, 2020.

Centers for Disease Control and Prevention: Injection Drug Use and HIV Risk. 2018e. Available at: https://www.cdc.gov/hiv/risk/idu.html. Accessed January 8, 2020.

Choopanya K, Martin M, Suntharasamai P, et al: Antiretroviral prophylaxis for HIV infection in injecting drug users in Bangkok, Thailand (the Bangkok Tenofovir Study): a randomised, double-blind, placebo-controlled phase 3 trial. Lancet 381(9883):2083–2090, 2013 23769234

De Pedro KT, Gilreath TD, Jackson C, et al: Substance use among transgender students in California public middle and high schools. J Sch Health 87(5):303–309, 2017 28382667

Deutsch MB, Green J, Keatley J, et al; World Professional Association for Transgender Health EMR Working Group: Electronic medical records and the transgender patient: recommendations from the World Professional Association for Transgender Health EMR Working Group. J Am Med Inform Assoc 20(4):700–703, 2013 23631835

Downing JM, Przedworski JM: Health of transgender adults in the U.S., 2014–2016. Am J Prev Med 55(3):336–344, 2018 30031640

Duncan DT, Zweig S, Hambrick HR, Palamar JJ: Sexual orientation disparities in prescription opioid misuse among U.S. adults. Am J Prev Med 56(1):17–26, 2019 30467089

Federal Bureau of Investigation: 2018 hate crimes statistics. 2018. Available at: https://ucr.fbi.gov/hate-crime/2018/topic-pages/victims. Accessed June 29, 2020.

Glick JL, Theall KP, Andrinopoulos KM, et al: The role of discrimination in care postponement among trans-feminine individuals in the U.S. National Transgender Discrimination Survey. LGBT Health 5(3):171–179, 2018 29589995

Gonzalez CA, Gallego JD, Bockting WO: Demographic characteristics, components of sexuality and gender, and minority stress and their associations to excessive alcohol, cannabis, and illicit (noncannabis) drug use among a large sample of transgender people in the United States. J Prim Prev 38(4):419–445, 2017 28405831

Hatzenbuehler ML, Keyes KM, Hasin DS: State-level policies and psychiatric morbidity in lesbian, gay, and bisexual populations. Am J Public Health 99(12):2275–2281, 2009 19833997

Hatzenbuehler ML, McLaughlin KA, Keyes KM, Hasin DS: The impact of institutional discrimination on psychiatric disorders in lesbian, gay, and bisexual populations: a prospective study. Am J Public Health 100(3):452–459, 2010 20075314

Hughes TL, Wilsnack SC, Kantor LW: The influence of gender and sexual orientation on alcohol use and alcohol-related problems: toward a global perspective. Alcohol Res 38(1):121–132, 2016 27159819

Johnson SE, Holder-Hayes E, Tessman GK, et al: Tobacco product use among sexual minority adults: findings from the 2012–2013 National Adult Tobacco Survey. Am J Prev Med 50(4):e91–e100, 2016 26526162

Kann L, Olsen EO, McManus T, et al: Sexual identity, sex of sexual contacts, and health-related behaviors among students in grades 9–12—United States and selected sites, 2015. MMWR Surveill Summ 65(9):1–202, 2016 27513843

Kerridge BT, Pickering RP, Saha TD, et al: Prevalence, sociodemographic correlates and DSM-5 substance use disorders and other psychiatric disorders among sexual minorities in the United States. Drug Alcohol Depend 170:82–92, 2017 27883948

Kidd JD, Dolezal C, Bockting WO: The relationship between tobacco use and legal document gender-marker change, hormone use, and gender-affirming surgery in a United States sample of trans-feminine and trans-masculine individuals: implications for cardiovascular health. LGBT Health 5(7):401–411, 2018a 30334686

Kidd JD, Jackman KB, Wolff M, et al: Risk and protective factors for substance use among sexual and gender minority youth. Curr Addict Rep 5(2):158–173, 2018b 30393591

Kidd JD, Levin FR, Dolezal C, et al: Understanding predictors of improvement in risky drinking in a U.S. multi-site, longitudinal cohort study of transgender individuals: implications for culturally tailored prevention and treatment efforts. Addict Behav 96:68–75, 2019 31039507

Klein A, Golub SA: Family rejection as a predictor of suicide attempts and substance misuse among transgender and gender nonconforming adults. LGBT Health 3(3):193–199, 2016 27046450

Lee JG, Griffin GK, Melvin CL: Tobacco use among sexual minorities in the USA, 1987 to May 2007: a systematic review. Tob Control 18(4):275–282, 2009 19208668

Levounis P, Anson AJ: Sexual identity in patient-therapist relationships, in The LGBT Casebook. Edited by Levounis P, Drescher J, Barber M. Washington, DC, American Psychiatric Association Publishing, 2012, pp 73–83

Medley G, Lipari RN, Bose J, et al: Sexual Orientation and Estimates of Adult Substance Use and Mental Health: Results From the 2015 National Survey of Drug Use and Health, 2016. Available at: https://www.samhsa.gov/data/sites/default/files/NSDUH-SexualOrientation-2015/NSDUH-SexualOrientation-2015/NSDUH-SexualOrientation-2015.htm. Accessed October 13, 2018.

Meyer IH: Prejudice, social stress, and mental health in lesbian, gay, and bisexual populations: conceptual issues and research evidence. Psychol Bull 129(5):674–697, 2003 12956539

National Academy of Medicine: The Health of Lesbian, Gay, Bisexual, and Transgender People: Building a Foundation for Better Understanding. Washington, DC, National Academies Press, 2011

New York City Commission on Lesbian, Gay, Bisexual, Transgender, and Questioning Runaway and Homeless Youth: All Our Children: Strategies to Prevent Homelessness, Strengthen Services, and Build Support for LGBTQ Youth. June 2010. Available at: http://www.nyc.gov/html/om/pdf/2010/pr267_10_report.pdf. Accessed January 8, 2020.

Parsons JT, Kelly BC, Wells BE: Differences in club drug use between heterosexual and lesbian/bisexual females. Addict Behav 31(12):2344–2349, 2006 16632210

Poteat VP, Heck NC, Yoshikawa H, et al: Gay-Straight Alliances as settings to discuss health topics: individual and group factors associated with substance use, mental health, and sexual health discussions. Health Educ Res 32(3):258–268, 2017 28472258

Rajasingham R, Mimiaga MJ, White JM, et al: A systematic review of behavioral and treatment outcome studies among HIV-infected men who have sex with men who abuse crystal methamphetamine. AIDS Patient Care STDS 26(1):36–52, 2012 22070609

Reback CJ, Peck JA, Fletcher JB, et al: Lifetime substance use and HIV sexual risk behaviors predict treatment response to contingency management among homeless, substance-dependent MSM. J Psychoactive Drugs 44(2):166–172, 2012 22880545

Rowe C, Santos GM, McFarland W, et al: Prevalence and correlates of substance use among trans female youth ages 16–24 years in the San Francisco Bay Area. Drug Alcohol Depend 147:160–166, 2015 25548025

Santos GM, Rapues J, Wilson EC, et al: Alcohol and substance use among transgender women in San Francisco: prevalence and association with human immunodeficiency virus infection. Drug Alcohol Rev 33(3):287–295, 2014 24628655

Scheim AI, Bauer GR, Shokoohi M: Heavy episodic drinking among transgender persons: disparities and predictors. Drug Alcohol Depend 167:156–162, 2016 27542688

Scheim AI, Bauer GR, Shokoohi M: Drug use among transgender people in Ontario, Canada: disparities and associations with social exclusion. Addict Behav 72:151–158, 2017 28411424

Slater ME, Godette D, Huang B, et al: Sexual orientation-based discrimination, excessive alcohol use, and substance use disorders among sexual minority adults. LGBT Health 4(5):337–344, 2017 28876167

Stevens P, Carlson LM, Hinman JM: An analysis of tobacco industry marketing to lesbian, gay, bisexual, and transgender (LGBT) populations: strategies for mainstream tobacco control and prevention. Health Promot Pract 5(3 suppl):129S–134S, 2004 15231106

Streed CG Jr, Harfouch O, Marvel F, et al: Cardiovascular disease among transgender adults receiving hormone therapy: a narrative review. Ann Intern Med 167(4):256–267, 2017 28738421

Swann G, Bettin E, Clifford A, et al: Trajectories of alcohol, marijuana, and illicit drug use in a diverse sample of young men who have sex with men. Drug Alcohol Depend 178:231–242, 2017 28667941

Talley AE, Gilbert PA, Mitchell J, et al: Addressing gaps on risk and resilience factors for alcohol use outcomes in sexual and gender minority populations. Drug Alcohol Rev 35(4):484–493, 2016 27072658

Thompson WK, Charo L, Vahia IV, et al: Association between higher levels of sexual function, activity, and satisfaction and self-rated successful aging in older postmenopausal women. J Am Geriatr Soc 59(8):1503–1508, 2011 21797827

van de Grift TC, Elaut E, Cerwenka SC, et al: Effects of medical interventions on gender dysphoria and body image: a follow-up study. Psychosom Med 79(7):815–823, 2017 28319558

Veldhuis CB, Drabble L, Riggle EDB, et al: "I fear for my safety, but want to show bravery for others": violence and discrimination concerns among transgender and gender-nonconforming individuals after the 2016 presidential election. Violence and Gender 5(1):26–36, 2018. Available at: https://www.liebertpub.com/doi/full/10.1089/vio.2017.0032. Accessed February 6, 2020.

Wight RG, LeBlanc AJ, de Vries B, et al: Stress and mental health among midlife and older gay-identified men. Am J Public Health 102(3):503–510, 2012 22390515

World Professional Association for Transgender Health: Standards of Care for the Health of Transsexual, Transgender, and Gender Nonconforming, 7th Edition. 2011. Available at: https://www.wpath.org/media/cms/Documents/SOC%20v7/SOC%20V7_English.pdf. Accessed January 8, 2020.

Zaazaa A, Bella AJ, Shamloul R: Drug addiction and sexual dysfunction. Endocrinol Metab Clin North Am 42(3):585–592, 2013 24011888

CHAPTER 40

Cross-Cultural Aspects of Substance-Related and Addictive Disorders

Nady el-Guebaly, M.D., D.Psych., D.P.H.

Hyoun S. Kim, M.A.

In our ever-shrinking global village, the need for cross-cultural sensitivity and clinical competence increases along with the pace of our contact with other cultures, either through travel or via permanent resettlement. Clinical cultural competence is a lifelong journey. In this chapter, we identify the clinically relevant variables of culture and their implications for assessment and management of addictions. Most of the recent scientific literature in English addresses culture in the context of our modern multiethnic societies in the United States, Great Britain, Canada, and Australia. The definition of *culture* has shifted in the past several decades. Whereas the term *culture* has traditionally referred to an individual's ethnicity or race, it has broadened to include such characteristics as a person's sexual orientation. The concept of *addictions* has also changed. Specifically, the fifth edition of the *Diagnostic and Statistical Manual of Mental Disorders* (DSM-5; American Psychiatric Association 2013) now includes behavioral addictions (gambling disorder and Internet gaming disorder) alongside traditional substance addictions such as alcohol, cannabis, and cocaine. Although the focus of this chapter remains primarily on psychoactive substances, we include behavioral addictions (gambling, gaming) when possible due to their rising relevance in psychiatry and clinical psychology (see also Chapter 42 in this volume, "Behavioral Addictive Disorders").

Concepts and Definitions

In multiethnic societies, the following definitions represent current attempts to explain cross-cultural terminology:

- *Culture* refers to systems of knowledge, concepts, rules, and practices that are learned and transmitted across generations (American Psychiatric Association 2013, p. 749).
- *Ethnicity* applies to people from diverse cultures who share a common background. *Background* refers to identity with a national and/or shared language of origin, religious practice, dress, diet, holidays or ceremonial events, traditional family rituals, use of disposable income, and leisure activities (Keyes 1976).
- *Subculture* refers to a distinct cultural group within a larger culture that is organized around shared values, beliefs, and other characteristics (e.g., sexuality, hobbies). Subcultures can also be organized around people's substance use, abuse, or dependence (in the context of addiction) (Bobakova et al. 2012). In addition, the term can be applied to groupings, such as affiliations with cocktail lounges, gambling outlets, or shooting galleries.
- *Acculturation* is the accumulative social learning process in which people assimilate the values of the host culture while retaining the values of the original culture (Thomson and Hoffman-Goetz 2009).
- *Cross-cultural* refers to the comparison of characteristics across cultural groups or, in the case of addiction, to treatment strategies addressing both clinician and patient differences in cultures.
- *Intersectionality* is the notion that an individual may hold more than one cultural identity, in which case the interaction of identities may result in more complex experiences (Nash 2008). For example, a nonheterosexual African American woman might have a different experience from that of a heterosexual African American woman.
- *Cultural humility* is "the ability to maintain an interpersonal stance that is other-oriented (or open to the other) in relation to the aspects of cultural identity that are most important to the [person]" (Hook et al. 2013, p. 2). Cultural humility promotes a "knowing and not knowing" stance by being aware of patients' cultural values and being open to understanding each individual's unique cultural experiences.

Operationally, in census gatherings or clinical surveys in the United States, the categorization of five major ethnic groups may represent an oversimplification. Hispanic or Latino ethnic groups have diverse roots traced to more than 20 countries with various phenotypic admixtures, divergent historical origins, and diverse social and educational levels and patterns of use of services. The same can be said of African American, Asian, Native American, and other ethnic groupings that are traditionally recorded at the introduction of any medical history or clinical presentation. The identification of ethnocultural groups also depends on national political priorities. In Canada, the study of cultures based on English and French languages has been prioritized; in the United Kingdom, particular attention has been paid to religious Muslim groups.

Historical Context

A testimony to the creativity of humans across civilizations is that different alcoholic beverages came to prominence in various times and places, first to address the need for a more palatable and safer alternative to brackish water, then to be used in religious rites, and also as a means of celebration and social bonding. The farming of cereal grains in the plains of the Near East some 10,000 years ago resulted in the appearance of a rudimentary form of beer. The early grain farming civilizations of Mesopotamia and Egypt instituted a wage system largely consisting of bread and beer (el-Guebaly and el-Guebaly 1981).

Ancient Greece popularized wine at drinking parties, called *symposia,* in which diluted wine was provided in a shared bowl. Originally from grapes grown in mountainous areas, wine became the basis of a vast Mediterranean seaborne trade. The Roman Empire embraced Greek wine drinking and adapted it to its elaborate hierarchical society. The quality of the wine became a symbol of social differentiation.

In the post-Renaissance era, from the fifteenth century onward, during the age of global exploration, refinement of the distillation process by Arab scholars provided alcohol in a more concentrated form, resulting in the creation of brandy, rum, and whiskey. These beverages became currencies with which people could buy slaves to develop newly discovered colonies in North America and other parts of the world.

During the eighteenth century, in the Age of Reason, coffee was introduced to Europe from the Middle East, and tea was imported from China. Carbonated beverages originated in Europe in the late eighteenth century but came to prominence in America a century later when coca leaves and caffeine-based kola nuts were added to soda water. In fact, Coca-Cola was first marketed as a stimulant medicine (Standage 2006).

Vegetation around the world was used for other psychoactive drugs, originally for medical purposes and eventually for elaborate religious rites. Neolithic archeological discoveries from around 6000 B.C. included opium pellets, marijuana seeds, and hallucinogens such as black henbane (*Hyoscyamus niger*) at burial sites in prehistoric Britain, and ergot (*Claviceps purpurea*) and hallucinogenic fungi (psilocybin) in ancient Greece. Archeological evidence documents the use of opium (*Papaver somniferum*) in the Mesopotamian civilization as far back as 3000 B.C. (Rudgley 1995).

Gambling has also existed for thousands of years, with the earliest evidence of gambling dating back as far as 4000 B.C. (Schwartz 2006). Gambling activities have been found throughout ancient civilizations and are mentioned in the ancient writings of Homer and Aristotle (Aasved 2003). Furthermore, gambling has existed in virtually every culture around the world (Aasved 2003; Schwartz 2006), speaking to its immense popularity.

Nowadays, human migration is often associated with the exportation of favorite drugs from the countries of origin. Khat (*Catha edulis*), for example, a mild stimulant derived from a flowering bush native to the Horn of Africa, is now used by migrant populations from the area (Griffiths et al. 2010). North American indigenous contributions to psychoactive drugs have included peyote buttons, which were once used mainly by Native Americans. In recent decades, the arrival of designer drugs (synthetic drugs concocted in laboratories rather than grown in plantations) has played an increasing role in the pursuit of intoxication. In regard to gambling, technological advances have increased the availability of gambling activities worldwide, and new gambling activities (e.g., gambling on video games [e-sports], daily fantasy sports) have been made available since the 2000s (Gainsbury et al. 2014). Throughout the ages, substance use and gambling have served as mechanisms of social integration and, when used in excess, as instruments of social disorganization.

Risk and Protective Factors Moderating the Impact of Culture

Given the multiplicity of ethnic groups, a listing of recorded differences is beyond the scope of this chapter. Assimilation of the related empirical literature is a complex undertaking, and to avoid stereotyping, one must exercise caution when interpreting results. Confounding variables, such as those outlined in the following subsections, are commonly noted to affect prevalence estimates comparing the impact of addiction between ethnic groups. Most studies to date, however, do not account for many of the confounding effects referred to herein; more prospective studies are required to tease out the relative impact of these variables.

Disentangling Sociodemographic Variables From Culture

It is crucial to control sociodemographic variables so that results can be reliably and effectively interpreted. Differences in age distribution must be taken into account. For example, the higher proportion of youth, a high-risk group for substance use, among Native Americans (Schinke et al. 2000) influences the prevalence of substance use disorder in that ethnic group. In another example, like the societal norms of many ethnic groups, Mexican societal attitudes are more negative toward women's alcohol consumption than toward men's (Alaniz et al. 1999); therefore, this societal norm is likely to have a protective effect on the prevalence estimates of women's alcohol consumption. Differences in family stability and the occurrence of domestic violence in a given ethnic group may also be a cause and/or consequence of the prevalence of substance use in that group. The same can be said about differences in socioeconomic status and work history.

Extent of Acculturation

The extent of recent migration in an ethnic group is viewed as both a risk and a protective factor. For example, first- and second-generation acculturation may create socioeconomic stressors, which increase the vulnerability to addiction (Lindström et al. 2013); however, a New York survey also shows that the stronger the ties are to Hispanic culture among persons born outside the United States who speak mostly Spanish, the less likely that group is to use drugs, compared with Hispanics born in the United States who speak mostly English (Frank et al. 1988). Additionally, Mexican Americans who had at least one parent born in the United States were more likely to have a substance use disorder than those who did not have at least one parent born in the States (Ortega et al. 2000). Hawaiian residents of Chinese and Japanese ancestry also were found to have lower levels of alcohol use if born in Asia than if born in Hawaii (Johnson et al. 1987). Acculturation may also have an effect on the rates of engagement in behavioral addictions. Indeed, the combination of permissive attitudes toward gambling in Asian culture and the increased access to gambling in Western countries may increase the rates of problem gambling among people of Asian descent living in those countries (Kim 2012).

Impact of Sampling and Other Survey Designs

The method of population selection is of importance in estimating the prevalence of substance use disorders in an ethnic group. For example, school survey results should account for potential ethnic differences in rates of school retention; however, the ethnicities of school dropouts are not reflected in school surveys. Furthermore, a group's urban-rural distribution may also confound estimates.

Language barriers also represent a variable that must be accounted for in research design to increase the accuracy of the estimation of rates of substance use in ethnic groups. Numerous challenges must be met to establish validity and reliability in research methodology that controls for variables such as language barriers for non-English-speaking groups and cultural biases for groups such as African Americans, immigrants, and Native Americans.

The timing of a survey is also relevant. Is the group experiencing an epidemic superimposed on traditional consumption? For example, from the sixteenth century onward, the gin epidemic in the United Kingdom and the opium epidemic across Asia heralded the onset of episodic epidemics of substance abuse. More recently, the fentanyl epidemic in Canada and the United States may temporarily affect the prevalence figures for designated ethnic groups (Fischer et al. 2018).

The selection of a particular addictive substance or behavior surveyed for a study will also affect ethnic differences. Certain Asian groups, for example, may report a lower prevalence of alcohol use but a higher prevalence of gambling and/or gaming behaviors (Caetano et al. 1998; Oei et al. 2008). These differences may have biological (e.g., deficiency in the liver aldehyde dehydrogenase) and/or cultural influences. For example, gambling is an important part of Chinese culture, specifically in regard to the concept of luck (Tse et al. 2010). Also, gaming is increasingly being integrated into the social fabric of Korean culture (Jin and Chee 2008), which may help explain the higher rates of video game addiction in Korea.

Legal Frameworks of Home and Host Countries

The traditional use of coca leaves in the Andes and of marijuana and hashish in India and the Middle East adds to the cultural disconnect felt by immigrants from these countries who arrive in a new community where *their* drug of use is illegal but other substances are socially promoted. Indeed, in North America, the criminalization of some drugs over others has been associated with the need to protect the majority from the habits of recently immigrated minorities. In the nineteenth century, temperance and abstinence movements may have originated as a reaction to the new Irish and German-Catholic immigrants' "wet" cultures, which presented a conflict for the original abstemious Protestant groups. Anti-opium legislation in Canada and the United States was originally enacted to protect the majority population from migrant Chinese railroad workers' opium dens. In the early twentieth century, the cocaine laws were spurred by the fear of use among African Americans. In the 1930s, the marijuana laws reflected similar concerns about the drug's use by Mexican migrant workers. Currently, there is a differential propensity for arrests, imprisonment, and treatment opportunities among minority groups in various countries (Alegria et al. 2011). Similar legal issues are also present regarding gambling disorder. In certain countries, gambling in any form is prohibited. In other countries, only certain forms of gambling, such as lottery tickets, are legalized, while other forms, such as electronic gaming machines, remain prohibited (Spapens 2014). For example, in Korea, although gambling is allowed for non-Koreans, it is prohibited for Korean citizens, except in one gambling venue (Jin 2015). In Brazil, gambling is prohibited with the exception of state-run lotteries and bingo (Tavares 2014).

Biological Factors and Physical Comorbidities

Studies have examined the impact of genetic factors on the predisposition toward substance use and the response to various pharmacological treatments among ethnic groups. For example, Aoki et al. (2017) reported that approximately 30%–40% of East Asians (Chinese, Japanese, Koreans) have a mutation in the liver aldehyde dehydrogenase 2 gene *ALDH2*, that leads to slower oxidation of acetaldehyde and a resulting "flushing reaction" following ingestion of alcohol. This mutation is considered to be a protective factor against alcohol abuse by Asians (Luczak et al. 2006). Coping with the reaction, however, can be learned in order to accommodate a Western lifestyle. The complexity of gene-environment interplay is being increasingly fleshed out (Bookman et al. 2011). Socioeconomic disadvantage also leads to differential health outcomes, including fatal and nonfatal overdoses, hepatitis B and C infection, AIDS, increased risk of pregnancy, and perinatal complications.

Psychological Factors

Cultures fostering shame and guilt as means of social control have been reported to facilitate alcohol use disorder. Low levels of self-esteem, self-confidence, and assertiveness as well as "loss of face" have all been related to the use of substances among adolescents in general and among adolescents in immigrant groups in particular (Bhattacharya 1998). The higher rate of suicide among Native American youths while under the influence of substances is the ultimate resulting tragedy (Resnik and Dizmang 1971). The general protective effect of norms and values in Asian cultures, including traditional values such as responsibility to others, interdependence, restraint, and group achievement, has also been investigated (Sue 1987).

Cultural Influences on DSM and ICD Nosological Classifications

Do current diagnoses, such as alcohol use disorder and gaming disorder, and their criteria have universal applicability, or are cultural influences strong enough to require reframing of these diagnoses and criteria (Room 2006)? So far, the answer to this question is mixed. Kraepelin (1902) was perhaps the first to use a universalistic approach to psychopathology. Jellinek (1960), in his conceptualization of alcoholism as a disease, recognized different subtypes whereby the "gamma" species derived from the Anglo-Saxon drinking pattern, the "delta" from the French drinking pattern, and the "epsilon" from the Finnish pattern.

Analyses of the applicability of the World Health Organization's Alcohol Use Disorders Identification Test (AUDIT) in diverse cultures elicited considerable cross-cultural generalizability (Reinert and Allen 2007). Site-specific cross-cultural analysis of the validity of DSM and International Classification of Diseases (ICD) classifications showed that the constructs of alcohol dependence items were more familiar to respondents in Sydney, Australia, than to respondents in Bangalore, India, thereby resulting in lower reliability (Chatterji et al. 1997).

The attribution of causality varies across cultures. A World Health Organization survey of key informants on the cross-cultural applicability of diagnostic criteria found differences as to when an item threshold was considered positive. For example, in Athens, Greece, and Santander, Spain, where regular drinking is normalized, problem thresholds were set much higher (Schmidt and Room 1999). Similarly, studies investigating heavy drinking in French populations found a need to utilize higher problem thresholds to account for the cultural effects of elevated alcohol consumption (Bataille et al. 2003). The value, moral judgment, and stigma associated with use of alcohol and other psychoactive substances also differ from society to society (Schomerus et al. 2011).

Stigmatization also influences the terminology used to describe substance use disorders. The term *addiction,* defined as compulsive drug-seeking behavior, was cast away in 1987 by the DSM-III-R committee in favor of the term *dependence,* which was perceived as being more neutral by a single majority vote (American Psychiatric Association 1987). More recently, *dependence* was perceived as being too closely associated with physical dependence and its consequent withdrawal symptoms (O'Brien et al. 2006). A lobbying effort to revert to *addiction* and its connotation of loss of control over intense urges despite negative consequences was not accepted for DSM-5; instead, the two diagnoses of abuse and dependence were collapsed into a single substance use disorder diagnosis (American Psychiatric Association 2013).

ICD-10's *harmful use* (World Health Organization 1992) shunned, in principle, negative social consequences or reactions of others to drug use as criteria, whereas DSM-IV-TR's *abuse* incorporated them (American Psychiatric Association 2000). British psychiatry took the view that social reactions and consequences did not belong in the definitions of diseases and disorders (Room 2006). The diagnosis of harmful use was retained in ICD-11 (World Health Organization 2019). Neither category—harmful use nor abuse—performed very well in test-retest studies. In the United States in 1992, half of the cases diagnosed as alcohol abuse were related to the criterion of hazardous use, as in "driving under the influence," raising the question of whether a culturally reprehensible and unwise behavior in isolation warranted a psychiatric diagnosis (Hasin et al. 1999). Indeed, the culturally laden criterion of "legal problems" has been removed altogether in DSM-5 (American Psychiatric Association 2013).

Differences in health care systems, from a national insurance to a more entrepreneurial fee-for-service system, may also influence the nosology, depending on a more or less assertive determination of the limits of practice through recognized diagnoses.

The differences in cultural views and understanding of addictions may partly explain the differing rates of substance use and gambling disorder in different cultures. For example, family attitudes toward addictions may have a bigger impact on prevalence levels in nonwhite populations, and integration of family members into treatment can lead to better patient outcomes (Gainsbury 2017). Similarly, popular therapies for majority populations have shown some evidence for decreased generalizability, particularly among marginalized cultures (Gainsbury 2017). In working with people from different cultures, sensitivity training, matching patients to native speakers of their languages, and modifying approaches to integrate with systems of belief can improve therapeutic outcomes.

Clinical Cultural Formulation

Through a cultural assessment, the clinician can obtain a better understanding of a patient's subjective view of the world, the meaning of the illness to the patient, and the patient's expected recovery process. The importance of working within a framework of cultural understanding was acknowledged in DSM-IV with the inclusion of the Outline for Cultural Formulation. This outline provided a framework for understanding patients' perceptions of their mental health or addiction. The Outline for Cultural Formulation contained the following five categories (American Psychiatric Association 2000):

- *Cultural identity of the individual.* The overarching ethnic group must be complemented by further descriptors, such as where the patient was raised and by whom, parents' and grandparents' ethnicity, and involvement with both culture of origin and host culture.
- *Cultural explanations of the individual's illness.* The predominant idioms of distress must be articulated, in addition to the meaning and perceived severity of the symptoms in relation to cultural norms. Traditionally, diagnostic evocation of culture has been associated with rare *culture-bound syndromes* rather than the much more common clinical presentations found in daily practice. Examples of common clinical presentations in daily practice include the following:
  - *Norm conflict.* Standards held desirable by a culture may conflict with the person's behavior.
  - *Normative versus deviant behavior.* Any substance use in an abstinence-based group would be considered deviant, but would not necessarily be called pathological from a health perspective.
  - *Socially prescribed use.* Use in religious rites may be replaced by secular use, often involving new routes of administration (e.g., from eating to smoking opium) and/or new forms of the substance (e.g., opium to heroin).
  - *Cultural change.* Changes in norms and values may occur through immigration and exposure to new norms.
- *Cultural factors related to psychosocial environment and levels of functioning.* The patient's interpretations of social stressors and available social supports, including religion and levels of functioning and disability, are elicited.

- *Cultural elements of the relationship between the individual and the clinician.* Similarities and differences between the clinician's and the patient's language, social context, and beliefs and behaviors of relevance to the clinical onset, course, and treatment create a set of dynamics that should be part of the cultural formulation. Transference and countertransference issues can be understood once underlying mechanisms, such as projection or stereotyping, become visible. Guidelines for training curricula are continuously being refined (Kirmayer et al. 2012; Westermeyer et al. 2006).
- *Overall cultural assessment for diagnosis and care.* Based on the overall assessment, diagnosis and treatment implications are discussed within the context of the cultural considerations.

A criticism of the DSM-IV Outline for Cultural Formulation was the lack of guidelines provided for its application. To address this gap, the DSM-5 Gender and Cross-Cultural Issues Subgroup created the Cultural Formulation Interview (CFI; Table 40–1), which provides a set of 16 questions aimed at assessing the first four domains of the DSM-IV Outline for Cultural Formulation summarized above. Although the CFI is a step forward in delivering culturally sensitive treatments, barriers to its implementation have been noted by both patients and clinicians, including the lack of buy-in (Aggarwal et al. 2013). Indeed, realistic clinical challenges arise when the largely open-ended socioanthropological conversation that is required to assess culture collides with the need for a clinical interview focused on making a diagnosis and establishing a treatment plan. An adequate cultural assessment may require several interviews to get to know the person behind the illness. Often, differing belief systems with regard to the nature of the behavior or diagnosis may affect treatment compliance, adding to the complexity of clinical care (Bhui and Bhugra 2002). Findings from a field trial with New York clinicians indicated that the CFI was helpful in building rapport, gathering data, and eliciting perspective, although ratings of usefulness differed according to respondent ethnicity as well as between patients and therapists (Aggarwal et al. 2015). In particular, confusing phrasing of certain questions was identified as a main area of weakness, whereas ability to build rapport was identified as the most consistent strength. Although these preliminary findings are promising, future research will help provide more information about the benefits and drawbacks of the CFI and strategies that may help to improve clinical care in a culturally sensitive manner.

Implications of Clinically Relevant Variables of Culture for Management of Addiction Risk

Empowering a community to manage its own risks for addiction is a complex but rewarding process—one that involves culturally sensitive public and private leadership and coordinated health, education, law enforcement, and social programming. Depending on community needs and values, goals may vary from emphasis on responsible drinking or gambling to a focus on reducing intoxication to the establishment of "dry" communities. A multigenerational healing process may be required, as has been successfully initiated in a number of Native American communities (Grayshield et al. 2015).

TABLE 40–1.   **Cultural Formulation Interview (CFI)**

Supplementary modules used to expand each CFI subtopic are noted in parentheses.

GUIDE TO INTERVIEWER	INSTRUCTIONS TO THE INTERVIEWER ARE *ITALICIZED*.
The following questions aim to clarify key aspects of the presenting clinical problem from the point of view of the individual and other members of the individual's social network (i.e., family, friends, or others involved in current problem). This includes the problem's meaning, potential sources of help, and expectations for services.	*INTRODUCTION FOR THE INDIVIDUAL:* I would like to understand the problems that bring you here so that I can help you more effectively. I want to know about *your* experience and ideas. I will ask some questions about what is going on and how you are dealing with it. Please remember there are no right or wrong answers.

CULTURAL DEFINITION OF THE PROBLEM

CULTURAL DEFINITION OF THE PROBLEM
(Explanatory Model, Level of Functioning)

Elicit the individual's view of core problems and key concerns. *Focus on the individual's own way of understanding the problem.* *Use the term, expression, or brief description elicited in question 1 to identify the problem in subsequent questions (e.g., "your conflict with your son").*	1. What brings you here today? *IF INDIVIDUAL GIVES FEW DETAILS OR ONLY MENTIONS SYMPTOMS OR A MEDICAL DIAGNOSIS, PROBE:* People often understand their problems in their own way, which may be similar to or different from how doctors describe the problem. How would *you* describe your problem?
Ask how individual frames the problem for members of the social network.	2. Sometimes people have different ways of describing their problem to their family, friends, or others in their community. How would you describe your problem to them?
Focus on the aspects of the problem that matter most to the individual.	3. What troubles you most about your problem?

CULTURAL PERCEPTIONS OF CAUSE, CONTEXT, AND SUPPORT

CAUSES
(Explanatory Model, Social Network, Older Adults)

This question indicates the meaning of the condition for the individual, which may be relevant for clinical care.	4. Why do you think this is happening to you? What do you think are the causes of your [PROBLEM]?
Note that individuals may identify multiple causes, depending on the facet of the problem they are considering.	*PROMPT FURTHER IF REQUIRED:* Some people may explain their problem as the result of bad things that happen in their life, problems with others, a physical illness, a spiritual reason, or many other causes.
Focus on the views of members of the individual's social network. These may be diverse and vary from the individual's.	5. What do others in your family, your friends, or others in your community think is causing your [PROBLEM]?

TABLE 40–1.	**Cultural Formulation Interview (CFI)** *(continued)*
Supplementary modules used to expand each CFI subtopic are noted in parentheses.	
GUIDE TO INTERVIEWER	**INSTRUCTIONS TO THE INTERVIEWER ARE** *ITALICIZED.*

STRESSORS AND SUPPORTS

(Social Network, Caregivers, Psychosocial Stressors, Religion and Spirituality, Immigrants and Refugees, Cultural Identity, Older Adults, Coping and Help Seeking)

Elicit information on the individual's life context, focusing on resources, social supports, and resilience. May also probe other supports (e.g., from co-workers, from participation in religion or spirituality).	6. Are there any kinds of support that make your [PROBLEM] better, such as support from family, friends, or others?
Focus on stressful aspects of the individual's environment. Can also probe, e.g., relationship problems, difficulties at work or school, or discrimination.	7. Are there any kinds of stresses that make your [PROBLEM] worse, such as difficulties with money, or family problems?

ROLE OF CULTURAL IDENTITY

(Cultural Identity, Psychosocial Stressors, Religion and Spirituality, Immigrants and Refugees, Older Adults, Children and Adolescents)

	Sometimes, aspects of people's background or identity can make their [PROBLEM] better or worse. By *background* or *identity*, I mean, for example, the communities you belong to, the languages you speak, where you or your family are from, your race or ethnic background, your gender or sexual orientation, or your faith or religion.
Ask the individual to reflect on the most salient elements of his or her cultural identity. Use this information to tailor questions 9–10 as needed.	8. For you, what are the most important aspects of your background or identity?
Elicit aspects of identity that make the problem better or worse.	9. Are there any aspects of your background or identity that make a difference to your [PROBLEM]?
Probe as needed (e.g., clinical worsening as a result of discrimination due to migration status, race/ethnicity, or sexual orientation).	
Probe as needed (e.g., migration-related problems; conflict across generations or due to gender roles).	10. Are there any aspects of your background or identity that are causing other concerns or difficulties for you?

CULTURAL FACTORS AFFECTING SELF-COPING AND PAST HELP SEEKING

SELF-COPING

(Coping and Help Seeking, Religion and Spirituality, Older Adults, Caregivers, Psychosocial Stressors)

Clarify self-coping for the problem.	11. Sometimes people have various ways of dealing with problems like [PROBLEM]. What have you done on your own to cope with your [PROBLEM]?

TABLE 40–1.   **Cultural Formulation Interview (CFI)** *(continued)*

Supplementary modules used to expand each CFI subtopic are noted in parentheses.

GUIDE TO INTERVIEWER	INSTRUCTIONS TO THE INTERVIEWER ARE *ITALICIZED.*
PAST HELP SEEKING (Coping and Help Seeking, Religion and Spirituality, Older Adults, Caregivers, Psychosocial Stressors, Immigrants and Refugees, Social Network, Clinician-Patient Relationship)	
Elicit various sources of help (e.g., medical care, mental health treatment, support groups, work-based counseling, folk healing, religious or spiritual counseling, other forms of traditional or alternative healing). *Probe as needed (e.g., "What other sources of help have you used?").* *Clarify the individual's experience and regard for previous help.*	12. Often, people look for help from many different sources, including different kinds of doctors, helpers, or healers. In the past, what kinds of treatment, help, advice, or healing have you sought for your [PROBLEM]? *PROBE IF DOES NOT DESCRIBE USEFULNESS OF HELP RECEIVED:* What types of help or treatment were most useful? Not useful?
BARRIERS (Coping and Help Seeking, Religion and Spirituality, Older Adults, Psychosocial Stressors, Immigrants and Refugees, Social Network, Clinician-Patient Relationship)	
Clarify the role of social barriers to help seeking, access to care, and problems engaging in previous treatment. *Probe details as needed (e.g., "What got in the way?").*	13. Has anything prevented you from getting the help you need? *PROBE AS NEEDED:* For example, money, work or family commitments, stigma or discrimination, or lack of services that understand your language or background?
CULTURAL FACTORS AFFECTING CURRENT HELP SEEKING	
PREFERENCES (Social Network, Caregivers, Religion and Spirituality, Older Adults, Coping and Help Seeking)	
Clarify individual's current perceived needs and expectations of help, broadly defined. *Probe if individual lists only one source of help (e.g., "What other kinds of help would be useful to you at this time?").* *Focus on the views of the social network regarding help seeking.*	Now let's talk some more about the help you need. 14. What kinds of help do you think would be most useful to you at this time for your [PROBLEM]? 15. Are there other kinds of help that your family, friends, or other people have suggested would be helpful for you now?
CLINICIAN-PATIENT RELATIONSHIP (Clinician-Patient Relationship, Older Adults)	
Elicit possible concerns about the clinic or the clinician-patient relationship, including perceived racism, language barriers, or cultural differences that may undermine goodwill, communication, or care delivery. *Probe details as needed (e.g., "In what way?").* *Address possible barriers to care or concerns about the clinic and the clinician-patient relationship raised previously.*	Sometimes doctors and patients misunderstand each other because they come from different backgrounds or have different expectations. 16. Have you been concerned about this and is there anything that we can do to provide you with the care you need?

An often-replicated research finding is that treatment resources available in Western countries are underused by minority ethnic groups (Guerrero et al. 2015). Legal prospective immigrants to these countries are required to undergo health screening in their home countries. In Canada, the discovery of an undeclared preexisting chronic illness in an individual who has not yet obtained citizenship may be grounds for deportation, a risk that discourages immigrants from using the health care system (Gainsbury 2017). Encounters with the health care system and/or the social welfare system and the intimacy involved in dealing with health care issues are fraught with wide-ranging cross-cultural challenges. Examples of potential cultural barriers to using the health care system include language (i.e., proficiency, fluency), the individual right to confidentiality versus the family expectation for information, the fear of rights being taken away, the ease of disclosure in a therapeutic group involving both sexes, and the use of condoms or needle exchange (Gainsbury 2017).

Challenges of Culturally Adapted Evidence-Based Interventions

Evidence-based treatments are developed within a particular linguistic and cultural context and are often manualized for the purpose of fidelity. However, questions remain regarding whether such treatments are appropriate for ethnocultural groups that do not share the same language and/or cultural values. The challenges include finding a balance between adherence to the treatment manual and clinical flexibility, as well as between attention to the therapeutic relationship and attention to the therapeutic technique. Mismatches may arise from group characteristics, characteristics of the program delivery staff, and/or administrative or community factors. Evidence regarding the effectiveness of culturally adapted interventions has been described as promising but mixed. Common adaptation efforts have involved inclusion of cultural values and concepts, use of the native language, and ethnic matching of clients to therapists, as well as clinics specifically serving clients from diverse cultural backgrounds (Castro et al. 2010). Some have expressed concern that studies conducted in the United States with minority groups may not reflect the experience with these groups in their nations of origin.

Despite these challenges, research has demonstrated that culturally adapted or culturally sensitive interventions produce beneficial effects and improved outcomes (Griner and Smith 2006). Generally speaking, use of culturally adapted evidence-based therapies may beneficially affect outcomes, including treatment retention, among diverse ethnic populations (Huey et al. 2014). Although the literature specifically focused on addiction treatments is sparse, there is some evidence to suggest that culturally sensitive treatment may help improve therapeutic outcomes and patient-clinician relationships among racial/ethnic minorities (Hodge et al. 2012), including youths (Gainsbury 2017). That said, more research is needed in this domain.

Alternative Models of Care

The increasing multiethnicity of Western English-speaking countries has sparked a debate about optimal models for culturally sensitive delivery of care. In this section, we examine some possible models.

Separate Services for Ethnic Minority Groups

In the United States, separate public and voluntary sector services for African Americans, Hispanic Americans, and Native Americans are common. Religious denominations sponsor certain hospitals and social services for members of the religion. Lending credibility to the argument for allowing creation of separate services are consistent research findings that show that members of ethnic minorities may experience increased coercive treatment and social encounters that promote their distrust in secular hospitals (Henderson et al. 2015). These experiences are often based on a mutual lack of knowledge of cherished cultural, spiritual, and religious beliefs, as well as a perceived slow pace of change. Operating against the idea of separate services are the fears of promoting "ghettoization" and further marginalization of many people who are already marginalized (Bhui and Sashidharan 2003).

Cultural Consultation Model

One concern is how major urban centers in which numerous languages are spoken can respond to health care needs. In Montreal, Quebec, a specialized multidisciplinary team brings together clinical experience with cultural knowledge and linguistic skills. A consultant who has relevant cultural expertise directly assesses the patient, a process that may take anywhere from 1 to 3 sessions. The cultural consultant then provides a brief report and immediate recommendations to the clinical team, which consists of psychiatrists, psychologists, social workers, psychiatric nurses, and medical anthropologists (Kirmayer et al. 2003).

A Melting Pot Approach for the Cultural Mosaic

In the melting pot approach, institutional factors promoting ethnic inequalities are addressed. Culturally influenced or culturally capable services are important to the mainstream delivery of services and not only to minority ethnic groups. In this approach, culture is not perceived as a problem or disability that requires specialized interventions for minority groups. Mainstream services are commonly enriched by responding to the needs of all cultural groups, guaranteeing equality of access, and ensuring rights for all individuals (Bhui and Sashidharan 2003).

An Individualized Approach

Advocates of an individualized strategy acknowledge, for example, that offering both prescribed medication and ethnic spiritual therapy may be the best hope for securing patient adherence to treatment (Griner and Smith 2006). This model also encourages a more honest discussion of the other therapies being tried and their potential interactions.

Two potent forces that can serve as instruments of change—family and religion—are commonly recognized in the cross-cultural treatment literature. The significance of *the family* as the conduit of cultural norms and values is recognized in most ethnically sensitive programs. Supporting the family foundation and home stability is a cherished goal in communities originating from cultures with a strong extended-family network that is threatened by the reduced family mosaic in our modern Western societies. A sensitive family assessment will take into account the individual roles of all family members and respect their potential impact on a positive outcome (Gainsbury 2017). *Religious affiliations and religious beliefs* also play a major positive role in the development of prevention networks for recovery and treatment adherence in many ethnic groups (Galanter 2006). The adaptation of 12-step programs to many cultures in various parts of the world is an example of the shared value placed on spiritual growth as an ingredient of recovery.

Cultural recovery may involve regaining a viable ethnic identity and developing a healthy affiliation with an individual's ethnic group; reacquiring a functional social network, as well as a religious or spiritual commitment; rebuilding social status in the recovering as well as the cultural community; and reestablishing vocational and recreational activities. Cultural recovery starts after physical and psychological recovery begins and often takes years (Westermeyer et al. 2006). Unreasonable cultural expectations, as well as cultural cues encouraging resumption of the addictive behavior, may delay recovery, whereas cultural abstinence-based programs may facilitate recovery.

Conclusion

The goal of this chapter has been to advance knowledge of how to provide optimal clinical care to individuals from varied cultures. The impact of ethnicity is moderated by a number of risk and protective factors. Sometimes everything is attributed to ethnicity or culture, whereas at other times the existence of cultural impact is completely denied. Concentration on cultural differences may lead to missed important diagnostic signs. Cultural sensitivity is not a fixation on culture, and it should not be a ready explanation for the unexplained. Currently, the methodological differences used in various studies lead to caution about the validity and reliability of the results. Many conclusions range from the subjective to the speculative.

A better understanding of the patient can be gained through a systematic cultural formulation, which includes the cultural aspects of the clinician-patient relationship. Minority groups underutilize psychiatric treatment and social services. Making these services more user friendly should be a first-order concern in multicultural societies when the subject of alternative models of care is addressed.

We provide the following key points to help clinicians be informed of the importance of working in a culturally sensitive manner:

- Culturally sensitive clinical care is required for individuals from different cultures.
- The impact of ethnicity is moderated by both risk and protective factors.
- Nosological classifications are influenced by culture.
- A cultural assessment provides a better understanding of the patient's subjective views.
- Culturally sensitive treatments can lead to improved outcomes in addiction treatment, although more research is needed in this domain.
- Culturally sensitive care can be delivered through separated services, a consultation model, a sensitized melting pot approach, or an individualized approach.

References

Aasved MJ: The Sociology of Gambling, Vol 2. Springfield, IL, Charles C Thomas, 2003

Aggarwal NK, Nicasio AV, DeSilva R, et al: Barriers to implementing the DSM-5 Cultural Formulation Interview: a qualitative study. Cult Med Psychiatry 37(3):505–533, 2013 23836098

Aggarwal NK, Desilva R, Nicasio AV, et al: Does the Cultural Formulation Interview for the fifth revision of the Diagnostic and Statistical Manual of Mental Disorders (DSM-5) affect medical communication? A qualitative exploratory study from the New York site. Ethn Health 20(1):1–28, 2015 25372242

Alaniz ML, Treno AJ, Saltz RF: Gender, acculturation, and alcohol consumption among Mexican Americans. Subst Use Misuse 34(10):1407–1426, 1999 10446767

Alegria M, Carson NJ, Goncalves M, et al: Disparities in treatment for substance use disorders and co-occurring disorders for ethnic/racial minority youth. J Am Acad Child Adolesc Psychiatry 50(1):22–31, 2011 21156267

American Psychiatric Association: Diagnostic and Statistical Manual of Mental Disorders, 3rd Edition, Revised. Washington, DC, American Psychiatric Association, 1987

American Psychiatric Association: Diagnostic and Statistical Manual of Mental Disorders, 4th Edition, Text Revision. Washington, DC, American Psychiatric Association, 2000

American Psychiatric Association: Diagnostic and Statistical Manual of Mental Disorders, 5th Edition. Arlington, VA, American Psychiatric Association, 2013

Aoki Y, Wehage SL, Talalay P: Quantification of skin erythema response to topical alcohol in alcohol-intolerant East Asians. Skin Res Technol 23(4):593–596, 2017 28513003

Bataille V, Ruidavets JB, Arveiler D, et al: Joint use of clinical parameters, biological markers and CAGE questionnaire for the identification of heavy drinkers in a large population-based sample. Alcohol Alcohol 38(2):121–127, 2003 12634258

Bhattacharya G: Drug use among Asian-Indian adolescents: identifying protective/risk factors. Adolescence 33(129):169–184, 1998 9583669

Bhui K, Bhugra D: Explanatory models for mental distress: implications for clinical practice and research. Br J Psychiatry 181:6–7, 2002 12091256

Bhui K, Sashidharan SP: Should there be separate psychiatric services for ethnic minority groups? Br J Psychiatry 182:10–12, 2003 12509312

Bobakova D, Madarasova Geckova A, Reijneveld SA, et al: Subculture affiliation is associated with substance use of adolescents. Eur Addict Res 18(2):91–96, 2012 22286898

Bookman EB, McAllister K, Gillanders E, et al: Gene-environment interplay in common complex diseases: forging an integrative model—recommendations from an NIH workshop. Genet Epidemiol 35(4):217–225, 2011 21308768

Caetano R, Clark CL, Tam T: Alcohol consumption among racial/ethnic minorities: theory and research. Alcohol Health Res World 22(4):233–241, 1998 15706749

Castro FG, Barrera M Jr, Holleran Steiker LK: Issues and challenges in the design of culturally adapted evidence-based interventions. Annu Rev Clin Psychol 6:213–239, 2010 20192800

Chatterji S, Saunders JB, Vrasti R, et al: Reliability of the alcohol and drug modules of the Alcohol Use Disorder and Associated Disabilities Interview Schedule—Alcohol/Drug-Revised (AUDADIS-ADR): an international comparison. Drug Alcohol Depend 47(3):171–185, 1997 9306043

el-Guebaly N, el-Guebaly A: Alcohol abuse in ancient Egypt: the recorded evidence. Int J Addict 16(7):1207–1221, 1981 7035380

Fischer B, Vojtila L, Rehm J: The "fentanyl epidemic" in Canada—some cautionary observations focusing on opioid-related mortality. Prev Med 107:109–113, 2018 29126920

Frank B, Marel R, Schmeidler J, et al: Statewide Household Survey of Substance Abuse, 1986: Illicit Substance Use Among Hispanic Adults in New York State. New York, State Division of Substance Abuse Services, 1988

Gainsbury SM: Cultural competence in the treatment of addictions: theory, practice and evidence. Clin Psychol Psychother 24(4):987–1001, 2017 27976434

Gainsbury SM, Russell A, Hing N, et al: The prevalence and determinants of problem gambling in Australia: assessing the impact of interactive gambling and new technologies. Psychol Addict Behav 28(3):769–779, 2014 24865462

Galanter M: Spirituality and addiction: a research and clinical perspective. Am J Addict 15(4):286–292, 2006 16867923

Grayshield L, Rutherford JJ, Salazar SB, et al: Understanding and healing historical trauma: the perspectives of Native American elders. Journal of Mental Health Counseling 37(4):295–307, 2015. Available at: https://meridian.allenpress.com/jmhc/article-abstract/37/4/295/83296/Understanding-and-Healing-Historical-Trauma-The?redirectedFrom=fulltext. Accessed July 3, 2020.

Griffiths P, Lopez D, Sedefov R, et al: Khat use and monitoring drug use in Europe: the current situation and issues for the future. J Ethnopharmacol 132(3):578–583, 2010 20452413

Griner D, Smith TB: Culturally adapted mental health intervention: a meta-analytic review. Psychotherapy (Chic) 43(4):531–548, 2006 22122142

Guerrero EG, Fenwick K, Kong Y, et al: Paths to improving engagement among racial and ethnic minorities in addiction health services. Subst Abus Treat Prev Policy 10:40, 2015 26503509

Hasin D, Paykin A, Endicott J, et al: The validity of DSM-IV alcohol abuse: drunk drivers versus all others. J Stud Alcohol 60(6):746–755, 1999 10606485

Henderson RC, Williams P, Gabbidon J, et al: Mistrust of mental health services: ethnicity, hospital admission and unfair treatment. Epidemiol Psychiatr Sci 24(3):258–265, 2015 24636750

Hodge DR, Jackson KF, Vaughn MG: Culturally sensitive interventions and substance use: a meta-analytic review of outcomes among minority youths. Social Work Research 36(1):11–19, 2012. Available at: https://academic.oup.com/swr/article-abstract/36/1/11/1646392?redirectedFrom=fulltext. Accessed February 6, 2020.

Hook JN, Davis DE, Owen J, et al: Cultural humility: measuring openness to culturally diverse clients. J Couns Psychol 60(3):353–366, 2013 23647387

Huey SJ Jr, Tilley JL, Jones EO, et al: The contribution of cultural competence to evidence-based care for ethnically diverse populations. Annu Rev Clin Psychol 10:305–338, 2014 24437436

Jellinek EM: The Disease Concept of Alcoholism. New Brunswick, NJ, Hillhouse Press, 1960

Jin CH: Research on the effects of integrated resorts in Korea on gambling addiction. J Exerc Rehabil 11(4):188–191, 2015 26331132

Jin DY, Chee F: Age of new media empires: a critical interpretation of the Korean online game industry. Games and Culture 3(1):38–58, 2008. Available at: https://journals.sagepub.com/doi/10.1177/1555412007309528. Accessed February 6, 2020.

Johnson RC, Nagoshi CT, Ahern FM, et al: Cultural factors as explanations for ethnic group differences in alcohol use in Hawaii. J Psychoactive Drugs 19(1):67–75, 1987 3585595

Keyes CF: Towards a new formulation of the concept of ethnic groups. Ethnicity 3:202–212, 1976. Available at: https://www.academia.edu/8631787/Towards_a_New_Formulation_of_the_Concept_of_Ethnic_Group. Accessed August 4, 2020.

Kim W: Acculturation and gambling in Asian Americans: when culture meets availability. International Gambling Studies 12(1):69–88, 2012

Kirmayer LJ, Groleau D, Guzder J, et al: Cultural consultation: a model of mental health service for multicultural societies. Can J Psychiatry 48(3):145–153, 2003 12728738

Kirmayer LJ, Fung K, Rousseau C, et al: Guidelines for training in cultural psychiatry. Can J Psychiatry 57 (3 suppl):1–16, 2012

Kraepelin E: Clinical Psychiatry. Adapted by Defendor AR. New York, Macmillan, 1902

Lewis-Fernández R, Aggarwal NK, Hinton L, et al (eds): DSM-5 Handbook on the Cultural Formulation Interview. Washington, DC, American Psychiatric Publishing, 2015

Lindström M, Modén B, Rosvall M: A life-course perspective on economic stress and tobacco smoking: a population-based study. Addiction 108(7):1305–1314, 2013 23432606

Luczak SE, Glatt SJ, Wall TL: Meta-analyses of ALDH2 and ADH1B with alcohol dependence in Asians. Psychol Bull 132(4):607–621, 2006 16822169

Nash JC: Re-thinking intersectionality. Feminist Review 89(1):1–15, 2008. Available at: https://journals.sagepub.com/doi/full/10.1057/fr.2008.4. Accessed February 6, 2020.

O'Brien CP, Volkow N, Li T-K: What's in a word? Addiction versus dependence in DSM-V. Am J Psychiatry 163(5):764–765, 2006 16648309

Oei TP, Lin J, Raylu N: The relationship between gambling cognitions, psychological states, and gambling: a cross-cultural study of Chinese and Caucasians in Australia. Journal of Cross-Cultural Psychology 39(2):147–161, 2008. Available at: https://journals.sagepub.com/doi/10.1177/0022022107312587. Accessed February 6, 2020.

Ortega AN, Rosenheck R, Alegría M, et al: Acculturation and the lifetime risk of psychiatric and substance use disorders among Hispanics. J Nerv Ment Dis 188(11):728–735, 2000 11093374

Reinert DF, Allen JP: The alcohol use disorders identification test: an update of research findings. Alcohol Clin Exp Res 31(2):185–199, 2007 17250609

Resnik HL, Dizmang LH: Observations on suicidal behavior among American Indians. Am J Psychiatry 127(7):882–887, 1971 5540333

Room R: Taking account of cultural and societal influences on substance use diagnoses and criteria. Addiction 101 (suppl 1):31–39, 2006 16930159

Rudgley R: The archaic use of hallucinogens in Europe: an archaeology of altered states. Addiction 90(2):163–164, 1995 7703811

Schinke SP, Tepavac L, Cole KC: Preventing substance use among Native American youth: three-year results. Addict Behav 25(3):387–397, 2000 10890292

Schmidt I, Room R: Cross-cultural applicability in international classifications and research on alcohol dependence. J Stud Alcohol 60(4):448–462, 1999 10463800

Schomerus G, Lucht M, Holzinger A, et al: The stigma of alcohol dependence compared with other mental disorders: a review of population studies. Alcohol Alcohol 46(2):105–112, 2011 21169612

Schwartz DG: Roll the Bones: The History of Gambling. New York, Gotham Books, 2006

Spapens T: Illegal gambling, in The Oxford Handbook of Organized Crime. Edited by Paoli L. Oxford, UK, Oxford University Press, 2014, pp 402–418

Standage T: A History of the World in 6 Glasses. Toronto, Canada, Random House, 2006, p 311

Sue D: Use and abuse of alcohol by Asian Americans. J Psychoactive Drugs 19(1):57–66, 1987 3585594

Tavares H: Gambling in Brazil: a call for an open debate. Addiction 109(12):1972–1976, 2014 24851676

Thomson MD, Hoffman-Goetz L: Defining and measuring acculturation: a systematic review of public health studies with Hispanic populations in the United States. Soc Sci Med 69(7):983–991, 2009 19525050

Tse S, Yu ACH, Rossen F, et al: Examination of Chinese gambling problems through a socio-historical-cultural perspective. Scientific World Journal 10:1694–1704, 2010 20842314

Westermeyer J, Mellman L, Alarcon R: Cultural competence in addiction psychiatry. Addictive Disorders and Their Treatment 5(3):107–119, 2006. Available at: https://insights.ovid.com/crossref?an=00132576-200609000-00001. Accessed February 6, 2020.

World Health Organization: International Statistical Classification of Diseases and Related Health Problems, 10th Revision. Geneva, World Health Organization, 1992

World Health Organization: International Statistical Classification of Diseases and Related Health Problems, 11th Revision. Geneva, World Health Organization, 2019

Recommended Readings

Bookman EB, McAllister K, Gillanders E, et al: Gene-environment interplay in common complex diseases: forging an integrative model—recommendations from an NIH workshop. Genet Epidemiol 35:217–225, 2011

Castro FG, Barrera M Jr, Holleran Steiker LK: Issues and challenges in the design of culturally adapted evidence-based interventions. Annu Rev Clin Psychol 6:213–239, 2010

Gainsbury SM: Cultural competence in the treatment of addictions: theory, practice and evidence. Clin Psychol Psychother 24(4):987–1001, 2017

Kirmayer LJ, Fung K, Rousseau C, et al: Guidelines for training in cultural psychiatry. Can J Psychiatry 57 (3 suppl):1–16, 2012

Room R: Taking account of cultural and societal influences on substance use diagnoses and criteria. Addiction 101 (suppl 1):31–39, 2006

Westermeyer J, Mellman L, Alarcon R: Cultural competence in addiction psychiatry. Addict Disord Their Treat 5:107–119, 2006

CHAPTER 41

Substance-Related Disorders in Older Adults

Maria A. Sullivan, M.D., Ph.D.

Although substance use disorders (SUDs) are often perceived as problems affecting primarily adolescents and younger adults, the increasing prevalence in the older population represents a significant public health concern (Han et al. 2009). At the same time, the world population of older adults is growing rapidly. It is estimated that persons ages 65 years and older will grow from 15% of the population in 2014 to 21% of the population in 2030, when the youngest "baby boomers" (a group defined as individuals born between 1946 and 1964) will be 66 years of age (U.S. Census Bureau 2014). In addition to these demographic changes, the cohort of aging baby boomers has higher rates of illicit drug use than preceding generations. Social changes and shifts in cultural attitudes toward authority have made this cohort more likely to have experimented with illicit drugs in their youth (Koechl et al. 2012), and addiction initiated in youth often persists into advanced age (Anderson and Levy 2003). This expanding group of aging elders has a greater need of treatment for SUDs than previous generations (Gross 2008). The prevalence of SUDs in older adults is often underreported and is certainly underestimated. This phenomenon of occult substance misuse by the older population has been referred to as an invisible epidemic.

To date, the clinical problem of SUDs in older adults has received relatively little attention as a research initiative and often goes unrecognized as a clinical focus. This pattern of underdiagnosis can be partly explained by the fact that among both family members and practitioners, cultural biases tend to minimize the extent of substance-related problems in older adults. Behavior considered a problem in younger adults does not engender the same sense of urgency in older adults. Relatives and practitioners may carry unexamined beliefs that older adults should be allowed to engage in whatever behaviors they choose at their age. However, it is also true that misuse of alcohol or other substances in older age is frequently a hidden phenomenon, because family members, friends, and coworkers are not present to observe the types of changes in behavior or personality by which SUDs are frequently identified in younger persons (Johnson 1989). Likewise, many screening instruments measure the presence of legal, social, and work-related problems and thus may not detect the presence of an SUD in older individuals. Older patients themselves may be reluctant to reveal SUDs because of the related feelings of shame and stigma that are heightened in this generational cohort.

Most primary care physicians and specialists do not routinely screen older adults for SUDs (Rothrauff et al. 2011), in spite of the risk factors of social isolation and poor physical health, as well as anxiety or depressive symptoms, that may predispose older adults to initiate or continue use of psychoactive substances. In addition, compared with previous generations, the current aging cohort has had more exposure to alcohol and addictive drugs due to cultural shifts that have taken place in the past 50 years. For the first time, the proportion of older adults entering SUD treatment is increasing relative to younger adults (Arndt et al. 2011). In addition, the number of older adults in the population continues to increase. Routine screening for alcohol and substance use in a sensitive manner related to health concerns, framing evidence-based recommendations, and referring to, or initiating, treatment can significantly improve health and quality of life in this older population.

Scope of the Problem

The current problem of limited clinical knowledge regarding the phenomenology of SUDs in later life is rendered more acute by the changing demographics of the U.S. population. Over the next decade, the rapidly growing cohort of aging adults will pose a significant challenge for the field of addiction treatment. By 2030, it is estimated that there will be about 72.1 million adults ages 65 years and older, representing 19.3% of the total population. Moreover, this cohort continues to use alcohol and psychoactive prescription medications at a higher rate than previous generations. For instance, about 50% of adults ages 65 years and older and 25% of individuals ages 85 years and older drink alcohol (Caputo et al. 2012). This considerable portion of the older population at potential risk for the development of alcohol use disorder (AUD) also incurs heightened risks from reduced activity of gastric antidiuretic hormone, leading to elevation of blood alcohol levels by up to 25% (Lieber 2005). Further highlighting the risk of AUD in this population, the National Survey on Drug Use and Health (NSDUH) for 2005–2006 revealed a relatively high level of binge drinking in men (14%) and women (3%) ages 65 years and older (Blazer and Wu 2009a).

Along with alcohol, psychoactive prescription drugs are the most frequently abused substances by older Americans (Weintraub et al. 2002). Approximately one-third of all prescription drugs in the United States are used by adults ages 65 years and older (National Institute on Drug Abuse 2011). Polypharmacy is a common clinical phenomenon among older adults, who tend to have multiple medical disorders. It is estimated that a rising proportion of older adults will experience prescription SUDs in the context of increased accessibility of prescription drugs (Dowling et al. 2008).

Historically, the use of illicit drugs has been relatively rare among older adults. In the 2004 NSDUH, only 1.8% of individuals ages 50 years and older reported use of illicit drugs (Huang and Lai 2006). That survey projected that by 2020, the percentage of individuals ages 50 years and older using any illicit drug would have increased from 2.2% (1.6 million) to 3.1% (3.5 million), and the percentage using psychoactive prescription drugs (opioids, sedatives, and stimulants) for nonmedical reasons would have increased from 1.2% (911,000) to 2.4% (2.7 million). Consistent with these predictions of increasing substance use by older Americans, data from the 2017 NSDUH indicated that the prevalence of illicit substance use (including marijuana, cocaine/crack, heroin, hallucinogens, inhalants, and methamphetamine) was 10.1%–15.0% among individuals ages 50–64 years and 5.3% among those ages 65 years and older (Substance Abuse and Mental Health Services Administration 2018b). Findings from the 2012 NSDUH indicated that past-month illicit drug use among adults ages 55–59 years had increased by more than 50% in the past 2 years, from 4.1% in 2010 to 6.6% in 2012 (Substance Abuse and Mental Health Services Administration 2012). Over the last decade, older adults have shown an increase in reported past-month use of alcohol (National Institute on Alcohol Abuse and Alcoholism 2015). Similarly, NSDUH survey results from 2012–2013 to 2015–2016 indicated an increased prevalence of past-year marijuana use by middle-aged (50–64 years) and older (age 65+) adults (Han and Palamar 2018). Cocaine and heroin use have increased among older adults entering SUD treatment (Arndt et al. 2011). The average age at treatment admission is increasing, and many older adults with opioid use disorder present for treatment for the first time at ages 50–70 years (Carew and Comiskey 2018). For older Americans, morbidity and mortality related to illicit substance use are expected to continue to rise.

Clinical Presentation and Assessment

Previous studies have shown that older adults are more likely than younger people to underreport their substance use, mainly in response to the stigma and discomfort of being assessed for drug use (Rockett et al. 2006). This behavior creates a barrier for older adult patients to honestly and openly discuss their substance use, thereby making it difficult for physicians to use standard procedures for recognizing and assessing substance use problems. Furthermore, recognizing SUDs in elderly patients can be challenging, because clinical indicators of these conditions in younger patients (e.g., unsteady gait, cognitive impairment, insomnia) may reflect other common medical or psychiatric problems in the older population. AUD may exacerbate underlying health problems, such as hypertension or diabetes, or may contribute to the onset of common diseases in older adults. Screening for SUDs should be conducted when older patients present with a new-onset cognitive or psychiatric disorder or a disorder potentially associated with alcohol or substance use, deterioration of a chronic disease, or decreased effectiveness of a pharmacological treatment (Caputo et al. 2012).

SUD diagnoses are often missed in primary care, family practice, and general psychiatry. Certain laboratory findings are suggestive of chronic alcohol consumption and should raise the possibility of an AUD diagnosis. Such findings include macrocytosis (increased mean corpuscular volume of the red blood cells), low vitamin B_{12} and folate, anemia, thrombocytopenia, and elevation of the hepatic enzymes aspartate aminotransferase, alanine aminotransferase, and γ-glutamyltransferase. Other common findings in AUD include increased bilirubin and albumin deficiency; the latter is present in 17% of alcohol-dependent patients ages 65 years and older, compared with 3% of those younger than 65 years (Caputo et al. 2012). In addition, deficiencies in calcium, magnesium, and phosphorus—resulting from decreased intake and malabsorption—should serve as possible markers of AUD in the older population.

The National Institute on Alcohol Abuse and Alcoholism (2014) recommended that adults ages 65 years and older consume no more than 7 drinks per week, and no more than 3 drinks on any single occasion. However, the concomitant use of prescription or nonprescription medication by 60%–78% of older adults means that a safe quantity of alcohol consumption should be established for each individual on a case-by-case basis. For most substances, it is generally recommended that acceptable levels of use be set at lower levels for older adults than for younger adults, or that abstinence be advised for older adults.

General Principles of Treatment

In the treatment of all SUDs in older adults, certain principles should be applied. Screening measures should be universally implemented in all primary care visits to identify older individuals who may be engaging in hazardous alcohol or substance use. Brief interventions may then be offered, consisting of education, advice, assessment of motivation for change, and, if warranted, referral for treatment. If group or individual therapies are initiated, it is important that these include age-specific content relevant to older adults. When pharmacotherapies are offered, it is advisable to begin prescribing cautiously at low dosages, and to make dosage adjustments gradually (i.e., "start low, go slow"). Age-related physiological changes, including decreased metabolism and decreased end-organ sensitivity, place older individuals at heightened risk for experiencing side effects from medications. Although pharmacotherapies are equally effective in older and younger patients, medication compliance and careful monitoring for adverse effects are especially important for aging patients, many of whom are taking multiple medications simultaneously.

Before offering an older individual treatment for an AUD or SUD, the clinician first needs to identify through screening whether a harmful pattern of drug use is present. A screening intervention is used to identify substance misuse that may not be evident or recognized by clinicians. Barriers to screening for substance use in older individuals include discomfort in patients and providers with discussing stigmatized behavior such as substance use, as well as the common perception of many older adults that the symptoms of SUDs are related to aging or another disease process, rather than the substance use itself. Screening and brief interventions can be carried out by any health care provider. Although standardized instruments may be used as screening measures to facilitate brief interventions, few screening instruments have been tested in older adults, so their validity in this population is uncertain (Kalapatapu and Sullivan 2010). Although computer-based self-report assessments have increased in popularity, use of these screening tools may be difficult for older adults with reduced visual acuity or inexperience with computers.

Although few substance use/misuse screening instruments have been evaluated in regard to their use in older adults, two exceptions with demonstrated high sensitivity and specificity in older adults are the CAGE questionnaire (Ewing 1984) and the Michigan Alcohol Screening Test—Geriatric Version (MAST-G), which focuses on stressors and behaviors common among older adults (Blow et al. 1992). Screening instruments based on criteria from the *Diagnostic and Statistical Manual of Mental Disorders,* 5th Edition (DSM-5) (American Psychiatric Association 2013), are generally considered the "gold standard," but some of these criteria (e.g., the impact of substance use on employment) may not be applicable to older adults (Kuerbis et al. 2014). Consideration of age-appropriate criteria (e.g., identifying at-risk, hazardous, problematic, or unhealthy use) is a better screening goal The Substance Use Brief Screen (SUBS) is a self-administered brief screener for tobacco, alcohol, and illegal and prescription drug use that has been validated in the primary care setting (McNeely et al. 2015). Universal screening will help identify patients who may be at risk for or who are currently engaging in unhealthy substance use behaviors.

Brief interventions typically include several features: 1) assessment of the substance misuse and its negative consequences; 2) feedback about the misuse and its negative consequences; 3) information or education about misuse, negative consequences, and options for reduction of misuse; 4) advice about treatment needs and resources, and about elimination of misuse; and 5) provision of self-help or other relevant materials (Babor et al. 2011). Most brief interventions are modeled on the techniques of motivational interviewing, employing a nonjudgmental approach that minimizes shame and highlights autonomy and collaboration. Brief interventions may include assessment of the patient's interest in and motivation for changing substance misuse behaviors. Education about the symptoms, behaviors, and negative consequences may warrant the inclusion of age-specific content for older adults (Kalapatapu and Sullivan 2010).

Brief interventions for older adults consist of structured interventions of relatively short duration in which the level of intervention is matched to the severity of the substance misuse: intervention alone, brief intervention leading to brief treatment (or referral for intensive treatment) (Babor et al. 2011). Assessments focused on symptoms, behaviors, and the negative consequences of substance misuse should include age-specific content for brief interventions for older adults. It is advisable to offer information about the harmful effects of substances, their potential for greater harm among older adults due to the effects of aging, the hazards of using more than one substance simultaneously, and the potential adverse effects of substances in combination with prescribed and over-the-counter medications. However, brief interventions targeting this population have not been well studied; there is little available evidence to guide substance-related brief interventions for older adults.

Preliminary studies suggest that older adults can reduce at-risk and heavy drinking and use of psychotropic medications (e.g., benzodiazepines) in response to a brief intervention (Tannenbaum et al. 2014). However, there is a need for more robust clinical trials of brief interventions in older adults, particularly with regard to illicit drugs. Future studies should examine whether the presence of age-specific content increases the success of these interventions. For instance, compared with younger adults, older adults tend to be more "backward-viewing"—reflecting on their life experiences. A foreshortened view of the future might reduce one's motivation to engage in changing behaviors. In conducting brief interventions, the practitioner should explore with older adults which perspective they primarily hold, in order to adapt the brief intervention accordingly. For instance, "forward-viewing" brief interventions might focus on the individual's motivations to change in anticipation of future events (e.g., the birth of a grandchild, upcoming family gatherings, retirement), whereas "backward-viewing" interventions might reflect on negative consequences, social mores from youth, role models for change, and other aspects from earlier life experiences (Merchant and Beaudoin 2016).

Treatment guidelines from the Substance Abuse and Mental Health Services Administration (2020) recommend age-specific treatment approaches for SUDs, including group therapy that can address losses and bereavement needs early in treatment and teach skills for rebuilding social support networks (for a more extensive discussion of this recommendation, see Briggs et al. 2011). It is important that staff be experienced in working with older adults and demonstrate respect, proceed at a slower pace using age-appropriate content, and offer a therapeutic context marked by nonconfrontational support for change. Primary care settings appear more effective than specialty substance treatment centers with respect to treatment retention outcomes for older adults. The Primary Care Research in Substance Abuse and Mental Health (PRISM) trial randomly assigned older at-risk drinkers (N=414) to either an integrated primary care intervention or referral to a specialty provider, such as a substance abuse clinic. The researchers found that older alcohol users who received the integrated intervention were more than twice as likely as those in the referral group to stay in treatment (Bartels et al. 2004).

At a time when precision medicine—a medical model that proposes to tailor medical decisions and treatments to the individual patient—is in the ascendancy, there is a significant current clinical need for additional research to develop screening instruments sensitive to SUDs in older patients. Similarly, brief interventions targeting older adults have not been well characterized, yet the inherent nonconfrontational approach of these behavioral therapies seems especially well suited to older individuals. Group and family therapies may be of particular benefit to older adults because of their emphasis on social support. These treatments could be enhanced by content tailored for older adults, including life experiences of loss and social isolation. Similar benefits may be derived from self-help groups, which can represent important sources of social support. Pharmacotherapies should be given consideration in older adults, as in younger patients, with the caveat that lower initial dosages may be needed, and close monitoring for potential adverse effects is recommended.

Alcohol

Excessive alcohol use by older adults is a growing public health concern. Alcohol is the most frequently used substance in older populations and can contribute to the leading causes of death in older adults: heart disease, cancer, and stroke. Age-related physiological changes make this group more vulnerable to the complications of acute and long-term alcohol use, yet historically, there has been less detection and treatment of AUD in older adults compared with the general population. Recent research has begun to examine the effectiveness of certain treatment approaches for identifying and addressing at-risk drinking in older patients (Duru et al. 2015; Kuerbis et al. 2015).

Screening for alcohol use is the first clinical step needed to address the problem of AUD in older adults. The U.S. Preventive Services Task Force recommends that all adults be screened for alcohol use (Moyer and Preventive Services Task Force 2013).

However, primary care physicians have been found to screen only 15.7% of all adults and only 9.3% of adults ages 65 years and older (McKnight-Eily et al. 2017). In a study of current drinkers ages 60 years and older who accessed primary care clinics, Barnes et al. (2010) found that at-risk drinking was present in 34.7% of the sample. White men ages 60–64 years and those with lower levels of education were most likely to engage in high-risk alcohol use (McKnight-Eily et al. 2017).

Among heavy drinkers, older adults are more likely than younger ones to suffer from alcoholic liver disease (ALD) because of age-related changes in alcohol distribution and metabolism. Common complications of ALD in later life include portal hypertension, ascites, and esophageal varices (Seitz and Stickel 2007). Older alcohol users are also at heightened risk for gastritis, ulcers, and upper gastrointestinal bleeding (Menninger 2002). Other medical conditions commonly caused by AUD are acute and chronic pancreatitis, chronic diarrhea, and electrolyte imbalances (Kristiansen et al. 2008). AUD is also associated with poorer control of diabetes and may increase the risk of hypoglycemia due to inhibition of gluconeogenesis. Chronic heavy drinking is a well-established cause of brain atrophy and dementia in late life (Topiwala and Ebmeier 2018) and has been found to increase the risk of incident depression and anxiety, as well as persistent depression among older women (Carvalho et al. 2018).

AUD is also a significant risk factor for accidents, falls, and bone fractures in the older population (Caputo et al. 2012). Sequelae of drinking, such as balance problems, orthostatic hypotension, neuropathies, myopathies, ataxia, and confusion, may render patients more vulnerable to accidents and falls. Another risk factor for falls and fractures in older patients with AUD is decreased bone density, especially when combined with other risk factors for osteoporosis (e.g., cigarette smoking) (Bikle et al. 1985).

Medication management is an option that should be discussed with older adults with AUD. In this treatment approach, the physician or prescriber seeks to optimize treatment outcomes by evaluating the patient's need for pharmacotherapy, providing psychoeducation to enhance compliance, formulating a medication treatment plan, and monitoring the patient's response to ensure safety and efficacy. Medications approved by the U.S. Food and Drug Administration (FDA) that may be helpful for older adults are naltrexone (oral and injectable) and acamprosate. Because of their benign side-effect profiles, both oral naltrexone and acamprosate are well suited as pharmacological agents for older individuals with AUD. Topiramate and gabapentin may also be useful for some patients and have been used off-label for treatment of AUD, although neither has been studied specifically in the population of older adults with AUD. Side effects that may pose a particular risk in elderly patients include cognitive impairment with topiramate or disequilibrium with gabapentin. Gabapentin confers one particular advantage for its use in older patients: it exerts no significant effects on other medications likely to be used by older adults, and its serum levels and metabolism rate are not affected by other medications (Leppik and Epilepsy Foundation of America 2005). More research is needed to develop and test drugs targeted for use in older adults with AUD and those with AUD and other comorbidities.

A large study of adults ages 60 years and older ($N=10,860$) in the addiction care system in Germany found that only 3% of these older patients with AUD were utilizing treatment services, compared with 10%–13% of individuals in the general population with AUD who sought help for an addiction (Dauber et al. 2018). Despite the low use of AUD services by the older adults, they had highly positive treatment outcomes, to a greater extent than younger adults (Dauber et al. 2018). This finding is consistent with findings from other research documenting that older age is associated with higher rates of successful treatment completion (Sahker et al. 2015) and better 6-month treatment outcomes for AUD (Wieben et al. 2018). Older adults are thus less likely to access treatment services than younger adults, despite the fact that the outcomes for treatment-seeking older adults surpass outcomes for the general population.

Benzodiazepines and Sedative-Hypnotics

Benzodiazepines are the most frequently prescribed class of psychotropic medication. Their prevalence of use increases linearly with age, and the rate of use among women is essentially twice that among men (Olfson et al. 2015). Until recently, few studies had examined benzodiazepine use disorder among older adults. The prevalence of benzodiazepine use among older community-dwelling adults ranges from 10% to 42% (Llorente et al. 2000). Compared with rates of benzodiazepine use in this general population, rates are generally higher among elderly patients who are homebound and are even higher among older adults who are institutionalized (Williams and Bogunovic 2016).

Indications for the use of benzodiazepines are the same for older patients as they are for younger patients: treatment of generalized anxiety disorder and other anxiety disorders, adjustment disorder, and insomnia. Among general adult populations from various countries, about 30% report one or more symptoms of insomnia (Ancoli-Israel and Roth 1999), but this prevalence increases with age and is estimated to be as high as 50% in older adults (Crowley 2011); thus, the presence of insomnia is an especially common indication for benzodiazepine use among older patients. Although benzodiazepines shorten sleep latency, reduce the number of awakenings, and increase total sleep time on a short-term basis, they do not improve the overall quality of sleep. Behavioral treatments for insomnia have been shown to provide superior results, and there is little evidence to support long-term use of benzodiazepines for insomnia among older patients (Williams and Bogunovic 2016).

Benzodiazepines are typically prescribed as the first-line treatment for anxiety in older patients, as well as for depression—which often presents with anxiety rather than classic mood symptoms in this population (Williams and Bogunovic 2016). However, the adverse-effect profile of benzodiazepines includes cognitive and psychomotor impairment, and their use in older patients can produce incoordination and lead to gait disturbances and falls, especially when given in combination with other medications. Serotonergic antidepressants are often a more appropriate choice for treatment of anxiety in this population because of their efficacy for many types of anxiety as well as for depression. Notably, both benzodiazepines and antidepressants, particularly selective serotonin reuptake inhibitors, are associated with a fall risk in older adults (Laberge and Crizzle 2019). Past-year benzodiazepine misuse, as well as opioid misuse, has been found to be associated with past-year suicidal ideation in older adults in the United States (Schepis et al. 2019).

The physiological and pharmacological effects of aging render older adults more sensitive to the potential side effects of benzodiazepines. Decreased albumin levels lead to an increase in the pharmacologically active free-drug fraction and thus to potentiation of benzodiazepine effects; reduced hepatic blood flow can increase peak concentrations; drug metabolism decreases as much as 30% with age; and plasma clearance of benzodiazepines is reduced. In older women in particular, the proportion of total body fat to lean mass is increased, which raises the volume of distribution, lowers peak plasma concentrations, and prolongs plasma half-life. Older patients are more likely to be on multiple classes of medications, leading to greater rates of drug–drug interactions. In addition, it is likely that in older individuals, age-related alterations in benzodiazepine receptors cause heightened sensitivity and increased sedation (Williams and Bogunovic 2016).

Several studies have found that benzodiazepine use in older populations can be associated with adverse health consequences, including at least a 50% increased risk of hip fractures related to the medication's effects on cognition, balance, and gait (Madhusoodanan and Bogunovic 2004). In addition, exposure to longer-half-life benzodiazepines in older drivers has been associated with a 30%–50% increase in motor vehicle accidents (Neutel 1995). Furthermore, in comparison with younger patients, older patients may exhibit atypical symptoms of benzodiazepine withdrawal. Among elderly medical inpatients, confusion and disorientation with or without hallucinations are predominant symptoms of benzodiazepine withdrawal following discontinuation (Foy et al. 1995). It is estimated that up to 10% of hospital admissions may be directly or indirectly linked to benzodiazepines (Williams and Bogunovic 2016).

A second commonly prescribed class of sedative-hypnotics is that of the nonbenzodiazepine α_1-selective γ-aminobutyric acid type A (GABA$_A$) receptor agonists—zolpidem, eszoplicone, and zaleplon, often referred to as the "Z-drugs." Each class of sedative-hypnotic binds to different architecture in the GABA$_A$ receptor complex. In general, pharmacological agents that show greater selectivity at the GABA receptor are associated with lower abuse liability. For example, zolpidem binds to α_1 subunits of the GABA receptor, affecting sedation, but has fewer anxiolytic or muscle-relaxant effects. By contrast, benzodiazepines are less selective; they bind to any of the GABA receptor α units containing histidine, including α_1, α_2, α_3, and α_5 (Williams and Bogunovic 2016), and therefore have high abuse liability.

Intoxication with benzodiazepines is typically dose dependent; symptoms can include sleepiness, lethargy, weakness, dizziness, ataxia, confusion, disorientation, and anterograde amnesia. Older women have been found to be at particularly heightened risk for prescription drug misuse (Kalapatapu and Sullivan 2010). Other risk factors in older women include increased rates of anxiety and mood disorders, particularly if these have gone untreated. Nonmedical use of sedative-hypnotics is more likely to occur in individuals with any additional mood, anxiety, or personality disorder (Huang and Lai 2006).

The DSM-5 criteria for sedative, hypnotic, or anxiolytic use disorder are less sensitive for an aging population, and underdiagnosis of prescription drug use disorders is a widespread problem for older individuals (Wetterling et al. 2002). It is important to assess for dysfunction in domains of life relevant to each patient's personal context (e.g., social functioning rather than job performance). Although the general treatment approach for sedative, hypnotic, or anxiolytic use disorder is similar for all adults, detoxification strategies often need to be tailored for older individuals, who may have had more prolonged exposure (i.e., decades of use) and may have greater difficulty ceasing use. Slower, longer tapers (e.g., over several months) should be considered to minimize rebound symptoms, withdrawal, and the risk of relapse. If an expedited taper is necessary, it is advisable to use a benzodiazepine with a shorter half-life and no active metabolites (e.g., lorazepam) for the detoxification regimen.

The American Geriatrics Society (2019) has cautioned against the use of any benzodiazepine or other sedative-hypnotic agent as initial treatment for insomnia, agitation, or delirium in older adults. Paradoxically, however, benzodiazepines are the most frequently prescribed drugs for insomnia and anxiety in older patients. These medications may have a helpful role in treating acute indications such as intense grief reactions, severe and time-limited anxiety, transient psychotic symptoms, and medical procedures, but they should be prescribed at low dosages and for short periods of time (2–4 weeks). If a benzodiazepine is needed for an older adult, shorter-acting agents (e.g., lorazepam, oxazepam) are usually recommended, because they are more rapidly cleared. Other classes of medications (e.g., selective serotonin reuptake inhibitors, serotonin-norepinephrine reuptake inhibitors, buspirone) may be more helpful for persistent symptoms (Crocco et al. 2018). In many cases, behavioral, psychosocial, and psychotherapeutic interventions can offer significant relief from anxiety or insomnia and serve to minimize unnecessary medication exposure and polypharmacy in older patients (Williams and Bogunovic 2016).

Substance use disorders related to benzodiazepine or other sedative-hypnotic use are serious and often unrecognized problems in elderly patients. Older adults who are also prescribed stimulants or opioids should be monitored for benzodiazepine misuse. More research is needed to identify specific risk factors and potential biomarkers for substance abuse in this population and to develop efficacious strategies for prevention, detection, and treatment.

Cannabis, Nicotine, and Stimulants

Cannabis Use in Older Adults

Cannabis or marijuana is not only one of the most widely used illicit drugs among all age groups in the United States (Substance Abuse and Mental Health Services Administration 2013) but also, after alcohol and tobacco, the most commonly used substance among older adults (Dinitto and Choi 2011). According to data from the 2012–2013 National Epidemiologic Survey on Alcohol and Related Conditions (NESARC-III; $N=14,715$ respondents age 50 years or older; Choi et al. 2016) and the 2006–2013 NSDUH cohorts (Han et al. 2017), the prevalence of past-year marijuana use in the older adult population ranged from 3.9% (Choi et al. 2016) to 4.8% (Han et al. 2017). After further stratification of the NSDUH data by population age, prevalences of past-year cannabis use from 2006–2007 to 2012–2013 among adults ages 50–64 years showed a 57.8% relative increase (linear trend $P<0.001$), and those among adults age 65 years or older showed a 250% relative increase (linear trend $P=0.002$) (Han et al. 2017). Given the current climate of greater acceptance of the medical benefits of marijuana and the widespread belief that it is relatively safe, particularly in comparison with alcohol, recreational use by older adults is expected to continue to rise.

In a secondary analysis of data from the last eight cohorts (2006–2013) of the NSDUH, Han et al. (2017) found that the majority of adults ages 50 years and older who reported regular marijuana use perceived either no risk or only slight risk associated with monthly cannabis use (85.3%) or weekly use (79%). However, marijuana use can lead to numerous negative health effects. For example, impairment in short-term memory, poor judgment, elevated blood pressure, increased heart and respiratory rates, anxiety, panic attacks, paranoid thinking, and hallucinations can occur with acute intoxication, and older users of cannabis are at greater risk for adverse cardiovascular events or cognitive impairment (Kuerbis et al. 2014). Similarly, upon abrupt discontinuation of cannabis, long-term users can experience unpleasant withdrawal symptoms, such as anger, aggression, anxiety, depressed mood, sleep disturbance, restlessness, decreased appetite, and weight loss. Compared with the younger population, older adults, who have less cognitive reserve (Stern and Barulli 2019), may be at greater risk of experiencing these effects. Evidence regarding the effects of marijuana use on the physical and mental well-being of older individuals is mixed. Han et al. (2017) found that older marijuana users reported an increased prevalence of two or more chronic diseases, yet in comparison with older nonusers or never users, marijuana users reported better overall health. However, older marijuana users display a high-risk profile, in that they report higher levels of psychological distress, depression, anxiety, and use of other substances (e.g., alcohol, tobacco) and illicit drugs (Dinitto and Choi 2011). Moreover, recent neuroimaging data suggest that older adults with a history of heavy cannabis use in adolescence show morphological brain changes (hippocampal cortical loss) that are not seen in older nonusers (Burggren et al. 2018).

These findings suggest that older adult marijuana users are a vulnerable population whose patterns of use need to be carefully assessed to determine whether a cannabis use disorder is present. If so, then treatment should be offered and tailored to their needs. Currently, no medications have FDA approval for use in the treatment of cannabis use disorder. Behavioral therapies targeting relapse prevention and motivational enhancement should be considered as part of any treatment plan until more-tailored interventions for older adults are developed.

Nicotine Use in Older Adults

Cigarette smoking is the leading cause of premature death among older adults. It is associated with a myriad of medical problems, increased health care costs, increased disability, greater rates of cognitive decline, and higher mortality rates. Although the frequency of tobacco use is lower in older individuals than in younger adults, data from the Centers for Disease Control and Prevention (2019) indicate that 16.3% of adults ages 45–64 years and 8.4% of those 65 years and older are current smokers. The combination of tobacco and alcohol use puts older individuals at risk for severe health-related consequences and places a greater burden on the health care system.

Compared with older adults who have never smoked, those who are current smokers report lower levels of social participation and intimacy, and those with higher severity of nicotine dependence report higher levels of fear and concern about death and pain before death than do older individuals with lower levels of dependence (Viana et al. 2019). Even in older adults who have smoked tobacco for several decades, smoking cessation is associated with dramatic improvements in health and reduction in the risk of premature death. For example, among older smokers who quit smoking at age 65 years, men were found to gain 1.4–2.0 years of life and women to gain 2.7–3.7 years of life (Taylor et al. 2002). Smoking cessation results in a markedly reduced risk of coronary events, improvement in respiratory symptoms and a slower decline in pulmonary function, improved quality of life, and increased ability to perform activities of daily living.

Multimodal interventions that include pharmacotherapy and behavioral treatment can help to increase cessation rates in older adults. Nicotine replacement therapy (NRT), bupropion, and varenicline are FDA-approved treatments for nicotine dependence and have repeatedly been shown to be effective for smoking cessation in the general population. NRT has been the primary agent studied in older smokers. In one study involving 940 participants (239 persons ≥60 years and 701 persons ≤59 years) in a smoking cessation program, NRT was significantly more effective in promoting cessation among older participants than among younger ones (41% vs. 35.4%) (Scholz et al. 2016). This study also showed that quitting success rates among older individuals using NRT alone were equal to or better than rates among those using bupropion or varenicline (Scholz et al. 2016). Similarly, in a meta-analysis of smoking cessation studies in adults ages 50 years and older, Chen and Wu (2015) found that multiple types of treatment, including pharmacological (NRT, bupropion, varenicline), nonpharmacological (cognitive-behavioral therapies, face-to-face interviews, self-help materials), and multimodal interventions (counseling plus NRT, bupropion/varenicline), resulted in significant treatment effects and higher cessation rates when compared with control groups. This review was useful because it quantitatively analyzed the relative effect sizes of different treatment modalities for smoking cessation in older individuals. Fixed-effects analysis showed significant treatment effects for pharmacological (relative risk [RR]=3.18; 95% confidence interval [CI]=1.89–5.36), nonpharmacological (RR=1.80; 95% CI=1.67–1.94), and multimodal interventions (RR=1.61; 95% CI=1.41–1.84) in comparison with control groups (Chen and Wu 2015). Estimations based on meta-regression suggested that pharmacological interventions (mean point prevalence abstinence rate [PPA]=26.10%; 95% CI=15.20–37.00) resembled nonpharmacological (PPA=27.97%; 95% CI=24.00–31.94) and multimodal interventions (PPA=36.64%; 95% CI=31.66–41.62) and that nonpharmacological and multimodal interventions produced higher PPAs than did the control group (PPA=18.80%; 95% CI=14.48–23.12) after adjustment for a number of trial and sample characteristics (Chen and Wu 2015). There is also evidence that motivational interviewing or motivational enhancement therapy targeting behavioral change is effective in promoting smoking cessation among older adults (Conigliaro et al. 2000).

Stimulant Use in Older Adults

The most commonly used stimulants among older adults are cocaine and prescription stimulants such as methylphenidate and dextroamphetamine; however, there is a paucity of research addressing psychostimulant use in older adults (Franzen 2012). A longitudinal analysis from 2000 to 2012 (Treatment Episode Data Set—Admissions) showed a 63% increase in admissions to publicly funded SUD treatment programs for older adults who used cocaine/crack (Substance Abuse and Mental Health Services Administration 2014). NSDUH data pooled from 2011 to 2015 showed a significant increase among adults ages 50 years and older in the prevalence of past-year cocaine use (0.30%–0.68%), as well as increased weekly cocaine use (0.11%–0.37%) and cocaine use disorder (0.07%–0.26%) (John and Wu 2017). A study of veterans ages 50 years and older found that 14.5% of those being treated for crack cocaine dependence first used the drug after age 50 years (Chait et al. 2010). These findings contradict prevailing misconceptions that substance use, and particularly cocaine use, is rare in older adults. Specific risk factors for cocaine use that have been identified in the older population include male sex, comorbid drug or alcohol use, retirement, chronic pain, loneliness, and stressful late-life events (Chait et al. 2010).

By increasing catecholamine levels in the brain (e.g., dopamine, norepinephrine), stimulants can increase blood pressure and heart rate, constrict blood vessels, and increase glucose. In older individuals, stimulant use may lead to severe hypertension, arrhythmias, gastrointestinal complications, unintentional weight loss, stroke, myocardial infarction, and seizures. Negative psychiatric effects include irritability; paranoia; psychosis; precipitation of anxiety and panic attacks; unexplained falls or injuries; and increased confusion and neurocognitive deficits. To minimize these risks, the clinician can use brief screening instruments to assess the level of substance misuse by elderly patients.

No specific medications have FDA approval for the treatment of stimulant use disorder, and treatment studies addressing stimulant use in the elderly population are lacking. Although dopaminergic agents, antidepressants, and anticonvulsants have been studied as treatment options for cocaine and methamphetamine dependence, conclusive evidence for their efficacy is lacking. Evidence-based behavioral interventions, such as motivational enhancement therapy and mindfulness-based cognitive-behavioral therapy, may address ongoing cravings and can help in reducing relapse in older adults.

Summary of Cannabis, Nicotine, and Stimulant Use in Older Adults

All clinicians who care for older adults must be alert for possible signs and symptoms of cannabis, nicotine, or stimulant use by older patients. Educational materials describing the health consequences of substance use and screening assessments to identify problematic use may be helpful preventive measures, while treatment referrals should include age-appropriate interventions and counseling. Treatment options targeting older populations are generally limited, in that few programs or health care settings offer tailored interventions for older adults. Current evidence-based therapies and medications may be useful and effective for treating substance use disorders involving cannabis, nicotine, and stimulants in older patients.

Opioids

In older patients, misuse and nonmedical use of prescription pain medications are important concerns (Wang and Andrade 2013). Prescription opioids (POs) account for a large proportion of medications used nonmedically today, and misuse of these prescription medications is growing among older adults. A study of chronic pain patients ages 50 years and older ($N=130$) found that 35% had misused POs (Chang 2017). Significant predictors of opioid misuse included education (higher), illicit drug use, depression (moderate level), and pain interference with normal work. Illicit opioid use is much less common in elderly adults than in younger cohorts (Denisco et al. 2008); data from the 2012 NSDUH (Substance Abuse and Mental Health Services Administration 2013) showed that 1.9% of adults ages 50 years and older reported prior lifetime heroin use, and 0.1% reported having used heroin in the past year. However, PO misuse is more prevalent than illicit opioid use in the older population; in 2005–2006, the prevalence of nonmedical use of POs was 1.4% (Blazer and Wu 2009b).

Among individuals who misuse POs, older adults are more likely than younger ones to obtain these drugs from legitimate sources. In a study of data from the NSDUH 2009–2014 cohorts (N=336,643 adults, of whom 24,384 [7.2%] were age 50–64 years and 15,177 [4.5%] were age 65 years or older), past-month PO misuse was reported by 597 adults ages 50–64 years and by 109 adults ages 65 years and older (Schepis et al. 2018). Physician sources for POs were reported by nearly half (47.7%) of those in the age 65+ group, in comparison with 39.2% of those in the age 50–64 group. Conversely, theft (5.3%), illicit purchases (8.5%), or friends/family (for free; 23.2%) were the least common PO sources reported by adults in the age 65+ group (Schepis et al. 2018). In a study carried out through focus groups of PO misusers, Inciardi et al. (2009) noted that a significant theme among these participants was that many older adults overstated their chronic pain to physicians in order to obtain opioids; although some reported abusing their drugs, the overwhelming majority diverted their medications for economic gain.

Risk factors for PO misuse by older patients include personal or family history of SUDs, comorbid psychiatric disorders, multiple medical problems, chronic pain, depression in the prior year, and American Indian/Alaskan Native ancestry (Blazer and Wu 2009b; Levi-Minzi et al. 2013). Furthermore, among middle-aged and older adults, PO abuse is more common among males; adults ages 50–64 years; misusers of prescription sedatives, stimulants, and tranquilizers; users of other substances (i.e., tobacco, marijuana, cocaine); and individuals with AUD (Han et al. 2019).

Age-related physiological changes in gastrointestinal, renal, and hepatic functions place older individuals at increased risk for experiencing side effects from opioids. Opioid-related adverse effects, which are more common in older adults, include constipation, fatigue, pruritus, anorexia, somnolence, mental status changes, and nausea (Burgos-Chapman et al. 2016). Apnea is a serious risk in older adults; for hospitalized patients, the risk of opioid-related respiratory depression increases steadily from the seventh to the ninth decades of life, rising from 2.8 to 8.7 times the risk in younger patients (Cepeda et al. 2003). Not all overdoses are accidental, and it is recognized that older adults, especially white males, have increased suicide rates. An analysis of Researched Abuse, Diversion and Addiction-Related Surveillance (RADARS) poison center program data from 2012 to 2013 revealed that the rates of death from opioid overdose for adults ages 60 years and older exceeded rates for those ages 20–59 years, and accidental overdose occurred to a significant degree (West et al. 2015). From 1999 to 2011, while adults ages 25–34, 35–44, and 45–54 years had higher opioid analgesic death rates than other age groups, the largest increase in accidental opioid overdose deaths occurred in White women ages 55–64 years (Chen et al. 2014). Following nearly a decade of rising numbers of opioid-involved overdose deaths in the United States between 2010 (21,088 deaths) and 2017 (47,600 deaths), the number in 2018 dipped slightly and remained steady, at 46,802 deaths (National Institute on Drug Abuse 2020). However, at the time of this writing in late 2020, the United States is experiencing a significant surge in opioid overdose deaths related to the COVID-19 pandemic. For example, the University of Baltimore Center for Drug Policy and Enforcement has documented, via real-time surveillance of overdose data nationally, a 17.6% increase in suspected drug overdoses when data from the weeks prior to and following the state-mandated stay-at-home orders were compared (Alter and Yeager 2020); and data from the Kentucky emergency medical services during the first months of COVID-19 revealed a 50% increase in runs for suspected opioid overdoses with deaths at the scene (Slavova et al. 2020). Both interruptions in drug supplies and lack of available treatment for opioid use disorder (OUD) have contributed to this trend.

In light of the chronic, relapsing course of OUD and the serious risks of infectious disease from intravenous opioid use and of death from opioid overdose, it is currently accepted that the "gold standard" for treatment includes medications for OUD. The FDA has approved three pharmacotherapies for OUD, including two opioid agonists (methadone, buprenorphine) and an opioid antagonist (extended-release injectable naltrexone), and all have demonstrated efficacy over placebo in preventing relapse in multiple randomized clinical trials (Substance Abuse and Mental Health Services Administration 2018a). Supportive counseling or behavioral therapy is recommended as part of a comprehensive treatment program to promote adherence to medications for OUD, and each of these pharmacotherapies may also be combined with self-help or 12-step group attendance.

PO misuse and OUD are challenging clinical issues in the older population. The prevalence of these conditions is likely to increase, given the growing numbers of older adults, the risk factors of the baby boomer generational cohort (see first paragraph of this chapter), and the current opioid epidemic. Although certain risk factors and the many adverse consequences of opioid use by older individuals are well recognized, little research to date has examined specific interventions or therapies targeting OUD in older adults.

Comorbid Psychiatric Disorders

The co-occurrence of SUDs with other psychiatric disorders is commonly referred to as dual diagnosis. The most common comorbidities with SUDs are mood disorders, especially depression. Along with environmental risks, a genetic predisposition is believed to underlie the development of comorbid disorders (Kessler 2004). Dual diagnosis is of great concern because it is often associated with higher disease severity; impaired physical and social functioning; and increased rates of psychiatric hospitalization (including emergency admissions), self-harm, and suicide (Torrens et al. 2006).

Data from the 2001–2002 NESARC (Lin et al. 2014) indicated strong associations between alcohol or tobacco use disorder and mood, anxiety, and personality disorders. Similarly, using 2005–2014 data from the NSDUH, Han et al. (2018) found that among adults ages 50 years and older ($N=61,240$), 14.4% reported past-month binge drinking. Binge drinkers were more likely to use tobacco and illegal drugs than were non–binge drinkers ($P<0.001$). In a study characterizing psychiatric comorbidity in older smokers, smokers without nicotine dependence were most likely to have a mood disorder, whereas older smokers with nicotine dependence were most likely to have an anxiety or substance use disorder (Sachs-Ericsson et al. 2011).

A recent study (Lane et al. 2018) found that among psychiatric inpatients ages 50 years and older (*N*=7,258), the overall SUD rate was 26%, with cocaine being the most common SUD (≈10%). SUD status and additional (non-SUD) comorbid psychiatric diagnoses were each significantly associated with longer lengths of stay (both *P*s<0.001). For individual SUDs, use disorders involving cocaine, marijuana, opiates, or alcohol were all significantly associated with longer lengths of stay (all *P*s<0.01), and barbiturates, opiates, and alcohol were all significantly associated with the presence of medical comorbidities (all *P*s<0.01). Thus, the combination of SUD and serious mental illness in older adults may increase the complexity of care and warrants further investigation into causal mechanisms and long-term outcomes.

Concurrent alcohol and drug use is highly prevalent among older adults. In a study of 153 adults (57 men and 96 women) ages 60 years and older seeking outpatient psychiatric care for depression (without SUD treatment), past-month alcohol use was reported by 53% of the men and 50% of the women; past-month cannabis use was reported by 12% of the men and 4% of the women; and past-month misuse of sedatives was reported by 16% of the men and 9% of the women. In a logistic regression, higher scores (denoting worse symptoms) on the Beck Depression Inventory–II (Dozois et al. 1998) were associated with cannabis use (odds ratio=15.8; 95% CI=2.0–734.0; *P*=0.003) (Satre et al. 2011).

Conclusion

In this chapter, we have reviewed the available literature on substance use disorders in older adults, a topic that has received relatively little attention to date. The number of older adults with SUDs was predicted to rise from 1.7 million in 2000–2001 to 4.4 million by 2020 (Gfroerer et al. 2003), an increase of more than 150%. This anticipated magnitude of increase in the prevalence of late-life illicit substance use was already evident in the 2012 NSDUH data (Substance Abuse and Mental Health Services Administration 2012), which showed that the rate of past-month illicit drug use had increased over the past decade from 3.4% (2002) to 7.2% (2012) for adults ages 50–54 years, from 1.9% to 6.6% for those ages 55–59 years, and from 1.1% to 3.6% for those ages 60–64 years. This pattern of expanding prevalence in SUDs among older adults partially reflects the aging of the cohort of baby boomers, who have had higher rates of illicit drug use than previous older cohorts (Substance Abuse and Mental Health Services Administration 2012).

However, SUDs in older adults are frequently unrecognized, for a variety of reasons, including unexamined biases about elderly people on the part of family members and providers, absence of behavioral disturbances or social "red flags," age-related metabolic changes that lead to negative consequences from drinking "the same amount as in the past," and patterns of inappropriate prescribing of benzodiazepines and opioids to treat anxiety and mood conditions in late life.

Physicians and other health care providers often neglect to ask older patients about alcohol use, because of the mistaken assumption that older individuals are not likely to be motivated to change their patterns of use (Sharp and Vacha-Haase 2011). Research, however, suggests the contrary—that older patients respond better than their younger counterparts to treatment, because they are more likely to adhere to treatment and therapy sessions, and therefore are less likely to relapse (Oslin et al. 2005).

Alcohol and psychoactive prescription drugs are the substances most frequently used by older adults, and cigarette smoking represents the leading cause of premature death in this population. While rates of illicit substance use are lower in older adults than in younger cohorts, the prevalence of late-life SUDs has been increasing over the past two decades, as the baby boomer cohort ages and the percentage of older adults in the U.S. population grows. Among illicit (or recently illicit) drugs, cannabis and cocaine are the substances most frequently used by older Americans, and their rates of use have been rising. In this chapter, we have considered some of the risk factors for SUDs in older adults, including concurrent mood or anxiety disorders, as well as some of the physiological, social, and cultural vulnerabilities that characterize this population.

Reliance on standard DSM criteria may result in a failure to detect SUD that presents with cognitive symptoms or physical injury, as well as the absence of work or social consequences. A validated screening measure can be an important diagnostic tool, and the presence of anxiety or affective disorders should raise concern about heightened risk for alcohol or other substance use. Older women in particular are vulnerable to psychoactive prescription drug misuse, especially misuse of benzodiazepines and opioid analgesics.

Brief interventions appear promising for older individuals. It is recommended that older individuals be referred to treatment settings that offer age-appropriate group therapy and nonconfrontational individual therapy focusing on late-life issues of loss and sources of social support. Older adults also deserve to receive full consideration for the potential benefits of medication management for SUDs. Although research to date has been limited regarding older adults, treatment outcomes for SUDs have been found to be superior in older adults compared with younger or middle-aged adults (Carew and Comiskey 2018). This encouraging finding appears to reflect older patients' better adherence to treatment and consequently lower relapse rates.

Addiction is an underrecognized and undertreated clinical problem in later life. The misuse of prescribed and illicit substances by older adults is a significant public health problem. As the general population continues to age, it will be increasingly important for clinicians to address the unique concerns of older adults with SUDs. Educating providers on the importance of universal screening for SUDs for patients ages 50 years and older is an important first step. In addition, prescribers should be informed of the risk of inappropriate prescribing of medications with abuse liability for older patients at risk for SUDs. An emerging literature on tailored treatments for older populations suggests the benefits of brief interventions and age-specific treatment services in both inpatient and outpatient settings, as well as generally favorable treatment outcomes for older patients. Current and future research will inform new methods of assessing SUDs and implementing effective treatments for older patients.

References

Alter A, Yeager C: COVID-19 Impact on US National Overdose Crisis. Overdose Detection Mapping Application Program, June 2020. Available at: http://www.odmap.org/Content/docs/news/2020/ODMAP-Report-June-2020.pdf. Accessed September 8, 2020.

American Geriatrics Society: Ten Things Physicians and Patients Should Question. July 1, 2019. Available at: http://www.choosingwisely.org/wp-content/uploads/2015/02/AMDA-Choosing-Wisely-List.pdf. Accessed January 10, 2020.

American Psychiatric Association: Diagnostic and Statistical Manual of Mental Disorders, 5th Edition. Arlington, VA, American Psychiatric Association, 2013

Ancoli-Israel S, Roth T: Characteristics of insomnia in the United States: results of the 1991 National Sleep Foundation Survey, I. Sleep 22 (suppl 2):S347–S353, 1999 10394606

Anderson TL, Levy JA: Marginality among older injectors in today's illicit drug culture: assessing the impact of ageing. Addiction 98(6):761–770, 2003 12780364

Arndt S, Clayton R, Schultz SK: Trends in substance abuse treatment 1998–2008: increasing older adult first-time admissions for illicit drugs. Am J Geriatr Psychiatry 19(8):704–711, 2011 21785290

Babor TE, McRee BG, Kassebaum PA, et al: Screening, Brief Intervention, and Referral to Treatment (SBIRT): toward a public health approach to the management of substance abuse. Journal of Lifelong Learning in Psychiatry 9(1):130–148, 2011. Available at: https://focus.psychiatryonline.org/doi/abs/10.1176/foc.9.1.foc130. Accessed February 6, 2020.

Barnes AJ, Moore AA, Xu H, et al: Prevalence and correlates of at-risk drinking among older adults: the Project SHARE study. J Gen Intern Med 25(8):840–846, 2010 20396975

Bartels SJ, Coakley EH, Zubritsky C, et al: Improving access to geriatric mental health services: a randomized trial comparing treatment engagement with integrated versus enhanced referral care for depression, anxiety, and at-risk alcohol use. Am J Psychiatry 161(8):1455–1462, 2004 15285973

Bikle DD, Genant HK, Cann C, et al: Bone disease in alcohol abuse. Ann Intern Med 103(1):42–48, 1985 2988390

Blazer DG, Wu LT: The epidemiology of at-risk and binge drinking among middle-aged and elderly community adults: National Survey on Drug Use and Health. Am J Psychiatry 166(10):1162–1169, 2009a 19687131

Blazer DG, Wu LT: Nonprescription use of pain relievers by middle-aged and elderly community-living adults: National Survey on Drug Use and Health. J Am Geriatr Soc 57(7):1252–1257, 2009b 19486199

Blow FC, Brower KJ, Schulenberg JE, et al: The Michigan Alcohol Screening Test—Geriatric Version (MAST-G): a new elderly specific screening instrument. Alcohol Clin Exp Res 16:372, 1992

Briggs WP, Magnus VA, Lassiter P, et al: Substance use, misuse, and abuse among older adults: implications for clinical mental health counselors. Journal of Mental Health Counseling 33(2):112–127, 2011. Available at: https://meridian.allenpress.com/jmhc/article-abstract/33/2/112/83170/Substance-Use-Misuse-and-Abuse-Among-Older-Adults?redirectedFrom=fulltext. Accessed July 29, 2020.

Burggren AC, Siddarth P, Mahmood Z, et al: Subregional hippocampal thickness abnormalities in older adults with a history of heavy cannabis use. Cannabis Cannabinoid Res 3(1):242–251, 2018 30547094

Burgos-Chapman I, Trevisan LA, Sevarino K: Abuse of opioids and prescription medications, in Addiction in the Older Patient. Edited by Sullivan MA, Levin FR. New York, Oxford University Press, 2016, pp 105–137

Caputo F, Vignoli T, Leggio L, et al: Alcohol use disorders in the elderly: a brief overview from epidemiology to treatment options. Exp Gerontol 47(6):411–416, 2012 22575256

Carew AM, Comiskey C: Treatment for opioid use and outcomes in older adults: a systematic literature review. Drug Alcohol Depend 182:48–57, 2018 29136566

Carvalho AF, Stubbs B, Maes M, et al: Different patterns of alcohol consumption and the incidence and persistence of depressive and anxiety symptoms among older adults in Ireland: a prospective community-based study. J Affect Disord 238:651–658, 2018 29957483

Centers for Disease Control and Prevention: Smoking and Tobacco Use: Current Cigarette Smoking Among Adults in the United States. November 18, 2019. Available at: https://www.cdc.gov/tobacco/data_statistics/fact_sheets/adult_data/cig_smoking/index.htm. Accessed July 11, 2020.

Cepeda MS, Farrar JT, Baumgarten M, et al: Side effects of opioids during short-term administration: effect of age, gender, and race. Clin Pharmacol Ther 74(2):102–112, 2003 12891220

Chait R, Fahmy S, Caceres J: Cocaine abuse in older adults: an underscreened cohort. J Am Geriatr Soc 58(2):391–392, 2010 20370870

Chang YP: Factors associated with prescription opioid misuse in adults aged 50 or older. Nursing Outlook 66(2):112–120, 2017 29523356

Chen D, Wu LT: Smoking cessation interventions for adults aged 50 or older: a systematic review and meta-analysis. Drug Alcohol Depend 154:14–24, 2015 26094185

Chen LH, Hedegaard H, Warner M: Drug-poisoning deaths involving opioid analgesics: United States, 1999–2011. NCHS data brief, no 166. Hyattsville, MD, National Center for Health Statistics, 2014. Available at: https://www.cdc.gov/nchs/products/databriefs/db166.htm. Accessed July 14, 2020.

Choi NG, DiNitto DM, Marti CN: Older-adult marijuana users and ex-users: comparisons of sociodemographic characteristics and mental and substance use disorders. Drug Alcohol Depend 165:94–102, 2016 27282425

Conigliaro J, Kraemer K, McNeil M: Screening and identification of older adults with alcohol problems in primary care. J Geriatr Psychiatry Neurol 13(3):106–114, 2000 11001132

Crocco EA, Jaramilo S, Cruz-Ortiz C, Camfield K: Pharmacologic management of anxiety disorders in the elderly. Curr Treat Options Psychiatry 4(1):33–46, 2018 28948135

Crowley K: Sleep and sleep disorders in older adults. Neuropsychol Rev 21(1):41–53, 2011 21225347

Dauber H, Pogarell O, Kraus L, et al: Older adults in treatment for alcohol use disorders: service utilisation, patient characteristics and treatment outcomes. Subst Abuse Treat Prev Policy 13(1):40, 2018 30400930

Denisco RA, Chandler RK, Compton WM: Addressing the intersecting problems of opioid misuse and chronic pain treatment. Exp Clin Psychopharmacol 16(5):417–428, 2008 18837638

Dinitto DM, Choi NG: Marijuana use among older adults in the U.S.A.: user characteristics, patterns of use, and implications for intervention. Int Psychogeriatr 23(5):732–741, 2011 21108863

Dowling GJ, Weiss SR, Condon TP: Drugs of abuse and the aging brain. Neuropsychopharmacology 33(2):209–218, 2008 17406645

Dozois DJA, Dobson KS, Ahnberg JL: A psychometric evaluation of the Beck Depression Inventory—II. Psychological Assessment 10(2):83–89, 1998. Available at: https://psycnet.apa.org/doiLanding?doi=10.1037%2F1040-3590.10.2.83. Accessed July 27, 2020.

Duru OK, Xu H, Moore AA, et al: Examining the impact of separate components of a multicomponent intervention designed to reduce at-risk drinking among older adults: the Project SHARE study. Alcohol Clin Exp Res 39(7):1227–1235, 2015 26033430

Ewing JA: Detecting alcoholism: the CAGE questionnaire. JAMA 252(14):1905–1907, 1984 6471323

Foy A, O'Connell D, Henry D, et al: Benzodiazepine use as a cause of cognitive impairment in elderly hospital inpatients. J Gerontol A Biol Sci Med Sci 50(2):M99–M106, 1995 7874596

Franzen JD: Psychostimulants for older adults. Current Psychiatry 11(1):23–32, 2012. Available at: https://www.mdedge.com/psychiatry/article/64585/depression/psychostimulants-older-adult. Accessed July 29, 2020.

Gfroerer J, Penne M, Pemberton M, et al: Substance abuse treatment need among older adults in 2020: the impact of the aging baby-boom cohort. Drug Alcohol Depend 69(2):127–135, 2003 12609694

Gross J: New generation gap as older adults seek help. The New York Times, March 6, 2008. Available at: https://www.nytimes.com/2008/03/06/us/06abuse.html. Accessed January 10, 2020.

Han BH, Palamar JJ: Marijuana use by middle-aged and older adults in the United States, 2015–2016. Drug Alcohol Depend 191:374–381, 2018 30197051

Han B, Gfroerer JC, Colliver JD, et al: Substance use disorder among older adults in the United States in 2020. Addiction 104(1):88–96, 2009 19133892

Han BH, Sherman S, Mauro PM, et al: Demographic trends among older cannabis users in the United States, 2006–13. Addiction 112(3):516–525, 2017 27767235

Han BH, Moore AA, Sherman SE, et al: Prevalence and correlates of binge drinking among older adults with multimorbidity. Drug Alcohol Depend 187:48–54, 2018 29627405

Han BH, Sherman SE, Palamar JJ: Prescription opioid misuse among middle-aged and older adults in the United States, 2015–2016. Prev Med 121:94–98, 2019 30763631

Huang WF, Lai IC: Potentially inappropriate prescribing for insomnia in elderly outpatients in Taiwan. Int J Clin Pharmacol Ther 44(7):335–342, 2006 16961163

Inciardi JA, Surratt HL, Cicero TJ, et al: Prescription opioid abuse and diversion in an urban community: the results of an ultrarapid assessment. Pain Med 10(3):537–548, 2009 19416440

John WS, Wu L-T: Trends and correlates of cocaine use and cocaine use disorder in the United States from 2011 to 2015. Drug Alcohol Depend 180:376–384, 2017 28961544

Johnson LK: How to diagnose and treat chemical dependency in the elderly. J Gerontol Nurs 15:22–26, 1989 2600367

Kalapatapu RK, Sullivan MA: Prescription use disorders in older adults. Am J Addict 19(6):515–522, 2010 20958847

Kessler RC: The epidemiology of dual diagnosis. Biol Psychiatry 56(10):730–737, 2004 15556117

Koechl B, Unger A, Fischer G: Age-related aspects of addiction. Gerontology 58(6):540–544, 2012 22722821

Kristiansen L, Grønbaek M, Becker U, et al: Risk of pancreatitis according to alcohol drinking habits: a population-based cohort study. Am J Epidemiol 168(8):932–937, 2008 18779386

Kuerbis A, Sacco P, Blazer DG, et al: Substance abuse among older adults. Clin Geriatr Med 30(3):629–654, 2014 25037298

Kuerbis AN, Yuan SE, Borok J, et al: Testing the initial efficacy of a mailed screening and brief feedback intervention to reduce at-risk drinking in middle-aged and older adults: the co-morbidity alcohol risk evaluation study. J Am Geriatr Soc 63(2):321–326, 2015 25643851

Laberge S, Crizzle AM: A literature review of psychotropic medications and alcohol as risk factors for falls in community dwelling older adults. Clin Drug Investig 39(2):117–139, 2019 30560350

Lane SD, da Costa SC, Teixeira AL, et al: The impact of substance use disorders on clinical outcomes in older-adult psychiatric inpatients. Int J Geriatr Psychiatry 33(2):e323–e329, 2018 29044798

Leppik IE; Epilepsy Foundation of America: Choosing an antiepileptic: selecting drugs for older patients with epilepsy. Geriatrics 60(11):42–47, 2005 16287341

Levi-Minzi MA, Surratt HL, Kurtz SP, et al: Under treatment of pain: a prescription for opioid misuse among the elderly? Pain Med 14(11):1719–1729, 2013 23841571

Lieber CS: Metabolism of alcohol. Clin Liver Dis 9(1):1–35, 2005 15763227

Lin JC, Karno MP, Grella CE, et al: Psychiatric correlates of alcohol and tobacco use disorders in U.S. adults aged 65 years and older: results from the 2001–2002 National Epidemiologic Survey of Alcohol and Related Conditions. Am J Geriatr Psychiatry 22(11):1356–1363, 2014 24021218

Llorente MD, David D, Golden AG, et al: Defining patterns of benzodiazepine use in older adults. J Geriatr Psychiatry Neurol 13(3):150–160, 2000 11001138

Madhusoodanan S, Bogunovic OJ: Safety of benzodiazepines in the geriatric population. Expert Opin Drug Saf 3(5):485–493, 2004 15335303

McKnight-Eily LR, Okoro CA, Mejia R, et al: Screening for excessive alcohol use and brief counseling of adults—17 states and the District of Columbia, 2014. MMWR Morb Mortal Wkly Rep 66(12):313–319, 2017 28358798

McNeely J, Strauss SM, Saitz R, et al: A brief patient self-administered substance use screening tool for primary care: two-site validation study of the Substance Use Brief Screen (SUBS). Am J Med 128(7):784.e9–784.e19, 2015 25770031

Menninger JA: Assessment and treatment of alcoholism and substance-related disorders in the elderly. Bull Menninger Clin 66(2):166–183, 2002 12141383

Merchant RC, Beaudoin FL: Brief interventions for substance-use disorder in older patients, in Addiction in the Older Patient. Edited by Sullivan MA, Levin FR. New York, Oxford University Press, 2016, pp 37–67

Moyer VA; Preventive Services Task Force: Screening and behavioral counseling interventions in primary care to reduce alcohol misuse: U.S. Preventive Services Task Force recommendation statement. Ann Intern Med 159(3):210–218, 2013 23698791

National Institute on Alcohol Abuse and Alcoholism: Older Adults. 2014. Available at: https://www.niaaa.nih.gov/alcohol-health/special-populations-co-occurring-disorders/older-adults. Accessed January 10, 2020.

National Institute on Alcohol Abuse and Alcoholism: NIH Study Finds Alcohol Use Disorder on the Increase. June 3, 2015. Available at: https://www.niaaa.nih.gov/news-events/news-releases/nih-study-finds-alcohol-use-disorder-increase. Accessed January 10, 2020.

National Institute on Drug Abuse: Prescription Drug Abuse. NIDA Research Report Series (NIH Publ No 05-4881). October 2011. Available at: https://www.drugabuse.gov/sites/default/files/rxreportfinalprint.pdf. Accessed January 10, 2020.

National Institute on Drug Abuse: Advancing Addiction Science: Overdose Death Rates. March 10, 2020. Available at: https://www.drugabuse.gov/drug-topics/trends-statistics/overdose-death-rates. Accessed July 13, 2020.

Neutel CI: Risk of traffic accident injury after a prescription for a benzodiazepine. Ann Epidemiol 5(3):239–244, 1995 7606314

Olfson M, King M, Schoenbaum M: Benzodiazepine use in the United States. JAMA Psychiatry 72(2):136–142, 2015 25517224

Oslin DW, Slaymaker VJ, Blow FC, et al: Treatment outcomes for alcohol dependence among middle-aged and older adults. Addict Behav 30(7):1431–1436, 2005 16022937

Rockett IR, Putnam SL, Jia H, et al: Declared and undeclared substance use among emergency department patients: a population-based study. Addiction 101(5):706–712, 2006 16669904

Rothrauff TC, Abraham AJ, Bride BE, et al: Substance abuse treatment for older adults in private centers. Subst Abus 32(1):7–15, 2011 21302179

Sachs-Ericsson N, Collins N, Schmidt B, et al: Older adults and smoking: characteristics, nicotine dependence and prevalence of DSM-IV 12-month disorders. Aging Ment Health 15(1):132–141, 2011 20924817

Sahker E, Schultz SK, Arndt S: Treatment of substance use disorders in older adults: implications for care delivery. J Am Geriatr Soc 63(11):2317–2323, 2015 26502741

Satre DD, Sterling SA, Mackin RS, et al: Patterns of alcohol and drug use among depressed older adults seeking outpatient psychiatric services. Am J Geriatr Psychiatry 19(8):695–703, 2011 21788921

Schepis TS, McCabe SE, Teter CJ: Sources of opioid medication for misuse in older adults: results from a nationally representative survey. Pain 159(8):1543–1549, 2018 29624517

Schepis TS, Simoni-Wastila L, McCabe SE: Prescription opioid and benzodiazepine misuse is associated with suicidal ideation in older adults. Int J Geriatr Psychiatry 34(1):122–129, 2019 30328160

Scholz J, Santos PC, Buzo CG, et al: Effects of aging on the effectiveness of smoking cessation medication. Oncotarget 7(21):30032–30036, 2016 27166253

Seitz HK, Stickel F: Alcoholic liver disease in the elderly. Clin Geriatr Med 23(4):905–921, viii, 2007 17923345

Sharp L, Vacha-Haase T: Physician attitudes regarding alcohol use screening in older adult patients. Journal of Applied Gerontology 30(2):226–240, 2011. Available at: https://journals.sagepub.com/doi/10.1177/0733464810361345. Accessed July 14, 2020.

Slavova S, Rock P, Bush HM, et al: Signal of increased opioid overdose during COVID-19 from emergency medical services data. Drug Alcohol Depend 214:108176, 2020 32717504

Stern Y, Barulli D: Cognitive reserve. Handb Clin Neurol 167:181–190, 2019 31753132

Substance Abuse and Mental Health Services Administration: Results From the 2011 National Survey on Drug Use and Health Services Administration. 2012. Available at: https://www.samhsa.gov/data/sites/default/files/2011MHFDT/2k11MHFR/Web/NSDUHmh-fr2011.htm. Accessed January 10, 2020.

Substance Abuse and Mental Health Services Administration: Results From the 2012 National Survey on Drug Use and Health: Summary of National Findings, Figure 2.10 (p. 22). NSDUH Series H-46, HHS Publ No SMA-13-4795. 2013. Available at: https://www.samhsa.gov/data/sites/default/files/NSDUHresults2012/NSDUHresults2012.pdf. Accessed July 20, 2020.

Substance Abuse and Mental Health Services Administration: Treatment Episode Data Set (TEDS): 2002–2012. National Admissions to Substance Abuse Treatment Services BHSIS Series S-71, HHS Publication No. (SMA) 14-4850. Rockville, MD, Substance Abuse and Mental Health Services Administration Center for Behavioral Health Statistics and Quality, 2014. Available at: https://www.samhsa.gov/data/sites/default/files/TEDS2012N_Web.pdf. Accessed February 16, 2020.

Substance Abuse and Mental Health Services Administration: Medications for Opioid Use Disorder. Treatment Improvement Protocol (TIP) Series 63 (full document). HHS Publication No. (SMA) 19-5063FULLDOC. Rockville, MD, Substance Abuse and Mental Health Services Administration, 2018a. Available at: https://www.ncbi.nlm.nih.gov/books/NBK535268/. Accessed July 29, 2020.

Substance Abuse and Mental Health Services Administration: Results From the 2017 National Survey on Drug Use and Health: Detailed Tables. Rockville, MD, Center for Behavioral Health Statistics and Quality, Substance Abuse and Mental Health Services Administration, September 7, 2018. Available at: https://www.samhsa.gov/data/sites/default/files/cbhsq-reports/NSDUHDetailedTabs2017/NSDUHDetailedTabs2017.pdf. Accessed July 11, 2020.

Substance Abuse and Mental Health Services Administration: Substance Use Treatment for Older Adults. April 30, 2020. Available at: https://www.samhsa.gov/homelessness-programs-resources/hpr-resources/substance-use-treatment-older-adults. Accessed July 5, 2020.

Tannenbaum C, Martin P, Tamblyn R, et al: Reduction of inappropriate benzodiazepine prescriptions among older adults through direct patient education: the EMPOWER cluster randomized trial. JAMA Intern Med 174(6):890–898, 2014 24733354

Taylor DH Jr, Hasselblad V, Henley SJ, et al: Benefits of smoking cessation for longevity. Am J Public Health 92(6):990–996, 2002 12036794

Topiwala A, Ebmeier KP: Effects of drinking on late-life brain and cognition. Evid Based Ment Health 21(1):12–15, 2018 29273599

Torrens M, Martin-Santos R, Samet S: Importance of clinical diagnoses for comorbidity studies in substance use disorders. Neurotox Res 10(3–4):253–261, 2006 17197374

U.S. Census Bureau: National Population Projections Tables. Table 3: Projections of the Population by Sex and Selected Age Groups for the United States: 2015 to 2060. 2014. Available at: https://www.census.gov/data/tables/2014/demo/popproj/2014-summary-tables.html. Accessed January 9, 2020.

Viana DA, Andrade FCD, Martins LC, et al: Differences in quality of life among older adults in Brazil according to smoking status and nicotine dependence. Health Qual Life Outcomes 17(1):1, 2019 30606205

Wang Y-P, Andrade LH: Epidemiology of alcohol and drug use in the elderly. Curr Opin Psychiatry 26(4):343–348, 2013 23689545

Weintraub E, Weintraub D, Dixon L, et al: Geriatric patients on a substance abuse consultation service. Am J Geriatr Psychiatry 10(3):337–342, 2002 11994222

West NA, Severtson SG, Green JL, et al: Trends in abuse and misuse of prescription opioids among older adults. Drug Alcohol Depend 149:117–121, 2015 25678441

Wetterling T, Backhaus J, Junghanns K: [Addiction in the elderly—an underestimated diagnosis in clinical practice?] (German). Nervenarzt 73(9):861–866, 2002 12215877

Wieben ES, Nielsen B, Nielsen AS, et al: Elderly alcoholics compared to middle-aged alcoholics in outpatient treatment—6-month follow-up. Nord J Psychiatry 72(7):506–511, 2018 30348042

Williams AR, Bogunovic OJ: Benzodiazepines and other sedative-hypnotics in the older adult, in Addiction in the Older Patient. Edited by Sullivan MA, Levin FR. New York, Oxford University Press, 2016, pp 159–172

CHAPTER 42

Behavioral Addictive Disorders

Mayumi Okuda, M.D.

Maria Alejandra Gallo Ruiz, M.D.

Matisyahu Shulman, M.D.

Although clinicians and laypeople refer to *behavioral addictions,* most of these "addictions" have not been officially classified in either the *Diagnostic and Statistical Manual of Mental Disorders* (DSM) or the *International Classification of Diseases* (ICD). Reservations about creating a scientific category for behavioral addictions, such as compulsive eating, sex, pornography use, Internet use, and exercise, were summed up during discussions about the inclusion of gaming disorder in ICD-10 (World Health Organization 1992). Concerns regarding classification of behavioral addictions include the following: 1) difficulties defining each disorder; 2) creating criteria that may lead to labeling as pathological some behaviors that are in the spectrum of normal; 3) the notion that pathological compulsive and repetitive behaviors can take almost an infinite number of manifestations; and 4) the idea that these compulsive behaviors could be subsumed under a more general personality or psychiatric condition that leads to the behaviors. As a result of these concerns, gambling disorder is considered the prototypical example of a behavioral addiction, and it is the only one that has been formally recognized in DSM-5 (American Psychiatric Association 2013). In light of the above, the remainder of this chapter focuses on the diagnosis, epidemiology, course, and treatment of gambling disorder. This chapter is based on studies using the DSM-IV (American Psychiatric Association 1994) classification of pathological gambling (requiring at least 5 of 10 listed diagnostic criteria) and problem gambling (meeting fewer than 5 of the criteria and generally considered a subsyndromal form of pathological gambling). Throughout the chapter, we use the term *gambling disorder* to denote both pathological and problem gambling.

Reclassification of Gambling Disorder as an Addictive Disorder

In DSM-IV, the diagnosis pathological gambling was included among the Impulse-Control Disorders Not Elsewhere Classified, but in DSM-5, the diagnosis was renamed gambling disorder and reclassified among the Substance-Related and Addictive Disorders (American Psychiatric Association 2013). The reclassification of gambling disorder in DSM-5 was based on substantial research demonstrating, among other things, that gambling disorder and substance use disorders (SUDs) have common etiological factors and biological markers and share similar features, including clinical presentations, cognitive deficits, and personality characteristics (Blanco et al. 2015). Disturbances in various domains (and neurotransmitter systems)—including behavior initiation and cessation (serotonin), arousal and excitement (norepinephrine), reward and reinforcement (dopamine), and pleasure and urges (opioids)—appear to influence both disorders (Potenza 2008). Other commonalities include similar findings in brain imaging data (e.g., changes in prefrontal function when exposed to gambling cues) and similarly high heritability (Davis et al. 2019).

Gambling disorder also appears to align more closely with SUDs than with other psychiatric disorders. The overlap of gambling disorder with substance-related addictive disorders is so great that roughly half of individuals with gambling disorder also suffer from an SUD, the latter of which is most frequently alcohol use disorder (AUD) or nicotine dependence (Petry et al. 2005; Spunt et al. 1998). Gambling disorder and SUDs also appear to affect each other in various ways. SUDs may play a role in the initiation, exacerbation, or perpetuation of an existing gambling disorder. Alcoholic beverages are available at casinos, racetracks, and sports bars, making alcohol consumption a frequent activity among gamblers (Corbin and Cronce 2017). Similarly, most casinos across the world continue to allow smoking. Negative consequences appear to be more frequent among individuals with both gambling disorder and an SUD as compared with individuals with only one or the other. For example, among individuals who consume alcohol daily, the odds of experiencing suicidal ideation increase as gambling problems become more severe (Kim et al. 2016). People with comorbid gambling disorder and cocaine use disorder appear more likely to have attention-deficit/hyperactivity disorder, nicotine dependence, and antisocial personality disorder, as well as to be unemployed, to have recently engaged in illegal activity for profit, and to have been incarcerated (Hall et al. 2000). Additionally, substance use paired with gambling is associated with riskier behaviors, larger average bets, more rapid money losses, and a higher risk of relapse after quitting gambling (Corbin and Cronce 2017).

Prevalence rates of other psychiatric disorders, such as mood, anxiety, or personality disorders, have been shown to be significantly higher in individuals with gambling disorder (Petry et al. 2005). As is the case for individuals with SUDs, individuals with gambling disorder have higher rates of suicide compared with rates in the general population (Moghaddam et al. 2015). In addition, effective treatments for gambling disorder have been based on treatments for SUDs. Finally, individuals with gambling disorder are more likely than individuals without the disorder to experience significant financial problems, including bankruptcy, loss of employment, and poverty; also, in parallel with the negative consequences of SUDs, individuals with gambling disorder are more likely to experience health problems, family dysfunction, and domestic violence, and (albeit more rarely) to engage in criminal behavior.

Diagnosis

Gambling disorder is a new DSM-5 diagnosis. Besides the name change from pathological gambling, other changes in DSM-5 involved 1) elimination of the criterion "has committed illegal acts such as forgery, fraud, theft, or embezzlement to finance gambling" and 2) reduction of the threshold for diagnosis from 5 out of 10 criteria to 4 out of 9 criteria (American Psychiatric Association 2013). Elimination of the "committing illegal acts" criterion was based on findings that such behavior was rare and virtually never occurred in the absence of the other criteria (Petry et al. 2013).

Symptoms of gambling disorder (Table 42–1) have similarities with symptoms of SUDs: compulsive pursuit of the behavior despite its serious negative consequences, craving or urges, neglect of other areas of life (increased preoccupation with gambling), loss of control (chasing losses and repeated unsuccessful attempts to control or stop the behavior), tolerance (betting increasing amounts of money to achieve the same level of excitement), and withdrawal symptoms (restlessness or irritability when unable to continue gambling).

Types of Gambling

A wide range of gambling forms, including online gambling, have emerged with the proliferation of legalized gambling activities throughout the world. Many individuals with gambling disorder have a specific type of gambling that is most problematic for them, and often the gambling form in which individuals engage is closely related to personal characteristics and the course of the gambling disorder. For example, in contrast to forms such as sports betting, card games (e.g., poker, blackjack), and betting on the stock market, in which skill or knowledge may have some impact on the outcome of the bet, other forms of gambling (e.g., slot machines, bingo) require no skill or little concentration. Studies suggest that some individuals gamble to seek a "rush" or for excitement, whereas others (women in particular) gamble to "escape" from personal or family problems. In fact, machine gambling is often referred to as "escape" gambling, given that this form facilitates dissociation (losing track of time and place). Gambling forms such as the lottery or scratch-off tickets may appeal to disadvantaged groups that have limited access to transportation or live in areas where there is wide availability. Some studies (McCreadie et al. 2001) have reported that scratch-off and lottery tickets are a common recreational activity for individuals with severe persistent mental illness (e.g., primary psychotic disorders such as schizophrenia), whereas other studies (Hendriks et al. 1997) have found that heavy lottery playing is associated with lower educational levels and lower socioeconomic status (Potenza et al. 2001). Online gambling is often considered one of the most dangerous forms of gambling because of its anonymity, accessibility, convenience, and 24-hour availability (Griffiths 1999). Epidemiological surveys and studies in selected samples of college students have found that among gamblers, those who gamble online have higher rates of gambling disorder (Petry and Gonzalez-Ibanez 2015).

TABLE 42–1.   **DSM-5 diagnostic criteria for gambling disorder**

A. Persistent and recurrent problematic gambling behavior leading to clinically significant impairment or distress, as indicated by the individual exhibiting four (or more) of the following in a 12-month period:

　　1.　Needs to gamble with increasing amounts of money in order to achieve the desired excitement.

　　2.　Is restless or irritable when attempting to cut down or stop gambling.

　　3.　Has made repeated unsuccessful efforts to control, cut back, or stop gambling.

　　4.　Is often preoccupied with gambling (e.g., having persistent thoughts of reliving past gambling experiences, handicapping or planning the next venture, thinking of ways to get money with which to gamble).

　　5.　Often gambles when feeling distressed (e.g., helpless, guilty, anxious, depressed).

　　6.　After losing money gambling, often returns another day to get even ("chasing" one's losses).

　　7.　Lies to conceal the extent of involvement with gambling.

　　8.　Has jeopardized or lost a significant relationship, job, or educational or career opportunity because of gambling.

　　9.　Relies on others to provide money to relieve desperate financial situations caused by gambling.

B. The gambling behavior is not better explained by a manic episode.

Specify if:

　Episodic: Meeting diagnostic criteria at more than one time point, with symptoms subsiding between periods of gambling disorder for at least several months.

　Persistent: Experiencing continuous symptoms, to meet diagnostic criteria for multiple years.

Specify if:

　In early remission: After full criteria for gambling disorder were previously met, none of the criteria for gambling disorder have been met for at least 3 months but for less than 12 months.

　In sustained remission: After full criteria for gambling disorder were previously met, none of the criteria for gambling disorder have been met during a period of 12 months or longer.

Specify current severity:

　Mild: 4–5 criteria met.

　Moderate: 6–7 criteria met.

　Severe: 8–9 criteria met.

Source.   Reprinted from American Psychiatric Association: *Diagnostic and Statistical Manual of Mental Disorders,* 5th Edition, Arlington, VA, American Psychiatric Association, 2013, pp. 585–586. Copyright © 2013, American Psychiatric Association. Used with permission.

After adjustment of data to control for demographic variables, Petry (2003) found that individuals seeking treatment for gambling disorder differed in the severity of their gambling, alcohol use, and psychiatric problems (based on their Addiction Severity Index score), depending on the gambling form that was most problematic for them. Sports gamblers were typically young and male, had intermediate-severity gambling problems, and had relatively high rates of current substance use, but had fewer psychiatric problems. Card gamblers spent low to moderate amounts of time and money in their gambling, and they generally reported fewer alcohol problems and lower psychiatric distress. Horse/dog racing gamblers were generally older, male, and less educated; were younger at the age of gambling initiation; and spent relatively large amounts of money on gambling. Slot machine players were more likely to be older and female, to have begun gambling later in life, and to have had higher rates of bankruptcy and psychiatric problems. Lastly, scratch-off/lottery gamblers spent the least amount of money gambling, but gambled the most frequently and had relatively severe alcohol and psychiatric symptoms (Petry 2003).

Epidemiology

Gambling activities are present in almost every culture and have been recorded throughout history, and gambling problems are found worldwide. Twelve-month prevalence rates of gambling disorder worldwide range from 0.2% to 5.3% (Hodgins et al. 2011). The largest national epidemiological survey found a 0.4% lifetime prevalence of gambling disorder in the United States (Petry et al. 2005); in this study, the prevalence of gambling disorder was 1.6% among individuals with any SUD and 1% among individuals with AUD. In treatment-seeking populations, around 4.3% of individuals with SUD had a lifetime gambling disorder, and an additional 7.2% endorsed problem gambling (Cowlishaw and Hakes 2015). Gambling prevalence rates can be quite high in populations with specific substance use problems. For instance, a study conducted with 313 outpatients receiving treatment for cocaine dependence (200 of them were also opioid dependent) found that the lifetime prevalence of gambling disorder was 8% (Hall et al. 2000). Another study conducted with 462 patients receiving treatment in two large methadone maintenance programs identified 21% of the patients as probable pathological gamblers and an additional 9% as having some gambling-related problems (Spunt et al. 1998).

Psychiatric Comorbidity

A significant percentage of individuals with gambling disorder meet criteria for another lifetime psychiatric disorder. A study analyzing data from the 2001–2002 National Epidemiologic Survey on Alcohol and Related Conditions, which used a general population sample, found that among people with DSM-IV pathological gambling (N=195), 61% reported a lifetime personality disorder, 50% a lifetime mood disorder, and 41% a lifetime anxiety disorder (Petry et al. 2005). A meta-analysis that included 26 studies suggested that approximately 14% of patients with SUDs have a comorbid gambling disorder (Cowlishaw et al. 2014).

 Compared with the general population, individuals with gambling disorder are more likely to experience suicidal ideation and to attempt suicide. In a study assessing individuals seeking treatment for DSM-IV pathological gambling (N=342), 32% reported having experienced suicidal ideation and 17% reported having made at least one suicide attempt (Petry and Kiluk 2002). According to a study analyzing data from the 2001–2002 National Epidemiologic Survey on Alcohol and Related Conditions, 49% of individuals with gambling disorder (N=120) had a lifetime history of suicidal ideation and 18% had made a lifetime suicide attempt (Moghaddam et al. 2015). Among these individuals with gambling disorder, those with a history of suicidal ideation or of suicide attempts reported earlier gambling initiation, greater debt, more criminal activity, and more severe gambling disorder symptoms (Moghaddam et al. 2015). In an analysis of 44 case records of suicides noted to be related to gambling problems, difficulties with finances, employment, and health were cited as reasons for the suicide (Blaszczynski and Farrell 1998).

Genetics

One meta-analysis estimated the heritability of gambling disorder to be approximately 16%, with at least 84% of the variance in gambling disorder probably non-genetic in nature (Walters 2001). Polymorphisms in the following genes have been suggested as possible risk factors for gambling disorder: *MAOA* (monoamine oxidase A), *5-HTTLPR* (5-hydroxytryptamine [5-HT; serotonin] transporter–linked polymorphic region), *DRD3* (dopamine receptor D_3), *DRD4* (dopamine receptor D_4), *HTR2A* (5-HT receptor 2A), and *COMT* (catechol-*O*-methyltransferase) (Nautiyal et al. 2017). Using data from twin studies, a genome-wide association study found that two single-nucleotide polymorphisms on chromosomes 9 and 12 were significantly associated with gambling disorder (Lind et al. 2013). Familial and twin studies have also demonstrated that overlapping genetic risk factors account for approximately half of the association in the risk for gambling disorder and AUD in both men and women (Slutske et al. 2000).

Risk Factors

Numerous studies have documented a broad range of risk factors for gambling disorder, including sociodemographic characteristics such as younger age and male gender. Neighborhood disadvantage and low socioeconomic status are important risk factors for the development of gambling disorder. Certain cultural groups appear to be more vulnerable to early gambling initiation and to the development of gambling disorder. In the United States, the prevalence of gambling disorder is greater among Native Americans, Asians, and blacks than among whites (Alegria et al. 2009). High rates of gambling disorder have also been found in other aboriginal groups and other minority groups across the world (Okuda et al. 2016). Risk factors for gambling disorder, such as socioeconomic disadvantage and a higher prevalence of psychiatric disorders, including SUDs, may be more prominent in certain cultural groups. Beliefs and values about gambling and availability and cultural acceptance of gambling also vary in different parts of the world. For immigrant groups, unemployment, language barriers, and social exclusion may contribute to increased gambling participation (Okuda et al. 2016). For example, although limited by a very small sample size (N=96) of refugees seeking services at community centers, one study (Petry et al. 2003) reported a 59% lifetime prevalence of gambling disorder in a group of Southeast Asian refugees who immigrated to the United States, a rate that is anywhere from 10 to 25 times higher than that in the general population. The high rates of gambling disorder in this specific sample may have been related to the higher load of risk factors (low income/ educational level, male gender, history of trauma) in this group (Petry et al. 2003).

Early exposure to and initiation of gambling activities as well as gambling availability are important risk factors that may also explain some of the cultural disparities in gambling disorder prevalence. For instance, self-reported convenient access to gambling venues or activities has been strongly associated with gambling disorder among Native American groups in the United States (Okuda et al. 2016). The establishment of casino gambling on several reservations through the 1988 Federal Indian Gaming Regulatory Act led to an increased exposure to gambling activities, which may partly explain the higher rates of gambling disorder in this population. Paralleling findings reported for SUDs, psychiatric comorbidities (including having another addiction), adverse childhood events, and a positive family history (of gambling disorder or SUDs) have also been identified as risk factors for the development of gambling disorder. Lastly, the high levels of stigma associated with seeking help or of barriers to accessing services may play a role in the perpetuation of gambling disorder in some groups (Okuda et al. 2009). Thus, racial and ethnic minority status may be a proxy for underlying adverse conditions (e.g., socioeconomic disadvantage, gambling availability, lack of treatment options, the stress related to immigrating to a new country) that increase the risk for development or perpetuation of gambling disorder. Cultural attitudes toward gambling can influence the initiation and maintenance of gambling disorder. Some cultures perceive gambling as a legitimate activity to make a profit, whereas other cultures (e.g., Muslims) prohibit and even condemn gambling (Raylu and Oei 2004).

The trait of sensation seeking has been consistently associated with problematic behaviors, including SUDs and gambling disorder. Individuals with sensation-seeking traits pursue situations and experiences that are varied, novel, complex, and intense, and they are willing to take physical, social, and financial risks for the sake of obtaining these experiences (Nower et al. 2004).

Finally, some neurological conditions or their treatments may place individuals at risk for gambling disorder. For example, individuals who take dopamine agonist medications to treat Parkinson's disease or restless legs syndrome are at increased risk of developing a syndrome characterized by repetitive compulsive behaviors, including excessive gambling, compulsive shopping, hypersexual behavior, or overeating. Up to 17% of patients treated with a minimally therapeutic dose of these medications may develop these behavioral addictions (Rabinak and Nirenberg 2010). Similarly, case reports of individuals who developed gambling disorder and other impulse-control disorders soon after taking aripiprazole, a partial dopamine receptor agonist, led the U.S. Food and Drug Administration (FDA) to issue a specific warning about this potential adverse outcome. In many cases of both dopamine replacement therapy–related and aripiprazole-related gambling disorder, gambling behaviors were reported to have stopped when the medication dosage was reduced or the medication was discontinued (if this was possible) (Olley et al. 2015).

Course and Prognosis

Most individuals have a gradual onset of gambling disorder, and problematic behaviors usually take several years to progress into a full-blown gambling disorder. Once developed, gambling disorder tends to have a chronic course similar to that of SUDs.

This course generally includes either continuous chronic episodic gambling or periods of abstinence of variable durations (weeks to years) followed by a single lapse (e.g., gambling one time after achieving a period of abstinence) or full-blown relapses (e.g., return to a cycle of gambling habits after a period of abstinence) (Seiger 2012). Although gambling is more common among men than among women, it has been suggested that the gender gap in the prevalence of gambling disorder may be closing. The pattern of progression of the disorder also differs by sex. Although gambling disorder in women may start later in life, the time elapsed between the age of regular involvement in the primary gambling activity and the age at onset of the disorder may be shorter, a course described as "telescoping," which has been extensively documented among women with SUDs (Potenza 2008). The speed of gambling disorder development may also depend on the gambling type. Machine gambling, for instance, may have a faster progression from initial engagement to gambling disorder; this more rapid progression appears to be related to the social, environmental, and structural characteristics of machine gambling (Breen and Zimmerman 2002). Machine gambling has a high event frequency (i.e., the number of opportunities to gamble in a given time period) and a short payout interval (i.e., the time between the bet and the winning payment) (Griffiths 1999). These and other structural characteristics appear to be critical in relation to whether some people might develop gambling disorder.

Screening

Fewer than 15% of individuals with gambling disorder receive treatment (Slutske 2006), and many barriers to care exist. The first step toward increasing the percentage of individuals with gambling disorder who are treated is to increase screening in medical, psychiatric, and SUD treatment settings. Gambling disorder has been called a "hidden addiction" because it is often unrecognized and is not typically assessed. Instruments to screen for gambling disorder include the Structured Clinical Interview for Pathological Gambling (SCI-PG), the South Oaks Gambling Screen (SOGS), the Diagnostic Interview for Gambling Severity (DIGS), the Gamblers Anonymous 20 Questions, the Massachusetts Gambling Screen (MAGS), and the Gambling Assessment Module (GAM-IV) (Seiger 2012). The Lie/Bet Questionnaire (Johnson et al. 1997) is a very simple and brief screening tool consisting of two questions—"Have you ever had to lie to people important to you about how much you gambled?" and "Have you ever felt the need to bet more and more money?"—that has demonstrated sensitivity and specificity in identifying individuals with problematic gambling.

Treatment

The mainstay of treatment for gambling disorder is psychosocial intervention. Many of the evidence-based approaches are modeled on similar approaches used to address SUDs. Cognitive-behavioral therapy (CBT) has proven to be the most efficacious treatment for gambling disorder (Cowlishaw et al. 2012). The theoretical underpinnings of the cognitive work included in this approach center on the notion that individuals with gambling disorder often have cognitive distortions that perpetuate their gambling behaviors (Petry 2005). CBT for gambling includes work on exploring these distortions and helping patients to more accurately understand the behaviors they are engaging in. CBT for gambling disorder also focuses on behavioral change, including acquisition of skills that facilitate lifestyle changes and restructure the environment to increase reinforcement from nongambling behaviors. In the initial stages of treatment, patients are encouraged to describe their gambling activities and to identify their external triggers for gambling—i.e., the places, times, activities, moods, and people that make them more likely to gamble (Okuda et al. 2009). Patients are also encouraged to practice alternative responses to cues or triggers and to engage in alternative activities that replace gambling.

Motivational interviewing, which has been found to be effective in treating SUDs, has also been found useful in treating gambling disorder (Cowlishaw et al. 2012; Grant et al. 2009). This approach, delivered either as a stand-alone treatment or in combination with CBT in the form of motivational enhancement therapy, has been shown both to decrease gambling frequency and to increase the likelihood of remission from gambling disorder (Cowlishaw et al. 2012). Motivational interviewing is a nonstructured and nondirective treatment approach based on the premise that it is patients themselves who have the most knowledge about what they need in order to change their behaviors, and the provider is tasked with enhancing each patient's intrinsic motivation to change by exploring and developing a discrepancy between the current addictive behavior and an alternative healthier behavior. This process strengthens the patient's self-efficacy and seeks to diminish the patient's resistance to changing the status quo, with the ultimate goal of eliciting "change talk" that can lead to behavioral change (Miller and Rose 2009).

Internet-based therapies for behavioral addictive disorders have the potential to make evidence-based interventions more widely accessible. Self-directed treatments, in the form of written materials provided in a workbook or an online format and based on CBT principles, are likewise becoming more readily available. Studies suggest that online self-guided interventions utilizing these components represent an efficacious option for individuals with gambling disorder (Carlbring et al. 2012; Gainsbury and Blaszczynski 2011).

Other approaches include brief personalized feedback or advice about gambling, but these brief interventions have not been shown to be superior to control conditions or CBT. Nonetheless, some of the brief treatments appear to offer some benefit to individuals who screen positive for gambling problems but who are not yet ready to engage in treatment (Petry et al. 2017).

Pharmacotherapy

Although no medications have yet received FDA approval for treating gambling disorder, opioid antagonists have shown the most promise among medications tested for this purpose. Naltrexone and nalmefene, two prototypical nonspecific opioid antagonists that have FDA approval for the treatment of AUD and opioid use disorder, have been examined in five randomized controlled trials (RCTs) for gambling disorder (Grant et al. 2014). In a fixed-effects meta-analysis, opioid antagonists demonstrated a small (effect size Cohen's $d=0.22$) but significant benefit compared with placebo. Some data suggest that these medications may be particularly helpful for individuals who experience intense gambling cravings and those who have a family history of AUD (Grant et al. 2008).

Large placebo effects have been noted in RCTs testing fluvoxamine, sertraline, and paroxetine for treatment of gambling disorder (Grant et al. 2008). Bupropion was also tested for gambling disorder in a 12-week RCT (Black et al. 2007); although a few differences were found between the group receiving bupropion ($n=18$) and the group receiving placebo ($n=21$) on primary and secondary outcome measures, participants in both groups experienced significant improvement (36% of patients given bupropion and 47% of those given placebo were classified as responders). A meta-analysis that included six RCTs examining the effects of antidepressants (fluvoxamine, paroxetine, sertraline, and bupropion) versus placebo failed to find a statistically significant benefit for antidepressants compared with placebo (Bartley and Bloch 2013). Other antidepressants, including clomipramine, fluoxetine, citalopram, and nefazodone, showed some positive outcomes in open-label studies (Grant et al. 2008). Altogether, these studies have been limited by their design, small size, high dropout rates, high placebo rates, and short follow-up periods.

An RCT suggested possible benefits with lithium in patients with gambling disorder and bipolar spectrum disorders (largely bipolar II disorder) (Hollander et al. 2005). Ten of the 12 patients taking lithium were responders, compared with only 5 of the 17 patients given placebo. Improvement in gambling severity was correlated with improvement in mania ratings. These findings are limited given the patient characteristics in the study. Topiramate, an anticonvulsant medication, was not superior to placebo in a 12-week RCT (Berlin et al. 2013). Another RCT comparing four sessions of CBT plus either topiramate or placebo found that individuals in both groups exhibited significant reductions over time in measurements of gambling cravings, time and money spent on gambling, cognitive distortions related to gambling, and social adjustment (de Brito et al. 2017). Two RCTs comparing the atypical antipsychotic olanzapine with placebo found no significant differences (Fong et al. 2008; McElroy et al. 2008).

Replications of study findings using larger RCTs with long-term follow-up are needed before definitive recommendations can be made. Until more information is available, the best approach might be to select a medication that is directed toward the patient's comorbid psychiatric disorder (e.g., another substance use, mood, or anxiety disorder).

Conclusion

Gambling disorder is a significant cause of morbidity, and only a portion of individuals with the disorder receive treatment. Gambling disorder and SUDs share common etiological factors and clinical characteristics. Logically, treatments for gambling disorder can be derived from those used for SUDs. Several studies support the use of psychotherapeutic interventions, such as CBT and motivational interviewing, and some pharmacological treatments used in SUDs (e.g., opiate antagonists) have shown promise in treating gambling disorder. In terms of treatment for gambling disorder, the availability of evidence-based treatments remains a key problem, lack of insurance coverage for gambling treatment is a common issue, and most professional treatment for gambling disorder tends to occur in specialized gambling treatment settings. Evidence-based interventions that use newer technologies may be the key to increasing dissemination of gambling disorder treatments and may represent a corresponding response to the increased availability of online forms of gambling. Self-directed treatments, in the form of written materials provided in a workbook or an online format and based on CBT principles, are becoming more readily available, and studies suggest that interventions utilizing these components represent an efficacious option for individuals with gambling disorder. Interventions of this type may offer an alternative that could address the treatment availability issues limiting patient access to evidence-based treatments. Increased knowledge on the prevalence and treatment of other proposed behavioral addictions is needed.

References

Alegria AA, Petry NM, Hasin DS, et al: Disordered gambling among racial and ethnic groups in the U.S.: results from the National Epidemiologic Survey on Alcohol and Related Conditions. CNS Spectr 14(3):132–142, 2009 19407710

American Psychiatric Association: Diagnostic and Statistical Manual of Mental Disorders, 4th Edition. Arlington, VA, American Psychiatric Association, 1994

American Psychiatric Association: Diagnostic and Statistical Manual of Mental Disorders, 5th Edition. Arlington, VA, American Psychiatric Association, 2013

Bartley CA, Bloch MH: Meta-analysis: pharmacological treatment of pathological gambling. Expert Rev Neurother 13(8):887–894, 2013 23952195

Berlin HA, Braun A, Simeon D, et al: A double-blind, placebo-controlled trial of topiramate for pathological gambling. World J Biol Psychiatry 14(2):121–128, 2013 21486110

Black DW, Arndt S, Coryell WH, et al: Bupropion in the treatment of pathological gambling: a randomized, double-blind, placebo-controlled, flexible-dose study. J Clin Psychopharmacol 27(2):143–150, 2007 17414236

Blanco C, Hanania J, Petry NM, et al: Towards a comprehensive developmental model of pathological gambling. Addiction 110(8):1340–1351, 2015 25879250

Blaszczynski A, Farrell E: A case series of 44 completed gambling-related suicides. J Gambl Stud 14(2):93–109, 1998 12766437

Breen RB, Zimmerman M: Rapid onset of pathological gambling in machine gamblers. J Gambl Stud 18(1):31–43, 2002 12050846

Carlbring P, Degerman N, Jonsson J, Andersson G: Internet-based treatment of pathological gambling with a three-year follow-up. Cogn Behav Ther 41(4):321–334, 2012 22620990

Corbin WR, Cronce JM: Effects of alcohol, initial gambling outcomes, impulsivity, and gambling cognitions on gambling behavior using a video poker task. Exp Clin Psychopharmacol 25(3):175–185, 2017 28493742

Cowlishaw S, Hakes JK: Pathological and problem gambling in substance use treatment: results from the National Epidemiologic Survey on Alcohol and Related Conditions (NESARC). Am J Addict 24(5):467–474, 2015 25950376

Cowlishaw S, Merkouris S, Dowling N, et al: Psychological therapies for pathological and problem gambling. Cochrane Database Syst Rev (11):CD008937, 2012 23152266

Cowlishaw S, Merkouris S, Chapman A, et al: Pathological and problem gambling in substance use treatment: a systematic review and meta-analysis. J Subst Abuse Treat 46(2):98–105, 2014 24074847

Davis CN, Slutske WS, Martin NG, et al: Genetic and environmental influences on gambling disorder liability: a replication and combined analysis of two twin studies. Psychol Med 49(10):1705–1712, 2019 30160223 de Brito AM, de Almeida Pinto MG, Bronstein G, et al: Topiramate combined with cognitive restructuring for the treatment of gambling disorder: a two-center, randomized, double-blind clinical trial. J Gambl Stud 33(1):249–263, 2017 27256372

Fong T, Kalechstein A, Bernhard B, et al: A double-blind, placebo-controlled trial of olanzapine for the treatment of video poker pathological gamblers. Pharmacol Biochem Behav 89(3):298–303, 2008 18261787

Gainsbury S, Blaszczynski A: A systematic review of Internet-based therapy for the treatment of addictions. Clin Psychol Rev 31(3):490–498, 2011 21146272

Grant JE, Kim SW, Hollander E, et al: Predicting response to opiate antagonists and placebo in the treatment of pathological gambling. Psychopharmacology (Berl) 200(4):521–527, 2008 18581096

Grant JE, Donahue CB, Odlaug BL, et al: Imaginal desensitisation plus motivational interviewing for pathological gambling: randomised controlled trial. Br J Psychiatry 195(3):266–267, 2009 19721120

Grant JE, Odlaug BL, Schreiber LR: Pharmacological treatments in pathological gambling. Br J Clin Pharmacol 77(2):375–381, 2014 22979951

Griffiths M: Gambling technologies: prospects for problem gambling. J Gambl Stud 15(3):265–283, 1999 12766464

Hall GW, Carriero NJ, Takushi RY, et al: Pathological gambling among cocaine-dependent outpatients. Am J Psychiatry 157(7):1127–1133, 2000 10873922

Hendriks VM, Meerkerk GJ, Van Oers HA, Garretsen HF: The Dutch instant lottery: prevalence and correlates of at-risk playing. Addiction 92(3):335–346, 1997 9219395

Hodgins DC, Stea JN, Grant JE: Gambling disorders. Lancet 378(9806):1874–1884, 2011 21600645

Hollander E, Pallanti S, Allen A, et al: Does sustained-release lithium reduce impulsive gambling and affective instability versus placebo in pathological gamblers with bipolar spectrum disorders? Am J Psychiatry 162(1):137–145, 2005 15625212

Johnson EE, Hamer R, Nora RM, et al: The Lie/Bet Questionnaire for screening pathological gamblers. Psychol Rep 80(1):83–88, 1997 9122356

Kim HS, Salmon M, Wohl MJ, et al: A dangerous cocktail: alcohol consumption increases suicidal ideations among problem gamblers in the general population. Addict Behav 55:50–55, 2016 26790140

Lind PA, Zhu G, Montgomery GW, et al: Genome-wide association study of a quantitative disordered gambling trait. Addict Biol 18(3):511–522, 2013 22780124

McCreadie R, Farrington S, Halliday J, et al: Leisure activities of people with schizophrenia: listening to music and playing the National Lottery. Psychiatric Bulletin 25(7):277–278, 2001. Available at: https://doi.org/10.1192/pb.25.7.277-b. Accessed July 17, 2020.

McElroy SL, Nelson EB, Welge JA, et al: Olanzapine in the treatment of pathological gambling: a negative randomized placebo-controlled trial. J Clin Psychiatry 69(3):433–440, 2008 18251624

Miller WR, Rose GS: Toward a theory of motivational interviewing. Am Psychol 64(6):527–537, 2009 19739882

Moghaddam JF, Yoon G, Dickerson DL, et al: Suicidal ideation and suicide attempts in five groups with different severities of gambling: findings from the National Epidemiologic Survey on Alcohol and Related Conditions. Am J Addict 24(4):292–298, 2015 25808267

Nautiyal KM, Okuda M, Hen R, et al: Gambling disorder: an integrative review of animal and human studies. Ann N Y Acad Sci 1394(1):106–127, 2017 28486792

Nower L, Derevensky JL, Gupta R: The relationship of impulsivity, sensation seeking, coping, and substance use in youth gamblers. Psychol Addict Behav 18(1):49–55, 2004 15008685

Okuda M, Balán I, Petry NM, et al: Cognitive-behavioral therapy for pathological gambling: cultural considerations. Am J Psychiatry 166(12):1325–1330, 2009 19952084

Okuda M, Liu W, Cisewski JA, et al: Gambling disorder and minority populations: prevalence and risk factors. Curr Addict Rep 3(3):280–292, 2016 28824833

Olley J, Blaszczynski A, Lewis S: Dopaminergic medication in Parkinson's disease and problem gambling. J Gambl Stud 31(3):1085–1106, 2015 25267527

Petry NM: A comparison of treatment-seeking pathological gamblers based on preferred gambling activity. Addiction 98(5):645–655, 2003 12751982

Petry NM: Pathological Gambling: Etiology, Comorbidity, and Treatment. Washington, DC, American Psychological Association, 2005

Petry NM, Gonzalez-Ibanez A: Internet gambling in problem gambling college students. J Gambl Stud 31(2):397–408, 2015 24337905

Petry NM, Kiluk BD: Suicidal ideation and suicide attempts in treatment-seeking pathological gamblers. J Nerv Ment Dis 190(7):462–469, 2002 12142848

Petry NM, Armentano C, Kuoch T, et al: Gambling participation and problems among South East Asian refugees to the United States. Psychiatr Serv 54(8):1142–1148, 2003 12883143

Petry NM, Stinson FS, Grant BF: Comorbidity of DSM-IV pathological gambling and other psychiatric disorders: results from the National Epidemiologic Survey on Alcohol and Related Conditions. J Clin Psychiatry 66(5):564–574, 2005 15889941

Petry NM, Blanco C, Stinchfield R, et al: An empirical evaluation of proposed changes for gambling diagnosis in the DSM-5. Addiction 108(3):575–581, 2013 22994319

Petry NM, Ginley MK, Rash CJ: A systematic review of treatments for problem gambling. Psychol Addict Behav 31(8):951–961, 2017 28639817

Potenza MN: Review. The neurobiology of pathological gambling and drug addiction: an overview and new findings. Philos Trans R Soc Lond B Biol Sci 363(1507):3181–3189, 2008 18640909

Potenza MN, Steinberg MA, McLaughlin SD, et al: Gender-related differences in the characteristics of problem gamblers using a gambling helpline. Am J Psychiatry 158(9):1500–1505, 2001 11532738

Rabinak CA, Nirenberg MJ: Dopamine agonist withdrawal syndrome in Parkinson disease. Arch Neurol 67(1):58–63, 2010 20065130

Raylu N, Oei TP: Role of culture in gambling and problem gambling. Clin Psychol Rev 23(8):1087–1114, 2004 14729424

Seiger B: Substance Dependence and Co-Occurring Psychiatric Disorders: Best Practices for Diagnosis and Clinical Treatment (2010), by Edward V. Nunes, Jeffrey Selzer, Petros Levounis, and Carrie A. Davies (book review). Journal of Social Work Practice in the Addictions 12(1):108–110, 2012. Available at: https://www.tandfonline.com/doi/abs/10.1080/1533256X.2012.648889. Accessed February 6, 2020.

Slutske WS: Natural recovery and treatment-seeking in pathological gambling: results of two U.S. national surveys. Am J Psychiatry 163(2):297–302, 2006 16449485

Slutske WS, Eisen S, True WR, et al: Common genetic vulnerability for pathological gambling and alcohol dependence in men. Arch Gen Psychiatry 57(7):666–673, 2000 10891037

Spunt B, Dupont I, Lesieur H, et al: Pathological gambling and substance misuse: a review of the literature. Subst Use Misuse 33(13):2535–2560, 1998 9818989

Walters GD: Behavior genetic research on gambling and problem gambling: a preliminary meta-analysis of available data. J Gambl Stud 17(4):255–271, 2001 11842524

World Health Organization: International Statistical Classification of Diseases and Related Health Problems, 10th Revision. Geneva, World Health Organization, 1992

PART VII

Psychiatric Comorbidity in
Substance-Related Disorders

CHAPTER 43

Epidemiology of Co-Occurring Psychiatric and Substance Use Disorders

Jeffrey D. Schulden, M.D.

Carlos Blanco, M.D., Ph.D., M.S.

Substance use disorders (SUDs) and other psychiatric disorders are well known to co-occur more commonly than would be expected by chance alone. This comorbidity, sometimes referred to as *dual diagnosis,* is often associated with greater symptom severity, worse long-term prognosis, and higher rates of service utilization (Brady et al. 2007; Jacobi et al. 2004; Lopez-Quintero et al. 2011; Morojele et al. 2012). It is critical that clinicians recognize how commonly SUDs and other psychiatric conditions co-occur and that they routinely assess clients for comorbidity. In order to most effectively serve dual-diagnosis populations, treatment strategies must simultaneously target the substance use problems and any psychiatric comorbidity. In this first chapter of Part VII, we provide an overview of the epidemiology of psychiatric comorbidity in substance-related disorders. Subsequent chapters examine in greater detail the comorbidity of SUDs with specific other psychiatric disorders (see Chapters 44–49).

Comorbidity in General Population Samples

Several large-scale epidemiological studies have examined the degree of co-occurrence between SUDs and other psychiatric disorders in general population samples. Seminal studies that have addressed these issues include the Epidemiologic Catchment Area (ECA) study, the National Comorbidity Survey (NCS), the NCS Replication (NCS-R), the National Epidemiologic Survey on Alcohol and Related Conditions (NESARC), the NESARC-III, and the World Mental Health (WMH) surveys. By recruiting participants from representative community population samples, these studies sought to avoid the sampling biases that can occur when samples are drawn primarily or exclusively from clinical populations. Clinical samples often overrepresent the prevalence of comorbidity, because individuals with multiple disorders are often more likely to be found in treatment settings, in part as a result of the greater severity of their symptoms. In addition, these seminal studies used standardized, validated diagnostic instruments to ensure the consistency and reliability of measures across study sites. Of note, the diagnostic categories utilized for most of these studies were from earlier editions of the *Diagnostic and Statistical Manual of Mental Disorders* (DSM), such as DSM-III, DSM-III-R, or DSM-IV (American Psychiatric Association 1980, 1987, 1994), which had separate diagnoses for substance abuse and substance dependence; the current edition, DSM-5 (American Psychiatric Association 2013) joins abuse and dependence into a single diagnosis, substance use disorder. For many findings presented in this section, the substance abuse and substance dependence categories were combined for analyses into a single substance use disorder category, but for some findings presented, the earlier diagnostic categories were used. In addition, these studies and subsequent psychiatric epidemiological studies have sometimes used differing time frames to define current diagnoses, most commonly using the past 6 months or past 12 months. Overall, despite variation in the prevalences found for specific disorders among different studies, due in part to these differences in research methodologies, studies have generally found strong positive associations between SUDs and other psychiatric disorders, including mood, anxiety, psychotic, and personality disorders.

The ECA study was conducted in the early 1980s and was one of the first large-scale population-based psychiatric studies, with over 20,000 participants across five U.S. communities (Regier et al. 1990). Its survey instrument was based on DSM-III diagnostic categories. The 6-month prevalence of any SUD in the ECA sample was 6.1%, and that of any other psychiatric disorder was 15.1%. The overall lifetime prevalence of any SUD was 16.7%, and the lifetime prevalence of any other psychiatric disorder was 22.5%. However, among those with any lifetime psychiatric disorder, the prevalence of any SUD was substantially higher, at 28.9%. Thus, a lifetime psychiatric disorder was found to be associated with more than twice the odds of having an SUD. Epidemiological research often quantifies the strength of an association as an odds ratio (OR), in this case comparing the odds of developing an SUD among persons with a psychiatric disorder with the odds among persons without a psychiatric disorder. The greater the OR value above 1.0, the greater the strength of the positive association. Here, the ECA study found a robust association (OR=2.7) for having a lifetime SUD among persons with a psychiatric disorder compared with those without. Similarly, the ECA study found that persons with a lifetime history of an SUD showed a substantially increased odds of also having a lifetime psychiatric disorder. Among persons with a lifetime history of an alcohol use disorder (AUD), more than a third (36.6%) also had a lifetime history of a psychiatric disorder (OR=2.3), and among those with a lifetime history of any other drug use disorder, over half (53.1%) also had a lifetime history of a psychiatric disorder (OR=4.5). Of note, among participants with a lifetime drug use disorder, 28.3% also had an anxiety disorder, 26.4% had a mood disorder, and 6.8% had schizophrenia. The ECA study found particularly high rates of comorbid SUDs among persons with several specific psychiatric disorders. Over half (56.1%) of participants with a lifetime diagnosis of bipolar disorder also had an SUD (OR=6.6); 47.0% of participants with schizophrenia or schizophreniform disorder also had an SUD (OR=4.6); and 35.8% of participants with panic disorder also had a lifetime SUD diagnosis (OR=2.9).

The initial wave of the NCS was conducted in the early 1990s. This wave included a probability sample of over 8,000 participants from the U.S. general population, and its survey instrument was based on DSM-III-R (Kessler et al. 1996). In addition, a new study, the NCS-R, was fielded in the early 2000s. The NCS-R recruited a new national sample of more than 9,000 participants and used a methodology similar to that of the original NCS, although its instrument incorporated diagnostic changes made in DSM-IV (Kessler et al. 2005a). The 12-month prevalence of any SUD in the NCS was 11.3%, and that of any psychiatric disorder was 24.0% (Kessler et al. 1996). The lifetime prevalence of any SUD was 26.6%, and that of any psychiatric disorder was 43.2%. Similar to findings in the ECA study, the NCS found substantial comorbidity between SUDs and other psychiatric disorders. Among persons with a lifetime history of any SUD, 51.4% also had "any psychiatric disorder" (further broken down into 29.7% with a mood disorder and 40.7% with an anxiety disorder). Persons with a lifetime history of an SUD had more than twice the odds of also having a lifetime psychiatric condition compared with persons without a history of an SUD (OR=2.4). Likewise, the NCS found that just over half (50.9%) of persons who reported a lifetime history of a psychiatric disorder also reported a lifetime history of an SUD. In the NCS, a lifetime history of mania was associated with a more than sixfold increased odds of having a comorbid SUD (OR=6.8), and a lifetime history of posttraumatic stress disorder (PTSD) was associated with a more than twofold increased odds of having a comorbid SUD (OR=2.5). Among persons with a lifetime history of a drug dependence diagnosis, 54.4% also had an anxiety disorder and 39.1% also had a mood disorder (Kessler et al. 1996). The NCS-R findings were generally consistent with findings from the NCS, showing a relatively high prevalence of disorders and a high degree of comorbidity between SUDs and other psychiatric disorders (Kessler et al. 2005a, 2005b). Among the entire sample, the lifetime prevalence of any SUD was 14.6%, that of any mood disorder was 20.8%, and that of any anxiety disorder was 28.8% (Kessler et al. 2005a). Kessler et al. (2005b) also found that comorbidity was generally associated with greater severity of illness.

The NESARC Wave 1 was conducted in 2001–2002 and included more than 40,000 participants from the U.S. general population (Grant et al. 2004). Its survey instrument was based on DSM-IV diagnostic criteria. A longitudinal follow-up, the NESARC Wave 2, was conducted in 2004–2005. In addition, the NESARC-III was conducted in 2012–2013 among a new sample of more than 36,000 participants; its survey instrument was based on DSM-5 categories (Grant et al. 2015). The NESARC baseline wave (i.e., Wave 1) reported the 12-month prevalence of any SUD as 9.4% (Grant et al. 2004). The 12-month prevalence of mood disorders was 9.2%, and that of anxiety disorders was 11.1%. Individuals with a 12-month history of any SUD had more than twice the odds of also having a 12-month history of any mood disorder (OR=2.8) and nearly twice the odds of also having a 12-month history of any anxiety disorder (OR=1.9).

Again, some of the strongest associations were seen for persons with a 12-month history of mania, who had an almost fourfold increased odds of also having a 12-month history of an SUD (OR=3.9), and for persons with a 12-month history of panic disorder with agoraphobia, who had more than three times the odds of also having a 12-month history of an SUD (OR=3.1). Among persons with a 12-month history of a drug use disorder, 25.4% also had an anxiety disorder and 31.8% also had a mood disorder (Grant et al. 2004). The NESARC-III found similarly high prevalences of alcohol and drug use disorder. The lifetime prevalence of AUD was 29.1%, and that of drug use disorder (DUD) was 9.9% (Grant et al. 2015, 2016). A lifetime AUD or DUD diagnosis was significantly associated with a lifetime diagnosis of any anxiety disorder (OR=1.3 for both AUD and DUD) and of any mood disorder (OR=1.5 for both). Table 43–1 highlights the strength of associations found between SUDs and selected psychiatric disorders in the ECA study, the NCS, the NESARC, and the NESARC-III, demonstrating an overall consistent trend of positive associations across studies. Table 43–2 presents prevalences of selected psychiatric disorders among persons with SUDs, and for comparison, Table 43–3 presents prevalences of any SUD among persons with selected psychiatric disorders. For example, in the NCS, 1.2% of persons with a lifetime SUD diagnosis also had a diagnosis of bipolar disorder (Table 43–2), whereas 71.1% of persons with a lifetime bipolar disorder diagnosis also had a diagnosis of any SUD (Table 43–3).

Similarly high rates of comorbidity have been found in non-U.S. epidemiological samples. The World Health Organization WMH surveys, with population-based samples from more than 20 countries, found wide variations in the prevalence of substance use and SUDs across countries, likely influenced by a range of demographic, social, policy, and research methodological factors (Degenhardt et al. 2008, 2018). In a recent analysis of WMH data, 7.7% of respondents across participating countries reported a lifetime AUD, and 3.3% reported a lifetime illicit drug use disorder (Degenhardt et al. 2018). Among WMH survey respondents with a lifetime history of psychosis, the lifetime prevalences of these SUDs was substantially higher: 17.1% for AUD and 8.2% for illicit drug use disorders. The European Study of the Epidemiology of Mental Disorders, a component of the WMH initiative for several European countries, found strong associations between 12-month alcohol dependence and major depressive disorder (OR=6.7), generalized anxiety disorder (OR=11.2), and PTSD (OR=3.1) (Alonso et al. 2004). Comorbid associations were reported as similar across the countries included, despite variations in prevalence rates for individual disorders. A British national household survey found that 12% of the population without any substance dependence had a psychiatric disorder (Farrell et al. 2003). However, among individuals with substance dependence, the rates of such disorders were much higher, with psychiatric comorbidity found in 22% of individuals with nicotine dependence, 30% of those with alcohol dependence, and 45% of those with drug dependence (Farrell et al. 2003). The German Health Interview and Examination Survey found that among persons with any 12-month SUD, 44.9% also met criteria for at least one other psychiatric diagnosis (Jacobi et al. 2004). Individuals with comorbid conditions were substantially more likely to be enrolled in some form of treatment. The Australian National Survey of Mental Health and Wellbeing found that among participants with a 12-month history of SUD, 21.4% also met criteria for a mood disorder, and 33.5% also met criteria for an anxiety disorder (Teesson et al. 2009).

TABLE 43–1.   **Co-occurrence (odds ratios) of substance use disorders and selected other psychiatric disorders: ECA, NCS, NESARC, and NESARC-III**

	ECA SUD	NCS SUD	NESARC SUD	NESARC-III AUD	NESARC-III DUD
Any mood disorder	2.6	2.3	2.8	1.5	1.5
Major depressive disorder	1.9	2.3	2.5	1.3	1.2
Dysthymia	2.4	1.9	2.2	1.3	1.3
Bipolar disorder/mania	6.6	6.8	3.9	2.0	1.4
Any anxiety disorder	1.7	2.1	1.9	1.3	1.3
Generalized anxiety disorder	–	2.1	2.3	1.2	1.3
Panic disorder	2.9	2.0	$3.1^a/2.1^b$	1.3	1.3
Posttraumatic stress disorder	–	2.5	–	1.3	1.5
Schizophrenia	4.6	–	–	–	–

Note. For ECA, NCS, and NESARC-III, odds ratios (ORs) presented are based on lifetime prevalences. For NESARC, ORs are based on 12-month prevalences. Note that instruments for studies were based on different DSM editions: ECA: DSM-III; NCS: DSM-III-R; NESARC: DSM-IV; and NESARC-III: DSM-5. For NESARC-III, ORs are presented separately for alcohol use disorder (AUD) and drug use disorder (DUD).
ECA=Epidemiologic Catchment Area study; NCS=National Comorbidity Survey; NESARC=National Epidemiologic Survey on Alcohol and Related Conditions; SUD=substance use disorder.
Dash (–) indicates that ORs were not reported or assessed in study.
[a]Panic disorder with agoraphobia.
[b]Panic disorder without agoraphobia.
Source.   ECA: Regier et al. 1990; NCS: Kessler et al. 1996; NESARC: Grant et al. 2004; NESARC-III: Grant et al. 2015, 2016.

As a part of understanding the relationship between comorbid SUDs and psychiatric disorders, epidemiological studies have sought to examine the temporal sequencing of co-occurring conditions to try to determine which came first. Overall, findings regarding temporal sequencing have varied, and there are important limitations to these findings (Hassan et al. 2017; Kessler et al. 1996). For example, large-scale studies have often asked participants to self-report their substance use and psychiatric history. Self-reported findings could be subject to reporting and/or recall biases, whereby participants might be systematically more likely to report or recall one disorder preceding another, regardless of the actual sequencing. Moreover, it is important to recognize that temporal sequencing alone does not necessarily suggest a causal pathway, as other independent factors could be at play. Nevertheless, with these caveats, findings on temporal sequencing contribute to our understanding of the complex factors that contribute to comorbidity. For example, an analysis of longitudinal data from a subsample of the ECA study suggested that the presence of either alcohol dependence or major depressive disorder significantly increased the odds of the other condition newly developing at 1-year follow-up, although baseline alcohol dependence seemed to more strongly predict comorbidity at follow-up than baseline major depressive disorder (Gilman and Abraham 2001).

Data from the NCS based on participants' retrospective self-reports suggested that the majority of individuals with comorbid lifetime substance use and psychiatric dis-

TABLE 43–2.   **Prevalences of selected psychiatric disorders among persons with SUDs: ECA, NCS, and NESARC**

	ECA		NCS	NESARC
	AUD (%)	DUD (%)	SUD (%)	SUD (%)
Any psychiatric disorder	36.6	53.1	51.4	–
Any mood disorder	13.4	26.4	29.7	19.7
Major depressive disorder	–	–	26.6	14.5
Dysthymia	–	–	4.5	3.5
Bipolar disorder/mania	–	–	1.2	4.9
Any anxiety disorder	19.4	28.3	40.7	17.7
Generalized anxiety disorder	–	–	8.3	4.2
Panic disorder	–	–	5.5	$1.5^a/2.9^b$
Posttraumatic stress disorder	–	–	12.9	–
Schizophrenia	3.8	6.8	–	–

Note.   For ECA and NCS, data are based on lifetime prevalences. For NESARC, data are based on 12-month prevalences. For ECA, data are presented for any alcohol use disorder (AUD) and any drug use disorder (DUD) separately. For NCS and NESARC, data are presented for prevalence of a combined "any substance use disorder (SUD)" category.
ECA=Epidemiologic Catchment Area study; NCS=National Comorbidity Survey; NESARC=National Epidemiologic Survey on Alcohol and Related Conditions.
Dash (–) indicates that prevalence data were not reported or assessed in study.
[a]Panic disorder with agoraphobia.
[b]Panic disorder without agoraphobia.
Source.   ECA: Regier et al. 1990; NCS: Kessler et al. 1996; NESARC: Grant et al. 2004.

orders describe the psychiatric symptoms as having emerged before the SUD (Kessler et al. 1996). In general, higher proportions of men than of women in the NCS reported a mood or anxiety disorder occurring prior to an SUD. Only AUD among men was more frequently reported to precede the onset of the mood disorder. In an analysis of baseline psychiatric disorders as risk factors for subsequent onset of new SUDs in a 10-year longitudinal follow-up survey to the NCS, having any anxiety disorder at the baseline interview was significantly associated with subsequently developing a new diagnosis of alcohol dependence with abuse (OR=3.2) or drug dependence with abuse (OR=3.5) (Swendsen et al. 2010). Baseline bipolar disorder was strongly associated with a subsequent new diagnosis of alcohol dependence with abuse (OR=3.6) or drug dependence with abuse (OR=5.1). Utilizing data from Wave 2 of the NESARC, Grant et al. (2009) examined the association between baseline disorders and the subsequent development of new disorders. After controlling for sociodemographic characteristics and other psychiatric disorders, they found that having SUDs at baseline did not predict the emergence of any new mood or anxiety disorders. Baseline bipolar I disorder predicted development of incident drug abuse, and baseline panic disorder was associated with later emergence of incident drug dependence. In a subsequent analysis of cross-sectional data from the NESARC-III, among participants who acknowledged any nonmedical use of opioid medications, those who reported PTSD symptoms at baseline were significantly more likely to develop an opioid use disorder (OUD) than

TABLE 43–3.   **Prevalences of SUDs among persons with selected other psychiatric disorders: ECA, NCS, and NESARC**

	ECA (%)	NCS (%)	NESARC (%)
Any psychiatric disorder	28.9	50.9	–
Any mood disorder	32.0	41.2	20.0
Major depressive disorder	27.2	41.4	19.2
Dysthymia	31.4	40.0	18.1
Bipolar disorder/mania	56.1	71.1	27.9
Any anxiety disorder	23.7	37.8	15.0
Generalized anxiety disorder	–	42.3	19.1
Panic disorder	35.8	41.2	24.2[a]/17.3[b]
Posttraumatic stress disorder	–	45.2	–
Schizophrenia	47.0	–	–

Note. For ECA and NCS, data are based on lifetime prevalences. For NESARC, data are based on 12-month prevalences. For all studies, data are presented for prevalence of a combined "any substance use disorder (SUD)" category.
ECA=Epidemiologic Catchment Area study; NCS=National Comorbidity Survey; NESARC=National Epidemiologic Survey on Alcohol and Related Conditions.
Dash (—) indicates that prevalence data were not reported or assessed in study.
[a]Panic disorder with agoraphobia.
[b]Panic disorder without agoraphobia.
Source.   ECA: Regier et al. 1990; NCS: Kessler et al. 1996; NESARC: Grant et al. 2004.

those who did not report PTSD (OR=1.6) (Hassan et al. 2017). The severity of the OUD was also greater for participants reporting PTSD than for those not reporting PTSD.

Comorbidity in Clinical Settings

Although rates of comorbidity are thus quite high in population-based samples, co-occurrence of SUDs and psychiatric disorders is generally even more common in treatment settings. This finding likely represents a form of selection bias in which persons with comorbidity are more likely to present in clinical settings. That is, there is an increased likelihood for treatment seeking among persons with comorbid conditions, who often have greater severity of symptoms than those with a single condition (Carton et al. 2018; Degenhardt et al. 2008; Kessler et al. 1996). A number of other factors can contribute to the variability in the prevalence of comorbidity found in studies utilizing clinical populations, including characteristics of the treatment settings, the patient population served, and the methods used for determining diagnoses. Nevertheless, it is important for clinicians to recognize how commonly comorbidity presents in treatment settings. For example, the NESARC found much higher rates of 12-month comorbidity among participants who had sought SUD treatment within the previous 12 months than among those who had not sought such treatment. Among participants who had sought treatment for a current AUD, 40.7% also had an independent mood disorder and 33.4% also had an independent anxiety disorder. Among participants who had sought treatment for a current drug use disorder, 60.3% also had an independent mood disorder and 42.6% also had an independent anxiety disorder (Grant et al. 2004).

A study examining comorbidity among clients receiving community mental health treatment or substance misuse treatment services at urban centers in the United Kingdom found that 44% of mental health treatment clients reported problematic substance use in the past 12 months (Weaver et al. 2003). Among substance treatment clients, 85% of alcohol service clients and 75% of drug service clients reported a 12-month history of a psychiatric disorder. A large proportion of these clients were only receiving care for either their substance use or their psychiatric condition. In another study of psychiatric outpatients at five Danish clinics, 33% of participants reported problematic alcohol use and 19% reported illicit drug use within the past month (Sørensen et al. 2018). The Sequenced Treatment Alternatives to Relieve Depression (STAR*D) trial, which enrolled more than 2,800 patients with major depressive disorder from primary care and psychiatric clinics, found that 6.9% of participants had a comorbid SUD and an additional 10.4% had both a comorbid anxiety disorder and a comorbid SUD (Howland et al. 2009). About two-thirds of the participants with a comorbid SUD were enrolled from psychiatric clinics as opposed to the primary care setting. Lower rates of response to treatment and of remission were found in participants with comorbidity. Similarly, a French study of more than 4,000 participants with major depressive disorder found that participants with comorbid AUD reported greater severity of symptoms—including greater frequency of psychotic features and greater frequency of history of suicide attempts—than did those without AUD (Carton et al. 2018).

In practice, diagnosing comorbid substance use and psychiatric disorders in clinical settings presents numerous challenges. Substance use, dependence, and withdrawal can all result in a wide range of psychiatric symptoms, including affective and psychotic spectrum symptoms. For individuals with a long-standing SUD, it can be challenging to tease out to what extent their psychiatric symptoms represent an independent psychiatric disorder as opposed to a disorder attributable to their substance use. Ideally, a clinician would want to observe an individual's symptoms during a period of prolonged abstinence from substances to assess whether the psychiatric symptoms appear to be independent of the substance use. In addition, in order to qualify for an independent disorder, the psychiatric symptoms should be substantially in excess of what would be expected from the substance use itself. Through a detailed history, a clinician can attempt to determine whether the psychiatric symptoms predated the onset of substance use and how severe the symptoms were during periods of abstinence or reduced use; however, in practice, this can often be difficult to tease out and is subject to recall and reporting biases.

In addition, treatment of persons with comorbid disorders can be especially difficult because these individuals often have greater severity of symptoms and a worse overall long-term prognosis compared with those without comorbid conditions (Blanco et al. 2012; Brady et al. 2007; Morojele et al. 2012). For example, in a study among outpatient alcohol treatment clients, those with comorbid anxiety and/or depression were found to be significantly more disabled and to drink more heavily than those without a comorbid psychiatric disorder at baseline and at follow-up (Burns et al. 2005). Among people with psychiatric disorders, comorbid substance use also has been found to be associated with shorter times to hospital readmission (Lin et al. 2007), higher rates of disability (Brière et al. 2014), and higher rates of mortality due to suicide and other causes (Yoon et al. 2011). Of particular concern are the high rates of smoking and heavier smoking among persons with psychiatric disorders, contributing to elevated rates of cancer, stroke, and cardiovascular and respiratory disease in this population (de Leon and Diaz 2005; Lawrence et al. 2009; Vanable et al. 2003). Among persons with schizophrenia, schizoaffective disorder, or bipolar disorder, rates of smoking are especially high, with the prevalence of current smoking often being more than two-thirds in these clients (Hartz et al. 2014; Ziedonis et al. 2003).

Comorbidity therefore further compounds the already elevated rates of morbidity and mortality observed among persons with noncomorbid psychiatric disorders or SUDs. The WMH surveys have sought to quantify the global burden of morbidity and mortality attributable to psychiatric and substance disorders (Kessler et al. 2009). Kessler and colleagues noted that because psychiatric disorders and SUDs are relatively common and have an earlier onset than many other chronic conditions, their overall contributions to lifetime adversity and disability are disproportionately high. The Global Burden of Disease (GBD) research program, a comprehensive initiative focused on measurement of disease and injury burden in populations worldwide, introduced a new metric—the disability-adjusted life year (DALY), a composite measure of the years of healthy life lost at the population level due to death, illness, or disability—to quantify the burdens and health effects associated with specific conditions. An analysis of GBD data from 2010 calculated that combined mental and substance use disorders accounted for 7.4% of global DALYs, and drug and alcohol use disorders accounted for 0.8% and 0.7%, respectively, of global DALYs (Murray et al. 2012). In higher-income regions, mental and substance use disorders accounted for 11% of DALYs. A component measure of the DALY is years lived with disability (YLD), which captures the disability attributable to a condition over the time lived with that condition at a population level. Because of the early age at onset of SUDs and psychiatric disorders, these conditions account for a high proportion of YLDs globally (Whiteford et al. 2016). The GBD study estimated that mental disorders and SUDs accounted for 18.9% and 3.9%, respectively, of YLDs globally. Whiteford and colleagues noted that the proportions of DALYs and YLDs attributable to mental and substance use disorders have been rising and are expected to continue to rise as treatments for other acute and chronic medical conditions improve.

Models of Comorbidity

The possible etiological underpinnings that contribute to the high co-occurrence rates for SUDs and other psychiatric disorders remain open questions for ongoing investigation. Continued research is needed to better understand to what extent shared underlying premorbid factors predispose an individual to both an SUD and another psychiatric disorder, to what extent psychiatric disorders predispose an individual to developing an SUD, and to what extent substance use increases one's risk for a psychiatric disorder. For example, it could be that a shared underlying diathesis of genetic/biological factors and/or psychological/environmental stressors may lead to a combined increased risk for both substance use and psychiatric illness. Alternatively, psychiatric symptoms could predispose a person to use substances and/or could increase the reinforcing effects of substances. This model would include what has sometimes been framed as the *self-medication hypothesis*—that is, the notion that individuals begin using substances to alleviate (i.e., self-treat) their psychiatric symptoms. It may be that use of a substance precipitates psychiatric symptoms and/or increases exposure to stressors that might increase the risk of a psychiatric disorder. For example, individuals who engage in substance use at an early age are less likely to complete higher-level education, a consequence that could indirectly exacerbate risk for subsequent psychiatric illness. Efforts to examine genetic factors that contribute to comorbidity for specific conditions have found some evidence for shared covariance from common genetic variations across some SUDs and psychiatric disorders, but these findings of genetic correlation do not allow for conclusions on the underlying mechanisms driving comorbidity (Agrawal et al. 2016; Polimanti et al. 2017; Reginsson et al. 2018). Additional research is needed to determine the role that shared genetic factors could play in explaining comorbidity. Furthermore, multiple different factors and mechanistic pathways could all operate at once, and differing etiological permutations could apply in different individuals and/or to different combinations of substances and psychiatric conditions.

For SUDs and psychiatric disorders, it is likely that in most instances, risk for illness arises from the complex interactions of myriad factors—genetic, biological, developmental, familial, social, and environmental, each of small effect on its own. Several researchers have examined advanced etiological models to explain such complex, multifactorial relationships between comorbid SUDs and psychiatric disorders. Neale and Kendler (1995) proposed several hypothetical explanations for comorbidity of multifactorial disorders. They described nuanced explanatory pathways that could contribute to comorbidity, beyond more general direct and indirect causal effects between disorders and shared underlying liabilities. For example, comorbidity could be observed if one disorder manifested as an *epiphenomenon* of the other, meaning that under certain conditions, the first disorder would generate symptoms of the second, independent of the risk for the second disorder itself. Alternatively, there could be a unique risk pathway for the comorbid state itself, independent of the specific risks for each of the disorders. In this model, the comorbid condition in essence constitutes a third disorder with a constellation of risk factors that is separate from and independent of the sets of risk factors associated with the first and second disorders. Neale and Kendler (1995) presented mathematical models that can be used to test these hypothetical pathways and compare them with observed findings. Continued research efforts to understand the unique and shared risks for psychiatric disorders and SUDs, including genetic, biological, and environmental factors, are needed to assess which of these etiological models best explains the patterns of comorbidity between SUDs and psychiatric disorders that are found in epidemiological studies (Anttila et al. 2018; Neale and Kendler 1995).

Conclusion

Comorbidity between SUDs and psychiatric disorders is highly prevalent and is associated with greater severity of illness. It is thus important that clinicians routinely assess clients for comorbidity and treat comorbid conditions in an integrated fashion. Ongoing research seeks to further illuminate several promising etiological models that may potentially explain the complex, multifactorial influences that contribute to the high rates of comorbidity observed. Clinical trials commonly exclude participation of individuals who have comorbidities because of the complexities of their clinical conditions; as a result, findings from these studies may support treatment options that are inappropriate or inadequate for patients with co-occurring psychiatric and substance use disorders. More research is needed to develop improved treatment strategies for dual-diagnosis populations.

References

Agrawal A, Edenberg HJ, Gelernter J: Meta-analyses of genome-wide association data hold new promise for addiction genetics. J Stud Alcohol Drugs 77(5):676–680, 2016 27588522

Alonso J, Angermeyer MC, Bernert S, et al: 12-Month comorbidity patterns and associated factors in Europe: results from the European Study of the Epidemiology of Mental Disorders (ESEMeD) project. Acta Psychiatr Scand Suppl (420):28–37, 2004 15128385

American Psychiatric Association: Diagnostic and Statistical Manual of Mental Disorders, Third Edition. Washington, DC, American Psychiatric Association, 1980

American Psychiatric Association: Diagnostic and Statistical Manual of Mental Disorders, Third Edition, Revised. Washington, DC, American Psychiatric Association, 1987

American Psychiatric Association: Diagnostic and Statistical Manual of Mental Disorders, Fourth Edition. Washington, DC, American Psychiatric Association, 1994

American Psychiatric Association: Diagnostic and Statistical Manual of Mental Disorders, Fifth Edition. Arlington, VA, American Psychiatric Association, 2013

Anttila V, Bulik-Sullivan B, Finucane HK, et al: Analysis of shared heritability in common disorders of the brain. Science 360(6395):eeap8757, 2018 29930110

Blanco C, Alegría AA, Liu SM, et al: Differences among major depressive disorder with and without co-occurring substance use disorders and substance-induced depressive disorder: results from the National Epidemiologic Survey on Alcohol and Related Conditions. J Clin Psychiatry 73(6):865–873, 2012 22480900

Brady KT, Verduin ML, Tolliver BK: Treatment of patients comorbid for addiction and other psychiatric disorders. Curr Psychiatry Rep 9(5):374–380, 2007 17915076

Brière FN, Rohde P, Seeley JR, et al: Comorbidity between major depression and alcohol use disorder from adolescence to adulthood. Compr Psychiatry 55(3):526–533, 2014 24246605

Burns L, Teesson M, O'Neill K: The impact of comorbid anxiety and depression on alcohol treatment outcomes. Addiction 100(6):787–796, 2005 15918809

Carton L, Pignon B, Baguet A, et al: Influence of comorbid alcohol use disorders on the clinical patterns of major depressive disorder: a general population-based study. Drug Alcohol Depend 187(187):40–47, 2018 29626745

Degenhardt L, Chiu WT, Sampson N, et al: Toward a global view of alcohol, tobacco, cannabis, and cocaine use: findings from the WHO World Mental Health surveys. PLoS Med 5(7):e141, 2008 18597549

Degenhardt L, Saha S, Lim CCW, et al: The associations between psychotic experiences and substance use and substance use disorders: findings from the World Health Organization World Mental Health surveys. Addiction 113(5):924–934, 2018 29284197

de Leon J, Diaz FJ: A meta-analysis of worldwide studies demonstrates an association between schizophrenia and tobacco smoking behaviors. Schizophr Res 76(2–3):135–157, 2005 15949648

Farrell M, Howes S, Bebbington P, et al: Nicotine, alcohol and drug dependence, and psychiatric comorbidity—results of a national household survey. Int Rev Psychiatry 15(1–2):50–56, 2003 12745310

Gilman SE, Abraham HD: A longitudinal study of the order of onset of alcohol dependence and major depression. Drug Alcohol Depend 63(3):277–286, 2001 11418232

Grant BF, Stinson FS, Dawson DA, et al: Prevalence and co-occurrence of substance use disorders and independent mood and anxiety disorders: results from the National Epidemiologic Survey on Alcohol and Related Conditions. Arch Gen Psychiatry 61(8):807–816, 2004 15289279

Grant BF, Goldstein RB, Chou SP, et al: Sociodemographic and psychopathologic predictors of first incidence of DSM-IV substance use, mood and anxiety disorders: results from the Wave 2 National Epidemiologic Survey on Alcohol and Related Conditions. Mol Psychiatry 14(11):1051–1066, 2009 18427559

Grant BF, Goldstein RB, Saha TD, et al: Epidemiology of DSM-5 alcohol use disorder: results from the National Epidemiologic Survey on Alcohol and Related Conditions III. JAMA Psychiatry 72(8):757–766, 2015 26039070

Grant BF, Saha TD, Ruan WJ, et al: Epidemiology of DSM-5 drug use disorder: results from the National Epidemiologic Survey on Alcohol and Related Conditions-III. JAMA Psychiatry 73(1):39–47, 2016 26580136

Hartz SM, Pato CN, Medeiros H, et al: Comorbidity of severe psychotic disorders with measures of substance use. JAMA Psychiatry 71(3):248–254, 2014 24382686

Hassan AN, Foll BL, Imtiaz S, Rehm J: The effect of post-traumatic stress disorder on the risk of developing prescription opioid use disorder: results from the National Epidemiologic Survey on Alcohol and Related Conditions III. Drug Alcohol Depend 179(179):260–266, 2017 28818717

Howland RH, Rush AJ, Wisniewski SR, et al: Concurrent anxiety and substance use disorders among outpatients with major depression: clinical features and effect on treatment outcome. Drug Alcohol Depend 99(1–3):248–260, 2009 18986774

Jacobi F, Wittchen H-U, Holting C, et al: Prevalence, co-morbidity and correlates of mental disorders in the general population: results from the German Health Interview and Examination Survey (GHS). Psychol Med 34(4):597–611, 2004 15099415

Kessler RC, Nelson CB, McGonagle KA, et al: The epidemiology of co-occurring addictive and mental disorders: implications for prevention and service utilization. Am J Orthopsychiatry 66(1):17–31, 1996 8720638

Kessler RC, Berglund P, Demler O, et al: Lifetime prevalence and age-of-onset distributions of DSM-IV disorders in the National Comorbidity Survey Replication. Arch Gen Psychiatry 62(6):593–602, 2005a 15939837

Kessler RC, Chiu WT, Demler O, et al: Prevalence, severity, and comorbidity of 12-month DSM-IV disorders in the National Comorbidity Survey Replication. Arch Gen Psychiatry 62(6):617–627, 2005b 15939839

Kessler RC, Aguilar-Gaxiola S, Alonso J, et al: The global burden of mental disorders: an update from the WHO World Mental Health (WMH) surveys. Epidemiol Psichiatr Soc 18(1):23–33, 2009 19378696

Lawrence D, Mitrou F, Zubrick SR: Smoking and mental illness: results from population surveys in Australia and the United States. BMC Public Health 9:285, 2009 19664203

Lin CH, Chen YS, Lin CH, et al: Factors affecting time to rehospitalization for patients with major depressive disorder. Psychiatry Clin Neurosci 61(3):249–254, 2007 17472592

Lopez-Quintero C, Hasin DS, de Los Cobos JP, et al: Probability and predictors of remission from life-time nicotine, alcohol, cannabis or cocaine dependence: results from the National Epidemiologic Survey on Alcohol and Related Conditions. Addiction 106(3):657–669, 2011 21077975

Morojele NK, Saban A, Seedat S: Clinical presentations and diagnostic issues in dual diagnosis disorders. Curr Opin Psychiatry 25(3):181–186, 2012 22449761

Murray CJ, Vos T, Lozano R, et al: Disability-adjusted life years (DALYs) for 291 diseases and injuries in 21 regions, 1990–2010: a systematic analysis for the Global Burden of Disease Study 2010. Lancet 380(9859):2197–2223, 2012 23245608

Neale MC, Kendler KS: Models of comorbidity for multifactorial disorders. Am J Hum Genet 57(4):935–953, 1995 7573055

Polimanti R, Agrawal A, Gelernter J: Schizophrenia and substance use comorbidity: a genome-wide perspective. Genome Med 9(1):25, 2017 28327175

Regier DA, Farmer ME, Rae DS, et al: Comorbidity of mental disorders with alcohol and other drug abuse. Results from the Epidemiologic Catchment Area (ECA) study. JAMA 264(19):2511–2518, 1990 2232018

Reginsson GW, Ingason A, Euesden J, et al: Polygenic risk scores for schizophrenia and bipolar disorder associate with addiction. Addict Biol 23(1):485–492, 2018 28231610

Sørensen T, Jespersen HSR, Vinberg M, et al: Substance use among Danish psychiatric patients: a cross-sectional study. Nord J Psychiatry 72(2):130–136, 2018 29117747

Swendsen J, Conway KP, Degenhardt L, et al: Mental disorders as risk factors for substance use, abuse and dependence: results from the 10-year follow-up of the National Comorbidity Survey. Addiction 105(6):1117–1128, 2010 20331554

Teesson M, Slade T, Mills K: Comorbidity in Australia: findings of the 2007 National Survey of Mental Health and Wellbeing. Aust N Z J Psychiatry 43(7):606–614, 2009 19530017

Vanable PA, Carey MP, Carey KB, et al: Smoking among psychiatric outpatients: relationship to substance use, diagnosis, and illness severity. Psychol Addict Behav 17(4):259–265, 2003 14640821

Weaver T, Madden P, Charles V, et al: Comorbidity of substance misuse and mental illness in community mental health and substance misuse services. Br J Psychiatry 183:304–313, 2003 14519608

Whiteford HA, Ferrari AJ, Degenhardt L, et al: Global burden of mental, neurological, and substance use disorders: an analysis from the Global Burden of Disease Study 2010, in Mental, Neurological, and Substance Use Disorders (Disease Control Priorities Series, Vol. 4), 3rd Edition. Edited by Patel V, Chisholm D, Dua T, et al. Washington, DC, The International Bank for Reconstruction and Development/The World Bank, 2016, pp 29–40 (PMID 27227244)

Yoon YH, Chen CM, Yi HY, et al: Effect of comorbid alcohol and drug use disorders on premature death among unipolar and bipolar disorder decedents in the United States, 1999 to 2006. Compr Psychiatry 52(5):453–464, 2011 21146814

Ziedonis D, Williams JM, Smelson D: Serious mental illness and tobacco addiction: a model program to address this common but neglected issue. Am J Med Sci 326(4):223–230, 2003 14557739

CHAPTER 44

Mood Disorders

Jonathan M. Wai, M.D.

Matisyahu Shulman, M.D.

Edward Nunes, M.D.

Mood disorders and substance use disorders (SUDs) frequently occur together, and this comorbidity poses a significant challenge for clinicians across clinical settings. Effective management of patients with this comorbidity requires a sound knowledge of the diagnosis and therapeutics of mood disorders and SUDs individually and of how the disorders may interact to complicate diagnosis and treatment.

Epidemiology

Prevalence of Co-Occurrence

Depressive disorders are second only to anxiety disorders as the mental disorder category that most commonly co-occurs with SUDs (Hasin et al. 2018). In large community surveys, such as the National Epidemiologic Survey on Alcoholism and Related Conditions (NESARC) (Hasin et al. 2018), the National Comorbidity Survey (NCS) (Kessler et al. 2005), and the Epidemiological Catchment Area (ECA) study (Regier et al. 1990), the presence of a depressive disorder has consistently been shown to more than double the risk of an alcohol or other substance use disorder. Depression is the most common co-occurring diagnosis in individuals seeking treatment for a substance use disorder, with a prevalence ranging from 15% to 50% (Hasin et al. 2004).

In the general population, bipolar and related disorders have a lower prevalence (between 1% and 3% [Blanco et al. 2017; Merikangas et al. 2007]) than depressive disorders, which have a lifetime prevalence of around 10% (Hasin et al. 2018); however, bipolar disorders have a stronger association with SUDs than do depressive disorders. In the large community surveys mentioned above, the presence of bipolar disorder has been shown to increase the odds of an alcohol use disorder or a drug use disorder by a factor of 4 of more (Blanco et al. 2017). Comorbid SUDs are highly prevalent among patients presenting with bipolar disorder in clinical settings, with co-occurrence rates estimated at 40% or greater (Cerullo and Strakowski 2007). Among patients seeking treatment for SUDs, bipolar disorder is less common than unipolar depressive disorder due to the low baseline prevalence of bipolar disorders.

Course and Prognosis

A comorbid diagnosis of current major depressive disorder has been shown to predict worse outcomes for SUD treatment among individuals with alcohol use disorder (Greenfield et al. 1998; Hasin et al. 2002), individuals with opioid use disorder (OUD) on methadone maintenance (Rounsaville et al. 1986), and individuals with cocaine use disorder (Carroll et al. 1993). In contrast, comorbid subsyndromal depressive symptoms, as measured by screening tools such as the Beck Depression Inventory or the Hamilton Depression Scale, do not consistently predict worse outcomes for SUD treatment (Greenfield et al. 1998; Hasin et al. 2004). In longitudinal studies, persistence of depression during treatment has been associated with worse outcomes for substance use (e.g., increased risk of relapse, heavier drinking) (Curran et al. 2000; Prisciandaro et al. 2012), while treatment of comorbid depression has been associated with better drinking outcomes (e.g., lower risk of relapse) (Greenfield et al. 1998). These findings suggest the importance both of taking a careful clinical history to establish a diagnosis of mood disorder among patients with SUDs and of providing treatment for co-occurring mood disorders.

Assessment and Diagnosis

Diagnostic Criteria

Prior to the advent of the fourth edition of the *Diagnostic and Statistical Manual of Mental Disorders* (DSM-IV; American Psychiatric Association 1994), there were no consensus criteria for the diagnosis of co-occurring substance use and other mental disorders, and the field was more polarized. Clinicians working in addiction treatment settings tended to view mood symptoms as simply a manifestation of the addictive disorder. The idea that a mood disorder could be diagnosed and treated in a patient with an SUD was not well accepted. Clinicians working in general psychiatric settings tended to view substance use as a manifestation of a mood or other psychiatric disorder, missing the opportunity to intervene directly against the SUD. In the pre-DSM-IV era, co-occurring mental disorders in the presence of SUDs were sometimes characterized as either *primary* or *secondary* on the basis of which disorder had the earlier onset (Nunes et al. 2004). These terms were also commonly used to denote an etiological relationship between SUDs and co-occurring mood disorders, with *primary* indicating that the mood disorder was the predominant problem, with substance use as a consequence, and *secondary* indicating that the SUD was predominant, with the mood syndrome being a consequence of the substance use.

  DSM-IV advanced the field by recognizing a distinction between an "independent" mood disorder in the presence of a SUD and a newly created diagnostic entity, "substance-induced mood disorder." This diagnosis should be used when the patient's mood symptoms cannot be better explained by an independent mood disorder and "are in excess of [symptoms] usually associated with the intoxication or withdrawal syndrome" characteristic of the particular substance and are "sufficiently severe to warrant clinical attention." This diagnosis in turn needs to be distinguished from the usual intoxication or withdrawal effects of the substance ingested (see Table 44–1). DSM-5 retained this distinction (American Psychiatric Association 2013); by definition, a substance/medication-induced disorder should resolve within a predictable period of time after abstinence from substance use, indicating a causal relationship (i.e., that the substance is causing the mood syndrome). However, in clinical practice, one often encounters patients with a mood syndrome and ongoing substance use, where it is unclear from the history whether the mood disorder can be called independent, and ongoing substance use does not afford observation of what would happen if abstinence were achieved. Alternatively, the clinician may encounter a patient who has just become abstinent—for example, upon admission to inpatient or residential treatment—and it is too soon to know what will happen over several weeks of abstinence. In this instance, the "substance/medication-induced" category provides a way to recognize a clinically significant mood syndrome that cannot be clearly established as "independent" but needs clinical attention and follow-up.

DSM-5 delineates diagnoses of "substance/medication-induced depressive disorder" and "substance/medication-induced bipolar and related disorder." A substance-induced mood disorder is a clinically significant syndrome that develops during active substance use and is characterized by symptoms in excess of those usually associated with the intoxication or withdrawal syndrome for the substance. Thus, the mood symptoms should not be better explained simply by intoxication or withdrawal syndromes. The symptoms should also not be better explained by an independent mood disorder, as indicated by symptoms of mood disorder that precede the onset of substance use or continue for 1 month after cessation. An important and sometimes overlooked point is that the substance must be capable of producing the observed symptoms, although the time course of symptom appearance may vary, depending on the substance and the mood symptoms associated with that substance. For example, stimulant-induced mania is well described and would be expected to appear soon after substance ingestion and to resolve within 1–2 days. On the other hand, corticosteroid-induced mania most often appears several days after steroid administration, and symptoms may last longer. Substance-induced depression in a patient with alcohol use disorder may take several weeks to fully resolve. Although most of the literature cited in this chapter comes from the DSM-IV era, for convenience we will refer to DSM-5 in the remainder of this chapter, given the close similarity between DSM-IV and DSM-5 with respect to mood disorders and the criteria for substance-induced disorders.

A new addition in DSM-5 was disruptive mood dysregulation disorder, a diagnosis given to children with prominent irritable mood and depressive symptoms (distinct from children on the bipolar spectrum). This disorder has its onset in childhood, prior to the age of risk for SUDs. However, as these children pass into adolescence, they may be more vulnerable to substance use. Recent reviews suggest that a serotonin reuptake inhibitor (SRI) should be the first-line treatment for disruptive mood dysregulation disorder (Bruno et al. 2019).

TABLE 44-1.   **DSM-5 diagnostic approach to evaluating co-occurring mood and substance use disorders**

- Independent (primary) mood disorder
  - Temporally independent from substance use (i.e., preceded onset of use or persisted for a substantial period after establishment of abstinence)
  - Ideally diagnosed during a period of abstinence under direct observation (e.g., during inpatient treatment) or with other evidence of abstinence (e.g., drug testing)
- Substance-induced mood disorder
  - Not temporally independent from substance use
  - Symptoms in excess of those usually associated with the intoxication or withdrawal syndrome for substance
- Usual effects of substances
  - See DSM-5 intoxication and withdrawal criteria

Source.   American Psychiatric Association 2013.

Diagnostic Challenges

Differentiation of Substance-Induced Versus Independent Mood Disorders

An understanding of both the DSM-5 criteria for the suspected mood disorder and the symptoms of substance intoxication and withdrawal syndromes is important for an accurate diagnosis. Table 44–2 provides a summary of mood symptoms that may occur as part of intoxication and withdrawal syndromes.

Mood disorders often co-occur with other psychiatric disorders in addition to SUDs. For example, borderline personality disorder may be difficult to distinguish from bipolar disorder or from a depressive disorder with prominent irritability or rejection sensitivity (Ruggero et al. 2010), or these disorders may co-occur. Symptoms of poor concentration or hyperactivity may occur as part of depression or hypomania, while attention-deficit/hyperactivity disorder (ADHD) often co-occurs with mood disorders (American Psychiatric Association 2013). A history of trauma or posttraumatic stress disorder (PTSD) is common in patients with SUDs. The symptoms of PTSD overlap those of depression. PTSD and anxiety disorders often co-occur with mood disorders.

The high comorbidity among mood disorders, SUDs, and other psychiatric disorders, illustrated in Figure 44–1, suggests an important principle for clinical assessment: *Among patients with substance use and depressive symptoms, look for co-occurring disorders,* particularly bipolar disorder (suggested by a history of mania or hypomania in a currently depressed patient), ADHD, anxiety disorders (e.g., social anxiety disorder, panic disorder, agoraphobia), PTSD, borderline personality disorder, or the conduct disorder/antisocial personality disorder spectrum. These disorders have distinct treatment indications and are thus important in treatment planning.

Clinical Evaluation of Patient History and Symptom Patterns

Guidelines for obtaining the clinical history for evaluating patients with co-occurring mood symptoms and substance use are outlined in Table 44–3. The *developmental history* should include school experiences and performance (which can reveal a picture

TABLE 44–2. Substance intoxication and withdrawal syndromes with symptoms that may overlap with symptoms of depressive or bipolar disorders

Substance/condition	Depressive symptoms	Manic symptoms	Other symptoms[a]
Alcohol intoxication	Impairment in attention or memory	Inappropriate sexual or aggressive behavior, mood lability, impaired judgment	Slurred speech, incoordination, unsteady gait, nystagmus, stupor or coma
Alcohol withdrawal	Insomnia, anxiety, psychomotor agitation	Insomnia, auditory hallucinations or illusions, psychomotor agitation	Autonomic hyperactivity, increased hand tremor, generalized tonic-clonic seizures, transient visual, tactile, or auditory hallucinations or illusions
Caffeine intoxication	Restlessness, nervousness, insomnia, psychomotor agitation	Excitement, insomnia, rambling flow of thought and speech, periods of inexhaustibility, psychomotor agitation	Flushed face, diuresis, gastrointestinal disturbance, muscle twitching, tachycardia or cardiac arrhythmia
Caffeine withdrawal	Marked fatigue or drowsiness, dysphoric mood, depressed mood, irritability, difficulty concentrating	—	Headache, flu-like symptoms
Cannabis intoxication	Increased appetite, anxiety, social withdrawal	Euphoria, impaired judgment	Conjunctival injection, dry mouth, tachycardia, sensation of slowed time, impaired motor coordination
Cannabis withdrawal	Nervousness or anxiety, sleep disturbances, decreased appetite or weight loss, restlessness, depressed mood	Irritability, anger, or aggression; sleep disturbances	Abdominal pain; shakiness/tremors; sweating; fever, chills, or headache
Phencyclidine (PCP) intoxication	—	Belligerence, assaultiveness, impulsiveness, unpredictability, psychomotor agitation, impaired judgment	Vertical or horizontal nystagmus, hypertension, tachycardia, numbness or diminished responsiveness to pain, ataxia, dysarthria, muscle rigidity, seizures, coma, hyperacusis

TABLE 44–2. Substance intoxication and withdrawal syndromes with symptoms that may overlap with symptoms of depressive or bipolar disorders (continued)

Substance/condition	Depressive symptoms	Manic symptoms	Other symptoms[a]
Other hallucinogen intoxication	Marked anxiety, depression	Ideas of reference, paranoid ideation, impaired judgment, hallucinations	Pupillary dilation, tachycardia, sweating, palpitations, blurring of vision, tremors, incoordination, subjective intensification of perceptions, depersonalization, derealization, illusions, synesthesia, fear of "losing one's mind"
Inhalant intoxication	Lethargy, psychomotor retardation, apathy	Euphoria, belligerence, assaultiveness, impaired judgment	Dizziness, nystagmus, incoordination, slurred speech, unsteady gait, depressed reflexes, tremor, generalized muscle weakness, blurred vision or diplopia, stupor or coma
Opioid intoxication	Impairment in attention or memory, apathy, dysphoria, psychomotor agitation or retardation	Euphoria, impaired judgment, psychomotor agitation	Drowsiness or coma, slurred speech
Opioid withdrawal	Dysphoric mood, insomnia	Insomnia	Nausea or vomiting; muscle aches; lacrimation or rhinorrhea; pupillary dilation, piloerection, or sweating; diarrhea; yawning; fever
Sedative-hypnotic intoxication	Impairment in attention and memory	Inappropriate sexual or aggressive behavior, mood lability, impaired judgment	Slurred speech, incoordination, unsteady gait, nystagmus, stupor or coma
Sedative-hypnotic withdrawal	Anxiety, insomnia	Auditory hallucinations, psychomotor agitation, insomnia, auditory hallucinations	Autonomic hyperactivity; tremor; nausea or vomiting; transient visual, tactile, or auditory hallucinations or illusions; seizures

TABLE 44–2. Substance intoxication and withdrawal syndromes with symptoms that may overlap with symptoms of depressive or bipolar disorders *(continued)*

Substance/condition	Depressive symptoms	Manic symptoms	Other symptoms[a]
Stimulant intoxication	Weight loss, psychomotor agitation or retardation, affective blunting, anxiety	Euphoria, changes in sociability, hypervigilance, interpersonal sensitivity, tension or anger, impaired judgment, psychomotor agitation	Tachycardia or bradycardia; pupillary dilation; elevated or lowered blood pressure; perspiration or chills; nausea or vomiting; muscular weakness; respiratory depression, chest pain, or cardiac arrhythmias; confusion; seizures; dyskinesias; dystonia; coma; stereotyped behaviors
Stimulant withdrawal	Dysphoric mood, fatigue, insomnia or hypersomnia, increased appetite, psychomotor retardation or agitation	Insomnia	Vivid, unpleasant dreams
Tobacco/nicotine withdrawal	Anxiety, difficulty concentrating, increased appetite, restlessness, depressed mood, insomnia	Insomnia; irritability, frustration, or anger	—

[a]"Other symptoms" column lists symptoms that are characteristic of substance intoxication and withdrawal but that do not typically appear in mood disorders. The presence of any of these symptoms should raise suspicion for ongoing substance use.

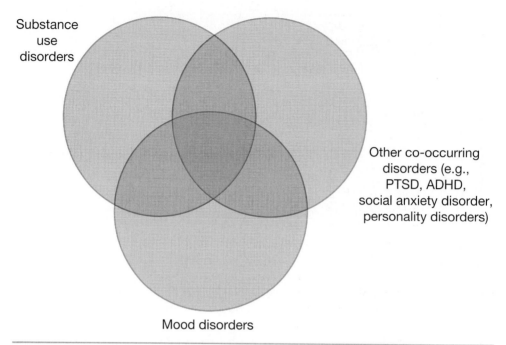

FIGURE 44–1.   Conceptual model of the comorbidity of substance use disorders with mood disorders and other disorders that commonly co-occur with them (not drawn to scale).
ADHD=attention-deficit/hyperactivity disorder; PTSD=posttraumatic stress disorder.

consistent with ADHD, social anxiety disorder, learning problems, or conduct disorder), abuse or other trauma, problems with irritability and getting into fights (which may indicate ADHD, disruptive mood dysregulation disorder, a mood disorder, or conduct disorder), or frequent sad mood (indicative of an early-onset mood disorder). A history of a syndrome that manifests first in childhood can be very helpful in clarifying the diagnosis because they typically occur well before the onset of substance use in a patient's lifetime and thus support a diagnosis of an independent rather than a substance-induced disorder.

An accurate assessment of the timing of the onset of symptoms is also important in distinguishing independent from substance-induced disorders. Thus, to obtain the *history of present illness,* the clinician should ascertain whether criteria for a DSM-5 mood disorder are met, whether the mood symptoms preceded or followed the onset of substance use in the current episode, and whether the mood symptoms are consistent in quality and time course with the known intoxication or withdrawal effects of the substance.

The *substance use and psychiatric history* should establish the age at onset of first regular substance use and use disorder in the patient's lifetime and the time course of substance problems, including any substantial periods of abstinence from substances across the lifetime. It is also useful to know whether such periods of abstinence coincided with particular treatment efforts, such as an inpatient or residential treatment (which enforces abstinence), outpatient treatment, 12-step meeting participation (which strongly encourages abstinence), or medication treatment (e.g., disulfiram or naltrexone for alcohol use disorder; methadone, buprenorphine, or naltrexone for

TABLE 44–3.   **Clinical guidelines for evaluating patient history in the context of co-occurring mood and substance use disorders**

History of present illness

- Review recent substance use and onset of use.
- Identify recent mood symptoms/syndrome and onset of symptoms.
- Ascertain the pattern of mood symptoms/syndrome in relation to substance intoxication and withdrawal.
- Ascertain whether the mood syndrome preceded the onset of the current substance use episode or persisted after abstinence was achieved.

Substance use and psychiatric history (including treatment history)

- Establish lifetime onset of substance use disorders.
- Identify substantial periods of abstinence lasting a month or more.
- Establish the onset and course of mood syndromes and map them onto the lifetime course of substance use disorder.
- Review the treatment history: Was treatment of the substance use disorder followed by improved mood symptoms? Was treatment of the mood disorder followed by improvement in substance use?
- Look for other co-occurring disorders (e.g., ADHD, PTSD, social anxiety disorder, panic disorder, agoraphobia).

Developmental history

- Review school experiences and performance: look for learning difficulties, ADHD, separation anxiety, social anxiety, depression, irritability, or frequent fights.
- Ascertain the presence of developmental stressors, trauma, or abuse.

Family history

- Review family history for mood, anxiety, and substance use disorders in family members.

Note.   ADHD=attention-deficit/hyperactivity disorder; PTSD=posttraumatic stress disorder.

OUD). Once the life course of SUD has been established, the history of the mood disorder and mood symptoms can be mapped onto this lifetime history. Did a mood syndrome begin before or after the first substance use? Or did a mood syndrome emerge or persist during past periods of abstinence lasting for a month or more? The presence of such historical features would suggest an independent mood disorder.

The *family history* can also be helpful in evaluating comorbidity. SUDs and mood disorders have strong inherited components. Thus, in a patient with a current SUD, a clear history of a mood or anxiety disorder in parents or siblings can raise the index of suspicion that a concurrent mood syndrome may represent an independent mood disorder.

Figure 44–2 illustrates various temporal patterns of mood and substance use syndromes in a current episode and corresponding diagnoses. Symptoms of substance intoxication should rapidly resolve upon substance discontinuation, with withdrawal symptoms usually resolving soon after. A substance-induced mood syndrome should also resolve after abstinence is established. This suggests another important clinical principle: *Always initiate treatment for the SUD as a first step.* The SUD needs to be treated in any case, and achievement of abstinence or substantial reduction in substance use may help clarify the diagnosis of comorbidity. DSM-5 suggests that a mood

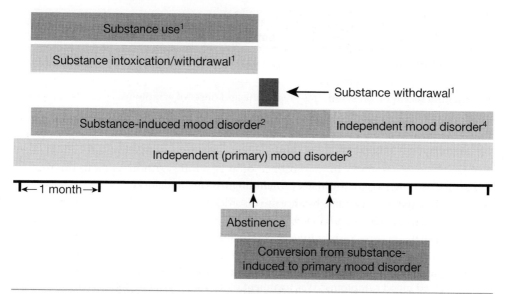

FIGURE 44–2. Representative timeline of the temporal relationships among substance use, substance-induced mood disorders, and primary mood disorders.

[1]*Substance intoxication and withdrawal* occur concurrently with active substance use and resolve shortly after cessation of substance use (abstinence).

[2]*Substance-induced mood disorder* occurs concurrently with active substance use but exceeds usual intoxication or withdrawal effects and should resolve within 1 month of abstinence.

[3]*Independent (primary) mood disorder* begins prior to the onset of substance use and persists after abstinence.

[4]*Substance-induced mood disorder* that persists beyond 1 month after abstinence can be rediagnosed as *independent mood disorder.*

Source. American Psychiatric Association 2013.

syndrome that persists for a month or more after abstinence be considered an independent disorder. However, in clinical practice, it is often not possible to convince the patient to stop using substances, or it may not seem advisable to wait for a month of abstinence in the setting of a severe or clear-cut mood syndrome. In these instances, an independent mood disorder may be diagnosed on the basis of the patient's lifetime history or the clinician's judgment.

When conducting the clinical evaluation, it is useful to bear in mind the multiple potential relationships between substance use and mood syndromes (Nunes and Weiss 2014), including the following: 1) substance use may cause a mood syndrome (substance-induced); 2) substance use may be partly an effort to obtain relief from mood symptoms (self-medication); 3) a substance use disorder and a mood disorder may co-occur because they stem from shared risk factors or vulnerabilities, such as stress; and 4) a substance use disorder and a mood disorder may simply be independent disorders.

Treatment

Depressive Disorders

An algorithm for the clinical approach to patients presenting with substance use and depression is suggested in Figure 44–3. Numerous studies have shown that among patients presenting for treatment for an SUD who have substantial depressive symptoms, the depression tends to improve or resolve within a short period (ranging from a few days to a few weeks) after abstinence is achieved—for example, after admission to an inpatient unit or initiation of a powerful outpatient treatment such as methadone maintenance (Brown et al. 1995; Liappas et al. 2002; Strain et al. 1991). Similarly, substantial improvement of depression has often been observed in the placebo groups in placebo-controlled trials of antidepressant medications for co-occurring depression and alcohol or drug use disorder, particularly if the placebo group is receiving a behavioral intervention targeting substance use (Nunes and Levin 2004). This evidence of improvement in the absence of active intervention leads to the recommendation that the first step with a patient presenting with co-occurring substance use and depression, as illustrated in Figure 44–3, should be to initiate treatment for the SUD (with the goal of patient abstinence from—or at least significant reduction in—alcohol or drug use) while taking a complete clinical history (see Table 44–3). If other likely independent disorders are revealed in the history (e.g., past episodes of substance-independent mania, hypomania combined with bipolar disorder, PTSD, ADHD, other anxiety disorders), specific treatment for those disorders should be considered. If a depressive syndrome (major depressive disorder or persistent depressive disorder [dysthymia]) is present, is clearly independent (per patient history), or is severe (e.g., suicidality), the clinician should consider initiating specific antidepressant treatment immediately. Otherwise, the patient should be observed over the first few days or weeks of substance treatment. Depression that resolves as the patient reduces or stops substance use is suggestive of a substance-induced depression. If depression persists, specific treatment for depression should be initiated.

Antidepressant Medication Targeting Major Depressive Disorder Co-Occurring With SUDs

Several placebo-controlled trials of antidepressant medications for treatment of depression/SUD comorbidity were conducted between the 1970s and early 2000s. Two meta-analyses (Nunes and Levin 2004; Torrens et al. 2005) concluded that antidepressants were effective in improving both mood disorders and substance use disorder, particularly in the following circumstances: 1) studies of alcohol use disorder; 2) studies of tricyclic antidepressants, although two studies from that era found strong results for other SRIs (fluoxetine and sertraline) among alcoholic individuals who were observed while abstinent prior to starting medication; 3) studies that required abstinence prior to confirming depression and initiating medication or otherwise made efforts via the clinical history to distinguish independent from substance-induced disorders; and 4) studies that did not offer a concurrent manual-guided behavioral therapy. The studies that showed effectiveness for antidepressants had low placebo response rates. High placebo response rates may reflect response to concurrent manual-guided behavioral therapies, which have general elements likely to benefit both disorders. More recent trials have tested SRIs in comorbid mood and substance use disorders, often yielding high placebo response rates and little evidence of efficacy (Nunes and Weiss 2014).

Taken together, these findings suggest the importance of efforts to establish the presence of an independent depressive disorder, preferably by treating the SUD and observing whether depression persists after abstinence or substantial reduction in

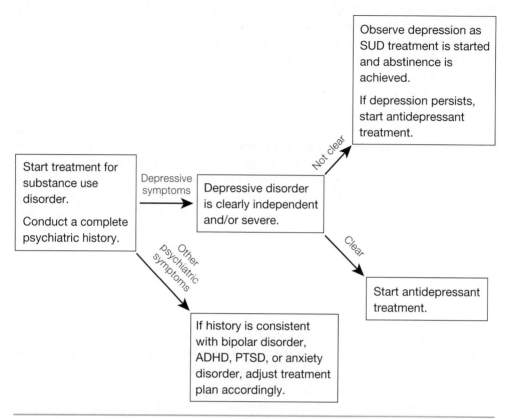

FIGURE 44–3. Algorithm for evaluation and treatment of co-occurring depression and substance use disorder.

ADHD=attention-deficit/hyperactivity disorder; PTSD=posttraumatic stress disorder.

substance use (Bennabi et al. 2019; National Institute for Health and Clinical Excellence 2011; Urness et al. 2016). However, in outpatient settings, it may be difficult to reduce substance use, and evaluation of the history and clinical judgment are needed to determine whether there is sufficient evidence of independent depression to start an antidepressant (Nunes and Weiss 2014; Tanguay et al. 2017).

Regarding choice of medication, SRIs can be considered the first-line treatment for an independent depressive disorder, given these agents' low side-effect burden and two positive trials with low placebo response rates showing efficacy (Cornelius et al. 1997; Roy-Byrne et al. 2000). Tricyclic antidepressants (TCAs) have the most evidence of efficacy but carry more risks and side effects in comparison with other SRIs. If an initial trial of an SRI fails to provide symptom improvement, a TCA or a newer-generation antidepressant, perhaps with a noradrenergic mechanism, should be considered, although more clinical trials investigating such medications are needed. Several trials among alcoholic patients *not* selected for depression have shown that SRIs may make drinking worse (Charney et al. 2015), particularly among individuals with the early-onset alcoholic subtype (Kranzler et al. 2012; Pettinati et al. 2000), characterized by onset before age 25 years. Although these trials did not enroll depressed patients, their findings suggest that patients being treated with an SRI should be carefully monitored for worsening of drinking.

The opioid epidemic and recent reports of the potential role of suicidal intent in opioid overdoses (Oquendo and Volkow 2018) suggest the importance of evaluating for and treating depression among patients with OUD. A meta-analysis examining treatments for depression or anxiety in patients receiving opioid agonist therapy (Hassan et al. 2017) raised concerns regarding the lack of evidence for efficacy in trials of antidepressants among patients with OUD, although many of these trials had high placebo response rates, and several trials of TCAs with lower placebo response rates showed efficacy. As in our suggested algorithm (see Figure 44–3), the approach to a patient with OUD and depression should emphasize initiating treatment with one of the effective medications for OUD (methadone, buprenorphine, or injection naltrexone) and obtaining a comprehensive clinical history (see Table 44–3), with antidepressant medication considered for patients whose depression does not resolve after initiation of medications for OUD.

Pharmacotherapy Targeting SUDs Co-Occurring With Depression

Pharmacological treatment of SUDs in patients with co-occurring major depressive disorder should follow typical substance treatment guidelines. Standard medications such as disulfiram, naltrexone, methadone, or buprenorphine should be started when indicated. Patients initiating methadone maintenance have been found to have substantially decreased depressive symptoms within the first 2 weeks of treatment (Strain et al. 1991), with symptoms of about half of the patients with depressive syndromes resolving within the initial weeks of treatment (Nunes et al. 1998). Medications for alcohol use disorder, such as naltrexone and disulfiram, have also been shown to be effective and safe for use with co-occurring major depressive disorder (Petrakis et al. 2005). Several small trials have also found that combining an antidepressant medication with naltrexone or disulfiram may be more effective than either as monotherapy (Nunes et al. 1993; Pettinati et al. 2010).

Psychotherapy for Co-Occurring Major Depressive Disorder and SUDs

As noted in the subsection "Antidepressant Medication for Co-Occurring Major Depressive Disorder and SUDs," the high placebo response rates in clinical trials that included concurrent manual-guided behavioral treatments for SUD suggest the potential utility of psychotherapeutic approaches. Cognitive-behavioral approaches for various disorders share common features, including teaching strategies for coping with unhelpful thoughts and painful feelings and fostering positive activities. Research on behavioral treatments specifically targeting depression among patients with SUDs is limited; however, studies have suggested the effectiveness of an integrated approach to SUD and depression (Baker et al. 2010) and of transdiagnostic approaches such as mindfulness-based psychotherapy, acceptance and commitment therapy, and behavioral activation (Martínez-Vispo et al. 2018; Vujanovic et al. 2017). Automated cognitive-behavioral interventions delivered either online or via a smartphone application have also shown promise (Elison et al. 2017; Kay-Lambkin et al. 2011).

Bipolar Disorder

Patients with co-occurring bipolar disorder in an acute manic episode will typically require inpatient treatment. The presence of mania with substance intoxication or withdrawal can produce significant mood instability and impulsivity, and the initial approach should focus on stabilization and safety. While bipolar disorder involves episodes of mania or hypomania, patients typically spend more time in depressive episodes—hence the importance of evaluating the history of a depressed patient for episodes of mania or hypomania. Substance use occurs more commonly during the manic or hypomanic phase than during the depressive periods of bipolar disorders (Weiss et al. 1988).

Pharmacotherapy Targeting Bipolar Disorder Co-Occurring With SUDs

Treatment of a bipolar disorder with a co-occurring SUD can generally follow guidelines for treatment of an independent bipolar disorder (Salloum and Brown 2017). Mood stabilizers (e.g., lithium, valproate) and second-generation antipsychotics are the main strategies. Antidepressants are often ineffective for the treatment of bipolar depression and may exacerbate mood instability. The available research suggests that the typical treatments for mood stabilization in bipolar disorder are also helpful in treating co-occurring SUDs. A randomized double-blind trial of patients with bipolar disorder and co-occurring alcohol use disorder showed that lithium and valproate were superior to lithium and placebo in reducing heavy-drinking days (Salloum et al. 2005). Lithium has also been shown to improve both mood and SUD symptoms in hospitalized adolescents with co-occurring bipolar disorder and SUDs (Geller et al. 1998). Carbamazepine was shown to decrease depressive symptoms in a placebo-controlled trial of patients with mood (depressive or bipolar) disorders who were also cocaine dependent (Brady et al. 2002). Lamotrigine (Brown et al. 2006b; Rubio et al. 2006), valproate (Brady et al. 1995; Salloum et al. 2007), and gabapentin (Perugi et al. 2002) have also shown evidence of tolerability and efficacy in open-label trials in individuals with co-occurring bipolar disorder and SUDs involving various substances of abuse.

Second-generation antipsychotics have become a mainstay of treatment in bipolar disorder and remain highly utilized in bipolar disorder with co-occurring substance use. Small open-label trials have shown promise for quetiapine (Brown et al. 2002) and aripiprazole (Brown et al. 2005). However, placebo-controlled trials of quetiapine have yielded mixed findings, with one trial showing its efficacy over placebo in combination with other mood stabilizers on depression outcomes but not on substance use measures (Brown et al. 2008) and other trials showing no effects on substance use (Brown et al. 2014; Stedman et al. 2010) or mood outcomes (Brown et al. 2014).

In summary, akin to the literature on antidepressant treatment in patients with unipolar depression and a co-occurring SUD (Nunes and Levin 2004), the literature suggests that pharmacological treatment of the mood disorder may improve substance use as well. However, treatment of the mood disorder without attention to the SUD is generally unlikely to adequately treat the SUD, and targeted SUD treatment should be instituted as well.

Pharmacotherapy Targeting SUDs Co-Occurring With Bipolar Disorder

The evidence for medications specifically targeting substance use with a co-occurring bipolar disorder is sparse. Generally, indicated medications for SUDs should be used cautiously, with careful monitoring. Disulfiram has been associated with rare cases of psychotic episodes, possibly due to its inhibition of dopamine beta-hydroxylase, leading to an increase in brain dopamine (Nunes and Quitkin 1987). However, it is not clear that bipolar disorder would increase the risk of disulfiram-induced psychosis, and the potential benefits of disulfiram in eliminating alcohol use (presuming adherence can be secured), probably outweigh the risks. Trials of naltrexone (Brown et al. 2006a, 2009) and acamprosate (Tolliver et al. 2012) have found them to be well tolerated, although with limited evidence of efficacy.

Psychotherapy for Co-Occurring Bipolar Disorder and SUDs

As for co-occurring depressive disorders and SUDs, behavioral strategies are needed to complement medication treatments for co-occurring bipolar disorder and SUD. In addition to standard behavioral strategies for SUDs, behavioral therapies specific to treatment for bipolar disorder may also be considered (Scott and Gutierrez 2004). Integrated group therapy, a cognitive-behavioral treatment–based group therapy focused on co-occurring bipolar disorder and SUDs, has shown evidence of efficacy in several clinical trials (Weiss et al. 2007, 2009). Integrated group therapy highlights the commonalities between both disorders by using the term "bipolar substance abuse" and emphasizes abstinence from substances, adherence to medication treatment, and maintenance of daily routines, including regular sleep schedules. For chronic severe bipolar illness, often involving substance use, assertive community treatment, which uses multidisciplinary treatment teams to deliver all required services, has strong evidence of efficacy (Drake et al. 2007).

Conclusion

Mood disorders are highly prevalent among patients with SUDs and are associated with worse outcomes. The clinical approach to a patient with the combination of an SUD and mood symptoms should include initiation of treatment for the substance use in an effort to achieve patient abstinence. This could be outpatient behavioral treatment (e.g., motivational interviewing, cognitive-behavioral treatment plus relapse prevention), inpatient treatment, and/or medication treatment. For OUD, initiation of one of the effective medications (methadone, buprenorphine, or injection naltrexone) is particularly important, given the risk of overdose in untreated OUD. A thorough clinical history should be taken to establish evidence of an independent depressive or bipolar disorder over the lifetime (versus a substance-induced mood disorder), and a search for other commonly co-occurring disorders with specific treatment indications, including ADHD, PTSD, and anxiety disorders, should be undertaken. Substantial evidence from clinical trials shows that independent depressive and bipolar disorders respond to medication treatment—namely, antidepressant medication and mood stabilizers, respectively—and that such treatment is associated with improvement in substance use as well as mood. The literature also contains negative antidepressant trials, typically with high placebo response rates, suggesting either selection of samples with predominantly substance-induced depression or depression that responds to the behavioral interventions offered as part of the trials. Behavioral treatments for substance and mood disorders share common elements, and some evidence supports integrated treatments for the comorbidity or transdiagnostic treatments. Thus, behavioral treatment is also an important part of treatment planning for patients with co-occurring mood disorders and SUDs.

References

American Psychiatric Association: Diagnostic and Statistical Manual of Mental Disorders, 4th Edition. Washington, DC, American Psychiatric Association, 1994
American Psychiatric Association: Diagnostic and Statistical Manual of Mental Disorders, 5th Edition. Arlington, VA, American Psychiatric Association, 2013
Baker AL, Kavanagh DJ, Kay-Lambkin FJ, et al: Randomized controlled trial of cognitive-behavioural therapy for coexisting depression and alcohol problems: short-term outcome. Addiction 105(1):87–99, 2010 19919594
Bennabi D, Yrondi A, Charpeaud T, et al: Clinical guidelines for the management of depression with specific comorbid psychiatric conditions French recommendations from experts (the French Association for Biological Psychiatry and Neuropsychopharmacology and the fondation FondaMental). BMC Psychiatry 19(1):50, 2019 30700272
Blanco C, Compton WM, Saha TD, et al: Epidemiology of DSM-5 bipolar I disorder: results from the National Epidemiologic Survey on Alcohol and Related Conditions—III. J Psychiatr Res 84:310–317, 2017 27814503
Brady KT, Sonne SC, Anton R, Ballenger JC: Valproate in the treatment of acute bipolar affective episodes complicated by substance abuse: a pilot study. J Clin Psychiatry 56(3):118–121, 1995 7883730
Brady KT, Sonne SC, Malcolm RJ, et al: Carbamazepine in the treatment of cocaine dependence: subtyping by affective disorder. Exp Clin Psychopharmacol 10(3):276–285, 2002 12233988
Brown SA, Inaba RK, Gillin JC, et al: Alcoholism and affective disorder: clinical course of depressive symptoms. Am J Psychiatry 152(1):45–52, 1995 7802119
Brown ES, Nejtek VA, Perantie DC, et al: Quetiapine in bipolar disorder and cocaine dependence. Bipolar Disord 4(6):406–411, 2002 12519101
Brown ES, Jeffress J, Liggin JD, et al: Switching outpatients with bipolar or schizoaffective disorders and substance abuse from their current antipsychotic to aripiprazole. J Clin Psychiatry 66(6):756–760, 2005 15960570
Brown ES, Beard L, Dobbs L, Rush AJ: Naltrexone in patients with bipolar disorder and alcohol dependence. Depress Anxiety 23(8):492–495, 2006a 16841344
Brown ES, Perantie DC, Dhanani N, et al: Lamotrigine for bipolar disorder and comorbid cocaine dependence: a replication and extension study. J Affect Disord 93(1–3):219–222, 2006b 16519947
Brown ES, Garza M, Carmody TJ: A randomized, double-blind, placebo-controlled add-on trial of quetiapine in outpatients with bipolar disorder and alcohol use disorders. J Clin Psychiatry 69(5):701–705, 2008 18312058
Brown ES, Carmody TJ, Schmitz JM, et al: A randomized, double-blind, placebo-controlled pilot study of naltrexone in outpatients with bipolar disorder and alcohol dependence. Alcohol Clin Exp Res 33(11):1863–1869, 2009 19673746
Brown ES, Davila D, Nakamura A, et al: A randomized, double-blind, placebo-controlled trial of quetiapine in patients with bipolar disorder, mixed or depressed phase, and alcohol dependence. Alcohol Clin Exp Res 38(7):2113–2118, 2014 24976394
Bruno A, Celebre L, Torre G, et al: Focus on disruptive mood dysregulation disorder: a review of the literature. Psychiatry Res 279:323–330, 2019 31164249

Carroll KM, Power ME, Bryant K, et al: One-year follow-up status of treatment-seeking cocaine abusers. Psychopathology and dependence severity as predictors of outcome. J Nerv Ment Dis 181(2):71–79, 1993 8426174

Cerullo MA, Strakowski SM: The prevalence and significance of substance use disorders in bipolar type I and II disorder. Subst Abuse Treat Prev Policy 2:29, 2007 17908301

Charney DA, Heath LM, Zikos E, et al: Poorer drinking outcomes with citalopram treatment for alcohol dependence: a randomized, double-blind, placebo-controlled trial. Alcohol Clin Exp Res 39(9):1756–1765, 2015 26208048

Cornelius, JR, Salloum IM, Ehler JG, et al: Fluoxetine in depressed alcoholics: a double-blind, placebo-controlled trial. Arch Gen Psychiatry 54(8):700–705, 1997 9283504

Curran GM, Flynn HA, Kirchner J, et al: Depression after alcohol treatment as a risk factor for relapse among male veterans. J Subst Abuse Treat 19(3):259–265, 2000 11027896

Drake RE, Mueser KT, Brunette MF: Management of persons with co-occurring severe mental illness and substance use disorder: program implications. World Psychiatry 6(3):131–136, 2007 18188429

Elison S, Jones A, Ward J, et al: Examining effectiveness of tailorable computer-assisted therapy programmes for substance misuse: programme usage and clinical outcomes data from Breaking Free Online. Addict Behav 74:140–147, 2017 28645092

Geller B, Cooper TB, Sun K, et al: Double-blind and placebo-controlled study of lithium for adolescent bipolar disorders with secondary substance dependency. J Am Acad Child Adolesc Psychiatry 37(2):171–178, 1998 9473913

Greenfield SF, Weiss RD, Muenz LR, et al: The effect of depression on return to drinking: a prospective study. Arch Gen Psychiatry 55(3):259–265, 1998 9510220

Hasin D, Liu X, Nunes E, et al: Effects of major depression on remission and relapse of substance dependence. Arch Gen Psychiatry 59(4):375–380, 2002 11926938

Hasin D, Nunes E, Meydan J: Comorbidity of alcohol, drug, and psychiatric disorders: epidemiology, in Dual Diagnosis and Psychiatric Treatment: Substance Abuse and Comorbid Disorders. Edited by Kranzler HR, Tinsley JA (Medical Psychiatry Series). New York, Marcel Dekker, 2004, pp 1–31

Hasin DS, Sarvet AL, Meyers JL, et al: Epidemiology of adult DSM-5 major depressive disorder and its specifiers in the United States. JAMA Psychiatry 75(4):336–346, 2018 29450462

Hassan AN, Howe AS, Samokhvalov AV, et al: Management of mood and anxiety disorders in patients receiving opioid agonist therapy: review and meta-analysis. Am J Addict 26(6):551–563, 2017 28675762

Kay-Lambkin FJ, Baker AL, Kelly B, et al: Clinician-assisted computerised versus therapist-delivered treatment for depressive and addictive disorders: a randomised controlled trial. Med J Aust 195(3):S44–S50, 2011 21806518

Kessler RC, Chiu WT, Demler O, et al: Prevalence, severity, and comorbidity of 12-month DSM-IV disorders in the National Comorbidity Survey Replication. Arch Gen Psychiatry 62(6):617–627, 2005 15939839

Kranzler HR, Feinn R, Armeli S, et al: Comparison of alcoholism subtypes as moderators of the response to sertraline treatment. Alcohol Clin Exp Res 36(3):509–516, 2012 21895712

Liappas J, Paparrigopoulos T, Tzavellas E, et al: Impact of alcohol detoxification on anxiety and depressive symptoms. Drug Alcohol Depend 68(2):215–220, 2002 12234651

Martínez-Vispo C, Martínez Ú, López-Durán A, et al: Effects of behavioural activation on substance use and depression: a systematic review. Subst Abuse Treat Prev Policy 13(1):36, 2018 30268136

Merikangas KR, Akiskal HS, Angst J, et al: Lifetime and 12-month prevalence of bipolar spectrum disorder in the National Comorbidity Survey replication. Arch Gen Psychiatry 64(5):543–552, 2007 17485606

National Institute for Health and Clinical Excellence: Guidance, in Alcohol-Use Disorders: Diagnosis, Assessment and Management of Harmful Drinking (High-Risk Drinking) and Alcohol Dependence. NICE Clinical Guideline 115. Leicester, UK, British Psychological Society and The Royal College of Psychiatrists, 2011, pp 4–31

Nunes EV, Levin FR: Treatment of depression in patients with alcohol or other drug dependence: a meta-analysis. JAMA 291(15):1887–1896, 2004 15100209

Nunes E, Quitkin F: Disulfiram and bipolar affective disorder. J Clin Psychopharmacol 7(4):284, 1987 3624520

Nunes EV, Weiss R: Co-occurring mood and substances use disorders, in The ASAM Principles of Addiction Medicine. Edited by Ries RK, Fiellin DA, Miller SC, et al. Philadelphia, PA, Lippincott Williams & Wilkins, 2014, pp 1300–1332

Nunes EV, McGrath PJ, Quitkin FM, et al: Imipramine treatment of alcoholism with comorbid depression. Am J Psychiatry 150(6):963–965, 1993 8494079

Nunes EV, Quitkin FM, Donovan SJ, et al: Imipramine treatment of opiate-dependent patients with depressive disorders. A placebo-controlled trial. Arch Gen Psychiatry 55(2):153–160, 1998 9477929

Nunes E, Hasin D, Blanco C: Overview of diagnostic methods: diagnostic criteria, structured and semi-structured interviews, and biological markers, in Dual Diagnosis and Psychiatric Treatment: Substance Abuse and Comorbid Disorders. Edited by Kranzler HR, Tinsley JA (Medical Psychiatry Series). New York, Marcel Dekker, 2004, pp 61–101

Oquendo MA, Volkow ND: Suicide: a silent contributor to opioid-overdose deaths. N Engl J Med 378(17):1567–1569, 2018 29694805

Perugi G, Toni C, Frare F, et al: Effectiveness of adjunctive gabapentin in resistant bipolar disorder: is it due to anxious–alcohol abuse comorbidity? J Clin Psychopharmacol 22(6):584–591, 2002 12454558

Petrakis IL, Poling J, Levinson C, et al: Naltrexone and disulfiram in patients with alcohol dependence and comorbid psychiatric disorders. Biol Psychiatry 57(10):1128–1137, 2005 15866552

Pettinati HM, Volpicelli JR, Kranzler HR, et al: Sertraline treatment for alcohol dependence: interactive effects of medication and alcoholic subtype. Alcohol Clin Exp Res 24(7):1041–1049, 2000 10924008

Pettinati HM, Oslin DW, Kampman KM, et al: A double-blind, placebo-controlled trial combining sertraline and naltrexone for treating co-occurring depression and alcohol dependence. Am J Psychiatry 167(6):668–675, 2010 20231324

Prisciandaro JJ, DeSantis SM, Chiuzan C, et al: Impact of depressive symptoms on future alcohol use in patients with co-occurring bipolar disorder and alcohol dependence: a prospective analysis in an 8-week randomized controlled trial of acamprosate. Alcohol Clin Exp Res 36(3):490–496, 2012 21933201

Regier DA, Farmer ME, Rae DS, et al: Comorbidity of mental disorders with alcohol and other drug abuse. Results from the Epidemiologic Catchment Area (ECA) study. JAMA 264(19):2511–2518, 1990 2232018

Rounsaville BJ, Kosten TR, Weissman MM, et al: Prognostic significance of psychopathology in treated opiate addicts. A 2.5-year follow-up study. Arch Gen Psychiatry 43(8):739–745, 1986 3729668

Roy-Byrne PP, Pages KP, Russo JE, et al: Nefazodone treatment of major depression in alcohol-dependent patients: a double-blind, placebo-controlled trial. J Clin Psychopharmacol 20(2):129–136, 2000 10770449

Rubio G, López-Muñoz F, Alamo C: Effects of lamotrigine in patients with bipolar disorder and alcohol dependence. Bipolar Disord 8(3):289–293, 2006 16696832

Ruggero CJ, Zimmerman M, Chelminski I, et al: Borderline personality disorder and the misdiagnosis of bipolar disorder. J Psychiatr Res 44(6):405–408, 2010 19889426

Salloum IM, Brown ES: Management of comorbid bipolar disorder and substance use disorders. Am J Drug Alcohol Abuse 43(4):366–376, 2017 28301219

Salloum IM, Cornelius JR, Daley DC, et al: Efficacy of valproate maintenance in patients with bipolar disorder and alcoholism: a double-blind placebo-controlled study. Arch Gen Psychiatry 62(1):37–45, 2005 15630071

Salloum IM, Douaihy A, Cornelius JR, et al: Divalproex utility in bipolar disorder with co-occurring cocaine dependence: a pilot study. Addict Behav 32(2):410–415, 2007 16814474

Scott J, Gutierrez MJ: The current status of psychological treatments in bipolar disorders: a systematic review of relapse prevention. Bipolar Disord 6(6):498–503, 2004 15541065

Stedman M, Pettinati HM, Brown ES, et al: A double-blind, placebo-controlled study with quetiapine as adjunct therapy with lithium or divalproex in bipolar I patients with coexisting alcohol dependence. Alcohol Clin Exp Res 34(10):1822–1831, 2010 20626727

Strain EC, Stitzer ML, Bigelow GE: Early treatment time course of depressive symptoms in opiate addicts. J Nerv Ment Dis 179(4):215–221, 1991 2007892

Tanguay RL, Lamba W, Fraser R, et al: Alcohol use disorder and depression: proposed rewording of Choosing Wisely recommendation. CMAJ 189(11):E442–E443, 2017 28385718

Tolliver BK, Desantis SM, Brown DG, et al: A randomized, double-blind, placebo-controlled clinical trial of acamprosate in alcohol-dependent individuals with bipolar disorder: a preliminary report. Bipolar Disord 14(1):54–63, 2012 22329472

Torrens M, Fonseca F, Mateu G, et al: Efficacy of antidepressants in substance use disorders with and without comorbid depression. A systematic review and meta-analysis. Drug Alcohol Depend 78(1):1–22, 2005 15769553

Urness D, Parker NJ, Rapoport MJ, et al: Choosing Wisely: wise choices in psychiatry. Can J Psychiatry 61(11):700–704, 2016 27310235

Vujanovic AA, Meyer TD, Heads AM, et al: Cognitive-behavioral therapies for depression and substance use disorders: an overview of traditional, third-wave, and transdiagnostic approaches. Am J Drug Alcohol Abuse 43(4):402–415, 2017 27494547

Weiss RD, Mirin SM, Griffin ML, et al: Psychopathology in cocaine abusers. Changing trends. J Nerv Ment Dis 176(12):719–725, 1988 3199107

Weiss RD, Griffin ML, Kolodziej ME, et al: A randomized trial of integrated group therapy versus group drug counseling for patients with bipolar disorder and substance dependence. Am J Psychiatry 164(1):100–107, 2007 17202550

Weiss RD, Griffin ML, Jaffee WB, et al: A "community-friendly" version of integrated group therapy for patients with bipolar disorder and substance dependence: a randomized controlled trial. Drug Alcohol Depend 104(3):212–219, 2009 19573999

CHAPTER 45

Anxiety Disorders

Kathleen T. Brady, M.D., Ph.D.
Sudie E. Back, Ph.D.

The relationship between substance use and anxiety disorders is complex, bidirectional, and multifaceted. As described in this chapter, epidemiological surveys as well as studies of treatment-seeking individuals indicate that anxiety disorders, symptoms of anxiety, and substance use disorders (SUDs) commonly co-occur. Anxiety disorders may be a risk factor for the development of an SUD. In many cases, anxiety symptoms emerge during the course of chronic intoxication and withdrawal from alcohol or drugs. Furthermore, substance use and SUDs modify the presentation and outcome of anxiety disorders, just as anxiety disorders modify the presentation and outcome of SUDs. The interplay of these variables is likely to differ among individual cases and between different anxiety disorders. In this chapter, the prevalence, etiological relationships, diagnostic considerations, and treatment options of co-occurring anxiety disorders and SUDs will be reviewed.

Epidemiology

Epidemiological studies conducted over the past 20 years in the United States have concluded that anxiety disorders and SUDs co-occur more commonly than would be expected by chance alone (Grant et al. 2004; Kessler et al. 1994, 1997; Regier et al. 1990). In Table 45–1, the prevalence rates for SUDs and anxiety disorders in the three largest epidemiological studies conducted in the United States are shown. The most recent and largest comorbidity study conducted to date is the National Epidemiologic Survey on Alcohol and Related Conditions (NESARC). Surveying more than 43,000 adults, NESARC was designed to distinguish between independent mood and anxiety disorders (i.e., those not attributed to withdrawal or intoxication) and substance-induced mood and anxiety disorders. Among individuals with any anxiety disorder in the past 12 months ($N=4{,}741$), approximately 15% had at least one co-occurring SUD, and more than 17% of respondents with an SUD in the prior 12 months met criteria for an independent anxiety disorder (Grant et al. 2004). The odds ratio (OR) measures the likelihood that an individual with one specific disorder (anxiety) will develop a second disorder (drug/alcohol use) compared with general population estimates of the disorder alone. The relationship between anxiety disorders and drug use disorders ($OR=2.8$) was stronger than the relationship between anxiety disorders and alcohol use disorder ($OR=1.7$). The relationships between SUDs and specific anxiety disorders were all significantly positive ($P<0.05$), with the ORs for women being more positive than those for men. Among individuals with anxiety disorders ($N=4{,}741$), the most common substance of misuse was marijuana (15.1%), followed by cocaine (5.4%), amphetamines (4.8%), hallucinogens (3.7%), and sedative-hypnotics (2.6%) (Conway et al. 2006).

A meta-analysis of epidemiological surveys investigating comorbid substance use and mood and anxiety disorders between 2000 and 2014 indicated a strong relationship between any anxiety disorder and illicit drug use ($OR=2.91$) or alcohol use disorder ($OR=2.11$) across studies. ORs for dependence were higher than ORs for abuse, irrespective of diagnosis (Lai et al. 2015).

Treatment-Seeking and Other Clinical Populations

Patients with anxiety disorders are more frequent users of all types of health services compared with individuals without anxiety disorders (Gurmankin Levy et al. 2007). A study of opioid users in a needle exchange program ($N=422$) found that approximately 15% had a lifetime anxiety disorder diagnosis: 12% in men and 21% in women (Kidorf et al. 2004). In a sample of patients attending SUD treatment clinics ($N=260$), 80% had at least one co-occurring anxiety disorder, and presence of comorbidity was significantly associated with overall mental distress at the initial interview and 6 years later (Bakken et al. 2005).

Order of Onset

The order of onset of co-occurring disorders can help in understanding the etiological connections. Analysis of data from the National Comorbidity Survey–Replication (NCS-R) indicated that the typical age at onset varies among different psychiatric disorders, with anxiety disorders tending to have an earlier onset than mood disorders (Kessler et al. 2005). A review by Kushner et al. (1990) indicated that among individuals with co-occurring anxiety and substance use disorders, order of onset differs for different anxiety disorders. Social phobia, panic, and agoraphobia generally precede SUDs. Findings regarding the typical onset of generalized anxiety disorder (GAD) were less clear but suggested that GAD tended to develop near the same time as or after alcohol problems (Kushner et al. 1990). The same pattern of results was found in a later study of SUD patients in treatment (Compton et al. 2000).

TABLE 45–1. Prevalence of substance use disorders and anxiety disorders in people in the United States

	ECA (%) (lifetime)	NCS-R (%) (lifetime)	NESARC (%) (12 months)
Alcohol abuse	5.6	13.2	4.7
Alcohol dependence	7.9	5.4	3.8
Drug abuse	2.6	7.9	1.4
Drug dependence	3.5	3.0	0.6
Generalized anxiety disorder	–	5.7	2.1
Social phobia	2.8	12.1	2.8
Panic disorder			
With agoraphobia	0.5	1.1	0.6
Without agoraphobia	–	3.7	1.6

Note. Dash indicates data not available. ECA=Epidemiologic Catchment Area study (Regier et al. 1990); NCS-R=National Comorbidity Survey–Replication (Kessler et al. 2006); NESARC=National Epidemiologic Survey on Alcohol and Related Conditions (Grant et al. 2004).

Neurobiological Connections Between Anxiety Disorders and SUDs

A growing body of evidence indicates that abnormalities in common neurobiological pathways underlie the link between anxiety and addictions. One bridging construct involves the role of stress. Corticotropin-releasing factor (CRF), a key hormone involved in the stress response, has been implicated in the pathophysiology of anxiety, mood, and addictive disorders (Brady and Sinha 2005; Koob and Kreek 2007). Preclinical evidence suggests that CRF and noradrenergic pathways are involved in stress-induced reinstatement of drug-seeking behavior among drug-dependent laboratory animals (Piazza and Le Moal 1998). Similarly, emotional stress and negative affect states increase drug craving in drug-dependent humans (Sinha 2008). In animal models, early-life stress and chronic stress result in long-term changes in the stress response, altering the sensitivity of the dopamine system to stress and increasing susceptibility to drug self-administration (Meaney et al. 2002). In humans as well, there is evidence of the deleterious effects of early-life stress, childhood maltreatment, and accumulated adversity on alterations in the CRF and hypothalamic-pituitary-adrenal (HPA) axis (CRF-HPA), the extrahypothalamic CRF, the autonomic arousal, and the central noradrenergic systems (Sinha 2008). Current models of addiction and anxiety posit that aberrant functioning and remodeling of neuronal circuits involving brain systems mediating fear and reward underlie the pathological behavior. Thus, a disease-defining experience (i.e., drug reward or stress) triggers specific forms of synaptic plasticity that can become persistent in susceptible individuals and lead to disease. These circuits involve diverse brain structures, such as the amygdala, ventral tegmental area, nucleus accumbens, and prefrontal cortices, and have functionally diverse neurons, including glutamatergic/GABAergic (γ-aminobutyric acid), endogenous opiate, noradrenergic, neuropeptide Y, nociceptin, and oxytocin (Lüthi and Lüscher 2014). New techniques, such as optogenetics, allow more precise exploration of this circuitry and will hopefully lead to new treatment strategies in the future.

Diagnostic Considerations

One concern in the area of comorbid anxiety disorders and SUDs is accurate diagnosis and differentiation between drug-induced states of anxiety and primary anxiety diagnoses. Active use of certain substances (e.g., marijuana, stimulants) is associated with anxiety symptoms, and withdrawal from other substances (e.g., opiates, benzodiazepines) is marked by anxiety states. It is also likely that chronic use of substances of abuse, which have powerful effects on neurotransmitter systems involved in the production of anxiety disorders, may unmask vulnerability or lead to neurobiological changes that manifest as anxiety disorders.

The best way to differentiate transient, substance-induced symptoms from true anxiety symptoms is through observation during a period of abstinence. A key issue is the duration of abstinence necessary for accurate diagnosis. The duration of abstinence needed for diagnostic purposes will vary by diagnosis and by the substance being used. For long-half-life drugs (e.g., some benzodiazepines, methadone), withdrawal symptoms may be quite protracted, and several weeks of abstinence may be required for accurate diagnosis. For shorter-acting substances (e.g., cocaine, short-half-life benzodiazepines), the durations of acute intoxication and withdrawal are likely to be briefer, and it may be possible to arrive at a diagnosis after shorter periods of abstinence. In cases where the diagnosis remains unclear, the following factors weigh in favor of an anxiety disorder diagnosis: onset of anxiety symptoms before the onset of the SUD, positive family history of anxiety disorders, and sustained anxiety symptoms during lengthy periods of abstinence.

Because anxiety is commonly seen in association with substance use, any patient presenting for treatment of anxiety should be screened for alcohol and other drug use. Brief screening tools for SUDs that have demonstrated usefulness in psychiatric settings include the Alcohol Use Disorders Identification Test (AUDIT; Bohn et al. 1995), the Michigan Alcohol Screening Test (MAST; Teitelbaum and Carey 2000), and the Drug Abuse Screening Test (DAST; Maisto et al. 2000). It is important to bear in mind that caffeine and some over-the-counter medications (e.g., pseudoephedrine, diet pills) can cause substantial anxiety, and although the use of these substances in an individual case might not constitute substance abuse, decreasing their use may be of enormous benefit in decreasing symptoms of anxiety.

The remainder of this chapter is divided into sections that address individual anxiety disorders. For each disorder, the prevalence of comorbidity with SUDs as well as diagnostic and treatment considerations will be discussed. For many of the disorders discussed, few data exist. Relatively more studies have been conducted that explore the relationship between anxiety disorders and alcohol use disorder. In areas where data are lacking, relevant studies concerning alcohol and anxiety disorders will be cited, and general principles guiding appropriate clinical management of patients with comorbidities will be reviewed.

Psychosocial Treatments

Among psychosocial treatments, cognitive-behavioral therapy (CBT) has been shown to decrease both anxiety symptoms in individuals with anxiety disorders and relapse in individuals with SUDs. Techniques such as relaxation, coping skills, behavioral activation therapy, problem solving, and sleep hygiene can assist patients with both disorders (McKeehan and Martin 2002). Nutritional counseling and regular exercise may also be useful in helping individuals learn alternative strategies for coping with anxiety, but empirical trials are lacking. Associative learning and classical conditioning are involved in the linking of drug craving (in SUDs) or fearful responses (in anxiety disorders) with cues and contextual stimuli. *Extinction learning* is an active process that reduces the value or salience of these conditioned cues and contexts, and it can be effective in reducing cue- and context-induced symptoms in addiction and anxiety, thereby improving outcomes (Kaplan et al. 2011). Convergent neurobiological evidence documents the central role of the prefrontal cortex in extinction of conditioned fear and drug reward behaviors. Future studies focused on extinction training and targeting both SUDs and anxiety disorders are needed, and the use of pharmacotherapeutic agents to facilitate extinction training warrants further investigation.

Co-Occurrence of SUDs in Specific Anxiety Disorders

Generalized Anxiety Disorder

Epidemiology

Second to major depressive disorder, SUD is the most common comorbid psychiatric disorder among individuals with GAD. An epidemiological study of 5,877 adults found that GAD was the anxiety disorder most often associated with use of alcohol or drugs to alleviate (i.e., self-medicate) symptoms (Bolton et al. 2006). Similarly, data from the NESARC showed a strong association between 12-month prevalence of GAD and alcohol use disorder (OR=2.0) or drug use disorders (OR=4.5) (Grant et al. 2005). The presence of comorbid GAD is associated with an accelerated progression from first use to the onset of dependence. For example, in a study examining childhood risk factors predictive of alcohol use and dependence among 1,269 adolescents and young adults (mean age=20.1 years), Sartor et al. (2007) found that the presence of GAD was associated with a 3.5-fold increase in the rate of progression from first drink to the onset of alcohol dependence. Furthermore, the presence of comorbid SUDs has been shown to significantly reduce the likelihood of recovery from GAD.

Differential Diagnosis

GAD is particularly hard to diagnose in the presence of SUDs because every symptom of GAD can be mimicked by substance use or withdrawal. To help ensure accurate diagnosis, the assessment of GAD should be delayed until intoxication or withdrawal has terminated. As mentioned earlier, for short-acting drugs (e.g., cocaine), it may be possible to assess GAD after 1 week of abstinence, but longer periods of time (e.g., 4–8 weeks) may be required for longer-acting drugs (e.g., methadone, valium). DSM-5 (American Psychiatric Association 2013) requires that a core number of anxiety symptoms be present for at least 6 months in order to meet diagnostic criteria for GAD. Substance use during those 6 months must be considered, and symptoms of GAD must have been present during times other than when the patient was using or recovering from alcohol or drugs. This can be challenging to assess, because many SUD patients presenting for treatment and complaining of anxiety will not have had 6 months of abstinence.

A nosological issue concerning the diagnosis of GAD is whether the symptoms reflect a true anxiety disorder or are the result of other comorbid psychiatric conditions (Grant et al. 2005). Because long-term heavy use of alcohol and drugs can result in occupational, interpersonal, and physical health impairments, it can be difficult to discern whether the anxiety symptoms resulting from such impairments represent a true anxiety disorder. These are complicated and difficult issues to resolve. Consultation with colleagues on a case-by-case basis is recommended to design appropriate treatment plans. In addition, following the patient and reassessing the diagnosis of GAD is important. As the patient becomes abstinent and his or her functioning improves, the course of anxiety symptoms will provide useful information regarding diagnosis.

Pharmacological Treatment

The treatment of GAD in the context of addiction can be challenging. Although benzodiazepines are effective in the treatment of GAD, their use in individuals with current or previous SUDs is controversial because of their abuse liability. Some authors (e.g., Posternak and Mueller 2001) posit, however, that the empirical evidence regarding the dangers of benzodiazepine treatment in individuals with SUDs is insufficient and that benzodiazepines may be safely used to treat anxiety disorders in some SUD patients. Buspirone, a partial agonist at the serotonin (5-hydroxytryptamine type 1A [5-HT$_{1A}$]) receptor with low abuse potential, has been shown to be efficacious in alcoholic patients with anxiety (Kranzler et al. 1994), but findings have been inconsistent. For example, Malcolm et al. (1992) found no between-group differences in anxiety or alcohol use severity among patients treated with buspirone or placebo. A randomized trial of buspirone among anxious opiate-dependent individuals found that buspirone was associated with a trend toward improvement in depressive symptomatology and a slower return to substance use, but no significant improvements in anxiety symptoms (McRae et al. 2004). Clearly, more research is needed to help clarify buspirone's spectrum of efficacy, but there is some evidence supporting the use of buspirone in SUD patients with GAD. Selective serotonin reuptake inhibitors (SSRIs) are efficacious in reducing GAD symptoms; however, no clinical trials of SSRIs in individuals with comorbid GAD and SUDs have been conducted.

Summary of Comorbid SUDs in Generalized Anxiety Disorder

SUDs and GAD commonly co-occur; therefore, all patients with GAD should be screened for alcohol and drug use disorders, for subsyndromal use of substances to self-medicate anxiety symptoms, and for the use of caffeine or over-the-counter substances that can induce anxiety (e.g., diet pills). Identifying substance use as a coping strategy before it becomes problematic is critical, because GAD is associated with significantly faster progression from initial use to addiction and because once an SUD has developed, the likelihood of recovery from GAD is significantly compromised. Care should be taken in diagnosing GAD among individuals with SUDs, given that intoxication or withdrawal can mimic GAD symptoms. Findings regarding the use of buspirone treatment among patients with SUDs and GAD are mixed, but some support for its efficacy exists. SSRIs, which are effective in treating GAD, have not been explored in patients with co-occurring SUDs and GAD. This would be a worthwhile area for future investigations. More research on the use of benzodiazepines and on the development of psychosocial treatments is needed to advance the treatment of comorbid GAD and SUDs.

Social Anxiety Disorder (Social Phobia)

Epidemiology

Alcohol is the most commonly abused substance among patients with social anxiety disorder (social phobia); individuals with social anxiety are two to three times more likely than those without the condition to develop an alcohol use disorder (Kushner et al. 1990). Social phobia is also associated with illicit drug use, with ORs from community samples ranging from 1.6 to 2.3 (Sareen et al. 2006). In particular, complex social phobia (which involves fear and avoidance of multiple social situations, not just public speaking) was associated with increased drug use (Sareen et al. 2006). Consistent with the self-medication model, SUDs generally follow the onset of social phobia symptoms (Carrigan and Randall 2003). Many socially anxious individuals report consuming alcohol or drugs to help reduce fear of criticism or embarrassment (Carrigan and Randall 2003). In the NCS data, 16.4% of socially phobic individuals ($N=5,877$) endorsed self-medicating with alcohol and drugs (Bolton et al. 2006).

Differential Diagnosis

In contrast to other anxiety disorders, social phobia does not require a period of abstinence to be reliably diagnosed in a patient with SUD, for several reasons. Because the average onset of social phobia is before adolescence, symptoms of social anxiety are often present before the initiation of alcohol or drug use. Also, the cardinal symptom of social phobia, fear of public scrutiny, is fairly specific and is not mimicked by substance use and withdrawal phenomena. Social anxiety symptoms that arise only in the context of acute intoxication or withdrawal are not sufficient to meet criteria for a diagnosis of social phobia.

Pharmacological Treatment

Randall et al. (2001a) examined the effectiveness of paroxetine, an SSRI, in a placebo-controlled trial in 15 outpatients with alcohol dependence and social phobia. In comparison with the placebo group, the paroxetine-treated group showed significant reductions in social phobia symptoms at the end of the 8-week trial. Although no significant group differences in measures of frequency or quantity of alcohol use were seen, the authors found significant improvement in overall functioning, as measured by scores on the Clinical Global Index, in the paroxetine group (Randall et al. 2001a).

Gabapentin is an anticonvulsant agent with demonstrated efficacy in a placebo-controlled, double-blind trial for the treatment of social phobia (Pande et al. 1999).

This is particularly noteworthy because gabapentin has also demonstrated efficacy in the treatment of alcohol withdrawal (Malcolm et al. 2001), and gabapentin has limited abuse potential compared with the benzodiazepines. However, there are no controlled trials examining the efficacy of gabapentin in co-occurring social phobia and SUDs. Future directions in the treatment of co-occurring social phobia and SUDs should include further exploration of anxiolytic anticonvulsant agents.

Psychosocial Treatment

Several controlled trials have examined psychosocial treatment for co-occurring social phobia and SUDs. In 93 outpatients with social phobia and alcohol dependence, Randall et al. (2001b) compared the efficacy of a 12-week manual-based CBT for alcohol dependence alone with an integrated manual-based CBT for both disorders. The authors had posited that patients' exposure to feared social situations during early recovery may have led to increases in alcohol use to cope; however, contrary to this hypothesis, patients who received the alcohol-dependence-only treatment evidenced better outcomes than those who received the integrated treatment. This finding suggests that for patients with this comorbidity, it may be preferable to focus solely on the alcohol use during the early stages of treatment.

Schadé et al. (2004) randomly assigned 96 individuals with alcohol dependence and comorbid social phobia and/or agoraphobia to receive either relapse prevention alone or relapse prevention plus CBT for the anxiety disorder. The majority (89 of 96) of the sample had social phobia. Both groups were offered concomitant SSRI pharmacotherapy (fluvoxamine), but more than half of the participants (53%) refused it. Individuals who received the combined psychosocial treatment (for alcohol dependence plus anxiety) showed significantly greater improvement in anxiety symptoms than those who received treatment addressing alcohol dependence only. No significant between-group differences in alcohol use severity were observed, and the use of fluvoxamine did not predict improved outcomes for social phobia or alcohol use severity (Schadé et al. 2004).

Summary of Comorbid SUDs in Social Anxiety Disorder

Individuals with social phobia often use alcohol or drugs to alleviate their anxiety symptoms (i.e., self-medication). In the majority of cases, social phobia precedes the development of SUDs—thus, preventive efforts are critical. SSRIs show promise in the treatment of co-occurring social phobia and alcohol dependence, but further research is needed. Gabapentin has also been shown in separate studies to decrease symptoms of social phobia and alcohol withdrawal. Examination of gabapentin among patients with this comorbidity would be a useful next step. Studies comparing psychosocial treatments of SUDs only and combined treatments addressing both SUDs and social phobia have shown mixed results, and it remains unclear whether and for whom integrated treatments are superior to single-diagnosis treatments.

Panic Disorder and Agoraphobia

Epidemiology

In the NESARC study (Grant et al. 2004), panic disorder with agoraphobia was the anxiety disorder with the strongest association with SUDs. The 12-month odds of experiencing panic disorder with agoraphobia were 1.4 with alcohol abuse, 3.6 with alcohol dependence, 3.5 with any drug abuse, and 10.5 with any drug dependence (Grant et al. 2004). The 12-month odds of having panic disorder without agoraphobia were 0.8 with alcohol abuse, 3.4 with alcohol dependence, 1.6 with any drug abuse, and 7.6 with any drug dependence (Grant et al. 2004).

The NCS-R study also indicated that limited panic attacks, in addition to full-blown panic disorder, are significantly associated with SUDs (Kessler et al. 2006). Among respondents with panic disorder only, agoraphobia only, or their combination (n=3,604), 37.3% had an alcohol use disorder and 20.6% had an illicit drug use disorder. Among respondents with a history of panic attacks without the full disorder (n=5,172), 19.3% had an alcohol use disorder and 13.0% had an illicit drug use disorder, indicating significant risk associated even with subsyndromal symptoms (Kessler et al. 2006).

The relationship between nicotine use and panic disorder is particularly interesting. Prospective data suggest that smoking increases the risk for panic attacks and panic disorder, and panic in turn may increase the risk for nicotine dependence (Breslau et al. 2004). A review of longitudinal epidemiological data from the National Household Survey on Drug Abuse (now called the National Survey on Drug Use and Health) indicated that the risk for panic attacks was increased more than threefold among adults who had used cocaine (O'Brien et al. 2005). A review examining 20 studies to clarify any direct links between panic disorder and alcohol use disorder concluded that panic disorder and alcohol use disorder can precipitate one another. These findings were attributed to heritability of comorbidity, the pharmacological properties of alcohol that reduce subjective and physiological panic symptoms, and the tendency for heavy alcohol use to increase carbon dioxide sensitivity, perhaps increasing the likelihood of a panic attack (Cosci et al. 2007).

Differential Diagnosis

Panic attacks can occur in many other psychiatric disorders (e.g., other anxiety disorders, psychotic disorders) and the ability of some substances to evoke panic-like symptoms highlights the need for a careful differential diagnosis when panic attacks are reported. As previously noted, heavy alcohol use increases sensitivity to carbon dioxide, thereby increasing the possibility of a panic attack in heavy drinkers (Cosci et al. 2007). Because of noradrenergic stimulation, stimulant drugs can induce panic attacks that are not necessarily diagnostic of panic disorder but may develop into full-blown panic disorder over time. MDMA (3,4-methylenedioxymethamphetamine; "ecstasy") has also been associated with the development of panic disorder in some clinical case studies (Pallanti and Mazzi 1992). One of the primary points to consider in the differential diagnosis of panic disorder in the context of another mental disorder is whether the panic attacks are ever untriggered or unexpected. The diagnosis also requires persistent worry about having an attack and symptoms that cause significant distress or impairment in at least one area of functioning (American Psychiatric Association 2013).

Pharmacological Treatment

Clinical trials for the treatment of anxiety disorders, including panic disorder, generally exclude participants with active SUDs. Thus, to date, there are no pharmacotherapy trials for the treatment of co-occurring panic disorder and SUDs. SSRIs, however, are U.S. Food and Drug Administration approved for the treatment of panic disorder.

Psychosocial Treatment

Two treatment studies have investigated psychosocial treatments for panic disorder in individuals with a co-occurring SUD. Among alcohol-dependent inpatients with panic disorder (with or without agoraphobia), Bowen et al. (2000) compared treatment as usual for alcohol dependence with a CBT-oriented group treatment for panic disorder plus treatment as usual. Although the combined treatment group received an additional 12 hours of treatment, no significant differences between groups were observed in anxiety symptoms or drinking measures (Bowen et al. 2000). Moreover, both groups showed improvement on measures of anxiety and alcohol abstinence up to 1 year after treatment completion. Among the hypothesized reasons for these findings were resistance from inpatient staff to the CBT intervention, limited cognitive skills and motivation for engagement among patients, and the severity of symptoms associated with inpatient populations (Bowen et al. 2000).

In a study conducted in a partial hospitalization program for addictions, a group cognitive-behavioral intervention for co-occurring panic and alcohol dependence was developed and tested (Kushner et al. 2006). The integrated treatment model was added to treatment as usual in an intensive program. The treatment contained three modules—psychoeducation, cognitive restructuring, and exposure—and explicitly addressed links among patients' alcohol use, panic symptoms, and agoraphobia. Despite the small sample (N=48), participants who completed the additional panic treatment were significantly less likely to meet criteria for panic disorder at the 4-month follow-up. Although relapse rates did not differ, patients who participated in the integrated treatment had less severe relapses (i.e., fewer drinks and fewer drinking binges) (Kushner et al. 2006).

Summary of Comorbid SUDs in Panic Disorder and Agoraphobia

Panic disorder is strongly associated with SUDs. Individuals with panic disorder and agoraphobia appear to be particularly vulnerable to increased substance use. Because acute intoxication or withdrawal from some substances of abuse can precipitate panic-like symptoms, careful assessment of SUD patients is required. To date, no pharmacological trials and only two psychosocial studies have examined the treatment of comorbid panic disorder and SUDs. Studies of integrated CBT approaches have yielded mixed findings, and further study is necessary. Several medications, particularly SSRIs, have proven efficacious for the treatment of panic disorder and may be useful in patients with SUDs, but this needs to be systematically studied. The high prevalence of panic disorder and SUD comorbidity and the lack of tested treatments present a tremendous opportunity for growth in the development of treatments in this area.

Behavioral Addictions and Anxiety

Much attention has recently been focused on the area of behavioral addictions (e.g., pathological gambling, problematic Internet use and online gaming, compulsive sexual behavior, compulsive buying, and exercising) and anxiety (Starcevic and Khazaal

2017). Behavioral addictions are themselves a controversial construct, with symptoms that straddle impulse-control disorders and SUDs, and the quality of research in this area varies, suffering from various methodological limitations, including diverse diagnostic criteria and conceptual heterogeneity of most behavioral addictions. Nevertheless, most studies show a strong but nonspecific relationship between behavioral addictions and anxiety (Starcevic and Khazaal 2017). Behavioral addictions are clearly common, and as they become better characterized, it will be important to further delineate their relationship to anxiety and anxiety disorders, as this may influence treatment course and outcome.

Opioid Use Disorder and Anxiety

The United States is currently in the midst of an opioid epidemic. The rate of opioid overdose deaths quadrupled between 1999 and 2008 and continues to rise every year, with more than 72,000 lives lost to overdose in 2017 (Scholl et al. 2018). Thus, the relationship of anxiety to opioid use disorder (OUD) is of particular interest. Both basic science and clinical studies demonstrate that the endogenous opioid system plays a critical role in the neural modulation of anxiety, and the activation of the opioid system leads to anxiolytic responses in healthy subjects and those with anxiety disorders (Colasanti et al. 2011). In the NESARC study, anxiety disorders were identified in approximately 61% of opioid-dependent subjects (Conway et al. 2006), and all associations between OUD and specific anxiety disorders were significant and strong. Of interest, opioid withdrawal states are characterized by noradrenergic overactivity and anxiety, and panic attacks are not infrequent. These aversive symptoms of opioid withdrawal may be exaggerated in individuals with anxiety disorders and could contribute to escalation to compulsive drug use. It is particularly important to screen individuals with OUD for anxiety disorders and to aggressively treat the anxiety, as this may be critical to successful recovery.

Conclusion

Interest in the co-occurrence of anxiety disorders and SUDs has grown tremendously in recent years. Co-occurrence of these disorders is common and has a significant impact on prognosis and treatment. Furthermore, treatment of anxiety disorders may be associated with decreased substance use. Increasing evidence concerning the common neurobiology of anxiety and SUDs combined with the development of new methodologies that allow investigation of specific neural circuitry may lead to new therapeutic approaches. Although there are promising developments in both pharmacotherapeutic and psychotherapeutic treatments that provide cause for considerable optimism, much work remains to be done.

References

American Psychiatric Association: Diagnostic and Statistical Manual of Mental Disorders, 5th Edition. Arlington, VA, American Psychiatric Association, 2013

Bakken K, Landheim AS, Vaglum P: Substance-dependent patients with and without social anxiety disorder: occurrence and clinical differences. A study of a consecutive sample of alcohol-dependent and poly-substance-dependent patients treated in two counties in Norway. Drug Alcohol Depend 80(3):321–328, 2005 15964156

Bohn MJ, Babor TF, Kranzler HR: The Alcohol Use Disorders Identification Test (AUDIT): validation of a screening instrument for use in medical settings. J Stud Alcohol 56(4):423–432, 1995 7674678

Bolton J, Cox B, Clara I, et al: Use of alcohol and drugs to self-medicate anxiety disorders in a nationally representative sample. J Nerv Ment Dis 194(11):818–825, 2006 17102705

Bowen RC, D'Arcy C, Keegan D, et al: A controlled trial of cognitive behavioral treatment of panic in alcoholic inpatients with comorbid panic disorder. Addict Behav 25(4):593–597, 2000 10972451

Brady KT, Sinha R: Co-occurring mental and substance use disorders: the neurobiological effects of chronic stress. Am J Psychiatry 162(8):1483–1493, 2005 16055769

Breslau N, Novak SP, Kessler RC: Daily smoking and the subsequent onset of psychiatric disorders. Psychol Med 34(2):323–333, 2004 14982138

Carrigan MH, Randall CL: Self-medication in social phobia: a review of the alcohol literature. Addict Behav 28(2):269–284, 2003 12573678

Colasanti A, Rabiner EA, Lingford-Hughes A, et al: Opioids and anxiety. J Psychopharmacol 25(11):1415–1433, 2011 20530588

Compton WM 3rd, Cottler LB, Phelps DL, et al: Psychiatric disorders among drug dependent subjects: are they primary or secondary? Am J Addict 9(2):126–134, 2000 10934574

Conway KP, Compton W, Stinson FS, et al: Lifetime comorbidity of DSM-IV mood and anxiety disorders and specific drug use disorders: results from the National Epidemiologic Survey on Alcohol and Related Conditions. J Clin Psychiatry 67(2):247–257, 2006 16566620

Cosci F, Schruers KR, Abrams K, et al: Alcohol use disorders and panic disorder: a review of the evidence of a direct relationship. J Clin Psychiatry 68(6):874–880, 2007 17592911

Grant BF, Stinson FS, Dawson DA, et al: Prevalence and co-occurrence of substance use disorders and independent mood and anxiety disorders: results from the National Epidemiologic Survey on Alcohol and Related Conditions. Arch Gen Psychiatry 61(8):807–816, 2004 15289279

Grant BF, Hasin DS, Stinson FS, et al: Prevalence, correlates, co-morbidity, and comparative disability of DSM-IV generalized anxiety disorder in the USA: results from the National Epidemiologic Survey on Alcohol and Related Conditions. Psychol Med 35(12):1747–1759, 2005 16202187

Gurmankin Levy A, Maselko J, Bauer M, et al: Why do people with an anxiety disorder utilize more nonmental health care than those without? Health Psychol 26(5):545–553, 2007 17845106

Kaplan GB, Heinrichs SC, Carey RJ: Treatment of addiction and anxiety using extinction approaches: neural mechanisms and their treatment implications. Pharmacol Biochem Behav 97(3):619–625, 2011 20723558

Kessler RC, McGonagle KA, Zhao S, et al: Lifetime and 12-month prevalence of DSM-III-R psychiatric disorders in the United States. Results from the National Comorbidity Survey. Arch Gen Psychiatry 51(1):8–19, 1994 8279933

Kessler RC, Crum RM, Warner LA, et al: Lifetime co-occurrence of DSM-III-R alcohol abuse and dependence with other psychiatric disorders in the National Comorbidity Survey. Arch Gen Psychiatry 54(4):313–321, 1997 9107147

Kessler RC, Berglund P, Demler O, et al: Lifetime prevalence and age-of-onset distributions of DSM-IV disorders in the National Comorbidity Survey Replication. Arch Gen Psychiatry 62(6):593–602, 2005 15939837

Kessler RC, Chiu WT, Jin R, et al: The epidemiology of panic attacks, panic disorder, and agoraphobia in the National Comorbidity Survey Replication. Arch Gen Psychiatry 63(4):415–424, 2006 16585471

Kidorf M, Disney ER, King VL, et al: Prevalence of psychiatric and substance use disorders in opioid abusers in a community syringe exchange program. Drug Alcohol Depend 74(2):115–122, 2004 15099655

Koob G, Kreek MJ: Stress, dysregulation of drug reward pathways, and the transition to drug dependence. Am J Psychiatry 164(8):1149–1159, 2007 17671276

Kranzler HR, Burleson JA, Del Boca FK, et al: Buspirone treatment of anxious alcoholics. A placebo-controlled trial. Arch Gen Psychiatry 51(9):720–731, 1994 8080349

Kushner MG, Sher KJ, Beitman BD: The relation between alcohol problems and the anxiety disorders. Am J Psychiatry 147(6):685–695, 1990 2188513

Kushner MG, Donahue C, Sletten S, et al: Cognitive behavioral treatment of comorbid anxiety disorder in alcoholism treatment patients: presentation of a prototype program and future directions. J Ment Health 15:697–707, 2006. Available at: https://www.tandfonline.com/doi/abs/10.1080/09638230600998946. Accessed February 13, 2020.

Lai HMX, Cleary M, Sitharthan T, Hunt GE: Prevalence of comorbid substance use, anxiety and mood disorders in epidemiological surveys, 1990-2014: a systematic review and meta-analysis. Drug Alcohol Depend 154:1–13, 2015 26072219

Lüthi A, Lüscher C: Pathological circuit function underlying addiction and anxiety disorders. Nat Neurosci 17(12):1635–1643, 2014 25402855

Maisto SA, Carey MP, Carey KB, et al: Use of the AUDIT and the DAST-10 to identify alcohol and drug use disorders among adults with a severe and persistent mental illness. Psychol Assess 12(2):186–192, 2000 10887764

Malcolm R, Anton RF, Randall CL, et al: A placebo-controlled trial of buspirone in anxious inpatient alcoholics. Alcohol Clin Exp Res 16(6):1007–1013, 1992 1335217

Malcolm R, Myrick H, Brady KT, et al: Update on anticonvulsants for the treatment of alcohol withdrawal. Am J Addict 10(s1 suppl):s16–s23, 2001 11268817

McKeehan MB, Martin D: Assessment and treatment of anxiety disorders and co-morbid alcohol/other drug dependency. Alcoholism Treatment Quarterly 20(1):45–59, 2002. Available at: https://www.tandfonline.com/doi/abs/10.1300/J020v20n01_03. Accessed February 13, 2020.

McRae AL, Sonne SC, Brady KT, et al: A randomized, placebo-controlled trial of buspirone for the treatment of anxiety in opioid-dependent individuals. Am J Addict 13(1):53–63, 2004 14766438

Meaney MJ, Brake W, Gratton A: Environmental regulation of the development of mesolimbic dopamine systems: a neurobiological mechanism for vulnerability to drug abuse? Psychoneuroendocrinology 27(1-2):127–138, 2002 11750774

O'Brien MS, Wu LT, Anthony JC: Cocaine use and the occurrence of panic attacks in the community: a case-crossover approach. Subst Use Misuse 40(3):285–297, 2005 15776977

Pallanti S, Mazzi D: MDMA (Ecstasy) precipitation of panic disorder. Biol Psychiatry 32(1):91–95, 1992 1356491

Pande AC, Davidson JR, Jefferson JW, et al: Treatment of social phobia with gabapentin: a placebo-controlled study. J Clin Psychopharmacol 19(4):341–348, 1999 10440462

Piazza PV, Le Moal M: The role of stress in drug self-administration. Trends Pharmacol Sci 19(2):67–74, 1998 9550944

Posternak MA, Mueller TI: Assessing the risks and benefits of benzodiazepines for anxiety disorders in patients with a history of substance abuse or dependence. Am J Addict 10(1):48–68, 2001 11268828

Randall CL, Johnson MR, Thevos AK, et al: Paroxetine for social anxiety and alcohol use in dual-diagnosed patients. Depress Anxiety 14(4):255–262, 2001a 11754136

Randall CL, Thomas S, Thevos AK: Concurrent alcoholism and social anxiety disorder: a first step toward developing effective treatments. Alcohol Clin Exp Res 25(2):210–220, 2001b 11236835

Regier DA, Farmer ME, Rae DS, et al: Comorbidity of mental disorders with alcohol and other drug abuse. Results from the Epidemiologic Catchment Area (ECA) study. JAMA 264(19):2511–2518, 1990 2232018

Sareen J, Chartier M, Paulus MP, et al: Illicit drug use and anxiety disorders: findings from two community surveys. Psychiatry Res 142(1):11–17, 2006 16712953

Sartor CE, Lynskey MT, Heath AC, et al: The role of childhood risk factors in initiation of alcohol use and progression to alcohol dependence. Addiction 102(2):216–225, 2007 17222275

Schadé A, Marquenie LA, Van Balkom AJ, et al: Alcohol-dependent patients with comorbid phobic disorders: a comparison between comorbid patients, pure alcohol-dependent and pure phobic patients. Alcohol Alcohol 39(3):241–246, 2004 15082462

Scholl L, Seth P, Kariisa M, et al: Drug and opioid-involved overdose deaths—United States, 2013–2017. MMWR Morb Mortal Wkly Rep 67(5152):1419–1427, 2018 30605448

Sinha R: Chronic stress, drug use, and vulnerability to addiction. Ann NY Acad Sci 1141:105–130, 2008 18991954

Starcevic V, Khazaal Y: Relationships between behavioural addictions and psychiatric disorders: what is known and what is yet to be learned. Front Psychiatry 8:53, 2017 28439243

Teitelbaum LM, Carey KB: Temporal stability of alcohol screening measures in a psychiatric setting. Psychol Addict Behav 14(4):401–404, 2000 11130159

CHAPTER 46

Eating Disorders

Therese K. Killeen, Ph.D., A.P.R.N.
Timothy D. Brewerton, M.D.

Eating disorders are associated with high mortality rates and often go undetected and unaddressed, particularly when comorbid with other psychiatric disorders, including alcohol use disorder (AUD) and substance use disorders (SUDs). Eating disorders defined in the fifth edition of the *Diagnostic and Statistical Manual of Mental Disorders* (DSM-5; American Psychiatric Association 2013) include anorexia nervosa (AN), bulimia nervosa (BN), and binge-eating disorder (BED), as well as the two categories *other specified feeding or eating disorder* (e.g., atypical AN, subthreshold BN and BED, purging disorder, night eating syndrome) and *unspecified feeding or eating disorder,* which replaced the former *eating disorders not otherwise specified* category. Table 46–1 summarizes the essential features of the most common DSM-5 eating disorders.

Epidemiology

In a systematic review of the prevalence of DSM-5 eating disorders assigned by diagnostic interview in nonclinical female populations, lifetime AN rates ranged from 0.8% to 1.9%, the lifetime BN rate was 2.6%, and lifetime BED rates ranged from 3.0% to 3.6% (Lindvall Dahlgren et al. 2017). Higher rates of DSM-5-defined AN and BN were expected, as the new criteria had been broadened to be more inclusive. The one reported lifetime prevalence for males was 2.1% for BED (Lindvall Dahlgren et al. 2017). Although eating disorders primarily affect females, males are increasingly being diagnosed with eating disorders, particularly BED and other specified feeding or eating disorder. Males with eating disorders may not have the presentations typical in females, and eating disorder characteristics may not fit the conventional female diagnostic criteria (see Table 46–1). For example, males may idealize a muscular body shape rather than the thinness idealized by females (Murray et al. 2017).

TABLE 46–1.   **Essential features of the most common DSM-5 eating disorders**

Anorexia nervosa	Bulimia nervosa	Binge-eating disorder
Restricted energy intake relative to requirements, leading to significantly low body weight in the context of age, sex, developmental trajectory, and physical health	Recurrent episodes of binge eating (i.e., eating large amounts of food in a short period of time)	Binge-eating episodes with no evidence of compensatory behaviors
Restricting type (anorexia nervosa, restricting type [AN-R]): weight loss accomplished primarily through dieting, fasting, and/or excessive exercise	Recurrent compensatory behavior (i.e., self-induced vomiting; misuse of laxatives, diuretics, diet pills, or other medications; fasting; excessive exercise)	
Binge-eating/purging type (anorexia nervosa, binge-eating/purging type [AN-BP]): engages in compensatory behavior to prevent weight gain	Both binge eating and compensatory behavior occurring at least once a week for 3 months	Binge eating occurring at least once a week for 3 months
Intense fear of gaining weight/becoming fat	Feelings of loss of control during episodes	Feelings of loss of control during episodes
Disturbance in how body weight or shape is experienced, undue influence of body weight or shape on self-evaluation, or lack of recognition of the seriousness of low body weight	Undue influence of body weight or shape on self-evaluation	Feelings of guilt, shame, and self-disgust

Note. Not shown in table are two new DSM-5 categories—*other specified feeding or eating disorder* and *unspecified feeding or eating disorder*—that can be applied to cases in which eating disorder symptoms are present but do not meet full diagnostic criteria for any of the DSM-5 eating disorders.
Source. Data from DSM-5 feeding and eating disorders (American Psychiatric Association 2013).

Etiology

Etiology of Eating Disorders

Biological, genetic, and environmental factors play a role in the development of eating disorders. Identification of risk factors is important for targeted preventive interventions. Twin studies provide the strongest evidence for genetic heritability as well as for shared and nonshared environmental influences. Females are 3–12 times more likely than males to have an eating disorder, and heritability accounts for about 52% (range 39%–74%) of the variance in liability to eating disorders, with both AN and BN having high genetic heritability (Bulik et al. 2016). Nonshared environmental effects generally account for the remaining variance (35%–45%), whereas shared environmental effects tended to be very low or insignificant (Wade and Bulik 2018).

Research showing environmental influence on gene expression has also been studied in the development, exacerbation, and progression of eating disorders. In individuals with genetic vulnerability, environmental factors likely influence the development of eating disorders or eating disorder behaviors, possibly via epigenetic mechanisms (Rozenblat et al. 2017; Steiger and Thaler 2016). Positive influences and social support may diminish the likelihood of developing eating disorder behaviors in individuals with genetic vulnerability. Alternatively, negative events and influences such as parental divorce, dysfunctional family relationships, and peer pressure/teasing may unmask eating disorder behaviors in genetically vulnerable individuals. Identified phenotypes associated with the development of eating disorders include perfectionism (more specific to AN), obsessionality, high harm avoidance, body image dissatisfaction, idealization of thinness, negative affect, impaired interpersonal functioning, overeating, dieting behavior, and impulsivity (Hilbert et al. 2014; Stice et al. 2017). Multiple types of child maltreatment have also been shown to be associated with all types of eating disorders. A study of risk factors for eating disorders in a community sample of middle-aged women found that women who had experienced childhood sexual abuse were 3.8–4.7 times more likely than those who had not experienced abuse to develop a binge-eating/purging–type eating disorder (Micali et al. 2017). Other risk factors in this population were unhappiness in childhood and low paternal bonding. Additional contributory environmental risk factors reported to increase the likelihood of developing an eating disorder included childhood eating and digestive problems; disordered eating behavior (e.g., excessive dieting, fasting, pica); weight and shape concerns; adverse life events, including neglect and abuse; low self-esteem; and psychiatric comorbidity (Jacobi et al. 2018).

Sociocultural influences, including globalization, urbanization, and cultural transitions, have also been notably observed in the development of eating disorders. Over the last several decades, there has been an increase in the rate of eating disorders in non-Western countries. Idealization of thinness in social media likely affects individuals' views about beauty and the ideal body. Peer pressure, teasing, and stigma associated with being overweight or obese in childhood or adolescence have adverse effects on eating attitudes and behaviors (Pike and Dunne 2015).

Shared Etiological Influences for Eating Disorders and Other Psychiatric Disorders

Shared environmental influences for and genetic heritability of eating disorders and other psychiatric disorders have been explored for overlapping risk factors. There is a significant genetic risk overlap between AN and anxiety disorders, obsessive-compulsive disorder, major depressive disorder, and suicidality. The shared genetic risk association between BN and AUD/SUDs is significant, at 35%–53% (Wade and Bulik 2018). The shared genetic risk is higher in binge-type eating disorders that involve compensatory behaviors. Baker et al. (2017) suggested that the role of genetics in the association between eating disorders and SUDs may be better explained by symptoms than by diagnoses. For example, early-onset alcohol use has been associated with subsequent bulimic behaviors, specifically binge eating and compensatory behaviors (Baker et al. 2017).

Genetic variants in the dopamine and serotonin systems have also been implicated in the development of both eating disorders and SUDs (Frank 2014; Rozenblat et al. 2017). Serotonin is involved in mood, anxiety, aggression, and appetite regulation, whereas dopamine is involved in reward, food/substance intake, emotion, and motivation.

Comorbidity

Comorbidity in Eating Disorders

Anxiety and mood disorders are the most common co-occurring disorders in individuals with an eating disorder. Other disorders commonly comorbid with eating disorders include posttraumatic stress disorder (PTSD), AUD/SUDs, attention-deficit/hyperactivity disorder, oppositional defiant disorder, and cluster B and C personality disorders and their traits, especially borderline, obsessive-compulsive, and avoidant personality disorders (Pearson et al. 2014). Obsessive-compulsive disorder is highly comorbid with AN (Cederlöf et al. 2015). The prevalence of lifetime PTSD in representative samples of individuals with an eating disorder is between 24% and 45% (Brewerton 2018; Hudson et al. 2007).

Eating Disorder and Substance Use Disorder Comorbidity

A World Health Organization Mental Health Survey found lifetime rates of any SUD in individuals with BN and with BED of 27.5% and 23.7%, respectively (Kessler et al. 2013). Rates of comorbidity are highest among individuals with BN and those with the binge-eating/purging subtype of AN. A recent meta-analysis of SUD comorbidity among individuals with eating disorders found a 21.9% lifetime and 7.7% current prevalence (Bahji et al. 2019). Alcohol and tobacco were the most common lifetime comorbid substances, with prevalences of 20.6% and 36.1%, respectively. Individuals with BN and those with binge-eating/purging behaviors were more likely to have a lifetime comorbid SUD, indicating the associated difficulties in emotional regulation and impulse control seen in both disorders. Several studies exploring current SUD subtype prevalence found cocaine, cannabis, tobacco, and opioids to be the most commonly used substances among individuals with an eating disorder (Bahji et al. 2019). In a group of college women reporting illicit substance use, those with eating disorder pathology were more likely to use illicit stimulants for appetite suppression and weight reduction than women without eating disorder pathology (Bruening et al. 2018). A few studies have explored the relationship between opioid use disorder (OUD) and disordered eating behaviors. About a third of individuals entering a methadone maintenance treatment program reported loss of control related to eating (Goldschmidt et al. 2018), and another study found that men entering treatment for OUD were three times more likely than age- and body mass index (BMI)–matched control subjects without OUD to report binge eating and food addiction (Canan et al. 2017). PTSD is commonly comorbid with both SUDs and eating disorders (Brewerton and Brady 2014). Individuals with eating disorders have higher rates of trauma, particularly interpersonal trauma, in comparison with individuals without eating disorders, and this trauma may be a common mediating link between eating disorders and SUDs (Mitchell et al. 2012).

Longitudinal studies have shed light on the temporal relationship between eating disorders and SUDs. Lu et al. (2017) studied a community sample to determine the prevalence of illicit substance use (ISU), recurrent binge eating (RBE), and comorbid RBE and ISU and the temporal course of these behaviors over 6 years. From year 2 to year 4, individuals with baseline ISU were more likely to develop RBE alone or RBE with ISU, but those with baseline RBE either remained unchanged or remitted and were unlikely to develop ISU. This finding supports the idea that binge eating may be an alternative compensatory coping mechanism in the absence of substance use, but substance use is less likely if RBE remits. Franko et al. (2008) followed a clinical sample over a 9-year span. In this study, several factors were predictive of developing an SUD in individuals with AN or BN. Psychiatric hospitalizations and suicide attempts predicted a subsequent SUD for individuals with AN, whereas for individuals with BN, high severity of bulimic symptoms predicted onset of an SUD. For both BN and AN, having AUD predicted onset of an SUD. Mustelin et al. (2016) followed a large cohort of women with eating disorders (N=182) in five waves spanning more than 22 years. At age 16 years, women with a lifetime eating disorder were twice as likely as those in a non–eating disorder control group to report harmful drinking. At wave 4 (ages 22–27 years) and wave 5 (ages 31–37 years), the odds ratios were higher for problematic drinking (2.4 and 3.06, respectively) and for harmful drinking (defined as drinking to intoxication one or more times per week) (1.9 and 2.4, respectively). Interestingly, individuals who had recovered from eating disorders at the wave 5 interview were 2.0–2.4 times more likely to report problematic drinking, suggesting possible continuation of one reinforcing behavior in the absence of the other. This may also suggest that harmful drinking may be less likely to adversely affect recovery from eating disorders (Franko et al. 2008). However, the reverse may not be true, in that individuals with AUD or an SUD complicated by a untreated eating disorder may be less likely to recover.

Although food addiction is not a DSM-5 diagnosis, research on food addiction has been evolving over the past decade. The Yale Food Addiction Scale (YFAS), developed by Gearhardt et al. (2009), uses DSM SUD criteria to identify individuals with problematic eating behavior. The prevalence of food addiction (as measured with the YEAS) in a nationally representative sample (N=986) was estimated at 15%, with the highest prevalences found among underweight and obese individuals (Schulte and Gearhardt 2018). Obese individuals with BED are more likely to screen positive on the YFAS than obese individuals without BED. There is disagreement in the eating disorder field on the validity of the idea of food addiction (Hebebrand et al. 2014). The debate centers on whether food addiction represents a loss of control of eating, a response to the addictive quality of highly palatable foods, or both (Munn-Chernoff and Baker 2016). The hedonic properties of alcohol/drugs of abuse combined with loss of control over behavior play an important role in the development of SUD.

SUDs and eating disorders have a number of commonalities and differences. Both disorders are highly stigmatized, such that pathological behaviors are secretive, associated with guilt and shame, and self-destructive. Substances and/or food are used to "self-medicate" negative affective states. Individuals with SUDs often use certain addictive substances, and individuals with eating disorders use food in an attempt to cope with or relieve anxiety and stress (Brewerton and Brady 2014). When strong cravings or urges to binge-eat (eating disorders) or to use substances (SUDs) occur, eating or use can relieve tension (momentarily) and provide an escape, whereas re-sisting the urge to engage in these behaviors increases anxiety (Cook et al. 2014).

Pauwels et al. (2018) explored similarities and differences in maladaptive person-ality traits among different subtypes of eating disorders and SUDs in female patients. Similarities included insufficient self-control, indicative of impulsivity, in both the binge-eating/purging subtype of eating disorders (ED-BP) and SUDs but not in the restricting subtype of eating disorders (ED-R). Patients with an eating disorder scored higher than patients with an SUD on scales of defectiveness, social undesirability, fail-ure to achieve, and unrelenting standards.

Individuals with eating disorders experience consequences similar to those experi-enced by individuals with SUDs. Interpersonal and family relationships are strained, employment/academic pursuits are compromised, and overall quality of life is re-duced. Psychosocial and medical mortality/morbidity are also common sequelae.

An important differentiation between SUDs and eating disorders is the presence of weight and body shape concerns as a driving symptom in eating disorders. However, low self-esteem is common in both disorders, and body shape concerns are linked to low self-esteem (Grossbard et al. 2009). Low self-esteem associated with poor body image is a predictor of alcohol/drug use among female adolescents (Wu et al. 2014). Several studies have explored weight and body image concerns in women recovering from SUDs (Killeen et al. 2015). Warren et al. (2013) surveyed 297 women in treatment for SUDs on measures of weight-related concerns and associated eating disorder pa-thology. About 5% reported a history of a past eating disorder diagnosis, and another 18% reported eating disorder symptoms. The majority of women endorsed weight concerns (70%), and almost half (43%) of the women thought that weight gain could trigger relapse to drugs. Women with weight-gain relapse concerns were significantly more likely than those without such concerns to report body dissatisfaction and eat-ing disorder behaviors ($P<0.01$; medium to large effect sizes). Therefore, weight and shape concerns among patients in recovery from SUDs may trigger cravings that are satisfied by palatable food or by relapse to alcohol and/or drug use to avoid subse-quent weight gain.

Assessment of Eating Disorders

Although the prevalence of eating disorders in the general population is relatively low in comparison with the prevalence of SUDs, there are high rates of comorbid medical and psychiatric disorders among people with eating disorders that warrant early identification and treatment referral to optimize outcomes (Hudson et al. 2007; Powers and Cloak 2014). Eating disorders are often overlooked by SUD and medical treatment providers, and individuals may be more likely to present with eating dis-order–related medical complications than to present for treatment of an eating disor-der. Medical problems associated with an eating disorder can be life-threatening and can include malnutrition, dehydration, electrolyte imbalances, gastrointestinal com-plications, and metabolic and cardiovascular problems. Unfortunately, these patients may leave medical treatment without detection of the underlying eating disorder. Individuals with an eating disorder often present to mental health or SUD treatment programs for help with mood, anxiety, or behavioral problems. Comorbid disorders, including SUDs, are more likely to be screened for and treated in eating disorder programs than in other types of treatment programs (Killeen et al. 2011). In non-eating-disorder treatment settings, screening for and assessment of eating disorders, through use of a number of well-validated self-report questionnaires and/or interviews, can be part of the routine intake process.

The gold standard for assessment and most commonly used instrument for eating disorder diagnosis is the Eating Disorder Examination (EDE; Cooper and Fairburn 1987), which can be administered as either a clinical interview or a self-report questionnaire (EDEQ). The EDE uses a calendar prompt to collect data on the frequency and intensity of various eating-related behaviors over the previous 28 days. There are four subscales: dietary restraint, weight concerns, shape concerns, and eating concerns. Behavioral measures include frequency of binge-eating episodes and compensatory behaviors. In a meta-analysis of the psychometric properties of the EDE and the EDEQ, both instruments demonstrated good internal consistency, test–retest and interrater reliability, and construct validity. In addition, the EDE and the EDEQ modified for DSM-5 have demonstrated good diagnostic concordance (Berg et al. 2012).

The Eating Disorder Assessment–5 (EDA-5) is a newer semistructured interview developed with consideration of the DSM-5 feeding and eating disorder diagnoses (Sysko et al. 2015). The number of items varies and depends on the answers given, in that some endorsed items prompt more questions. Diagnostic agreement between the EDE and the EDA-5 was between 0.65 and 0.77. Sensitivity was between 0.65 and 1.0, specificity was between 0.83 and 0.96, and diagnostic accuracy was between 0.88 (other specified and unspecified feeding or eating disorders) and 0.90 (BED). An electronic format has also been developed for the EDA-5, which can reduce administrative time.

A number of other eating disorder assessments are available; examples include the Eating Attitudes Test (EAT), the Bulimia Test—Revised (BULIT-R), the Eating Disorder Diagnostic Scale (EDDS), the Eating Disorder Inventory (EDI), and the SCOFF (Sick, Control, One [stone; 14 lb], Fat, Food) questionnaire (Rodgers and Franko 2015).

Treatment of Eating Disorders

Practice guidelines for the treatment of eating disorders have been published (Lock et al. 2015; National Institute for Health and Care Excellence 2017). Treatment for eating disorders initially involves weight stabilization and management of medical problems associated with disordered eating behaviors. Goal weight attainment and medical stabilization are important initial targets for individuals with an eating disorder, particularly AN, in which starvation and malnutrition are life-threatening. Treatment outcomes associated with recovery from an eating disorder include remission of pathological eating behaviors and thought patterns (including body image concerns) and use of more adaptive coping strategies. Similar to treatment for SUDs, treatment for eating disorders is characterized by cycles of remission and relapse. Disordered eating behaviors such as the restrictive dieting seen in AN can be extremely resistant to treatment.

Psychotherapy

There are limited studies that address treatment for comorbid eating disorders and SUDs. The sequential treatment model, wherein the most problematic disorder is treated first, is more typical. However, evidence has shown that in SUDs comorbid with other disorders, an integrated treatment model is preferred. If left unaddressed, eating disorder symptoms may be exacerbated in recovery from SUDs, and substance use may become more problematic during eating disorder recovery. Cognitive-behavioral therapy (CBT) is an evidence-based therapy used in the treatment of both eating disorders and AUD/SUDs. The most widely used therapy for the treatment of eating disorders is CBT-BN, developed by Fairburn in 1981. CBT-BN has the greatest amount of evidence-based support and is considered the gold standard treatment. This manualized structured therapy consists of approximately 19 individual or group sessions that are implemented in stages. Over the years, CBT-BN has been enhanced (CBT-E) to improve outcomes and adapted to include AN and BED (Cooper and Fairburn 2011). CBT-E addresses the psychological and physiological aspects of pathological eating behaviors, as well as the mechanisms that maintain such behaviors, including low self-esteem, perfectionism, emotional dysregulation, and interpersonal problems (Fursland and Byrne 2015). Initial sessions are focused on establishing a regular eating pattern so that individuals gain a sense of self-control. For patients with AN, a 5- to 10-pound weight-gain goal that ensures medical stability, including normalization of gonadal hormonal function, is established. Therapeutically, food is considered "medicine" in that type of food, portion sizes, and timing of meals are monitored and titrated. The therapist and the dietitian work together with the patient to gradually introduce healthful foods or previously avoided eating situations through use of exposure techniques (Steinglass et al. 2014).

For patients with BED who are obese, the goal is to reduce or eliminate binge-eating episodes; there is less focus on weight reduction. Dieting is likely to perpetuate binge eating. Weight reduction may be addressed once the individual has better control over eating behavior. Self-monitoring of eating behavior and of emotional triggers for binge eating can inform patients about their specific eating and thought patterns and what changes are indicated. The therapist also encourages lifestyle changes, such as finding activities that can replace the reinforcement derived from food.

The percentage of patients treated with CBT for eating disorders who achieve long-term recovery (5–6 years) is estimated at 52% for AN and 55% for BN. However, rates of long-term recovery for patients with BED are variable and are more likely to decline with time, with reported rates ranging from 19% to 32% over 4–6 years (Smink et al. 2013).

Although CBT has been shown to be effective in both SUDs and eating disorders separately, its effectiveness in the comorbid population has not been established. Given the shared common relapse triggers (i.e., impulsivity, shame, guilt, denial, obsessive thinking, loss of control, dysfunctional thoughts, isolation, hopelessness, low self-esteem), an integrated CBT model would likely be the most helpful approach. Both substances and food are used for coping with negative emotions. Development of coping skills that can address both eating disorder and SUD behaviors may improve treatment outcomes. The high prevalence of PTSD in both SUDs and eating disorders suggests that integrated approaches addressing PTSD symptoms may be beneficial. Evidence-based integrated treatments are now available for SUDs and PTSD, but research is limited in eating disorder and PTSD comorbidity (Back et al. 2015; Brewerton 2018).

Dialectical behavioral therapy (DBT), another effective therapy commonly used for binge-type eating disorders, has the potential to be effective in SUD and eating disorder comorbidity (Federici and Wisniewski 2013). This skills training approach has the advantage of addressing common features of both eating disorders and SUDs, including impulsivity, emotional dysregulation, and poor interpersonal skills. One report indicated that DBT was effective for eating disorder patients with significant comorbidity, including SUDs and PTSD (Courbasson et al. 2012). A 3-month DBT skills training program for patients with alcohol dependence ($N=244$) reported that 73% of patients were abstinent at the end of treatment, mediated in part by improvements in emotional regulation (Maffei et al. 2018).

Motivational interviewing, an established evidence-based treatment approach for SUDs, is also effective in the treatment of eating disorders (Killeen et al. 2014). In this approach, the therapist helps the patient to identify important life goals and values and explores how current eating disorder behavior may be interfering with achieving these values. The goal of motivational interviewing is for the patient to resolve his or her ambivalence about behavior change. The therapist uses motivational interviewing skills to elicit "change and commitment talk," which is a precursor to actual behavior change.

Family inclusion is an important component of both SUD and eating disorder treatment, particularly for younger patients. Ideally, family support and involvement are essential to the recovery of all patients with eating disorders and SUDs at any age. Family approaches are considered vital evidence-based approaches for eating disorders, specifically AN (Murray et al. 2014). Common family goals are as follows: decrease risks related to dysfunction and enhance protective factors; promote/encourage expression of love and commitment toward the significant other, instill hope, and improve parenting and communication practices; change interaction patterns among family members and replace eating disorder and SUD behaviors with more adaptive ways of functioning; improve skills to assist parents/significant others in establishing clear benefits and consequences for positive/negative behaviors; and encourage interaction with peers who engage in prosocial behaviors and discourage interaction with nonsupportive peers.

Although SUDs and eating disorders are often comorbid, eating disorders are rarely identified and/or addressed in SUD treatment, and SUDs are rarely identified and/or addressed in eating disorder treatment (Killeen et al. 2011). Individuals with comorbid eating disorders and SUDs have a more complex clinical presentations, including life-threatening medical comorbidities, and lower rates of successful outcomes in comparison with individuals with either disorder alone (Franko et al. 2013; Harrop and Marlatt 2010). Although there are no evidence-based integrated models for co-treating eating disorders and SUDs, similar therapeutic approaches are used in the treatment of each disorder. Cognitive-behavioral treatment, motivational interviewing, and contingency management are commonly used in both disorders. In one study, a 12-week group intervention, Healthy Steps to Freedom, that addressed body image, weight concerns, and eating pathology was implemented in several SUD treatment programs (Lindsay et al. 2012). From preintervention to postintervention, women reported reductions in binge-purge behaviors, body dissatisfaction, and concerns that weight would trigger drug use (Lindsay et al. 2012). Greenfield (2016) developed a women's SUD recovery group manual that addresses common problems encountered by women in recovery, including disordered eating and weight and body image concerns.

Pharmacotherapy

Although psychotherapy is the treatment of choice for all eating disorders, several psychopharmacological agents have been shown to be effective in double-blind, placebo-controlled trials. Notably, in controlled studies, the efficacy of medications for the treatment of eating disorders is generally weaker than that of psychotherapy, and dropout rates are higher in pharmacological studies. The most efficacious agent in the treatment of AN is the antipsychotic olanzapine, which has been shown in several randomized controlled trials to facilitate weight gain and/or to reduce obsessional anxiety or ruminations (Brewerton 2012). It also may significantly alleviate symptoms of depression or other mood disturbances. A recent randomized placebo-controlled trial enrolled 160 patients with AN, who received either olanzapine (initiated at 2.5 mg/day for 2 weeks and titrated to 10 mg/day at 4 weeks) or placebo. At 16 weeks, patients in the olanzapine group had significantly increased their weight (increased BMI=0.259 kg/m^2 [SD=0.053] per month in treatment) compared with patients in the placebo group (increased BMI=0.095 kg/m^2 [SD=0.051] per month in treatment) (Attia et al. 2019).

Antidepressants have been efficacious in both SUDs and eating disorders in treating other comorbid conditions, including mood and anxiety disorders and PTSD. For the binge-type eating disorders (i.e., BN, BED), antidepressants (in particular, higher dosages of fluoxetine [i.e., 60 mg/day]) may be very helpful in reducing binge eating as well as associated comorbidity (Arnold et al. 2002). Despite the significant alterations in serotonin in AN, fluoxetine is not effective in the low-weight state, but once a patient's weight is restored, relapse may be significantly reduced with fluoxetine. However, there have been no pharmacological studies in patients with comorbid eating disorders and SUDs.

Several medications used to reduce consumption and craving in AUD/SUDs have shown efficacy in eating disorders, particularly when used to target food craving and binge eating. In a small randomized crossover study, baclofen, a γ-aminobutyric acid (GABA) agonist, titrated to 60 mg/day, was shown to reduce binge-eating frequency in patients with BN and BED (McElroy 2017). Naltrexone SR (32 mg), an opioid receptor antagonist used in the treatment of OUD and AUD, combined with bupropion SR (360 mg) has been approved by the U.S. Food and Drug Administration for weight reduction in obese individuals (Billes et al. 2014). Naltrexone-bupropion combination was compared with a comprehensive lifestyle intervention program in a large open-label randomized study exploring binge eating in overweight and obese individuals (N=242) (Halseth et al. 2018). At 26 weeks, 91% of the individuals treated with the naltrexone-bupropion combination (n=153) showed reductions in binge eating, compared with only 18% of the individuals enrolled in the comprehensive lifestyle intervention program (*n*=89). However, use of bupropion is contraindicated in individuals with BN because of a higher risk for seizures. A case report of a 46-year-old man with severe AUD and BED treated with naltrexone (100 mg/day divided into two doses) noted significant reductions in both alcohol cravings and binge eating (from 3–4 times per day to once per week) and a 3-kg weight loss over 4 weeks (Leroy et al. 2017). Acamprosate, an *N*-methyl-D-aspartate (NMDA) receptor antagonist medication used in the treatment of AUD, was found to be superior to placebo in reducing binge-eating frequency, food craving, obsessive-compulsive binge eating, and body weight in patients with BED (Amodeo et al. 2019). Although opioid agonist therapy (methadone, buprenorphine) for the treatment of OUD is not contraindicated in eating disorders, there are no studies that demonstrate any outcomes specific to eating disorders. When using maintenance medications for OUD in patients with co-occurring eating disorders, monitoring for prolongation of the QTc interval and hypotension is particularly important.

Anticonvulsants used for impulse-control deficits have been found to be useful in both eating disorders and SUDs. Topiramate, which has shown efficacy in reduction of alcohol and cocaine craving, was associated with weight loss and reduced binge-eating frequency in patients with BED (Amodeo et al. 2019). Topiramate has also been shown to enhance the efficacy of CBT in patients with BED (McElroy 2017).

Tobacco use disorder is one of the most common comorbid SUDs in persons with eating disorders. There is a high dropout rate in smoking cessation programs, secondary to weight gain after smoking cessation. Typically, smoking cessation programs using nicotine replacement therapy and behavioral counseling are the treatment of choice (Simioni and Cottencin 2016). Few studies have explored pharmacotherapy for smoking cessation in individuals with eating disorders alone or comorbid with AUD/SUDs. Because bupropion is contraindicated in individuals with BN, comparative studies using bupropion largely exclude patients with eating disorders. There are no studies on the use of varenicline in this population.

Conclusion

Eating disorders are serious, potentially life-threatening psychiatric disorders that are commonly comorbid with SUDs and other psychiatric disorders. Eating disorders comorbid with SUDs typically have a more complex clinical presentation than either disorder alone, including higher rates of morbidity and mortality. Although there is little research dedicated to treatment of comorbid eating disorders and SUDs, detection and treatment of the eating disorder may be necessary to improve SUD outcomes. Eating disorders and substance use disorders share common phenotypes, including impulsivity, low self-esteem, and negative emotionality. Food addiction, although not a DSM-5 disorder, may be linked to SUDs through similar effects on the brain reward systems of highly palatable food. Body image concerns have been found in women recovering from SUDs and may be a significant relapse trigger. Because of these similarities in the psychopathology of SUDs and eating disorders, integrated interventions that address both disorders are warranted.

References

American Psychiatric Association: Diagnostic and Statistical Manual of Mental Disorders, 5th Edition. Arlington, VA, American Psychiatric Association, 2013

Amodeo G, Cuomo A, Bolognesi S, et al: Pharmacotherapeutic strategies for treating binge eating disorder. Evidence from clinical trials and implications for clinical practice. Expert Opin Pharmacother 20(6):679–690, 2019 30696303

Arnold LM, McElroy SL, Hudson JI, et al: A placebo-controlled, randomized trial of fluoxetine in the treatment of binge-eating disorder. J Clin Psychiatry 63(11):1028–1033, 2002 12444817

Attia E, Steinglass JE, Walsh BT, et al: Olanzapine versus placebo in adult outpatients with anorexia nervosa: a randomized clinical trial. Am J Psychiatry 176(6):449–456, 2019 30654643

Back SE, Foa EB, Killeen TK, et al: Concurrent Treatment of PTSD and Substance Use Disorders Using Prolonged Exposure (COPE). New York, Oxford University Press, 2015

Bahji A, Mazhar MN, Hudson CC, et al: Prevalence of substance use disorder comorbidity among individuals with eating disorders: a systematic review and meta-analysis. Psychiatry Res 273:58–66, 2019 30640052

Baker JH, Munn-Chernoff MA, Lichtenstein P, et al: Shared familial risk between bulimic symptoms and alcohol involvement during adolescence. J Abnorm Psychol 126(5):506–518, 2017 28691841

Berg KC, Stiles-Shields EC, Swanson SA, et al: Diagnostic concordance of the interview and questionnaire versions of the eating disorder examination. Int J Eat Disord 45(7):850–855, 2012 21826696

Billes SK, Sinnayah P, Cowley MA: Naltrexone/bupropion for obesity: an investigational combination pharmacotherapy for weight loss. Pharmacol Res 84:1–11, 2014 24754973

Brewerton TD: Antipsychotic agents in the treatment of anorexia nervosa: neuropsychopharmacologic rationale and evidence from controlled trials. Curr Psychiatry Rep 14(4):398–405, 2012 22628000

Brewerton TD: An overview of trauma-informed care and practice for eating disorders. Journal of Aggression, Maltreatment and Trauma 28(4):455–462, 2018. Available at: https://www.tandfonline.com/doi/full/10.1080/10926771.2018.1532940. Accessed February 13, 2020.

Brewerton TD, Brady K: The role of stress, trauma, and PTSD in the etiology and treatment of eating disorders, addictions, and substance use disorders, in Eating Disorders, Addictions, and Substance Use Disorders: Research, Clinical and Treatment Perspectives. Edited by Brewerton TD, Dennis AB. New York, Springer, 2014, pp 379–404

Bruening AB, Perez M, Ohrt TK: Exploring weight control as motivation for illicit stimulant use. Eat Behav 30:72–75, 2018 29886378

Bulik CM, Kleiman SC, Yilmaz Z: Genetic epidemiology of eating disorders. Curr Opin Psychiatry 29(6):383–388, 2016 27532941

Canan F, Karaca S, Sogucak S, et al: Eating disorders and food addiction in men with heroin use disorder: a controlled study. Eat Weight Disord 22(2):249–257, 2017 28434177

Cederlöf M, Thornton LM, Baker J, et al: Etiological overlap between obsessive-compulsive disorder and anorexia nervosa: a longitudinal cohort, multigenerational family and twin study. World Psychiatry 14(3):333–338, 2015 26407789

Cook BJ, Wonderlich SA, Lavender JM: The role of negative affect in eating disorders and substance use disorders, in Eating Disorders, Addictions, and Substance Use Disorders: Research, Clinical and Treatment Perspectives. Edited by Brewerton TD, Dennis AB. New York, Springer, 2014, pp 363–378

Cooper Z, Fairburn C: The eating disorder examination: a semi-structured interview for the assessment of the specific psychopathology of eating disorders. International Journal of Eating Disorders 6(1):1–8, 1987. Available at: https://onlinelibrary.wiley.com/doi/abs/10.1002/1098-108X%28198701%296%3A1%3C1%3A%3AAID-EAT2260060102%3E3.0.CO%3B2-9. Accessed February 13, 2020.

Cooper Z, Fairburn CG: The evolution of "enhanced" cognitive behavior therapy for eating disorders: learning from treatment nonresponse. Cognit Behav Pract 18(3):394–402, 2011 23814455

Courbasson C, Nishikawa Y, Dixon L: Outcome of dialectical behaviour therapy for concurrent eating and substance use disorders. Clin Psychol Psychother 19(5):434–449, 2012 21416557

Fairburn C: A cognitive behavioural approach to the treatment of bulimia. Psychol Med 11(4):707–711, 1981 6948316

Federici A, Wisniewski L: An intensive DBT program for patients with multidiagnostic eating disorder presentations: a case series analysis. Int J Eat Disord 46(4):322–331, 2013 23381784

Frank GKW: The role of neurotransmitter systems in eating and substance use disorders, in Eating Disorders, Addictions, and Substance Use Disorders: Research, Clinical and Treatment Perspectives. Edited by Brewerton TD, Dennis AB. New York, Springer, 2014, pp 47–70

Franko DL, Dorer DJ, Keel PK, et al: Interactions between eating disorders and drug abuse. J Nerv Ment Dis 196(7):556–561, 2008 18626296

Franko DL, Keshaviah A, Eddy KT, et al: A longitudinal investigation of mortality in anorexia nervosa and bulimia nervosa. Am J Psychiatry 170(8):917–925, 2013 23771148

Fursland A, Byrne SM: Cognitive behavioral therapy for the treatment of eating disorders, in The Wiley Handbook of Eating Disorders. Edited by Levine JM, Smolak L. New York, Wiley, 2015, pp 771–787

Gearhardt AN, Corbin WR, Brownell KD: Preliminary validation of the Yale Food Addiction Scale. Appetite 52(2):430–436, 2009 19121351

Goldschmidt AB, Cotton BP, Mackey S, et al: Prevalence and correlates of loss of control eating among adults presenting for methadone maintenance treatment. Int J Behav Med 25(6):693–697, 2018 30259293

Greenfield S: Treating Women With Substance Use Disorders: The Women's Recovery Group Manual. New York, Guilford, 2016

Grossbard JR, Lee CM, Neighbors C, et al: Body image concerns and contingent self-esteem in male and female college students. Sex Roles 60(3–4):198–207, 2009 28959088

Halseth A, Shan K, Gilder K, et al: Quality of life, binge eating and sexual function in participants treated for obesity with sustained release naltrexone/bupropion. Obes Sci Pract 4(2):141–152, 2018 29670752

Harrop EN, Marlatt GA: The comorbidity of substance use disorders and eating disorders in women: prevalence, etiology, and treatment. Addict Behav 35(5):392–398, 2010 20074863

Hebebrand J, Albayrak Ö, Adan R, et al: "Eating addiction," rather than "food addiction," better captures addictive-like eating behavior. Neurosci Biobehav Rev 47:295–306, 2014 25205078

Hilbert A, Pike KM, Goldschmidt AB, et al: Risk factors across the eating disorders. Psychiatry Res 220(1–2):500–506, 2014 25103674

Hudson JI, Hiripi E, Pope HG Jr, et al: The prevalence and correlates of eating disorders in the National Comorbidity Survey Replication. Biol Psychiatry 61(3):348–358, 2007 16815322

Jacobi C, Hutter K, Fittig E: Psychosocial risk factors for eating disorders, in The Oxford Handbook of Eating Disorders. Edited by Agras WS, Robinson A. New York, Oxford University Press, 2018, pp 106–125

Kessler RC, Berglund PA, Chiu WT, et al: The prevalence and correlates of binge eating disorder in the World Health Organization World Mental Health Surveys. Biol Psychiatry 73(9):904–914, 2013 23290497

Killeen TK, Greenfield SF, Bride BE, et al: Assessment and treatment of co-occurring eating disorders in privately funded addiction treatment programs. Am J Addict 20(3):205–211, 2011 21477048

Killeen TK, Cassin SE, Geller J: Motivational interviewing in the treatment of substance use disorders, addictions, and eating disorders, in Eating Disorders, Addictions, and Substance Use Disorders: Research, Clinical and Treatment Perspectives. Edited by Brewerton TD, Dennis AB. New York, Springer, 2014, pp 491–508

Killeen T, Brewerton TD, Campbell A, et al: Exploring the relationship between eating disorder symptoms and substance use severity in women with comorbid PTSD and substance use disorders. Am J Drug Alcohol Abuse 41(6):547–552, 2015 26366716

Leroy A, Carton L, Gomajee H, et al: Naltrexone in the treatment of binge eating disorder in a patient with severe alcohol use disorder: a case report. Am J Drug Alcohol Abuse 43(5):618–620, 2017 28301250

Lindsay AR, Warren CS, Velasquez SC, Lu M: A gender-specific approach to improving substance abuse treatment for women: the Healthy Steps to Freedom program. J Subst Abuse Treat 43(1):61–69, 2012 22154034

Lindvall Dahlgren C, Wisting L, Rø Ø: Feeding and eating disorders in the DSM-5 era: a systematic review of prevalence rates in non-clinical male and female samples. J Eat Disord 5:56, 2017 29299311

Lock J, La Via MC; American Academy of Child and Adolescent Psychiatry (AACAP) Committee on Quality Issues (CQI): Practice parameter for the assessment and treatment of children and adolescents with eating disorders. J Am Acad Child Adolesc Psychiatry 54(5):412–425, 2015 25901778

Lu HK, Mannan H, Hay P: Exploring relationships between recurrent binge eating and illicit substance use in a non-clinical sample of women over two years. Behav Sci (Basel) 7(3):E46, 2017 28718830

Maffei C, Cavicchioli M, Movalli M, et al: Dialectical behavior therapy skills training in alcohol dependence treatment: findings based on an open trial. Subst Use Misuse 53(14):2368–2385, 2018 29958050

McElroy SL: Pharmacologic treatments for binge-eating disorder. J Clin Psychiatry 78 (suppl 1):14–19, 2017 28125174

Micali N, Martini MG, Thomas JJ, et al: Lifetime and 12-month prevalence of eating disorders amongst women in mid-life: a population-based study of diagnoses and risk factors. BMC Med 15(1):12, 2017 28095833

Mitchell KS, Mazzeo SE, Schlesinger MR, et al: Comorbidity of partial and subthreshold PTSD among men and women with eating disorders in the national comorbidity survey–replication study. Int J Eat Disord 45(3):307–315, 2012 22009722

Munn-Chernoff MA, Baker JH: A primer on the genetics of comorbid eating disorders and substance use disorders. Eur Eat Disord Rev 24(2):91–100, 2016 26663753

Munn-Chernoff MA, Grant JD, Agrawal A, et al: Genetic overlap between alcohol use disorder and bulimic behaviors in European American and African American women. Drug Alcohol Depend 153:335–340, 2015 26096536

Murray SB, Labuschagne Z, Le Grange D: Family and couples therapy for eating disorders, substance use disorders, and addictions, in Eating Disorders, Addictions, and Substance Use Disorders: Research, Clinical and Treatment Perspectives. Edited by Brewerton TD, Dennis AB. New York, Springer, 2014, pp 563–586

Murray SB, Nagata JM, Griffiths S, et al: The enigma of male eating disorders: a critical review and synthesis. Clin Psychol Rev 57:1–11, 2017 28800416

Mustelin L, Latvala A, Raevuori A, et al: Risky drinking behaviors among women with eating disorders: a longitudinal community-based study. Int J Eat Disord 49(6):563–571, 2016 27038220

National Institute for Health and Care Excellence: Eating Disorders: Recognition and Treatment (NICE Guideline No 69). London, National Institute for Health and Care Excellence, 2017

Pauwels E, Dierckx E, Schoevaerts K, et al: Early maladaptive schemas: similarities and differences between female patients with eating versus substance use disorders. Eur Eat Disord Rev 26(5):422–430, 2018 29882613

Pearson CM, Guller L, Smith GT: Dimensions of personality and neuropsychological function in eating disorders, substance use disorders, and addictions, in Eating Disorders, Addictions, and Substance Use Disorders: Research, Clinical and Treatment Perspectives. Edited by Brewerton TD, Dennis AB. New York, Springer, 2014, pp 107–126

Pike KM, Dunne PE: The rise of eating disorders in Asia: a review. J Eat Disord 3:33, 2015 26388993

Powers PS, Cloak NL: Medical complications of eating disorders, substance use disorders, and addictions, in Eating Disorders, Addictions, and Substance Use Disorders: Research, Clinical and Treatment Perspectives. Edited by Brewerton TD, Dennis AB. New York, Springer, 2014, pp 323–362

Rodgers RF, Franko DL: Screening for eating disorders: an updated guide, in The Wiley Handbook of Eating Disorders. Edited by Levine JM, Smolak L. New York, Wiley, 2015, pp 507–523

Rozenblat V, Ong D, Fuller-Tyszkiewicz M, et al: A systematic review and secondary data analysis of the interactions between the serotonin transporter 5-HTTLPR polymorphism and environmental and psychological factors in eating disorders. J Psychiatr Res 84:62–72, 2017 27701012

Schulte EM, Gearhardt AN: Associations of food addiction in a sample recruited to be nationally representative of the United States. Eur Eat Disord Rev 26(2):112–119, 2018 29266583

Simioni N, Cottencin O: Screening for eating disorders in outpatient smoking cessation: feasibility, pertinence, and acceptance of referral to specific treatment. Int J Eat Disord 49(11):1018–1022, 2016 27218668

Smink FR, van Hoeken D, Hoek HW: Epidemiology, course, and outcome of eating disorders. Curr Opin Psychiatry 26(6):543–548, 2013 24060914

Steiger H, Thaler L: Eating disorders, gene-environment interactions and the epigenome: roles of stress exposures and nutritional status. Physiol Behav 162:181–185, 2016 26836275

Steinglass JE, Albano AM, Simpson HB, et al: Confronting fear using exposure and response prevention for anorexia nervosa: a randomized controlled pilot study. Int J Eat Disord 47(2):174–180, 2014 24488838

Stice E, Gau JM, Rohde P, et al: Risk factors that predict future onset of each DSM-5 eating disorder: predictive specificity in high-risk adolescent females. J Abnorm Psychol 126(1):38–51, 2017 27709979

Sysko R, Glasofer DR, Hildebrandt T, et al: The eating disorder assessment for DSM-5 (EDA-5): development and validation of a structured interview for feeding and eating disorders. Int J Eat Disord 48(5):452–463, 2015 25639562

Wade TD, Bulik CM: Genetic influences on eating disorders, in The Oxford Handbook of Eating Disorders. Edited by Agras WS, Robinson A. New York, Oxford University Press, 2018, pp 80–105

Warren CS, Lindsay AR, White EK, et al: Weight-related concerns related to drug use for women in substance abuse treatment: prevalence and relationships with eating pathology. J Subst Abuse Treat 44(5):494–501, 2013 23107389

Wu CS, Wong HT, Shek CH, et al: Multi-dimensional self-esteem and substance use among Chinese adolescents. Subst Abuse Treat Prev Policy 9:42, 2014 25269693

CHAPTER 47

Attention-Deficit/ Hyperactivity Disorder

Timothy E. Wilens, M.D.

Tamar A. Kaminski, B.S.

An estimated 6%–8% of children (ages 2–18 years) in the United States are diagnosed with attention-deficit/hyperactivity disorder (ADHD), making this syndrome the most common neurobehavioral disorder presenting in childhood (Thomas et al. 2015). It is now widely recognized that ADHD persists into adulthood in one-half to two-thirds of cases (Wilens and Spencer 2010), with estimates from epidemiological data indicating that 4%–5% of adults struggle with ADHD (for a review, see Adler et al. 2015). ADHD is characterized by inattention and/or hyperactive and impulsive behaviors that are persistent across multiple settings to a degree that is inconsistent with developmental level and that give rise to social, familial, emotional, interpersonal, educational, or work performance difficulties. Compared with their non-ADHD peers, individuals with the diagnosis are also at increased risk for co-occurring learning disorders and psychiatric disorders, such as mood, anxiety, oppositional, conduct, and substance use disorders (for a review, see Adler et al. 2015).

Substance use disorders (SUDs) share many features with ADHD. SUDs commonly begin in childhood, with data suggesting onset before age 18 years in one-half of cases and onset by young adulthood in three-quarters of cases (Compton et al. 2007). Approximately 10% of adolescents have SUDs (Merikangas et al. 2010); among adults, epidemiological data show that 9.9% of adults have had a lifetime drug use disorder and 29.3% of adults have had a lifetime alcohol use disorder (Grant et al. 2015). Like ADHD, SUDs are considered to be chronic disorders with substantial individual, family, and public health consequences. Large-scale epidemiological surveys have linked SUDs to comorbid psychiatric disorders. Among mental disorders overlapping with SUDs, ADHD has been one of the most studied conditions, with evidence of bidirectionality (Charach et al. 2011; van Emmerik-van Oortmerssen et al. 2012; Wilens and Morrison 2011).

ADHD as a Risk Factor for Substance Use Disorders

Because ADHD first manifests in early childhood, by definition, it generally precedes substance use or SUDs. The chronological relationship between these disorders allows us to investigate ADHD as a risk factor for SUDs, and a large amount of evidence suggests that ADHD is associated with cigarette smoking and problematic substance use, as well as earlier initiation of substance use. In fact, a meta-analytic review reported that children with ADHD were 1.5 times more likely to develop an SUD and had a 2.4-fold greater risk of initiating cigarette smoking compared with their non-ADHD peers (Charach et al. 2011). Among youths with ADHD, cigarette smoking may be a marker for and/or may set in motion the later development of SUDs (Biederman et al. 2006; Molina et al. 2018). For instance, in one study among adolescents with ADHD, those who smoked cigarettes were significantly more likely than those who were nonsmokers to go on to develop SUDs (Biederman et al. 2006).

In the same way that ADHD is predictive of cigarette smoking, individuals with ADHD are more likely than their non-ADHD peers to begin drinking alcohol and smoking marijuana at a young age (Estévez et al. 2016). In a case–control study, Kousha et al. (2012) found that in comparison with their peers, adolescents with ADHD initiated cigarette smoking and substance use at an earlier age and developed abuse and dependence within a shorter period of time. Additionally, substance use in these adolescents with ADHD was both more severe (for cigarettes, marijuana, heroin, and benzodiazepines) and associated with greater functional impairment compared with substance use in their non-ADHD peers (Kousha et al. 2012). Estévez et al. (2016) reported similar findings in a sample of 5,677 Swiss men, in which ADHD was positively associated with the risky use of alcohol, nicotine, and marijuana as well as with the early initiation of use of all three substances. Additionally, an ADHD diagnosis was found to be a predictor of alcohol use disorder, cannabis dependence, and nicotine dependence (Estévez et al. 2016).

A history of ADHD has implications for onset and severity of SUDs; our group previously reported longer durations of psychoactive SUD and slower remission rates in adults with an SUD and ADHD in comparison with adults with an SUD without ADHD (Wilens et al. 1998). Similarly, others have found that an ADHD diagnosis in patients at an outpatient addiction treatment center was associated with earlier onset of SUD and multiple SUDs (Fatséas et al. 2016). These findings highlight the interconnected nature of ADHD, risky substance use, and SUDs, as well as the severity, complexity, and chronicity of SUDs.

Increased Rates of ADHD in Substance Use Disorder Populations

ADHD has been found in large numbers of both adolescents and adults with SUDs. Among adolescents (ages 12–17 years) with SUDs in a drug treatment program (N=4,939), between 61% and 64% reported six or more symptoms of inattention and hyperactivity and/or a diagnosis of ADHD (Chan et al. 2008). Similarly, in the Cannabis Youth Treatment Study, out of 600 adolescent participants who met DSM-IV (American Psychiatric Association 1994) criteria for cannabis abuse or dependence, 38% also met DSM-IV criteria for ADHD (Dennis et al. 2004). Although these findings vary greatly for a number of reasons (e.g., diverse criteria for ADHD, substance use severity, age groups), they consistently document increased rates of ADHD in adolescents with SUDs in comparison with the general adolescent population.

A similar pattern has been documented in adult populations. A meta-analysis conducted by van Emmerik-van Oortmerssen et al. (2012) reported that nearly one out of every four patients with an SUD met DSM-IV criteria for ADHD. On the basis of data from the International ADHD in Substance Use Disorder Prevalence (IASP) study, of 1,205 adults seeking SUD treatment from 10 countries, 13.9% met DSM-IV criteria for ADHD based on the Conners' Adult ADHD Diagnostic Interview (van Emmerik-van Oortmerssen et al. 2014). Notably, the IASP data were quite variable among countries, with rates of ADHD between 4% and 22% in patients seeking alcohol use disorder treatment and between 5% and 52% in patients seeking drug use disorder treatment (van de Glind et al. 2014). Even so, the underidentification of ADHD in the addiction treatment setting continues to be problematic, with some studies reporting less than 5% of adolescent substance users carrying a formal ADHD diagnosis in their medical record (McAweeney et al. 2010), suggesting the need for consistent ADHD screening in SUD populations.

Associations Between ADHD and Substance Use Disorders

Research suggests that the association between ADHD and SUDs might be due to a combination of developmental, behavioral, biological, and genetic factors (Table 47–1). From a psychosocial perspective, SUDs might be the outcome of the low academic performance, risky decision making, and social dysfunction highly correlated with ADHD symptoms. For example, individuals with ADHD often suffer from poor academic performance throughout the elementary school, middle school, high school, and college years, even with adequate intellectual capabilities (for a review, see Adler et al. 2015). Academic underachievement continues to be a risk factor for SUDs. It may also be that some individuals with ADHD are drawn to substance use as way to self-medicate in response to ADHD symptoms and/or the sequelae of ADHD (Mariani et al. 2014; Wilens et al. 2007).

A neurobiological link may exist between ADHD and SUDs on the basis of studies suggesting overlapping abnormalities in brain structure. In support of this finding, changes in the dopaminergic system and striatal involvement are also implicated in both disorders (van Wingen et al. 2013). More recently, Adisetiyo and Gray (2017) suggested that perturbations in the frontal/cortical oversight of the deeper limbic motivation-reward structures in ADHD patients might lead to dysregulation, resulting in greater risky substance use and SUDs.

Other factors that have been implicated in the link between ADHD and SUDs include familial contributions and prenatal exposure to parental substance use. Several studies have linked maternal smoking or other maternal exposure to nicotine to

TABLE 47–1. Overlap of attention-deficit/hyperactivity disorder (ADHD) and substance use disorders (SUDs) throughout development

Perinatal	⇒	Child (age 0–12 years)	⇒	Adolescent (age 12–18 years)	⇒	Young adult (age 18–26 years)	⇒	Adult (age 26+ years)
• Genetic and familial factors are associated with risk of ADHD and SUDs • Alcohol, nicotine, or illicit drug exposure in utero increases risk for ADHD • Symptoms associated with perinatal substance exposure may persist multigenerationally		• ADHD diagnosis is predictive of SUDs • ADHD (and psychiatric comorbidity) is associated with earlier onset of cigarette smoking, alcohol use, and marijuana use • Academic underachievement due to ADHD is associated with later SUDs • Earlier initiation of stimulant treatment for ADHD reduces risk of later substance use		• ADHD (and psychiatric comorbidity) is associated with earlier onset of cigarette smoking and substance use • Risky decision making, low academic performance, and social dysfunction in ADHD are associated with later SUDs • Pharmacotherapy for ADHD may reduce risk of cigarette smoking and SUDs		• ADHD is associated with cigarette smoking • ADHD is associated with more severe and chronic substance use and SUD • SUDs and ADHD worsen functional impairment • Individual may initiate "self-medication" of ADHD symptoms with substances		• Concurrent ADHD predicts path of more severe and chronic SUDs • ADHD treatment reduces risk of SUDs • Treatment of SUDs in patients in recovery decreases risk of ADHD and SUDs • Treatment of adults with ADHD + SUDs with higher stimulant dosages improves outcomes for both SUDs and ADHD • Earlier stimulant misuse is linked to higher risk for SUDs

ADHD in offspring (de Zeeuw et al. 2012). In a retrospective case–control study, individuals with ADHD ($n=280$) were 2.1 times more likely than control individuals without ADHD ($n=242$) to have experienced prenatal nicotine exposure (17% of ADHD case subjects vs. 7% of non-ADHD control subjects) and 2.5 times more likely to have experienced prenatal alcohol exposure (4% of ADHD cases vs. 2% of non-ADHD controls); these findings were unaffected by adjustment for familial ADHD and other psychopathology (Mick et al. 2002). Interestingly, Zhang et al. (2018) showed in animal models that exposure to nicotine in utero resulted in ADHD-like symptoms in the offspring that even persisted into the next generation of animals (McCarthy et al. 2018). Prenatal exposure to illicit drugs has also been found to be associated with an increased risk of childhood ADHD when other predictors of ADHD were adjusted for (Sagiv et al. 2013). These findings suggest that prenatal exposure to nicotine and other substances probably increases the risk of ADHD.

Co-Occurring Disorders as Mediators of ADHD and Substance Use Disorder Comorbidity

The connection between ADHD and SUDs has often been examined in the context of co-occurring disorders. Accordingly, it appears that patients with co-occurring SUDs and ADHD are more likely to present with additional co-occurring disorders, including antisocial personality disorder, borderline personality disorder, depression, anxiety, and hypomania (van Emmerik-van Oortmerssen et al. 2014; Wilens et al. 2005). Among boys diagnosed with ADHD in childhood, rates of conduct disorder have generally ranged from 25% to 30% (Molina 2011). On the basis of a meta-analysis by Lee et al. (2011), a few studies have suggested that the association between SUDs and ADHD may disappear after controlling for conduct disorder and other comorbid disorders. Findings from a meta-analysis by Serra-Pinheiro et al. (2013) suggested that ADHD does not show an impact on illicit substance use after adjustment for comorbid conduct and oppositional defiant disorders. However, other studies have found that ADHD and conduct disorder may interact to form an additive effect, conferring a higher risk for substance use when both disorders are present than occurs with either disorder alone. In a case–control follow-up study of ADHD, we reported that ADHD alone placed individuals at 1.6-fold increased risk for SUDs, whereas those with ADHD and concurrent conduct disorder at baseline had a 2.5-fold greater risk for SUDs (Wilens et al. 2011b). Hence, developmentally comorbid psychopathology with ADHD drives a higher risk for SUDs over the risk observed with noncomorbid ADHD. Therefore, when evaluating patients with comorbid ADHD and SUDs, clinicians must conduct a thorough assessment to look for other comorbidities.

Diagnosis of ADHD and Substance Use Disorders

Diagnostic clarity of ADHD can be challenging when individuals present with problematic drug or alcohol use; thus, it is important to conduct a thorough diagnostic workup that includes all aspects of the individual's life span course. Diagnosis of

ADHD involves review of past performance, testing results, and medical/neurological histories—and, if possible, use of standardized tools such as self-, parent-, or observer-completed ADHD rating scales (for a review, see Adler et al. 2015; Levin 2007). Notably, substance use may result in behavioral and functioning deficits that mirror ADHD symptomatology, such as withdrawal, hyperactivity, executive functioning impairment, and inattention. Additionally, active SUDs may exacerbate ADHD symptoms by as much as 30% (Wilens et al. 2011a). For transitional-age youth (individuals 16–26 years of age) with comorbid ADHD and SUDs, a careful assessment of the patient should include psychiatric, addiction, social, cognitive, educational, medical, and family evaluations. If possible, a period of abstinence or stable reduced substance use might be needed to clarify true ADHD symptoms and impairment.

A recent consensus statement on the treatment of comorbid ADHD and SUDs called for routine ADHD screening in SUD populations because of the consistent overlap between the two disorders (Crunelle et al. 2018). Screening for ADHD is generally not common practice in drug and alcohol treatment programs (McAweeney et al. 2010), even though SUD patients with comorbid ADHD have worse treatment outcomes and a higher risk of relapse compared with SUD patients without ADHD (Upadhyaya 2007). As a result of this lack of screening, the debilitating effects of ADHD are often overlooked, underappreciated, and unaddressed. An implementation study reported that challenges to recognition and treatment of ADHD in adults with SUDs include lack of validated ADHD instruments appropriate for use in SUD populations, lack of ADHD expertise in SUD treatment programs, and the potential for ADHD medication misuse (Matthys et al. 2014). Similar to the recommendations in our previous examination of this issue (Wilens and Kaminski 2018), Matthys et al. (2014) suggested an integrated approach to treatment of patients with comorbid SUDs and ADHD that includes both psychotherapy and medication.

Treatment Plan

Psychotherapy

Psychotherapy is often helpful for achieving stable low-level use of substances and/or abstinence that will enhance the efficacy of pharmacotherapeutics for ADHD. Interestingly, randomized placebo-controlled medication trials for ADHD and SUDs showing overall improvement in all groups for SUDs and ADHD often include adjunctive psychotherapies, a finding suggesting that use of structured psychotherapies may be related to response (Wilens and Kaminski 2018).

Our own group (Wilens and Kaminski 2018) recommends a psychotherapy regimen that implements motivational interviewing and/or motivational enhancement therapy to facilitate behavioral change and encourage patients to explore and resolve their ambivalence about making a change. Follow-up sessions might use standard cognitive-behavioral therapy (CBT) to help patients identify triggers for substance use, develop effective coping skills, and determine treatment goals. The remaining portion of treatment should then continue CBT, but with increased specificity to symptom reduction in either disorder.

CBT has demonstrated success in reducing ADHD symptom and SUD severity when the disorders are treated separately; however, research is still limited regarding the potential benefit of psychotherapy for individuals who have both disorders. Although implementing an adapted CBT is compelling, these findings suggest the need for further research on integrated CBT for co-occurring SUDs and ADHD, such as the protocol suggested by van Emmerik-van Oortmerssen et al. (2013), and on strategies for improving treatment adherence in these populations.

Psychopharmacological Interventions

Although medication interventions for ADHD have been shown to effectively reduce symptoms, improve daily functioning and quality of life, and result in long-term benefit (Adler et al. 2015), less is known regarding patients with both ADHD and active SUDs. Trials of atomoxetine have reported improvement in ADHD symptoms and reductions in the intensity, frequency, and duration of heavy drinking and cravings (but not relapse), but these studies targeted recently abstinent adults rather than adults with currently active SUDs (Wilens et al. 2008). Of interest, no clinically meaningful adverse effects were noted with atomoxetine in the context of heavy drinking (Adler et al. 2010). Studies of atomoxetine in adolescents with ADHD and current SUDs failed to show improvement in either the ADHD or the SUD (Thurstone et al. 2010).

Although outcomes of earlier studies of stimulant treatment of both ADHD and SUDs were generally not optimistic, it is notable that more recent studies employing higher stimulant dosages have resulted in improved outcomes (Konstenius et al. 2014; Levin et al. 2015), questioning the possible role of alterations to the dopaminergic system with current substance use that negates the effectiveness of more typical moderate, therapeutic doses of stimulants for ADHD. In a long-term follow-up naturalistic study among 60 male patients with ADHD and comorbid severe SUDs, the patients who received ADHD pharmacotherapy exhibited less frequent SUD relapses and compulsory care, while also being more successful in obtaining supportive housing and having a higher employment rate compared with the nontreated group (Bihlar Muld et al. 2015). In a well-conducted placebo-controlled study investigating the efficacy of 60 mg/day and 80 mg/day dosages of extended-release mixed amphetamine salts in adults with co-occurring ADHD and cocaine use disorder, more patients in the medication groups achieved at least a one-third reduction in ADHD symptom severity (Levin et al. 2015). In addition, rates of continuous abstinence and the odds of a cocaine-negative week were greater in the medicated groups. Konstenius et al. (2014) similarly found that incarcerated subjects with ADHD and amphetamine dependence who, upon release, received osmotic-release oral methylphenidate at a mean dosage of 108 mg/day had greater reductions in ADHD symptoms ($P=0.011$), more drug-negative urine tests ($P=0.047$), and better retention in treatment ($P=0.032$) than the placebo group over a period of 24 weeks.

Clearly, further understanding of the role of appropriate dosing of stimulants in the context of current or very recent SUDs is necessary. Moreover, Carpentier and Levin (2017) further emphasized the need to better account for various factors (e.g., ADHD severity, psychiatric comorbidity) in future studies to improve the ability to prescribe the most appropriate pharmacotherapy in clinical practice.

Early Pharmacological Treatment for ADHD and Risk of Future Substance Use Disorders

Although stimulant medications have a known potential for misuse, there is no evidence that stimulant treatment increases the likelihood of later SUDs. Several meta-analyses have found that stimulant treatment for ADHD had either a protective or a negligible effect on later SUDs (Humphreys et al. 2013; Wilens 2003). In a separate study, Lichtenstein et al. (2012) reported on 25,656 Swedish patients with ADHD from 2006 through 2009 in the largest study to date focused on long-term outcomes associated with ADHD treatment. They determined that during periods when patients received ADHD medication, compared with nonmedicated periods, there was a 32% and a 41% reduction in the criminality rate for men and women, respectively, with a significant decrease in drug-related offenses (a proxy for drug use disorders) specifically (odds ratio [OR]=0.6). Similarly, at the conclusion of a 3-year naturalistic follow-up of a 52-week methylphenidate trial, Ginsberg et al. (2015) reported that stimulant treatment was associated with reductions in ADHD symptoms, functional impairment, criminality, and substance misuse. In a review of 2,993,887 health care claims from U.S. patients processed between 2005 and 2014, Quinn et al. (2017) found that male patients had a 35% reduced likelihood of substance-related events (i.e., SUD-related emergency department visits) during the period they were receiving ADHD medication compared with periods in which they did not take ADHD medication, and 2 years after receiving medication, the odds of substance-related events were reduced by 19% (Figure 47–1). In a study using data from the self-report survey responses of 40,358 U.S. high school seniors participating in the Monitoring the Future study, McCabe et al. (2016a) found that patients who began ADHD treatment with stimulant medication at a younger age had a reduced likelihood of substance use in adolescence compared with patients for whom stimulant treatment was initiated later. In fact, youth who began stimulant treatment before age 9 years and who remained on long-term stimulant medication were similar to healthy control subjects in their substance use. These aggregate data, particularly in the very large, more recent claims data (see Figure 47–1) and the national survey and registry data, strongly support the conclusion that stimulant treatment of ADHD initiated at an early age and continued long term is associated with a reduced risk for subsequent substance use and SUDs.

Stimulant Misuse

Although stimulant medications are considered a safe and effective treatment for ADHD, a number of studies have documented notable rates of misuse and diversion among transitional-age youth (McCabe et al. 2016b). Rates of prescription stimulant misuse and diversion peak in late adolescence, with roughly one in six college students engaging in misuse (McCabe et al. 2016b). These rates are magnified among certain specific student populations, such as those attending competitive institutions and living in social fraternities and sororities, in whom a 2015 study found signifi-

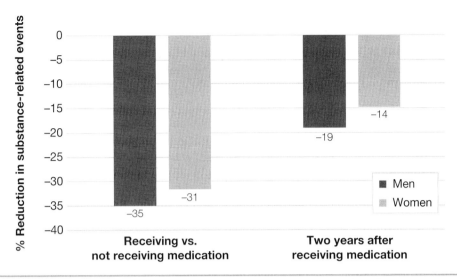

FIGURE 47–1. Pharmacological ADHD treatment and substance-related events.

Analysis of 2,994,887 health care claims from patients with attention-deficit/hyperactivity disorder (ADHD) between 2005 and 2014, using within-individual comparisons of risk of concurrent substance-related events during months patients were receiving stimulant medication or atomoxetine and months not receiving medication, as well as within-individual comparisons of risk of concurrent substance-related events 2 years after the medication period began, demonstrated reductions in both instances for male and female patients. *Substance-related events* included emergency department visits with a substance use disorder diagnosis.

Source. Based on data from Quinn et al. (2017).

cantly increased rates of stimulant misuse (Kilmer et al. 2015). Furthermore, youths who misuse stimulants report easily procuring stimulants for nonmedical purposes and report perceiving misuse as widespread and as not being associated with negative consequences for physical or mental health (Kilmer et al. 2015). Motivations cited by study participants for their stimulant misuse have consistently been found to include achieving better grades, increasing productivity, and self-treating subthreshold or undiagnosed ADHD (Wilens et al. 2016), which are not reasons commonly associated with risky use of alcohol or other drugs (Wilens et al. 2017).

In a controlled study of college students (N=298), we found that more than one-third of participants who reported nonmedical use of prescription stimulants met criteria for either a threshold or a subthreshold stimulant use disorder, and half met criteria for an SUD (Wilens et al. 2016). These data suggest that nonmedical stimulant use may not be an isolated occurrence or inconsequential scenario and more frequently occurs in individuals with SUDs (Arria et al. 2013). Peoples who misuse stimulants often have other mental and substance use disorders. Multiple studies have shown an overrepresentation of SUDs, depression, and neuropsychological dysfunction among individuals who misuse stimulants (Arria et al. 2013; Wilens et al. 2016, 2017). Hence, these individuals need to be evaluated for SUDs and other psychopathology, including ADHD.

Individuals who misuse stimulants also appear to be at heightened risk for longer-term adverse outcomes—even in adulthood. For instance, in a 17-year follow-up study using data from a Monitoring the Future national survey of 8,362 high school students, McCabe et al. (2017) found a higher likelihood of current substance use and substance-related problems in students who reported nonmedical use of stimulant medication in adolescence compared with students who reported either no use or only appropriate use of stimulant medication for ADHD.

If pharmacological treatment to control ADHD symptoms is indicated, providers should carefully consider the medication type and formulation. Given that the non-stimulants used to treat ADHD lack abuse liability, have demonstrated effectiveness in ADHD (and/or SUDs), and are effective in comorbid conditions, these medications are often the initial choice of treatment. Atomoxetine, bupropion, and tricyclic anti-depressants should be considered in adolescents and adults with ADHD plus SUDs. Stimulants continue to be the most effective class of agents used for the treatment of ADHD. If stimulants are prescribed, data suggest that extended-release preparations have a lower abuse liability (Spencer et al. 2006), even in placebo-controlled studies of adolescent and adult cigarette smokers and/or more severe SUD (Riggs et al. 2011; Winhusen et al. 2011). Given that recent data (Konstenius et al. 2014; Levin et al. 2015) suggest that higher stimulant dosages may be necessary to achieve symptom reductions in both ADHD and SUDs, practitioners should seriously consider prescribing relatively higher dosages for best outcomes.

Monitoring of pill counts, prescribing only the amount of medication necessary, providing instructions on safe storage (e.g., not in medicine cabinets), educating patients about ethical/legal issues surrounding misuse and diversion, and recognizing premature refill requests are suggested when prescribing stimulants. Close monitoring of substance use and of cravings and urges, as well as appropriate management of medication, is required when treating patients with comorbid ADHD and SUDs.

Conclusion

There continues to be a great deal of research regarding comorbid ADHD and SUDs, both in terms of how the disorders are linked mechanistically and in terms of prevention and the best course of action for treatment. Studies have shown that ADHD increases the risk of SUDs and that comorbid ADHD is present in 38%–64% of adolescents with SUDs (Chan et al. 2008; Dennis et al. 2004) and 4%–52% of adults with SUDs (van Emmerik-van Oortmerssen et al. 2014; van de Glind et al. 2014); however, most SUD populations are not screened or treated for ADHD. Early initiation of pharmacotherapy for ADHD reduces the future risk of both cigarette smoking and SUDs. In individuals with ADHD and current SUDs, clinicians should consider strategies that include structured psychotherapies, such as CBT, and pharmacotherapy, specifically nonstimulants and extended-release stimulants. More research on the mechanisms of overlap between the disorders, preventive effects of early ADHD treatment on SUDs, stimulant misuse- and abuse-deterrent stimulant preparations, and concurrent psychotherapeutic and pharmacological treatments for ADHD and SUDs are necessary.

References

Adisetiyo V, Gray KM: Neuroimaging the neural correlates of increased risk for substance use disorders in attention-deficit/hyperactivity disorder: a systematic review. Am J Addict 26(2):99–111, 2017 28106934

Adler L, Guida F, Irons S, et al: Open label pilot study of atomoxetine in adults with ADHD and substance use disorder. Journal of Dual Diagnosis 6(3–4):196–207, 2010. Available at: https://www.tandfonline.com/doi/abs/10.1080/15504263.2010.537224. Accessed February 13, 2020.

Adler L, Spencer T, Wilens T (eds): Attention-Deficit Hyperactivity Disorder in Adults and Children. Cambridge, UK, Cambridge University Press, 2015

American Psychiatric Association: Diagnostic and Statistical Manual of Mental Disorders, 4th Edition. Washington, DC, American Psychiatric Association, 1994

Arria AM, Wilcox HC, Caldeira KM, et al: Dispelling the myth of "smart drugs": cannabis and alcohol use problems predict nonmedical use of prescription stimulants for studying. Addict Behav 38(3):1643–1650, 2013 23254212

Biederman J, Monuteaux MC, Mick E, et al: Is cigarette smoking a gateway to alcohol and illicit drug use disorders? A study of youths with and without attention deficit hyperactivity disorder. Biol Psychiatry 59(3):258–264, 2006 16154546

Bihlar Muld B, Jokinen J, Bölte S, et al: Long-term outcomes of pharmacologically treated versus non-treated adults with ADHD and substance use disorder: a naturalistic study. J Subst Abuse Treat 51:82–90, 2015 25491733

Carpentier PJ, Levin FR: Pharmacological treatment of ADHD in addicted patients: what does the literature tell us? Harv Rev Psychiatry 25(2):50–64, 2017 28272130

Chan YF, Dennis ML, Funk RR: Prevalence and comorbidity of major internalizing and externalizing problems among adolescents and adults presenting to substance abuse treatment. J Subst Abuse Treat 34(1):14–24, 2008 17574804

Charach A, Yeung E, Climans T, et al: Childhood attention-deficit/hyperactivity disorder and future substance use disorders: comparative meta-analyses. J Am Acad Child Adolesc Psychiatry 50(1):9–21, 2011 21156266

Compton WM, Thomas YF, Stinson FS, et al: Prevalence, correlates, disability, and comorbidity of DSM-IV drug abuse and dependence in the United States: results from the national epidemiologic survey on alcohol and related conditions. Arch Gen Psychiatry 64(5):566–576, 2007 17485608

Crunelle CL, van den Brink W, Moggi F, et al: International consensus statement on screening, diagnosis and treatment of substance use disorder patients with comorbid attention deficit/hyperactivity disorder. Eur Addict Res 24(1):43–51, 2018 29510390

Dennis M, Godley SH, Diamond G, et al: The Cannabis Youth Treatment (CYT) Study: main findings from two randomized trials. J Subst Abuse Treat 27(3):197–213, 2004 15501373

de Zeeuw P, Zwart F, Schrama R, et al: Prenatal exposure to cigarette smoke or alcohol and cerebellum volume in attention-deficit/hyperactivity disorder and typical development. Transl Psychiatry 2:e84, 2012 22832850

Estévez N, Dey M, Eich-Höchli D, et al: Adult attention-deficit/hyperactivity disorder and its association with substance use and substance use disorders in young men. Epidemiol Psychiatr Sci 25(3):255–266, 2016 25989844

Fatséas M, Hurmic H, Serre F, et al: Addiction severity pattern associated with adult and childhood attention deficit hyperactivity disorder (ADHD) in patients with addictions. Psychiatry Res 246:656–662, 2016 27842945

Ginsberg Y, Långström N, Larsson H, et al: Long-term treatment outcome in adult male prisoners with attention-deficit/hyperactivity disorder: three-year naturalistic follow-up of a 52-week methylphenidate trial. J Clin Psychopharmacol 35(5):535–543, 2015 26284932

Grant BF, Goldstein RB, Saha TD, et al: Epidemiology of DSM-5 alcohol use disorder: results from the National Epidemiologic Survey on Alcohol and Related Conditions III. JAMA Psychiatry 72(8):757–766, 2015 26039070

Humphreys KL, Eng T, Lee SS: Stimulant medication and substance use outcomes: a meta-analysis. JAMA Psychiatry 70(7):740–749, 2013 23754458

Kilmer JR, Geisner IM, Gasser ML, et al: Normative perceptions of non-medical stimulant use: associations with actual use and hazardous drinking. Addict Behav 42:51–56, 2015 25462654

Konstenius M, Jayaram-Lindström N, Guterstam J, et al: Methylphenidate for attention deficit hyperactivity disorder and drug relapse in criminal offenders with substance dependence: a 24-week randomized placebo-controlled trial. Addiction 109(3):440–449, 2014 24118269

Kousha M, Shahrivar Z, Alaghband-Rad J: Substance use disorder and ADHD: is ADHD a particularly "specific" risk factor? J Atten Disord 16(4):325–332, 2012 22127397

Lee SS, Humphreys KL, Flory K, et al: Prospective association of childhood attention-deficit/hyperactivity disorder (ADHD) and substance use and abuse/dependence: a meta-analytic review. Clin Psychol Rev 31(3):328–341, 2011 21382538

Levin FR: Diagnosing attention-deficit/hyperactivity disorder in patients with substance use disorders. J Clin Psychiatry 68 (suppl 11):9–14, 2007 18307376

Levin FR, Mariani JJ, Specker S, et al: Extended-release mixed amphetamine salts vs placebo for comorbid adult attention-deficit/hyperactivity disorder and cocaine use disorder: a randomized clinical trial. JAMA Psychiatry 72(6):593–602, 2015 25887096

Lichtenstein P, Halldner L, Zetterqvist J, et al: Medication for attention deficit/hyperactivity disorder and criminality. N Engl J Med 367(21):2006–2014, 2012 23171097

Mariani JJ, Khantzian EJ, Levin FR: The self-medication hypothesis and psychostimulant treatment of cocaine dependence: an update. Am J Addict 23(2):189–193, 2014 25187055

Matthys F, Soyez V, van den Brink W, et al: Barriers to implementation of treatment guidelines for ADHD in adults with substance use disorder. J Dual Diagn 10(3):130–138, 2014 25392286

McAweeney M, Rogers NL, Huddleston C, et al: Symptom prevalence of ADHD in a community residential substance abuse treatment program. J Atten Disord 13(6):601–608, 2010 19365086

McCabe SE, Dickinson K, West BT, et al: Age of onset, duration, and type of medication therapy for attention-deficit/hyperactivity disorder and substance use during adolescence: a multi-cohort national study. J Am Acad Child Adolesc Psychiatry 55(6):479–486, 2016a 27238066

McCabe SE, Kloska DD, Veliz P, et al: Developmental course of non-medical use of prescription drugs from adolescence to adulthood in the United States: national longitudinal data. Addiction 111(12):2166–2176, 2016b 27338559

McCabe SE, Veliz P, Wilens TE, et al: Adolescents' prescription stimulant use and adult functional outcomes: a national prospective study. J Am Acad Child Adolesc Psychiatry 56(3):226–233, 2017 28219488

McCarthy DM, Morgan TJ Jr, Lowe SE, et al: Nicotine exposure of male mice produces behavioral impairment in multiple generations of descendants. PLoS Biol 16(10):e2006497, 2018 30325916

Merikangas KR, He JP, Burstein M, et al: Lifetime prevalence of mental disorders in U.S. adolescents: results from the National Comorbidity Survey Replication—Adolescent Supplement (NCS-A). J Am Acad Child Adolesc Psychiatry 49(10):980–989, 2010 20855043

Mick E, Biederman J, Faraone SV, et al: Case-control study of attention-deficit hyperactivity disorder and maternal smoking, alcohol use, and drug use during pregnancy. J Am Acad Child Adolesc Psychiatry 41(4):378–385, 2002 11931593

Molina BS: Delinquency and substance use in ADHD: adolescent and young adult outcomes in developmental context, in Treating Attention Deficit Hyperactivity Disorder: Assessment and Intervention in Developmental Context. Edited by Evans SW, Hoza B. Kingston, NJ, Civic Research Institute, 2011, pp 19-2–19-42

Molina BSG, Howard AL, Swanson JM, et al: Substance use through adolescence into early adulthood after childhood-diagnosed ADHD: findings from the MTA longitudinal study. J Child Psychol Psychiatry 59(6):692–702, 2018 29315559

Quinn PD, Chang Z, Hur K, et al: ADHD medication and substance-related problems. Am J Psychiatry 174(9):877–885, 2017 28659039

Riggs PD, Winhusen T, Davies RD, et al: Randomized controlled trial of osmotic-release methylphenidate with cognitive-behavioral therapy in adolescents with attention-deficit/hyperactivity disorder and substance use disorders. J Am Acad Child Adolesc Psychiatry 50(9):903–914, 2011 21871372

Sagiv SK, Epstein JN, Bellinger DC, et al: Pre- and postnatal risk factors for ADHD in a nonclinical pediatric population. J Atten Disord 17(1):47–57, 2013 22298092

Serra-Pinheiro MA, Coutinho ES, Souza IS, et al: Is ADHD a risk factor independent of conduct disorder for illicit substance use? A meta-analysis and metaregression investigation. J Atten Disord 17(6):459–469, 2013 22344318

Spencer TJ, Biederman J, Ciccone PE, et al: PET study examining pharmacokinetics, detection and likeability, and dopamine transporter receptor occupancy of short- and long-acting oral methylphenidate. Am J Psychiatry 163(3):387–395, 2006 16513858

Thomas R, Sanders S, Doust J, et al: Prevalence of attention-deficit/hyperactivity disorder: a systematic review and meta-analysis. Pediatrics 135(4):e994–e1001, 2015 25733754

Thurstone C, Riggs PD, Salomonsen-Sautel S, Mikulich-Gilbertson SK: Randomized, controlled trial of atomoxetine for attention-deficit/hyperactivity disorder in adolescents with substance use disorder. J Am Acad Child Adolesc Psychiatry 49(6):573–582, 2010 20494267

Upadhyaya HP: Managing attention-deficit/hyperactivity disorder in the presence of substance use disorder. J Clin Psychiatry 68 (suppl 11):23–30, 2007 18307378

van de Glind G, Konstenius M, Koeter MWJ, et al: Variability in the prevalence of adult ADHD in treatment seeking substance use disorder patients: results from an international multicenter study exploring DSM-IV and DSM-5 criteria. Drug Alcohol Depend 134:158–166, 2014 24156882

van Emmerik-van Oortmerssen K, van de Glind G, van den Brink W, et al: Prevalence of attention-deficit hyperactivity disorder in substance use disorder patients: a meta-analysis and meta-regression analysis. Drug Alcohol Depend 122(1–2):11–19, 2012 22209385

van Emmerik-van Oortmerssen K, Vedel E, Koeter MW, et al: Investigating the efficacy of integrated cognitive behavioral therapy for adult treatment seeking substance use disorder patients with comorbid ADHD: study protocol of a randomized controlled trial. BMC Psychiatry 13:132, 2013 23663651

van Emmerik-van Oortmerssen K, van de Glind G, Koeter MW, et al: Psychiatric comorbidity in treatment-seeking substance use disorder patients with and without attention deficit hyperactivity disorder: results of the IASP study. Addiction 109(2):262–272, 2014 24118292

van Wingen GA, van den Brink W, Veltman DJ, et al: Reduced striatal brain volumes in non-medicated adult ADHD patients with comorbid cocaine dependence. Drug Alcohol Depend 131(3):198–203, 2013 23726981

Wilens TE: Does the medicating ADHD increase or decrease the risk for later substance abuse? Br J Psychiatry 25(3):127–128, 2003 12975683

Wilens TE, Kaminski TA: The co-occurrence of ADHD and substance use disorders. Psychiatric Annals 48:328–332, 2018. Available at: https://www.healio.com/psychiatry/journals/psycann/2018-7-48-7/%7Be07b328f-5cef-4334-9ba1-4eec9eadf23e%7D/the-co-occurrence-of-adhd-and-substance-use-disorders. Accessed February 13, 2020.

Wilens TE, Morrison NR: The intersection of attention-deficit/hyperactivity disorder and substance abuse. Curr Opin Psychiatry 24(4):280–285, 2011 21483267

Wilens TE, Spencer TJ: Understanding attention-deficit/hyperactivity disorder from childhood to adulthood. Postgrad Med 122(5):97–109, 2010 20861593

Wilens TE, Biederman J, Mick E: Does ADHD affect the course of substance abuse? Findings from a sample of adults with and without ADHD. Am J Addict 7(2):156–163, 1998 9598219

Wilens TE, Kwon A, Tanguay S, et al: Characteristics of adults with attention deficit hyperactivity disorder plus substance use disorder: the role of psychiatric comorbidity. Am J Addict 14(4):319–327, 2005 16188712

Wilens TE, Adamson J, Sgambati S, et al: Do individuals with ADHD self-medicate with ciga-
    rettes and substances of abuse? Results from a controlled family study of ADHD. Am J Ad-
    dict 16 (suppl 1):14–21, quiz 22–23, 2007 17453603

Wilens TE, Adler LA, Weiss MD, et al: Atomoxetine treatment of adults with ADHD and co-
    morbid alcohol use disorders. Drug Alcohol Depend 96(1–2):145–154, 2008 18403134

Wilens TE, Adler LA, Tanaka Y, et al: Correlates of alcohol use in adults with ADHD and co-
    morbid alcohol use disorders: exploratory analysis of a placebo-controlled trial of atomox-
    etine. Curr Med Res Opin 27(12):2309–2320, 2011a 22029549

Wilens TE, Martelon M, Joshi G, et al: Does ADHD predict substance-use disorders? A 10-year
    follow-up study of young adults with ADHD. J Am Acad Child Adolesc Psychiatry
    50(6):543–553, 2011b 21621138

Wilens T, Zulauf C, Martelon M, et al: Nonmedical stimulant use in college students: associa-
    tion with attention-deficit/hyperactivity disorder and other disorders. J Clin Psychiatry
    77(7):940–947, 2016 27464314

Wilens TE, Carrellas NW, Martelon M, et al: Neuropsychological functioning in college stu-
    dents who misuse prescription stimulants. Am J Addict 26(4):379–387, 2017 28494131

Winhusen TM, Lewis DF, Riggs PD, et al: Subjective effects, misuse, and adverse effects of os-
    motic-release methylphenidate treatment in adolescent substance abusers with attention-
    deficit/hyperactivity disorder. J Child Adolesc Psychopharmacol 21(5):455–463, 2011
    22040190

Zhang L, Spencer TJ, Biederman J, et al: Attention and working memory deficits in a perinatal
    nicotine exposure mouse model. PLoS One 13(5):e0198064, 2018 29795664

CHAPTER 48

Trauma- and Stressor-Related Disorders

Skye Fitzpatrick, Ph.D.

Amber Jarnecke, Ph.D.

Sudie Back, Ph.D.

Elizabeth Straus, Ph.D.

Sonya Norman, Ph.D.

Denise A. Hien, Ph.D.

A convergence of epidemiological, clinical, genetic, and neurobiological research has led to increased recognition of the co-occurrence of substance use disorders (SUDs), including alcohol use disorder (AUD), with traumatic stress and related posttraumatic stress disorder (PTSD) (e.g., Norman et al. 2012; Smith and Randall 2012). PTSD and trauma exposure are highly prevalent among individuals receiving treatment for SUDs; in one study involving 423 patients with SUDs, 36.6% scored positive for current PTSD, and 97.4% reported having been exposed to trauma at some point in their lives (Gielen et al. 2012). Shared mechanisms underlie both sets of conditions, such as dysregulation in neural circuitry, neurotransmitters, and noradrenergic sensitivities, including hypothalamic-pituitary-adrenal axis dysregulation as well as genetic factors (e.g., Norman et al. 2012; Sartor et al. 2011). Clinically, patients with comorbid PTSD and SUDs typically have a poor course of treatment, including higher rates of dropout; more clinically severe consequences, such as suicidal ideation and attempts; higher rates of additional comorbidities (e.g., depression, anxiety, psychotic symptoms, medical problems); greater need for multiple medications; and more difficulty maintaining abstinence (e.g., Smith and Randall 2012). In a maladaptive, reciprocally reinforcing process, PTSD symptoms can trigger substance use or misuse, which leads to cyclical increases in PTSD symptoms (e.g., Back et al. 2006; Hien et al. 2010). Because causal relationships and mechanisms have been identified between

PTSD and the development of SUDs, treatment of PTSD may help these patients to achieve abstinence and maintain recovery (Back et al. 2006; Hien et al. 2010). In this chapter, we highlight the importance of proper diagnostic and treatment strategies for individuals who present with a trauma history and PTSD in substance use treatment settings.

Posttraumatic Stress Disorder Diagnosis

PTSD first appeared in the *Diagnostic and Statistical Manual of Mental Disorders* in its third edition, released in 1980 (DSM-III; American Psychiatric Association 1980). Since that time, the criteria for and symptoms of PTSD have undergone several modifications. The most recent DSM edition (DSM-5) defines a qualifying traumatic event as "exposure to actual or threatened death, serious injury, or sexual violence" (American Psychiatric Association 2013, p. 271). Exposure to a traumatic event may take the form of directly experiencing it, witnessing it in person, learning that a relative or close friend was exposed to the event, or experiencing exposure to aversive details of the event (e.g., in professional duties as a military service member or first responder).

An individual meeting criteria for PTSD also must endorse symptoms within each of the four clusters. *Reexperiencing* includes unwanted memories of the events, nightmares, flashbacks, and emotional or physiological distress when reminded of the trauma. *Avoidance* refers to avoiding trauma-related thoughts, feelings, or reminders. *Negative thoughts or feelings* may include inability to recall aspects of the traumatic event, negative thoughts about oneself or the world, exaggerated blame of self or others for the trauma, negative affect, decreased interest in significant activities, feeling isolated, and difficulty experiencing positive emotions. *Alterations in arousal* involve irritability or aggression, reckless behavior, hypervigilance, heightened startle response, difficulty concentrating, and difficulty sleeping. The symptoms must cause significant distress and impairment; must not be associated with medication, substance use, or illness; and must be present for more than 1 month. PTSD diagnoses also may include a dissociative specifier (i.e., indicating that the individual experiences high levels of trauma-related depersonalization or derealization) and a delayed specifier (i.e., indicating that full diagnostic criteria were not met until at least 6 months posttrauma).

Posttraumatic Stress Disorder Assessment

A thorough evaluation of trauma exposure and related symptoms is crucial to the accurate diagnosis and treatment of PTSD. Assessment of PTSD may involve multiple steps, including screening, diagnostic interview, and self-report questionnaires. Several assessment tools that are aligned with current DSM-5 criteria have been developed to facilitate diagnosis and monitoring of PTSD in adults (Table 48–1). Screening tools typically assess exposure to traumatic events or PTSD symptoms. Structured clinical interviews help determine whether an individual meets diagnostic criteria for PTSD. The Clinician-Administered PTSD Scale for DSM-5 is the gold standard for

PTSD assessment and has excellent psychometric properties (Weathers et al. 2013a); however, the interview does not assess for psychiatric comorbidities, such as SUDs. The Structured Clinical Interview for DSM-5 also has excellent psychometric properties and can be used for assessing a range of psychiatric disorders in addition to PTSD (First et al. 2016). Self-report questionnaires can aid in evaluating symptom severity and treatment progress. The most commonly used measures include the PTSD Checklist for DSM-5 (Weathers et al. 2013b) and the Posttraumatic Diagnostic Scale for DSM-5 (Foa et al. 2016a).

Effect of Posttraumatic Stress Disorder on Substance Use Disorder and Vice Versa

There are associations between the symptoms and the consequences of PTSD and SUDs. For instance, intoxication and withdrawal from a substance can mimic PTSD symptoms such as sleep disturbance, irritability, concentration difficulties, social withdrawal, lack of interest, and feeling socially disconnected. Given the overlap between PTSD and substance use, an individual's particular constellation of PTSD symptoms may affect his or her drug of choice, because substances can differentially alleviate PTSD symptoms through their mechanism of action (e.g., stimulating or depressing the central nervous system). One study found that individuals with greater arousal symptoms were more likely to use alcohol, whereas those with more severe avoidance and reexperiencing symptoms were more likely to use cocaine (Saladin et al. 1995). Another investigation suggested that individuals with more severe arousal symptoms and less severe avoidance symptoms had a greater likelihood of having an opioid use disorder, as compared with an alcohol or cocaine use disorder (Tull et al. 2010). PTSD symptoms and severity are also associated with substance use severity in comorbid populations. For instance, veterans with more reexperiencing, negative thoughts and feelings, and arousal reported more severe alcohol misuse (Walton et al. 2018). Together, these findings point to the importance of understanding the severity and heterogeneity of PTSD in SUD populations.

Differential Diagnosis and Key Comorbidities for Individuals With Posttraumatic Stress Disorder and Substance Use Disorders

PTSD and SUDs commonly co-occur with other psychiatric disorders—in particular, major depressive disorder and anxiety disorders (e.g., Gielen et al. 2012; McGovern et al. 2015; Ruglass et al. 2017). One concern with these comorbidities is accurate diagnosis and differentiation between substance-induced symptoms or states and primary depressive or anxiety disorders. The chronic use of alcohol and illicit drugs can have profound effects on neurotransmitter systems involved in regulating mood and affect and may either unmask vulnerability or facilitate neurobiological changes that manifest as depression or anxiety. For example, use of stimulants is associated with in-

TABLE 48–1.   Selected posttraumatic stress disorder (PTSD) assessment measures for adults

Assessment measure	Number of items	Features assessed	Reference
Screening measures			
Primary Care PTSD Screen for DSM-5	5	Effect of trauma over the past month	Prins et al. 2016
Stressful Life Events Screening Questionnaire	13	Frequency/duration of trauma and associated injuries	Goodman et al. 1998
Traumatic Life Events Questionnaire	23	Adulthood trauma exposure	Kubany et al. 2000
Short Posttraumatic Stress Disorder Rating Interview	8	Core symptoms of PTSD	Connor and Davidson 2001
Brief Trauma Questionnaire	10	Trauma exposure	Schnurr et al. 2002
Trauma History Screen	14	Frequency; contextual, subjective details of trauma	Carlson et al. 2011
Trauma History Questionnaire	24	Frequency of trauma and age(s) of trauma exposure	Hooper et al. 2011
Diagnostic interview assessments			
Structured Clinical Interview for DSM-5		Semistructured interview for DSM-5 diagnoses	First et al. 2016
Mini-International Neuropsychiatric Interview 7.0.2		Brief semistructured interview assessing 17 common DSM-5 psychiatric diagnoses	Sheehan et al. 1998
Clinician-Administered PTSD Scale for DSM-5		Structured interview assessing current and lifetime PTSD diagnoses and past-week PTSD symptoms	Weathers et al. 2013a
PTSD Symptom Scale Interview for DSM-5		Semistructured interview assessing DSM-5 criteria for PTSD and PTSD symptoms over the past month	Foa et al. 2016b
Self-report symptom monitoring measures			
PTSD Checklist for DSM-5	20	DSM-5 symptoms of PTSD	Weathers et al. 2013b
Posttraumatic Diagnostic Scale for DSM-5	26	Severity of DSM-5 PTSD symptoms	Foa et al. 2016a

creased anxiety symptoms, and withdrawal from certain substances (e.g., alcohol, opioids, benzodiazepines) is marked by anxiety states. Excessive alcohol use may contribute to behaviors that mimic or overlap with DSM-5 criteria for major depressive disorder, such as significant weight loss or gain, insomnia or hypersomnia, fatigue, and difficulty concentrating. Withdrawal from substances of abuse can also manifest as dysphoria, anhedonia, depressed mood, or suicidal ideation (Quello et al. 2005).

One way to differentiate substance-induced, transient symptoms from primary depression or anxiety disorders is through observation during abstinence. The appropriate minimum duration of abstinence necessary for accurate diagnosis varies, depending on the diagnosis under consideration and the substance being used. For substances with a long half-life (e.g., diazepam, methadone), withdrawal symptoms may be protracted, and several weeks of abstinence may be necessary in order to make an accurate diagnosis. For shorter-acting compounds (e.g., alcohol, cocaine), the duration of acute intoxication and withdrawal is briefer, and a shorter period of abstinence may be necessary for accurate diagnosis.

For anxiety, it is important to inquire about the use of caffeine and over-the-counter medications (e.g., pseudoephedrine, diet pills) that may increase anxiety (Kendler et al. 2006). Although the use of these substances in an individual case may not constitute an SUD, decreasing use may result in clinical improvement. Generalized anxiety disorder (GAD) is particularly challenging to diagnose in the presence of SUDs, because substance use or withdrawal can mimic every GAD symptom. For accurate diagnosis, GAD assessment should be delayed until intoxication and withdrawal have terminated, with the duration of this delay depending on how long substances remain active (McKeehan and Martin 2002). When the diagnosis of depression or anxiety disorders remains unclear, the following factors weigh in favor of a primary diagnosis of depression or anxiety and not the lingering effects of a substance: 1) family history of mood or anxiety disorders, 2) symptoms of depression or anxiety that predate the initiation of substance use or SUD onset, 3) severity of symptoms that exceeds what is typically seen in intoxication and withdrawal, and 4) sustained symptoms following extended abstinence.

Personality disorders are often present in individuals with PTSD and SUDs—in particular, antisocial personality disorder and borderline personality disorder. Acute and chronic use of alcohol and drugs can influence and exacerbate symptoms of antisocial personality disorder (e.g., unlawful behavior, repeated lying, impulsivity, reckless disregard for safety, repeated fights or assaults). To determine whether these behaviors and characteristics represent a primary personality disorder or are secondary to an SUD, clinicians should note that the diagnostic criteria for antisocial personality disorder require that the individual must have met criteria for conduct disorder before the age of 15 years. In addition, if the unlawful behavior is related only to the substance use (e.g., stealing money to buy drugs, drug-related criminal charges, lying about use) or to the trauma(s) (e.g., getting into fights because of anger about being a victim of trauma), the behavior would not count toward the diagnosis of antisocial personality disorder.

Excessive substance use can have a negative impact on affect regulation (e.g., irritability, uncontrolled anger, intense mood fluctuations, feelings of emptiness, dysphoria) and can contribute to a pattern of unstable relationships, as well as an unstable sense of self, which are characteristic of borderline personality disorder (American

Psychiatric Association 2013). Impulsivity, a feature of both SUDs and borderline personality disorder, can be exacerbated by intoxication. In addition, individuals with PTSD often struggle with interpersonal relationships. This can be a result of, for example, issues related to trust and safety, as well as the numbing of feelings, which may make it difficult to connect with others. Individuals with borderline personality disorder have high rates of early life trauma (e.g., childhood sexual abuse), and approximately half of the individuals with borderline personality disorder also have PTSD (e.g., Scheiderer et al. 2015). The overlapping clinical presentations of PTSD, SUDs, and borderline personality disorder can make differential diagnosis challenging. Observing the patient over an extended period of abstinence can assist with accurate diagnosis. In addition, examination of the temporal order of onset of symptoms as well as the pervasiveness of symptoms can help inform the diagnosis.

Trajectory of Substance Use Disorder and Posttraumatic Stress Disorder Development

Researchers have developed several theories to explain the etiology of co-occurring PTSD and SUDs. Some models propose a causal pathway between PTSD and SUDs, whereas others suggest that the association between the two disorders is noncausal and instead can be accounted for by shared vulnerabilities. One of the most widely accepted causal models is the *self-medication hypothesis* (Khantzian 1985), which posits that PTSD increases the risk for developing SUDs because individuals with PTSD have a propensity to use substances to alleviate their PTSD symptoms. Furthermore, the hypothesis suggests that the relationship between the two disorders is maintained through a cycle of negative reinforcement, whereby the temporary alleviation of PTSD symptoms (e.g., sleep disturbances, intrusive memories, hyperarousal) through substance use leads to further problematic use. The self-medication hypothesis has received strong empirical support from longitudinal, clinical, and laboratory studies (e.g., Back et al. 2006).

Despite the substantial support for the self-medication hypothesis, other longitudinal studies have failed to find evidence of a causal pathway linking PTSD to the subsequent development of SUDs (e.g., Najdowski and Ullman 2009). Alternative etiological models for PTSD and SUD comorbidity include the *high-risk hypothesis* and the *susceptibility hypothesis,* which theorize that preexisting SUDs enhance the risk for developing PTSD. The high-risk hypothesis postulates that SUDs confer risk for developing PTSD by increasing the likelihood of trauma exposure, whereas the susceptibility hypothesis suggests that individuals with SUDs are more vulnerable to the negative correlates associated with trauma exposure (e.g., problematic substance use may interfere with the emotional processing necessary to recover from trauma or may increase PTSD-related distress as a result of withdrawal symptoms). Studies investigating these hypotheses have produced mixed findings. Some studies have found support for the high-risk hypothesis only (e.g., Bromet et al. 1998), whereas other studies have found support for the susceptibility hypothesis only (Acierno et al. 1999). Taken together, these findings highlight the need to examine factors that moderate the relationship between the two disorders.

In contrast to the causal models, the *shared vulnerability hypothesis* proposes that the high rate of PTSD–SUD comorbidity is the result of shared risk factors. A large body of research shows that the two disorders have common genetic, neurobiological, and environmental risk factors (e.g., Norman et al. 2012; Sartor et al. 2011). Furthermore, several studies showed that a range of environmental factors are linked with both PTSD and SUDs, including parental psychiatric disorders and adverse childhood experiences.

Although some studies suggest that neurobiological changes associated with PTSD may subsequently increase risk for SUDs (Enman et al. 2014), PTSD and SUDs also may have neurobiological mechanisms that reciprocally confer risk for developing this comorbidity. For instance, various neurotransmitter systems have been implicated in both disorders—namely, dopamine, norepinephrine, and serotonin (Norman et al. 2012). Moreover, brain structure abnormalities, including decreased hippocampal volume and increased regional cerebral blood flow within the amygdala, are associated with comorbid PTSD and SUDs (for a review, see Norman et al. 2012). Notably, study findings regarding structural abnormalities have been mixed. For instance, although some studies show reduced hippocampal volume in both disorders (Norman et al. 2012), others indicate structural changes in PTSD only (Hull 2002). In summary, these models reflect a complex relationship between PTSD and SUDs and suggest that multiple pathways may lead to the development and maintenance of these disorders.

Treatment of Posttraumatic Stress Disorder in Individuals With Substance Use Disorders

When working with patients with PTSD and SUDs, clinicians must decide whether to treat the two disorders sequentially or concurrently. Clinicians may be hesitant to treat PTSD in patients with active SUDs, and addressing the SUD first may be important in some circumstances (e.g., if a patient is in withdrawal or is too severely intoxicated to attend treatment regularly or to engage in trauma work). However, the research reviewed in the following subsection suggests that treating PTSD in the context of an active SUD can be safe and efficacious, and improvements in PTSD symptoms can facilitate subsequent improvements in SUD treatment outcomes (e.g., Hien et al. 2010). Thus, in addition to being feasible, targeting PTSD in these populations may lead to long-lasting positive SUD outcomes. Given the mutually exacerbating effects of the two disorders, concurrent treatment may be the most efficient and effective method of addressing PTSD, SUDs, and their exacerbating influence on each other; however, no research has directly compared concurrent treatment with sequential treatment for this group. Regardless of treatment strategy, clinicians should consider ways to increase patient engagement and reduce the high treatment dropout rates that occur in the treatment of both disorders (e.g., Roberts et al. 2015).

Treatments for comorbid PTSD and SUDs are typically based on existing evidence-based models of treatment for either PTSD or SUDs, with adaptations incorporated to address the comorbid disorder. Alternatively, treatments may reflect new integrated interventions designed specifically for this comorbidity. We discuss both of these approaches in the next subsection.

Evidence-Based PTSD Psychotherapies Applied to PTSD and Substance Use Disorders

Prolonged exposure (PE; Foa and Rothbaum 1998) is an empirically supported PTSD treatment based on the notion that fearful experiences are mentally stored as fear structures that incorporate information about the situation, appropriate responses to it (e.g., fighting, fleeing), and its meaning. Fear structures become pathological in PTSD because they are activated by many nonthreatening situations, eliciting disproportionate fear responses that are not based in reality (e.g., a veteran hears a car backfire and reacts as if it were a bomb exploding). Among individuals with PTSD, avoidance of trauma memories and reminders prevents pathological fear structures from being modified by realistic information (e.g., learning that a car backfiring is not dangerous [Foa and Kozak 1986]). PE thus targets PTSD by activating and updating the fear structures through systematic, gradual *exposure* to trauma memories and reminders (Foa and Rothbaum 1998). Meta-analyses have supported the robust efficacy of PE in reducing PTSD symptoms (e.g., Cusack et al. 2016).

PE has been integrated into treatments that blend it with psychoeducation and relapse prevention therapy for SUD (i.e., Concurrent Treatment of PTSD and SUDs Using PE [Mills et al. 2012]). PE has also been paired with SUD outpatient and inpatient treatments (for a review, see Roberts et al. 2015) and medication (Foa et al. 2013). Although there are exceptions (Foa et al. 2013), findings from studies that included PE have generally indicated that interventions incorporating PE produced superior PTSD treatment outcomes in comparison with the same or similar interventions that did not include PE or other control conditions (e.g., Roberts et al. 2015; Ruglass et al. 2017). In addition, most SUD treatments with PE produced comparable or, more rarely, superior (Foa et al. 2013) SUD outcomes by posttreatment or follow-up in comparison with SUD treatments without PE (e.g., Roberts et al. 2015; Ruglass et al. 2017).

Cognitive processing therapy (CPT; Resick et al. 2016) is an evidence-based PTSD treatment based on the theory that trauma does not readily integrate with the individual's existing beliefs. For example, a belief such as "I am in control" does not clearly align with a random assault. In the wake of a traumatic experience, individuals may change their interpretation of the traumatic event (e.g., "This happened because I gave up control") or may alter their beliefs (e.g., "I never have control") to reconcile the discrepancy. These inaccurate or extreme trauma beliefs are thought to lead to negative emotions (e.g., shame) that obstruct the natural recovery of PTSD. Avoidance of traumatic memories and reminders further maintains PTSD by preventing individuals from taking in more accurate information that could correct their distorted beliefs. Therefore, CPT uses cognitive therapy to modify trauma-related beliefs and to help patients approach, rather than avoid, trauma memories (Resick et al. 2016). CPT is often 12 sessions long, and meta-analyses showed that CPT reduced PTSD symptoms more than did control conditions (e.g., Cusack et al. 2016). A recent study showed that a CPT-based day program for PTSD and SUDs reduced PTSD symptom severity and trauma-cue-induced craving for substances (Peck et al. 2018), and other studies have found that the presence of AUD (Kaysen et al. 2014) or of substance misuse (McDowell and Rodriguez 2013) did not alter CPT outcomes. These preliminary studies suggest that CPT is tolerable and efficacious for PTSD in patients receiving treatment for an SUD; however, CPT's effects on SUD outcomes are as yet unclear.

Notably, some studies blend cognitive and exposure techniques (i.e., cognitive-behavioral therapy [CBT]) to treat comorbid PTSD and SUDs. One study showed that CBT for PTSD paired with CBT for SUDs resulted in improved PTSD, and similar SUD treatment outcomes, compared with CBT for SUDs alone (van Dam et al. 2013). Another study showed that CBT for PTSD and AUD resulted in twice the rate of clinically significant change in PTSD symptoms compared with CBT for AUD alone, but only in individuals who attended at least one exposure session. However, comparisons of the effects of these two treatments on AUD outcomes suggested that CBT for AUD alone resulted in superior AUD outcomes compared with CBT for both PTSD and AUD (Sannibale et al. 2013). CBT for PTSD thus may be efficacious in SUD groups if individuals engage in at least some exposure therapy. However, the effects of these CBT approaches on SUDs are mixed (Sannibale et al. 2013; van Dam et al. 2013).

Novel PTSD and Substance Use Disorder Interventions

Several integrated treatments for PTSD and SUDs do not explicitly focus on trauma. Of these, Seeking Safety (Najavits 2002) has received the most empirical attention. Seeking Safety is premised on the notion that patients require safety and stability and emphasizes the acquisition of coping skills informed by CBT models (e.g., grounding techniques, self-care) to manage SUDs and PTSD-associated distress. Trauma memories and beliefs are not directly addressed, and traumatic experiences are not discussed. Several Seeking Safety pilot studies with small sample sizes of various populations, such as outpatient, inpatient, homeless, and incarcerated men and women, have shown promising PTSD and SUD outcomes (for a review, see Najavits and Hien 2013). However, results from randomized controlled trials (RCTs) were less encouraging. RCTs suggested that Seeking Safety resulted in PTSD symptom reduction comparable to that produced with nontrauma treatments such as relapse prevention, treatment as usual, and psychoeducation (for a review, see Roberts et al. 2015). Study results were mixed with respect to SUD treatment outcomes. A systematic review and meta-analysis showed some benefit for Seeking Safety relative to control treatments from pre- to posttreatment but not at follow-up time points (Roberts et al. 2015). Collectively, rigorous studies of Seeking Safety have generally suggested that it is not more effective than inactive control conditions or nontrauma treatments in reducing PTSD symptoms and that it may produce SUD treatment outcomes comparable to those produced with existing SUD interventions. Indeed, the meta-analysis conducted by Roberts et al. (2015) concluded that Seeking Safety had little empirical support in study samples with comorbid PTSD and SUDs (Roberts et al. 2015). Efficacious PTSD treatments share a common emphasis on approaching, rather than avoiding, trauma memories and beliefs (e.g., Foa and Rothbaum 1998; Resick et al. 2016). Such approach behaviors are not encouraged in Seeking Safety, which may explain the RCT findings.

Notably, another integrated CBT intervention (McGovern et al. 2009) for PTSD and SUDs that does not involve engagement with trauma memories or beliefs has been developed and shows mixed findings for PTSD and SUDs (McGovern et al. 2011, 2015) compared with current SUD interventions or treatment as usual. More research is needed to examine the efficacy of this integrated intervention in treating PTSD and SUDs.

Medications

Several medications, such as naltrexone, disulfiram, paroxetine, sertraline, topiramate, prazosin, and some combinations, used in the treatment of PTSD and SUDs have been examined (for a review, see Petrakis and Simpson 2017). Although there are some exceptions, findings generally suggest that these medications are equivalent to one another or to placebo in their effects on PTSD symptoms and are superior to placebo or combinations of active medicine in improving AUD outcomes (e.g., Petrakis and Simpson 2017). A review of medications for PTSD and AUD suggested that although the evidence for the efficacy of medications for either disorder was inconclusive and weak, these medications could be safely prescribed (Petrakis and Simpson 2017). However, some studies have shown support for the use of specific medications, such as topiramate and N-acetylcysteine, in improving both PTSD and SUDs (Back et al. 2016; Petrakis and Simpson 2017). Therefore, further investigation into the effects of these medications is warranted, especially in populations with comorbid PTSD and SUDs (rather than AUD only).

Conclusion and Key Points

PTSD and SUDs are overlapping disorders that reflect a complex interplay of distressing symptoms that reinforce and exacerbate each other. In closing, we offer the following summary of key points from this chapter:

- Proper screening and assessment of traumatic exposure and PTSD diagnosis are critical among individuals with SUDs.
- Common comorbidities of PTSD and SUDs include anxiety disorders, mood disorders, sleeping disturbances, and personality disorders.
- Shared underlying neurobiological vulnerabilities such as hypothalamic-pituitary-adrenal axis dysregulation are linked to features of both PTSD and SUDs, suggesting the need to treat both conditions.
- Determining selection of treatment approaches for PTSD should include factors such as SUD severity, patient preferences, and access to social support.
- Clinicians can consider combination therapy with evidence-based behavioral models and medications that are deemed best practices for each condition separately or cognitive-behavioral interventions for which empirical evidence supports addressing both disorders concurrently.

References

Acierno R, Resnick H, Kilpatrick DG, et al: Risk factors for rape, physical assault, and posttraumatic stress disorder in women: examination of differential multivariate relationships. J Anxiety Disord 13(6):541–563, 1999 10688523

American Psychiatric Association: Diagnostic and Statistical Manual of Mental Disorders, 3rd Edition. Washington, DC, American Psychiatric Association, 1980

American Psychiatric Association: Diagnostic and Statistical Manual of Mental Disorders, 5th Edition. Arlington, VA, American Psychiatric Association, 2013

Back SE, Brady KT, Sonne SC, et al: Symptom improvement in co-occurring PTSD and alcohol dependence. J Nerv Ment Dis 194(9):690–696, 2006 16971821

Back SE, McCauley JL, Korte KJ, et al: A double-blind, randomized, controlled pilot trial of N-acetylcysteine in veterans with posttraumatic stress disorder and substance use disorders. J Clin Psychiatry 77(11):e1439–e1446, 2016 27736051

Bromet E, Sonnega A, Kessler RC: Risk factors for DSM-III-R posttraumatic stress disorder: findings from the National Comorbidity Survey. Am J Epidemiol 147(4):353–361, 1998 9508102

Carlson EB, Smith SR, Palmieri PA, et al: Development and validation of a brief self-report measure of trauma exposure: the Trauma History Screen. Psychol Assess 23(2):463–477, 2011 21517189

Connor KM, Davidson JRT: SPRINT: a brief global assessment of post-traumatic stress disorder. Int Clin Psychopharmacol 16(5):279–284, 2001 11552771

Cusack K, Jonas DE, Forneris CA, et al: Psychological treatments for adults with posttraumatic stress disorder: a systematic review and meta-analysis. Clin Psychol Rev 43:128–141, 2016 26574151

Enman NM, Zhang Y, Unterwald EM: Connecting the pathology of posttraumatic stress and substance use disorders: monoamines and neuropeptides. Pharmacol Biochem Behav 117:61–69, 2014 24333548

First MB, Williams JBW, Karg RS, et al: Structured Clinical Interview for DSM-5 Disorders, Clinician Version (SCID-5-CV). Arlington, VA, American Psychiatric Association, 2016

Foa EB, Kozak MJ: Emotional processing of fear: exposure to corrective information. Psychol Bull 99(1):20–35, 1986 2871574

Foa EB, Rothbaum BO: Treating the Trauma of Rape: Cognitive-Behavioral Therapy for PTSD. New York, Guilford, 1998

Foa EB, Yusko DA, McLean CP, et al: Concurrent naltrexone and prolonged exposure therapy for patients with comorbid alcohol dependence and PTSD: a randomized clinical trial. JAMA 310(5):488–495, 2013 23925619

Foa EB, McLean CP, Zang Y, et al: Psychometric properties of the Posttraumatic Diagnostic Scale for DSM-5 (PDS-5). Psychol Assess 28(10):1166–1171, 2016a 26691504

Foa EB, McLean CP, Zang Y, et al: Psychometric properties of the Posttraumatic Stress Disorder Symptom Scale Interview for DSM-5 (PSSI-5). Psychol Assess 28(10):1159–1165, 2016b 26691507

Gielen N, Havermans RC, Tekelenburg M, et al: Prevalence of post-traumatic stress disorder among patients with substance use disorder: it is higher than clinicians think it is. Eur J Psychotraumatol 3(1):17734, 2012 22893849

Goodman LA, Corcoran C, Turner K, et al: Assessing traumatic event exposure: general issues and preliminary findings for the Stressful Life Events Screening Questionnaire. J Trauma Stress 11(3):521–542, 1998 9690191

Hien DA, Jiang H, Campbell ANC, et al: Do treatment improvements in PTSD severity affect substance use outcomes? A secondary analysis from a randomized clinical trial in NIDA's Clinical Trials Network. Am J Psychiatry 167(1):95–101, 2010 19917596

Hooper LM, Stockton P, Krupnick JL, et al: Development, use, and psychometric properties of the Trauma History Questionnaire. Journal of Loss and Trauma 16(3):258–283, 2011. Available at: https://www.tandfonline.com/doi/full/10.1080/15325024.2011.572035. Accessed February 26, 2020.

Hull AM: Neuroimaging findings in post-traumatic stress disorder: systematic review. Br J Psychiatry 181:102–110, 2002 12151279

Kaysen D, Schumm J, Pedersen ER, et al: Cognitive processing therapy for veterans with comorbid PTSD and alcohol use disorders. Addict Behav 39(2):420–427, 2014 24035644

Kendler KS, Myers J, Gardner CO: Caffeine intake, toxicity and dependence and lifetime risk for psychiatric and substance use disorders: an epidemiologic and co-twin control analysis. Psychol Med 36(12):1717–1725, 2006 16893482

Khantzian EJ: The self-medication hypothesis of addictive disorders: focus on heroin and cocaine dependence. Am J Psychiatry 142(11):1259–1264, 1985 3904487

Kubany ES, Haynes SN, Leisen MB, et al: Development and preliminary validation of a brief broad-spectrum measure of trauma exposure: the Traumatic Life Events Questionnaire. Psychol Assess 12(2):210–224, 2000 10887767

McDowell J, Rodriguez J: Does substance abuse affect outcomes for trauma-focused treatment of combat-related PTSD? Addiction Research & Theory 21(5):357–364, 2013. Available at: https://www.tandfonline.com/doi/abs/10.3109/16066359.2012.746316. Accessed February 26, 2020.

McGovern MP, Lambert-Harris C, Acquilano S, et al: A cognitive behavioral therapy for co-occurring substance use and posttraumatic stress disorders. Addict Behav 34(10):892–897, 2009 19395179

McGovern MP, Lambert-Harris C, Alterman AI, et al: A randomized controlled trial comparing integrated cognitive behavioral therapy versus individual addiction counseling for co-occurring substance use and posttraumatic stress disorders. J Dual Diagn 7(4):207–227, 2011 22383864

McGovern MP, Lambert-Harris C, Xie H, et al: A randomized controlled trial of treatments for co-occurring substance use disorders and post-traumatic stress disorder. Addiction 110(7):1194–1204, 2015 25846251

McKeehan MB, Martin D: Assessment and treatment of anxiety disorders and co-morbid alcohol/other drug dependency. Alcoholism Treatment Quarterly 20(1):45–59, 2002. Available at: https://www.tandfonline.com/doi/abs/10.1300/J020v20n01_03. Accessed February 26, 2020.

Mills KL, Teesson M, Back SE, et al: Integrated exposure-based therapy for co-occurring posttraumatic stress disorder and substance dependence: a randomized controlled trial. JAMA 308(7):690–699, 2012 22893166

Najavits LM: Seeking Safety: A Treatment Manual for PTSD and Substance Abuse. New York, Guilford, 2002

Najavits LM, Hien D: Helping vulnerable populations: a comprehensive review of the treatment outcome literature on substance use disorder and PTSD. J Clin Psychol 69(5):433–479, 2013 23592045

Najdowski CJ, Ullman SE: Prospective effects of sexual victimization on PTSD and problem drinking. Addict Behav 34(11):965–968, 2009 19501469

Norman SB, Myers US, Wilkins KC, et al: Review of biological mechanisms and pharmacological treatments of comorbid PTSD and substance use disorder. Neuropharmacology 62(2):542–551, 2012 21600225

Peck KR, Coffey SF, McGuire AP, et al: A cognitive processing therapy-based treatment program for veterans diagnosed with co-occurring posttraumatic stress disorder and substance use disorder: the relationship between trauma-related cognitions and outcomes of a 6-week treatment program. J Anxiety Disord 59:34–41, 2018 30248534

Petrakis IL, Simpson TL: Posttraumatic stress disorder and alcohol use disorder: a critical review of pharmacologic treatments. Alcohol Clin Exp Res 41(2):226–237, 2017 28102573

Prins A, Bovin MJ, Smolenski DJ, et al: The Primary Care PTSD Screen for DSM-5 (PC-PTSD-5): development and evaluation within a veteran primary care sample. J Gen Intern Med 31(10):1206–1211, 2016 27170304

Quello SB, Brady KT, Sonne SC: Mood disorders and substance use disorder: a complex comorbidity. Sci Pract Perspect 3(1):13–21, 2005 18552741

Resick PA, Monson CM, Chard KM: Cognitive Processing Therapy for PTSD: A Comprehensive Manual. New York, Guilford, 2016

Roberts NP, Roberts PA, Jones N, et al: Psychological interventions for post-traumatic stress disorder and comorbid substance use disorder: a systematic review and meta-analysis. Clin Psychol Rev 38:25–38, 2015 25792193

Ruglass LM, Lopez-Castro T, Papini S, et al: Concurrent treatment with prolonged exposure for co-occurring full or subthreshold posttraumatic stress disorder and substance use disorders: a randomized clinical trial. Psychother Psychosom 86(3):150–161, 2017 28490022

Saladin ME, Brady KT, Dansky BS, et al: Understanding comorbidity between PTSD and substance use disorders: two preliminary investigations. Addict Behav 20(5):643–655, 1995 8712061

Sannibale C, Teesson M, Creamer M, et al: Randomized controlled trial of cognitive behaviour therapy for comorbid post-traumatic stress disorder and alcohol use disorders. Addiction 108(8):1397–1410, 2013 25328957

Sartor CE, McCutcheon VV, Pommer NE, et al: Common genetic and environmental contributions to post-traumatic stress disorder and alcohol dependence in young women. Psychol Med 41(7):1497–1505, 2011 21054919

Scheiderer EM, Wood PK, Trull TJ: The comorbidity of borderline personality disorder and posttraumatic stress disorder: revisiting the prevalence and associations in a general population sample. Borderline Personal Disord Emot Dysregul 2:11, 2015 26401313

Schnurr PP, Spiro A, Vielhauer MJ, et al: Trauma in the lives of older men: findings from the Normative Aging Study. Journal of Clinical Geropsychology 8(3):175–187, 2002. Available at: https://link.springer.com/article/10.1023/A:1015992110544. Accessed February 26, 2020.

Sheehan DV, Lecrubier Y, Sheehan KH, et al: The Mini-International Neuropsychiatric Interview (M.I.N.I.): the development and validation of a structured diagnostic psychiatric interview for DSM-IV and ICD-10. J Clin Psychiatry 59 (suppl 20):22–33, quiz 34–57, 1998 9881538

Smith JP, Randall CL: Anxiety and alcohol use disorders: comorbidity and treatment considerations. Alcohol Res 34(4):414–431, 2012 23584108

Tull MT, Gratz KL, Aklin WM, et al: A preliminary examination of the relationships between posttraumatic stress symptoms and crack/cocaine, heroin, and alcohol dependence. J Anxiety Disord 24(1):55–62, 2010 19767174

van Dam D, Ehring T, Vedel E, et al: Trauma-focused treatment for posttraumatic stress disorder combined with CBT for severe substance use disorder: a randomized controlled trial. BMC Psychiatry 13(1):172, 2013 23782590

Walton JL, Raines AM, Cuccurullo LJ, et al: The relationship between DSM-5 PTSD symptom clusters and alcohol misuse among military veterans. Am J Addict 27(1):23–28, 2018 29251380

Weathers FW, Blake DD, Schnurr PP, et al: The Clinician-Administered PTSD Scale for DSM-5 (CAPS-5). 2013a. Available at: https://www.ptsd.va.gov/professional/assessment/adult-int/caps.asp. Accessed January 14, 2020.

Weathers FW, Litz BT, Keane TM, et al: The PTSD Checklist for DSM-5 (PCL-5). 2013b. Available at: https://www.ptsd.va.gov/professional/assessment/adult-sr/ptsd-checklist.asp. Accessed January 14, 2020.

CHAPTER 49

Schizophrenia Spectrum and Other Psychotic Disorders

Elizabeth K.C. Schwartz, M.D., Ph.D.

Mary F. Brunette, M.D.

Alan I. Green, M.D.

Schizophrenia, characterized by hallucinations, delusions, and disorganized thinking and behavior, occurs in approximately 1% of the population. Almost 50% of individuals diagnosed with schizophrenia also have had a substance use disorder (SUD) at some time in their life (such comorbidity is often called *dual diagnosis*)—a rate two to three times higher than that in the general population (Brunette et al. 2018a; Regier et al. 1990). Alcohol, cannabis, and stimulants, in that order, are the most commonly abused substances among this population, and 50%–90% of patients with schizophrenia smoke tobacco, in comparison with 15.5% of the general U.S. population (Correll et al. 2014). Although the prevalence of opioid use disorders has increased in the United States, it is unclear how common this problem is in schizophrenic patients.

Most SUDs not only are more prevalent among patients with schizophrenia but also tend to worsen the course of the psychotic illness. Compared with patients with schizophrenia who do not abuse substances, patients with both schizophrenia and an SUD tend to report more symptoms, are less treatment adherent, have more hospitalizations, and are more likely to be homeless. They also have more medical morbidity; are at greater risk for HIV, hepatitis B, and hepatitis C infection; and are more likely

Dr. Green's research is partially supported by National Institute on Drug Abuse (NIDA) grants R21DA044501 and R01DA034699.

759

to die at a younger age from illnesses such as cancer, heart disease, vascular disease, and lung disease, because these conditions are often caused or exacerbated by substance use.

Many theories have been advanced to explain the high prevalence of SUD and schizophrenia comorbidity. The self-medication hypothesis suggests that substance use in individuals with schizophrenia aims to decrease symptoms or lessen side effects of antipsychotic medication. Numerous studies, however, have been unable to confirm this clinical hypothesis. Other theories, including a stress-diathesis hypothesis, a primary addiction hypothesis, and a reward deficiency syndrome hypothesis, also have been proposed. Our group has presented a unifying hypothesis that takes into account recent data, as well as the previously mentioned hypotheses (Khokhar et al. 2018). This unifying hypothesis proposes a shared vulnerability for substance use in persons with schizophrenia (or even in those at risk) because of a dysfunctional dopamine-mediated mesocorticolimbic brain reward circuit. It explains why even prepsychotic individuals may use substances at a high rate and how the substance use itself could trigger the onset of psychosis in such people or perpetuate their continued substance use. This hypothesis also implies that the substance use, through its effects on brain reward circuitry, may ameliorate some of the circuit dysfunction, even though it can worsen the course of schizophrenia.

Substance-Specific Factors In Schizophrenia

Although a common circuitry may underlie the propensity toward increased substance use in individuals with schizophrenia, drug-specific factors are also important. Nicotine is by far the most common substance used by individuals with schizophrenia—at the time of the first episode of psychosis, approximately 50% of patients smoke tobacco (Correll et al. 2014). Nicotinic acetylcholine receptors are found throughout the brain, and nicotine facilitates a wide variety of cognitive processes, including attention, executive function, learning, and memory. Patients with schizophrenia have been shown to have fewer—and fewer functional—nicotinic receptors in the brain. Increased activation of these receptors via nicotine may, by increasing dopaminergic transmission, potentially improve cognition in schizophrenia, providing additional reinforcement for smoking in this group (Rezvani and Levin 2001). However, findings from studies investigating the ability of nicotine treatment to improve cognition in individuals with schizophrenia have been mixed (Boggs et al. 2018a).

Alcohol use disorder is also more prevalent among this population. In an animal model of schizophrenia, even minimal alcohol use during adolescence led to disinhibited control of alcohol intake in adulthood (Jeanblanc et al. 2015). Although this finding suggests that patients with schizophrenia may be more vulnerable to alcohol addiction after priming with early alcohol use in adolescence (Jeanblanc et al. 2015), epidemiological studies have not supported this association (Hiemstra et al. 2018). Nevertheless, people with schizophrenia may be more vulnerable to the detrimental effects of alcohol.

Cannabis is the most prevalent illicit drug used among individuals with schizophrenia. With the expanding legalization of medical and recreational marijuana in the United States, use of this drug is increasing, and interest in its therapeutic use is high.

Tetrahydrocannabinol (THC), the primary psychoactive component of marijuana, not only causes feelings of relaxation and "high" but also may cause or worsen psychotic symptoms and cognitive impairments in schizophrenia (D'Souza et al. 2016). Heavy use of cannabis with high THC potency early in adolescence has been associated with increased vulnerability for the development of schizophrenia (Marconi et al. 2016). Continued cannabis use is associated with relapses of psychosis and more hospitalization (Schoeler et al. 2016). Use of THC is hypothesized to lead to or exacerbate psychosis by impairing the ability to correctly attribute salience to environmental stimuli (Wijayendran et al. 2018). Paradoxically, however, data from pilot studies (which have yet to be confirmed) suggest that cannabis with low THC potency may improve the functioning of brain reward circuits (Fischer et al. 2014). Nonetheless, because the level of THC in street marijuana has increased dramatically over the past 30 years, use of street marijuana or of any cannabis product containing THC remains highly problematic for people with schizophrenia.

Cannabidiol (CBD), a component of cannabis that is not thought to be psychoactive, may be less harmful or even potentially helpful in patients with schizophrenia. Some studies have indicated that CBD may play a role in antipsychotic treatment, as described later in this chapter (see "Cannabidiol" in section "Pharmacological Treatment Options"). Cannabis containing high levels of CBD is associated with fewer psychotic symptoms than cannabis containing low levels of CBD (Schubart et al. 2011). THC and CBD were shown to have opposite effects on functional connectivity in regions important for the processing of attentional salience, a cognitive process thought to underpin symptoms in schizophrenia (Bhattacharyya et al. 2015).

Detection and Management of Substance Use Disorders in Individuals With Schizophrenia

SUDs in individuals with schizophrenia are frequently both underdetected and undertreated in mental health and in addiction treatment. Clinicians from different settings provide different messages to patients about their disorders, and care provided by multiple providers is often fragmented. To improve detection, clinicians should routinely assess and discuss substance use with all patients at regular intervals. Use of standardized screening measures such as the web-based National Institute on Drug Abuse (NIDA)–Modified Alcohol, Smoking, and Substance Involvement Screening Test (NM-ASSIST; www.drugabuse.gov/nmassist) or instruments specifically developed for patients with mental illness (e.g., Dartmouth Assessment of Lifestyle Instrument [Rosenberg et al. 1998], Clinician Rating Scales for alcohol use and for drug use [Mueser et al. 1995]) can facilitate screening and assessment. In addition to using these self-report assessments, clinicians should monitor their patients for behaviors consistent with substance misuse (e.g., frequent missed appointments, difficulty managing components of daily life, financial or legal problems) and seek collateral information from family members and other treatment providers. To detect risky prescription drug use, clinicians should check prescription drug monitoring program websites.

Clinicians can also conduct a functional analysis, which incorporates the individual's experience of both the positive and the negative aspects of substance use and how these may help or complicate his or her life. Patients can be actively involved in this assessment process, which provides the foundation for cognitive-behavioral substance abuse counseling. Clinicians should have a nonjudgmental attitude, which reinforces honest communication about substance use and improves detection and treatment.

Pharmacological Treatment Options

Antipsychotic Medications

Antipsychotic medications reduce symptoms of psychosis, disorganization, anxiety, and depression. Whether these medications also affect co-occurring SUDs is a question of great interest. First-generation antipsychotics, including potent antagonists of dopamine type 2 (D_2) receptors such as haloperidol, may actually increase substance use in some patients with schizophrenia. Additionally, prospective studies indicate that patients with a dual diagnosis of an SUD and another mental disorder may not respond as well to first-generation antipsychotics compared with patients with psychosis who do not have an SUD.

Second-generation antipsychotics with lower levels of dopamine D_2 receptor occupancy (e.g., clozapine) may be more helpful than first-generation agents for the treatment of schizophrenia in patients who are using substances. Green and colleagues proposed that clozapine—a second-generation antipsychotic that weakly blocks dopamine D_2 receptors, potently blocks α_2-noradrenergic receptors, and also increases norepinephrine levels—may normalize the signal detection capability of dysfunctional mesocorticolimbic brain reward circuits, leading to reduced substance use in individuals with schizophrenia (Khokhar et al. 2018). Open and naturalistic trials of clozapine and several small randomized controlled trials (RCTs) have reported beneficial effects of clozapine on alcohol and cannabis use. In one RCT comparing switching to clozapine with continuing current treatment among 31 individuals with co-occurring schizophrenia and cannabis use, the clozapine group used less cannabis over 12 weeks of treatment (Brunette et al. 2011). In another RCT of 28 patients with schizophrenia and cannabis use disorder, those taking clozapine reported less cannabis craving and showed reduced bilateral insula activation during a Stroop Test compared with those taking risperidone (Machielsen et al. 2014). However, no definitive trial of clozapine for substance use in schizophrenia has been performed, and concerns about clozapine's side effects, including risk for agranulocytosis and the consequent required white blood cell count monitoring for patients taking clozapine continue to limit its use.

Research examining the efficacy of other second-generation antipsychotics for substance use among people with schizophrenia and SUDs is mixed. Quetiapine, a medication that shares with clozapine a relatively low blockade of dopamine D_2 receptors (and produces a metabolite that is a norepinephrine reuptake inhibitor), reduced substance abuse severity and number of days drinking in small open trials among patients with co-occurring schizophrenia and alcohol use disorder (e.g., Brunette et al. 2009). Although an RCT in people with alcohol use disorder without psychosis (Litten et al. 2012) showed that quetiapine did not reduce alcohol use, to our knowledge, no RCT has examined the effect of quetiapine in people with alcohol use disorder and schizophrenia.

Open trials also have suggested that patients with schizophrenia and co-occurring SUDs may respond to olanzapine. However, controlled prospective trials did not show differences between olanzapine and haloperidol in the number of cocaine-positive urine drug screen results (Smelson et al. 2006) or between olanzapine and risperidone in reduction of cannabis use in patients with schizophrenia and co-occurring SUDs (Sevy et al. 2011).

Two small open-label trials found that the partial dopamine D_2 receptor agonist aripiprazole reduced cocaine and alcohol cravings. One trial found reduced cocaine-positive urine test results (Beresford et al. 2005), but the other did not show a reduction in cocaine use (Brown et al. 2005) among patients with schizophrenia and cocaine use disorder. In a separate open-label trial of 139 patients with schizophrenia and tobacco use disorder, the group randomly assigned to aripiprazole treatment had less tobacco craving and nicotine dependence compared with the groups assigned to haloperidol, risperidone, or olanzapine (Kim et al. 2010).

Long-acting injectable formulations of antipsychotics simplify medication taking and allow clinicians to know when a patient is nonadherent, which may be particularly advantageous in patients with schizophrenia. Additionally, these formulations provide the antipsychotic at a steady state, which may permit use of a lower dose that is more tolerable and results in a lower level of dopamine D_2 receptor blockade. Evidence from large population-based studies suggests modestly better outcomes overall for individuals who take long-acting injectable antipsychotics compared with oral antipsychotics (Tiihonen et al. 2017). Several studies showed beneficial effects of long-acting injectable risperidone on alcohol use or ratings of alcohol-related problems in patients with schizophrenia and alcohol use disorder (Green et al. 2015; Rosenheck et al. 2011; Rubio et al. 2006). In an RCT of 95 patients with schizophrenia and alcohol use disorder comparing oral with long-acting injectable risperidone, patients receiving the long-acting injectable form of risperidone reported fewer drinking days (Green et al. 2015). In two trials among veterans with schizophrenia, Addiction Severity Index scores were modestly better among patients assigned to long-acting injectable risperidone than among those receiving oral risperidone (Leatherman et al. 2014; Rosenheck et al. 2011).

To our knowledge, no reports have been published on the effect of ziprasidone, lurasidone, iloperidone, or cariprazine on SUDs in schizophrenia.

U.S. Food and Drug Administration–Approved Adjunctive Treatments

The U.S. Food and Drug Administration (FDA) has approved drugs for the treatment of alcohol use disorder, opioid use disorder, and tobacco use disorder, all of which appear to be relatively safe and effective for use in patients with schizophrenia and co-occurring SUDs, as reviewed in the following sections. Although there are no FDA-approved medications for the treatment of cannabis use disorder, research is ongoing in this area (see "Cannabidiol" subsection below).

Medications for alcohol use disorder.   Disulfiram inhibits aldehyde dehydrogenase, causing flushing, sweating, nausea, and vomiting after drinking alcohol. Use of this medication with monitoring increases abstinence from alcohol. Although it was initially suggested that disulfiram might increase psychotic symptoms in patients with schizophrenia, a retrospective chart review found that disulfiram reduced alcohol use in dual-diagnosis patients without causing significant psychiatric symptoms and also decreased hospitalization days (Mueser et al. 2003).

Naltrexone, a μ-opioid receptor antagonist initially used to treat opioid addiction, is also approved by the FDA as a treatment for alcohol use disorder. Naltrexone is hypothesized to decrease the rewarding effects of alcohol via inhibition of the mesolimbic reward circuit. Findings from multiple studies indicate that this medication is safe and effective for the treatment of alcohol use disorder in schizophrenia. In a subset of veterans with psychotic symptoms and alcohol use disorder ($n=66$ of 185) enrolled in a randomized trial comparing naltrexone, disulfiram, and the combination of these two medications with placebo, Petrakis et al. (2006) found that participants in all active treatment arms showed greater reductions in drinking compared with participants receiving placebo. In a small placebo-controlled study in a sample of patients with schizophrenia and comorbid alcohol use disorder, these same authors found that patients receiving naltrexone with weekly cognitive-behavioral therapy (CBT) demonstrated reductions in alcohol use in comparison with those receiving placebo, with no exacerbation of psychotic symptoms (Petrakis et al. 2004). A separate controlled trial in 19 individuals with schizophrenia found that three-times-a-week monitored oral naltrexone—with doses of 100 mg (twice a week) and 150 mg (once a week)—resulted in a significant trend for fewer drinks per week in the group taking naltrexone compared with their drinks per week before naltrexone treatment (Batki et al. 2009). In a 12-week open-label prospective study examining the effects of a monthly long-acting 380-mg injection of naltrexone among participants with alcohol use disorder plus another serious mental illness, including 6 with schizophrenia and 11 with schizoaffective disorder, those given three monthly depot injections showed reduced drinking compared with their earlier use (Batki et al. 2010).

Acamprosate, which has been suggested to decrease both alcohol craving and the rewarding effects of alcohol, also has been observed to reduce relapse risk after detoxification from alcohol and to increase total abstinence time. However, a small RCT investigating this medication's effects on alcohol consumption in patients with co-occurring schizophrenia did not find reduced drinking with acamprosate as compared with placebo (Ralevski et al. 2011).

Varenicline, which is FDA approved for treating tobacco use disorder and is safe for use in schizophrenia (Anthenelli et al. 2016), has been found to reduce drinking in people with alcohol use disorder. One small trial of varenicline in people with schizophrenia and alcohol use disorder ($N=10$) showed promising results but was limited by the low tolerability of varenicline (Meszaros et al. 2013).

Medications for opioid use disorder.　Case reports (Kern et al. 2014) and a retrospective study (Unglaub et al. 2003) have suggested that medication-assisted treatment with methadone or buprenorphine within an integrated treatment program can be beneficial for individuals with co-occurring opioid use disorder and schizophrenia. Naltrexone is also a first-line treatment for opioid use disorder. Nonetheless, to our knowledge, none of the medications used for the treatment of opioid use disorder has been tested prospectively in people with schizophrenia.

Medications for tobacco use disorder.　FDA-approved medications for smoking cessation have been shown to be safe and effective in patients with schizophrenia and tobacco use disorder, particularly when combined with behavioral cessation therapy. A longitudinal study found that 8 weeks of nicotine patch use increased rates of smoking abstinence compared with the no-treatment control group (Chou et al. 2004), and a large placebo-controlled trial determined that a nicotine patch was superior to a placebo patch in helping patients with psychotic disorders to quit smoking (23.2% abstinence vs. 4.1%; odds ratio [OR]=3.40; 95% CI=0.74–15.61) (Evins et al. 2019). Although the combination of a daily nicotine patch with as-needed use of nicotine gum or lozenges has been shown to be more effective than use of the patch alone in smokers in the general population in the early phases of quitting, comparative effectiveness studies of different doses and delivery modalities of nicotine replacement therapies have not been reported in smokers with schizophrenia.

Bupropion, also approved by the FDA as an antidepressant medication, has been found to decrease smoking in patients with schizophrenia. Four small placebo-controlled trials showed that bupropion and CBT, with or without nicotine replacement therapy, reduced smoking or led to smoking cessation (Evins et al. 2005, 2007; George et al. 2002, 2008). As has been shown in smokers without mental illness, the combination of bupropion with nicotine replacement therapy was superior to nicotine replacement therapy alone (George et al. 2008). On discontinuing bupropion after a 12-week treatment, many patients rapidly relapse back to smoking; thus, longer-term pharmacotherapy should be considered.

Varenicline, a selective $\alpha_4\beta_2$ partial nicotinic receptor agonist, is thought to decrease smoking cravings by regulating dopamine release in the ventral tegmental area and striatum after nicotine exposure. Three RCTs, two for cessation (Anthenelli et al. 2016; Williams et al. 2012) and one for relapse prevention (Evins et al. 2017), have shown the efficacy of varenicline among smokers with schizophrenia. For example, in a 12-week trial of varenicline with supportive counseling, varenicline was associated with a smoking cessation rate of 19%, compared with 4.7% for placebo—without significant differences in adverse events, mood symptoms, or psychotic symptoms between groups (Williams et al. 2012). In an RCT of maintenance treatment with varenicline plus CBT in patients with bipolar disorder or schizophrenia who had achieved abstinence in an initial open-label phase, those assigned to the varenicline maintenance group were less likely to relapse to smoking compared with those assigned to placebo (Evins et al. 2014). Given varenicline's effects on nicotinic receptors, researchers also have investigated whether this medication can improve cognitive performance in patients with schizophrenia who smoke; however, results have been mixed. Although varenicline has been shown to be as safe as and more effective than the other FDA-approved treatment options for smoking cessation (Anthenelli et al. 2016), its use remains less common in general practice, perhaps because of concerns about side effects and limitations imposed on insurance coverage by "prior authorization" requirements.

Alternative strategies are also being investigated. Although nicotine delivery via electronic cigarettes is not FDA approved for smoking cessation, many smokers use e-cigarettes for this purpose, with mixed success. Several small studies have shown that use of e-cigarettes with nicotine reduced smoking and increased abstinence rates among smokers with schizophrenia (Pratt et al. 2016). Reducing the nicotine content in combustible cigarettes is a strategy being considered by the FDA to reduce the addictiveness of cigarettes and to extinguish nicotine craving among smokers. One small controlled study found that use of cigarettes with very low nicotine content safely reduced craving as well as reducing the use of regular brand cigarettes in smokers with schizophrenia (Tidey et al. 2013).

Cannabidiol

Because the dopamine system is, in part, modulated by the endocannabinoid system, targeting cannabinoid receptor activity has potential for treating addiction. As described earlier, CBD and THC may have counteractive effects through their opposing activity in the striatum, hippocampus, and prefrontal cortex (Iseger and Bossong 2015). Despite the potential of CBD in schizophrenia, prospective studies of CBD thus far have provided negative results for addressing cannabis use disorder in this population and mixed results for treating psychosis. A small case series in which antipsychotic-treated inpatients with co-occurring schizophrenia and cannabis use disorder (N=7) received substitution therapy with a medicinal low-THC/high-CBD cannabis variant concluded that this formulation was neither appealing to patients with schizophrenia nor effective in reducing their cannabis use (Schipper et al. 2018). When given with antipsychotic medication, CBD reduced psychotic symptoms compared with treatment with an antipsychotic and placebo (McGuire et al. 2018), and CBD given without an antipsychotic was as effective as the potent antipsychotic amisulpride in reducing psychotic symptoms but had a more benign side-effect profile than that agent (Leweke et al. 2012). However, at least one RCT found that oral CBD given with antipsychotic medication did not provide any benefit for psychotic symptoms and cognitive impairment in comparison with placebo and antipsychotic medication (Boggs et al. 2018b).

Anticonvulsants and Benzodiazepines

Although some reports indicated that certain anticonvulsants can decrease heavy drinking and increase time to relapse (Johnson et al. 2007), to our knowledge, the effects of anticonvulsants in dual-diagnosis individuals have not been studied.

Although prescription benzodiazepines are effective for alcohol withdrawal, outpatient use of benzodiazepines does not appear to improve outcomes for SUDs, is associated with increased risk of mortality (Tiihonen et al. 2016), and is also associated with the development of benzodiazepine use disorder in people with schizophrenia and co-occurring SUDs (Brunette et al. 2003). Thus, benzodiazepines should be avoided in this population.

Tricyclic Antidepressants

Two small studies noted that tricyclic antidepressant medications may help reduce substance use in individuals with schizophrenia when used with first-generation antipsychotics (Green et al. 2008). Interestingly, in an animal model with alcohol-drinking hamsters, desipramine combined with risperidone reduced alcohol intake more than either drug alone, suggesting an interesting pharmacological treatment approach that warrants further investigation (Gulick et al. 2014).

Neurostimulation

Preliminary studies suggested that transcranial magnetic stimulation, particularly over the dorsolateral prefrontal cortex, can reduce cravings in individuals with SUDs, but small studies have yielded mixed results for transcranial magnetic stimulation in reducing cigarette smoking in patients with schizophrenia (Kozak et al. 2018).

Nonpharmacological and Behavioral Interventions

Because SUDs lead to problems with symptom management, social and family interactions, employment, housing, and health among patients with schizophrenia, an array of social and psychological services should be provided, in addition to pharmacological treatments, to address the psychosis, the SUDs, and other areas of need. Outreach and practical help may be needed to engage people in treatment, but once people are engaged, education can raise awareness about the adverse effects of their substance use. Motivational interventions then can be used to begin to build interest in change. Once people are ready to reduce and stop substance use, behavioral interventions can help them learn new skills and stay motivated to avoid using substances. Use of a team-based, integrated approach has been shown to be most effective in engaging and working with people with co-occurring schizophrenia and SUDs.

Many types of behavioral addiction interventions have been tested among patients with schizophrenia, mostly with mixed results. Preliminary, mixed evidence indicates that motivational interviewing reduces substance use in people with a dual diagnosis. For example, in a small RCT, participants assigned to four to six sessions of motivational interviewing had decreased cannabis use at 3- and 6-month follow-ups, but not at the 12-month follow-up (Bonsack et al. 2011). Motivational interviewing is typically incorporated into more comprehensive behavioral interventions. Evidence to support this approach is mixed for motivational interviewing combined with CBT for patients with schizophrenia and cannabis use disorder (Madigan et al. 2013). In a trial in stabilized outpatients meeting DSM criteria for drug dependence (cocaine, heroin, or cannabis) and serious mental illness (schizophrenia or schizoaffective disorder, major mood disorder), a group treatment approach that combined motivational interviewing, social skills training, and monetary rewards for abstinence was found to be more effective than a group psychoeducational approach (Bellack et al. 2006).

Family interventions alone or added to other treatments can be helpful for patients who interact regularly with family members. For example, an RCT of a family intervention for dual-diagnosis individuals (77% of whom had a schizophrenia spectrum diagnosis) found that family psychoeducation, skills training, and stage-wise intervention delivered to individual families and in multifamily groups improved substance abuse outcomes compared with an extended-family psychoeducational protocol (Mueser et al. 2013).

People with severe SUDs and housing instability benefit from residential treatment that addresses their housing needs, helps them learn skills to maintain independent housing in the future, and provides intensive SUD and psychiatric treatment in a supportive environment. Long-term, tailored residential treatment is more effective than short-term residential treatment for patients with schizophrenia and co-occurring disorders (Brunette et al. 2001).

Contingency management, in which tangible rewards reinforce verifiable behaviors, has been shown to be effective in multiple RCTs among people with a dual diagnosis. Studies have shown efficacy for tobacco use disorder (Brunette et al. 2018b), alcohol use disorder (McDonell et al. 2017), stimulant use disorder (McDonell et al.

2013), and injection drug use (McDonell et al. 2013) among people with serious mental illness and comorbid SUDs.

Case Management and Assertive Community Treatment

Because people with a dual diagnosis often need many types of services and supports, case management, which links people with needed services and supports, is often used. By contrast, Assertive Community Treatment (ACT) is a team-based, intensive, and comprehensive care model in which all services, including pharmacological treatment, counseling, case management, supported employment, and substance use treatment, are provided by the ACT team, often using mobile outreach. Evidence is mixed as to whether ACT is superior to case management for reducing substance use in people with a dual diagnosis, but ACT is often used for people with frequent hospitalizations or homelessness because this service has been reported to improve community tenure (Essock et al. 2006).

Integrated Treatment

Patients with schizophrenia and comorbid SUDs are better able to access and remain in treatment when it is integrated and delivered by a multidisciplinary team that provides a consistent message about both disorders. A comprehensive approach, combining pharmacological, behavioral, and psychosocial interventions for both schizophrenia and the SUD, can improve treatment adherence and outcomes for both disorders. Attention to employment supports and housing needs may be essential for some patients. Despite the fact that inadequate treatment of either the psychotic disorder or the SUD can interfere with recovery, most people still receive treatment aimed at only one or the other of their disorders; and only approximately 18% of addiction treatment centers and 9% of mental health programs are adequately equipped to provide treatment for co-occurring disorders (McGovern et al. 2014). Thus, ongoing efforts are needed to improve access to and quality of care for people with a dual diagnosis of an SUD and another mental disorder.

Summary and Conclusion

SUDs are common in patients with schizophrenia and can have devastating effects on the illness course, quality of life, cost of care, and family burden in this population. For optimal effectiveness, treatment for dual-diagnosis individuals should be delivered in an integrated manner that addresses the needs of both conditions concurrently. In terms of pharmacological options, antipsychotic treatment is paramount. Clozapine shows promise in reducing substance use, but further studies are needed. Several FDA-approved adjunctive medications have been shown to be effective in reducing substance use among dual-diagnosis patients. In terms of nonpharmacological options, intensive combination therapy delivered in a group setting or interventions that include contingency management have yielded the highest success rates in dual-diagnosis populations. Further studies are needed to develop and evaluate effective, scalable treatment approaches for individuals with schizophrenia and co-occurring SUDs.

References

Anthenelli RM, Benowitz NL, West R, et al: Neuropsychiatric safety and efficacy of varenicline, bupropion, and nicotine patch in smokers with and without psychiatric disorders (EAGLES): a double-blind, randomised, placebo-controlled clinical trial. Lancet 387(10037):2507–2520, 2016 27116918

Batki SL, Dimmock JA, Ploutz Snyder R, et al: Directly monitored naltrexone reduces heavy drinking in schizophrenia: preliminary analysis of a controlled trial (abstract 133A). Alcohol Clin Exp Res 33 (suppl 1):11A–346A, 2009. Available at: https://onlinelibrary.wiley.com/doi/abs/10.1111/j.1530-0277.2009.01001.x. Accessed February 26, 2020.

Batki SL, Dimmock JA, Meszaros ZS, et al: Extended-release naltrexone for alcohol dependence in patients with serious mental illness (abstract 176A). Alcohol Clin Exp Res 33 (suppl 2):11A–301A, 2010. Available at: https://onlinelibrary.wiley.com/doi/abs/10.1111/j.1530-0277.2010.01208.x. Accessed February 26, 2020.

Bellack AS, Bennett ME, Gearon JS, et al: A randomized clinical trial of a new behavioral treatment for drug abuse in people with severe and persistent mental illness. Arch Gen Psychiatry 63(4):426–432, 2006 16585472

Beresford TP, Clapp L, Martin B, et al: Aripiprazole in schizophrenia with cocaine dependence: a pilot study. J Clin Psychopharmacol 25(4):363–366, 2005 16012280

Bhattacharyya S, Falkenberg I, Martin-Santos R, et al: Cannabinoid modulation of functional connectivity within regions processing attentional salience. Neuropsychopharmacology 40(6):1343–1352, 2015 25249057

Boggs DL, Surti TS, Esterlis I, et al: Minimal effects of prolonged smoking abstinence or resumption on cognitive performance challenge the "self-medication" hypothesis in schizophrenia. Schizophr Res 194:62–69, 2018a 28392208

Boggs DL, Surti T, Gupta A, et al: The effects of cannabidiol (CBD) on cognition and symptoms in outpatients with chronic schizophrenia: a randomized placebo controlled trial. Psychopharmacology (Berl) 235(7):1923–1932, 2018b 29619533

Bonsack C, Gibellini Manetti S, Favrod J, et al: Motivational intervention to reduce cannabis use in young people with psychosis: a randomized controlled trial. Psychother Psychosom 80(5):287–297, 2011 21646823

Brown ES, Jeffress J, Liggin JD, et al: Switching outpatients with bipolar or schizoaffective disorders and substance abuse from their current antipsychotic to aripiprazole. J Clin Psychiatry 66(6):756–760, 2005 15960570

Brunette MF, Drake RE, Woods M, et al: A comparison of long-term and short-term residential treatment programs for dual diagnosis patients. Psychiatr Serv 52(4):526–528, 2001 11274501

Brunette MF, Noordsy DL, Xie H, et al: Benzodiazepine use and abuse among patients with severe mental illness and co-occurring substance use disorders. Psychiatr Serv 54(10):1395–1401, 2003 14557527

Brunette MF, Dawson R, O'Keefe C, et al: An open label study of quetiapine in patients with schizophrenia and alcohol disorders. Mental Health and Substance Use 2(3):203–211, 2009. Available at: https://www.tandfonline.com/doi/abs/10.1080/17523280903156073. Accessed February 26, 2020.

Brunette MF, Dawson R, O'Keefe CD, et al: A randomized trial of clozapine vs. other antipsychotics for cannabis use disorder in patients with schizophrenia. J Dual Diagn 7(1–2):50–63, 2011 25914610

Brunette MF, Mueser KT, Babbin S, et al: Demographic and clinical correlates of substance use disorders in first episode psychosis. Schizophr Res 194:4–12, 2018a 28697856

Brunette MF, Pratt SI, Bartels SJ, et al: Randomized trial of interventions for smoking cessation among Medicaid beneficiaries with mental illness. Psychiatr Serv 69(3):274–280, 2018b 29137560

Chou K-R, Chen R, Lee J-F, et al: The effectiveness of nicotine-patch therapy for smoking cessation in patients with schizophrenia. Int J Nurs Stud 41(3):321–330, 2004 14967189

Correll CU, Robinson DG, Schooler NR, et al: Cardiometabolic risk in patients with first-episode schizophrenia spectrum disorders: baseline results from the RAISE-ETP study. JAMA Psychiatry 71(12):1350–1363, 2014 25321337

D'Souza DC, Radhakrishnan R, Sherif M, et al: Cannabinoids and psychosis. Curr Pharm Des 22(42):6380–6391, 2016 27568729

Essock SM, Mueser KT, Drake RE, et al: Comparison of ACT and standard case management for delivering integrated treatment for co-occurring disorders. Psychiatr Serv 57(2):185–196, 2006 16452695

Evins AE, Cather C, Deckersbach T, et al: A double-blind placebo-controlled trial of bupropion sustained-release for smoking cessation in schizophrenia. J Clin Psychopharmacol 25(3):218–225, 2005 15876899

Evins AE, Cather C, Culhane MA, et al: A 12-week double-blind, placebo-controlled study of bupropion SR added to high-dose dual nicotine replacement therapy for smoking cessation or reduction in schizophrenia. J Clin Psychopharmacol 27(4):380–386, 2007 17632223

Evins AE, Cather C, Pratt SA, et al: Maintenance treatment with varenicline for smoking cessation in patients with schizophrenia and bipolar disorder: a randomized clinical trial. JAMA 311(2):145–154, 2014 24399553

Evins AE, Hoeppner SS, Schoenfeld DA, et al: Maintenance pharmacotherapy normalizes the relapse curve in recently abstinent tobacco smokers with schizophrenia and bipolar disorder. Schizophr Res 183:124–129, 2017 27956009

Evins AE, Benowitz NL, West R, et al: Neuropsychiatric safety and efficacy of varenicline, bupropion, and nicotine patch in smokers with psychotic, anxiety, and mood disorders in the EAGLES trial. J Clin Psychopharmacol 39(2):108–116, 2019 30811371

Fischer AS, Whitfield-Gabrieli S, Roth RM, et al: Impaired functional connectivity of brain reward circuitry in patients with schizophrenia and cannabis use disorder: effects of cannabis and THC. Schizophr Res 158(1–3):176–182, 2014 25037524

George TP, Vessicchio JC, Termine A, et al: A placebo controlled trial of bupropion for smoking cessation in schizophrenia. Biol Psychiatry 52(1):53–61, 2002 12079730

George TP, Vessicchio JC, Sacco KA, et al: A placebo-controlled trial of bupropion combined with nicotine patch for smoking cessation in schizophrenia. Biol Psychiatry 63(11):1092–1096, 2008 18096137

Green AI, Noordsy DL, Brunette MF, et al: Substance abuse and schizophrenia: pharmacotherapeutic intervention. J Subst Abuse Treat 34(1):61–71, 2008 17574793

Green AI, Brunette MF, Dawson R, et al: Long-acting injectable vs oral risperidone for schizophrenia and co-occurring alcohol use disorder: a randomized trial. J Clin Psychiatry 76(10):1359–1365, 2015 26302441

Gulick D, Chau DT, Khokhar JY, et al: Desipramine enhances the ability of risperidone to decrease alcohol intake in the Syrian golden hamster. Psychiatry Res 218(3):329–334, 2014 24836200

Hiemstra M, Nelemans SA, Branje S, et al: Genetic vulnerability to schizophrenia is associated with cannabis use patterns during adolescence. Drug Alcohol Depend 190:143–150, 2018 30031300

Iseger TA, Bossong MG: A systematic review of the antipsychotic properties of cannabidiol in humans. Schizophr Res 162(1–3):153–161, 2015 25667194

Jeanblanc J, Balguerie K, Coune F, et al: Light alcohol intake during adolescence induces alcohol addiction in a neurodevelopmental model of schizophrenia. Addict Biol 20(3):490–499, 2015 24725220

Johnson BA, Rosenthal N, Capece JA, et al; Topiramate for Alcoholism Advisory Board; Topiramate for Alcoholism Study Group: Topiramate for treating alcohol dependence: a randomized controlled trial. JAMA 298(14):1641–1651, 2007 17925516

Kern AM, Akerman SC, Nordstrom BR: Opiate dependence in schizophrenia: case presentation and literature review. J Dual Diagn 10(1):52–57, 2014 25392062

Khokhar JY, Dwiel LL, Henricks AM, et al: The link between schizophrenia and substance use disorder: a unifying hypothesis. Schizophr Res 194:78–85, 2018 28416205

Kim SH, Han DH, Joo SY, et al: The effect of dopamine partial agonists on the nicotine dependency in patients with schizophrenia. Hum Psychopharmacol 25(2):187–190, 2010 20033907

Kozak K, Sharif-Razi M, Morozova M, et al: Effects of short-term, high-frequency repetitive transcranial magnetic stimulation to bilateral dorsolateral prefrontal cortex on smoking behavior and cognition in patients with schizophrenia and non-psychiatric controls. Schizophr Res 197:441–443, 2018 29486960

Leatherman SM, Liang MH, Krystal JH, et al: Differences in treatment effect among clinical subgroups in a randomized clinical trial of long-acting injectable risperidone and oral antipsychotics in unstable chronic schizophrenia. J Nerv Ment Dis 202(1):13–17, 2014 24375206

Leweke FM, Piomelli D, Pahlisch F, et al: Cannabidiol enhances anandamide signaling and alleviates psychotic symptoms of schizophrenia. Transl Psychiatry 2:e94, 2012 22832859

Litten RZ, Fertig JB, Falk DE, et al; NCIG 001 Study Group: A double-blind, placebo-controlled trial to assess the efficacy of quetiapine fumarate XR in very heavy-drinking alcohol-dependent patients. Alcohol Clin Exp Res 36(3):406–416, 2012 21950727

Machielsen MW, Veltman DJ, van den Brink W, et al: The effect of clozapine and risperidone on attentional bias in patients with schizophrenia and a cannabis use disorder: an fMRI study. J Psychopharmacol 28(7):633–642, 2014 24646809

Madigan K, Brennan D, Lawlor E, et al: A multi-center, randomized controlled trial of a group psychological intervention for psychosis with comorbid cannabis dependence over the early course of illness. Schizophr Res 143(1):138–142, 2013 23187069

Marconi A, Di Forti M, Lewis CM, et al: Meta-analysis of the association between the level of cannabis use and risk of psychosis. Schizophr Bull 42(5):1262–1269, 2016 26884547

McDonell MG, Srebnik D, Angelo F, et al: Randomized controlled trial of contingency management for stimulant use in community mental health patients with serious mental illness. Am J Psychiatry 170(1):94–101, 2013 23138961

McDonell MG, Leickly E, McPherson S, et al: A randomized controlled trial of ethyl glucuronide-based contingency management for outpatients with co-occurring alcohol use disorders and serious mental illness. Am J Psychiatry 174(4):370–377, 2017 28135843

McGovern MP, Lambert-Harris C, Gotham HJ, et al: Dual diagnosis capability in mental health and addiction treatment services: an assessment of programs across multiple state systems. Adm Policy Ment Health 41(2):205–214, 2014 23183873

McGuire P, Robson P, Cubala WJ, et al: Cannabidiol (CBD) as an adjunctive therapy in schizophrenia: a multicenter randomized controlled trial. Am J Psychiatry 175(3):225–231, 2018 29241357

Meszaros ZS, Abdul-Malak Y, Dimmock JA, et al: Varenicline treatment of concurrent alcohol and nicotine dependence in schizophrenia: a randomized, placebo-controlled pilot trial. J Clin Psychopharmacol 33(2):243–247, 2013 23422399

Mueser KT, Drake RE, Clark RE, et al: Evaluating Substance Abuse in Persons With Severe Mental Illness. Cambridge, MA, Human Services Research Institute, 1995. Available at: https://www.researchgate.net/publication/255596243_Evaluating_Substance_Abuse_in_Persons_with_Severe_Mental_Illness. Accessed September 28, 2020.

Mueser KT, Noordsy DL, Fox L, et al: Disulfiram treatment for alcoholism in severe mental illness. Am J Addict 12(3):242–252, 2003 12851020

Mueser KT, Glynn SM, Cather C, et al: A randomized controlled trial of family intervention for co-occurring substance use and severe psychiatric disorders. Schizophr Bull 39(3):658–672, 2013 22282453

Petrakis IL, O'Malley S, Rounsaville B, et al: Naltrexone augmentation of neuroleptic treatment in alcohol abusing patients with schizophrenia. Psychopharmacology (Berl) 172(3):291–297, 2004 14634716

Petrakis IL, Nich C, Ralevski E: Psychotic spectrum disorders and alcohol abuse: a review of pharmacotherapeutic strategies and a report on the effectiveness of naltrexone and disulfiram. Schizophr Bull 32(4):644–654, 2006 16887890

Pratt SI, Sargent J, Daniels L, et al: Appeal of electronic cigarettes in smokers with serious mental illness. Addict Behav 59:30–34, 2016 27043170

Ralevski E, O'Brien E, Jane JS, et al: Treatment with acamprosate in patients with schizophrenia spectrum disorders and comorbid alcohol dependence. J Dual Diagn 7(1–2):64–73, 2011 26954912

Regier DA, Farmer ME, Rae DS, et al: Comorbidity of mental disorders with alcohol and other drug abuse: results from the Epidemiologic Catchment Area (ECA) Study. JAMA 264(19):2511–2518, 1990 2232018

Rezvani AH, Levin ED: Cognitive effects of nicotine. Biol Psychiatry 49(3):258–267, 2001 11230877

Rosenberg SD, Drake RE, Wolford GL, et al: Dartmouth Assessment of Lifestyle Instrument (DALI): a substance use disorder screen for people with severe mental illness. Am J Psychiatry 155(2):232–238, 1998 9464203

Rosenheck RA, Krystal JH, Lew R, et al: Long-acting risperidone and oral antipsychotics in unstable schizophrenia. N Engl J Med 364(9):842–851, 2011 21366475

Rubio G, Martínez I, Ponce G, et al: Long-acting injectable risperidone compared with zuclopenthixol in the treatment of schizophrenia with substance abuse comorbidity. Can J Psychiatry 51(8):531–539, 2006 16933590

Schipper R, Dekker M, de Haan L, et al: Medicinal cannabis (Bedrolite) substitution therapy in inpatients with a psychotic disorder and a comorbid cannabis use disorder: a case series. J Psychopharmacol 32(3):353–356, 2018 29039260

Schoeler T, Monk A, Sami MB, et al: Continued versus discontinued cannabis use in patients with psychosis: a systematic review and meta-analysis. Lancet Psychiatry 3(3):215–225, 2016 26777297

Schubart CD, Sommer IE, van Gastel WA, et al: Cannabis with high cannabidiol content is associated with fewer psychotic experiences. Schizophr Res 130(1–3):216–221, 2011 21592732

Sevy S, Robinson DG, Sunday S, et al: Olanzapine vs. risperidone in patients with first-episode schizophrenia and a lifetime history of cannabis use disorders: 16-week clinical and substance use outcomes. Psychiatry Res 188(3):310–314, 2011 21636134

Smelson DA, Ziedonis D, Williams J, et al: The efficacy of olanzapine for decreasing cue-elicited craving in individuals with schizophrenia and cocaine dependence: a preliminary report. J Clin Psychopharmacol 26(1):9–12, 2006 16415698

Tidey JW, Rohsenow DJ, Kaplan GB, et al: Separate and combined effects of very low nicotine cigarettes and nicotine replacement in smokers with schizophrenia and controls. Nicotine Tob Res 15(1):121–129, 2013 22517190

Tiihonen J, Mittendorfer-Rutz E, Torniainen M, et al: Mortality and cumulative exposure to antipsychotics, antidepressants, and benzodiazepines in patients with schizophrenia: an observational follow-up study. Am J Psychiatry 173(6):600–606, 2016 26651392

Tiihonen J, Mittendorfer-Rutz E, Majak M, et al: Real-world effectiveness of antipsychotic treatments in a nationwide cohort of 29,823 patients with schizophrenia. JAMA Psychiatry 74(7):686–693, 2017 28593216

Unglaub W, Kandel M, Zenner D, et al: [Neuroleptic treatment of opiate addicts with a comorbid schizophrenia in a methadone maintenance program]. Psychiatrische Praxis 30 (suppl 2):121–124, 2003 13130354

Wijayendran SB, O'Neill A, Bhattacharyya S: The effects of cannabis use on salience attribution: a systematic review. Acta Neuropsychiatr 30(1):43–57, 2018 27866486

Williams JM, Anthenelli RM, Morris CD, et al: A randomized, double-blind, placebo-controlled study evaluating the safety and efficacy of varenicline for smoking cessation in patients with schizophrenia or schizoaffective disorder. J Clin Psychiatry 73(5):654–660, 2012 22697191

PART VIII

Special Topics

CHAPTER 50

Testing for Substances of Abuse

David A. Gorelick, M.D., Ph.D., DLFAPA, FASAM

This chapter provides a brief overview of testing for substances of abuse in clinical settings and contexts, as part of the identification and diagnosis of substance use disorders (SUDs) or of monitoring the progress of or adherence to treatment for SUDs. More detailed information on testing can be found in clinical guidelines, such as those issued by the American Society of Addiction Medicine (American Society of Addiction Medicine 2017; Jarvis et al. 2017). Testing in forensic and workplace settings is considered elsewhere in this volume (see Chapter 51, "Forensic Addiction Psychiatry," and Chapter 53, "Addiction in the Workplace"); testing in sports and athletic settings has been reviewed elsewhere (e.g., Thevis et al. 2016, 2019). This chapter is divided into two major sections: "General Principles" and "Specific Substances." The section on general principles covers concepts and methods that apply to all types of substances, such as pharmacokinetic principles, biological matrices being tested, and testing (assay) methods and characteristics. The section on specific substances provides information relevant to each of the substances covered in this textbook, in the order presented in Part III.

General Principles

Testing in Clinical Settings

Testing for substances of abuse is defined as assaying a biological sample to detect the presence or absence of a specific drug or drugs (and/or their metabolites) (Jarvis et al. 2017). Testing in clinical settings is usually done as a component of one of four tasks: screening (i.e., identification of individuals using a particular substance), assessment for a possible SUD, monitoring of treatment for an SUD, and treatment (e.g., contingency management). Because testing alone is almost never sufficient to accomplish these tasks, it should always be accompanied by other relevant components of clinical care, especially patient self-report. Any discordance between a test result and patient self-report should be used as a point of nonjudgmental engagement between clinician and patient, rather than an immediate assumption that the patient is lying. For example, the patient may not have been aware of what he or she ingested. This is often the case with illicitly manufactured substances, which are often sold on the illicit market either unlabeled or mislabeled. Conversely, an individual who recently used a substance might provide a positive self-report but produce a negative test because testing was done outside the window of detection for that substance or the individual used an amount of substance that was below the limit of detection of the assay. The typical window of detection (or detection time) for many commonly abused substances in urine, oral fluid, and blood is shown in Table 50–1.

Assays can be broadly grouped into two categories: *presumptive* (often termed *screening* or *preliminary*) and *definitive* (often termed *confirmatory*) (American Society of Addiction Medicine 2017; Jarvis et al. 2017). Presumptive assays have lower costs and more rapid turnaround times than definitive assays, but with less sensitivity and specificity (i.e., higher rates of false-negative and false-positive results). Thus, presumptive assays are most commonly used in high-volume settings (e.g., for screening purposes) and at the point of collection (i.e., point of care). In contrast, definitive assays are more expensive and time-consuming, but are more accurate and can identify specific substances within a class. Thus, definitive assays are often used to confirm the result of a presumptive assay, especially when significant clinical decisions are at stake, such as referral to or retention in treatment, or when significant legal or occupational consequences may flow from the assay result.

Regardless of the assay or the test context, a positive test result indicates only that the individual has used the substance within the window of detection for that substance. A positive test result does not indicate that the substance was responsible for any of the patient's current signs and symptoms, nor does it indicate a diagnosis of an SUD. An SUD diagnosis is always a clinical decision based on a careful assessment of the patient's behavior over time. The *Diagnostic and Statistical Manual of Mental Disorders*, 5th Edition (DSM-5; American Psychiatric Association 2013) diagnostic criteria for SUDs do not require any particular duration, frequency, or intensity of substance use. Thus, a positive test for a substance does not necessarily indicate an SUD, and a negative test does not automatically rule out an SUD.

In choosing the appropriate test, the clinician must take into account several variables: the substance(s) being tested for, the biological matrix to be tested, and the assay to be used (American Society of Addiction Medicine 2017). When interpreting the test result, the clinician must take into account the pharmacokinetics of the substance (especially the window of detection) in the biological matrix being tested and the characteristics of the assay (e.g., limit of detection, sensitivity, specificity) as applied to the substance being tested for. These variables are discussed below.

Pharmacokinetic Principles

Testing for any substance is significantly influenced by the pharmacokinetic characteristics of the substance, especially its half-life (i.e., how rapidly the parent com-

TABLE 50–1. **Typical time window of detection (in days) for commonly abused substances in urine, oral fluid, and blood**

Substance	Detection window (days)[a]		
	Urine	Oral Fluid	Blood
Alcohol	0.5	1	—
Amobarbital	3 [100]	—	—
Amphetamine	1–4 [100, 500, 1,000]	1–2 [100]	2 [4]
Buprenorphine	7 [0.5]	—	—
Butalbital	7 [100]	—	—
Cannabis (THC)	1–3 [15, 50, 100]	0.5–2 [0.5, 15]	0.2 [10]
Cocaine (BZE)	2–4 [150, 300]	0.5–3	0.5–2
Codeine	1–4 [300]	0.3–1.5 [2.5, 40]	—
Diazepam	2–10 [100, 300, 500]	1–3	—
Fentanyl	1–3 [0.2, 5]	—	—
GHB	0.5 [10,000]	0.2 [4,000]	0.2 [4,000]
Heroin (6-MAM)	1–3 [10, 300]	0.3 [1]	—
Hydrocodone	1–3 [0.2, 5]	—	—
Hydromorphone	1–4 [25, 300]	0.25 [1]	—
LSD	1–1.5 [0.2, 0.5]	—	—
MDMA	1–3 [20, 25]	—	—
Methadone	2–7 [100, 300]	1–3 [5, 20]	—
Methamphetamine	1–5 [500, 1,000]	1 [2.5]	2 [3]
Morphine	1–5 [25, 300]	0.5–1.5 [0.6, 1]	—
Oxycodone	1–1.5 [100]	—	—
Oxymorphone	1.5–2.5 [100]	—	—
Pentobarbital	3–8 [300]	—	—
Phencyclidine	1.5–10 [25]	—	—
Phenobarbital	15 [100]	—	—

Note. Typical detection time (days) for parent compound (unless otherwise indicated) after single or intermittent use; detection time will be longer with heavy or chronic use, if assay includes metabolites, for extended-release formulations, or with lower cutoff values.
[a]Cutoff value(s) (ng/mL) shown in brackets.
—=no data provided; BZE=benzoylecgonine; GHB=γ-hydroxybutyrate; LSD=lysergic acid diethylamide; 6-MAM=6-monoacetylmorphine; MDMA=3,4-methylenedioxymethamphetamine ("ecstasy"); THC=Δ⁹-tetrahydrocannabinol.
Source. Adapted from American Society of Addiction Medicine 2017.

pound is broken down) and the presence or absence of detectable metabolites. These pharmacokinetic characteristics help determine the window of detection for the substance—that is, the amount of time after the substance was ingested during which it can be detected. Substances whose parent compound has a long half-life and/or detectable metabolites will have longer windows of detection compared with substances whose parent compound has a short half-life and no detectable metabolites.

Biological Matrices

Substances of abuse can be detected in a variety of biological matrices, including urine, blood (whole blood, plasma, or serum), oral fluid, hair, exhaled breath, and sweat (American Society of Addiction Medicine 2017). Several other biological matrices used only in specific clinical settings or under evaluation are not covered in this chapter. These include meconium and umbilical cord blood, used for substance testing during the perinatal period (Concheiro et al. 2017); dried blood spots, which can be collected by capillary sampling (Sadones et al. 2014); and nails (Hill et al. 2018).

The choice of matrix for any particular test depends on several factors, including the pharmacokinetic characteristics of the substance in the matrix and the cost and convenience of collecting a specimen from the patient. Available matrices differ in these characteristics. Blood is the matrix that most closely reflects the current concentration of a substance in the central nervous system, the presumed major site of action of psychoactive substances. Blood concentrations are more closely correlated with the pharmacodynamic effects of the substance and more likely to reflect recent ingestion. Concentrations in oral fluid, a filtrate of blood, also reflect recent ingestion, although the blood:oral fluid concentration ratio is not necessarily 1:1 (Gjerde et al. 2014). Therefore, blood and oral fluid are the preferred matrices when the goal of testing is to detect recent substance use or to correlate use with pharmacodynamic effects. In contrast, urine and hair concentrations reflect long-term exposure to the substance and the degree to which the substance is stored in the body after ingestion. Therefore, urine and hair are the preferred matrices when the goal of testing is to identify patterns of long-term use and/or when the time of the most recent ingestion is not important.

Ease of collection, the resources needed, and the costs involved are often key factors in choosing a biological matrix for testing (American Society of Addiction Medicine 2017). Blood (typically collected from a peripheral vein) is the most difficult and expensive matrix to collect. Blood collection is an invasive procedure that requires a trained health professional and sterile technique, making it impractical for either nonclinical or low-intensity clinical settings. Blood collection also has the possibility of clinically significant harm not associated with other biological matrices. For this reason, blood is less often used for presumptive (screening) purposes but more often used for definitive testing. In contrast, collection of other matrices is not considered invasive, does not require a health professional, and poses no physical harms. However, urine collection has disadvantages in comparison with collection of oral fluid, breath, sweat, and hair: it requires a private collection area and staff observation (to ensure validity), which increase costs and pose a loss of privacy and risk of embarrassment.

Urine

Urine is the most widely used and studied biological matrix for testing in clinical settings, and has the greatest body of supporting evidence, especially for presumptive testing (American Society of Addiction Medicine 2017; Moeller et al. 2017; Nelson et al. 2016). Both parent substances and their metabolites appear in urine. In general, the window of detection for substances in urine runs from about 2 hours to 1–4 days after ingestion. The window of detection depends on several factors, including the individual's recent fluid intake and overall level of hydration, which influence the concentration of substances in the urine; the pH of the urine, which influences the degree to which substances are transported into or out of the urine; and the time interval between urine collection and last voiding, which influences the amount of substance accumulated in the bladder.

Urine has two major disadvantages compared with other matrices. First, because it is not directly derived from blood, but rather reflects processing in the kidneys, it is less likely to contain the parent substance that was ingested and more likely to contain mostly metabolites of the substance. Second, it is relatively easy to compromise the validity of a urine specimen. This could be done in one of three ways: diluting the sample so that the concentration of the substance is below the limit of detection or cutoff threshold for that assay, adulterating the sample to interfere with the ability of the assay to detect the substance (Fu 2016), or substituting another specimen (either urine or synthetic urine) for the individual's own specimen (Jaffee et al. 2007). Dilution can be attempted by drinking large quantities of water over several hours before collection and/or by taking a diuretic to enhance urine flow. Adulteration can be done either in vivo (e.g., by ingesting something before urine collection) or ex vivo (i.e., by adding something to the specimen after collection). Commonly used ex vivo adulterants include strong oxidants that can break down the drug molecule.

Several techniques help to prevent specimen tampering. The most effective and commonly used method is to have a staff member directly observe the urine collection. To minimize patient embarrassment, observation is typically done by a staff member of the same gender as the patient, and preferably from behind a one-way mirror. When direct observation is not possible, the urine collection procedure should be arranged to minimize the opportunity for specimen substitution or tampering; recommendations include prohibiting the carrying of personal items into the collection area; keeping potential adulterants, such as soap, out of the area; adding brightly colored dye to the toilet; and shutting off all water sources.

Every urine specimen should be checked for signs of possible tampering, especially when not collected under direct observation. Common signs of a possibly invalid urine specimen include an unusual smell (e.g., of vinegar or alcohol), color (very pale color suggests dilution), or appearance (e.g., soapy [from addition of soap], floating particles [from addition of salt or another adulterant]), or a temperature outside the range of plausible body temperature (which should be about 90°–100°F within 4 minutes of collection). If specimen tampering is suspected, several simple measures to evaluate specimen validity can be taken (Kirsh et al. 2015); these are sometimes built into point-of-collection or testing material (e.g., temperature-sensitive strips on the side of the collection cup). Such specimen validity measures include creatinine concentration (<20 mg/dL indicates a dilute urine), pH (normal range= 4.5–8.0; abnormal values suggest dilution or addition of a strongly alkaline [e.g., bleach] or acidic [e.g., vinegar] adulterant), specific gravity (normal range=1.003– 1.030; values below normal range suggest dilution, whereas values above normal range suggest addition of an adulterant, such as salt), and temperature (cooler than expected temperature suggests dilution with a cool liquid; warmer than expected temperature suggests heating of a cool diluent). There are also standardized chemical tests (some available for point-of-collection use) to detect some commonly used adulterants, such as glutaraldehyde, nitrates, and pyridinium chlorochromate (Fu 2016).

However, some commonly used adulterants, such as tetrahydrozoline (found in some medicated eye drops), are not detected by most such tests.

Blood

Blood is used as a biological matrix primarily when definitive testing or a quantitative substance concentration is needed (American Society of Addiction Medicine 2017). Its use for presumptive testing or screening is discouraged by the expense and invasiveness, including the need for universal precautions when handling the specimen. Blood has two advantages over urine: a very low likelihood of tampering and a greater likelihood of detecting the parent compound.

Oral Fluid

Oral fluid, commonly termed saliva, actually includes fluid excreted by cells of the oral mucosa and gingival crevice, as well as the salivary glands (American Society of Addiction Medicine 2017). Substances enter oral fluid from the blood primarily by passive diffusion. Therefore, oral fluid concentrations are usually highly correlated with blood concentrations. A major exception is when a substance has recently been taken orally. Direct contact with and adsorption onto the oral mucosa may result in very high substance concentrations that do not reflect actual blood concentrations. To avoid such misleading results, oral fluid specimens should not be collected within 2 hours of oral intake of the substance(s) targeted for testing.

Oral fluid, like urine, is widely used for presumptive testing. It sometimes replaces urine because of two advantages. First, although collection is under direct observation, thereby minimizing the possibility of specimen tampering, collection is less intrusive because there is no need for toilet facilities, and no privacy issues are involved. Second, oral fluid is more likely than urine to contain the parent compound because oral fluid is directly derived from blood.

Hair

Hair absorbs substances from two sources: blood flowing through the hair follicle and sweat that collects around the base of the hair shaft (American Society of Addiction Medicine 2017; Frederick 2012). A major advantage of using hair is the long window of detection compared with all other biological matrices, although hair does not detect recent use. Substances can generally be detected in hair from about 8 days after ingestion, the time it takes the hair shaft to grow from the follicle to above the skin, where it can be collected. Because substances in hair gradually degrade over time, detection is less reliable after 3 months. Substance absorption varies somewhat based on hair characteristics such as pigmentation and texture. The concentration of melanin in hair may affect absorption of drugs such as cocaine, but there is little evidence that race itself influences drug absorption (Cuypers and Flanagan 2018).

Two potential sources of invalid results from hair testing are external contamination of the hair shaft by drugs in the environment (but not ingested by the individual) and use of hair treatments (Cuypers and Flanagan 2018). External contamination can be minimized by washing or decontaminating the hair sample before analysis. However, this process itself may alter assay results, and the degree of decontamination may vary with hair characteristics. One approach to minimizing false-positive hair test results is to assay for drug metabolites (presumably generated by in vivo drug metabolism) rather than for the parent drug. However, testing for drug metabolites may require more sophisticated assays that are more expensive and not as widely available as assays for the parent compound.

Hair testing may also be affected by chemical treatments, such as straightening and bleaching. Some treatments may alter hair characteristics in ways that change the rate at which substances are absorbed into or eliminated from hair (Marrinan et al. 2017; Pritchett and Phinney 2015). For example, some hair treatments favored by specific racial/ethnic groups increase drug concentrations in hair, albeit in all hair types (Kidwell et al. 2015). There is little evidence supporting the effectiveness of products sold to help evade hair testing (Marrinan et al. 2017).

Because analysis of hair specimens is time-consuming and expensive, it is typically reserved for situations requiring a long window of detection or a determination of patterns of substance use. Hair specimens are usually collected from the scalp, but can also be collected from the face, axilla, and pubic areas. Because hair on the body grows more slowly than hair on the head, body hair may provide a longer window of detection, potentially up to 12 months. Individuals should be questioned about their use of chemical hair treatments so that an alternate collection site can be used, if necessary.

Breath

Substances that volatilize at body temperature, such as alcohol (ethanol), can be assayed in exhaled breath (American Society of Addiction Medicine 2017). Breath testing is used almost exclusively for alcohol, which appears in exhaled air by diffusion from pulmonary capillaries into the pulmonary alveoli. Most testing for alcohol is done in this way; breath alcohol concentration directly reflects the blood alcohol concentration. Numerous small, portable devices have been developed that can be used at the point of collection or in forensic settings (e.g., roadside testing to detect driving under the influence of alcohol).

Nonvolatile substances might be detectable in exhaled breath to the extent that they are absorbed onto aerosolized microparticles in exhaled breath (Beck et al. 2016; Trefz et al. 2017). These particles can be condensed after exhalation and then assayed for substances. Relatively little research and few systematic studies have evaluated testing for nonvolatile substances in exhaled breath. One comparison of breath and urine testing for cannabis, opioids, stimulants, and benzodiazepines in 112 patients found breath testing to be less sensitive than urine testing (i.e., only 58% of patients positive in urine were also positive in breath) (Carlsson et al. 2015). However, there were no false-positive breath tests. The drugs found in urine that were least likely to be detected in breath were cannabis (0%) and benzodiazepines (16%). This pattern of findings could be due, in part, to the fact that urine has a longer window of detection for the drugs tested than does breath.

In most circumstances, especially forensics, breath alcohol testing is considered presumptive, rather than definitive, largely because of two limitations. First, recent oral ingestion of alcohol from other sources, such as in food or oral hygiene products, will generate a falsely high test result. Second, an insufficient volume of exhaled breath may limit assay validity.

Sweat

Ingested substances appear in sweat by at least two possible mechanisms: diffusion from blood vessels surrounding the sweat glands and excretion from sebaceous glands on the skin (American Society of Addiction Medicine 2017; De Giovanni and Fucci 2013). The exact mechanisms remain unclear. A sweat specimen is collected on an absorbent pad, often termed a "sweat patch," that is held tightly against the skin by an overlying adhesive film. Environmental contamination of the collection pad is prevented by the overlying film. The substance concentration represents the amount accumulated over the duration that the patch was worn, typically 1–2 weeks. This concentration includes drugs ingested from about 24 hours before the patch was applied until 24 hours before the patch is removed. Sweat, like hair, offers a relatively long window of detection. The sweat patch can also be applied prospectively as a deterrent to future substance use. Another advantage of the sweat patch is that it collects both parent drug and any metabolites that appear in blood, allowing identification of parent drugs that may share the same metabolite (e.g., codeine and heroin). The major limitations of sweat collection are loss of the patch, either inadvertently from loss of adhesion or intentionally by patient removal; inability to determine when an identified drug was actually ingested; and cost. Tampering is usually evident in the form of wrinkles, creases, rips, needle holes, or discoloration of the adhesive covering or the absorbent pad. Commercially available sweat pads are roughly comparable in cost to point-of-collection urine test devices, but there are additional costs for assay of the sweat specimen at a laboratory.

There are relatively few studies evaluating the test characteristics or effectiveness of sweat testing in realistic clinical settings. Thus, sweat testing is not as commonly used in clinical settings as other biological matrices such as urine and oral fluid.

Test Methods

The assays used for substance testing vary in several important characteristics, such as limit of detection, sensitivity, specificity, and cross-reactivity (American Society of Addiction Medicine 2017). *Limit of detection* refers to the lowest concentration (smallest amount) of a substance that can be detected (identified) by the assay. This is the major factor determining the sensitivity of a test—that is, the likelihood that the test will detect a substance that is actually present in the specimen being tested (generating a true-positive result).

Sensitivity is calculated as the number of true-positive tests divided by the number of all truly positive specimens (i.e., true positives plus false negatives). A negative result in a test with high sensitivity likely rules out the presence of the substance, because the likelihood of a false-negative result is low. For example, if a drug test has 90% sensitivity, then 90% of positive test results are true positives (i.e., the drug is actually present); only 10% of positive results are false negatives (i.e., negative test results when the drug is actually present).

Specificity refers to the likelihood that a negative test result reflects the true absence of that substance (i.e., is not a false negative). Specificity is calculated as the number of true negative tests divided by the number of all truly negative specimens (i.e., true negatives plus false positives). A positive result in a test with high specificity likely means that the substance is present, because the likelihood of a false-positive result is low. For example, if a drug test has 90% specificity, then 90% of negative test results are true negatives (i.e., the drug is actually absent); only 10% of negative results are false positives (i.e., positive test results when the drug is actually absent).

Cross-reactivity refers to the extent to which the chemicals or antibodies in the assay react with substances other than the intended target of the test. This is a major factor in determining the specificity of a test.

Assays used for drug testing vary widely in their chemical methods. Immunoassays use antibodies directed against specific substances (both parent compounds and metabolites) to trigger an enzyme reaction whose intensity corresponds to the concentration of the substances in the specimen. Commonly used varieties of immunoassays include the enzyme-multiplied immunoassay technique (EMIT), the enzyme-linked immunosorbent assay (ELISA), the cloned enzyme donor immunoassay (CEDIA), and the fluorescence polarization immunoassay (FPIA). Immunoassays generally (but not always) react with a range of substances with similar chemical structures, which would lower assay specificity. Dozens of legal prescription and over-the-counter medications cross-react with common immunoassays to produce false-positive test results (Saitman et al. 2014). Immunoassays provide only qualitative results, typically as a dichotomous "present" or "absent" result based on whether the substance's concentration is above or below a prespecified cutoff value. The cutoff value is chosen as a compromise between sensitivity and specificity, which are reciprocally related. The lower the cutoff value is, the better the test sensitivity but the poorer the test specificity. Conversely, the higher the cutoff value is, the better the test specificity but the poorer the test sensitivity. For these reasons, immunoassays are generally used as presumptive (screening) tests, rather than definitive tests.

Immunoassays have several practical advantages. Because of their low cost, they can be used in high-volume settings. They generate test results within minutes of adding the specimen. They have been automated in small, lightweight units, so they are commonly used as point-of-collection tests (Wiencek et al. 2017). Therefore, they provide prompt results for the clinician and avoid the delay, expense, and possible specimen loss involved in sending specimens to a testing laboratory. Point-of-collection immunoassays, especially for urine, are usually packaged as a panel that tests for several substances at the same time. The most commonly used panel is probably the five-drug panel mandated by federal workplace drug testing regulations (known as the SAMHSA 5 or the NIDA 5 [referring to the Substance Abuse and Mental Health Services Administration and the National Institute on Drug Abuse]), which screens for cannabis (detects Δ^9-tetrahydrocannabinol [THC] and its metabolite THC-9-carboxylic acid), cocaine (detects the metabolite benzoylecgonine [BZE]), amphetamines, opiates (detects morphine), and phencyclidine (PCP). A variety of more extensive panels are also available, including some that test for up to 15 substances. The clinician should choose a panel that tests for the substances most expected in a particular clinical setting.

Chromatographic tests use the physical and chemical properties of compounds held in a stationary column to separate the substances in a heated specimen (in vaporized or liquid phase) as they flow through the column. The specimen is carried through the column by either a gas (gas chromatography) or a liquid (liquid chromatography). Because of differential binding to compounds in the column, substances travel through the column at different rates, and thus leave the column at different times. As substances leave the column, they are identified by mass spectrometry (MS). MS splits the molecules into ionized atoms and passes them through an electric field. This separates the ions by their electric charge, with more highly charged ions traveling faster. The stream of ions then passes through a magnetic field, which bends the ions from the stream, with the degree of bending dependent on their weight and charge. Heavier and more negatively charged ions bend less than lighter and more positively charged ions. This process generates a spectrum of ions separated by their differing weight/charge ratios. Each substance generates a unique MS spectrum, but its identification depends on matching the observed MS spectrum with a known MS spectrum associated with a specific substance.

Chromatographic tests are considered to be definitive tests because of their high sensitivity and specificity. They also provide quantitative results, which may be useful in correlating substance concentrations with pharmacodynamic effects. A major disadvantage of chromatographic tests is their requirement for expensive equipment and trained technicians. Therefore, chromatographic tests are performed in laboratories and are not available for point-of-collection testing.

Specific Substances

Alcohol

Because alcohol (ethanol) is a volatile chemical at body temperature, it is commonly measured in exhaled breath, as well as in blood, oral fluid, and urine (American Society of Addiction Medicine 2017). For all matrices except urine, ethanol itself is most commonly measured. In urine testing, measurement of alcohol metabolites (conjugates), such as ethyl glucuronide and ethyl sulfate, allows a much longer window of detection, typically 1–2 days, than does measurement of alcohol itself.

Alcohol is eliminated from the body by a constant amount per unit of time, independent of the concentration (i.e., zero-order kinetics), except at very low alcohol concentrations (Cederbaum 2012). Almost all other substances of clinical interest follow first-order kinetics—that is, their concentration decreases as a proportion of the current concentration. The "typical" 70-kg (154-lb) individual eliminates alcohol at a rate of 7 g/hour. Because alcohol is not stored in the body, this fairly constant rate allows back-estimation of the time at which alcohol was last ingested. However, there is up to fourfold individual variation around this "typical" elimination rate, in part because of genetic variability in the enzyme alcohol dehydrogenase, the first step in the alcohol metabolic pathway. Women eliminate alcohol faster than men, even after correction for lean body mass.

Stimulants

Cocaine and its major metabolite, BZE, are readily detected in blood, urine, and oral fluid. Cocaine is an ester that is readily metabolized by enzymes throughout the body, and also spontaneously at body temperature and pH. Therefore, the window of detection for the parent substance is relatively short; most urine tests identify BZE rather than cocaine. The windows of detection for cocaine and BZE in urine are 24 hours and

2–4 days, respectively; in blood, 12 hours and 2 days, respectively; and in oral fluid, 8–12 hours and 1–2 days, respectively. In chronic, heavy users of cocaine, BZE may be detected in urine (300 ng/mL cutoff) up to 2 weeks after the last use (Preston et al. 2002). Cocaine can also be detected in hair (Felli et al. 2005) and sweat (Uemura et al. 2004), but these matrices are rarely used in clinical settings because results may vary depending on methodological aspects of specimen collection and varying rates of cocaine disappearance from the matrix after cessation of use.

Amphetamines are readily detected in urine, blood, and oral fluid, with windows of detection of 2–4 days in urine (7–10 days for heavy users), 1–2 days in oral fluid, and 2 days in blood (American Society of Addiction Medicine 2017). Immunoassays for amphetamines have limited specificity, as they generally target only amphetamine. They do not distinguish between amphetamine and methamphetamine, because the former is a metabolite of the latter. Amphetamine tests are more likely than tests for other substances to generate false-positive results, because amphetamines and structurally similar compounds are found in legally available medications, such as those used to treat attention-deficit/hyperactivity disorder, as well as in over-the-counter preparations for respiratory conditions (e.g., Vicks® inhaler). Amphetamine immunoassays have some cross-reactivity with cathinone (the stimulant compound in khat) and limited cross-reactivity with synthetic cathinones ("bath salts") (Dasgupta 2017). Identification of specific stimulant compounds requires laboratory-based definitive testing.

Opioids

Opioids can be detected in blood, urine, oral fluid, and hair, but most presumptive tests identify opioids as a group rather than specific individual opioids (American Society of Addiction Medicine 2017). Standard presumptive immunoassays for opioids target morphine, so a positive test could be due to ingestion of heroin, codeine, and/or morphine itself (which is a metabolite of heroin and codeine). Standard presumptive immunoassays also show some cross-reactivity with semisynthetic opioids derived from morphine, such as hydrocodone and hydromorphone, but show little cross-reactivity with semisynthetic opioids derived from thebaine, such as oxycodone and oxymorphone. They show little to no cross-reactivity with synthetic opioids such as methadone, buprenorphine, meperidine, and fentanyl. Detection of a specific opioid requires a test targeted specifically to that opioid or to a metabolite generated only by that opioid (e.g., 6-monoacetylmorphine [6-MAM] from heroin, sometimes termed 6-acetylmorphine [6-AM]).

Heroin has a very short half-life (10–30 minutes), so tests for heroin actually target its specific metabolite 6-MAM, which has a window of detection of 1–8 hours in oral fluid and 1–3 days in urine. Morphine, a metabolite of 6-MAM, has a window of detection of 12–24 hours in oral fluid and 1–5 days in urine. Codeine, which is metabolized to morphine, has a window of detection of 7–24 hours in oral fluid and 1–3 days in urine. Semisynthetic opioid analgesics, such as hydrocodone, hydromorphone (a metabolite of hydrocodone), oxycodone, and oxymorphone (a metabolite of oxycodone), have windows of detection of 2–4 days in urine; extended-release formulations may have even longer windows. The synthetic opioid methadone has a window of detection of 1–3 days in oral fluid and 2–7 days in urine. When taken daily on a long-term basis (as in treatment for opioid use disorder), methadone has a window of detection of 3–5 days in oral fluid and up to 11 days in urine. Buprenorphine, also used in the treatment of opioid use disorder, has a window of detection of 5 days in oral fluid and up to 7 days in urine.

Hallucinogens, Club Drugs, and Designer Drugs

Hallucinogens (e.g., lysergic acid diethylamide [LSD], mescaline), club drugs (e.g., 3,4-methylenedioxymethamphetamine [MDMA; "ecstasy," "molly"], inhalants), and designer drugs (e.g., synthetic cannabinoids ["spice"], synthetic cathinones ["bath salts"]) are difficult to identify with commonly used presumptive tests such as immunoassays (Dasgupta 2017; Liu et al. 2018), for several reasons. First, many of these substances are highly potent, so concentrations in biological matrices may be below the limit of detection. Second, standard immunoassays have limited sensitivity and specificity for these substances. Because of their chemical structures, these substances may be completely undetected or may cross-react as a more common substance. For example, synthetic cannabinoids are not detected by immunoassays for THC (plant cannabis). Common cross-reactivities include cathinone (khat), synthetic cathinones, and psilocybin with immunoassays for amphetamines. Thus, detection of these substances requires either a targeted immunoassay or a definitive test such as gas or a liquid chromatography. Targeted immunoassays have recently been developed for some common synthetic cannabinoids and synthetic cathinones. Development of a definitive test for a new designer drug lags behind the drug's appearance on the illicit market because test development requires identification of the compound's chemical structure and synthesis of the compound for use as an internal standard.

Cannabis

Cannabis is most commonly detected via urine testing but can also be detected in blood, oral fluid, and hair (American Society of Addiction Medicine 2017; Musshoff and Madea 2006). Testing for cannabis usually measures THC and/or its major (inactive) metabolite 11-nor-9-carboxy-THC. Regardless of the testing matrix, cannabidiol and other clinically relevant cannabinoids are detected with less sensitivity or not at all.

THC has a complex pharmacokinetic profile, which complicates interpretation of tests (Huestis and Smith 2018). THC is highly lipophilic and is stored in fatty tissue throughout the body. Therefore, regular or heavy users may test positive long after their last use (e.g., THC is detectable for several weeks in urine), as a result of the gradual release of THC from body stores as blood concentrations decline; this makes it impossible to confidently determine the time since last cannabis ingestion by testing of a single specimen. Several algorithms have been developed to help calculate the time of last ingestion based on ratios of THC metabolites to parent compound, but these algorithms are not practical for routine clinical use. This extended THC release from body stores also results in a poor correlation between THC concentrations in biological matrices (especially urine) and the degree of current cannabis effects.

Tobacco (Nicotine)

Nicotine, the primary psychoactive constituent of tobacco, has a half-life of about 2 hours, so it is not useful as a marker of tobacco use in clinical settings (Benowitz et al.

2009). The common target for testing is cotinine, the major metabolite of nicotine, which has a half-life of about 16 hours. Cotinine can be measured in blood, oral fluid, and urine, with a window of detection of 3–4 days. Measurement of 3-hydroxy-cotinine, the primary metabolite of cotinine, provides an even longer window of detection (about an additional 6 hours). The cotinine concentration cutoff values generally used to identify whether a patient has abstained from tobacco smoking are 3 ng/mL in serum, 12 ng/mL in oral fluid, and 50–200 ng/mL in urine (Kim 2016).

Nicotine replacement therapies will also generate a positive test for nicotine or cotinine (Benowitz et al. 2009). In the context of nicotine replacement therapy, recent tobacco use can be identified by measuring anatabine in urine. Anatabine is a minor alkaloid in tobacco with a half-life of 10–16 hours.

Benzodiazepines and Other Sedative-Hypnotics

Benzodiazepines are typically measured in blood, urine, and oral fluid (American Society of Addiction Medicine 2017). Many immunoassays for benzodiazepines have low sensitivity and specificity, largely because of their poor cross-reactivity with the urinary metabolites of some commonly used benzodiazepines (Nelson et al. 2016). For example, they may not detect clonazepam, which appears in very low concentrations at therapeutic doses. Many immunoassays specifically target diazepam metabolites, such as oxazepam and nordiazepam, and therefore may not detect other benzodiazepines such as alprazolam and lorazepam. The window of detection for benzodiazepines in urine varies depending on the half-life of the parent benzodiazepine and of its metabolites. Short-acting benzodiazepines, such as midazolam and triazolam, are detectable for 1–2 days. Intermediate-acting benzodiazepines, such as alprazolam, clonazepam, and lorazepam, are detectable for 2–5 days. The long-acting benzodiazepines chlordiazepoxide and diazepam also have long-lived metabolites, so they may be detected in urine for 5 days to 3 weeks.

Barbiturates are typically measured in blood, urine, and oral fluid (American Society of Addiction Medicine 2017; Fritch et al. 2011). Many immunoassays primarily target secobarbital but have good cross-reactivity with other barbiturates (Nelson et al. 2016). With barbiturates, as with benzodiazepines, the window of detection in urine varies with the half-life of the parent compound and of its metabolites. Short-acting barbiturates, such as secobarbital, are detectable for 3–5 days. Intermediate-acting barbiturates, such as amobarbital, butabarbital, and pentobarbital, are detectable for 3–8 days. Long-acting barbiturates, such as phenobarbital, are detectable for 10–30 days.

Conclusion

A variety of immunoassays and chromatographic tests for detecting abused substances in biological matrices are available to help guide the diagnosis and treatment of SUDs. The clinician should choose a test based on several factors: the goal of testing (e.g., presumptive/screening vs. definitive/confirmatory), the window of detection needed, the cost and acceptability of collecting the biological matrix to be tested, and the need for a prompt result (e.g., point-of-collection vs. laboratory testing). Another relevant factor is whether the substance being tested for is known in advance (i.e., targeted vs. untargeted testing). The continuing appearance on the illicit drug market of abused substances with new chemical structures (so-called designer drugs or new psychoactive substances) means that the testing field must continually develop new assays and methods to help the clinician.

Key clinical points on this topic are listed below:

- Clinicians should choose a test based on the targeted substance(s), the goal of testing, and the ease and cost of specimen collection.
- Testing for substances of abuse can be done in several biological matrices, including blood, oral fluid, urine, hair, breath, and sweat.
- Tests can be either presumptive (e.g., for screening) or definitive (e.g., to identify a specific compound).
- Windows of detection for substances can range from hours to weeks, depending on the biological matrix, the sensitivity of the assay, and the pharmacokinetics of the substance.
- Point-of-collection tests are quick and inexpensive, but are usually only presumptive.
- Laboratory tests are expensive and time-consuming, but are definitive.
- Urine is the biological matrix most vulnerable to specimen tampering.

References

American Psychiatric Association: Diagnostic and Statistical Manual of Mental Disorders, 5th Edition. Arlington, VA, American Psychiatric Association, 2013

American Society of Addiction Medicine: Consensus Statement: Appropriate use of drug testing in clinical addiction medicine. 2017. Available at: https://www.asam.org/docs/default-source/quality-science/appropriate_use_of_drug_testing_in_clinical-1-(7).pdf?sfvrsn=2. Accessed January 16, 2020.

Beck O, Olin A-C, Mirgorodskaya E: Potential of mass spectrometry in developing clinical laboratory biomarkers of nonvolatiles in exhaled breath. Clin Chem 62(1):84–91, 2016 26578691

Benowitz NL, Hukkanen J, Jacob P 3rd: Nicotine chemistry, metabolism, kinetics and biomarkers. Handb Exp Pharmacol 192(192):29–60, 2009 19184645

Carlsson S, Olsson R, Lindkvist I, et al: Application of drug testing using exhaled breath for compliance monitoring of drug addicts in treatment. Scand J Clin Lab Invest 75(2):156–161, 2015 25562730

Cederbaum AI: Alcohol metabolism. Clin Liver Dis 16(4):667–685, 2012 23101976

Concheiro M, Lendoiro E, de Castro A, et al: Bioanalysis for cocaine, opiates, methadone, and amphetamines exposure detection during pregnancy. Drug Test Anal 9(6):898–904, 2017 27595432

Cuypers E, Flanagan RJ: The interpretation of hair analysis for drugs and drug metabolites. Clin Toxicol (Phila) 56(2):90–100, 2018 28938866

Dasgupta A: Challenges in laboratory detection of unusual substance abuse: issues with magic mushroom, peyote cactus, khat, and solvent abuse. Adv Clin Chem 78:163–186, 2017 28057187

De Giovanni N, Fucci N: The current status of sweat testing for drugs of abuse: a review. Curr Med Chem 20(4):545–561, 2013 23244520

Felli M, Martello S, Marsili R, et al: Disappearance of cocaine from human hair after abstinence. Forensic Sci Int 154(2–3):96–98, 2005 16182955

Frederick DL: Toxicology testing in alternative specimen matrices. Clin Lab Med 32(3):467–492, 2012 22939303

Fritch D, Blum K, Nonnemacher S, et al: Barbiturate detection in oral fluid, plasma, and urine. Ther Drug Monit 33(1):72–79, 2011 21099741

Fu S: Adulterants in urine drug testing. Adv Clin Chem 76:123–163, 2016 27645818

Gjerde H, Langel K, Favretto D, et al: Estimation of equivalent cutoff thresholds in blood and oral fluid for drug prevalence studies. J Anal Toxicol 38(2):92–98, 2014 24451086

Hill VA, Stowe GN, Paulsen RB, et al: Nail analysis for drugs: a role in workplace testing? J Anal Toxicol 42(6):425–436, 2018 29554333

Huestis MA, Smith ML: Cannabinoid markers in biological fluids and tissues: revealing intake. Trends Mol Med 24(2):156–172, 2018 29398403

Jaffee WB, Trucco E, Levy S, et al: Is this urine really negative? A systematic review of tampering methods in urine drug screening and testing. J Subst Abuse Treat 33(1):33–42, 2007 17588487

Jarvis M, Williams J, Hurford M, et al: Appropriate use of drug testing in clinical addiction medicine. J Addict Med 11(3):163–173, 2017 28557958

Kidwell DA, Smith FP, Shepherd AR: Ethnic hair care products may increase false positives in hair drug testing. Forensic Sci Int 257:160–164, 2015 26338354

Kim S: Overview of cotinine cutoff values for smoking status classification. Int J Environ Res Public Health 13(12):1236–1240, 2016 27983665

Kirsh KL, Christo PJ, Heit H, et al: Specimen validity testing in urine drug monitoring of medications and illicit drugs: clinical implications. J Opioid Manag 11(1):53–59, 2015 25750165

Liu L, Wheeler SE, Venkataramanan R, et al: Newly emerging drugs of abuse and their detection methods: an ACLPS critical review. Am J Clin Pathol 149(2):105–116, 2018 29385414

Marrinan S, Roman-Urrestarazu A, Naughton D, et al: Hair analysis for the detection of drug use—is there potential for evasion? Hum Psychopharmacol 32(3):e2587, 2017 28568705

Moeller KE, Kissack JC, Atayee RS, et al: Clinical interpretation of urine drug tests: what clinicians need to know about urine drug screens. Mayo Clin Proc 92(5):774–796, 2017 28325505

Musshoff F, Madea B: Review of biologic matrices (urine, blood, hair) as indicators of recent or ongoing cannabis use. Ther Drug Monit 28(2):155–163, 2006 16628124

Nelson ZJ, Stellpflug SJ, Engebretsen KM: What can a urine drug screening immunoassay really tell us? J Pharm Pract 29(5):516–526, 2016 25917168

Preston KL, Epstein DH, Cone EJ, et al: Urinary elimination of cocaine metabolites in chronic cocaine users during cessation. J Anal Toxicol 26(7):393–400, 2002 12422991

Pritchett JS, Phinney KW: Influence of chemical straightening on the stability of drugs of abuse in hair. J Anal Toxicol 39(1):13–16, 2015 25298521

Sadones N, Capiau S, De Kesel PM, et al: Spot them in the spot: analysis of abused substances using dried blood spots. Bioanalysis 6(17):2211–2227, 2014 25383733

Saitman A, Park HD, Fitzgerald RL: False-positive interferences of common urine drug screen immunoassays: a review. J Anal Toxicol 38(7):387–396, 2014 24986836

Thevis M, Geyer H, Tretzel L, et al: Sports drug testing using complementary matrices: advantages and limitations. J Pharm Biomed Anal 130:220–230, 2016 27040951

Thevis M, Kuuranne T, Geyer H: Annual banned-substance review: analytical approaches in human sports drug testing. Drug Test Anal 11(1):8–26, 2019 30488582

Trefz P, Kamysek S, Fuchs P, et al: Drug detection in breath: non-invasive assessment of illicit or pharmaceutical drugs. J Breath Res 11(2):024001, 2017 28220762

Uemura N, Nath RP, Harkey MR, et al: Cocaine levels in sweat collection patches vary by location of patch placement and decline over time. J Anal Toxicol 28(4):253–259, 2004 15189676

Wiencek JR, Colby JM, Nichols JH: Rapid assessment of drugs of abuse. Adv Clin Chem 80:193–225, 2017 28431640

CHAPTER 51

Forensic Addiction Psychiatry

Elie G. Aoun, M.D.

Jungjin Kim, M.D.

Forensic psychiatry is the psychiatric subspecialty in which psychiatric knowledge is applied to legal issues (Rappeport 1982). Forensic psychiatrists are in essence general psychiatrists with additional training in the intersection between psychiatry and the law. Practitioners become involved in forensic evaluations in which they may be asked to provide an expert opinion on a question posed by a legal authority, such as the court, or a civil body, such as a professional board of licensure or an insurance company. Additionally, they are regarded as experts in correctional mental health, providing specialized psychiatric evaluations and treatment for incarcerated individuals.

In the practice of addiction psychiatry, forensic issues frequently arise in a multitude of contexts. Examples include criminal responsibility evaluations for persons with substance use disorders (SUDs), malpractice litigation, drug courts, and treatment of incarcerated individuals with SUDs. Given that psychiatric expertise is often vital for informed judicial decision making, it is essential for the involved clinicians to be adequately equipped with the psychoforensic knowledge to interact with the legal system. In this chapter we provide a concise, synthesized overview of the approach to forensic addiction psychiatry for both general and addiction psychiatrists.

Basic Approach to Forensic Addiction Psychiatry

When serving as a *fact witness*, a clinician is requested to produce records (often via subpoena) or to testify on what he or she observed clinically *without* producing an expert opinion. In contrast, an *expert witness* opines on psychiatric issues arising during the course of criminal or civil litigation. Unlike the fact witness, the expert witness is asked to offer an expert opinion that may help the judicial system better understand a clinical situation or improve a judge's ability to tailor sentencing conditions to the circumstances of an individual defendant and the crime committed. The forensic clinician must clearly understand the role the court expects of him or her.

As an expert witness, the forensic clinician should strive to provide a clinical opinion that is both objective and honest. This emphasis on objective evaluation and opinion giving is disparate from the conventional doctor–patient relationship in that a forensic clinician working as an expert witness has no doctor-patient fiduciary relationship. Therefore, the clinician should inform the evaluees of the limits of confidentiality in forensic settings. Sometimes forensic clinicians may be asked to serve as expert witnesses in cases involving their own patients. Agreeing to do this is almost never recommended, because it runs the risk of creating an ethically prohibited dual agency that may interfere with the provision of an honest, objective opinion. Given the high stakes of forensic evaluations, clinicians should always strive to practice ethically, in accordance with the guidelines outlined by the American Academy of Psychiatry and the Law (2005).

Communicating With the Legal System

Forensic experts must be able to discuss their opinions in a way that is understandable to a nonclinical audience of juries, judges, and attorneys using diagnostic terms accepted by all parties. In the United States, the *Diagnostic and Statistical Manual of Mental Disorders,* 5th Edition (DSM-5; American Psychiatric Association 2013), is the standard for establishing the diagnosis of SUDs in both the clinical and the legal worlds (Norko and Fitch 2014). Whereas previous DSM editions divided SUDs into separate categories of *substance abuse* and *dependence,* DSM-5 uses a single diagnosis of *substance use disorder,* with severity specified as mild, moderate, or severe, according to the number of symptom criteria met over the past 12 months.

In the legal literature, including statutory law and judicial opinions, terms such as *addiction, alcoholism,* and *substance abuse* are used frequently and inconsistently, with significant consequential impact. Despite the potential criminal or civil implications of whether or not such terms apply to a given individual, lawmakers have been reluctant to establish firm definitions. Therefore, when these words come up, it is incumbent on the forensic expert to educate and assist the courts. Historically, some legal experts sought an equivalence between the term *addiction* and the DSM-IV (American Psychiatric Association 1994) diagnosis of substance dependence, which would be roughly equivalent to moderate to severe substance use disorder in DSM-5 (Aoun et al. 2017). Some clinicians may also use the term *addiction* to describe any compulsive or difficult-to-control behavior, such as gambling. The forensic expert needs to be careful in the use of language to avoid ambiguity and to be very clear in the definition of the clinical terminology being used.

Clinical Assessment for the Legal System

A forensic psychiatrist begins an assessment with the particular forensic question in mind. The psychiatrist may find it helpful to think through the questions outlined in Table 51–1 (Ash and Benedek 2017). History collected from evaluees should be cross-checked, because substance use–related self-reports are often fraught with bias and misinformation.

The forensic psychiatrist may supplement the clinical evaluation with results from standardized instruments. Examples of commonly used instruments in addiction psychiatry include the Addiction Severity Index (ASI; Kosten et al. 1983) and the Alcohol Use Disorders and Associated Disabilities Interview Schedule (AUDADIS; Hasin et al. 2015). The forensic psychiatrist must be aware of the advantages and disadvantages of any instrument used, must understand the instrument's general features, and must be able to explain its relevance in the context of the particular psycholegal question. Additionally, the expert needs to consider whether an instrument used in an evaluation has been validated for use in forensic settings.

Laboratory tests to detect substance use are often critically important, especially when making specific recommendations regarding monitoring. For example, commonly tested biomarkers for alcohol use include whole-blood phosphatidyl ethanol, serum carbohydrate-deficient transferrin, urinary ethyl glucuronide, and ethyl sulfate. The forensic psychiatrist needs to be familiar with each test's sensitivity, specificity, potential for false-positive or false-negative results, and detection time frame, as well as the clinical significance of positive or negative results.

A Brief Overview of the U.S. Legal System

The U.S. judicial approach is adversarial, with opposing parties pitted against each other in the presence of an impartial fact finder (judge or jury) who attempts to resolve disputes. The U.S. legal system relies on three sources of guidance: statutes, regulations, and case law. *Statutes* are written laws passed by federal or state legislatures; *regulations* offer technical guidance on the conduct of organizations; and *case laws* are a collection of appellate decisions that provide precedent materials for settling disputes arising from lower-court rulings. These complement and reinforce each other within the framework of the U.S. Constitution.

Legal proceedings are initiated when a complaint is filed (in civil cases) or an arrest occurs (in criminal cases). The rulings are fact based and grounded in evidence gathered from pretrial interrogatories, depositions, subpoenas, or the trial itself. An *interrogatory* is an extensive set of probing queries that is required of opposing parties and the forensic psychiatrist. Depositions usually occur after the opposing legal counsels review the interrogatory responses. *Depositions* are out-of-court, sworn oral testimonies of expert witnesses called to testify in a trial. Depositions provide an opportunity for the opposing legal counsels to size up what forensic clinicians might testify in a trial, these clinicians' level of expertise, and their ability to communicate in an often-adversarial atmosphere. *Subpoenas* are writs requiring the forensic expert to testify in court and/or requiring presentation of certain evidentiary documents. Whether forensic psychiatric evidence is admissible at trial in a particular jurisdiction is often governed by the statutes of that jurisdiction, and the involved forensic clinician needs to be aware of these rules.

In criminal matters, individuals suspected of a crime on the basis of probable cause are taken into custody. Arrested individuals are typically detained pending arraignment. If sufficient grounds exist, the suspect may be charged with a crime by the officer, but in some situations, a grand jury may be required. During pretrial proceedings,

TABLE 51–1.	Questions to be considered by the forensic consultant before beginning the evaluation

1. What is the forensic question that needs to be answered?
2. Who is requesting the evaluation?
3. Who is to be interviewed?
4. Who will give informed consent for the evaluation?
5. What are the limits of confidentiality in the evaluation?
6. To whom will the report be sent?
7. What are the arrangements for paying the fees?

Source. Adapted from Ash and Benedek 2017

defendants may be arraigned, wherein they are formally advised of the charges against them, and may enter a plea. If a not-guilty plea is entered, a trial ensues. If found guilty by trial or by plea, offenders may be sentenced to serve prison or probation time. Individuals who are incarcerated may benefit from receiving reentry programming before their release to facilitate their reintegration into society following release. Upon completion of their prison sentence, individuals may be released on parole or unconditionally. Both probation and parole are considered conditional releases, meaning that the released individuals may live freely in the community granted that they abide by certain conditions. One such condition may be abstinence from drugs and alcohol.

Criminal Process

SUDs, Violence, and Criminal Behavior

The connection between SUDs and violence is well established, as reflected in the exponential increase in academic publications studying this link over the past two decades (Duke et al. 2018). A meta-analysis of 32 studies identified a significant effect of drug or alcohol use on violence perpetration across different models of violence, including intimate partner violence, community violence, violent crimes, and laboratory-based models of aggression (Duke et al. 2018). Male gender and co-occurring psychotic illnesses were thought to increase the risk of violence even further. Maladaptive alcohol use was also associated with being the victim of violence. These findings are consistent with data from the Epidemiologic Catchment Area study, indicating a significant interaction between SUDs and other major mental illnesses as predictors of violence (Swanson et al. 1990). Data from the MacArthur Violence Risk Assessment Study (Monahan et al. 2005) indicated that persons with nonaddictive psychiatric disorders are more likely to be the victims than the perpetrators of violence, and their risk of perpetrating violence is likely lower than that in the general population. However, having a co-occurring SUD increases this risk dramatically (Steadman et al. 1998; Swartz et al. 1998). The risk of perpetrating violence is further increased among individuals who are actively using substances while also failing to adhere to their psychopharmacotherapy regimen (Torrey 1994).

Moreover, the connection between SUDs and criminal behavior leads to an overrepresentation in the U.S. justice system of individuals with SUDs, including those detained in jails and prisons and those on parole or probation (Bronson and Stroop 2017). According to survey data from the Bureau of Justice Statistics (2008), 4 in 10 arrestees were in a state of intoxication at the time of their offense and 1 in 3 committed their offense to obtain money to purchase drugs. Similarly, data from the National Crime Victimization Survey indicated that in 2007, more than 750,000 violent crimes were committed by offenders who were intoxicated (Bureau of Justice Statistics 2008). Overall, it appears that use of alcohol more than use of illegal drugs is associated with violent crimes such as murder, rape, assault, domestic violence, and child abuse. Use of other drugs (e.g., opiates, cocaine), however, is more commonly associated with robberies and property crimes (Pierce et al. 2015).

Valuable insight into the direction of causality comes from studies examining rates of criminal offense both prior to and following initial drug use. The majority of studies have shown that criminal behaviors increase following drug use (Hayhurst et al. 2017). Studies have also found through retrospective analysis that individuals who subsequently developed SUDs were more likely to have had a history of criminal behaviors preceding their initial drug use compared with those who never developed SUDs (Pierce et al. 2017). Therefore, initiation of drug use was thought to exacerbate existing levels of criminal offense, and this effect was greater for women than for men.

To better understand the relationship between substance use and criminal behavior, Paul Goldstein (1985) developed a taxonomy framework to examine the temporal relationship between crime and substance use and to identify common driving factors for both. Goldstein described three models that explain how drugs and crimes are related:

1. Economically compulsive crimes (or economic-related crimes): The crime is seen as a means of generating money to fund the use of substances.
2. Psychopharmacological crime (or use-related crime): Substance use leads to impairments in cognitive functioning (when the effects of the substance lead to criminal behaviors or when a person uses substances to become more disinhibited or to have the courage to commit the crime).
3. Systemic crime (or system-related crime): Crimes are associated with the production, manufacture, transportation, and/or sale of substances.

Substance Use as the Basis of an Insanity Defense

Two key elements are required for the establishment of a defendant's criminal liability: *actus reus* and *mens rea*. *Actus reus* (Latin for "guilty act") refers to the specific criminal activity, whereas *mens rea* (Latin for "guilty mind") refers to the level of intent and knowledge of the alleged criminal activity. Generally, both are required, although exceptions exist. Crimes such as driving under the influence are "strict liability crimes" that do not require *mens rea* to establish the defendant as guilty; *actus reus* (i.e., intoxication) alone is sufficient.

The defendant may seek lessened criminal responsibility by invoking an insanity defense (pleading to impaired mental capability at the time of the crime, which makes appreciation of the nature and quality of wrongfulness of the alleged crime difficult)

(Insanity Defense Reform Act of 1984). Substance involvement is often used for this defense, and the forensic expert may help the legal decision-making process by parsing out addiction's role in the criminal act or intent.

As can be inferred, *insanity* is a legal rather than a clinical term that may be used to lessen criminal culpability. Jurisdictions vary greatly in how they define *insanity*, especially when it comes to insanity as a result of SUDs. Almost all jurisdictions prohibit voluntary intoxication as the sole mental disorder used to justify an insanity defense. Certain jurisdictions may allow substance-related insanity defenses on the basis of the following conditions: 1) idiosyncratic intoxication, 2) involuntary intoxication, and 3) settled insanity. *Idiosyncratic intoxication* is a diminished mental capacity as a result of an unforeseeable and disproportionate intoxication with a small amount of drug or alcohol. Drugs that have well-established adverse sequelae, such as cocaine and methamphetamines, usually do not qualify for an idiosyncratic intoxication defense. *Involuntary intoxication* occurs when the defendant is unaware of or forced into the consumption of alcohol or drugs and therefore is not responsible for the adverse mental status sequelae of intoxication that led to the criminal act. *Settled insanity* refers to a permanent psychiatric or neurocognitive disorder as a result of substance use long past the intoxication period. Alcohol-related dementia is one such example.

Certain jurisdictions require an evaluation of the presence or absence of criminal intent *before* the consumption of the substance. In the absence of criminal intent before the consumption, *voluntary intoxication* may be used as a defense against criminal intent, because under the influence, the defendant could not have had the mental capacity to formulate criminal intent.

In intoxication defenses, alcohol-induced blackouts are often misused to reduce criminal culpability. The scientific basis to support the use of blackout phenomena for criminal exculpatory purposes is weak. The addiction expert needs to be knowledgeable about the jurisdiction-specific guidelines and precedents regarding intoxication defense when approaching topics such as alleged alcohol-induced blackouts.

Once the defendant has been established as guilty, the addiction expert may continue to provide important recommendations for substance-related treatment during and after the completion of the sentence.

Landmark Cases That Shaped the State of SUDs in the Justice System

There are three landmark rulings pertaining to SUDs: *Robinson v. California* (1962), *Powell v. Texas* (1968), and *Traynor v. Turnage* (1988). In 1962, the case of *Robinson v. California* was appealed to the U.S. Supreme Court. In this case, the defendant was arrested by a law enforcement officer, who observed track marks on his arms, under a California law making it a misdemeanor to be "addicted to the use of narcotics." The court ruled that it was unconstitutional to criminalize an individual with an SUD in light of the Eighth Amendment of the U.S. Constitution, which prohibits cruel and unusual punishments. This was a pivotal decision wherein the legal world embraced the medical disease model of SUD; Justice Potter Stewart famously wrote in the majority opinion that even "one day in prison for the 'crime' of having a common cold" would be cruel and unusual.

A subsequent case in the Supreme Court clarified that substance-related misconduct may be subject to both civil and criminal prosecutions. Notably, in *Powell v. Texas* (1968), the defendant had been charged with public intoxication and sought appeal on the grounds that he could not be arrested for being an alcoholic. The court recognized a dichotomy between having an SUD and substance-related misconduct and ruled that the precedent ruling in *Robinson v. California* does not protect individuals from the consequences of misconduct in which the person engages as a result of having an SUD.

In *Traynor v. Turnage* (1988), plaintiffs were seeking VA benefits under the GI bill even though they were discharged dishonorably from the military because they had alcohol use disorder. The Supreme Court denied their claim, opining that the behavior that led to their discharge was caused by "willful misconduct." In the majority opinion, Justice Byron White wrote, "Even among many who consider alcoholism a 'disease' to which its victims are genetically predisposed, the consumption of alcohol is not regarded as wholly involuntary." Had the court determined that individuals with SUDs are unable to control their drug or alcohol use, punishing them would have meant penalizing their SUD status, thereby violating the cruel and unusual punishments clause of the Eighth Amendment of the Constitution. Such cases provide the legal precedent for why alcohol use disorder would not be a legitimate defense to a charge of driving under the influence.

SUDs in the Criminal Justice System

As noted earlier, individuals with SUDs are overrepresented in the justice system. The most recent data from the Bureau of Justice Statistics (Bronson and Stroop 2017) show that close to two-thirds of convicted inmates in jails and prisons meet diagnostic criteria for SUDs. Similarly, persons on parole or probation are three times more likely than the general population to have SUDs.

Justice-involved persons with SUDs rarely seek medical help to treat their SUDs in the community. Therefore, when these persons come into contact with the justice system, medical professionals have a unique opportunity to steer them to treatments targeting their SUD, as well as to identify and treat co-occurring psychiatric illnesses and to address psychosocial factors that serve to maintain their addiction. Failing to do so constitutes a missed opportunity to improve the individuals' drug- and alcohol-using outcomes, improve their ability to function in their communities, lower criminal recidivism, and overall reduce the public health burden on society.

Criminal Diversion

Arrested individuals with SUDs may be eligible for diversion in lieu of arraignment, adjudication, or sentencing. Individuals are incentivized with the opportunity to not face criminal charges, to have their charges dropped or reduced, or to not be incarcerated if they comply with diversion conditions. These conditions typically include obtaining treatment for SUD and remaining free of drug and alcohol use. The Sequential Intercept Model (SIM) was introduced by Munetz and Griffin (2006) as a framework mapping the different opportunities for diversion along the justice continuum. The SIM seeks to "prevent individuals with mental illness from entering or penetrating deeper into the criminal justice system" (p. 544). The model identifies five interception points where diversion may be offered: 1) law enforcement and emergency services; 2) initial detention and initial hearings; 3) jail, courts, forensic evaluations, and forensic commitments; 4) reentry from jails, state prisons, and forensic hospitalization; and 5) community corrections and community support. The model may be adapted and applied to specific subpopulations, such as offenders with SUDs.

Prebooking Diversion

During an individual's encounter with law enforcement, the officers involved may use their discretional authority to identify eligible offenders with SUDs for diversion. Qualifying individuals are linked with a community treatment facility and are assigned case managers. Acceptable participation in the program may lead to not having the charges filed, or having them dropped or reduced. Diverted individuals are less likely to be rearrested and hospitalized, and are more likely to receive outpatient treatment services, even following completion of the program (Steadman and Naples 2005).

Judicial-Level Diversion

Preadjudication or initial hearing diversion.   Justice-involved individuals who have been arraigned may still be found to qualify for a preprosecution diversion via two pathways (Shafer et al. 2004):

1. Release on conditions: Qualifying individuals awaiting trial may be released from jail in order to engage in community-based SUD treatment.
2. Deferred prosecution: Judges may offer to hold off on moving forward with the legal proceedings and release the individual to the community under probation-like conditions (in these situations, the judge notes that the facts of the case may be sufficient to adjudicate the person guilty but does not move forward with the adjudication). Conditions of release typically include abstaining from substance use, engaging in community-based SUD treatment, and cooperation with close monitoring by case managers and the court. Successful completion of the program leads to dismissal of the criminal charges.

Probation: postadjudication diversion.   Individuals adjudicated guilty may still qualify for diversion. These individuals are offered traditional probation and conditional release in lieu of incarceration and are required to submit to regular supervision by a probation officer, maintain sobriety from drugs and alcohol, and participate in treatment as clinically recommended for a set period of time instead of serving a prison sentence.

Drug courts: preadjudication or postadjudication diversion.   Drug courts are voluntary, nonadversarial, special-jurisdiction courts in which eligible persons with SUDs who were charged with a crime may be offered diversion. In this setting, complying with the program set forth by the court (typically involving SUD treatment, abstinence, and close monitoring) affords individuals the opportunity to have their charges dropped (for preadjudication programs) or their punishment reduced (for postadjudication programs). Subspecialty drug courts have been developed for juveniles, individuals charged with driving while intoxicated, veterans, and individuals with comorbid SUDs and other mental disorders (Mitchell et al. 2012; National Association of Drug Court Professionals 1997).

A meta-analysis examining the effectiveness of drug courts showed that participation was associated with significant reductions in criminal recidivism, which persisted for years after successful completion of the program. However, there are no clear data supporting the effect of drug courts on improving substance use outcomes (Mitchell et al. 2012).

SUD Management in Correctional Settings

Discovery of individuals' SUDs may occur at any point in the incarceration process, and psychiatrists must be prepared to advise on screening and treatment in facilities. Arrested individuals may not disclose their use of drugs or alcohol, but may have been intoxicated at the time of arrest or experienced withdrawal soon thereafter. The initial intake is a crucial phase for the physician to identify at-risk individuals and offer appropriate treatment to reduce the potential for associated morbidity and mortality, including the risk of overdose when individuals consume their remaining drugs immediately upon arrest.

The vast majority of incarcerated individuals with SUDs do not receive appropriate treatment. A survey of 153,137 inmates in jails and prisons indicated that fewer than 15% of those requiring treatment received it while incarcerated (Bronson and Stroop 2017). SUD treatment offered to inmates varies widely, with a range of treatment options available in different facilities. Options include boot camps, self-help groups, counseling programs, cognitive-behavioral therapy–based individual or group therapy, and prison-based therapeutic communities.

Mitchell et al. (2012) conducted a meta-analysis examining the efficacy of incarceration-based SUD treatment programs in reducing postrelease recidivism and drug relapse. These investigators concluded that overall these programs were associated with a 15%–17% reduction in criminal recidivism and relapse to drugs or alcohol following participant release. Mitchell and colleagues noted, however, that prison-based therapeutic communities were associated with the best outcomes, counseling programs had mixed effects, and boot camps had a negligible impact on both future criminal behavior and future substance use.

Some correctional facilities across the United States have started using medication-assisted treatment for the maintenance treatment of opioid use disorder (OUD) (Brinkley-Rubinstein et al. 2019). Such practices are consistent with the World Health Organization's (2009) recommendations that medications for the treatment of SUDs be made available to incarcerated individuals. Unfortunately, limited published data are available regarding the use of medications approved by the U.S. Food and Drug Administration to treat alcohol or tobacco use disorder in correctional settings.

Studies have found that for inmates with OUD who were receiving methadone prior to their arrest, being maintained on methadone while incarcerated (as opposed to undergoing forced detoxification) leads to better postrelease SUD outcomes (Brinkley-Rubinstein et al. 2018; Rich et al. 2015) and lower rates of criminal recidivism (Westerberg et al. 2016). Also, studies of inmates with OUD who were not on maintenance treatment found that initiating treatment with buprenorphine during the incarceration period increased the likelihood that these individuals would continue treatment after their release (Magura et al. 2009). Similar outcomes are noted when facilities use medication-assisted treatment as part of reentry programming. Studies show that the initiation of methadone (Kinlock et al. 2009) or buprenorphine (Gordon et al. 2017) prior to individuals' release from incarceration leads to improved SUD outcomes and increased engagement in postrelease treatment.

Since the introduction of extended-release injectable naltrexone, correctional settings have shown interest in using this medication. Its appeal in these settings is likely because it is an opioid antagonist without diversion potential. Initiating this treatment immediately before release appears to be associated with improved treatment retention and opioid use outcomes (Lee et al. 2015; Lincoln et al. 2018).

Prisoners have high rates of comorbidity of psychiatric disorders and SUDs (Butler et al. 2011). Because the presence of psychiatric comorbidity has been shown to lead to recidivism and premature mortality following release (Chang et al. 2015), sustained efforts to address both SUDs and co-occurring psychiatric disorders are important.

In 2016, the American Psychiatric Association (APA) released a position statement on treating SUDs in individuals in the criminal justice system. APA recommends the use of evidence-based practices, including screening for SUDs and co-occurring psychiatric and infectious illnesses; training correctional staff in recognizing substance withdrawal and overdose; and providing medically supervised withdrawal treatment and overdose reversal with appropriate medication. Furthermore, APA supports the use of pharmacological as well as nonpharmacological treatment interventions for SUDs, including medication-assisted treatment, and recommends treatment-oriented reentry and community reintegration planning. The APA position statement also highlights the importance of making diversion courts available to eligible individuals, as well as the judicious use of parole or probation to further monitor sobriety following release (American Psychiatric Association 2016).

Civil Forensic Addiction Psychiatry

Civil law is a system of law concerned with settling disputes arising from interactions between noncriminal members of society. In civil cases, as in criminal cases, the psychiatrist may be asked to play the role of fact or expert witness. The forensic addiction psychiatrist may be asked to assess future risk based on an individual's past behaviors. In this section, we discuss essential topics within the domains of civil law, including civil commitment for SUDs, child custody disputes, personal injury and tort law, psychiatric disability, fitness for duty, and professional liability of addiction psychiatric practice.

Civil Commitment for Substance Use Disorder

Civil commitment for substance use disorder refers to a legal mechanism that allows family members or health care providers to seek court-mandated treatment for individuals with SUDs. The state's authority to commit individuals with SUDs is based on the principle of *parens patriae*, which views persons with SUDs as vulnerable, requiring the state to protect their interests. Unlike with drug courts, this process is independent of any criminal justice system involvement. Specific state statutes may mandate inpatient or outpatient treatment (in some cases, both are acceptable avenues). In the United States, 33 states have enacted statutes allowing for civil commitment, although there is significant variability in the extent to which states apply the statutes, with a majority of states rarely or never applying to civilly commit individuals with SUDs. Florida and Massachusetts stand out as high utilizers of these statutes (Christopher et al. 2015).

Despite the appeal of involuntary civil commitment for SUD, it remains a highly debated topic because of a lack of outcome data, ethical concerns, and unresolved questions about the importance of motivation in treatment for SUDs and long-term outcomes.

Child Custody Disputes

In custody or child safety disputes, psychiatrists are often asked to comment on the nature and severity of substance use by parents and its effects on the child. Custody disputes, by nature, are often fiercely adversarial and emotionally charged. Forensic experts must strive to maintain calm and objectivity while ensuring a thorough evaluation of all involved parties. A parent's SUD does *not* automatically mean that the individual lacks parental qualifications, but an SUD would be one of the important factors weighed in determining custody. Most child custody cases are settled around the "best interest of the child" standard (Child Welfare Information Gateway 2019). This standard advocates for the adjudication of the custodial arrangement that affords the child the best chance to grow into healthy adulthood. The parents sometimes pursue interests other than the best interest of the child, and in this case, the forensic expert should inform the court of such dynamics and advocate for an adjudication accordingly.

Personal Injury and Tort Law

The forensic addiction expert may be asked to evaluate the relative role and import of substance use in personal injury cases. Tort law is a subsection of civil law that provides remedies for personal injury caused by another party. Personal injury claims can be made on the basis of psychic or physical harm. In a personal injury dispute, the opposing side may allege that the other party was under the influence at the time of the injury. A thorough evaluation of both sides of the claim, sometimes complemented by psychometric testing and laboratory tests, is needed. The possibility of malingering should always be considered in a personal injury claim.

Psychiatric Disability

Addiction psychiatrists are often asked to evaluate disability claims based on SUDs. In the context of Social Security Disability Insurance and/or Social Security Insurance, *disability* is defined as "the inability to engage in any substantial gainful activity by reason of any medically determinable physical or mental impairment(s) which can be expected to result in death or…to last for a continuous period of not less than 12 months." While disability from independent disorders caused by substance use (e.g., depression or psychosis associated with a long history of drug or alcohol use) is covered by Social Security requirements for disability, disabilities related solely to drug and alcohol use are not.

The Americans With Disabilities Act (ADA) of 1990 and the ADA Amendments Act (2008) provide legal grounds for prohibiting discrimination against individuals with disabilities and for mandating that employers provide reasonable accommodations to enable a qualified individual with a disability to perform job functions. SUD, albeit a psychiatric disorder recognized in DSM-5, affords limited protections under the ADA. Therefore, persons "currently engaging in the illegal use of drugs" (we note that this exclusion does not apply to the current use of alcohol) may not be considered disabled and as such may not benefit from ADA protections. The ADA defines "currently" loosely, and it is unclear how long a period of sobriety is necessary for a person to qualify for protections. Furthermore, the ADA contains a provision holding that employers may hold employees with SUDs to the same standards as those without SUDs. In practice, this provision undermines the requirement to provide eligible employees with reasonable accommodations and makes it almost impossible for those with SUDs to establish a case of discrimination under the ADA. That is because potential defendants would be required to demonstrate that their SUD does not make them less qualified for the position, yet by doing so, they would be undermining their claim that the SUD causes substantial limitations in major life activities (Aoun and Appelbaum 2019).

Fitness for Duty

Occupations with significant public safety implications, such as medical professionals and law enforcement officers, are commonly subject to fitness-for-duty evaluations (FFDEs). The individual physician may have a duty to report an impaired peer, although there is considerable variability in state laws that govern this duty.

FFDEs may occur before or after employment begins, or before return to work when the employee has been out of the workforce for an extended period. FFDEs start with a review of the written account of the incident(s) of concern, the employee's job description and required work skills, the institutional regulations or statutes relating to substance use, the employment records, and the employee's medical and psychiatric records. These records should be supplemented by collateral information from supervisors, coworkers, close social contacts, and treatment providers. The assessment should focus *specifically* on how the individual's substance use affects performance of specific occupational duties.

Liability for Addiction Psychiatrists

Professional Liability

To win a malpractice claim against a psychiatrist, the plaintiff must prove that the psychiatrist had a duty and that the psychiatrist breached that duty, resulting in harm to the patient as a direct result of this breach. Contrary to popular belief, forensic addiction psychiatrists are not shielded from malpractice liability, even in the absence of a treatment relationship. Liability from forensic evaluations often relates to matters such as defamation and ordinary negligence in forming the forensic opinion.

There are ways to protect one's practice from liability, including being vigilant about potential high-risk practices and seeking expert consultation when questions arise. Although far from rendering the clinician invulnerable, these measures substantially mitigate the hazards of professional liability. Finally, the addiction psychiatrist involved in forensic activities must confirm coverage of those activities with insurers, because insurance policies do not always cover forensic activities.

Liability Associated With Prescribing Controlled Substances

Misuse of prescription medications has become increasingly problematic in recent years. A sound prescribing practice entails obtaining informed consent from patients, checking the prescription drug monitoring program, and properly documenting the prescription process. Part of the informed consent process involves educating the patient on the responsible handling and disposing of controlled medications. The psychiatrist needs to explain up front any stipulations regarding the stopping of medications, the escalation of level of monitoring or care, and the seeking of potential referrals (e.g., to a pain specialist) as deemed clinically necessary. Newer patients may be observed more closely, with initial limitation of emergency supplies until adequate clinical information is gathered. Prescription drug monitoring programs allow physicians to check the dispensation of controlled substances for their patients. Checking the monitoring program is a sound clinical practice that warrants documentation as part of the treatment plan.

Maintaining Confidentiality

Given the stigma associated with SUDs, maintaining patient confidentiality is critical for practicing addiction psychiatry. Several federal regulations are worth noting in this regard. The Health Insurance Portability and Accountability Act of 1996 (HIPAA) established the first federal minimum privacy standards for patient health information. Many states also have their own confidentiality and privilege laws, which may be stricter or more lenient than HIPAA. The Confidentiality of Alcohol and Drug Abuse Patient Records regulations of 1972 (amended in 2017) were enacted to provide stricter federal privacy standards for SUD treatment records than for psychiatric health treatment records.

It is important to remember that although confidentiality is an important ethical duty of the physician to his or her patients, it is far from absolute. Clinicians should be familiar with exceptions to patient confidentiality, including issues affecting the safety of members of the public or an identified third party. When the patient makes threats to an identified third party, the clinician should not be hesitant to initiate hospitalization of the patient, warn the identified target, and contact law enforcement.

Telepsychiatry

Telepsychiatry, or the provision of psychiatric treatment through interactive videoconferencing, has been gaining popularity among patients and clinicians. Cautions when using telepsychiatry include ensuring that the selected software and hardware meet HIPAA standards for patient privacy. Any telepsychiatry use carries with it inherent privacy risks, and the clinician should obtain the evaluee's informed consent prior to the use of such technology. The Ryan Haight Online Pharmacy Consumer Protection Act (2008) was created to regulate the prescribing of medications online and thereby further regulates the practice of telepsychiatry. The act requires prescribers to conduct an in-person medical evaluation at least once every 24 months if prescribing a controlled substance.

Conclusion

With the increasing prevalence of SUDs in civil and criminal populations, more and more psychiatrists may have to deal with legal entanglements. Working in a forensic role starts with acquiring basic knowledge of the legal landscape and clarifying one's role within the legal system. A forensic role may be very different from a fiduciary doctor-patient relationship, and it is critically important to be clear about one's obligation to the evaluee and to the legal system. Following ethical and clinical guidelines where appropriate and asking for consultation from peers, a local medical society, or an attorney are ways to safeguard one's forensic practice. As discussed in this chapter, there are many unmet needs for addiction psychiatrists in civil, criminal, and correction settings. Working within the legal system can offer both challenges and rewards, and, most importantly, an opportunity to better equip the legal system to address the growing epidemic of SUDs.

References

American Academy of Psychiatry and the Law: Ethics Guidelines for the Practice of Forensic Psychiatry. May 2005. Available at: http://www.aapl.org/ethics-guidelines. Accessed January 16, 2020.

American Psychiatric Association: Diagnostic and Statistical Manual of Mental Disorders, 4th Edition. Washington, DC, American Psychiatric Association, 1994

American Psychiatric Association: Diagnostic and Statistical Manual of Mental Disorders, 5th Edition. Arlington, VA, American Psychiatric Association, 2013

American Psychiatric Association: Position Statement on Treatment of Substance Use Disorders in the Criminal Justice System. Washington, DC, American Psychiatric Association, 2016

Americans with Disabilities Act of 1990, Pub L No 101-336, 104 Stat 328 (1990)

Americans with Disabilities Act Amendments Act of 2008, Pub L No 110-325, 122 Stat 3553 (2008)

Aoun EG, Appelbaum PS: Ten years after the ADA Amendment Act (2008): the relationship between ADA employment discrimination and substance use disorders. Psychiatr Serv 70(7):596–603, 2019 30991909

Aoun EG, Fusick A, Wagoner R: What's in a name? Deciphering the meaning of the word "addiction." American Academy of Psychiatry and the Law Newsletter 42(2):22, 31, 2017. Available at: https://www.aapl.org/docs/newsletter/April%202017.pdf. Accessed February 19, 2020.

Ash P, Benedek E: Forensic evaluations of children and adolescents, in The American Psychiatric Association Publishing Textbook of Forensic Psychiatry. Edited by Gold LH, Frierson RL. Arlington, VA, American Psychiatric Association Publishing, 2017, pp 359–372

Brinkley-Rubinstein L, McKenzie M, Macmadu A, et al: A randomized, open label trial of methadone continuation versus forced withdrawal in a combined U.S. prison and jail: findings at 12 months post-release. Drug Alcohol Depend 184:57–63, 2018 29402680

Brinkley-Rubinstein L, Peterson M, Clarke J, et al: The benefits and implementation challenges of the first state-wide comprehensive medication for addictions program in a unified jail and prison setting. Drug Alcohol Depend 205:107514, 2019 31614328

Bronson J, Stroop J: Drug Use, Dependence, and Abuse Among State Prisoners and Jail Inmates, 2007–2009. June 2017. Available at: https://www.bjs.gov/content/pub/pdf/dudaspji0709.pdf. Accessed January 16, 2020.

Bureau of Justice Statistics: Criminal Victimization in the United States, 2007. Washington, DC, U.S. Department of Justice, 2008

Butler T, Indig D, Allnutt S, et al: Co-occurring mental illness and substance use disorder among Australian prisoners. Drug Alcohol Rev 30(2):188–194, 2011 21355926

Chang Z, Lichtenstein P, Larsson H, et al: Substance use disorders, psychiatric disorders, and mortality after release from prison: a nationwide longitudinal cohort study. Lancet Psychiatry 2(5):422–430, 2015 26360286

Child Welfare Information Gateway: Parental substance use and the child welfare system. Washington, DC, U.S. Department of Health and Human Services, Administration for Children and Families, Children's Bureau, 2019. Available at: https://www.childwelfare.gov/pubs/factsheets/parentalsubabuse/. Accessed February 29, 2020.

Christopher PP, Pinals DA, Stayton T, et al: Nature and utilization of civil commitment for substance abuse in the United States. J Am Acad Psychiatry Law 43(3):313–320, 2015 26438809

Confidentiality of Substance Use Disorder Patient Records, 82 FR 6052, January 18, 2017

Duke AA, Smith KMZ, Oberleitner LMS, et al: Alcohol, drugs, and violence: a meta-meta-analysis. Psychology of Violence 8(2):238–249, 2018. Available at: https://psycnet.apa.org/doiLanding?doi=10.1037%2Fvio0000106. Accessed February 19, 2020.

Goldstein P: The drugs/violence nexus: a tripartite conceptual framework. Journal of Drug Issues 15:493–506, 1985. Available at: https://journals.sagepub.com/doi/10.1177/002204268501500406. Accessed February 19, 2020.

Gordon MS, Kinlock TW, Schwartz RP, et al: A randomized clinical trial of buprenorphine for prisoners: findings at 12-months post-release. Drug Alcohol Depend 172:34–42, 2017 28107680

Hasin DS, Greenstein E, Aivadyan C, et al: The Alcohol Use Disorder and Associated Disabilities Interview Schedule-5 (AUDADIS-5): procedural validity of substance use disorders modules through clinical re-appraisal in a general population sample. Drug Alcohol Depend 148:40–46, 2015 25604321

Hayhurst KP, Pierce M, Hickman M, et al: Pathways through opiate use and offending: a systematic review. Int J Drug Policy 39:1–13, 2017 27770693

Health Insurance Portability and Accountability Act of 1996, Pub L No 104-191, 110 Stat 1936 (1996)

Insanity Defense Reform Act of 1984, 18 U.S.C. § 17 (West 2016)

Kinlock TW, Gordon MS, Schwartz RP, et al: A randomized clinical trial of methadone maintenance for prisoners: results at 12 months postrelease. J Subst Abuse Treat 37(3):277–285, 2009 19339140

Kosten TR, Rounsaville BJ, Kleber HD: Concurrent validity of the addiction severity index. J Nerv Ment Dis 171(10):606–610, 1983 6619823

Lee JD, McDonald R, Grossman E, et al: Opioid treatment at release from jail using extended-release naltrexone: a pilot proof-of-concept randomized effectiveness trial. Addiction 110(6):1008–1014, 2015 25703440

Lincoln T, Johnson BD, McCarthy P, et al: Extended-release naltrexone for opioid use disorder started during or following incarceration. J Subst Abuse Treat 85:97–100, 2018 28479011

Magura S, Lee JD, Hershberger J, et al: Buprenorphine and methadone maintenance in jail and post-release: a randomized clinical trial. Drug Alcohol Depend 99(1–3):222–230, 2009 18930603

Mitchell O, Wilson DB, Eggers A, et al: Assessing the effectiveness of drug courts on recidivism: a meta-analytic review of traditional and non-traditional drug courts. Journal of Criminal Justice 40(1):60–71, 2012. Available at: https://www.sciencedirect.com/science/article/pii/S0047235211001255?via%3Dihub. Accessed February 19, 2020.

Monahan J, Steadman HJ, Robbins PC, et al: An actuarial model of violence risk assessment for persons with mental disorders. Psychiatr Serv 56(7):810–815, 2005 16020812

Munetz MR, Griffin PA: Use of the Sequential Intercept Model as an approach to decriminalization of people with serious mental illness. Psychiatr Serv 57(4):544–549, 2006 16603751

National Association of Drug Court Professionals: Defining Drug Courts: The Key Components. Washington, DC, Bureau of Justice Assistance, 1997

Norko MA, Fitch WL: DSM-5 and substance use disorders: clinicolegal implications. J Am Acad Psychiatry Law 42(4):443–452, 2014 25492070

Pierce M, Hayhurst K, Bird SM, et al: Quantifying crime associated with drug use among a large cohort of sanctioned offenders in England and Wales. Drug Alcohol Depend 155:52–59, 2015 26361712

Pierce M, Hayhurst K, Bird SM, et al: Insights into the link between drug use and criminality: lifetime offending of criminally active opiate users. Drug Alcohol Depend 179:309–316, 2017 28837946

Powell v. Texas, 392 U.S. 514, 88 S. Ct. 2145 (1968)

Rappeport JR: Differences between forensic and general psychiatry. Am J Psychiatry 139(3):331–334, 1982 7058947

Rich JD, McKenzie M, Larney S, et al: Methadone continuation versus forced withdrawal on incarceration in a combined U.S. prison and jail: a randomised, open-label trial. Lancet 386(9991):350–359, 2015 26028120

Robinson v. California, 370 U.S. 660, 82 S. Ct. 1417, 8 L. Ed. 2d 758 (1962)

Ryan Haight Online Pharmacy Consumer Protection Act of 2008, Pub. L. No. 110-425, sec. 3(k)(1)

Shafer MS, Arthur B, Franczak MJ: An analysis of post-booking jail diversion programming for persons with co-occurring disorders. Behav Sci Law 22(6):771–785, 2004 15386559

Steadman HJ, Naples M: Assessing the effectiveness of jail diversion programs for persons with serious mental illness and co-occurring substance use disorders. Behav Sci Law 23(2):163–170, 2005 15818607

Steadman HJ, Mulvey EP, Monahan J, et al: Violence by people discharged from acute psychiatric inpatient facilities and by others in the same neighborhoods. Arch Gen Psychiatry 55(5):393–401, 1998 9596041

Swanson JW, Holzer CE 3rd, Ganju VK, et al: Violence and psychiatric disorder in the community: evidence from the Epidemiologic Catchment Area surveys. Hosp Community Psychiatry 41(7):761–770, 1990 2142118

Swartz MS, Swanson JW, Hiday VA, et al: Violence and severe mental illness: the effects of substance abuse and nonadherence to medication. Am J Psychiatry 155(2):226–231, 1998 9464202

Torrey EF: Violent behavior by individuals with serious mental illness. Hosp Community Psychiatry 45(7):653–662, 1994 7927289

Traynor v. Turnage, 485 U.S. 535 (1988)

Westerberg VS, McCrady BS, Owens M, et al: Community-based methadone maintenance in a large detention center is associated with decreases in inmate recidivism. J Subst Abuse Treat 70:1–6, 2016 27692182

World Health Organization: Guidelines for the psychosocially assisted pharmacological treatment of opioid dependence. Geneva, World Health Organization, 2009. Available at: https://www.who.int/substance_abuse/publications/opioid_dependence_guidelines.pdf. Accessed February 19, 2020.

CHAPTER 52

Medical Education on Addiction

Jeffrey J. DeVido, M.D., M.T.S., FASAM

Ellen L. Edens, M.D., M.P.E., M.A.

Robert Werner, M.D.

Elizabeth F. Howell, M.D., M.S., DLFAPA, DFASAM

Addiction education for health care providers has advanced substantially over the past several decades, due to its greater integration into medical school and postgraduate training curricula as well as the expansion of specialty fellowship and board certification opportunities in addiction psychiatry and addiction medicine. Educational advancements in the field of addiction medicine were catalyzed by the 1971 federally sponsored Career Teacher Program and were subsequently fostered through crucial support from various federal agencies (e.g., Substance Abuse and Mental Health Services Administration [SAMHSA], National Institutes of Health [NIH]) and specialty societies and organizations (e.g., American Society of Addiction Medicine [ASAM], Association for Multidisciplinary Education and Research in Substance use and Addiction [AMERSA], American Psychiatric Association [APA], American Academy of Addiction Psychiatry [AAAP]). Despite these early efforts, a lack of faculty members with expertise to teach about addiction persists, and education about addiction is lacking in comparison with education on other chronic medical conditions (Ayu et al. 2015; Committee on Crossing the Quality Chasm 2006; Isaacson et al. 2000; Rasyidi et al. 2012).

The tragedy of the national opioid epidemic has exposed the urgent need for rapid development of a health care workforce more highly trained in addiction evaluation and treatment. A significant addiction *treatment gap* exists; only 11% of the 22 million Americans with addiction receive specialty addiction treatment (Lipari et al. 2016; Tetrault and Petrakis 2017). This gap is exacerbated by the lack of well-trained addiction treatment providers as well as the lack of adequate remuneration for addiction services (O'Connor et al. 2014).

Scientific, educational, and policy leaders have urged a conceptual shift to bring addiction evaluation and treatment responsibility squarely into mainstream medicine (U.S. Department of Health and Human Services, Office of the Surgeon General 2016; Volkow 2015; Wood et al. 2013). National leaders across multiple disciplines have also called for improved parity in access to treatment, provider reimbursement, and provider education (Lipari et al. 2016). In the past decade, health care reform under the Patient Protection and Affordable Care Act of 2010, as well as legislative efforts such as the Comprehensive Addiction and Recovery Act of 2016, have created additional opportunities and mandates for integrating addiction care into "mainstream" health care systems (Pating et al. 2012). The confluence of these public health needs, health care reform, and legislative efforts has facilitated increased interest in, study on, and funding for addiction education in undergraduate, medical, postgraduate medical, and continuing medical professional training programs.

Despite these efforts to expand the field, a significant addiction *education gap* persists. The education gap manifests across all disciplines at all levels of training. Examples include persistently low numbers of curricular hours devoted to addiction training; siloed curricular content; and inadequate knowledge about, poor attitudes toward, and disorganized practice habits around patients with addictions. Much additional work is needed to fully expand and integrate addiction training into medical education in order to meet our national needs.

In this chapter, we provide an overview of educational strategies to advance addiction knowledge, improve attitudes, and encourage skill development for physicians in various specialties and stages of training. We hope that expansion of effective addiction education for clinicians at all levels of training will lead to improvements in patient care.

Knowledge, Attitudes, and Clinical Practice Habits

Substance-related and addictive disorders remain stigmatized and poorly understood by the general lay public and even within the health care system. Separation of addiction treatment from mainstream health care, use of pejorative language to describe both individuals with addiction and addiction treatment itself, and outdated moral-deficit/willful-choice models of addiction all contribute to the persistence of stigma within health care systems (Wakeman and Rich 2018). Stigma within health care systems leads trainees to experience greater therapeutic nihilism, decreased role responsibility, and less satisfaction caring for patients with addictions (Geller et al. 1989; Lindberg et al. 2006). The following can contribute to medical students' worsened attitudes: inadequate curricula, exposure to end-stage addiction, lack of confidence in ability to communicate with patients about addictions, negative and cynical attitudes by senior clinicians, and lack of faculty expertise (Geller et al. 1989; Miller et al. 2001; van Boekel et al. 2013). As a result of insufficient provider education, addiction is underrecognized, underdiagnosed, and undertreated. In addition, even among the minority of individuals with substance use disorders (SUDs) who recognize the need for treatment, internalized stigma can perpetuate a sense of shame that poses a barrier to seeking treatment and confounds the recovery process (Matthews et al. 2017). Lack of provider sensitivity to and training in addictions compounds a scenario in which providers, much like individuals with addiction, may minimize or fail to recognize symptoms and signs of a substance-related disorder.

Clinician attitudes may be starting to change. Health care providers increasingly recognize their role in the genesis of the recent opioid epidemic, and efforts to adjust prescribing practices have decreased prescription numbers and volume (Barnett et al. 2017; Losby et al. 2017; Osborn et al. 2017). Consequently, health care providers and trainees are increasingly interested in education on the evaluation and management of addictions. Medical student groups are demanding better training in addiction, medical school and graduate medical education addiction training programs are expanding, health systems are developing comprehensive overdose prevention policies, clinicians are being trained in the prevention of overdoses and good stewardship of controlled substance prescribing and management, technological support tools are expanding, and some state medical licensing boards are requiring documentation of training in pain management and/or addiction treatment (Devries et al. 2017; Federation of State Medical Boards 2019; Wickramatilake et al. 2017). In the sections that follow, we take a closer look at how this increased interest in addiction training translates into expanded educational opportunities at various levels of medical training.

Integration of SUD Training Into Medical School Curricula

In March 2016, the Office of National Drug Control Policy encouraged all medical schools to sign a pledge to ensure that all medical students would graduate with an understanding of addiction and safe opioid prescribing and stewardship (The White House, Office of the Press Secretary 2016). Sixty-one of 170 medical schools across the nation signed the pledge. Unfortunately, this pledge did not contain specific guidance on how to develop and implement these goals.

Curricular requirements and corresponding medical school accreditation are governed by the Association of American Medical Colleges (AAMC). In 2018, the AAMC's research team published the results of a telephone survey of medical school deans to explore the state of opioid and addiction training in accredited medical schools in the United States (Howley et al. 2018). Respondents identified three areas of particular challenge to providing and/or expanding their institutions' opioid and addiction curricula: 1) unclear faculty and resident development pathways, 2) lack of time within the curricula to add new content, and 3) uncertainty about how to assess students' skills. However, survey respondents also identified several potential opportunities to address these challenges: 1) sharing and making use of existing resources, 2) teaching interprofessionally and engaging community partners, 3) integrating content throughout the curricula across the continuum in developmentally appropriate ways, 4) optimizing experiential training methods such as case-based teaching and simulation, and 5) building faculty capacity to teach and model evidence-based practices (e.g., Screening, Brief Intervention, and Referral to Treatment [SBIRT]).

In addition to AAMC efforts, some states have undertaken legislative efforts to concomitantly support achieving the same goals. For example, between 2015 and 2018, Massachusetts passed legislation incentivizing the development of core competencies for safe prescribing of opioids and SUD treatment, and providing implementation funding (Moss 2018). The Massachusetts Medical Education Working Group, consisting of representatives from the state's four medical schools, the Massachusetts Medical Society, and the Massachusetts Department of Public Health, developed 10 core competencies for all medical students to learn about safe prescribing of opioids and treatment of addiction (Bharel and Dorkin 2017; Table 52–1).

A number of other medical schools across the country have undertaken their own efforts to revamp their curricula to accommodate more addiction training. For example, Duke University School of Medicine developed an interprofessional SUD curriculum that begins during the preclinical years and extends through clinical clerkships (Muzyk et al. 2017). During their psychiatry clerkship, medical students are enrolled in an interprofessional course covering neurobiology, pharmacology, motivational interviewing, and cultural competency as the topics pertain to substance use. Medical students are also required to attend 12-step meetings and to reflect on their experience.

Similar programmatic efforts have evolved at other medical schools, including those at University of Kentucky, Harvard University, Michigan State University, Beaumont Health, West Virginia University, Indiana University, University of Utah, Boston University, Brown University, Columbia University, and Dartmouth University, to name a few (Hoffman 2018; Sokol and Kunz 2018).

Political and institutional will bent toward addressing the education gap is an important force of change. It remains challenging, however, to provide clinical training expertise, evidence-based curricular content, and additional educational opportunities for medical students, particularly in institutions without advanced addiction training programs (i.e., fellowship programs in addiction medicine and/or addiction psychiatry). Fortunately, myriad organizations, including those listed in Table 52–2, provide training programs and educational materials relating to substance use and addiction. It is beyond the scope of this chapter to highlight every educational resource and opportunity, but perusal of the organizations' websites (listed in Table 52–3) can provide information on their specific training opportunities.

One organization that specifically targets medical student training in addictive disorders is the Alcohol Medical Scholar Program (AMSP; www.alcoholmedical-scholars.org). As stated on the website, AMSP aims to "promote optimal education in medical schools regarding the identification and care of people with alcohol use disorder and other substance-related problems" by offering training opportunities for medical school faculty. Medical school faculty who receive a 2-year AMSP scholarship develop skills pertaining to education about alcohol and drugs of abuse. In addition, the Course on Addiction and Recovery Education (www.hazeldenbettyford.org/education/medical-professional-education/course-addiction-recovery-education) is an online curriculum developed by Hazelden Betty Ford Foundation in collaboration with MedU, ASAM, and the Treatment Research Institute to expand access to medical education about SUDs, and content is available for a fee for each continuing medical education (CME) unit.

Medical students have opportunities outside their medical school curriculum to engage in clinical rotations at nationally recognized substance use treatment facilities. The Hazelden Betty Ford Foundation offers the Summer Institute for Medical Students in which medical students experience immersion training in addiction at one of

TABLE 52–1. **Massachusetts Medical Education Working Group: medical education core competencies for prevention and management of prescription drug misuse and suggested education models**

Primary prevention domain—preventing prescription drug misuse and screening, evaluation, and prevention

1. Evaluate a patient's pain using age, gender, and culturally appropriate evidence-based methodologies.

2. Evaluate a patient's risk for substance use disorders by utilizing age, gender, and culturally appropriate evidence-based communication skills and assessment methodologies, supplemented with relevant available patient information, including but not limited to health records, family history, prescription dispensing records (e.g., the Prescription Drug Monitoring Program, or "PDMP"), drug urine screenings, and screenings for commonly co-occurring psychiatric disorders (especially depression, anxiety disorders, and PTSD [posttraumatic stress disorder]).

3. Identify and describe potential pharmacological and nonpharmacological treatment options including opioid and non-opioid pharmacological treatments for acute and chronic pain management, along with patient communication and education regarding the risks and benefits associated with each of these available treatment options.

Secondary prevention domain—treating patients at risk for substance use disorders

4. Describe substance use disorder treatment options, including medication-assisted treatment, as well as demonstrate the ability to appropriately refer patients to addiction medicine specialists and treatment programs for both relapse prevention and co-occurring psychiatric disorders.

5. Prepare evidence-based and patient-centered pain management and substance use disorder treatment plans for patients with acute and chronic pain with special attention to safe prescribing and recognizing patients displaying signs of aberrant prescription use behaviors.

6. Demonstrate the foundational skills in patient-centered counseling and behavior change in the context of a patient encounter, consistent with evidence-based techniques.

Tertiary prevention domain—managing substance use disorders as a chronic disease and recognizing the risk factors for, and signs of, opioid overdose and demonstrating the correct use of naloxone rescue

7. Describe substance use disorder treatment options, including medication-assisted treatment, and demonstrate the ability to appropriately refer patients to addiction medicine specialists and treatment programs for both relapse prevention and co-occurring psychiatric disorders.

8. Prepare evidence-based and patient-centered pain management and substance use disorder treatment plans for patients with acute and chronic pain with special attention to safe prescribing and recognizing patients displaying signs of aberrant prescription use behaviors.

9. Demonstrate the foundational skills in patient-centered counseling and behavior change in the context of a patient encounter, consistent with evidence-based techniques.

10. Identify and incorporate relevant data regarding social determinants of health into treatment planning for substance use disorders.

TABLE 52–1.   **Massachusetts Medical Education Working Group: medical education core competencies for prevention and management of prescription drug misuse and suggested education models** *(continued)*

Recommended evidence-based methodologies for the prevention and management of prescription drug misuse

In the appropriate setting, and across all prevention areas, it is recommended that the graduating medical student have operational knowledge of:

- Diagnosis-Intractability-Risk-Efficacy (DIRE)
- Motivational Interviewing (MI)
- Opioid Risk Tool (ORT)
- Safe Prescribing "Universal Precautions"
- Screening, Brief Intervention, and Referral to Treatment (SBIRT)
- Screener and Opioid Assessment for Patients with Pain (SOAPP)
- Screening Tool for Addiction Risk (STAR)

Source.   Reprinted from Bharel and Dorkin 2017. Public Domain.

Hazelden Betty Ford's two clinical sites (www.hazeldenbettyford.org/education/medical-professional-education/summer-institute-medical-students). Another similar opportunity is offered through the APA's Externship in Addiction Psychiatry; interested medical students can apply to partner with a mentoring psychiatrist and spend a summer shadowing him or her and learning about treating patients with addiction (www.psychiatry.org/residents-medical-students/medical-students/medical-student-programs/addiction-psychiatry-externship).

Medical student interest and advocacy groups also serve an important role in mobilizing medical student educational agendas. Medical student addiction interest groups have sprung up in many institutions across the country, some of which have lobbied effectively for increased addiction training in medical schools (Bailey 2016). The Psychiatry Student Interest Group Network (www.PsychSIGN.org), an APA-sponsored international network of medical students interested in psychiatry, has helped to connect medical students to faculty and mentors specializing in addiction psychiatry. Additionally, these interest groups provide an organizational structure for medical students to engage in legislative and social justice addiction advocacy efforts, experiences that represent an increasingly important aspect of work in health care.

Buprenorphine waiver training represents a very specific and potentially invaluable aspect of medical student training. Several medical schools are now offering this training as part of their medical curriculum. Early exposure to treatment modalities such as buprenorphine for the treatment of opioid use disorder increases the likelihood that providers will feel comfortable with and use these treatments with their patients throughout their careers. In Rhode Island, for example, Brown University partnered with state authorities to ensure that all medical students received the buprenorphine waiver training prior to graduation, enabling them to apply for the waiver directly after graduation (McCance-Katz et al. 2017).

Medical school curricula focused on recognizing and treating all forms of substance use and misuse are more important than ever for providing future physicians with a well-rounded medical education, as well as for decreasing the stigma many feel toward patients seeking access to care for substance-related issues.

TABLE 52–2. Psychiatry residency longitudinal curricula

Institution	Reference	Description
Massachusetts General Hospital (MGH)/ McLean Hospital Adult Psychiatry Residency Training Program	Iannucci et al. 2009	A six-part curriculum, phased in over 3 years, that includes the following: 1. Faculty training in fundamentals of diagnosis and treatment 2. Two comprehensive training binders for use in PGY1 and PGY3 rotations 3. One-month full-time inpatient addiction psychiatry rotation during PGY1 4. Integration of addiction psychiatry teaching and inpatient services during PGY2 5. Ten-hour-per-week, 2-month substance abuse consultation and outpatient supervision rotation required during PGY3 6. Substance abuse electives including chief residency in addiction psychiatry during PGY4

Canadian Psychiatric Association	Crockford et al. 2015	A 4-year curriculum including didactic seminar material and supervised clinical experiences to meet the 2007 Royal College of Physicians and Surgeons of Canada Specialty Training Requirements, which outline expectations from psychiatry residency training programs to ensure graduates' proficiency in substance-related and addictive disorder evaluation and management:
		1. Didactic seminar material
		  a. PGY1 or PGY2: three hours or more in basic principles of addiction psychiatry (e.g., substances' mechanisms of action, typical intoxication/withdrawal presentations, biopsychosocial etiology of addiction, screening principles)
		  b. PGY2–PGY5: six hours or more of advanced principles of addiction psychiatry (e.g., epidemiology of addictions, further exploration of biopsychosocial basis of addiction, further exploration of neurobiology of addiction, pharmacotherapies for addiction)
		  c. PGY2–PGY5: integration of psychotherapies for substance-related and addictive disorders into core psychotherapy training didactics

TABLE 52–2. **Psychiatry residency longitudinal curricula** *(continued)*

Institution	Reference	Description

Canadian Psychiatric Association *(continued)*		2. Supervised clinical experience
		
		   a. PGY2: intensive 1-month substance-related and addictive disorders experience in program with a primary clinical focus on addictions
		
		   b. PGY2–PGY5: longitudinal substance-related and addictive disorder experience (e.g., management of patients with addictions in multiple different clinical settings in addition to 2a above), and/or "blended" model in which, once a week for 12 months (half-day) or 6 months (full day), residents would attend to patients who are at inpatient, residential, or structured outpatient programs

Yale School of Medicine	Arnaout et al. 2018	A 6-week rotation based at a Veterans Affairs hospital's detoxification service, with the following components: 1. Learn to manage detoxification from a range of substances, and to address co-occurring mental illnesses. 2. Spend a half-day each week in the hospital's buprenorphine clinic, and another half-day at the opioid treatment program. 3. Attend 12-step meetings and participate in a half-day per week of outpatient rehabilitation day treatment programming. 4. Meet regularly with the rotation director. 5. Read several seminal papers on management of addictions.

TABLE 52–2. **Psychiatry residency longitudinal curricula** (*continued*)

Institution	Reference	Description
Boston University Medical Center	Renner 2004	A substance abuse core curriculum that is integrated throughout the general psychiatry residency program and utilizes various educational formats, such as lectures, clinical work, and reading assignments, requiring: 1. A minimum of 20 hours (spanning PGY1–PGY4) of instruction covering screening, diagnosis, epidemiology, the neurobiology of addiction, risk factors and genetic vulnerability for substance use disorders, stages of change and motivational theory, symptoms of intoxication and withdrawal, detoxification treatment, self-help programs, and addiction psychopharmacology. 2. A broader seminar series that introduces basic concepts in psychiatric research. 3. A recognition on the part of residents that the standard of care in the management of dual-diagnosis patients involves taking professional responsibility for both the substance use disorder and any comorbid psychiatric disorder(s).

Note. PGYt=postgraduate year.

TABLE 52–3. Organizations offering resources related to addiction training

Organization	Website/URL	Annotated content available
Addiction Treatment Coordinating Center (ATCC) (U.S. Department of Veterans Affairs)	www.va.gov/oaa/ specialfellows/programs/sf_ advaddictiontreatment.asp?p=17	• Provides Interprofessional Advanced Fellowship in Addiction Treatment • Bi-weekly "E-Blasts" on addiction topics
Addiction Technology Transfer Center Network (ATTC) (Substance Abuse and Mental Health Services Administration)	ATTCNetwork.org	• Training and events calendar • Online free training modules/presentations/enduring materials with focus on evidenced-based practice and systems of care integration practices • Addiction e-newsletter
Alcohol Medical Scholar Program (AMSP)	alcoholmedicalscholars.org	• Scholars program that includes medical school faculty attendance at annual meeting with goal of better integration of addiction training in medical schools • Online curriculum
American Academy of Addiction Psychiatry (AAAP)	AAAP.org	• Fellowships for medical students, residents, and fellows to attend annual meeting • Board preparation course materials • MOC resources and CME credit materials • Annual meeting • Mentorship program • Patient resources • Peer-reviewed journal • Buprenorphine waiver training (through Provider Clinical Support System—see below)

TABLE 52–3. Organizations offering resources related to addiction training *(continued)*

Organization	Website/URL	Annotated content available
American Academy of Family Physicians (AAFP)	AAFP.org	• CME webinars targeting addiction and pain management in primary care • Patient educational materials on a range of addiction and pain topics • Clinical toolkits and practice guidelines • Legislative advocacy updates and opportunities
American Association of Directors of Psychiatric Residency Training (AADPRT)	AADPRT.org	• Educational mentorship • Peer-reviewed model curricula (alcohol and addiction) (login required)
American College of Academic Addiction Medicine (ACAAM)	ACAAM.org	• Repository of addiction medicine fellowship information, from how to start one to lists of active programs • Library of MOC materials and resources with education portal (subscription required) • Board examination preparation materials • Annual meeting
American College of Surgeons (ACS)	FACS.org	• Repository of state-mandated CME content requirements
American Psychiatric Association (APA)	psychiatry.org	• CME and MOC materials and resources • Multiple annual meetings and travel fellowship opportunities • Online learning center (some materials require subscription/membership) • Advocacy updates and opportunities for involvement • Policy statements • Practice guidelines • Peer-reviewed journal • Buprenorphine waiver training

TABLE 52–3. Organizations offering resources related to addiction training *(continued)*

Organization	Website/URL	Annotated content available
American Society of Addiction Medicine (ASAM)	ASAM.org	<ul><li>Annual meeting and annual review course for board examination preparation</li><li>CME and MOC resources and materials</li><li>Advocacy updates and opportunities for involvement/online legislative tracker</li><li>"E-learning center"/learning hub (subscription required for some materials)</li><li>Policy statements</li><li>Practice guidelines</li><li>Patient resources</li><li>Peer-reviewed journal</li><li>Addiction e-newsletter</li><li>Buprenorphine waiver training</li></ul>
Association for Multidisciplinary Education and Research in Substance Use and Addiction (AMERSA)	AMERSA.org	<ul><li>Annual meeting</li><li>Special interest groups/forums for nursing, social work, physicians, adolescents, and young adults, and those interested in MAT</li><li>Project MAINSTREAM program and curriculum repository (to foster faculty development in addictions)</li><li>Links to resources on MAT and harm reduction/overdose prevention</li></ul>
Boston University Chief Resident Immersion Training (CRIT) Program in Addiction Medicine	bumc.bu.edu/care/education-and-training-programs/crit/	<ul><li>Links to CME opportunities</li><li>Program information and immersion program application</li></ul>
Boston University Fellow Immersion Training (FIT) Program in Addiction Medicine	bumc.bu.edu/care/education-and-training-programs/fellow-immersion-training-fit-program/	<ul><li>Immersion program application</li><li>Links to CME requirements</li></ul>

TABLE 52–3. Organizations offering resources related to addiction training *(continued)*

Organization	Website/URL	Annotated content available
California Society of Addiction Medicine (CSAM)	CSAM-ASAM.org	• Annual meeting and travel fellowship opportunities • Review course and enduring materials • Newsletter • Online education center (subscription required for some materials) • White papers and policy platform library • Board certification examination review materials
Center on Addiction (formerly Center on Addiction and Substance Abuse)	centeronaddiction.org	• National survey results and reports • Patient and family resources • Online learning center (registration required) • Repository of position statements and opinion pieces
Extension for Community Healthcare Outcomes (ECHO)	Echo.unm.edu	• Links to join online learning collaboratives on a range of medical, pain, and addiction topics
Hazelden Betty Ford Foundation	hazeldenbettyford.org	• Application materials for various clinical training programs • Curated abstract list of recent research publications • Online searchable addiction research library • Continuing education (webinar archive) and event calendar • Podcast archive
Institute for Research, Education, and Training in Addictions (IRETA)	IRETA.org	• Online courses, webinars • Application materials for medical student fellowship
Medical Education Research Foundation (MERF) for the Treatment of Addiction	MERFWeb.org	• Fellowships for California clinicians to have mentored experience at annual California Society of Addiction Medicine meeting (see above)

TABLE 52–3.   Organizations offering resources related to addiction training *(continued)*

Organization	Website/URL	Annotated content available
Opioid Response Network (ORN) (formerly State Targeted Response Technical Assistance Consortium)	opioidresponsenetwork.org	• Online request portal for obtaining vetted technical assistance in expanding addiction treatment (individuals, agencies, and systems of care are all eligible to apply)
Provider Clinical Support System (PCSS)	PCSSnow.org	• Webinars, archived materials • Treatment "success stories" repository • Clinical and professional mentoring • Clinical resources and tools • Buprenorphine waiver training
Substance Abuse and Mental Health Services Administration (SAMHSA)	SAMHSA.gov	• Repository of searchable national data • Links to SAMHSA-sponsored clinical training initiatives (e.g., ATTC, ORN, PCSS—see above) • Evidence-Based Practices Resource Center • Clinical practice guidelines and support information • Links to treatment-related statutes, regulations, and guidelines • Training calendars, archived webinars/summits/workshops
University of California San Francisco, Substance Use Warmline	nccc.ucsf.edu/clinician-consultation/substance-use-management/california-substance-use-line	• For California clinicians: real-time clinical curbside consultations • For all clinicians: substance use resource repository

Note.   This list is not comprehensive; rather, it preferentially highlights the organizations discussed in this chapter. CME=continuing medical education; MAT=medication-assisted treatment; MOC=maintenance of certification.

Incorporation of SUD Training Into Residency Programs

Similar expansions in addiction education are needed in postgraduate residency training programs. Many residency programs have undertaken a range of innovative approaches to enhance addiction training, and an array of professional and governmental organizations have expanded their offerings for residents seeking additional training in addictions. Regulatory agencies have concomitantly allotted structural time within graduate medical education to enhance addiction training experiences. In this section, we review efforts to enhance addiction training at the residency level, with particular emphasis on psychiatry residency training.

A residency program provides a critical developmental experience in which the individual forms and solidifies clinical skills, professional identities, and (importantly) attitudes toward patients, treatments, and peers and colleagues. Data suggest that psychiatry residents hold more stigmatizing attitudes toward patients with SUDs than toward patients without SUDs, and these attitudes become more negative over the course of residency training, indicating that there is significant room for improvement in education about addictions provided during residency training in psychiatry (Avery et al. 2017). Fortunately, several strategic approaches are being undertaken to address stigma and negative attitudes. For instance, residency regulatory bodies have mandated the provision of addiction training during psychiatry residencies. In 2001, the Residency Review Committee of the Accreditation Council for Graduate Medical Education (ACGME) issued a first-of-its-kind requirement that all psychiatry residency programs provide at least 1 month of full-time equivalent training in addiction psychiatry (Accreditation Council for Graduate Medical Education 2020d; Patil and Andry 2017) (Table 52–4).

Additionally, ACGME program requirements for child and adolescent psychiatry fellowship programs mandate that programs provide "instruction and experience in pain management if applicable for the subspecialty, including recognition of the signs of addiction" [Section IV.C.2] (Accreditation Council for Graduate Medical Education 2020a). Furthermore, it is stipulated that graduating fellows "demonstrate competence in evaluation and treatment…of substance use disorders" [Section IV.B.1.b.(1).(a).(i)] (Accreditation Council for Graduate Medical Education 2020a) and that early enrollment (also known as "fast tracking") into a child and adolescent psychiatry fellowship does not forgive the 1-month addiction training requirement.

Despite the ACGME mandate, tremendous variability exists in terms of curricular content and access to expert supervision, resulting in challenges for developing and assessing competency (Welsh et al. 2019). For consultation-liaison psychiatry (formerly psychosomatic medicine) fellowships, ACGME guidelines indicate that upon graduation, fellows must "demonstrate competence in their knowledge of substance use and its impact on the assessment and treatment of patients in the medical setting" [Section IV.B.1.c.(1).(c)] (Accreditation Council for Graduate Medical Education 2020b). The ACGME guidelines likewise require that geriatric psychiatry fellows must demonstrate "proficiency in diagnosis and treatment of…substance-related disorders" [Section IV.B.1.b.(1).(a)] (Accreditation Council for Graduate Medical Education

TABLE 52–4. **Accreditation Council for Graduate Medical Education program requirements for graduate medical education in psychiatry**

Section	Description
IV.C.3.j	Resident experience in addiction psychiatry must include one month FTE of organized experience focused on the evaluation and clinical management of patients with substance abuse/dependence problems, including dual diagnosis. [(Core)]
IV.C.3.j.(1)	Residents must have experience with treatment modalities that include:
IV.C.3.j.(1).(a)	• detoxification, overdose management, and maintenance pharmacotherapy; [(Core)]
IV.C.3.j.(1).(b)	• the use of therapeutic techniques that address the psychological and social consequences of addiction, to include confronting and intervening in chronic addiction rehabilitation used in recovery stages from pre-contemplation to maintenance; and [(Core)]
IV.C.3.j.(1).(c)	• self-help groups. [(Core)]

Note. FTE=full time equivalent.
Source. Reprinted from Accreditation Council for Graduate Medical Education: ACGME Program Requirements for Graduate Medical Education in Psychiatry (ACGME-approved focused revision: June 13, 2020; effective July 1, 2020). 2020d. Available at: https://www.acgme.org/Portals/0/PFAssets/ProgramRequirements/400_Psychiatry_2020.pdf?ver=2020-06-19-123110-817. Accessed August 9, 2020. Used with permission.

2020c). Because "fast-tracking" is not an option in consultation-liaison, forensic, and geriatric psychiatry, fellows in these programs will have fulfilled the mandated addiction clinical experience prior to fellowship matriculation. However, as with general psychiatry training, there is little guidance on how to achieve and assess "competency" in substance-related disorders in these psychiatric subspecialties, making fellowship clinical experiences highly variable. We discuss addiction-specific fellowship training in more detail in the next section (see "Addiction Psychiatry Fellowships and Board Certification" under "Postresidency Training").

Today, nearly 20 years after the ACGME first issued its program requirement, significant variability remains across programs in terms of the timing of this training mandate within the residency program, the availability of clinical training sites, and access to addiction specialty supervision (Shorter and Dermatis 2012). A 2017 survey of psychiatry training programs highlighted that most addiction training happens not in specialty addiction treatment sites but rather in general psychiatry settings such as inpatient units and consultation-liaison psychiatry services, thereby limiting the exposure to minimal if any longitudinal clinical exposure. Curricular content and clinical experiences varied widely across programs, and limited faculty were available to supervise and teach residents (Schwartz et al. 2018). These survey results, combined with the data indicating that psychiatry residents' attitudes toward patients with addiction deteriorate over the course of training (Avery et al. 2017), highlight that ACGME requirements are necessary but not sufficient to meet the training needs of psychiatry residents regarding addictions.

Although not a substitute for sound clinical exposure and supervision, both the Psychiatry Resident-In-Training Examination® (PRITE®; American College of Psychiatrists 2020; Dingle et al. 2018) and the American Board of Psychiatry and Neurology (ABPN) certification examinations (American Board of Psychiatry and Neurology 2019b) have portions dedicated to questions regarding substance-related and addictive disorders for which examinees must necessarily prepare. Many programs are using the Objective Structured Clinical Examination (OSCE) to assess residents through simulated experiences with patients with substance use concerns; in addition to providing management skill training, assessment, and immediate feedback, the OSCE also provides structured opportunities for addiction education (Parish et al. 2006, 2013).

Given the heterogeneity of implementation of addiction training in general psychiatry residency programs described above, several programs have sought to develop innovative curriculum programing to both meet the ACGME requirements and provide top-notch training that prepares graduates for working with patients with addictions and co-occurring disorders. Polydorou et al. (2008) has provided a useful framework of general principles for designing maximally helpful curricula to improve physician training in SUDs (Table 52–5).

In an attempt to provide comprehensive psychiatry resident training in the evaluation and treatment of individuals with SUDs, several programs have developed and implemented comprehensive curricula for this purpose. Implementation challenges remain, however, including insufficient time within residency programs to follow patients longitudinally, limited availability of qualified addiction supervision, and ongoing stigma (Iannucci et al. 2009). Largely, those programs that have developed longitudinal, comprehensive psychiatry resident training experiences in addictions benefit from having access to faculty and training sites around which they can build their residents' training. Programs with less robust faculty or training sites will need to develop creative ways of expanding their residents' access to training opportunities. In addition to the organizational educational opportunities outlined in the previous section on medical student education, several innovative approaches are outlined below.

Williams et al. (2019) at Rutgers Robert Wood Johnson Medical School describe the innovative use of an online webinar-type experience to educate residents about the recognition and management of tobacco use disorder, with posttest results indicating a significant increase in knowledge about diagnosis and treatment (Williams et al. 2019). The Yale Primary Care Internal Medicine Residency Program developed the Addiction Recovery Clinic to help meet addiction training needs of its internal medicine residents. Residents work one half-day per week at the clinic, which provides treatment of opioid use disorder (OUD) with buprenorphine; behavioral counseling; alcohol use disorder pharmacotherapy; tobacco use disorder treatment (if needed in addition to another substance presentation); and referrals for clinical services that are not directly provided (e.g., methadone maintenance) (Holt et al. 2017). Similarly, Sanchez-Ramirez et al. (2016) described the use of an addiction-focused intensive outpatient treatment setting as a nontraditional venue in which to effectively educate psychiatry senior residents. Agrawal et al. (2016) described an innovative approach to educating psychiatry residents about addictions and recovery by pairing service

TABLE 52–5. **Summary findings of substance abuse training programs for physicians**

- Brief, skills-based curricula can improve physician knowledge, attitudes, and practices.
- Combined interactive, experiential, and didactic curricula are preferable to didactics alone.
- Expert faculty in addiction are needed to serve as role models and provide support.
- Feedback to trainees should be integrated into training programs.
- Reinforcement of training improves outcomes.

Source. Reprinted from Polydorou S, Gunderson EW, Levin FR: "Training Physicians to Treat Substance Use Disorders." *Current Psychiatry Reports* 10(5):399–404, 2008.

users with lived experience with senior psychiatry residents. In addition, Avery et al. (2019) described a novel online training module on stigma related to individuals with SUDs. This training module presents information illustrating how clinicians' attitudes toward individuals with SUDs are worse than their attitudes toward individuals with other conditions, as well as information on the moral-failing model of addiction versus the brain disease model, videos of individuals in recovery and family members of individuals with SUDs, and resources for further information. Ballon and Skinner (2008) noted that incorporation of educational reflection techniques (journaling, group processing meetings, and composition of reflection paper) into the first-year resident curriculum at the University of Toronto has had a positive impact on residents' attitudes toward individuals with SUDs.

The list of organizations providing training opportunities to psychiatric and medical residents is rapidly expanding, with many having been previously highlighted above (see also Table 52–3). For example, Project ECHO® (Extension for Community Healthcare Outcomes), started in 2003, aims to "de-monopolize knowledge and amplify local capacity that provides best-practice care for underserved people all over the world" (University of New Mexico School of Medicine 2020). Project ECHO® brings together experts and community providers in case-based conversations over a telehealth platform, and the model has been recognized for some success (Komaromy et al. 2016); however, recent studies also suggest that although participants appreciate the content of these training programs, there are significant structural impediments to uptake of the platform (Salvador et al. 2019). Additionally, since 2003, SAMHSA has provided funding for 17 residency cooperatives (in two cohorts) aimed at providing assistance in the development of SBIRT programs at the participating grantees' organizations. A major thrust of these grants has been the improvement and provision of training around addiction recognition and treatment (see www.samhsa.gov/sbirt/grantees). SAMHSA has also funded the State Targeted Response Technical Assistance Consortium (STR-TA), renamed the Opioid Response Network (ORN), in collaboration with AAAP to provide and promote education and training for evidence-based practices in the prevention of, treatment of, and recovery from OUDs. In addition, several organizations, such as AAAP and ASAM, offer opportunities for subsidized travel and waived conference registration fees for participation in their organizations' annual meetings.

Fostering leadership skills is a critical component of building a health care workforce confident in and capable of addressing the needs of patients with addictive disorders. Chief residents, for example, play a key leadership role in training the future physician workforce. Boston University's Chief Resident Immersion Training (CRIT) Program aims to develop chief resident competency with the "scientific foundation of addiction medicine and state-of-the-art substance use diagnosis and management skills, in order to facilitate integration of [substance use] content into residency program curricula and [chief resident] teaching" (Alford et al. 2009, p. 41). The CRIT Program brings together chief residents from internal medicine and family medicine for a 4-day immersion training program in state-of-the-art methods of diagnosing, managing, and teaching about addiction medicine, as facilitated by leaders in the fields of addiction medicine and psychiatry.

Training residents on the use of buprenorphine for the treatment of OUD would be a practical addition to residency programs (Suzuki et al. 2016). A survey study of residency program directors in psychiatry, internal medicine, and family medicine revealed that only 22.6% of these training programs encourage or require completion of buprenorphine waiver training, even though the majority of the responding programs indicated that they believed such training to be important (88.1%) (Tesema et al. 2018). Moreover, data from 2012 suggested that only 16% of psychiatrists had obtained a buprenorphine waiver, and the numbers of those who had waivers and actually prescribed buprenorphine were likely much lower (Rosenblatt et al. 2015). Given the pivotal role that psychiatrists play in addressing the national opioid epidemic, some advocates and researchers have called for buprenorphine waiver training and clinical experiences in the prescribing of buprenorphine to be *mandated* in psychiatry residency training programs (Morris and Bentzley 2019; Muvvala et al. 2019).

Postresidency Training

Addiction Psychiatry Fellowships and Board Certification

Expansion of opportunities for postgraduate specialty training is a critical part of enhancing clinician expertise and expanding the health care workforce to meet the addiction needs of the public. Since 1993, addiction psychiatry has been recognized as a medical subspecialty by the American Board of Medical Specialties (ABMS) under the auspices of the ABPN. Board certification in addiction psychiatry requires 1) completion of an adult psychiatry residency and/or child and adolescent psychiatry fellowship, 2) completion of an ACGME-accredited addiction psychiatry fellowship, and 3) a passing grade on a clinical knowledge board examination. In its 2019 annual report, the ABPN noted that 2,665 individuals have been granted board certification in addiction psychiatry since the specialty's inception in 1993, with 1,164 holding currently active certification (American Board of Psychiatry and Neurology 2019a). Furthermore, the ACGME lists 50 accredited addiction psychiatry fellowship programs as being active during academic year 2018–2019 in the United States (Accreditation Council for Graduate Medical Education 2019). In addiction psychiatry, as in other medical specialties, continued board certification requires ongoing maintenance of certification (MOC), including continuing medical education, self-assessment education, and performance improvement projects, as well as completion of a knowledge-based examination during each 10-year MOC cycle.

Initiating an addiction psychiatry training fellowship program is complex. In addition to satisfying the ACGME Common Program Requirements, addiction psychiatry fellowship programs must have two faculty members who are board-certified in addiction psychiatry, adequate faculty and clinical rotations, meaningful didactic education in addiction psychiatry, capacity for scholarly activities, and other components to meet the program-specific requirements. Each year at the AAAP annual meeting, education workshops such as "How to Start an Addiction Psychiatry Fellowship" bring together program leaders and resources for those interested in starting an addiction psychiatry fellowship at their training institution.

To help address trainees' questions about the utility of fellowship training in addiction psychiatry, the American Association of Directors of Psychiatric Residency Training has compiled a useful resource guide, "Addiction Psychiatry Fellowship: How and Why to Apply" (available at: www.aadprt.org/application/files/7615/9122/0825/Addiction_Psychiatry_Fellowship_How_and_Why_to_Apply.pdf), that addresses many of the pros and cons of fellowship training.

Addiction Medicine Fellowships and Board Certification

Until 2016, addiction medicine was not an ABMS-recognized medical subspecialty. From 1986 to 2009, ASAM administered a knowledge-based certification examination in addiction medicine. Between 2009 and 2016, physicians could earn certification in addiction medicine by meeting specific practice criteria and by passing a knowledge-based examination administered through the American Board of Addiction Medicine (ABAM), which was established in 2007. The Addiction Medicine Foundation (TAMF), the education arm of ABAM, began to accredit addiction medicine fellowship programs in 2011. In 2016, ABAM achieved addiction medicine's recognition by ABMS as a multispecialty subspecialty, and starting in 2017, the addiction medicine certification examination was administered by the American Board of Preventive Medicine (ABPM). The ACGME began to accredit addiction medicine fellowships in 2018. TAMF was subsequently reorganized under the name American College of Academic Addiction Medicine (ACAAM) to continue its support for addiction medicine fellowship training. Readers interested in an extensive discussion of the evolution of the addiction psychiatry and addiction medicine specialties are referred to the detailed overview by Nunes et al. (2020).

As of September 2020, ACAAM lists a total of 91 addiction medicine fellowships available in the United States (79 accredited by ACGME and 12 accredited by ACAAM itself), all of which are described in the ACAAM Directory of Addiction Medicine Fellowship Programs (accessible through the ACAAM website at: www.acaam.org/accreditedfellowships/). Physicians from any primary ABMS specialty are eligible to take the addiction medicine certification examination if they have a primary board certification from an ABMS member board and have completed an ACGME-accredited addiction medicine fellowship. Notably, a practice pathway exists through 2021, during which time physicians meeting specific clinical practice criteria are permitted to sit for the ABPM addiction medicine board examination without having completed an ACGME-accredited addiction medicine fellowship.

MOC requirements in addiction medicine parallel the requirements of other ABPM specialties and subspecialties (American Board of Preventive Medicine 2018).

Comparisons Between Addiction Psychiatry and Addiction Medicine

There are some key similarities between the subspecialties of addiction psychiatry and addiction medicine: 1) specialists in both have overlapping membership and missions, 2) both are now ABMS certified, 3) both are growing their numbers of fellowship programs, and 4) both serve significant educational and research support functions.

Nonetheless, some important differences exist. Addiction psychiatry has clearly articulated interest and expertise in co-occurring mental illness and addictions, whereas addiction medicine takes a more explicit aim at evaluation and management of addictions in a wide variety of medical settings (e.g., primary care, internal medicine, pain, interventional practices). These distinctions, however, when viewed in aggregate, provide complementary functions. There exists a tremendous collaborative potential between the fields of addiction medicine and addiction psychiatry due to the similarities and overlap in clinician expertise, treatment approaches used, and patient populations served.

Support for Addiction Psychiatry and Addiction Medicine Fellowship Programs

In late 2019, the U.S. Health Resources and Service Administration (HRSA) Bureau of Health Workforce released a Notice of Funding Opportunity for the Addiction Medicine Fellowship (AMF) Program, a 5-year training grant open to accredited Addiction Psychiatry and Addiction Medicine fellowships. The goals of the AMF program are to "increase the number of board-certified addiction medicine specialists and addiction psychiatry subspecialists; collaborate and establish formal relationships with community treatment sites in underserved areas to provide training of program fellows; and develop or enhance training for faculty on opioid and substance use disorder prevention and treatment" (Health Resources and Services Administration 2019). In June 2020, HRSA awarded a total of $20,337,564 to 44 Addiction Psychiatry and Addiction Medicine fellowship training programs, with funding starting July 1, 2020 (Health Resources and Services Administration 2020).

Programs Targeting Addiction Fellows-in-Training

Several programs focused on addiction fellows-in-training are available. The Fellow Immersion Training (FIT) Program in Addiction Medicine at Boston University runs concomitantly with the CRIT Program (described earlier in chapter; see "Incorporation of SUD Training Into Residency Programs"). FIT offers a "four-day intensive immersion training that equips incoming and current clinical subspecialty fellows with state-of-the-art skills and content to integrate addiction medicine into clinical research" (www.bumc.bu.edu/care/fellow-immersion-training-fit-program/). Funded by a 5-year SAMHSA grant awarded to the AAAP in 2018, the Recognizing and Eliminating disparities in Addiction through Culturally informed Healthcare (REACH) program aims to "(1) increase the overall number of racial and ethnic underrepresented minority (URM) addiction specialists in the Addiction Psychiatry and Addiction Medicine workforce, and (2) increase the number of addiction specialists adequately trained to work with racial and ethnic URM patients with substance use disorders" (https://reachgrant.org/about/goals/). Based with Yale University's addiction medicine and psychiatry programs, REACH offers 1-week intensive training programs to participants, as well as mentorship and scholarly support. In addition, the National Institute on Drug Abuse (NIDA) and the National Institute on Alcohol Abuse and Alcoholism (NIAAA) offer a number of research fellowships for addiction fellows.

Programs Targeting Medical School Faculty

AMERSA, founded in 1976 as a nonprofit professional organization, offers interdisciplinary leadership in substance use education, research, clinical care, and policy. AMERSA's activities and resources can be of great value to health care providers who are interested in furthering their own or their organization's expertise in managing addictive disorders. AMERSA developed Project MAINSTREAM (the MultiAgency INitiative on Substance abuse TRaining and Education for AMerica) as an interdisciplinary approach to incorporation of sustainable curricular improvements at academic health centers in the United States. Project MAINSTREAM's collection of training modules represents a valuable model curriculum for individuals and organizations looking to build or enhance their addiction training programs (Madden et al. 2006), and modules are available for free on the organization's website (https://amersa.org/resources/project-mainstream/). In addition to AMERSA's pioneering efforts, the AMSP (described earlier in chapter; see "Integration of SUD Training Into Medical School Curricula") and the faculty development program described by Bigby and Barnes (1993) have helped set the stage for the changes necessary to integrate addiction training more fully into residency training programs.

Continuing Professional Education

Opioid Risk Management and Opioid Addiction Treatment Education

One approach to educating providers about safe opioid prescribing practices has been the issuance of prescribing guidelines to help guide clinicians' clinical decision making. The effectiveness of guidelines to shape clinician behavior and clinical decision making is not clear-cut, but evidence suggests that guidelines can improve clinical care by summarizing current medical knowledge and promoting safe, effective, and efficient practices (Grimshaw et al. 2004; Woolf et al. 1999). For example, in 2016, the Centers for Disease Control and Prevention (CDC) issued its first-ever "CDC Guideline for Prescribing Opioids for Chronic Pain" (Dowell et al. 2016a). To facilitate clinician implementation of these recommendations, the CDC supplemented the guideline document with checklists and other guideline tools, such as patient information sheets, webinars, a mobile app, and pocket reference cards (Centers for Disease Control and Prevention 2016; Dowell et al. 2016b). However, a number of unintended consequences have occurred as a result of misinterpretation and misapplication of the CDC guideline. Clinicians have used the guideline to rapidly taper and discontinue opioids and to refer or dismiss patients from care. The authors of the 2016 guideline clarified their concerns about misuse of the guideline's recommendations in 2019 (Dowell et al. 2019).

Another approach promoting clinician education around safe opioid prescribing and pain management involves tying educational mandates to medical license renewals. Many state medical boards, for example, have adopted specific content requirements for CME credits to include training in pain management, opioid prescribing, and patient safety. A summary of state requirements can be found on the American College of Surgeons website (www.facs.org/education/cme/state-mandates). By tying medical licensing to specific training in pain management and/or OUD treatment, medical boards provide external incentives toward closing the "education gap" discussed at the beginning of this chapter.

The use of buprenorphine in the treatment of OUD requires physicians, nurse practitioners, or physician assistants to undergo intensive training in order to be waivered by the U.S. Department of Justice Drug Enforcement Agency (DEA). Although some trainees are now undergoing this training as part of residency or medical school (see earlier sections in this chapter), the training of practicing clinicians in the use of buprenorphine remains a nationwide priority and goal (U.S. Department of Health and Human Services, Office of the Surgeon General 2016). To facilitate education about this treatment modality for practicing clinicians, SAMHSA and other agencies (APA, ASAM, AAAP, Providers Clinical Support System [PCSS]) have produced regulatory-compliant waiver training programs that are available at little or no cost to interested providers. Unfortunately, despite these widespread training efforts, those who have undertaken the requisite training underutilize buprenorphine prescribing (Jones and McCance-Katz 2019). Factors contributing to low rates of prescribing include time constraints, lack of institutional support, concerns about or lack of comfort with regulations, lack of addiction specialty referral options, and lack of confidence in managing patients with OUD. Several of these perceived barriers are remediable through education and supervision. Recognizing this need, several national and local agencies now collaborate in offering mentorship and education guidance to interested providers, in the hopes that increasing competence and confidence in treating OUD with buprenorphine will increase the availability of the treatment to patients in need. Examples of this direct provider support include the ORN (see earlier section "Incorporation of SUD Training Into Residency Programs") and several direct mentorship programs, such as those provided free of charge by PCSS, ASAM, and AAAP.

Continuing Medical Education

CME remains an integral part of ongoing maintenance of certification of a physician's medical license, as well as an opportunity to offer and incentivize (through CME credit) ongoing training for physicians in the field of substance-related and addictive disorders. Although many CME programs are didactic in nature, other offerings are increasingly innovative in their approach to providing evidence-based training, such as through the use of interactive webinars, self-assessment materials, and quality improvement projects. Ongoing educational reinforcement is imperative to improving the impact of CME programs (el-Guebaly et al. 2000).

Coupling Educational Interventions With Practice Prompts

Another approach to improving clinician practices in relation to substance use is pairing brief educational training with system-based clinical prompts. For instance, clinicians are given prompts in the actual clinical setting, such as through chart-based reminders or electronic health record–generated reports, which have been shown to improve clinician practices in treating tobacco use disorder, as one example (Unrod et al. 2007). Similarly, prompting primary care faculty and house staff with patients' alcohol screening results and specific recommendations for intervention may improve physician counseling and alcohol-related patient outcomes (Saitz et al. 2003).

Other Postgraduate Training Opportunities

The U.S. Department of Veterans Affairs (VA) has offered advanced fellowships in addiction treatment since 1994. Specifically, the Interprofessional Advanced Fellowship in Addiction Treatment provides 2 years of postresidency, postdoctoral research, education, and clinical learning opportunities to eligible physicians and associated health professionals and is coordinated by the VA's Addiction Treatment Coordinating Center in Pittsburgh, Pennsylvania.

The SAMHSA-funded Addiction Technology Transfer Center (ATTC) Network is an international multidisciplinary resource for professionals in the addiction treatment and recovery services field. ATTC offers an up-to-date, curated clearinghouse for local and national training events, as well as extensive educational products and resources.

Loan Repayment/Incentive Programs

Although not directly related to education activities themselves, education loan repayment programs tied to working with patients with addictions can provide significant incentives for pursuing further education in treating addictions. Established in 1970 through the Emergency Health Personnel Act (P.L. 91-623) and administered by the Health Resources and Services Administration, the National Health Service Corps (NHSC) provides educational loan forgiveness to clinicians who opt to work in underserved areas as designated by the NHSC (Heisler 2018). In 2018, H.R.6, the Substance Use-Disorder Prevention that Promotes Opioid Recovery and Treatment (SUPPORT) for Patients and Communities Act, amended the Public Health Services Act to authorize eligible loan forgiveness up to $250,000 to clinicians opting to practice either in a mental health professional shortage area or in a county with an overdose rate higher than the most recent available national average and working in a substance use treatment setting (H.R.6—SUPPORT for Patients and Communities Act 2018).

Impact of COVID-19 on Professional Health Care Education

Since its emergence in late 2019, the global coronavirus disease 2019 (COVID-19) pandemic caused by severe acute respiratory syndrome coronavirus 2 (SARS-CoV-2) has impacted nearly every facet of life, including how health care professionals are educated and trained. Hospitals were required to shift clinical services to contain virus spread while simultaneously care for a growing number of COVID-19 patients as well as continue care for patients with ongoing medical illnesses. To comply with required social distancing, health care professional schools undertook a range of measures to mitigate virus spread, including sending students home, shifting learning online, and delaying clinical rotations.

Simultaneously, postgraduate training programs transitioned along with the rest of the health care system to tele-clinical services and moved case discussions, team meetings, and didactics online as much as possible. While "flipping" the classroom to provide individualized asynchronous instruction and minimize in-class lectures existed prior to COVID-19, the pandemic accelerated this form of instructional design and further moved educational discussions online (Rose 2020). Fortuitously, in late 2019, the AAAP received a SAMHSA grant to develop and disseminate a foundational SUD curriculum to health care professional schools nationally. Partnering with the Yale School of Medicine, a massive open online course (MOOC) titled "Addiction Treatment: Clinical Skills for Healthcare Professionals" (Edens et al. 2020a) was launched in late 2019, just as the pandemic was emerging. Through this program, students from two dozen schools have accessed and explored this course's foundational, evidence-based materials on SUD prevention and treatment. Nearly 900 students were enrolled and actively engaged in the course during the first 6 months, and participation numbers further spiked after the March 2020 "stay at home" orders went into effect (Edens et al. 2020b).

Beyond content typically reserved for the classroom, clinical examinations and simulation training with standardized patients have also made their way out of the office and into the online "cloud." The ultimate impact of the SARS-CoV-2 pandemic on medical education will take time to understand, but pandemic-triggered changes may represent a permanent transformation in how we educate, disseminate, and collaborate on curriculum and clinical skills training in health professional programs.

Conclusion

Addiction research, our understanding of addictive diseases, and our treatment options for addiction have expanded tremendously over the past several decades. In addition, national rising trends in substance use, especially the national opioid epidemic, have highlighted significant gaps in treatment as well as in education. Educational efforts are needed to prepare and develop a health care workforce capable of handling the challenges posed by the rising rates of substance use. Fortunately, programs designed to tackle pernicious stigma and raise clinical acumen have arisen at all levels of medical training—from medical school through residency, and during postgraduate professional life. National organizations, such as SAMHSA, NIDA, NIAAA, AAAP, ASAM, American Psychiatric Association, Veterans Affairs, and others, as well as individual academic programs and health care systems, have risen to the challenge and developed innovative and state-of-the-science training tools and educational curricula to facilitate collective efforts aimed at raising awareness and enhancing treatment of addictive disorders. The effects of and treatment options for addiction are widespread and multifaceted, and therefore efforts at education necessitate cross-agency and cross-discipline collaboration in order to be effective. Finally, further research is needed in addiction education approaches and implementation strategies to most fully meet our national needs.

References

Accreditation Council for Graduate Medical Education: Addiction Psychiatry Programs, Academic Year 2018–2019, United States. April 5, 2019. Available at: https://www.aaap.org/wp-content/uploads/2019/04/2019_PublicListProgramsBySpecialty.pdf. Accessed on July 27, 2020.

Accreditation Council for Graduate Medical Education: ACGME Program Requirements for Graduate Medical Education in Child and Adolescent Psychiatry (ACGME-approved focused revision: June 13, 2020; effective July 1, 2020). 2020a. Available at: https://www.acgme.org/Portals/0/PFAssets/ProgramRequirements/405_ChildAdolescentPsychiatry_2020.pdf?ver=2020-06-19-130331-607. Accessed July 27, 2020.

Accreditation Council for Graduate Medical Education: ACGME Program Requirements for Graduate Medical Education in Consultation-Liaison Psychiatry (ACGME-approved focused revision: June 13, 2020; effective July 1, 2020). 2020b. Available at: https://www.acgme.org/Portals/0/PFAssets/ProgramRequirements/407_GeriatricPsychiatry_2020.pdf?ver=2020-06-19-131406-230. Accessed July 27, 2020. Accessed January 17, 2020.

Accreditation Council for Graduate Medical Education: ACGME Program Requirements for Graduate Medical Education in Geriatric Psychiatry (ACGME-approved focused revision: June 13, 2020; effective July 1, 2020). 2020c. Available at: https://www.acgme.org/Portals/0/PFAssets/ProgramRequirements/409_ConsultationLiaisonPsychiatry_2020.pdf?ver=2020-06-19-132534-420. Accessed July 27, 2020.

Accreditation Council for Graduate Medical Education: ACGME Program Requirements for Graduate Medical Education in Psychiatry (ACGME-approved focused revision: June 13, 2020; effective July 1, 2020). 2020d. Available at: https://www.acgme.org/Portals/0/PFAssets/ProgramRequirements/400_Psychiatry_2020.pdf?ver=2020-06-19-123110-817. Accessed August 9, 2020.

Agrawal S, Capponi P, López J, et al: From surviving to advising: a novel course pairing mental health and addictions service users as advisors to senior psychiatry residents. Acad Psychiatry 40(3):475–480, 2016 27056051

Alford DP, Bridden C, Jackson AH, et al: Promoting substance use education among generalist physicians: an evaluation of the Chief Resident Immersion Training (CRIT) Program. J Gen Intern Med 24(1):40–47, 2009 18937015

American Board of Preventive Medicine: News & Announcements: The American Board of Preventive Medicine (ABPM) Maintenance of Certification Requirements for Those Diplomates Certified by the ABPM in Addiction Medicine. Chicago, IL, August 24, 2018. Available at: https://www.theabpm.org/2018/08/24/the-american-board-of-preventive-medicine-abpm-maintenance-of-certification-requirements-for-those-diplomates-certified-by-the-abpm-in-addiction-medicine/. Accessed October 20, 2020.

American Board of Psychiatry and Neurology: 2019 Annual Report. 2019a. Available at: https://www.abpn.com/wp-content/uploads/2020/05/ABPN_2019_Annual_Report.pdf. Accessed July 27, 2020.

American Board of Psychiatry and Neurology: Certification Examination in Psychiatry. 2020 ABPN Content Specifications in Psychiatry Certification. October 30, 2019b. Available at: https://www.abpn.com/wp-content/uploads/2019/10/2020_Psychiatry_CERT_Content_Specifications.pdf. Accessed July 27, 2020.

American College of Psychiatrists: Psychiatry Resident-In-Training Examination® (PRITE®). 2020. Available at: https://www.acpsych.org/prite. Accessed July 27, 2020.

Arnaout B, Muvvala S, Rohrbaugh R, et al: Description of a comprehensive addiction rotation at a psychiatry residency program. Acad Psychiatry 42(2):313–316, 2018 29302930

Avery J, Han BH, Zerbo E, et al: Changes in psychiatry residents' attitudes towards individuals with substance use disorders over the course of residency training. Am J Addict 26(1):75–79, 2017 27749984

Avery J, Knoepflmacher D, Mauer E, et al: Improvement in residents' attitudes toward individuals with substance use disorders following an online training module on stigma. HSS J 15(1):31–36, 2019 30863230

Ayu AP, Schellekens AFA, Iskandar S, et al: Effectiveness and organization of addiction medicine training across the globe. Eur Addict Res 21(5):223–239, 2015 25966903

Bailey M: Medical Students Demand Better Training to Tackle Opioid Crisis. May 17, 2016. Available at: https://www.statnews.com/2016/05/17/opioid-addiction-medical-schools/. Accessed January 17, 2020.

Ballon BC, Skinner W: "Attitude is a little thing that makes a big difference": reflection techniques for addiction psychiatry training. Acad Psychiatry 32(3):218–224, 2008 18467479

Barnett ML, Olenski AR, Jena AB: Opioid-prescribing patterns of emergency physicians and risk of long-term use. N Engl J Med 376(7):663–673, 2017 28199807

Bharel M (Commissioner, Massachusetts Department of Public Health), Dorkin HL (President, Massachusetts Medical Society): Medical Education Core Competencies for the Prevention and Management of Prescription Drug Misuse and Suggested Education Modules. May 4, 2017. Available at: http://www.massmed.org/Physicians/Residents-and-Fellows/Medical-Education-Core-Competencies-for-the-Prevention-and-Management-of-Prescription-Drug-Misuse-and-Suggested-Education-Modules/#.Xk1Z82hKjq4. Accessed February 19, 2020.

Bigby J, Barnes HN: Evaluation of a faculty development program in substance abuse education. J Gen Intern Med 8(6):301–305, 1993 8320573

Centers for Disease Control and Prevention: Guideline Resources: CDC Guideline for Prescribing Opioids for Chronic Pain. 2016. Available at: https://www.cdc.gov/drugoverdose/prescribing/resources.html. Accessed January 17, 2020.

Committee on Crossing the Quality Chasm: Improving the Quality of Health Care for Mental and Substance-Use Conditions. Washington, DC, National Academies Press, 2006

Crockford D, Fleury G, Milin R, et al: Training in substance-related and addictive disorders, part 2: updated curriculum guidelines. Can J Psychiatry 60(12):1–12, 2015 26720815

Devries J, Rafie S, Polston G: Implementing an overdose education and naloxone distribution program in a health system. J Am Pharm Assoc 57(2 suppl):S154–S160, 2017 28233681

Dingle AD, Boland R, Travis M: The PRITE examinations: background and future directions. Acad Psychiatry 42(4):498–502, 2018 29204756

Dowell D, Haegerich TM, Chou R: CDC guideline for prescribing opioids for chronic pain—United States, 2016. JAMA 315(15):1624–1645, 2016a 26977696

Dowell D, Haegerich TM, Chou R: Checklist for Prescribing Opioids for Chronic Pain. 2016b. Available at: https://stacks.cdc.gov/view/cdc/38025. Accessed January 17, 2020.

Dowell D, Haegerich T, Chou R: No shortcuts to safer opioid prescribing. N Engl J Med 380(24):2285–2287, 2019 31018066

Edens EL, Drew S, Heimer R, et al: Addiction Treatment: Clinical Skills for Healthcare Providers [MOOC]. Coursera, 2020a. Available at: https://www.coursera.org/learn/addiction-treatment. Accessed July 27, 2020.

Edens EL, Platt B, Moore B, et al: Transforming and Expanding Substance Use Disorder Education for Healthcare Programs, Yale Medical Education Day Poster Session, June 2020b. Available at: https://medicine.yale.edu/tlc/mededday/virtualposters/category/innovation/ (Note: Material is free but requires user registration and creation of a login). Accessed July 27, 2020.

el-Guebaly N, Toews J, Lockyer J, et al: Medical education in substance-related disorders: components and outcome. Addiction 95(6):949–957, 2000 10946443

Federation of State Medical Boards: Continuing Medical Education by State. November 20, 2019. Available at: https://www.fsmb.org/siteassets/advocacy/key-issues/continuing-medical-education-by-state.pdf. Accessed January 17, 2020.

Geller G, Levine DM, Mamon JA, et al: Knowledge, attitudes, and reported practices of medical students and house staff regarding the diagnosis and treatment of alcoholism. JAMA 261(21):3115–3120, 1989 2716143

Grimshaw JM, Thomas RE, MacLennan G, et al: Effectiveness and efficiency of guideline dissemination and implementation strategies. Health Technol Assess 8(6):iii–iv, 1–72, 2004 14960256

Health Resources and Services Administration: Addiction Medicine Fellowship Program. 2019. Available at: https://www.hrsa.gov/grants/find-funding/hrsa-20-013. Accessed July 28, 2020.

Health Resources and Services Administration: Addiction Medicine Fellowship FY 2020 Awards. 2020. Available at: https://bhw.hrsa.gov/grants/medicine/addiction/fellowship-awards-fy20. Accessed July 28, 2020.

Heisler EJ: The National Health Services Corps (7-5700, R44970). Washington, DC, Congressional Research Service, April 26, 2018. Available at: https://fas.org/sgp/crs/misc/R44970.pdf. Accessed July 28, 2020.

Hoffman J: Most Doctors Are Ill-Equipped to Deal With the Opioid Epidemic. Few Medical Schools Teach Addiction. September 10, 2018. Available at: https://www.nytimes.com/2018/09/10/health/addiction-medical-schools-treatment.html. Accessed January 17, 2020.

Holt SR, Segar N, Cavallo DA, et al: The addiction recovery clinic: a novel, primary-care-based approach to teaching addiction medicine. Acad Med 92(5):680–683, 2017 28441678

Howley L, Whelan A, Rasouli T: Addressing the Opioid Epidemic: U.S. Medical School Curricular Approaches. Analysis in Brief, 2018. Available at: https://www.aamc.org/system/files/reports/1/january2018addressingtheopioidepidemicu.s.medicalschoolcurricul.pdf. Accessed January 17, 2020.

H.R.6—SUPPORT for Patients and Communities Act of 2018, Pub. L. No. 115-271. Available at: https://www.congress.gov/bill/115th-congress/house-bill/6. Accessed January 17, 2020.

Iannucci R, Sanders K, Greenfield SF: A 4-year curriculum on substance use disorders for psychiatry residents. Acad Psychiatry 33(1):60–66, 2009 19349447

Isaacson JH, Fleming M, Kraus M, et al: A national survey of training in substance use disorders in residency programs. J Stud Alcohol 61(6):912–915, 2000 11188498

Jones CM, McCance-Katz EF: Characteristics and prescribing practices of clinicians recently waivered to prescribe buprenorphine for the treatment of opioid use disorder. Addiction 114(3):471–482, 2019 30194876

Komaromy M, Duhigg D, Metcalf A, et al: Project ECHO (Extension for Community Healthcare Outcomes): a new model for educating primary care providers about treatment of substance use disorders. Subst Abus 37(1):20–24, 2016 26848803

Lindberg M, Vergara C, Wild-Wesley R, et al: Physicians-in-training attitudes toward caring for and working with patients with alcohol and drug abuse diagnoses. South Med J 99(1):28–35, 2006 16466119

Lipari RN, Park-Lee E, Van Horn S: America's Need for and Receipt of Substance Use Treatment in 2015: National Survey on Drug Use and Health, The CBHSQ Report, September 29, 2016. Rockville, MD, Center for Behavioral Health Statistics and Quality, Substance Abuse and Mental Health Services Administration. Available at: https://www.samhsa.gov/data/sites/default/files/report_2716/ShortReport-2716.html. Accessed January 17, 2020.

Losby JL, Hyatt JD, Kanter MH, et al: Safer and more appropriate opioid prescribing: a large healthcare system's comprehensive approach. J Eval Clin Pract 23(6):1173–1179, 2017 28707421

Madden TE, Graham AV, Straussner SLA, et al: Interdisciplinary benefits in Project MAINSTREAM: a promising health professions educational model to address global substance abuse. J Interprof Care 20(6):655–664, 2006 17095443

Matthews S, Dwyer R, Snoek A: Stigma and self-stigma in addiction. J Bioeth Inq 14(2):275–286, 2017 28470503

McCance-Katz EF, George P, Scott NA, et al: Access to treatment for opioid use disorders: medical student preparation. Am J Addict 26(4):316–318, 2017 28394437

Miller NS, Sheppard LM, Colenda CC, et al: Why physicians are unprepared to treat patients who have alcohol- and drug-related disorders. Acad Med 76(5):410–418, 2001 11346513

Morris NP, Bentzley BS: Requiring buprenorphine waivers for psychiatry residents. Acad Psychiatry 43(1):131–134, 2019 30414072

Moss B: Governor Baker Signs Second Major Piece of Legislation to Address Opioid Epidemic in Massachusetts. Mass.gov, August 14, 2018. Available at: https://www.mass.gov/news/governor-baker-signs-second-major-piece-of-legislation-to-address-opioid-epidemic-in. Accessed January 17, 2020.

Muvvala SB, Edens EL, Petrakis IL: What role should psychiatrists have in responding to the opioid epidemic? JAMA Psychiatry 76(2):107–108, 2019 30484813

Muzyk AJ, Tew C, Thomas-Fannin A, et al: An interprofessional course on substance use disorders for health professions students. Acad Med 92(12):1704–1708, 2017 28537951

Nunes EV, Kunz K, Galanter M, O'Connor PG: Addiction psychiatry and addiction medicine: the evolution of addiction physician specialists. Am J Addict 29(5):390–400, 2020 32902056

O'Connor PG, Sokol RJ, D'Onofrio G: Addiction medicine: the birth of a new discipline. JAMA Intern Med 174(11):1717–1718, 2014 25201642

Osborn SR, Yu J, Williams B, et al: Changes in provider prescribing patterns after implementation of an emergency department prescription opioid policy. J Emerg Med 52(4):538–546, 2017 28111065

Parish SJ, Ramaswamy M, Stein MR, et al: Teaching about substance abuse with objective structured clinical exams. J Gen Intern Med 21(5):453–459, 2006 16704387

Parish SJ, Stein MR, Hahn SR, et al: Teaching and assessing residents' skills in managing heroin addiction with Objective Structured Clinical Exams (OSCEs). Subst Abuse 34(4):350–355, 2013 24159905

Patil D, Andry T: Molding young minds: the importance of residency training in shaping residents' attitudes toward substance use disorders. Am J Addict 26(1):80–82, 2017 28000984

Pating DR, Miller MM, Goplerud E, et al: New systems of care for substance use disorders: treatment, finance, and technology under health care reform. Psychiatr Clin North Am 35(2):327–356, 2012 22640759

Polydorou S, Gunderson EW, Levin FR: Training physicians to treat substance use disorders. Curr Psychiatry Rep 10(5):399–404, 2008 18803913

Rasyidi E, Wilkins JN, Danovitch I: Training the next generation of providers in addiction medicine. Psychiatr Clin North Am 35(2):461–480, 2012 22640766

Renner JA Jr: How to train residents to identify and treat dual diagnosis patients. Biol Psychiatry 56(10):810–816, 2004 15556127

Rose S: Medical student education in the time of COVID-19. JAMA 323(21):2131–2132, 2020 32232420

Rosenblatt RA, Andrilla CH, Catlin M, et al: Geographic and specialty distribution of U.S. physicians trained to treat opioid use disorder. Ann Fam Med 13(1):23–26, 2015 25583888

Saitz R, Horton NJ, Sullivan LM, et al: Addressing alcohol problems in primary care: a cluster randomized, controlled trial of a systems intervention. The screening and intervention in primary care (SIP) study. Ann Intern Med 138(5):372–382, 2003 12614089

Salvador J, Bhatt S, Fowler R, et al: Engagement with project ECHO to increase medication-assisted treatment in rural primary care. Psychiatr Serv 70(12):1157–1160, 2019 31434561

Sanchez-Ramirez JP, Gakhal R, Oakman SA: Addiction psychiatry in PGY-3: use of the intensive outpatient treatment setting to train senior residents. Acad Psychiatry 40(3):517–519, 2016 26108398

Schwartz AC, Frank A, Welsh JW, et al: Addictions training in general psychiatry training programs: current gaps and barriers. Acad Psychiatry 42(5):642–647, 2018 30073538

Shorter D, Dermatis H: Addiction training in general psychiatry residency: a national survey. Subst Abus 33(4):392–394, 2012 22989284

Sokol RJ, Kunz K: Training Future Physicians to Address Opioid Crisis. September 19, 2017; updated May 5, 2018. Available at: https://www.aamc.org/news-insights/training-future-physicians-address-opioid-crisis. Accessed August 11, 2020.

Suzuki J, Ellison TV, Connery HS, et al: Training in buprenorphine and office-based opioid treatment: a survey of psychiatry residency training programs. Acad Psychiatry 40(3):498–502, 2016 26017618

Tesema L, Marshall J, Hathaway R, et al: Training in office-based opioid treatment with buprenorphine in U.S. residency programs: a national survey of residency program directors. Subst Abus 39(4):434–440, 2018 29513136

Tetrault JM, Petrakis IL: Partnering with psychiatry to close the education gap: an approach to the addiction epidemic. J Gen Intern Med 32(12):1387–1389, 2017 28766126

University of New Mexico School of Medicine: Project ECHO®: Our Story. 2020. Available at: https://echo.unm.edu/about-echo/ourstory. Accessed July 27, 2020.

Unrod M, Smith M, Spring B, et al: Randomized controlled trial of a computer-based, tailored intervention to increase smoking cessation counseling by primary care physicians. J Gen Intern Med 22(4):478–484, 2007 17372796

U.S. Department of Health and Human Services, Office of the Surgeon General: Facing Addiction in America: The Surgeon General's Report on Alcohol, Drugs, and Health. 2016. Available at: https://store.samhsa.gov/system/files/surgeon-generals-report.pdf. Accessed January 17, 2020.

van Boekel LC, Brouwers EP, van Weeghel J, et al: Stigma among health professionals towards patients with substance use disorders and its consequences for healthcare delivery: systematic review. Drug Alcohol Depend 131(1–2):23–35, 2013 23490450

Volkow N: Can the science of addiction help reduce stigma? Advances in Addiction and Recovery 25(3):16–20, 2015. Available at: https://www.naadac.org/AAR-archive/#Fall2014. Accessed February 19, 2020.

Wakeman SE, Rich JD: Barriers to medications for addiction treatment: how stigma kills. Subst Use Misuse 53(2):330–333, 2018 28961017

Welsh JW, Schwartz AC, DeJong SM: Addictions training in child and adolescent psychiatry fellowships. Acad Psychiatry 43(1):13–17, 2019 30066242

The White House, Office of the Press Secretary: Fact Sheet: Obama Administration Announces Additional Actions to Address the Prescription Opioid Epidemic. March 29, 2016. Available at: https://obamawhitehouse.archives.gov/the-press-office/2016/03/29/fact-sheet-obama-administration-announces-additional-actions-address. Accessed July 20, 2020.

Wickramatilake S, Zur J, Mulvaney-Day N, et al: How states are tackling the opioid crisis. Public Health Rep 132(2):171–179, 2017 28152337

Williams JM, Poulsen R, Chaguturu V, et al: Evaluation of an online residency training in tobacco use disorder. Am J Addict 28(4):277–284, 2019 30993797

Wood E, Samet JH, Volkow ND: Physician education in addiction medicine. JAMA 310(16):1673–1674, 2013 24150462

Woolf SH, Grol R, Hutchinson A, et al: Clinical guidelines: potential benefits, limitations, and harms of clinical guidelines. BMJ 318(7182):527–530, 1999 10024268

CHAPTER 53

Addiction in the Workplace

Laurence M. Westreich, M.D.

Alcohol and drugs exert powerful effects in the workplace, whether that workplace is a factory, an office, an athletic field, or the cockpit of a passenger airliner. This chapter is designed for clinicians who treat people with substance use disorders, as well as for clinicians who design workplace testing programs, employee assistance programs, and occupational drug and alcohol policies. Understanding the legal and practical aspects of addiction in the occupational sphere is mandatory for any clinician who treats patients who have been fired from a job, are looking for a job, or aspire to have a job in the future.

One marker of workplace drug use—and of the attitudes of the employees using those drugs—is the rate of drug-positive results in workplace drug testing. An analysis of more than 10 million employment drug tests from 2017 by a major laboratory for workplace drug testing showed that although the nationwide rate of opioid-positive results (0.39%) was lower than the rate in 2016 (0.47%), rates of drug-positive results had increased for cocaine (from 0.28% to 0.30%) and for methamphetamine (oral fluid) (from 0.42% to 0.43%) (Quest Diagnostics 2019). Nationwide, the rates of marijuana-positive results increased from 2.5% to 2.6%, with the most obvious increases seen in states where new legalization statutes were in place, such as Nevada, Massachusetts, and California. From 2013 to 2017, employee drug testing, as measured by Quest Diagnostics, revealed increases in drug-positive tests for marijuana and cocaine, and decreases in drug-positive tests for opioids (Figure 53–1).

In addition to the human suffering demonstrated by these results, businesses suffer from their employees' use of addictive substances. One study estimated that nonmedical use of prescription opioids alone was associated with an annual economic cost of $53.4 billion, of which 79% ($42 billion) was attributable to lost productivity (Hansen et al. 2011). Misuse of OxyContin, oxycodone, hydrocodone, propoxyphene, and methadone accounted for two-thirds of the total cost.

The decriminalization of cannabis in many states and the ongoing opioid epidemic have roiled the seas of workplace regulations, customs, and case law. Because of this

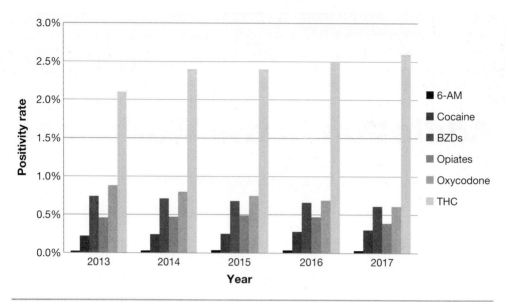

FIGURE 53–1.   Percentage of positive urine tests, by drug category,[a] U.S. workforce, 2013–2017.

6-AM=6-acetylmorphine metabolite of heroin; BZDs=benzodiazepines; THC=tetrahydrocannabinol (marijuana).
[a]Positivity rates by drug category as a percentage of all such tests in 2017 (N=6.2 million).
Source.   Data from Quest Diagnostics 2019.

rapidly changing environment, as well as the complexities of disability law, any person with questions about substance use in the workplace should seek advice from an attorney knowledgeable about the particular jurisdiction in which the question arises. Although psychiatrists should deliver state-of-the-art treatment and have productive interactions with employers and employees, legal advice must be left to those attorneys who are competent to dispense such information.

Workplace programs related to drugs and alcohol have a coercive aspect to them (Nace et al. 2007), even in businesses that maintain an impermeable firewall between treatment providers and the employer. The employer's obligations to maintain safety, focus on production, and avoid legal liability can promote at least the perception, on the part of employees, that these programs will be compulsory and lacking in confidentiality protections. However, coercion is an effective and sometimes necessary part of most entrances to treatment, and an employer's testing, workplace rules, and provision of treatment can help many employees enter into long-term sobriety or reduction of use, which benefits employer and employee alike, both on and off the job.

Role of the Workplace Psychiatrist

In addition to rendering treatment, workplace psychiatrists can design programs for random drug testing, educate employees about addiction, and monitor employees who have been found to have a problem with substances. However, the roles of "clinician" and "monitor" necessarily clash, in that any person with a drug or alcohol problem will naturally feel reluctant to discuss substance use if that information might eventually be disclosed to a work supervisor. Some businesses separate entirely the role of the clinician from any reporting duties for exactly that reason. Whatever the protocol, however, the psychiatrist must model absolute transparency about confidentiality requirements, even if an employee has signed off on a release of information to his or her employer.

The clinician should also exemplify a respectful, beneficent attitude toward the employee who misuses substances or has an addiction problem. Even though the language used to discuss addiction remains in flux, some uses of language definitively demonstrate a respectful attitude toward the addicted person and his or her struggles (Broyles et al. 2014). For instance, using "person-first" language by avoiding labeling human beings as addicts or alcoholics, and by eschewing pejorative terms such as "dirty" urine and "abuser," can go a long way toward identifying the substance use disorders as medical problems rather than a weakness or an immoral act. Using the clinical terminology contained in the *Diagnostic and Statistical Manual of Mental Disorders,* 5th Edition (DSM-5; American Psychiatric Association 2013), also promotes a respectful and compassionate attitude toward people with addiction problems.

Legal Structures for Addressing Addiction in the Workplace

Federal and state laws attempt to protect employees and others from the effects of addiction in the workplace, while also respecting the civil rights of those employees and avoiding discrimination or unreasonable intrusions on their privacy. These efforts are, of necessity, reactive to current societal conditions, and the evolution of these statutes and laws reflects those conditions and (arguably) an increasingly sophisticated response to addiction.

The Drug-Free Workplace Act of 1988 (P.L. 111-350), which was put into place by President Ronald Reagan, required federal contractors and those who received federal grants to provide a drug-free workplace. Although it applied only to those two groups, the act provided a procedural structure for other programs in both public and private sectors. Among the requirements laid out in the act were creation of a policy statement about the consequences for distribution or possession of drugs in the workplace, establishment of an awareness program about drug use, notification of the employee about the potential for job termination for criminal drug violation in the workplace, and mandatory participation in addiction treatment if needed. Although the act was focused on getting drugs out of the U.S. workplace, it did make a good-faith, if minimal, effort to acknowledge the rights and needs of the employee who is found to have violated the act.

By contrast, the Americans With Disabilities Act, as amended in 2009 (ADA; P.L. 110-325), is entirely designed to protect the rights of disabled persons, including those with drug or alcohol problems. Importantly, the ADA required that disabled persons be given "reasonable accommodations" to be able to participate in the workplace; these accommodations were especially meaningful for persons with addictions, who might need them to avoid venues in which they would be prone to relapse, to relinquish safety-sensitive tasks when necessary, or to take daily time off to attend a methadone program. Although the ADA has certainly improved national awareness of the rights and needs of people with disabilities, much work remains to be done, because people with disabilities still face substantial discrimination and prejudice in the workplace (Peacock et al. 2015).

Unfortunately, that discrimination occurs in regard to addiction more so than other impairments, as demonstrated by the fact that the ADA protections granted to people with addictions have been slowly weakened by case law over the years (Westreich 2002). One case that demonstrates a typical successful discrimination case under the ADA is *EEOC (Equal Employment Opportunity Commission) v. Randstad* (2015). A methadone-maintained woman, April Cox, applied for a laborer position with a Maryland staffing agency, Randstad, Inc. She appeared to have all of the necessary qualifications for the position and was moving forward with the hiring process when she was asked to provide a urine sample for a preemployment drug test. At that point, Cox disclosed her participation in a medically supervised methadone program, and the hiring manager replied, "I'm sure we don't hire people on methadone, but I will contact my supervisor." Following that conversation, Cox never heard back from Randstad, despite multiple attempts to contact them, and was eventually told that she could not be hired because of her methadone use. There was not even an allegation of inability to fulfill the job requirement, only the employer's demonstrably unfair bias. The EEOC sued Randstad on her behalf and won a settlement in which Randstad signed a consent decree and paid Cox $50,000 in damages. Although Randstad was within its rights to require the drug test, the court ruled that Randstad's rejection of Cox's job application was illegal because Randstad acted *merely based on Cox's participation in a legitimate treatment program.*

Confidentiality and Its Limits in the Workplace

Although confidentiality is important in addiction treatment, even more so than in general medical or psychiatric treatment, some specific limits to confidentiality exist in the occupational sphere. Generic exceptions to confidentiality with any licensed mental health clinician of course survive in the workplace; in states that use the *Tarasoff* standard (*Tarasoff v. Regents of the University of California* 1976), the clinician must protect the threatened victim of a patient, and in all jurisdictions, harm or threatened harm to a child requires immediate action by the clinician. However, in less starkly obvious situations, workplace addiction programs are complicated by the clinician's conflicting obligations to the patient/employee, the patient/employee's colleagues, and the company's management.

Safety-Sensitive Job Positions

Workplace addiction programs can reasonably differentiate between job positions that are so excruciatingly safety sensitive that no chances can be taken (pilots) and job positions in which physical safety is barely an issue at all (office clerk). The middle ground between these two extremes is occupied by most employees, whose minute-to-minute decisions do not immediately endanger others, but who could conceivably harm another if they are impaired on the job. The Connecticut Department of Labor, for instance, lists about 500 "high-risk or safety-sensitive occupations" (Connecticut

Department of Labor 2010), including the obvious "driller/explosives handler," but also "sprinkler apprentice" and "warehouse/shipping clerk."

An instructive case involving state employees demonstrates how the courts have often viewed the question of safety-sensitive versus non-safety-sensitive positions, at least for the imposition of random drug tests, based on the Fourth Amendment's prohibition against unreasonable search and seizure. In *American Federation of State, County and Municipal Employees (AFSCME) Council 79 v. Scott* (2013), Florida Governor Rick Scott was sued by the American Civil Liberties Union on behalf of a large union, the AFSCME. Scott's executive order required all state employees to have a suspicionless drug test as a condition of their employment. The Eleventh Circuit Court of Appeals had extended a previous case's "special needs" analysis to include pilots, police officers, firefighters, and corrections officers who interact with parolees or inmates. However, the Appeals Court found the Scott order to be overbroad because it would require testing of many state employees who were not members of the "special needs" class. Furthermore, the Supreme Court declined to hear the case in April 2014, leaving the state to put together a very specific list of "special needs" employees for whom preemployment drug tests and suspicionless on-the-job tests could be reasonably requested. It is important to note that state employees in this group are distinct from the employees of private companies, who are often given much less leeway in avoiding suspicionless drug tests.

U.S. Department of Transportation

The U.S. Department of Transportation (DOT) has developed a robust set of regulations for monitoring transportation workers for drug use. These regulations are often seen as a gold standard for other industries in maintaining an effective and fair system for detecting impairment from drug use and getting the employee to treatment. Because the DOT oversees commercial motor carriers (truck drivers), the Federal Aviation Administration, the Federal Railroad Administration, the Federal Transit Administration, the Pipeline and Hazardous Materials Safety Administration, and the U.S. Coast Guard, the DOT's rules cover drug testing and the response to that testing for about 8 million employees (Swotinsky 2015).

The DOT now requires alcohol tests in addition to drug tests and uses split-sample collections to allow for a retest if the employee denies having used the substance. Certified substance abuse professionals make addiction assessments and determine when and whether a return to work is appropriate. The most recent iteration of the DOT's source document (U.S. Department of Transportation 2020) describes the sophisticated procedures that would be expected for an agency that deals with thousands of positive tests, numerous disputes about its procedures, and public sentiment that demands safety on the nation's roads.

Elite Sports

The workplace of professional and elite amateur sports contains several distinct characteristics that affect those involved and are often of significant interest to those outside of the sport. The enormous attention paid to athletes and the projection of societal values upon them make the athletes (rightly or wrongly) supposed exemplars of values that eschew the use of drugs, both addictive and performance enhancing. The outsized influence of actual and potential earnings focuses attention on athletes' performance in a way that few other employees can imagine and can lead to use of performance-enhancing drugs, often contrary to the athlete's own values.

In the investigation of a notorious doping scandal related to the State-sponsored doping and evasion of drug testing by Russian athletes, it became clear that there were "high levels of collusion among athletes, coaches, doctors, regulatory officers, and sports agencies to systematically provide Russian athletes performance enhancing drugs" (World Anti-Doping Agency 2015). Although the athletes involved were putatively amateurs and stood to gain little financially from their performance (juiced or otherwise), they nevertheless went along with the doping scheme, which undermined the values of their sports and likely put them at risk of morbidity from substances they ingested. Given the notorious damage done to Russian athletes of a previous generation, the athletes' acquiescence suggests that the pressures put upon them were quite powerful.

A common workplace issue in elite sports organizations is the necessity of allowing certain athletes to take medications that are otherwise banned when these athletes have legitimate reasons for taking the medications. This issue most commonly relates to stimulant medications for the treatment of attention-deficit/hyperactivity disorder, but it can also occur with testosterone, diuretic medications, β-agonists, and antiestrogens. Although policies across professional sports, the Olympics, and amateur athletics differ somewhat as to the particular banned substances and the procedures for obtaining an exemption, all attempt to strike a fair balance between maintaining a level playing field for all the athletes and allowing appropriately diagnosed athletes to use the medications for which they have a documented medical need.

The National Collegiate Athletic Association (NCAA), for instance, has a "medical exception" policy that "allows exception to be made for those student-athletes with a documented medical history demonstrating the need for treatment with a banned medication" (National Collegiate Athletic Association 2020). Some medications that are banned, but for which student-athletes may obtain exceptions, include stimulants, β-blockers, β-agonists, anabolic agents, and anti-estrogens. Interestingly, the PowerPoint Slide Deck distributed to NCAA student-athletes makes the point that "because [marijuana] is an 'illicit drug' there is no 'medical exception' waver available" (NCAA 2018, slide 21).

Behavioral Addictions in the Workplace

Compulsive behaviors, including addictive relationships with food, sex, gambling, and shopping, occur in the workplace and can certainly lead to negative consequences for the sufferers. In light of the heightened sensitivity to sexual harassment in all its forms, individuals who demonstrate sexually compulsive behaviors risk criminal charges, job termination, and personal embarrassment for their behavior, notwithstanding the fact that the offensive behavior may have an underlying compulsive component and therefore be less volitional than it might appear.

A particularly insidious behavioral addiction is loosely called "Internet addiction" but is also referred to in the literature as Internet addiction disorder, pathological Internet use, compulsive computer use, and virtual addiction. DSM-5 includes Internet gaming disorder in the section titled "Conditions for Further Study" (American Psychiatric Association 2013). Because consistent Internet use is a hallmark of most modern jobs, Internet addiction can be a bit hard to differentiate from the assiduousness one would hope to have in an employee. One clinician (Young 2004) has suggested the following markers as being helpful in distinguishing pathological from non-pathological use of the Internet:

- Feeling preoccupied with Internet use
- Being unable to control Internet use
- Feeling restless, moody, depressed, or irritable when not online
- Jeopardizing a relationship, a job, or an educational or career opportunity because of the Internet
- Lying to others to conceal the extent of involvement with the Internet
- Using the Internet as a way of escaping problems or of relieving a dysphoric mood

Opioids in the Workplace

The ongoing opioid epidemic has of course reached into the workplace. Many families and offices have been touched by opioid dependence, overdose, or death. An expanding national consensus on the seriousness of opioid addiction has led to a decrease in needlessly prescribed prescription opioids, but opioid-related overdoses have continued apace, with many of them related to fentanyl-laced heroin.

One survey of 501 human resources specialists (National Safety Council 2017) found that 80% of these specialists considered abuse or misuse of prescription opioids to be a sign of addiction, and 71% thought that this misuse or abuse should be treated like any other chronic medical condition. Regarding their own companies, 39% felt that prescription drug misuse and abuse was endangering their workforce, and 36% felt that these phenomena were lowering productivity.

Although standard workplace substance use disorder interventions should be used, some more directed strategies for opioid problems are necessary, simply because of the lethality of opioid addiction. The easy availability of naloxone kits, in a form deployable by nonclinicians, is vital as a public health measure. Just as automatic electronic defibrillators are now ubiquitous in most workplaces and public gathering places, naloxone should be available. In addition, education about some easily recognizable signs of opioid use (e.g., lethargy, pinpoint pupils, absenteeism) should be delivered to supervisors and coworkers, who might then be able to save the life of an employee with a caring intervention long before naloxone resuscitation is needed.

Cannabis in the Workplace

Because 33 states and the District of Columbia have broadly legalized marijuana in some form, and recreational use is permitted in 11 states and the District of Columbia

(Governing.com 2019), U.S. employers and employees face myriad legal, business, and practical challenges. Most important are the numerous tricky ethical and public policy questions that face our nation, especially the dialectic between the public policy good and the individual harm many see associated with marijuana decriminalization and legalization, and the constraints on civil liberties implied in the prohibition of a widely used substance. These are important issues for all to address, but for the practical purposes of employees and employers, one must focus on the rapidly changing cannabis-related federal and state laws, case law, and administrative protocols for employers and employees.

Employees question whether medical marijuana recommended by a licensed physician will be exempted from the usual drug testing protocols. Employers must manage a rapidly changing set of legal obligations concerning safety-sensitive positions, potential ADA lawsuits, confidentiality, and the notoriously long-lasting tetrahydrocannabinol (THC) molecule in drug tests. Relatively sparse data exist on workplace accidents or lost productivity associated with cannabis, the effects of instituting drug testing programs for cannabis, and the cost/benefit ratios of these testing and treatment programs. Most importantly, businesses must grapple with the briskly changing case law and cultural ethos regarding cannabis, as well as the present discordance between federal law and states' laws regarding medicinal and recreational cannabis use. Only data-based and collaborative discussions about the issue will promote the most effective and legally defensible policies regarding cannabis in the workplace.

Cannabis use varies across age groups, geographic locations, and socioeconomic levels, as well as across occupations. A survey in Colorado, sponsored by the Centers for Disease Control and Prevention and published by the Colorado Department of Public Health and Environment (Smith et al. 2018), revealed that in 2014–2015, individuals working in the accommodation and food services industry and the arts and entertainment industry were on the high end of acknowledged marijuana users, whereas those working in the education, public administration, and mining industries were on the low end (Figure 53–2).

Whether cannabis use in the workplace causes workplace accidents is an open question. One recent review found "insufficient evidence to support or refute a statistical association between general, non-medical cannabis use and occupational accidents or injuries" (National Academies of Sciences-Engineering-Medicine 2017, p. 227).

A study of 3,365 high school students with part-time jobs (Shipp et al. 2005) found that students who acknowledged marijuana use in the previous 30 days had a significantly increased risk of nonfatal occupational injury compared with students who had not used marijuana in the previous 30 days, even after variables such as year in high school, gender, and ethnicity were controlled. Compared with their nonusing peers, students who smoked heavily—defined as smoking marijuana more than 40 times in the previous 30 days—were more than twice as likely to sustain a nonfatal occupational injury.

A larger epidemiological study (Dong et al. 2015) using data on 12,686 participants in the 1988–2000 National Longitudinal Survey of Youth studied construction workers between ages 14 and 22 years and divided them into three groups: those who had never used marijuana, those who had used marijuana between 1 and 10 times over their lifetime, and a final group who had used marijuana 11 or more times in their life.

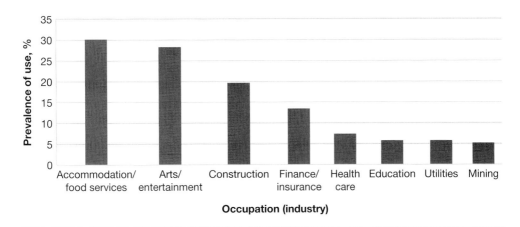

FIGURE 53–2.   Prevalence of current[a] marijuana use among employed adults,[b] by occupation: Behavioral Risk Factor Surveillance System, Colorado, 2014 and 2015.

[a]Current use was defined as use on at least 1 day during the preceding 30 days.

[b]Adults ages 18 years and older (N=10,169) who responded to the "current marijuana use" question.

Source.   Data from Smith et al. 2018.

In comparison with the never-used-marijuana group, neither of the marijuana-using groups showed higher rates of occupational injury or illness.

Although state laws regarding the medical and recreational use of cannabis vary widely, only 19 states (Arizona, Arkansas, Connecticut, Delaware, Illinois, Maine, Maryland, Massachusetts, Minnesota, Montana, Nevada, New Jersey, New Mexico, New York, Oklahoma, Pennsylvania, Rhode Island, Vermont, and West Virginia) explicitly protect employees with medical exemptions for their marijuana use (California NORML 2020). However, most states have no clear protections for individuals who test positive for THC in a preemployment test or on the job, even if that state has decriminalized or legalized medical and/or recreational use of marijuana. This lack of protection for their employment, even if marijuana is "legal" in their state, is an important and often-missed point for many employees.

No employer is expected to accept an intoxicated employee in the workplace, or one who uses drugs on the worksite. However, in the new atmosphere of increasing legal and cultural permissiveness about cannabis use, state courts have delineated a general understanding that private employers may still terminate or decline to hire individuals who use cannabis for medical or recreational purposes. Public employers, however, are held more tightly to the expectation that only employees with safety-sensitive positions may be held to account for their off-hours use of cannabis. Courts have varied widely in their findings about the details of suspicionless drug testing, certificates for medical marijuana use, and the definition of "safety sensitive."

In *Ross v. RagingWire Telecommunications, Inc.* (2008), the California Supreme Court held that employers are not required to accommodate an employee's medicinal marijuana use, irrespective of the Compassionate Use Act of 1996 (Health and Safety Code Section 11362.5), which provides that persons using marijuana under the care of a physician are not subject to criminal prosecution by the state. The court commented that the Compassionate Use Act does not grant marijuana the same status as legal prescription drugs and noted that marijuana remains illegal under federal law, and therefore cannot be "completely legalize[d] for medical purposes."

Drug and Alcohol Testing in the Workplace

For a more detailed review of clinical drug testing, see Chapter 50, "Testing for Substances of Abuse," and for a description of practicing forensic psychiatry in the addiction sphere, see Chapter 51, "Forensic Addiction Psychiatry."

Forensic tests, the focus of this section, are expressly designed to withstand scrutiny in court or in a hearing chamber. These legally defensible workplace testing programs, which result from a collaboration of medical, scientific, and legal professionals, have a clearly defined goal or set of goals. Preventing workplace accidents, assisting employees with addiction problems, satisfying federally mandated guidelines, and generating good publicity are all reasonable goals, but they must be intentionally set forth before the testing plan is put together.

Drug testing used in a legal or employment setting must be of forensic quality, with a clear chain of custody between the testee, collector, laboratory, and reporter. That is, everyone involved with the testing must be prepared to defend under cross-examination the provenance of the sample being tested, the security of its transportation and storage, and the scientific bases of the testing methods used. Consultation with a toxicologist and a labor attorney knowledgeable about drug testing and health care law is mandatory before putting a testing program into place; consideration of likely future challenges to the program by employees and their attorneys can avoid needless consternation.

In addition, there must be a clear protocol in place for choosing when to test, whom to test, and what body tissue to test. Any discrimination against a person or class of people discredits the entire process and calls into question the validity of a test result. For instance, preemployment testing, which is not considered medical testing and is therefore allowable under the ADA, should be applied fairly and with a clear protocol for which potential employees are tested.

Effects of Workplace Addiction Prevention and Treatment Programs

Research on the efficacy and cost-effectiveness of workplace addiction monitoring programs shows that these programs are generally very useful, as well as financially beneficial. Walton and Hall (2016) reviewed 12 different studies evaluating workplace addiction treatment programs, involving a total of more than 3,000 participants in both conventional employment and supported employment. They found that 11 of the 12 studies documented a positive relationship between workplace interventions and substance abuse treatment outcomes as measured by substance use, employment, and housing status (in those studies in which housing was recorded). In explaining this outcome, the authors hypothesized a bidirectional effect in which addiction treatment and employment enhance each other:

Individuals who are in recovery and are employed are provided with an alternative set of reinforcers that support both their livelihood and their recovery. Such reinforcement might be especially important in early recovery, when individuals could still experience strong craving, estrangement from family, social isolation, and other risks for relapse. These findings suggest interesting opportunities for collaboration between substance abuse professionals and those within the career counseling field. (Walton and Hall 2016, p. 377)

Conclusion

Employment-related responses to addiction represent opportunities for promoting needed treatment of employees while protecting the legitimate interests of employers; a healthy, sober workforce is to the advantage of both. One paradigm, promoted by New Hampshire Governor Chris Sununu (Recovery Friendly Workplace 2019) in response to the opioid epidemic and his state's difficulty in filling needed jobs, focused on making the workplace "Recovery Friendly," in the sense that having employees in recovery was seen as a strength that could support business goals. Rather than merely tolerating the person in recovery from addiction, the Recovery Friendly Workplace paradigm encouraged support and retention of employees in recovery, with the stated goal of collaborating to "create positive change and eliminate barriers for those impacted by addiction."

These sorts of active, intentionally constructed programs respect both the recovery needs of the employed individual suffering from addiction and the business needs of the employer. Beneficent coercion by an employer can work wonders in constructing a workplace that effectively manages both employee addiction problems and the necessities of production and effectiveness in a competitive economic environment.

References

American Federation of State, County, and Municipal Employees (AFSCME) Council 79 v. Scott, 717 F3d 851, 2013

American Psychiatric Association: Diagnostic and Statistical Manual of Mental Disorders, 5th Edition. Arlington, VA, American Psychiatric Association, 2013

Broyles LM, Binswanger IA, Jenkins JA, et al: Confronting inadvertent stigma and pejorative language in addiction scholarship: a recognition and response. Subst Abus 35(3):217–221, 2014 24911031

California NORML: State Laws Protecting Marijuana Users' Employment Rights. 2020. Available at: https://www.canorml.org/employment/state-laws-protecting-medical-marijuana-patients-employment-rights. Accessed July 12, 2020.

Connecticut Department of Labor: List of Occupations Designated as High-Risk or Safety-Sensitive by the Labor Commissioner of the State of Connecticut. March 2010. Available at: https://www.ctdol.state.ct.us/wgwkstnd/laws-regs/HRSSOccupationsList.pdf. Accessed January 17, 2020.

Dong XS, Wang X, Largay JA: Occupational and non-occupational factors associated with work-related injuries among construction workers in the USA. Int J Occup Environ Health 21(2):142–150, 2015 25816923

Drug-Free Workplace Act of 1988, Pub. L. No. 111-350, 41 U.S. Code § 8102

EEOC v. Randstad, US, LP, Civil Action No. RDB-15-3354 (2015)

Governing.com: State Marijuana Laws in 2019 Map. 2019. Available at: https://www.governing .com/gov-data/safety-justice/state-marijuana-laws-map-medical-recreational.html. Accessed July 13, 2020.

Hansen RN, Oster G, Edelsberg J, et al: Economic costs of nonmedical use of prescription opioids. Clin J Pain 27(3):194–202, 2011 21178601

Nace EP, Birkmayer F, Sullivan MA, et al: Socially sanctioned coercion mechanisms for addiction treatment. Am J Addict 16(1):15–23, 2007 17364417

National Academies of Sciences-Engineering-Medicine: The Health Effects of Cannabis and Cannabinoids: The Current State of Evidence and Recommendations for Research. Washington, DC, National Academies Press, 2017

National Collegiate Athletic Association: What Student-Athletes Need to Know About Marijuana. Modified October 2018. Available at: http://www.ncaa.org/sport-science-institute/ topics/what-student-athletes-need-know-about-marijuana. Accessed July 13, 2020.

National Collegiate Athletic Association: Medical Exceptions Procedures. Sport Science Institute. Updated June 23, 2020. Available at: http://www.ncaa.org/sport-science-institute/ medical-exceptions-procedures. Accessed July 13, 2020.

National Safety Council: Prescription Drugs and the U.S. Workforce: A Presentation for the National Safety Council by B2B International. January 2017. Available at: https://www.nsc.org/ portals/0/documents/newsdocuments/2017/national-employer-addiction-survey-methodology.pdf. Accessed January 17, 2020.

Peacock G, Iezzoni LI, Harkin TR: Health care for Americans with disabilities—25 years after the ADA. N Engl J Med 373(10):892–893, 2015 26225616

Quest Diagnostics: Workforce Drug Testing Positivity Climbs to Highest Rate Since 2004, According to New Quest Diagnostics Analysis. Secaucus, NJ, Quest Diagnostics, April 11, 2019. Available at: http://www.questdiagnostics.com/home/physicians/health-trends/ drug-testing/. Accessed May 6, 2020.

Recovery Friendly Workplace: Recovery Friendly Workplaces. 2019. Available at: https:// www.recoveryfriendlyworkplace.com/initiative. Accessed January 17, 2020.

Ross v. RagingWire Telecommunications, Inc, Defendant and Respondent, Supreme Court of California No. S138130 (2008)

Shipp EM, Tortolero SR, Cooper SP, et al: Substance use and occupational injuries among high school students in South Texas. Am J Drug Alcohol Abuse 31(2):253–265, 2005 15912715

Smith R, Hall KE, Etkind P, et al: Current marijuana use by industry and occupation—Colorado, 2014–2015. MMWR Morb Mortal Wkly Rep 67(14):409–413, 2018 29649186

Swotinsky R: The Medical Review Officer's Manual. Beverley Farms, MA, OEM Press, 2015

Tarasoff v. Regents of the University of California, 17 Cal. 3d 425, 131 Cal. Rptr. 14, 551 P.2d 334 (1976)

U.S. Department of Transportation: Title 49: Transportation, Part 40—Procedures for Transportation Workplace Drug and Alcohol Testing Programs. 2020. Available at: https:// www.ecfr.gov/cgi-bin/text-idx?SID=44edbc0e557a4cc5ff03365810ee5b1c&mc= true&node=pt49.1.40&rgn=div5. Accessed January 17, 2020.

Walton MT, Hall MT: The effects of employment interventions on addiction treatment outcomes: a review of the literature. Journal of Social Work Practice in the Addictions 16(4):358–384, 2016. Available at: https://www.tandfonline.com/doi/abs/10.1080/ 1533256X.2016.1235429?journalCode=wswp20. Accessed February 19, 2020.

Westreich LM: Addiction and the Americans With Disabilities Act. J Am Acad Psychiatry Law 30(3):355–363, 2002 12380414

World Anti-Doping Agency: Independent Commission Investigation No 1: Final Report. November 9, 2015. Available at: https://www.wada-ama.org/sites/default/files/resources/ files/wada_independent_commission_report_1_en.pdf. Accessed January 17, 2020.

Young KS: Internet addiction: a new clinical phenomenon and its consequences. American Behavioral Scientist 48(4):402–415, 2004. Available at: https://journals.sagepub.com/doi/ 10.1177/0002764204270278. Accessed July 17, 2020.

Index

Page numbers printed in **boldface** *type refer to tables and figures.*

Buprenorphine *(continued)*
 treatment costs, **98**
 waiver program, **98,** 101, 106, 108, 812,
  825, 829
Bupropion
 adverse effects, 287
 contraindications, 725
 gender differences, 549
 pharmacology of, 286, 287
 treatment applications
  for ADHD, 740
  for behavioral addictive disorders, 660
  for cannabis use disorder, 255
  for eating disorders, 724–725
  for stimulant-related disorders, 167, 168
  for tobacco-related disorders, 284–285,
   286–287, 288, 516, 552, 570, 640,
   765
Buspirone, 256, 550, 706
Butabarbital, 787
Butalbital, 301, **777**

CAGE Adapted to Include Drugs (CAGE-
 AID), 83
CAGE questionnaire, 79, 81–83, 133, 569,
 632–633
California Society of Addiction Medicine
 (CSAM), **819**
CAM (complementary and alternative
 medicine) treatments, 284, 454–456.
 See also Mindfulness practices
CAMP response element–binding protein
 (CREB), 11, 12–13, 150–151
Canada, 491, **494,** 621
Canadian Psychiatric Association, **813–814**
Cancer pain, 245
Cannabidiol (CBD)
 pharmacology of, 242, 243–244, 252, 259
 precautions and contraindications, 761,
  766
 treatment applications, 245, 579–580
Cannabis and cannabis-related disorders
 about
  historical context, 610
  overview and summary, 241, 248, 251,
   260–261
 adverse effects, 487, 639
 comorbidity
  psychiatric disorders, 27, 260, 732–733
  substance use disorders, 155–156, 482,
   760–761

DSM-5 diagnostic criteria, 51, **53–54,** 56
 future directions for, 260–261
 gender differences, **545,** 550
 genetics and, 27
 legislative and regulatory issues, 481–482,
  483–484, 485–491
 modes of use, 251–252, 489–491
 neurobiology of
  binge/intoxication stage, 5, **6**
  chronic use and, 252, 253
  cognition and brain development,
   242–244
  endocannabinoid system, 241–242.
   See also Endocannabinoid system
  stress response and, 247–248
 prevention, 530
 recreational use, **484,** 488, 489–491
 "risky" amounts of cannabis, 79
 in special populations
  adolescents, 40–41, **41,** 253, 490–491,
   544, **545,** 564, 565, **565,** 732–733,
   761, 844–845
  adolescent treatments, 254, 257–258,
   570
  older adults, 631, 638–639
  pregnant women, **553,** 554
  SGM population, **594,** 595, 597
  women, 542
 testing for, **777,** 786
 treatment applications
  medical cannabis programs, **483,**
   485–489, 580
  pain relief, 244–245
  sleep disturbances, 245–247, 257
 treatments for cannabis use disorder
  digitally delivered therapies, 437, 438,
   440
  pharmacotherapies, 253–260, 762, 767
  psychosocial treatments, 253–255, 347,
   366–367, **553,** 554
 withdrawal, 252, 253
 in the workplace, 837–838, 843–846, **845**
Cannabis Approach Avoidance Task, 254
Cannabis sativa, 242
Cannabis Youth Treatment Study, 254,
 732–733
Can Reduce, 439
CANreduce web tool, 255
CARA (Comprehensive Addiction and
 Recovery Act) of 2016, 206
Carbamazepine, 137–138, 309, 694